医学英语常用词辞典

A Dictionary of Common Words in Medical English

第 3 版

主　编　洪班信

副主编　刘向前　王群英

编　者　丁静民　王　曦　尹丙姣　叶嗣颖
向　明　艾继辉　吴河水　余　涛
陈　璟　周　强　郝　燕　曾繁典
鲁文清　董　慧　管思明

人民卫生出版社

图书在版编目（CIP）数据

医学英语常用词辞典：英汉对照/洪班信主编.
—3版. —北京：人民卫生出版社，2013
ISBN 978-7-117-18033-7

Ⅰ.①医… Ⅱ.①洪… Ⅲ.①医学-英语-词典
Ⅳ.①R-61

中国版本图书馆 CIP 数据核字(2013)第 236123 号

医学英语常用词辞典
第 3 版

主　　编：洪班信
出版发行：人民卫生出版社（中继线 010-59780011）
地　　址：北京市朝阳区潘家园南里 19 号
邮　　编：100021
E - mail：pmph @ pmph. com
购书热线：010-59787592　010-59787584　010-65264830
印　　刷：三河市宏达印刷有限公司
经　　销：新华书店
开　　本：850×1168　1/32　**印张**：36　**字数**：2157 千字
版　　次：1997 年 5 月第 1 版　2014 年 1 月第 3 版
2025 年 5 月第 3 版第14次印刷（总第 20 次印刷）
标准书号：ISBN 978-7-117-18033-7/R · 18034
定　　价：88. 00 元
打击盗版举报电话：010-59787491　E-mail：WQ @ pmph. com
（凡属印装质量问题请与本社市场营销中心联系退换）

第 2 版编者名单

主　编　**洪班信**

副主编　**张强华　张三才**

编　者　王应杰　邓　华　付四清　刘应宏
陈罗绮　吴植恩　张开平　张宏清
黄　毅　董　慧　蔡志坚　蔡红梅

第3版前言

本辞典于1997年5月出第1版，颇受读者欢迎，经多次印刷，7年后的2004年6月出第2版，现在又过8年，迎来了它的第3版。辞典收词的起点是排除大学四级考试要求掌握的4 000词（即该4 000最基本的词不收），在此基础上，主要收录常用的医学术语及少量医学文献中需要使用的普通词汇（包括名词、动词、形容词和个别副词）。收录的词条数量第1版约为3 300个，第2版增加3 700个，第3版又增加3 000个，总共大约达到10 000个，连同一般读者早已掌握的大学英语4 000个基础词汇，总数可达约14 000个；这个词汇范围对阅读一般医学书刊比较实用。

医学科学在不断发展，新的医学术语也随之不断涌现。第3版在增加词条数量时，除继续丰富医学常用术语外，特别将重点放在近十年来出现的一些新术语上。在给术语词条选择例句时，也尽量选用那些反映医学较新进展内容的英语句例。这次的15位编委均系我校基础和临床各科的教授专家，为实现上述目的创造了有利条件。

这本辞典从1版到3版，规模从小型逐步过渡到中型。它的编写方式不同于一般辞典，其特点表现在每个词条后面除音标、词性和基本词义外，一般配有两个医学例句和中文翻译，通过词在句中的使用可以帮助读者更深刻地了解该词的词义，句子的语境可加深读者对该词的印象，从而更容易地记住该词。不少读者体会到仔细阅读词条例句对他们的英语写作有启发和借鉴作用，对照阅读例句的中译文对翻译也有一定体会。总之，词条下的例句不仅深化了词义的理解和掌握，而且还能使读者猎取语言学习多方面的收获。这或许是本词典为什么受到读者欢迎和多次印刷的原因所在。

附录部分也是本辞典的一大特色，具体内容这里不作赘述，请参看目录。其中有关英语医学术语的特征和拉丁语的点滴介绍，不仅扩展和丰富了读者关于英语词汇的理论知识，而且给读者在医学阅读中遇到的词语障碍提供了一些有益的帮助，希望能引起读者的重视，善于利用。

词典的编写是一项繁重而细致的工作，它需要内部团队的合作和集体智慧的凝聚，也需要外力的扶持。在我们过去的工作中，先后得到了学校一些领导部门的关心和支持。这次，我们要特别感谢华中科技大学科学技术开发院陈建国副院长给我们的关心和帮助。另外，我校教师管汉雄、曲宝丽、何平和谌丁艳参加了部分编写工作，严娇同学承担了书稿电脑录入及编排的部分工作任务，在此对他们表示衷心的感谢。尽管我们在编写过程中尽了最大努力，但疏漏和错误在所难免，恳请同行专家和读者不吝给予指正。

编　者

2013 年 5 月

第 1 版序

现在已是 20 世纪 90 年代中期，医学科学与其他自然科学一样正在日新月异、突飞猛进地向前发展。医学科学工作者与医务工作者都应及时地掌握医学信息才能跟上时代的步伐。要掌握医学信息必须具备两个条件，其一是要有信息交流的载体，当今信息高速公路的开通为国内外医学信息交流奠定了良好的物质基础；其二是要掌握信息交流的语言文字工具，而世界通用的外语是英语，因此掌握好医学专业英语是进行世界医学信息交流必不可少的手段。

近 20 年来高等医学院校都普遍重视对医学生的英语教学，特别是全国四、六级英语统考对大学生公共英语水平的提高起了良好的导向和激励作用，公共英语教学质量都有明显的提高。但也必须指出当前医学生，也包括研究生的医学专业英语水平还很不够，要适应 21 世纪的医学信息交流，没有扎实的医学专业英语基础是难以胜任的。近年在国际医学专业会议上个别中国专家因受到专业英语限制，影响了学术交流。现在培养的医学生应该是医学信息交流的能手，因此高等医学院校加强医学专业英语教学已迫在眉睫。

学好医学专业英语的关键是要在学好公共英语的基础上，正确理解、牢固掌握医学英语常用词汇；并要多阅读英语医学书刊，很好地熟悉医学专业英语的表达形式。洪班信教授主编的《医学英语常用词辞典》是他数十年来从事医学英语教学的经验积累，以及与其他几位外语教师共同努力的结晶。该书中每个词汇都附有一个或一个以上来源于英语医学原文的例句，这是本书有别于其他医学词汇书籍的可贵之处，有助于读者深入地理解词汇，准确地运用词汇，牢固地掌握词汇。我深信，这本辞典对医学生、研究生、医学科学工作者、医务工作者在学习医学英语时将会起到良师益友的作用。

裘法祖

1996 年 · 仲冬 · 武汉

第2版前言

《医学英语常用词辞典》自1997年出版后，经过多次重印，深受读者欢迎。这次增订再版，充实了内容，词条由原来的3 300个扩大到7 000个，例句由原来的8 000条增至17 000条。将大学英语四级教学要求掌握的4 000单词，加上本辞典精选的7 000个常用词（包括医学各科较常用的专门术语和普通词汇），共计约11 000个词，基本上可满足医学读者系统学习和查阅之用。本辞典收集的词汇主要限于医学常用词，这次再版同时还注意增选了一些较新的常用医学术语，例句内容也加强了反映医学新的进展。每个词条下面的例句均为英汉对照，加深了对该词词义的理解及其在医学文献中的使用情况，对词汇的记忆和医学文章的阅读理解均有帮助。

这次再版除基本保留原有的编者外，增加了医学专业的教授和讲师数人，加强了编写力量，使辞典无论在内容的篇幅扩大和质量的提高上均得到了较好保证。

辞典这次的增订再版工作，得到了学校有关领导，特别是教务部马建辉部长和基础医学院陈长玲副院长的支持和鼓励，在此特向他们表示衷心的感谢。此外，夏世钧教授、向明副教授、李清芬博士和曹丽云硕士等同志参加了部分编写工作，刘向前硕士承担了全部新增词条的电脑录入，这些都使我们的再版准备工作得以顺利完成，谨此向他们表示深深的谢意。尽管如此，辞典仍然可能存在这样或那样的疏漏和缺点，敬祈同行专家和读者给予批评指正。

编　者

2004年3月9日

第 1 版前言

随着我国医药卫生事业的发展和国际科学技术交流的日益频繁，语言工具的作用显得愈来愈重要。广大医学生和青年医生为了学习新知识，了解国外的医学进展，吸取其中有益的经验，直接阅读英语医学文献和资料是最基本的方式。经过大学英语课程的学习，简明系统的语法知识和运用能力已基本具备，但要想比较顺利地进行阅读，关键的一环是要解决词汇问题。本辞典在大学英语四级教学（要求学生掌握基本词汇 4 000 个）的基础上，提供常用的医学词汇（包括少量医学书籍中常用的普通词汇）3 300 个，使学生的词汇量达到 7 000 以上，这将为顺利地进行医学阅读创造有利的条件。

本辞典所收词汇系选自英美出版的医学教科书，包括医学基础课程和临床课程共十余学科，并根据编者长期从事医学英语教学积累的常用词表和教学经验而加以确定的。尽管难以做到尽善尽美，但从整体来说所选词汇都是医学各科的常用词，具有较高出现率。因此，一旦掌握这些词汇，无论阅读哪一种参考书，均将发挥其重要作用。使读者在词汇的学习和掌握上避免了盲目性和精力的浪费，是本辞典的最大特点。在收词上，凡属四级范围内词汇，本辞典一般不予重复，个别词条虽四级已有，但遇新的“义项”也收。如 shock 的词义四级有“震惊”，但无“休克”；episode 四级有“事件”、“插曲”，但无“（疾病的）发作”；failure 四级有“失败”，但无“衰竭”；等等。

本辞典的另一特点是每一词条均有 1 ~ 2 个例句，少数词条有 3 ~ 4 个例句，表现其具体使用和不同用法，而且每个例句均附汉语译文，以助确切理解。词条例句的多少系根据单词不同的情况而定，单义的医学术语其中一部分仅给一个例句，有的给二个例句，多义的医学词和普通词一般均给二个以上的例句。词汇多例的作用可有：①阐明多种词义，如 confinement 限制，分娩；lens 透镜，镜片，晶体；indication 指标，指征，表现，适应证；②提供多种汉译表达，如 lesion 损害，病变，病灶，疾病；identify 确认，发现，鉴定，辨明；③显示不同语法特征，如单复数词义有变化（irregularity，spectacle），须与一定介词搭配（如 indicative，predispose）；④展现不同内容的英语写作表达方式（如 dressing，incidence）等等。总之，通过多个例句从不同角度加强对词义的理解和记忆。

附录部分是本辞典的第三个特点。“英语医学术语的特征”从六个方面作了介绍，重点放在医学术语的构词分析上，列出了常用的拉丁和希腊词根60个，前缀45个和后缀30个，并且配以相应的例词。将近300个例词可以扩大读者的医学术语学习范围。而且，在记熟词根、前缀和后缀这些构词词素及其含义后，对于一个医学术语可根据其结构能较容易地理解和记住它的词义，并可通过不同的排列组合无形地会认识上千个其他医学术语。因此，这一介绍向读者提供了一个有效的学习和记忆医学术语的科学方法和快速扩大医学词汇数量的捷径。附录部分提供的常用英语短语、常用缩写词、常用拉丁短语，以及一些不能从字面机械理解的双词医学术语均对读者的医学阅读理解有一定的帮助。

本辞典在编写过程中得到了同济医科大学教务处处长陆定中教授和科研处处长向继洲教授的鼓励和指导，同时，也得到了医大外语部领导的大力支持，特在此一并表示衷心的感谢。另外，医学硕士熊革在本辞典编辑中热情地给予了技术性的帮助，青年教师张晓君、戴芳和敖晓梅在书稿的计算机输入编排过程中，积极地承担了部分校对工作，在此也向他（她）们表示深深的谢意。由于编者水平有限，书中肯定存在不少缺点和错误，敬请读者批评指正，以便进一步修订。

编　者

1996年12月

体 例 说 明

1. 本辞典所收词条按外文字母顺序排列，均用黑正体。

2. 每个词条后面均有国际音标、词性和汉语对应词。词性的省略符号表示如下：*n.* 名词，*v.* 动词，*a.* 形容词，*ad.* 副词，*prep.* 介词。

3. 沿用希腊语和拉丁语特殊复数形式的英语医学名词，均在词条的国际音标后面加以注明。

4. 有些名词、动词和形容词须与一定的介词搭配使用，应搭配的介词用圆括号标明，放在英语词条后面。

5. 在单词的汉语对应词和句子的汉语译文中，圆括号“（ ）”表示可省略部分，有时起解释作用；方括号“[ ]”表示可换用部分。

6. 汉语译名同义词用逗号分开，异义词用分号分开。

7. 对有两种拼写形式的医学术语，本辞典均采用较通用的一种，即下面列举的后一种形式：

1） ae→e

如：aetiology→etiology
anaemia→anemia
haematoma→hematoma
haemoglobin→hemoglobin

2） oe→e

如：oedema→edema
diarrhoea→diarrhea

3） s→z

如：hydrolyse→hydrolyze
sterilisation→sterilization

4） c→k

如：leucocyte→leukocyte
leucemia→leukemia

5） ph→f

如:sulphate→sulfate

sulphonamide→sulfonamide

8. 英语词条具有两种词性的,以较常用的一种排在前,另一种排在后,分别给以例句说明其用法;极个别情况下仅就其中一种词性提供例句。

目　　录

正文

附录

A

Abacavir [ə'bækəviə] *n.* 阿巴卡韦(抗病毒药)

Abacavir is a nucleoside analog reverse transcriptase inhibitor (NRTI) used to treat HIV and AIDS.

阿巴卡韦是一种用于治疗 HIV 和 AIDS 的核苷类似物反转录酶抑制剂(NRTI)。

Abacavir is an oral medication that is used for the treatment of infections with the human immunodeficiency virus (HIV).

阿巴卡韦是一种用于治疗人类免疫缺陷病毒(HIV)感染的口服药。

abacterial [ˌeibæk'tiəriəl] *a.* 非细菌性的

The wound had been cleaned and was now considered an abacterial injury.

伤口已经被清洗干净,现在可认为是无菌损伤。

Chronic abacterial prostatitis is a condition where you have pain or discomfort in your genital and/or pelvic area for a period of at least three months, but there is no evidence of infection.

慢性无菌性前列腺炎的表现是生殖器和(或)盆腔的疼痛或不适持续至少 3 个月,但没有感染的证据。

abandon [ə'bændən] *v.* 放弃,抛弃

As long as there is a bit of hope, the doctor should not abandon treatment for the patient.

只要还有一线希望,医生不应放弃对病人的治疗。

Those rules and regulations of the hospital which are not in keeping with the patients' interests should be abandoned.

医院里那些不符合病人利益的规章制度应予废除。

It is natural that a good mother will not abandon her baby.

很自然,一位好的母亲不会遗弃她的婴儿。

abate [ə'beit] *v.* 减少,减退,减轻

After splenectomy, symptoms usually abate, the RBC count rises and the reticulocyte count returns to normal.

脾切除后,症状通常可以缓解,伴有红细胞计数上升及网织红细胞计数恢复正常。

After more than 1 week, acute symptoms usually subside; diarrhea may abate earlier.

急性期症状通常在一周多以后逐渐消退,其中腹泻的减轻可能早些。

Effective arterial blood volumes decline, and the stimuli to retain salt and water are not abated.

有效动脉血容量降低,但对水、钠潴留的刺激并不会减弱。

abdomen ['æbdəmen, əb'dəumen] *n.* 腹(部)

Abdomen is the portion of the body which lies between the thorax and the pelvis.

腹部是位于胸部和骨盆之间的身体部分。

The acute abdomen is defined as any abdominal disease process requiring immediate evaluation and treatment.

急腹症被解释为任何需要立即评估和处理的腹部疾患过程。

This child had a pain in his abdomen and felt that he might vomit.

这个小孩患腹痛并感觉要呕吐。

abdominal [æb'dɔminəl] *a.* 腹(部)的

The internal organs inside the thoracic and abdominal cavities are often called viscera.

位于胸腔及腹腔的内部器官,常称为内脏。

The abdominal X-ray can help identify suspected problems in the urinary system such as a kidney stone, or a blockage or perforation in the intestine.

腹部 X 线摄影可帮助鉴别泌尿系统的可疑问题，如肾结石、肠道阻塞或穿孔。

abduct [æb'dʌkt] *v.* 外展

The lid may elevate when the patient attempts to look down or may drop when the eye is abducted.

当患者欲下视时眼睑可能上抬，或者当眼球外展时眼睑可能下垂。

abduction [æb'dʌkʃən] *n.* 外展；诱拐

Raising the arms laterally, to the sides, is an example of abduction.

将两手臂沿侧面举起至身体两边，即是外展的一个实例。

When you move your legs sideways away from your body like for a leg lift or side kick you are doing hip abduction.

当你的腿部向侧面移动远离你的身体，就像要摆腿或侧踢，即是在做髋外展。

abductor [æb'dʌktə] *n.* 外展肌

One of the main problems is dislocation due to the lack of abductor function and soft tissue attachment.

主要问题之一是由于外展肌功能和软组织附着的缺陷而导致脱位。

The principal abductors of the vocal folds are the posterior cricoarytenoid muscles.

主要声襞展肌是环杓后肌。

aberrant [æ'berənt] *a.* 异常的，畸变的

Organs and tissues found in abnormal sites are called aberrant organs or tissues such as thyroid tissue which may be found at the upper end of the thyroglossal duct.

存在于异常部位的器官或组织称为异位器官或组织，如甲状腺组织可存在于甲状舌管的上端。

aberration [ˌæbə'reiʃən] *n.* 失常，畸变，脱离常轨

One type of immunologic aberration has been implicated in an extremely wide and varied group of diseases.

有一种类型的免疫失常与极为广泛且多种多样的疾病有关。

Abnormal chromosome numbers and structural chromosomal aberrations are invariably found in the cells of malignant tumours.

染色体数目异常和染色体结构畸变常见于恶性肿瘤细胞。

Any pathological deviation from normal mental activity is called mental aberration.

任何病理性偏离正常精神活动可称为精神错乱。

abiogenesis [ˌeibaiəu'dʒenisis] *n.* 自然发生说

In the natural sciences, abiogenesis is the study of how life on Earth could have arisen from inanimate matter.

在自然科学中，自然发生说是研究地球上的生命如何从无生命物质中产生。

Most premature deliveries are abiogenesis.

多数早产为自然发生。

abiotic [ˌeibai'ɔtik] *a.* 无生命的；非生物的

Abiotic factors include climate, chemical pollution, geographical features, etc.

非生物的因素包括气候、化学污染、地理特征等。

The preservation of the world's natural biological diversity and natural habitats is closely associated with the abiotic factors.

对世界上自然生物多态性和自然栖息地的保护与这些非生物因素息息相关。

abiotrophy [ˌæbi'ɔtrəfi] *n.* 生活力缺乏

Retinal abiotrophy is progressive degeneration of the retina leading to impaired vision, occurring in genetic disorders such as retinitis pigmentosa.

视网膜活力缺乏是视网膜的进行性变性,可导致视力损害,见于色素性视网膜炎等遗传性疾病。

ablate [æbˈleit] *v.* 切除,摘除,清除

These considerations are secondary to the need to ablate the cancer.

这些考虑都要从属于切除癌肿的需要。

PDT has recently been adopted to ablate metastatic tumors in the spine in preclinical animal models.

PDT 最近已经用于临床前期动物模型的脊柱转移瘤清除。

(PDT = photodynamic therapy 光动力疗法)

High-intensity focused ultrasound has been applied to internal organs from outside the body to ablate tissue.

高强度聚焦超声已经用于内脏从身体外面来消融组织。

ablation [æbˈleiʃən] *n.* 消融,消蚀

Radio-frequency ablation is most successful on small tumours of less than 3 centimetres in diameter.

射频消蚀技术用于治疗直径在 3cm 以下的小肿瘤是最为有效的。

Marrow transplantation after marrow ablation by radiotherapy has been successfully achieved.

在采用放射疗法消融病变骨髓后进行骨髓移植现已有成功的经验。

Microwave ablation of tumor is a new approach to tumor treatment that is restricted by the property of microwave.

微波消融治疗肿瘤是利用微波的性能而开发的一种治疗肿瘤新的方法。

ablepsia [əˈblepsiə] *n.* 失明,视觉缺失

The research points out that smoking may increase the risk of ablepsia, brain damage in old people, and Alzheimer's disease.

研究表明吸烟可能增加视觉缺失、老年人脑损伤和阿尔茨海默病的风险。

A trained guide dog can help a person who suffers from ablepsia.

经过训练的导盲犬可以在生活中帮助失明患者。

abnormal [æbˈnɔːməl] *a.* 不正常的,异常的

Significant deviations from these growth rates appear to indicate abnormal development.

在这些成长速度方面存在的显著差异似乎表明发育异常。

Abnormal lymph nodes are generally enlarged, rounded, and easily palpable.

异常淋巴结一般表现为肿大,呈圆形,并易于触及。

abnormality [ˌæbnɔːˈmæliti] *n.* 异常,畸形

The fetal heart rate is counted for a full minute, and any abnormality of rate and rhythm is noted.

计数一分钟的胎心率,注意是否有胎心率和节律的异常。

Among the skeletal abnormalities noted are prominent occiput and maxillary underdevelopment.

骨骼畸形中可见枕骨隆凸和上颌骨发育不良。

abnormally [æbˈnɔːməli] *ad.* 异常地

Abnormally high serum uric acid is an early sign of toxemia of pregnancy.

异常高的血清尿酸浓度是妊娠毒血症的早期征象。

Both children were big at birth but were not abnormally large.

这两个孩子出生时都比较大,但并非异常的大。

abolish [əˈbɔliʃ] *v.* 废除,取消

Treatment is aimed at ridding the patient of oedema and abolishing the proteinuria.

治疗目标是消除病人的水肿和蛋白尿。

In vomiting, the normal peristaltic motions of the oesophagus and stomach are abolished.

在呕吐过程中,食管和胃的正常蠕动均消失。

abortifacient [əˌbɔːtiˈfeiʃənt] *n.* 堕胎药

Prostaglandins, by causing uterine contraction, are abortifacients.
由于能引起子宫收缩，前列腺素属堕胎药。

a. 堕胎的

The abortifacient woman was a sufferer of chronic hepatitis B.
堕胎的妇女是一个慢性乙型肝炎患者。

abortion [əˈbɔːʃən] *n.* 流产，小产

Free contraceptives, sterilization and induced abortion are methods commonly used in the practice of family planning.
免费避孕药物(用具)、绝育和人流是实施计划生育中常用的方法。

A reduction in the length of the menstrual cycle is sometimes seen in the early months of marriage or after abortion.
月经周期缩短有时见于婚后几个月或流产以后。

abortive [əˈbɔːtiv] *a.* 夭折的，流产的，无结果的

Menstruation is therefore the outward sign of the end of an abortive cycle and the optimistic commencement of the next.
月经是一个无结果的周期结束和下一个周期良好开端的外在征象。

Abortive transduction is the transduction in which the genetic fragment from the donor bacterium is not integrated in the genome of the recipient bacterium, and, when the latter divides, is transmitted to only one of the daughter cells.
流产性转导是指转导过程中供体菌的遗传物质没有整合到受体菌的基因组中，当受体菌进行分裂时遗传物质只传递给其中的一个子细胞。

abound [əˈbaund] *v.* 丰富，大量存在

Microvilli abound in the epithelial lining of the small intestine.
小肠上皮内膜富含微绒毛。

News headlines abound about complaints of drug side effects, so intelligent people take the least amount of pharmaceutical products possible.
如今关于药物毒副作用投诉的新闻标题比比皆是，所以明智的人们都尽可能少地采用医药用品。

abrasion [əˈbreiʒən] *n.* 擦破，磨损

An abrasion is the displacement of epidermis by friction or by crushing.
擦损系由于摩擦或挤压使上皮移位。

An abrasion of the skin, which may be minute, allows the organisms to reach the subcutaneous tissues in which they multiply.
皮肤擦伤，即使很微小，也会让病原体到达皮下组织，在此繁殖。

abrupt [əˈbrʌpt] *a.* 突然的，意外的

In lobar pneumonia, the onset is often abrupt.
患大叶性肺炎时常突然发病。

Influenza is characterized by the abrupt onset of headache, fevers, chills, cough and sore throat.
流感的特征有突发的头痛、发热、寒战、咳嗽和咽痛。

An abrupt attack of vomiting usually ushers in this disease, along with irritability, general weakness and discomfort.
此病通常以呕吐的突然发作作为先兆，并伴有激动、全身无力和不适的症状。

abruption [əˈbrʌpʃən] *n.* 突然分离，分裂，断裂

Hypertension, particularly from preeclampsia, may be a cause or an effect of abruption.
高血压，特别是先兆子痫引起的高血压，可能是胎盘早剥的原因或结果。

Placenta praevia and placental abruption are of great clinical importance as causes of antepartum haemorrhage.
前置胎盘和胎盘早剥是临床上分娩前出血的重要原因。

abscess [ˈæbsis] *n.* 脓肿

A brain abscess is a localized area of suppuration within the cerebrum or cerebellum.

脑脓肿是大脑或小脑内的局限化脓区域。

Intra-abdominal abscess is the most frequent serious complication of peritonitis.

腹内脓肿是腹膜炎最常见的严重合并症。

absolute [ˈæbsəljuːt, ˈæbsəluːt] *a.* 绝对的，完全的

The essential chemical elements are present in varying absolute quantities, in varying relative quantities, and in varying combinations.

基本的化学元素是以不同的绝对量、不同的相对量和不同的化合方式而存在。

Many laboratories report both the relative and absolute values for leukocyte differentials.

许多实验室对白细胞分类计数的报告既有相对值又有绝对值。

If absolute diagnostic knowledge is required, cardiac catheterization with coronary angiography serves as the gold standard.

如果需要完整的诊断资料，心导管冠脉造影术的报告可作为金标准。

absolutely [ˈæbsəljuːtli] *ad.* 绝对地，完全地

Early detection is absolutely essential if any possibility of a cure for a lung cancer is to be maintained.

要想治愈肺癌，早期发现是完全必要的。

These drug treatments are relatively or absolutely contraindicated in the opposite situations.

在相反的情况下，这些药物疗法是相对或绝对禁忌的。

absorb [əbˈsɔːb] *v.* 吸收，吸引

The major portion of aspirin is absorbed in the upper small intestine.

大部分阿司匹林是在小肠上部被吸收的。

Drugs are mostly absorbed from the upper part of the small intestine.

大多数药物由小肠上部吸收。

absorbable [əbˌsɔːbəbl] *a.* 可吸收的

Weak bases will be highly ionized in the acidic gastric juice and therefore not generally absorbable.

弱碱基在酸性胃液中有高度电离化的特性，所以一般不易被吸收。

absorbance [əbˈsɔːbəns] *n.* 吸收率，吸光度

Absorbance is an expression of the amount of light absorbed by a solution.

吸光度是表达光被某种溶液吸收的量度。

absorbent [əbˈsɔːbent] *a.* 有吸收力的

Don't use absorbent cotton on an open burn-it will leave particles of cotton in the wound.

不要将脱脂棉用于开放性烧伤创面，因为会在伤口上留下棉花的碎屑。

Absorbent cotton may be used to apply medications to a tender burn in which skin is intact.

对皮肤无破损的轻微烧伤创面，敷药时可以使用脱脂棉。

absorptiometry [əbsɔːpʃiˈɔmitri] *n.* 吸收测量仪

Dual x-ray absorptiometry was used to measure bone mineral density.

双能 X 线吸收测量法被用来测量骨矿物质密度。

Calcium deposition in the cells was measured by atomic absorptiometry.

应用原子吸收测量法检测细胞内钙的沉积。

absorption [əbˈsɔːpʃən] *n.* 吸收（作用）

If rapid absorption is desired, drugs should be taken on an empty stomach.

若期望药物迅速吸收，应在空腹时服用。

The blood urea may rise to 15 ~ 25mmol/l due to absorption of protein from the gut.

由于肠道内蛋白被吸收，血清尿素可升高至 15 ~ 25mmol/l。

absorptive [əbˈsɔːptiv] *a.* 吸收的，有吸收力的

The total absorptive area of the small intestine and its microvilli has been estimated to be greater than $200m^2$.

据估计小肠和小肠绒毛的总吸收面积超过 $200m^2$。

abstain [əbˈstein] *v.* 戒,避免

The patient should abstain from smoking and alcoholic drink.

该病人应当戒烟、戒酒。

Rats that are forced to abstain from morphine or alcohol have decreased extracellular dopamine in the nucleus accumbens.

被强迫戒掉吗啡或酒精的大鼠已经出现伏核中胞外多巴胺水平的下降。

abstinence [ˈæbstinəns] *n.* 节制,禁戒

On abrupt withdrawal of methadone, the abstinence syndrome develops more slowly than that of morphine.

突然停药后,美沙酮的戒断症状比吗啡出现慢。

The only effective treatment usually is total abstinence from alcohol.

惟一有效的治疗通常是彻底戒酒。

abstract [æbˈstrækt] *v.* 提取

A gland is a group of cells which abstract certain materials from the blood and make new substances.

腺是从血液中提取某些原料并用其制造新的物质的一群细胞。

n. 摘要

An abstract is a short summary of your completed research.

摘要是对整个研究的一个简要概括。

abstraction [æbˈstrækʃən] *n.* 抽象;抽象概念

As a scientist the doctor may deal in abstractions and generalizations and isolated phenomena, but as a clinician he deals with people.

作为科学家,医生可以研究抽象概念、概括性原理和孤立的现象,而作为临床医生,他研究的是人。

abstruse [æbˈstruːs] *a.* 难解的,深奥的

Some of the view points are clear while others are frankly abstruse.

一些观点是很清楚的,而其他一些则相当难以理解。

absurd [əbˈsəːd] *a.* 不合理的,荒谬的

This may sound absurd at present, but work is still under way.

这在目前听起来是荒谬的,但工作依然在进行中。

abundance [əˈbʌndəns] *n.* 丰富,充裕

Some citrus fruits have vitamin C in great abundance.

有些柑橘属水果含有大量的维生素 C。

abundant [əˈbʌndənt] *a.* 丰富的,充裕的;充分的

Water is the most abundant constituent of cells and constitutes about two thirds of body weight.

细胞内含量最多的组成成分是水,约占体重的三分之二。

Eccrine sweat units are most abundant on the palms, soles, forehead and axillae.

外泌汗腺单位在掌、跖、前额和腋窝等部位最为丰富。

abuse [əˈbjuːs] *n.* 滥用

In adolescents, drug and alcohol abuse may complicate affective symptomatology.

在少年身上,滥用药物和酒精可使情感疾病症状更为复杂。

v. [əˈbjuːz] 滥用

Prominent among the substances used or abused are alcohol, cigarettes, and narcotics.

在能应用又能滥用的物质中,主要的有酒精、烟和麻醉剂。

academic [ˌækəˈdemik] *a.* 学术的

The academic debate will continue for years as to the exact definition or standards for intrauterine growth retardation.

关于宫内生长迟缓确切的定义及诊断标准，学术上的争论将会继续许多年。

academy [ə'kædəmi] *n.* 研究院；学会

Professor Wu has participated in a symposium sponsored by the Chinese Academy of Medical Sciences.

吴教授已参加了中国医学科学院主办的一次学术讨论会。

In order to establish a single childhood immunization schedule, the American Academy of Pediatrics have unified their vaccine recommendations.

为了制订一份儿童免疫接种时间表，美国儿科学会已统一了他们的疫苗计划。

acalculia [ˌækæl'kjuːliə] *n.* 计算力缺失；失算

Acalculia is associated with lesions of the parietal lobe (especially the angular gyrus) and the frontal lobe and can be an early sign of dementia.

失算与顶叶（尤其是角回）和额叶病变有关，并且可能是痴呆症的早期迹象。

Acalculia is sometimes observed as a "pure" defect, but is commonly observed as one of a constellation of symptoms, including agraphia and finger agnosia.

失算有时是单一缺陷，但通常是一组症状之一，包括失写和手指失认。

acanthocytosis [əˌkænθəusai'təusis] *n.* 刺状红细胞增多

The mortality rate of acanthocytosis caused by abetalipoproteinemia is still not fully described by any studies.

由无 β 脂蛋白血症引起的刺状红细胞增多症的死亡率目前尚无充分的研究。

acanthopanax [əˌkænθə'peinæks] *n.* 刺五加

Is there any contraindication if acanthopanax pieces are used with oryzanol?

刺五加片和谷维素合用有禁忌么？

We should explore the therapeutic mechanism of acanthopanax root saponin (ASS) in treating diabetes mellitus.

我们需要探讨刺五加叶皂甙（ASS）治疗糖尿病的作用机制。

acariasis [ˌækə'raiəsis] *n.* 螨病

It concludes that metronidazole is very efficient for the treatment of the experimental pulmonary acariasis.

结论甲硝唑在治疗实验性肺螨病中有很好的疗效。

The objective of this study is to evaluate the practical value of indirect fluorescent antibody test (IFAT) in diagnosis of intestinal acariasis.

本文的目的是探讨间接荧光抗体试验在肠螨病诊断中的应用价值。

acatalepsia [ə'kætəˌlepziə] *n.* 领悟不能；诊断不明

Patients with chronic abdominal pain need laparoscopic approach because of acatalepsia.

诊断不明的慢性腹痛患者有必要行腹腔镜检查。

Bronchial provocation test and bronchial dilation test are valuable diagnostic methods which could reduce asthma acatalepsia.

支气管激发试验和支气管扩张试验在哮喘的诊断中有重要价值，可减少哮喘诊断不足现象。

accelerate [æk'seləreit] *v.* 加速，促进

Lack of oxygen accelerates the heart beat, the degree of acceleration is related to the severity of the anoxia.

缺氧可加速心脏跳动，加速的程度与缺氧的严重程度有关。

The pulse is only slightly, if at all, accelerated in the early stage.

早期脉搏即使加速，也只是轻微的。

This procedure accelerates wound healing.

这个方法可促进创伤的治愈。

acceleration [ækˌseləˈreiʃən] *n.* 加速,促进

Recent studies suggest that there is an acceleration of age-related impairment of renal function in association with chronic low-level lead exposure.

现代的研究提出,慢性低浓度铅暴露具有一种加速肾功能随年龄而损伤的作用。

The pooling of blood in the lower parts of the body is prevented by reflex acceleration of the heart by means of aortic and carotid reflexes.

血液通过主动脉弓和颈动脉窦反射引起的反射性心跳加快可避免身体下部血液淤滞。

accelerator [ækˈseləreitə] *n.* 加速器

The more usual modern radiotherapeutic practice is to employ external beam of radiation from high energy linear accelerators.

现代更常用的放射治疗是应用来自高能线性加速器的外放射线。

accentuate [ækˈsentjueit] *v.* 增强,加重

The condition of varicose veins of the legs in this patient has been accentuated.

这个患者下肢静脉曲张的病情已有加重。

The first symptom is usually pain accentuated by deep breathing.

第一个症状通常是深呼吸时疼痛加剧。

The importance of muscle fatigue in accentuating respiratory failure has been recently emphasized.

肌肉疲劳对加重呼吸衰竭的重要性最近得到了强调。

acceptable [ækˈseptəbl] *a.* 可接受的,可取的

If this therapeutic scheme is not acceptable, doctors may suggest others.

如果此治疗方案未被接受,医师们可建议其他方案。

Here, only the most accurate quantitative methods for noninvasive evaluation are acceptable.

这里惟有最精确的非损伤性评估定量方法可以采用。

acceptor [ækˈseptə] *n.* 受体,受器

Copper is an essential metal, acting as an electron donor or acceptor in many enzymatic reactions.

铜是一种必需的金属,在很多酶反应中都起着电子供体或受体的作用。

access [ˈækses] *n.* 接近;(进入的)方法;(有权)使用

The skin is a fertile soil for the development of cancer because of its easy access to irritation.

皮肤由于容易接触刺激,因而是癌症孕育的肥沃土壤。

Direct laryngoscopy provides access for instrumental removal of the foreign body.

直接喉镜检查提供了用器械取出异物的途径。

v. [计] 存取,访问,取得

This scientist accessed enormous different files to find the correct information.

这位科学家在计算机上调阅了大量的不同文件以找寻所要的信息。

All the researchers can access the central database.

所有研究人员都能访问中央数据库。

accessibility [ækˌsesəˈbiliti] *n.* 易接近

Accessibility, informality, familiarity and continuity of care are proclaimed as features unique to general practice.

就医方便、不拘形式、亲切随和及持续照顾被宣称为全科医疗独有的特征。

accessible (to) [ækˈsesəbl] *a.* 易接近的,能进去的,可获得的

This is the rationale for primary health care accessible to all in a spirit of social equality.

这一点正是社会公平精神下人人皆可享受的基本卫生保健的理论基础。

The accessible population is defined using inclusion criteria and exclusion criteria for clinical trial.

临床试验通过使用入选标准和排除标准来确定纳入人群。

accessory [æk'sesəri] *a.* 附属的，副的，辅助的

One detects the involvement of these small accessory glands by the velvety condition of the urethra.

通过触摸尿道的柔软性可以判断这些小的附属腺体是否受到影响。

The muscles of respiration comprise three groups: the diaphragm, the intercostal and accessory muscles, and the muscles of the abdomen.

呼吸肌包括有三个部分：即膈肌、肋间肌和辅助肌、腹肌。

In addition to lymphocytes and phagocytes, there are a number of accessory cells.

除了淋巴细胞和吞噬细胞外，还有大量的辅助细胞。

In the human, each kidney is supplied only by a single renal artery, although one or more accessory renal arteries are not uncommon.

虽然具有一支或多支副肾小动脉者并不少见，但人体的每个肾脏仅由一根肾动脉供血。

accident ['æksidənt] *n.* 事故，意外伤害

Accident and emergency medicine (A and E) is evolving as a specialized area of patient care.

事故与急症(A 与 E)正在发展为医护中的一门专门的学科。

Accidents in older persons can result in disability and impairment far greater than an equivalent injury in younger persons.

受同等事故伤害的老年人出现的伤残者比年轻人要重得多。

The leading causes of death among young women in the United States are accidents and suicide.

在美国青年女性中首要的死亡原因是意外事故和自杀。

accidental [ˌæksi'dentl] *a.* 偶然的，突发的

Accidental perforation of the uterus can happen even in experienced hands.

子宫的意外穿孔，即使在有经验的人(医生)手上也会发生。

Acute placental failure may result from accidental antepartum haemorrhage.

急性胎盘功能衰竭可因突发性产前出血所引起。

acclimatization [əˌklaimətai'zeiʃən] *n.* 环境适应

Given time, their bodies adapt to less oxygen by means of adjustments collectively called acclimatization.

如果有时间，他们的身体通过总称为环境适应的一系列调节方式可适应少氧的情况。

accommodate [ə'kɔmədeit] *v.* 容纳；使适应，调节

As urine accumulates in the bladder the latter relaxes to accommodate it.

当尿液积聚在膀胱内时，膀胱可以松弛以便容纳。

accommodation [əkɔmə'deiʃən] *n.* 适应性调节

Sustained increases in SNGFR would require accommodation of the autoregulatory mechanisms that normally govern renal plasma flow.

持续性的 SNGFR 分泌增加需要平时控制肾血流量的自我调节机制产生适应性的变化。

accompany [ə'kʌmpəni] *v.* 陪同；伴随

The director of the hospital accompanied the foreign guests in visiting the surgical building.

医院院长陪同外宾们参观外科大楼。

Nausea often precedes or accompanies vomiting.

恶心通常出现于呕吐之前或伴随呕吐同时出现。

Reflex nausea and vomiting may accompany the onset of pain in acute appendicitis.

在急性阑尾炎病例中反射性恶心和呕吐可伴随疼痛的发作同时产生。

The intake of food also is accompanied by increased heat production.

摄食也伴有产热过程的增加。

Acute severe hemolysis may be accompanied by chills, fever, pain in the back and abdomen, prostration, and shock.

急性严重溶血可能伴有寒战、发热、背部和腹部疼痛、虚脱和休克。

accomplish [əˈkɔmpliʃ] *v.* 完成；达到

Sterilization may be accomplished by physical, chemical or mechanical processes.

灭菌可以通过物理、化学或机械的处理来达到。

This is accomplished by reducing the amount of the amino acid phenylalanine in the diet of the patient.

这要通过减少病人饮食中的苯丙氨酸量而实现。

Dihydromorphinone is able to accomplish the same degree of analgesia in a dose of 2mg.

二氢吗啡酮只需给予 2mg 剂量即可产生同样的镇痛效果。

accord [əˈkɔːd] *v.*, *n.* 符合，一致

These medical instruments do not accord with the demands.

这些医疗器械不符合要求。

First-degree burns will not cause scarring and will heal of their own accord.

一度烧伤将不会形成瘢痕而且会自行愈合。

accordance [əˈkɔːdəns] *n.* 一致；符合；in ~ with 按照，根据

For the bacterial type of pharyngitis, penicillin in certain forms can be given by mouth very effectively in accordance with a physician's directions.

对于细菌型的咽炎，有些类型的青霉素遵照医嘱口服很有效。

Combined application of transabdominal and transvaginal sonography can improve the diagnostic accordance of placenta previa.

经腹与经阴道超声联合应用能够提高前置胎盘诊断的符合率。

account (for) [əˈkaunt] *v.* 说明，是…的原因；占…

Benign adenomas account for about 4 percent of lung primary tumours.

良性腺瘤约占肺原发性肿瘤的 4% 。

Fatal heart attacks account for around 500,000 deaths in the US yearly.

美国每年有约 50 万人因致命的心脏病发作而丧生。

Cancer accounts as the fourth most expensive disease in terms of costs, according to study estimates based on 2005 data.

基于 2005 年数据的研究估计，癌症在花费最高的疾病中排列第四位。

accredit [əˈkredit] *v.* 相信，认可

He should be a member of the staff of at least one accredited hospital, and he should belong to the local medical society.

他应该至少是一所合格医院的成员，因而也是当地医学会的会员。

accretion [æˈkriːʃən] *n.* 增加物，粘连；增加

Despite the steady accretion of evidence tying physical activity to longevity, people today exercise no more than they did a decade ago.

尽管体育锻炼能促进健康长寿的证据在稳步增加，但现在人们并不比十年前锻炼更多。

The patient successfully received the accretion-lysis by laparoscope and there was no complication after the operation.

该患者成功地进行了腹腔镜粘连松解术并且无术后并发症发生。

accumulate [əˈkjuːmjuleit] *v.* 积累，集聚，蓄积

Through such anecdotal experiences we have accumulated some knowledge of the natural history of various diseases.

通过这样一些趣闻般的经历，我们积累了多种疾病自然病史的一些知识。

Heat, if there were no means of getting rid of it, would accumulate and the temperature of the body would rapidly rise.

如果没有方法将热从体内排出，它就会蓄积起来，使得体温迅速上升。

Raw materials coming to the cell may remain unprocessed and therefore accumulate in visible form.

到达细胞的原料可能仍呈未加工状态，因而集聚成可见的形态。

accumulation [əˌkjuːmjuˈleiʃən] *n.* 蓄积，累积

In alcoholism, fat accumulation continues, and cirrhosis of the liver may ensue.

酒精中毒则脂肪持续沉积，并可能导致肝硬化。

Traditional Chinese medicine is an accumulation of the knowledge and experience acquired by countless numbers of common people in combating diseases in the past.

传统的中医学是许许多多普通人在过去与疾病作斗争中获得的知识与经验的积累。

The accumulation of carbon dioxide produces a marked stimulation in respiration.

二氧化碳的积聚能对呼吸产生明显刺激作用。

accuracy [ˈækjurəsi] *n.* 准确，精确

The accuracy of diagnosis in thyroiditis may be as high as 90%.

诊断甲状腺炎的准确性可高达 90%。

I have concluded the book with tables of Normal Values and this has been checked for accuracy by Dr. Tom Hargreaves.

我在此书后面附有各种正常值的表格，这些表格均经 Tom Hargreaves 医生查核，务必准确无误。

accurate [ˈækjurit] *a.* 精确的，准确的

Effective treatment of genetic disorders requires accurate diagnosis.

有效地治疗遗传病需要对疾病进行准确的诊断。

The IgM-FTA-ABS test has proved less accurate than a positive VDRL test in rising titers.

采用 IgM 荧光螺旋体抗体吸收试验已经证实其上升的滴度不如 VDRL 试验显示阳性时准确。

An accurate record of all drugs given and the duration of treatment should now be regarded as an essential part of any patient's case-sheet.

全部用药及其持续时间的精确记录如今都应作为病历的重要组成部分。

accurately [ˈækjuritli] *ad.* 精确地，准确地

A count of the thrombocytes is done occasionally, but it is difficult to do accurately.

血小板计数是偶尔才做的，但很难做得准确。

Under the right conditions, plasma concentrations of an indicator can accurately reflect glomerular filtration rate.

在适当的条件下，一种标记物在血浆中的浓度可以准确地反映肾小球的滤过率。

accuse [əˈkjuːz] *v.* 指责

It is not right that the patient's relatives accuse the doctor.

该病人的家属指责医生的这种做法是不对的。

You should never accuse anyone without proof.

你千万不要在无证据的情况下去指责任何人。

acellular [eiˈseljulə] *a.* 无细胞的，非细胞的

The new acellular vaccines only contain select parts of the organism and its toxins.

新的无细胞疫苗只含有细菌及其毒素的某些选择部分。

acetabuloplasty [ˌæsəˈtæbjuləuˌplæsti] *n.* 髋臼成形术

Percutaneous acetabuloplasty appears to be safe and effective for improving the pain and decreased mobility secondary to metastatic lesions of the acetabulum.

经皮髋臼成形术对治疗髋臼继发性转移病灶的疼痛和灵活性降低是安全有效的方法。

Our report about long-term outcomes of acetabuloplasty was comparable to other reports.

我们报道的髋臼成形术的远期效果与其他文献报道的相似。

acetabulum [ˌæsiˈtæbjuləm] *n.* 髋臼

Acetabular index is a useful tool for the assessment of acetabulum of the hip joint.

髋臼指数是评估髋关节髋臼的一种有用方法。

acetaminophen [ˌæsiˈtæminəufen, ˌæsətəˈminəfən] *n.* 对乙酰氨基酚

Acetaminophen or aspirin may be used to reduce temperature and pharyngeal pain.

对乙酰氨基酚或阿司匹林可用于降温和减少咽部疼痛。

Currently acetaminophen is the most common cause of acute liver failure in both United States and United Kingdom.

目前，对乙酰氨基酚是美国和英国引起急性肝功能衰竭的最常见原因。

N-acetylcysteine is the most effective drug to prevent progression to liver failure from acetaminophen hepatotoxicity.

N-乙酰半胱氨酸是阻止对乙酰氨基酚肝毒性进展到肝衰竭的最有效药物。

acetate [ˈæsiteit] *n.* 乙酸盐，醋酸盐

Useful measures are wet dressings or soaks with solutions such as solution of aluminum acetate, one part to 20 parts of water.

有利的措施是用一些溶液湿敷或用溶液浸泡，如采用醋酸铝溶液一份加水 20 份配成的溶液。

Suitable wet dressings and lotions include aluminium acetate lotion 5% in sterile water and calamine lotion.

适宜的湿敷和洗剂包括含 5% 醋酸铝洗剂的无菌水和炉甘石洗剂。

acetazolamide [ˌæsitəˈzɔləmaid] *n.* 乙酰唑胺

Acetazolamide is the only carbonic anhydrase inhibitor with significant diuretic effects.

乙酰唑胺是唯一的有显著利尿作用的碳酸酐酶抑制药。

Acetazolamide can, however, correct the significant metabolic alkalosis which occasionally occurs with loop diuretic therapy.

然而，乙酰唑胺能够纠正袢利尿药治疗中偶发的严重的代谢性碱中毒。

acetic [əˈsiːtik] *a.* 醋的，醋酸的

Acetic acid is the shortest of the fatty acids.

醋酸是脂肪链最短的脂肪酸。

Acetic acid can cause iritis.

醋酸可引起虹膜炎。

acetone [ˈæsitəun] *n.* 丙酮

The urine is found to contain acetone.

发现小便内有丙酮。

An excess of acetone bodies in the urine is called acetonuria.

尿中含过多的丙酮体称为丙酮尿。

acetonuria [ˌæsitəuˈnjuəriə] *n.* 丙酮尿

Particular attention was directed toward the occurrence of acetonuria.

对丙酮尿的发生给予了特别的注意。

Acetonuria occurs in diabetes, fever, starvation and digestive disorders.

丙酮尿发生于糖尿病、发热、饥饿和一些消化疾病。

acetyl [ˈæsitil] *n.* 乙酰(基)

Acetyl-CoA is an important intermediate in the citric acid cycle.

乙酰辅酶 A 是柠檬酸循环中一个重要的中间产物。

acetylator [əˌsetiˈleitə] *n.* 乙酰化者，乙酰化个体

Peripheral neuropathy and encephalopathy occur in slow acetylators.

外周神经病和脑病常发生于慢性乙酰化者。

acetylcholine [ˌæsitilˈkəuliːn] *n.* 乙酰胆碱

Acetylcholine, causing bradycardia, is an agonist.

引起心动过缓的乙酰胆碱是一种激动药。

Acetylcholine receptors are critical to chemical transmission of the nerve impulse at the neuromuscular junction.

乙酰胆碱受体对神经肌肉接头处神经冲动的化学传导至关重要。

acetylcholinesterase [ˌæsitilˌkəuliˈnestəreis] *n.* 乙酰胆碱酯酶

Acetylcholinesterase levels correlate more closely with the degree of symptoms.

乙酰胆碱酯酶的水平与中毒症状的程度有更密切的关系。

Acetylcholinesterase splits acetylcholine into an acetate ion and choline.

乙酰胆碱酯酶将乙酰胆碱裂解为乙酸根离子和胆碱。

acetylcysteine [ˌæsitilˈsistiin] *n.* 乙酰半胱氨酸

N-acetylcysteine is a precursor of glutathione.

N-乙酰半胱氨酸为谷胱甘肽的前体。

The objective of this article is to investigate whether antioxidant N-L-acetylcysteine (NAC) can protect the cochlea from impulse noise trauma.

本文的目的是研究抗氧化剂 L-乙酰半胱氨酸是否能保护耳蜗免受脉冲噪声的伤害。

acetylsalicylic [ˌæsitilˌsæliˈsilik] *a.* 乙酰水杨酸的

Buffered acetylsalicylic acid preparations are dissolved faster and absorbed better chiefly in the intestine.

缓冲的乙酰水杨酸制剂主要在小肠中溶解得快些,吸收得好些。

Symptomatic therapy of viral pneumonia includes bed rest, acetylsalicylic acid for fever, and the use of humidity for younger children and infants.

病毒性肺炎的对症治疗包括卧床休息、乙酰水杨酸解热以及对幼童和婴儿使用蒸气吸入。

acetyltransferase [ˌæsitilˈtrænsfəreis] *n.* 转乙酰酶,乙酰基转移酶

On the other hand, people with more efficient acetyltransferase require larger doses of isoniazid to obtain its therapeutic effect.

另一方面,有较高效率转乙酰酶的人群常需要较大剂量的异烟肼才能取得治疗效果。

achalasia [ˌækəˈleiziə] *n.* 失弛缓性,弛缓不能

The objective of our study is to assess the role of ultrasonography in the diagnosis of esophageal achalasia.

我们研究的目的是探讨超声在食管失弛缓症诊断中的作用。

The motor pattern of esophageal body of achalasia was aperistalsis.

贲门失弛缓症患者的食管体部运动模式是无蠕动。

achieve [əˈtʃiːv] *v.* 达到,完成

Since phosphorus is present in milk and in meat, the daily intake of 2mg is readily achieved.

既然磷存在于牛奶和肉类中,每日 2 毫克的摄入量是容易达到的。

achlorhydria [ˌeiklɔːˈhaidriə] *n.* 胃酸缺乏

An ulcer which is found in the presence of true achlorhydria is almost surely a malignant ulcer.

在有真性胃酸缺乏时发现的溃疡,几乎可以肯定是恶性溃疡。

achondroplastic [əˌkɔndrəuˈplæstik] *a.* 软骨发育不全的

We have reported zinc deficiency in achondroplastic children and their parents.

我们曾报道过软骨发育不全的儿童及其父母有锌的缺乏。

achylia [əˈkailiə] *n.* 胃液缺乏

Pernicious anemia is characterized by megaloblastic anemia, achylia gastrica, and neurologic damage.

恶性贫血的特征为巨成红细胞性贫血、胃液缺乏和神经损伤。

acid [ˈæsid] *a.* 酸性的;*n.* 酸

Acid rain is caused by emissions of carbon dioxide, sulfur dioxide and nitrogen oxides which react with the water molecules in the atmosphere to produce acids.

酸雨是排入到大气中的二氧化碳、二氧化硫和氮氧化物作用于大气中的水分子来产生酸而形成的。

The enzymes of these microbes are denatured (changed in shape so they no longer function) by the acid.

这些微生物的酶在酸性条件下变性(形状发生改变,不再起作用)。

acidemia [ˌæsiˈdiːmiə] *n.* 酸血(症)

Some authors prefer to use the terms acidemia to indicate those situations in which the pH of the plasma is altered.

有些作者喜欢用“酸血症”一词表示血浆 pH 值有改变的某些情况。

acid-fast [ˈæsidfɑːst] *a.* 抗酸的,耐酸的

Acid-fast stain is used mainly to detect organisms that cause tuberculosis and leprosy.

抗酸染色主要用于检测那些可引起结核和麻风病的致病微生物。

The acid-fast stain is employed for sputum, gastric aspirates, tissue samples, or other fluids when acid-fast bacilli are suspected.

若怀疑有抗酸杆菌存在时,即可对痰液、胃液、组织取样以及其他体液进行抗酸染色。

acidic [əˈsidik] *a.* 酸的,酸性的

Acetylsalicylic acid is best absorbed when the pH of the stomach is highly acidic.

乙酰水杨酸在胃高酸性 pH 环境中吸收最好。

acidification [əˌsidifiˈkeiʃən] *n.* 变酸,酸化

In amphetamine toxicity, acidification of urine with ammonium chloride will be required.

在苯丙胺中毒时,需要用氯化铵酸化尿液。

acidify [əˈsidifai] *v.* 使酸化

Cerumen, secreted by glands, acidifies the canal and suppresses bacterial growth.

由腺体分泌的耳垢使外耳道酸化,并抑制细菌的生长。

acidity [əˈsiditi] *n.* 酸度,酸性,酸味

The stomach's acidity keeps the number of microorganisms at a minimum (103-105/mg of contents).

胃内的酸度使细菌保持在最低量(103 ~ 105/毫克内容物)。

Some patients with proven ulcers in a stage of symptoms may show only low levels of gastric acidity during their actual pain.

有些病人已证明有溃疡,并处于有症状期,但在实际疼痛时其胃液的酸度却处于低水平。

acidophilic [ˌæsidəuˈfilik] *a.* 嗜酸性的

It is not unusual to find the bronchiolar and alveolar walls bordered by a homogeneous acidophilic hyaline membrane.

常可见到在细支气管壁和肺泡壁上形成同质嗜酸性透明膜边。

acidosis [æsiˈdəusis] *n.* 酸中毒

In the presence of acidosis there is an increase in the blood concentration of glucose.

酸中毒时,血内葡萄糖浓度增加。

When the hydrogen ion concentration is higher than normal, the person is said to have acidosis.

当氢离子浓度高于正常时,我们说该患者有酸中毒。

aciduria [ˌæsiˈdjuəriə] *n.* 酸尿

All had significant elevation of CK levels but no hypovolemia or aciduria and subsequently zero cases of acute renal failure.

所有病例有血 CK 水平的明显升高,但是没有低血容量或酸性尿以及继发的急性肾功能衰竭。

This kind of aciduria is caused by a defect in the peroxisomal enzyme-alanine glyoxylate aminotransferase.

这种酸尿是源于过氧化物酶-丙氨酸乙醛酸转氨酶的缺陷。

acinar [ˈæsinə] *a.* 腺泡的

In distal acinar (periacinar) emphysema, the distal part of the acinus is involved, but the proxi-

mal portion is normal.
在腺泡远端型(腺泡周围型)肺气肿,腺泡远端部分受累,而近端部分正常。
Alpha-fetoprotein (AFP)-producing acinar cell carcinoma of the pancreas is a rare neoplasm.
分泌甲胎蛋白的胰腺腺泡细胞癌是一种很罕见的肿瘤。

acinebacter [eiˌsiniˈbæktə] *n.* 不动杆菌属
Acinebacter increased dramatically from 0 to 8 strains.
不动杆菌显著增长,由 0 株增加到 8 株。
High rate of drug resistance was found in pseudomonas and acinebacter.
假单胞菌和不动杆菌的耐药率高。

acinetobacter [eiˌsinitəuˈbæktə] *n.* 不动杆菌属
Acinetobacter, like other gram-negative bacteria, has an outer membrane and a cytoplasmic membrane.
像其他革兰阴性菌一样,不动杆菌属也有一层外膜和胞质膜。
However, there is a growing threat from a new family of bacterial infection including acinetobacter, which affects around 1,000 patients each year.
然而,一个新的细菌感染家族包括不动杆菌的威胁正在日益增长,每年影响大约 1000 名患者。

acinus [ˈæsinəs] *pl.* acini [ˈæsinai] *n.* 腺泡
The cells of the acini appear non-granular and distended or granular.
腺泡细胞显现出非颗粒状和膨胀状(或颗粒状)。
The acinus is composed of the respiratory bronchioles, the alveolar duct, the atria, and the terminal alveolar sac.
肺腺泡由呼吸性细支气管、肺泡管、肺泡前房和终末肺泡囊组成。
The acinus is the functional unit of the liver.
(肝)腺泡是肝脏的功能单位。

acknowledge [əkˈnɔlidʒ] *v.* 承认;对…表示感谢
The doctor openly acknowledged his fault in the process of treatment.
这位医生公开承认他在治疗过程中的错误。
It should be acknowledged that such identification is of largely epidemiologic and academic interest.
应该承认这样的鉴定对流行病学和学术研究大有裨益。
The author wishes to acknowledge the technical assistance of Mr. Smith.
作者在此对史密斯先生在技术上的帮助表示感谢。
His advice, encouragement and active participation in the investigation are greatly acknowledged.
在本研究中对他的建议、鼓励和协助深表感谢。

acknowledgement [əkˈnɔlidʒmənt] *n.* 感谢,致谢
For encouragement and general comments, grateful acknowledgement is due to Professor Johnson.
对于约翰逊教授所给予的鼓励和提出的意见,在此表示深切的感谢。

acleistocardia [əˌklaistəˈkɑːdjə] *n.* 卵圆孔未闭
Acleistocardia is a condition in which the foramen ovale of the heart fails to close.
卵圆孔未闭是一种心脏卵圆孔不能闭合的现象。
The most common associated deformities were chonechondrosteron, ankyloglossum and acleistocardia.
最常见的相关畸形是漏斗胸,舌系带过短和卵圆孔未闭。

acme [ˈækmi] *n.* (病的)极期
At the acme of the uterine contraction the patient may complain of a sudden sharp pain in the abdomen.

当子宫强烈的收缩至极期时，病人会主诉腹部有突发性剧痛。

acne [ˈækni] *n.* 痤疮，粉刺

Acne is a disease of the oil glands of the skin.

痤疮是一种皮脂腺的疾病。

Common acne is found most often in individuals between the ages of 14 and 25.

寻常型痤疮最常见于 14 ~ 25 岁年龄段的人。

The most common location for acne is the face, but the chest and back may be involved.

痤疮最常发生于面部，但胸背部也会出现。

aconitase [əˈkɔniteis] *n.* 顺乌头酸酶

The team detected the effect by examining the metabolic enzyme aconitase.

研究小组通过测定代谢的顺乌头酸酶来检测这种效应。

Aconitase is susceptible to damage from ROS.

顺乌头酸酶对活性氧的损伤。

aconitine [əˈkɔnitiːn] *n.* 乌头碱

The average recoveries of aconitine were 93.3%.

乌头碱平均回收率为 93.3%。

More doses of ouabain or aconitine to induce arrhythmia are needed in SAOH group than those in contrast group.

SAOH 组与对照组相比，需要更大剂量的哇巴因和乌头碱来诱发心律失常。

acquaint [əˈkweint] *v.* 使了解，使熟悉

It should be possible to determine the origin of the swelling if the examiner is acquainted with the anatomy of the region.

如果检查者熟悉这一部位的解剖，就可以确定肿胀的原发位置。

The patient is so well acquainted with the major symptoms resulting from these disorders that he may attribute many noncardiac complaints to cardiovascular disease.

病人对这些疾病引起的主要症状如此的熟悉，以致于他会将许多非心脏疾病的主诉归于心血管系统疾病。

acquire [əˈkwaiə] *v.* 获得，得到

Diphtheria may occur at any age, it is rarely seen before one year old, because immunity is acquired from the mother.

白喉可发生于任何年龄，但在一周岁前很少见，因为婴儿可从母体获得免疫（抗体）。

Fetal infection may also occur if the mother was inadequately treated for early acquired syphilis.

如果母亲以前患上的梅毒未经充分治疗，胎儿也有可能受到感染。

acquired [əˈkwaiəd] *a.* 后天的，获得的

Acquired chromosome abnormalities arise in most malignant neoplasms.

后天的染色体异常可出现在大多数患有恶性肿瘤的患者。

In contrast to innate immunity, acquired immunity is brought about actively by previous contact with the infecting microbe or its products.

与先天免疫形成对照，后天免疫是通过和感染微生物或其排泄物的预先接触而主动获得的。

The rare congenital form of anemia is best characterized and can be used to describe some aspects of this anemia in the acquired form.

罕见的先天性贫血最具特点，可用以描述这种获得性贫血的某些方面。

Epilepsy developing in childhood after the first year of life may be due to the congenital or acquired lesions.

1 岁以后儿童发生的癫痫可能 是由于先天性或后天获得性病变所致。

acquisition [ækwiˈziʃən] *n.* 获得；掌握

Severe sensory-motor impairments are usually present, and acquisition of speech is not possible.
通常出现严重的感觉运动性障碍，并且不可能有掌握语言的能力。
How can infection by these viruses lead to the acquisition of a stable inherited trait in the recipient cell?
这些病毒的感染如何能够使受体细胞获得一个稳定的遗传性状呢？
Later maternal acquisition of cytomegalovirus may be accompanied by the delivery of an uninfected infant.
妊娠后期获得巨细胞病毒感染的母亲可分娩出不受感染的婴儿。

acroanesthesia [ˌækrəˌænisˈθiːziə] *n.* 肢端麻木；四肢麻木
Some workers exposed to hexane had the following symptoms or signs: headache, dizziness, fatigue, acroanesthesia, decreased muscle strength, etc.
一些接触己烷的工人可出现下列症状和体征：头痛、头晕、疲劳、肢端麻木、肌力下降等。
The medicine is used for curing acroanesthesia, ache and limited activity.
这个药物用来治疗肢端麻木、疼痛和活动受限。

acrocentric [ˌækrəuˈsentrik] *a.* （染色体）近端着丝的
An acrocentric chromosome has a centromere near one end.
近端着丝粒染色体的着丝粒靠近一端。
Y chromosome has two types of polymorphism: metacentric (or submetacentric) and acrocentric chromosomes.
Y染色体有两种类型的多态性，即中间着丝粒（或亚中间着丝粒）和近端着丝粒染色体。

acrocyanosis [ˌækrəusiəˈnəusis] *n.* 肢端发绀症；手足发绀
While the best definitions of acrocyanosis focus on clinical description, there is no uniform definition of acrocyanosis.
虽然关于肢端发绀症的最好定义都集中于临床描述，但仍然没有统一定义。
In a single city in Chile with well-documented increased arsenic exposure in the community, acrocyanosis was present in 36.8% of people.
在智利单单一个城市里，有完善记录的砷超标环境影响下肢端发绀症人群的发生率是36.8%。

acrognosis [ˌækrəgˈnəusis] *n.* 肢体感；肢体感觉缺失
There were mild hypoaesthesia, hypoalgesia, acrognosis and reduced muscle strength in her left arm and leg.
她的左臂和腿有轻微的感觉迟钝、痛觉减退、肢体感觉缺失和肌力下降。
Cervical spondylopathy is manifested as pain on the head, neck, shoulder, arms and front chest, acrognosis and dyskinesia, and even paralysis of extremities.
颈椎疾病表现为头、颈、肩、臂、前胸的疼痛，肢体感觉缺失和运动障碍，甚至是四肢麻痹。

acromegaly [ˌækrəuˈmegəli] *n.* 肢端肥大症
Secondary forms of diabetes occurs in chronic pancreatitis, acromegaly and Cushing's syndrome.
继发性糖尿病多出现于慢性胰腺炎、肢端肥大症和库欣综合征。
Acromegaly is caused by excessive production of growth hormone by specific cells of the anterior pituitary gland.
肢端肥大症是由垂体前叶的特殊细胞过多地分泌生长激素所引起的。
Excess secretion of the growth hormone in adults may produce acromegaly.
成年人过度分泌生长激素可导致肢端肥大症。

acromion [əˈkrəumiən] *n.* 肩峰
In this article, we report on our experience with a patient who sustained a fracture of the acromion after reverse shoulder arthroplasty.
在这篇文章中，我们报道了一例我们接诊的反肩关节成形术后肩峰骨折的患者。
Aneurysmal bone cysts are rarely located in the scapula and are especially rare in the acromion.

动脉瘤样骨囊肿很少发生于肩胛骨,发生在肩峰的尤为罕见。

acropachy ['ækrəuˌpæki] *n.* 杵状指

Thyroid acropachy describes clubbing in association with Graves disease with additional swelling of the fingers and periosteal new bone formation.

甲状腺杵状指是指与甲状腺功能亢进症相关的指端杵状改变,伴有手指肿胀和骨膜的新骨形成。

The association of acropachy with pulmonary disease has been confirmed by numerous doctors.

很多医生已经证实了杵状指与肺部疾病的关联性。

acrosome ['ækrəusəum] *n.* 顶体

The acrosome reaction consists of two parts.

顶体反应由两部分组成。

actigraphy ['æktigrəfi] *n.* 活动记录检查,活动记录仪

Actigraphy recordings indicated that the average sleep duration was 8 hours.

活动记录仪显示平均睡眠时间持续 8 小时。

We assessed the duration and severity of tremor in patients by actigraphy.

我们用活动记录仪对病人震颤的严重性和持续性进行了评估。

actin ['æktin] *n.* 肌动蛋白

Chemicals that bind to tubulin or actin impair the assembly and/or disassembly of these cytoskeletal proteins.

结合到微管蛋白或肌动蛋白上的化学物质能损伤这些细胞骨架蛋白的装配和(或)分解。

actinobacillus [ˌæktinəubə'siləs] *n.* 放线杆菌属

Infections caused by Actinobacillus may occur following bites by horses or sheep.

放线杆菌感染可发生于马或羊咬伤之后。

actinobacteria [ˌæktinəuˌbæk'tiəriə] *n.* 放线菌门,放线细菌

Actinobacteria are a group of Gram-positive bacteria with high guanine and cytosine content.

放线细菌是一类富含鸟嘌呤和胞嘧啶的革兰阳性细菌。

Actinobacteria are well known as secondary metabolite producers and hence of high pharmacological and commercial interest.

放线菌是众所周知的次级代谢物质的制造者,因而具有高度的药物和商业价值。

actinomycete [ˌæktinəu'maisiːt] *n.* 放线菌

Actinomycetes are bacteria, not fungi.

放线菌是一种细菌,而不是真菌。

The actinomycetes include species that make antibiotics.

放线菌中包含有能产生抗生素的菌种。

The higher actinomycetes include Streptomyces and Micromonospora.

高级放线菌包括链霉菌属和单孢丝菌属。

actinomycin [ˌæktinəu'maisin] *n.* 放线菌素

Actinomycin can suppress the immue reaction.

放线菌素能抑制免疫反应。

Actinomycin D is the first effective antitumor antibiotic.

放线菌素 D 是第一个有效的抗肿瘤的抗生素。

actinomycosis [ˌæktinəumai'kəusis] *n.* 放线菌病

Actinomycosis is most commonly caused by Actinomyces israelli, an anaerobic gram-positive bacillus.

放线菌病绝大多数是由伊氏放线菌(一种革兰阳性厌氧杆菌)引起的。

Actinomycosis is a chronic bacterial infection that induces both a suppurative and granulomatous inflammatory response.

放线菌病是一种慢性的细菌感染,能诱发化脓性及肉芽肿性炎症两种反应。

Pulmonary actinomycosis develops when aspirated material reaches an area of lung with decreased oxygenetion (such as in atelectasis, infection).
当吸入物到达氧合减少(如肺不张、感染)的肺组织就易发生肺放线菌病。

action ['ækʃən] *n.* 行动,行为,作用
Rapid action is needed if we will try to save this patient.
如果我们要争取抢救这个病人,就得迅速行动。
The character of an effect produced by a drug is called the mode of action of that drug.
一种药物产生某效应的特性称为该药的作用方式。

activate ['æktiveit] *v.* 激活
Complement may be activated with formation of complexes.
补体经形成复合物而被激活。
An activated nerve fibre maintains a state of chemical stability.
激活的神经纤维可保持化学稳定状态。

activation [ˌækti'veiʃən] *n.* 激活,活性反应,活性化作用
These factors include products of activation and interaction of four major cascade systems.
这些因子包括四个主要连锁系激活和相互作用的产物。
Endotoxin activation of these mediators occurs in a matter of minutes.
这些介体的内毒素活性反应在几分钟内便可产生。
An enzyme lowers the activation energy required to achieve a transition state.
酶能降低达到变迁态所需的活化能。

activator ['æktiˌveitə] *n.* 促动剂,活化剂
Inorganic substances that tend to increase the activity of enzymes are called activators.
能增强酶活力的无机物称为促动剂。
Isoproterenol is a potent activator of beta-adrenergic receptors.
异丙肾上腺素为一高效 β 肾上腺素能受体激动剂。

active ['æktiv] *a.* 活性的,积极的,有效的
The living, active germs are capable of transmitting disease.
活的、活跃中的细菌能传播疾病。
People should play an active part in the choice of care and the protection of their own health.
人们应在选择保健措施和保护自身健康中起积极的作用。
By these routes of administration the active ingredient is absorbed into the venous circulation.
通过这些途径,有效成分被吸收进入静脉循环。

activity [æk'tiviti] *n.* 活性,活动(度)
Chlorpromazine reduces the syntheses of DNA by inhibiting the activity of thymidine kinase.
氯丙嗪抑制胸苷酸激酶的活性,从而减少 DNA 的合成。
Morphine reduces the activity of the entire gastrointestinal tract.
吗啡可降低整个胃肠道的运动。

actually ['æktjuəli] *ad.* 实际上,事实上
There are actually 6×10^9 bp of DNA in each human somatic cell.
事实上,每个人体细胞中的 DNA 分子均含有 6×10^9 碱基对。
A few drugs, such as antibiotics, actually cure some diseases.
一些药物,如抗生素,确实能治好某些疾病。
Active naturally acquired immunity can be acquired by actually having the disease.
有活力的自然的获得性免疫可通过实际患病而获得。

acuity [ə'kjuːiti] *n.* 尖锐,严重,剧烈;敏度(尤指视力)
The acuity level of patients in ICU (intensive care unit) is much higher than that in ordinary wards.
重症监护病房病人病情的严重程度比普通病房要厉害得多。

Macular oedema may develop, especially in the elderly NIDDM patient, and reduce visual acuity.
特别是老年非胰岛素依赖型糖尿病患者,可发生黄斑水肿而使视力减退。

acumen [ə'kjuːmen] *n.* 敏锐;聪明

Clinical acumen and experience are often required to discern the real reason behind the patient's chief complaint.
要从病人的主诉中找出真正的病因需要具有丰富的临床经验和慧眼识别的能力。

acupoint ['ækjupɔint] *n.* 穴,穴位,经穴

There are numerous acupoints distributed over the human body.
人体全身分布有许多穴位。

acupuncture ['ækjuˌpʌŋktʃə] *n.* 针刺(疗法)

Acupuncture anaesthesia does not require complicated apparatus or heavy doses of drugs.
针刺麻醉不需要复杂的仪器或大剂量的药物。

I found it useful treating the patient with acupuncture.
我发现用针刺法治疗这位患者是有效的。

Acupuncture is often used for relieving pain and some other therapeutic purposes.
针刺疗法常用来缓解疼痛和其他治疗目的。

acupuncturist [ˌækju'pʌŋktʃərist] *n.* 针灸医师

Acupuncturists in the West may be medically qualified but many are not.
针灸医师在西方有些具备行医资格,而多数并无此资格。

acute [ə'kjuːt] *a.* 急性的

Examples of this are seen in many acute inflammatory lesions.
这类例子也见于许多急性炎症性病变。

Except for acute pulmonary edema, narcotics are rarely needed in heart failure.
除了急性肺水肿,心力衰竭时很少需要麻醉剂。

acutely [ə'kjuːtli] *ad.* 急性地

The disease may develop acutely, with rapid development of symptoms.
这种病可以急性地产生,症状迅速发展。

acyanotic [eˌsaiə'nɔtik] *a.* 非紫绀性的

Coarctation of aorta is a kind of acyanotic congenital cardiovascular disease.
主动脉缩窄是一种非紫绀性先天性心血管病。

acyclovir [ei'saikləvi(r)] *n.* 阿昔洛韦,无环鸟苷(抗病毒药)

Prospective studies comparing acyclovir and adenoside arabinoside have not been completed.
无环鸟苷与阿糖腺苷的前瞻性对照研究尚未完成。

Intravenous acyclovir also has been reported to be effective in the therapy of immunocompromised children with chickenpox.
曾有报道当接受免疫抑制治疗的儿童患水痘时,静脉用阿昔洛韦有效。

adapt [ə'dæpt] *v.* 使适应,使适合

In subacute or chronic closed-angle glaucoma there may be only an ache, the eye becoming gradually adapted to high intraocular pressure.
患有亚急性或慢性闭角型青光眼的患者可能仅有疼痛,眼睛可逐渐适应增高的眼内压。

The small intestine is especially adapted for absorption.
小肠特别具有吸收的功能。

This method was well adapted to the conditions of the patient who had only six percent of the body—the crown of her head and the soles of her feet—free from serious burns.
这种方法对于全身只剩下6%体表即头顶和脚底未受严重烧伤的病人的情况很适合。

adaptation [ˌædæp'teiʃən] *n.* 适应,适合

Such evolution is an adaptation to a variety of living conditions.
这种进化是对不同生存条件的适应。

Pernicious anemia is often more profound than would be expected from the symptoms, because its slow evolution can elicit physiological adaptation.
恶性贫血的状况经常比症状所反映的要严重，因为它进展缓慢，使机体在生理上产生了适应。
In many cases, cells appear to be shaped as an adaptation for performing a specific function.
在很多情况下，细胞往往表现出与其所执行的特殊功能相适应的形状。

adaptin [ə'dæptin] *n.* 衔接蛋白
The association of ATM with β-adaptin in vesicles indicates that ATM may play a role in protein transport mechanisms.
ATM 与小囊泡内 β-衔接蛋白的连接，表明 ATM 可能在蛋白质转运机制中发挥作用。
There are several types of adaptin, each related to a different group of membrane-bound receptors.
衔接蛋白有几种，每一种分别与结合在细胞膜上的受体群类相关联。

adaptive [ə'dæptiv] *a.* 适应的，获得的
Such inability could result from an environment that changes beyond the inherent limits of human adaptive potential.
这种无能为力的原因可能是环境的变化超出了人类适应潜能的极限。
The two key features of the adaptive immune response are specificity and memory.
获得性免疫应答的两个关键特征是特异性和记忆性。

adaptor [ə'dæptə] *n.* 接合体（分子），转接器，连接物
Adaptor proteins are non-enzymatic proteins that form physical links between members of a signaling pathway.
接头蛋白是一种没有酶活性的蛋白质，只在信号转导通路的成员之间起物理连接作用。
MyD88 is an adaptor protein in the hToll/IL-1 receptor family signaling pathways.
MyD88 是 hToll/IL-1 受体家族信号通路中的一种接头蛋白。

add [æd] *v.* 增加，添加
They add sodium salicylate powder to water to make a colourless solution.
他们将水杨酸钠粉末加入水中制造一种无色溶液。

addict [ə'dikt] *v.* 使吸毒成瘾
The children of narcotic-addicted mothers will be born addicted to narcotics.
对麻醉剂成瘾的母亲所生的新生儿也对麻醉剂成瘾。
n. ['ædikt]（吸毒）有瘾的人
Strategies for dealing with drug addicts vary from country to country.
对待吸毒上瘾的人各个国家都有自己的策略。

addiction [ə'dikʃən] *n.* 瘾，癖嗜，成瘾
Pentazocin causes tolerance and addiction.
镇痛新可产生耐受性和成瘾性。
Potent analgesics result in addiction and dependence.
强效镇痛药可导致成瘾和依赖。
The use of morphine was not encouraged for fear that the patient should develop addiction.
不鼓励使用吗啡，因恐病人上瘾。

addition [ə'diʃən] *n.* 增加
The addition of a low-potency steroid cream during the initial three to five days of therapy will decrease irritation rapidly.
在治疗的最初 3 ~ 5 天中增加低强度的皮质类固醇霜应用，可迅速减少刺激。
In addition the skin performs an essential sensory function, receiving many impulses from the external environment.
此外，皮肤还具有重要的感觉功能，可接受来自外界环境的多种刺激。

In addition to relief of pain, treatment designed to prevent and care for shock should not wait until the burn can be properly dressed.
除了解除疼痛之外,防治休克的治疗亦不应等到烧伤创面敷裹之后才进行。

additional [ə'diʃənəl] *a.* 附加的,额外的
Further opportunities for additional basic and clinical research were identified.
明确了未来进行更多的基础研究和临床研究的时机。
Nevertheless, we must drink additional water to obtain adequate fluid for the body functions.
然而,我们必须增加饮水,以得到维持身体功能所需的足够的液体。
This is an additional drawback to the use of tetracycline.
这是应用四环素的又一缺点。

additive ['æditiv] *a.* 附加的
The presence of systemic and local disease is generally additive in determining the probability of death during hospitalization.
全身疾病和局部疾病的存在,通常是在推测住院期间死亡或然率方面的一个附加因素。
n. 添加剂
Color additives are very safe when used properly.
色素添加剂如果正确使用的话是非常安全的。
Some food additives are regarded as beneficial by the manufacturer.
生产厂家认为有些食品添加剂是有益的。

adduct [ə'dʌkt] *n.* 加合物
An adduct is a product of a direct addition of two or more distinct molecules, resulting in a single reaction product containing all atoms of all components.
加合物是指两个以上不同分子直接加合后形成的单一产物,该产物涵括所有组分的原子。
Diesel exhaust (DE) has been recognized as a noxious mutagen and/or carcinogen, because its components can form DNA adduct.
鉴于柴油尾气的组分可形成 DNA 加合物,其被公认为有毒的致突变物和(或)致癌物。

adduction [ə'dʌkʃən] *n.* 引用,引证;内转;内收作用
This article mainly uses the contrast analysis method and adduction analysis method, making use of the related finance and management knowledge.
本文主要采用对比分析和引用分析方法,运用金融学和企业管理学的相关知识来撰写。
Adduction of the wrist is called ulnar deviation.
手腕的内收被称为尺侧偏斜。
What's the effect of stiffness-variable walking shoes on knee adduction movement?
可变硬度的休闲鞋对膝关节内收运动的作用影响是什么?

adductor [ə'dʌktə] *n.* 内收肌群
The jaw adductors of horse are in relation to body size, diet and ingested food volume.
马的颌内收肌群与身体大小、饮食及摄食量有关。

adenemphraxia [əˌdinem'fræksiə] *n.* 腺梗阻
Adenemphraxia is defined as the obstruction of the discharge of a glandular secretion.
腺梗阻被定义为腺状分泌物的排出被阻碍。
No hemorrhage, acute respiratory obstruction, and adenemphraxia occurred after operation.
手术后没有出现出血、急性呼吸道梗阻、腺梗阻等并发症。

adenine ['ædəniːn] *n.* 腺嘌呤
Both DNA and RNA contain the purine nitrogen adenine and guanine and the pyrimidine cytosine.
DNA 和 RNA 两者都含有腺嘌呤、鸟嘌呤和胞嘧啶。
Every molecule of DNA contains equal amounts of adenine and thymine.
每个 DNA 分子都含有等量的腺嘌呤和胸腺嘧啶。

adenitis [ˌædiˈnaitis] *n.* 腺炎

The most common causes of acute adenitis are group A streptococcus and staphylococcus aureus.
急性淋巴结炎最常见的病因是 A 组链球菌和金黄色葡萄球菌。

adenocarcinoma [ˌædinəuˌkɑːsiˈnəumə] *n.* 腺癌

Adenocarcinoma is the most common type of peripheral primary lung cancer.
腺癌是一种最常见的周围型原发性肺癌。

Adenocarcinoma of duodenum is rare, but is more common than lymphoma.
十二指肠腺癌很少见，但比淋巴瘤要常见。

Sister Joseph's nodules arise most commonly from a metastasizing gastric adenocarcinoma.
约瑟夫结节最常见于转移性胃腺癌。

adenohypophysis [ˌædinəuhaiˈpɔfisis] *n.* 腺垂体

ACTH (adrenocorticotropic hormone) is synthesized in the adenohypophysis.
ACTH（促肾上腺皮质激素）在腺垂体中合成。

adenoid [ˈædinɔid] *a.* 腺样的

The most common minor salivary gland tumor is adenoid cystic carcinoma.
最常见的不严重的唾液腺肿瘤是囊腺样癌。

n. (*pl.*) 腺样体（指小儿的咽扁桃体）

The lymphatic tissues of the adenoids and tonsils enlarge during this period.
在此期间，腺样体和扁桃体的淋巴组织增生。

adenoidectomy [ˌædinɔiˈdektəmi] *n.* 腺样体切除术

Adenoidectomy is the surgical removal of the adenoids due to chronic infections.
腺样体切除术是手术切除因慢性感染而肥大的腺样体。

Adenoidectomy is not often performed on children aged 1-6, as adenoids are helpful to the body's immune system.
在儿童 1 ~6 岁期间通常不进行肥大腺样体切除术，因为腺样体可以辅助人体的免疫系统。

adenoiditis [ˌædinɔiˈdaitis] *n.* 增殖腺炎

We focus on the effect of endoscopic surgery of adenoid in the treatment for adult chronic adenoiditis.
我们关注内镜下手术治疗成人慢性增殖腺炎的疗效。

Immunologic movements, which accompany development of adenoiditis, are a serious problem.
伴随着增殖腺炎发展而进展的免疫反应是一个严重的问题。

adenoma [ˌædiˈnəumə] *n.* 腺瘤

An adenoma is a glandular tumor.
腺瘤是一种腺体（自身的）肿瘤。

At autopsy, a small 0.5cm papillary renal cortical adenoma with focal areas of calcification was identified.
在尸检中，发现一处有钙化集中点的 0.5cm 的小乳头状肾皮质腺瘤。

adenomatosis [ˌædinəuməˈtəusis] *n.* 腺瘤病

This article describes the pathological and RT-PCR diagnosis of sheep pulmonary adenomatosis.
本文描述绵羊肺腺瘤病的病理学及 RT-PCR 诊断。

Adenomatosis is a condition characterized by multiple adenomas within an organ or in several related organs.
腺瘤病是指在一个或数个相关器官内存在多个腺瘤为特征的病理状态。

adenomatous [ˌædiˈnəumətəs] *a.* 腺瘤的

Such adenomatous lesions are morphologically similar or identical to larger renal adenocarcinomas that metastasize when they are so small.
这种腺瘤样病变在形态上与在很小时就可转移的较大的肾腺瘤相似或相同。

adenomyoma [ˌædinəumaiˈəumə] *n.* 腺肌瘤

Adenomyoma, a type of complex and mixed tumor, includes components derived from glands and muscle.

子宫腺肌瘤是一种比较复杂的混合性肿瘤，其成分是从腺体和肌肉演化而来的。

An adenomyoma is an abnormal growth within the muscle tissue lining of the uterus.

子宫腺肌瘤是在子宫内肌组织层上异常生长的一种肿瘤。

adenomyosis [ˌædinəumaiˈəusis] *n.* 子宫内膜异位，子宫腺肌症

The development and extension of endometrial tissue into the myometrium is termed adenomyosis.

子宫内膜组织生长并延伸进入子宫肌层的现象，称为子宫内膜异位。

The sensitivity of CA125 and CA19-9 for adenomyosis were 57. 70% and 15. 4% , and the difference was significant (P<0. 05).

子宫腺肌症 CA125 及 CA19-9 的敏感性分别为 57. 7% 和 15. 4% ，有明显的差异（P<0. 05）。

adenopathy [ˌædiˈnɔpəθi] *n.* 腺病（腺肿大，尤指淋巴结肿大）

Hemophilus influenzae and streptococcus pneumoniae rarely cause suppurative or nonsuppurative adenopathy.

流感嗜血杆菌和肺炎链球菌极少引起化脓性或非化脓性淋巴结肿大。

adenosarcoma [ˌædinəusɑːˈkəumə] *n.* 腺肉瘤

Endometrial adenosarcoma usually presents as a large broad-based polypoid mass.

子宫内膜腺肉瘤通常表现为大的广基的息肉样肿物。

Adenosarcoma is a group of malignant stromal tumor of endometrium with benign glands.

腺肉瘤是一组含有良性腺体的恶性子宫内膜间质瘤。

adenosine [əˈdenəsiːn] *n.* 腺苷

Mitochondria are the primary site of energy generation in the cell, producing adenosine triphosphate.

线粒体是细胞产生能量的基地，即产生三磷酸腺苷。

adenosis [ˌædiˈnəusis] *n.* 腺病

Breast adenosis presents as a focal lump like fibroadenoma.

乳腺腺病像纤维腺瘤一样表现为局部的肿块。

The acini are compressed and distorted because of the dense stroma in the sclerosing adenosis.

硬化性腺病中，因为间质致密，腺泡受压变形。

adenosquamous [ˌædinəuˈskweiməs] *a.* 腺鳞的

Adenosquamous carcinoma is composed of mixed malignant glandular and malignant squamous epithelium.

腺鳞癌由混合的恶性腺上皮和恶性鳞状上皮构成。

Pulmonary adenosquamous carcinoma needs to be differentiated with mucoepidermoid carcinoma.

肺的腺鳞癌需要与黏液表皮样癌鉴别。

adenovirus [ˌædinəuˈvaiərəs] *n.* 腺病毒

If significant conjunctivitis is also present, the most likely causative agent is an adenovirus.

如果还出现严重的结膜炎，其病因最有可能是腺病毒。

A fourfold rise in serological titers from the acute to the convalescent serum is highly suggestive of adenovirus infection.

自急性期到恢复期血清滴度升高 4 倍，很可能表示腺病毒感染的存在。

adept [ˈædept, əˈdept] *a.* 擅长于…的，精于…的

The surgeon is adept in plastic surgery.

这位外科医生擅长于整形外科手术。

Mr. Eden is adept in thoracic surgery.

伊登先生擅长于胸外科。

adequacy ['ædikwəsi] *n.* 适当,足够

The adequacy of circulating blood volume needs to be evaluated.

需估计循环血容量是否充足。

The well-being of each individual cell is dependent on the adequacy of its environment to furnish nutrition and carry away metabolites.

每个细胞的健康有赖于其周围环境充分供应营养和运走代谢产物。

adequate ['ædikwit] *a.* 适当的,足够的,充足的

Recurrence usually does not take place when adequate amounts of griseofulvin have been taken.

用了足量的灰黄霉素之后一般不会复发。

Anyone who doesn't maintain an adequate fluid balance is susceptible.

没有保持适当体液平衡的任何人都易受感染。

The nurse must also determine whether a clients' hygiene practices are adequate.

护士必须确定病人的卫生习惯是否合适。

If calcium intake is not adequate, bone disease may occur.

如果钙摄入不足,骨病就会发生。

adequately ['ædikwitli] *ad.* 充分地,足够地;适当地

If the swelling is not adequately and promptly treated, suppuration is bound to happen.

如果肿胀得不到充分和及时的治疗,就一定会化脓。

All significant specific complaints and physical findings should be adequately evaluated.

所有明显的特异主诉和体检所见都应充分评估。

Many of the larger hospitals have discovered that the increasing number of patients cannot be cared for adequately in a single unit.

许多较大的医院感到在仅有一个监护室的情况下数量越来越多的病人不能得到充分的照顾。

adhere (to) [əd'hiə] *v.* 附着; 坚持

Family planning is a matter that concerns the interests of every household and the method of persuasion and education should be adhered to.

计划生育关系千家万户的利益,应坚持说服与教育的方法。

To eliminate invasive microorganisms, leukocytes must adhere to endothelial cells and migrate from the blood through the endothelial barrier and the extracellular matrix to sites of infection and tissue injury.

为了清除侵入的微生物,白细胞必须黏附到内皮细胞,并通过内皮屏障和细胞外基质从血液迁移到感染和组织损伤部位。

adherence [əd'hiərəns] *n.* 依附; 坚持

His adherence to the old habits is much to be regretted.

他守旧的习惯使人感到很遗憾。

adherent [əd'hiərənt] *a.* 粘连的,附着的

The surface of the papular syphilid is smooth, sometimes shiny, at other times covered with a thick adherent scale.

丘疹性梅毒疹表面光滑,有时发亮,有时有厚的黏着性鳞屑覆盖。

Adherent cells are counted under the microscope.

附壁细胞可在显微镜下计数。

adhesion [əd'hiːʒən] *n.* 粘连,黏附物

If much fluid is present, recovery may occur without pericardial fibrous adhesions.

如果渗出液较多,痊愈后可不引起心包纤维性粘连。

Non-specific adhesions usually follow previous surgical intervention.

非特异性粘连通常继发于既往的外科手术。

adhesive [əd'hiːsiv] *a.* 黏着的，有附着力的

Neither erythrocytes nor leucocytes are adhesive.

红细胞和白细胞都没有黏着性。

The result is chronic adhesive pericarditis.

其结果是慢性粘连性心包炎。

ad hoc [æd'hɔk] *a.* 专门的，特别的　*adv.* 特别地

Ad hoc studies are studies that require primary data collection.

特别研究是一类需要收集基本数据的调查研究。

Ad hoc studies can be designed to be able to collect such information.

可设计一些专门的研究项目用于收集此类信息。

adipocyte ['ædipəu,sait] *n.* 脂肪细胞

Resveratrol regulates human adipocyte number and function.

藜芦可调节人脂肪细胞的数目和功能。

Adipocytes play critical roles in the modulation of metabolic homeostasis.

脂肪细胞在体内代谢平衡方面扮演着重要角色。

adipocytokine [ˌædipəu'saitəukain] *n.* 脂肪细胞因子

The release of the adipocytokine visfatin is regulated by glucose and insulin.

脂肪细胞因子内脂素的释放要受到血糖和胰岛素的调节。

Anthocyanin enhances adipocytokine secretion and adipocyte-specific gene expression in isolated rat adipocytes.

花青素可促进离体大鼠脂肪细胞因子的分泌和脂肪细胞特异性基因的表达。

adipokines ['ædipəukains] *n.* 脂肪因子

Prof. Shelley made a report on Progress About Adipokines and Nonalcoholic Fatty Liver Disease.

谢利教授做了一个题为“脂肪因子与非酒精性脂肪性肝病研究进展”的报告。

Adipose tissue participate in the regulation of energy homeostasis as an important endocrine organ that secretes a number of biologically active “adipokines”.

脂肪组织，作为分泌大量具有生物活性脂肪因子的一个重要内分泌器官，参与能量代谢稳定的调节。

adiponectin [ˌædipəu'nektin] *n.* 脂联素；脂肪连接蛋白

Adiponectin also has antidiabetic properties, and plasma adiponectin level has correlation positively with insulin sensitivity.

脂联素具有抗糖尿病的作用；血浆脂联素水平和胰岛素敏感性呈正比。

Adiponectin encoded by the APM1 gene is one of the adipocyte-expressed proteins and its function is to control glucose, lipid, and energy metabolism.

被 APM1 基因编码的脂联素是脂肪细胞表达的蛋白之一，其功能为控制血糖、血脂和能量代谢。

adipose ['ædipəus] *a.* 脂肪的

Adipose tissue can provide insulation and energy storage.

脂肪组织能隔热和贮存能量。

Evidence has been presented recently that the above pathway is significant only in adipose tissue.

近来有证据表明，上述途径仅在脂肪组织中较显著。

adiposis [ˌædi'pəusis] *n.* 肥胖病

This article discusses the application of acupuncture in treating adiposis.

该文探讨针灸在肥胖病治疗中的应用。

The present study was based on the summary of the previous understandings and the recent achievement on adiposis and constipation.

本项研究建立在对肥胖病和便秘的前期认识及最新研究成果的总结基础上。

adiposity [ˌædiˈpɔsiti] *n.* 肥胖

He didn't explain clearly the relationship between infants growth and children's simple adiposity.

他没有解释清楚婴儿生长发育与儿童单纯性肥胖之间的关系。

With the standard of living improved, people had less and less interests in exercise, adiposity has been a problem that people have to be up against all over the world.

随着人民生活水平的提高,运动锻炼意识的日益淡化,肥胖已成为困扰现代社会的问题。

adjacent [əˈdʒeisənt] *a.* 邻近的

Each has a number of branches to adjacent muscles, to the skin and to the spinal cord.

每一(动脉)有许多分支达到邻近的肌肉、皮肤和脊髓。

The outward growth of the neoplasm can affect adjacent structure.

肿瘤向外生长可波及邻近结构。

adjoin [əˈdʒɔin] *v.* 贴近,毗连

Placenta previa means that the placenta develops in the lower uterine segment and either covers or adjoins the internal cervical os.

前置胎盘是指胎盘在子宫下段发育,且覆盖或毗连宫颈内口。

adjudication [əˌdʒuːdiˈkeiʃən] *n.* 裁定

Data monitoring committee or adjudication committee for clinical trail may be established with the primary role of periodically reviewing the data as they are generated by the registry.

可以建立临床试验数据监测委员会或裁定委员会,其主要任务是定期审查登记产生的数据。

adjunct [ˈædʒʌŋkt] *n.* 附件

In some cases, additional tests have been devised as an adjunct in the evaluation process.

有时,也设计其他测验作为评估的附加内容。

Rest and sedation are helpful adjuncts to the treatment.

休息和镇静是对治疗有益的辅助方法。

adjunctive [əˈdʒʌŋktiv] *a.* 附属的,辅助的

This is widely accepted as an effective adjunctive measure.

这个作为有效的辅助方法已被广泛承认。

Treatment of congestive heart failure is aimed at improving cardiac output, chiefly by pharmacologic means with certain adjunctive supportive measures.

对充血性心衰的治疗,目标应针对改善心输出量,主要通过药物途径加上某些辅助的支持措施。

adjust [əˈdʒʌst] *v.* 调节,调整

Uterine circulation adjusts itself well to the growing uterus.

子宫血循环能很好地自行调节以适应增大的子宫。

The maintenance dose is adjusted to produce a leukocyte count of 2000-5000/mm^3.

调节维持剂量以达到白细胞计数为每立方毫米 2000 ~ 5000 个。

adjustment [əˈdʒʌstmənt] *n.* 调节,调整

Mild side effects are occasionally observed and may be controlled by adjustment of dosage.

轻度副作用偶尔能见到,可以通过调整剂量来控制。

Disturbances of conduct are distinguished from an adjustment reaction by a longer duration and by a lack of close relationship in time and content to stress.

传导行为障碍与调节反应的区别是前者时程较长,以及对应激刺激在时间和内容上缺乏密切的联系。

adjuvant [ˈædʒuvənt] *a.* 辅助的

Adjuvant chemotherapy can prolong the disease-free period in women with breast cancer after radical mastectomy.

患乳腺癌的妇女，在根治性乳腺切除术后，用辅助性化疗可延长无病期。

n. 佐药

PAS (para-aminosalicylic acid) is a valuable adjuvant to streptomycin and dihydrostreptomycin in the treatment of tuberculosis.

治疗结核病，对氨基水杨酸钠是链霉素和双氢链霉素的良好佐药。

ad libitum [æd'libitəm] *ad.* 随意，任意

It was assumed that ad libitum feeding not only would satisfy the nutritional needs of the test animals, but also would reduce husbandry costs.

设想认为随意饲养不仅能满足受试动物的营养需要，而且可减少动物管理的费用。

administer [əd'ministə] *v.* 实施，用(药等)

Several important steps must be taken before anesthesia is administered.

有几个重要步骤必须在实施麻醉前采取。

Laxative was administered to the patient every morning for two days.

接连两天每天早晨都给病人服轻泻药。

Oxygen is administered in an effort to relieve cyanosis and the rising respiratory rate.

进行输氧以缓解发绀和呼吸率升高。

If an immediate onset of action is required, drugs must be administered directly into the general circulation.

如果需要药物立即发挥作用，必须将药物直接注入体循环。

administration [əd,minis'treiʃən] *n.* (药的) 服法，用法，给予

The physiochemical nature of certain drugs may exclude the oral route of administration.

某些药物的理化性质使其不能口服给药。

The administration of preoperative medication should be verified.

术前应核实药物的使用。

This potential danger should not preclude its administration.

这种潜在的危险性不应排除投药。

administrative [əd'ministrətiv] *a.* 行政的，管理的

The administrative task of running a modern hospital can be very complex.

现代医院运作中的管理工作是很复杂的。

A hospital administrator obviously cannot perform all of the administrative tasks in a hospital.

医院的院长显然不能一个人处理一个医院的所有管理事务。

To assure that this is possible, the hospital must have a qualified administrative staff.

为了确保这一切可能，医院必须有一个能胜任此项工作的管理队伍。

administratively [əd'ministrətivli] *ad.* 行政上

The dean is administratively responsible to the president of the university and, through him, to the board.

院长在行政上对大学校长负责，并通过校长向董事会负责。

admission [əd'miʃən] *n.* (入会，入学，入院) 许可，收留 (住院)

The need for hospital admission for the severely ill elderly is not usually in dispute.

患有严重疾病的老年患者需住院治疗，对此通常没有争议。

On admission to our hospital, the patient was kept under close observation for symptoms of lung cancer.

收住我院以后，严密地观察病人有无肺癌的症状。

admit [əd'mit] *v.* 许可(人或物)进入，容纳

The patient was admitted for cerebral hemorrhage.

病人因大脑出血住院。

This laboratory is small and admits only 10 people.

该实验室很小，只能容纳 10 人。

admonition [ˌædməu'niʃən] *n.* 忠告,训诫

Parental admonitions to eat those vegetables will likely take effect.

父母有关吃那些蔬菜的告诫似乎会产生效果。

adnexa [æd'neksə] *n.* 附件,附器

Melanocytes and other cells which are seen in the adult epidermis can be found within the adnexa.

黑素细胞和见于成人表皮中的其他细胞能在皮肤附属器内见到。

adnexal [æd'neksəl] *a.* 附件的(尤指子宫附件)

Because any solid ovarian mass may represent a malignant tumor,the description of any adnexal lesion must be accurately recorded.

由于任一卵巢实性肿块都有可能是恶性肿瘤,故所有的附件病变均应准确记录。

adnexitis [ˌædnek'saitis] *n.* 子宫附件炎

In complicated gonorrhea,liberation of gonococci into the bloodstream can occur,e. g. ,in parenchymatous gonococcal prostatitis or gonococcal adnexitis.

在淋病的并发症中可能发生淋球菌释放入血液的现象,如淋菌性实质性前列腺炎或淋菌性附件炎。

adolescence [ˌædəu'lesns] *n.* 青春期

The paranasal sinuses enlarge during childhood and adolescence.

鼻旁窦在童年和青春期增大。

When chronic or reactivation tuberculosis occurs during adolescence,it usually has a more acute clinical course than in adults.

当青少年期出现慢性或复发性结核时,常较成人有更急性的病程。

adolescent [ˌædəu'lesnt] *a.* 青春期的

The disease usually strikes adolescent girls who have no reason to diet.

此种病经常侵袭无理由节食的青春期女孩。

Currently,the adolescent population in the United States is the group least likely to have health insurance.

现在,美国人群中最少享有健康保险的是青少年。

n. 青少年

Aplastic anemias are most common in adolescents and young adults.

再生障碍性贫血最常见于少年和青年。

adopt [ə'dɔpt] *v.* 采用;领养

However,she admits the fate of this and other devices in development is tied to whether states adopt a low-carbon policy.

不过她也承认此装置以及其他在开发中的类似装置的命运和国家是否采取低碳政策紧密相关。

The best way to change your figure permanently is to adopt sensible eating and exercise habits.

长期改变体型的最佳办法就是养成合理的饮食和锻炼的习惯。

Recent studies of adopted children of alcoholics indicate that 30 to 40 percent become alcoholics themselves.

最近对酗酒者领养的孩子的研究表明,这些孩子自身有 30% ~40% 也成为酗酒者。

adoptive [ə'dɔptiv] *a.* 继承性的;采用的

Adoptive immunization refers to the transfer of immunity by the transfer of immune cells.

继承性免疫是指通过输注免疫细胞而获得了免疫能力。

adrenal [ə'driːnl] *a.* 肾上腺的 *n.* 肾上腺

Adequate treatment of patients with adrenal insufficiency includes the administration of glucocorticoids.

对肾上腺功能不全病人的适宜治疗包括使用糖皮质激素。

Conversely, adrenal hemorrhage during bacterial sepsis may cause glucocorticoid production to cease.

相反,细菌性脓毒病感染时,肾上腺出血可导致糖皮质激素生成停止。

adrenalectomy [əˌdriːnə'lektəmi] *n.* 肾上腺切除术

If the disease is primarily adrenal, bilateral adrenalectomy is followed by replacement therapy.

假如该病是肾上腺原发的,则行双侧肾上腺切除术,继以替代治疗。

adrenalin [ə'drenəlin] *n.* 肾上腺素

Adrenalin is not only the most effective drug for acute urticaria, but it works with great rapidity.

肾上腺素对急性荨麻疹不仅是最有效的药物,而且作用也很快。

adrenergic [ˌædre'nəːdʒik] *a.* 肾上腺素能的

This increased activity of the adrenergic neurons supports ventricular contractility in congestive heart failure.

充血性心力衰竭时,肾上腺素能神经元活性增加可以增加心室收缩力。

Neurotransmitter receptors include the cholinergic, α- and β-adrenergic, dopamine, opiates, and histamine receptors.

神经递质受体包括胆碱能受体、α 和 β 肾上腺素能受体、多巴胺受体、阿片受体和组胺受体。

adrenocortical [əˌdriːnəu'kɔːtikəl] *a.* 肾上腺皮质的

Adrenocortical steroids of a third group regulate water and salt balance.

第三类肾上腺皮质类固醇可以调节水和盐的平衡。

adrenocorticoid [əˌdriːnəu'kɔːtikɔid] *n.* 肾上腺皮质激素类

Adrenocorticoid or trace element values are useful for evaluating progression of chronic infection.

肾上腺皮质激素和痕量元素值对测定慢性感染的进展有用。

adrenocorticosteroid [əˌdriːnəuˌkɔːtikəu'stiərɔid] *n.* 肾上腺皮质激素

Adrenocorticosteroid therapy may also cause a false negative tuberculin skin reaction.

肾上腺皮质激素治疗也可引起结核菌素皮肤反应假阴性。

adrenocorticotropic [əˌdriːnəukɔːtikəu'trɔpik] *a.* 促肾上腺皮质激素的

In Cushing's disease, excessive pituitary production of adrenocorticotropic hormone (ACTH) causes adrenal cortical hyperplasia and excessive corticosteroid secretion.

库欣病是垂体产生过多的促肾上腺皮质激素(ACTH)引起肾上腺皮质增生和过多的皮质类固醇分泌。

These tumors sometimes are associated with syndromes of excess ACTH (adrenocorticotropic hormone) or ADH (antidiuretic hormone) production.

这些肿瘤有时与促肾上腺皮质激素或抗利尿激素的过多分泌综合征有联系。

adrenocorticotropin [əˌdriːnəuˌkɔːtikəu'trɔpin] *n.* 促皮质素,促肾上腺皮质激素

Adrenocorticotropin (ACTH) exerts a number of physiological actions including maintenance of the adrenal gland and stimulation of adrenal corticosteroid secretion.

促肾上腺皮质激素(ACTH)有多种生理功能,包括维持肾上腺素的分泌和刺激肾上腺皮质类固醇激素的分泌。

There are also endogenous antipyretic substances, such as adrenocorticotropin and corticotropin-releasing hormone.

也有内源性抗致热原物质,如促肾上腺皮质激素和促肾上腺皮质激素释放激素。

adrenodoxin [əˌdrenə'dɔksin] *n.* 皮质铁氧还蛋白

Substrate (cholesterol) binding to cytochrome P-450scc promotes the binding of the free adrenodoxin to the cytochrome.

底物(胆固醇)和细胞色素 P-450scc 结合能促进游离皮质铁氧还蛋白与细胞色素的结合。

They alter the oxidation-reduction potential of adrenodoxin.

他们改变了皮质铁氧还蛋白的氧化还原电位。

adrenogenital [əˌdrinəu'dʒenitəl] *a.* 肾上腺(性)生殖器的

It is also a feature of the adrenogenital syndrome in young infants, and Addison's disease.

这也是幼婴肾上腺性征综合征和艾迪生病的一个特征。

The adrenogenital syndrome is caused by a tumour or hyperplasia of the adrenal cortex.

肾上腺性征综合征系由肾上腺皮质肿瘤或增生引起。

adriamycin [ˌeidriə'maisin] *n.* 阿霉素(抗肿瘤药)

Adriamycin has the greatest potential for cardiac toxicity.

阿霉素有很强的潜在性的心脏毒性。

adsorption [æd'sɔːpʃən] *n.* 吸附

Several modifications have been designed to remove these substances before analysis, including deproteinization with specific adsorption.

已设计了几种改进的方法可以在分析之前去除这些物质,包括使用特殊的吸附剂去除蛋白。

adult ['ædʌlt, ə'dʌlt] *a.* 成年人的,成熟的

The adult spleen is about 13cm×8cm in size and weighs about 180-250g.

成年人的脾脏大小约为13cm×8cm,重量约为180～250g。

Normal adult hemoglobin consists of two identical alpha and two identical beta chains.

正常成年人的血红蛋白含有两条相同的α链和两条相同的β链。

n. 成人,成年;成虫

Adult respiratory distress syndrome (ARDS) may develop in adults with severe malaria.

患严重疟疾的成人可发生成人呼吸窘迫综合征(ARDS)。

In parasitic worms, the life cycle is generally divided into three stages—egg, larva and adult.

寄生虫的生活周期一般分为三个阶段——卵、幼虫和成虫。

adulterant [ʌ'dʌltərənt] *n.* 掺杂物

Drugs are purchased in powdered form and often contain adulterants such as quinine, talc, and dextrose.

所购的药物成粉状,常含有掺杂物如奎宁、滑石粉和葡萄糖。

advance [əd'vɑːns] *n.* 进展

This procedure extends previous advances in the diagnosis and therapy of coronary artery disease.

这一方法扩大了以前诊断和治疗冠心病进展的影响。

v. 推进,进展;提出

Many theories to explain enzyme actions have been advanced.

许多说明酶的作用的学说已被提出。

Diabetes as a rule advances comparatively slowly except in the young.

一般说来,糖尿病进展比较缓慢,但年轻人除外。

advanced [əd'vɑːnst] *a.* 晚期的;老年的;高级的;先进的

Because the onset of pulmonary tuberculosis is often insidious, many cases are not diagnosed until they have reached an advanced stage.

由于肺结核的发病常是隐性的,很多病例直到晚期才被诊断出来。

Magnetic resonance is a kind of advanced equipment.

磁共振是一种先进的设备。

Advanced life support means definitive emergency medical care that includes defibrillation, airway management, and use of drugs and medications.

高级生命维持措施是指提供起决定性作用的急救医疗,包括去纤颤、导气管和药物的使用。

The young doctor who has obtained a doctorate degree will go abroad for advanced study.

刚获得博士学位的这位年轻医生将去国外进修。

advantage [əd'vɑːntidʒ] *n.* 优点,有利条件

An advantage of the Y-U operation is the simplicity of its performance.
Y-U 幽门成形术的优点是简便易行。
The technique also had the advantage that it could be repeated without causing damage.
此技术还有一个优点，即可以重复进行而不造成损伤。
DNA vaccines have potentially a number of advantages over traditional methods of vaccination.
DNA 疫苗与传统方法制备的疫苗相比有许多潜在的优势。

advantageous [ˌædvən'teidʒəs] *a.* 有利的，有助的
How does such diversity manifest itself and how is it advantageous to the host?
这种多样性本身是如何展示的，对宿主有何好处？

advent ['ædvent] *n.* 来临
With the advent of the electron microscope a beautiful world of intracellular organization and architecture was revealed.
随着电子显微镜的问世，细胞内组织结构的绝妙境界被显示出来。

adverse ['ædvəːs] *a.* 逆的，有害的，不利的
Several types of antibodies neutralize the adverse effects of the parasite multiplication.
有几种类型的抗体可中和寄生虫繁殖所产生的有害作用。
In inherited subaortic stenosis, digitalis may cause an adverse drug reaction.
在遗传性主动脉瓣下狭窄时，洋地黄可引起不良的药物反应。
Sometimes, there are adverse factors in a person's physical, emotional, or social environment that are damaging to health.
在一个人的身心或社会环境中可能会有些有损健康的不利因素。

adversely ['ædvəsli] *ad.* 不利地，相反地
The fetal metabolism is adversely affected in this situation.
胎儿的代谢在这种情况下会受到不利的影响。

adversity [æd'vəːsiti] *n.* 逆境，灾难
People with positive attitude towards wellness have tremendous ability to bounce back from adversity.
那些对康复持积极态度的人有从逆境中恢复过来的惊人的能力。

advisable [əd'vaizəbl] *a.* 可取的，适当的
Penicillin treatment is particularly advisable for scarlet fever.
青霉素疗法特别适用于治疗猩红热。
It is advisable to admit a child to hospital after a first epileptic seizure in order to exclude the diagnosis of meningitis.
为了排除脑膜炎的诊断，第一次癫痫发作后将患儿收进医院是适宜的。
It is advisable to be on the alert for untoward reactions which may not have been described before.
应警惕以前没有记载过的不良反应。

advocate ['ædvəkeit] *v.* 提倡，主张
Preoperative irradiation has been advocated by some, but it is generally not employed.
有些人主张术前放疗，但一般不采用。
Some surgeons advocate conservative treatment with antibiotics for an attack of uncomplicated acute cholecystitis.
有些外科医生主张用抗生素对无并发症的急性胆囊炎发作进行保守治疗。

adynamic [ˌædai'næmik] *a.* 虚弱的，无力的
After a serious illness, he looked rather adynamic.
一场重病之后，他看上去很虚弱。

aeration [ˌeiə'reiʃən] *n.* 换气，充气
This baby appears to be perfectly normal on physical examination with good aeration throughout

both lung fields.
此婴儿体格检查看来完全正常，两肺野充气良好。

aerial [ˈɛəriəl] *a.* 空气的；空中的；航空的

The culture grossly shows profuse, fuzzy, cottony aerial mycelia tending to become powdery in the center.
培养的菌落粗略地显示出丰盛的、绒毛棉花样的气生菌丝，其中心部位往往变成粉末状。

aeroallergen [ˌɛərəuˈælədʒen] *n.* 空气中过敏原，空气中变应原

Aeroallergen is a substance in the air that causes or induce an allergy, such as floating pollen.
空气中能诱发变态反应的物质称为空气中变应原，如飘浮的花粉。

aerobe [ˈɛərəub] *n.* 需氧菌

Microbes that require oxygen for growth are called aerobes.
需要氧气以供生长的细菌被称为需氧菌。
Samples of sinus secretions should be cultured for anaerobes, aerobes and fungi.
窦道的分泌物样本应进行厌氧菌、需氧菌和真菌的培养。

aerobic [ɛəˈrəubik] *a.* 需氧的

Glycolysis can be both aerobic and anaerobic.
糖酵解可以是有氧和无氧代谢。
If you want to reduce your body fat, you have to do aerobic exercises very often.
如果你想减少身体的脂肪，你就得经常做有氧运动。

aerococcaceae [ˌɛərəukɔˈkeisiiː] *n.* 气球菌科

The Aerococcaceae are a family of Gram-positive lactic acid bacteria.
气球菌科是革兰阳性乳酸菌成员。
Aerococcaceae are ubiquitous in every habitat on Earth, growing in soil, acidic hot springs, radioactive waste, water, and deep in the Earth's crust.
气球菌在地球上无处不在，它们生长在土壤、酸性热温泉、放射性废物、水、甚至地壳深处。

aerogel [ˈɛərədʒel] *n.* 气凝胶

The synthesized aerogel was calcined at 500℃ to produce nanoparticle solids.
这种合成的气凝胶在500℃煅烧以生产出纳米颗粒。
Aerogel materials have myriad scientific and technological applications due to their large intrinsic surface areas and ultralow densities.
气凝胶材料由于其较大的固有表面积和超低密度而被广泛应用于科学技术领域。

aerosil [ˈɛərəsil] *n.* 微粉硅胶

Aerosil is amorphous nonporous silica with particle dimensions from 4 to 40nm.
微粉硅胶是粒径在4～40nm之间的无定形、无空隙二氧化硅。
Aerosil is a good adsorption medium in the tableting of oily and moist substance.
在油性和湿性物质压片时，微粉硅胶是良好的吸附介质。
Aerosil can be used as disintegrant, glidant, lubricant and loading agent in pharmaceutics.
微粉硅胶在药剂学中可用作崩解剂、助流剂、润滑剂和填充剂。

aerosol [ˈɛərəusɔl] *n.* 气雾剂，气溶胶

It is also given as an aerosol inhalant and is used in ointments, lotions, and troches.
它也用作气雾吸入剂，并用于药膏、洗剂和药片中。
Immediate relief can be obtained if the drug is inhaled from a pressurised aerosol or as a dry powder.
如果通过压力喷雾吸入或干粉状吸入药物，病情可立即缓解。
Relative humidity (RH) affects the liquid water content of an aerosol, altering its scattering and absorption of visible light.
相对湿度影响气溶胶的液态水含量，改变其对可见光的散射和吸收。

aesculetin [iːskju'letin] *n.* 七叶素,秦皮素

After being processed by different methods, the aesculetin contents of semen Euphorbia all decreased.

经不同方法加工炮制后,千金子的七叶素的含量均有所下降。

The crude and 5 kinds of different processed products of semen Euphorbia were determined by TLC scanning and aesculetin as control sample.

以七叶素为对照品,应用薄层扫描法(TLC)对千金子生品及5种不同炮制加工品进行了含量测定。

aetiological→etiological

aetiology→etiology

afebrile [ei'fiːbrail] *a.* 无热(度)的

Classically, the children are afebrile.

典型情况是患儿不发烧。

The dose may be reduced to 2g/d when the patient becomes afebrile.

如果病人停止发热,(应用的)剂量可以减至每日2克。

affect [ə'fekt] *v.* 影响;(疾病)侵袭

Anything that influences your nervous system affects the rest of your body.

累及神经系统的任何东西也会影响身体的其余部位。

Water pollution affects plants and organisms living in these bodies of water.

水污染可影响生活在这些水体中的植物和微生物。

His right lung is affected by tuberculosis.

他的右肺患有肺结核。

Bronchitis, especially chronic bronchitis, is a common disease affecting the health of many old persons.

支气管炎,特别是慢性支气管炎,是影响许多老年人的常见疾病。

Autoimmune hemolytic anemia affects women more than men, and most commonly those <50 years old.

自身免疫性溶血性贫血患者中女性多于男性,且多为50岁以下的人。

affect ['æfekt] *n.* 感情,情感

An infectious affect is characteristic of mania.

感染性情感是躁狂的特点。

Grief is mostly the affect resulting from bereavement.

悲伤主要是源于丧亲的那种情感。

affected [ə'fektid] *a.* 受(疾病等)侵袭的;感染的;受影响的

The most important first aid care of fractures is prevention of movement of the affected part.

骨折最重要的急救是防止受损部位的挪动。

In vitiligo, the affected skin becomes white because of destruction of melanocytes.

在白癜风患者,其受累皮肤的变白是由于皮肤的黑素细胞被破坏所致。

Rub Whitfield's ointment into the affected areas morning and night.

早晚用惠氏软膏涂擦受感染的区域。

Affected patients are strongly predisposed to both venous and arterial thrombi, a common cause of death.

受影响的病人极易发生静脉和动脉两者的血栓,这是常见的死因。

affection [ə'fekʃən] *n.* 疾患,病,病变;影响

Numerous affections of the nails make a firm diagnosis of onychomycosis difficult unless fungi are actually demonstrated.

很多指甲的疾患使甲真菌病确诊很困难,除非确实查到了真菌。

affective [ə'fektiv] *a.* 感情的,情感的

Twenty to thirty five percent of major affective disorders follow a chronic course.

20% ~35% 的严重情感障碍具有慢性病程。

Bipolar disorder is a form of phasic affective illness with both manic and depressive phenomena.

双相障碍是一种兼有躁狂和抑郁现象的时相性情感障碍。

afferent [ˈæfərənt] *a.* 传入的

The ANS (autonomic nervous system) also receives afferent impulses from these parts of the body.

自主神经系统亦接受来自身体这些部位的传入冲动。

Blood enters the glomerulus by way of an afferent arteriole of the renal artery.

血液通过肾动脉的输入小动脉进入肾小球。

affiliate [əˈfilieit] *v.* 使隶属,附属

He is a doctor of the Second Affiliated Hospital of Tongji Medical University.

他是同济医科大学附属第二医院的医生。

The objective of the study is to identify feeding practices and nutritional status of Mexican children affiliated to the Medical Insurance for a New Generation.

此研究的目的是确认隶属于"新一代医疗保险"项目的墨西哥儿童的喂养方式和营养状况。

n. [əˈfiliit] 分支机构

Its national affiliates have been in the front lines of this fight and will play a vital role in the years to come.

它在各国的分支机构一直战斗在第一线,并将在未来的岁月里起举足轻重的作用。

affiliation [əˌfiliˈeiʃən] *n.* 联合

Affiliation between the medical school and one or more hospitals provides facilities for practical work in the clinical subjects.

医学院与一个或多个医院建立合作关系,便于安排临床课的实习。

affinity [əˈfiniti] *n.* 亲和力

The plasma proteins have a high affinity for binding drugs.

血浆蛋白对药物有高度的亲和力。

There is a special affinity of streptomycin for the vestibular nerve.

链霉素对前庭神经有一种特殊的亲和力。

afflict [əˈflikt] *v.* 使苦恼,折磨

The mother is greatly afflicted by the loss of her child.

这位母亲因失去孩子而痛苦不堪。

These patients are seriously afflicted with heart diseases.

这些病人都受到心脏病的折磨。

affliction [əˈflikʃən] *n.* 苦恼,折磨

Facial paralysis is a terrible affliction, for it deprives the victim of emotional expression.

面神经麻痹是一种可怕的折磨,因为它剥夺了患者的表情能力。

afford [əˈfɔːd] *v.* 担负得起;提供,给予

For those patients who have spasmodic dysmenorrhoea, the use of the pill affords them relief.

对于那些痉挛痛经的病人,用这种药丸可提供缓解作用。

Although these drugs afford some benefit in experimental models of ischemic ARF, their efficacy has not been proven in clinical trials.

虽然这些药物在(动物)实验性缺血性急性肾衰(ARF)模型上有某些用途,但它的有效性在临床实践中尚未得到证实。

affordability [əˌfɔːdəˈbiliti] *n.* 个人可支付,负担能力,可负担性

The results of such an evaluation should take into account feasibility and affordability.

这一评估的结果应该考虑可行性和负担能力。

Empirical study of affordability of the essential medicines in the regional provinces of China has been performed.
中国部分地区对基本药物可负担性的实证研究已经完成。

affront [əˈfrʌnt] *n.* 蔑视，伤害
A result of these technologies was accompanied by ethical concerns about the potential for affronts to personal dignity.
这些技术的一个结果是伴有潜在伤害个人尊严的伦理学忧虑。
Such behavior is an affront to social morality.
这种行为是对社会公德的蔑视。

afibrinogenemia [ˌeifaiˌbrinədʒəˈniːmiə] *n.* 纤维蛋白原缺乏血症
Congenital afibrinogenemia is a rare autosomal recessive disorder, characterized by the complete absence or extremely reduced level of fibrinogen.
先天性纤维蛋白原缺乏血症是一种罕见的常染色体隐性遗传病，表现为纤维蛋白原水平极度降低或缺乏。
Congenital afibrinogenemia is a bleeding disorder caused by impairment of the blood clotting process.
先天性纤维蛋白原缺乏血症是一种凝血过程受损引起的出血性疾病。

aflatoxicosis [æfləˌtɔksiˈkəusis] *n.* 黄曲霉毒素中毒
The doctor signed his name on the report of pathological diagnosis on the complicating disease cases with aflatoxicosis.
医生已在黄曲霉毒素中毒并发病例的病理学诊断报告上签字了。
Attention should be paid to aflatoxicosis of sows to avoid big damage.
应注意预防母猪黄曲霉毒素中毒以避免产生大的损失。

aflatoxin [ˌæfləˈtɔksin] *n.* 黄曲霉毒素
Aflatoxin is thought to cause certain cancers in animals as well as abnormalities in human chromosomes.
黄曲霉毒素被认为可以使动物产生某些癌症以及人体产生染色体异常。

afterbirth [ˈɑːftəˌbəːθ] *n.* 胞衣，胎盘胎膜
When placenta is expelled following the birth of the baby, it is commonly called the afterbirth.
当胎盘随着婴儿的出生而娩出时，它通常被称作胞衣。

afterbrain [ˈɑːftəˌbrein] *n.* 后脑
The forebrain, the midbrain and the afterbrain make up the brain.
前脑、中脑和后脑组成了大脑。

afterload [ˈɑːftəˌləud] *n.* 后负荷
The peripheral vascular resistance forms the afterload of the heart.
外周血管阻力形成心脏的后负荷。

afterward(s) [ˈɑːftəwəd(z)] *ad.* 后来，以后
Gumma of the brain or spinal cord should be treated surgically first, and for syphilis afterward.
脑或脊髓部位的梅毒瘤，应该先行手术治疗，然后再作驱梅毒治疗。

agalactia [egəˈlæktiəˌægə-] *n.* 乳汁不足
Did you observe the effect of Xia Ru Yong Quan Powder on agalactia caused by low spirit?
你观察过下乳涌泉散对因不良情绪乳汁不足产妇的催乳效果吗？
The minimal bactericidal concentration(MBC) of Streptococcus agalactia was 25.00mg/ml.
无乳链球菌的最小杀菌浓度为25.00mg/ml。

agammaglobulinemia [əˌgæməˌglɔbjuliˈniːmiə] *n.* 无丙种球蛋白血症
Patients with sex-linked congenital agammaglobulinemia have absence of circulating mature B lymphocytes in the peripheral blood.
患性联锁先天性无丙种球蛋白血症的患者，外周血中缺乏循环的成熟 B 淋巴细胞。

agar ['ɑːgɑː] *n.* 琼脂

Agar slant cultures of some bacteria, yeasts, and molds are customarily stored for long periods of time.

一些细菌、酵母菌、霉菌的琼脂斜面培养物通常可长期保存。

agastache [ə'gæstaːʃ] *n.* 藿香

He says a flowering plant called agastache is also popular in gardens.

他说一种叫藿香的开花植物也很流行。

The agastache has great value in medicine, eating, spice, etc.

藿香兼具药用、食用、香料等多方面应用价值。

age [eidʒ] *v.* 变老,老化

With continued advancements in health care, the world's population is aging.

随着卫生保健事业的不断发展,世界人口在逐渐老化。

As a person ages, there take place characteristic changes in the over-all activity of his body cells.

当一个人年岁增大时,其全身细胞全面活动的特别明显的变化随之发生。

aged ['eidʒid] *a.* 年老的,…岁的

The fracture of a bone takes considerably longer time to heal in an aged person than in a young one.

老年人骨折后其愈合的时间比年轻人所需的要长得多。

agency ['eidʒənsi] *n.* 机构

Affiliation of the medical schools with government agencies and with nonofficial social and health agencies helps to further develop the medical and health cause of the country.

医学院校与政府机构、非官方的社会卫生事业机构的合作关系有助于进一步发展这个国家的医疗卫生事业。

agenesis [ei'dʒenisis] *n.* 发育不全

Agenesis of one thyroid lobe may occur.

可能发生一叶甲状腺发育不全。

Agenesis can refer to any part of the body.

发育不全可以出现在身体的任何部位。

agent ['eidʒənt] *n.* (药)剂,药物;因子

Not all agents are produced by chemical synthesis.

不是所有药品都是用化学合成法生产的。

Drugs may alter the protein binding of other agents.

有些药物可以改变另一些药物的蛋白结合率。

Acute inflammation is the immediate and early response of the organism to an injurious agent.

急性炎症是机体对有害因子的立即和早期反应。

agglomerate [ə'glɔməreit] *n.* 团块,聚结物

The invention relates to a method of producing an agglomerate of drug and solid binder.

本发明涉及制备药物和固体黏合剂的聚结物的方法。

v. 凝聚,成块

In general, fine particles tend to clump and agglomerate if they are moist or tacky.

通常潮湿和黏性的微细颗粒易于聚集和结块。

agglutinate [ə'gluːtineit] *v.* (使)凝集

Rheumatoid factor agglutinates sensitized sheep red cells.

类风湿因子可以凝集敏感化了的羊红细胞。

Lectins will agglutinate many kinds of cell.

外源凝集素可使多种细胞凝集。

IgM is much more efficient at agglutinating particles or cells.

IgM 在凝集颗粒和细胞上有效得多。

agglutination [əˌgluːtiˈneiʃən] *n.* 凝集作用，凝集反应

Precipitation and agglutination have also been adapted for development of several useful assays.
沉淀作用和凝集反应也可用来建立几种有用的测定方法。

Agglutination is clumping or close association of red cells caused by a specific antibody or antigen present on the cells.
凝集作用是由细胞表面上的特异性抗体或抗原使红细胞出现凝块或呈现聚集。

In a transfusion, donor and recipient should be of the same blood group to prevent agglutination.
输血时供血者与受血者应是同一血型以防止凝集反应。

agglutinin [əˈgluːtinin] *n.* 凝集素

Antibodies that form visible clumps, or agglutinate, with their specific antigens are called agglutinins.
能与特异性抗原形成可见凝块（即凝集）的抗体则被称为凝集素。

An O agglutinin titer of ≥1∶80 or a fourfold rise supports a diagnosis of typhoid fever.
抗原凝集素 O 的滴度≥1∶80 或升高 4 倍可支持伤寒的诊断。

agglutinogen [ˌægluːˈtinədʒən] *n.* 凝集原

When neither A nor B agglutinogen is present, the blood group is group O.
当既无 A 凝集原又无 B 凝集原时，则血型为 O 型。

aggravate [ˈægrəveit] *v.* 加重，使恶化

Cortisol has an antiinsulin effect and aggravates diabetes mellitus.
氢化可的松有抗胰岛素的作用，从而加重糖尿病。

The necrosis is usually aggravated by trauma and bacterial infection.
这种坏死常由于外伤和细菌感染而恶化。

Aggravating factors are azotemia, prolonged endotracheal intubation, and severe associated infection.
加重因素有氮血症、长期气管内置管以及严重的复合感染。

aggravation [ˌægrəˈveiʃən] *n.* 加速，恶化

A history of intense aggravation by coughing will usually point toward the pleura and pericardium as the site.
咳嗽明显加重的病史通常提示病变部位在胸膜和心包。

In early heart failure, dyspnea is observed only during activity, when it may simply represent an aggravation of the breathlessness that occurs normally.
在心力衰竭早期，呼吸困难仅见于活动时，此时它仅表现为正常发生的呼吸困难加重。

aggregate [ˈægrigit] *n.* 聚合体，聚合物

The violet basic dye and the iodine form a large aggregate within the heat-fixed cell.
紫色的碱性染料与碘在加热固定的菌细胞内形成大的聚合物。

a. 总数的，总计的

Aggregate analyse suggests that an adverse event is associated with exposure to a drug.
总计分析提示不良事件与药物的暴露有关。

aggregation [ˌægriˈgeiʃən] *n.* 聚集，集合（物），凝聚反应

PGE_1 (prostaglandin E_1) inhibits platelet aggregation whereas TXA_2 (thromboxane A_2) induces platelet aggregation.
前列腺素 E_1 抑制血小板聚集，而血栓烷 A_2 则导致血小板聚集。

aggressive [əˈgresiv] *a.* 攻击性的；强力的；有进取心的

An aggressive dosage of penicillin as high as 40000000 units per day is recommended.
建议给以每日高达 4000 万单位青霉素的冲击剂量（大剂量）。

The recurrent otitis media did not respond to prolonged aggressive medical treatment.
长程强力的药物治疗对复发性中耳炎无效。

The reaction is none the stronger for all the aggressive therapy.

治疗虽然积极，反应却毫不强烈。

aggressiveness [ə'gresivnis] *n.* 侵略；攻击

Disturbances of conduct are disorders mainly involving aggressiveness and distructive behaviour.

行为障碍主要包括攻击和破坏行为的病状。

aging ['eidʒiŋ] *n.* 衰老，老化

The aging process is of considerable interest biologically.

衰老过程具有重要的生物学意义。

An abrupt decline in any system or function is always due to disease and not to "normal aging".

任何系统或机体功能突然出现衰退，都由疾病引起而不是正常的衰老。

agitate ['ædʒiteit] *v.* 鼓动，搅动

We usually make the turns gently that they may not agitate the painful part.

通常我们（把病人）转动得很轻柔，以便不致刺激疼痛部位。

Add the sodium thiasulfate solution while continuously agitating the liquid.

在连续搅拌液体时，加入硫代硫酸钠溶液。

agitation [ædʒi'teiʃən] *n.* 振荡；焦虑不安

The acute reaction to stress may manifest a predominant psychomotor disturbance, e. g. agitation or stupor.

急性应激反应可表现为突出的精神运动障碍如焦虑不安或木僵。

Clinical manifestations of the uremic syndrome include neuropsychiatric disturbances, such as confusion, coma, and agitation.

尿毒症患者的临床表现包括有神经精神异常，如意识模糊、昏迷或兴奋。

agnosia [æg'nəusiə] *n.* 失认症

Agnosia is a loss of ability to recognize objects, persons, sounds, shapes, or smells.

失认症指患者丧失了对各类物体、人、声音、形状或气味的识别能力。

Agnosia can result from stroke, dementia, or other neurological disorders.

失认症可由卒中、痴呆或其他神经疾病所致。

agonist ['ægənist] *n.* 激动剂；主动肌

Drugs that interact with a receptor and elicit a response are called agonists.

凡作用于受体并产生效应的药物称为促效药。

agonize ['ægənaiz] *v.* 苦恼，折磨

The survey revealed that many men were unbothered by battle injuries that would have produced agonizing pain in civilian patients.

调查发现许多男性不理会战争创伤，这些创伤对于平民病人而言可引起巨大的苦恼。

agonizing ['ægənaiziŋ] *a.* 使人极度痛苦的

Agonizing pain denotes serious or advanced disease.

极度疼痛意味着存在严重的或晚期的疾病。

agony ['ægəni] *n.* 剧痛，极度痛苦

The patient has suffered agonies with toothache.

病人遭受过牙痛的痛苦。

agranulocyte [ei'grænjuləusait] *n.* 无粒（白）细胞

Agranulocytes are a category of white blood cells characterized by the absence of granules in their cytoplasm.

无粒白细胞是一类以细胞质中缺少颗粒为特点的白细胞。

There are two types of agranulocytes: lymphocytes and monocytes.

无粒白细胞分为两种类型：淋巴细胞和单核细胞。

agranulocytosis [əˌgrænjuləusai'təusis] *n.* 粒细胞缺乏症

Agranulocytosis is fortunately quite rare.

粒细胞缺乏症幸而相当罕见。

The most serious side effect of neuroleptic drugs is agranulocytosis.
精神抑制药的最严重的副作用是粒细胞缺乏症。

agraphesthesia [ə,grɑːfiːs'θiːziə] *n.* 书写感知不能

Agraphesthesia is a disorder of directional cutaneous kinesthesia or disorientation in cutaneous space.
书写感知不能是指皮肤定向运动觉障碍或皮肤空间定向障碍。
Patients with cortico-basal ganglionic degeneration often have agraphesthesia in the hand suffering from apraxia.
皮层基底节变性的病人失用的手经常表现书写感知不能。

agreement [ə'griːmənt] *n.* 同意

There is general agreement that early shock is usually due to a decrease in blood volume, or an increase in the capacity of the vascular space, or both.
一致的看法是早期休克是由于血量减少,或血管腔容量增大,或二者同时存在所致。

agricultural [ˌægri'kʌltʃərəl] *a.* 农业的;农艺的;农学的

Poisoning generally occurs as an accidental exposure in children, contamination in agricultural workers, or intentionally in suicide attempts.
农药中毒发生于偶然接触农药的儿童、受污染的农业工作者或有自杀倾向的人。
Ringworm of the beard occurs chiefly among those in agricultural pursuits, especially those in contact with farm animals.
须癣主要出现于从事农业的人群中,特别是那些经常接触农场动物者。

agrimophol [ˌægri'mɔːfəl] *n.* 仙鹤草酚

Agrimophol, a new phloroglucinol derivative with taenifuge activity, was isolated from the root sprout of a widely distributed Chinese herb—Agrimonia pilosa Ledeb.
仙鹤草酚(一种新的具有驱绦虫作用的间苯三酚衍生物)是从广泛分布的中草药——仙鹤草的根芽中分离出来的。
Owing to the low therapeutic effect of Agrimophol, it could not be used alone.
由于仙鹤草酚疗效不高,不适宜于单独使用。

aid [eid] *v.* 援助,帮助

X-ray examination of the chest aids in the differential diagnosis.
胸部 X 线检查有助于鉴别诊断。
Biopsy findings and serologic testing may aid in the diagnosis.
活检结果和血清学试验皆有助于诊断。
This patient can hear well with a hearing aid.
该患者使用了助听器之后听得清楚。
He pulled the drowning man from the water and gave him first aid.
他把溺水者从水中拖起并对他进行急救。
The WHO offered food and medical aid to the African countries.
世界卫生组织向非洲国家提供食品和医疗援助。

AIDS [eidz] *n.* 艾滋病(获得性免疫缺陷综合征)

AIDS(acquired immune deficiency syndrome) was first recognized as a distinct disease entity among homosexual men in the United States in 1981.
艾滋病于 1981 年首次在美国被公认为男性同性恋者中一种独特的病种。
AIDS is essentially a sexually transmitted disease, either homosexually or heterosexually.
艾滋病基本上是一种同性或异性间的性传播疾病。
Currently AIDS is considered to be fatal, although the type and length of illness preceding death varies considerably.
目前认为艾滋病可致命,虽然死亡前的类型和病程均有很大差异。

ailment ['eilmənt] *n.* (轻微)疾病,失调

Such ailments are often due to old age.
这种疾病常因年老所致。
Headache is one of the most common ailments of human beings.
头痛是人类最常见的疾病之一。
The family physician treats minor ailments so that they will not become serious.
家庭医生为病人治小毛病，不使其发展为严重的疾病。

ainhum ['einhəm] *n.* 自发性断趾病
Radiograph of the right fifth toe showed absorption of the proximal and intermediate phalanges, and a diagnosis of ainhum was made.
X 线片显示右脚第五趾的近端和中间段趾骨有吸收，因而作出自发性断趾病的诊断。
Ainhum is a rare condition of unknown etiology in which a groove or fissure of constricting tissue forms around the proximal end of the fifth toe.
自发性断趾病是一种原因不明的罕见疾病，以第五趾近端周围压缩组织裂隙或者凹槽形成为特征。

air [ɛə] *n.* 空气
Air condition disease is very common in hot summer.
空调病是炎热夏季常见的疾病。
Air pollution is one of the major problems of the modern world.
空气污染是当代世界的主要问题之一。

airborne ['ɛəbɔːn] *a.* 空气传播的，气载的
Infection with rhinoviruses is believed to occur by the airborne route.
一般认为鼻病毒感染是经空气传播发生的。
Dust clouds containing high levels of airborne spores (fungi and bacteria) posed a potential exposure problem for persons with hypersensitivity.
含有大量飘浮孢子（霉菌和细菌）的飘尘对过敏体质的人带来潜在的接触危害。

airspace ['ɛəspeis] *n.* 气腔，气囊
Emphysema refers to the irreversible enlargement of the airspaces distal to the terminal bronchiole in the lung.
肺气肿是指肺内终末细支气管以远的肺组织不可逆性的扩张。
With advanced emphysema, there are even larger abnormal airspaces in the apex of the lung.
随着肺气肿的进展，肺尖部甚至会有更大的异常气肿囊腔。

airway ['ɛəˌwei] *n.* 气道
Airway obstruction may be either partial or complete.
气道阻塞可以是部分阻塞或完全阻塞。
The treatment of the reversible component of airway obstructions is important.
治疗气道阻塞的可逆部分具有重要意义。

akathisia [ˌækə'θiːziə, eikæ'θiʒiə] *n.* 静坐不能
Non-compliance is likely to be increased in patients suffering from the unpleasant symptoms of akathisia.
患有静坐不能不适症状的病人的非依从性可能增加。
Akathisia can also, to a lesser extent, be caused by Parkinson's disease and related syndromes, and likely other neurological diseases.
在较小程度上，静坐不能可由帕金森病和相关综合征引起，也可能由其他神经系统疾病引起。

akebiaquinata [ˌækbiə'kuinətə] *n.* 木通
Isolation purification and analysis of polysaccharide from akebiaquinata decne are very important.
木通多糖的分离纯化及分析是非常重要的。

A new triterpene was found from akebiaquinata stem.
从木通茎中发现了一个新的三萜烯成分。

akin [əˈkin] *a.* 同类的,相近似的

Closely akin to this condition is acute pulmonary edema.
完全类似这种状态的有急性肺水肿。

akinesia [ˌeikaiˈniːziə] *n.* 运动不能

Absence of spontaneous movement is called akinesia.
自主运动能力丧失称为运动不能。

Local akinesia of free ventricular wall often indicates myocardial infarction.
自然的心室壁局部运动功能降低提示患有心肌梗死。

ala [ˈeilə] (pl:alae [ˈeiliː]) *n.* [拉] 翼,翼膜

Split papules are hypertrophic and fissured papules that form in the creases of the alae nasi and at the oral commissures.
裂开丘疹是顶端肥大和开裂的丘疹,多发生在鼻颊皱襞和口唇连合处(等部位)。

alarmingly [əˈlɑːmiŋli] *ad.* 使人吃惊地

The incidence of chronic obstructive pulmonary emphysema has increased alarmingly.
慢性阻塞肺气肿的发病率已升高到令人吃惊的地步。

albinism [ˈælbinizəm] *n.* 白化病(皮肤、毛发、眼睛先天性色素缺乏)

Albinism is an autosomal recessive disease.
白化病是一种常染色体隐性遗传病。

The frequency of the gene for albinism in a population is known to be 1/190.
群体中白化病基因的频率是1/190。

The reduction of hair and skin pigment in albinism is obvious.
白化病人的头发和皮肤的色素明显减少。

Examples include instruction to patients with albinism to limit sun exposure.
举例包括教导白化病病人要限制被日光照射的时间等。

albumin [ˈælbjuːmin] *n.* 白蛋白

Sodium-poor albumin infusions may be helpful in inducing diuresis.
低钠白蛋白输入可能有利于利尿。

Proteins which are soluble in water and also in dilute and moderately concentrated salt solutions are referred to as albumins.
能溶于水,也能溶于稀的和中等浓度的盐溶液的蛋白质称为白蛋白。

albuminoid [ælˈbjuːminɔid] *n.* 类白蛋白

The albuminoids are a special group of proteins, characterized by being essentially insoluble in most common reagents.
类白蛋白是一类特殊的蛋白质,其特征是基本不溶于最常用的试剂中。

albuminous [ælˈbjuːminəs] *a.* 白蛋白的

Being a manifestation of a disturbance of protein metabolism, cloudy swelling is also called albuminous degeneration.
混浊肿胀是一种蛋白质代谢紊乱的表现,也叫做白蛋白变性。

albuminuria [ælˌbjuːmiˈnjuəriə] *n.* 蛋白尿

Milder albuminuria is called an asymptomatic urinary abnormality.
轻度蛋白尿称为无症状性泌尿异常。

Gastrointestinal loss of albumin is compounded by albuminuria.
胃肠道白蛋白的丢失常伴有蛋白尿。

Albuminuria is not always associated with disease, it may occur after strenuous exercise or after a long period of standing (orthostatic albuminuria).
蛋白尿有时与疾病无关,可发生在紧张的锻炼或长时间站立之后(直立性蛋白尿)。

Alcaligenes [ˌælkəˈlidʒəniːz] *n.* 产碱杆菌属

Alcaligenes may also be found in the respiratory tracts of cystic fibrosis patients, where they cause clinical symptoms of pulmonary disease.

产碱杆菌属也存在于囊性纤维症病人的呼吸道中，引起肺病的临床症状。

Alcaligenes is a genus of Gram-negative, pathogenic, opportunistic bacteria.

产碱杆菌属是一类革兰阴性、致病性和机会致病性的细菌。

alcohol [ˈælkəhɔl] *n.* 酒精，乙醇

Alcohol interferes with intermediate metabolism of folic acid and probably its absorption as well.

酒精妨碍叶酸的中间代谢，而且也可能妨碍其吸收。

Blood alcohol levels are higher in women than in men after drinking equivalent amounts of alcohol.

喝相同量的酒之后，在女性血液中的酒精浓度要高于男性。

Blood drug concentrations, particularly alcohol, do tend to correlate with the patient's physiological condition.

血中药物的浓度，特别是乙醇，与病人的生理状况密切相关。

Alcoholic psychosis is an organic psychotic state due mainly to excessive consumption of alcohol.

酒精中毒性精神病主要是由于过量饮酒引起的器质性精神病状态。

alcoholase [ˈælkəhɔleis] *n.* 醇酶

Alcoholase will break down these monoses into alcohol and carbon dioxide.

醇酶将这些单糖分解为乙醇和二氧化碳。

Alcoholase makes alcohol, it does not break it down.

醇酶产生酒精，而不分解酒精。

alcoholic [ˌælkəˈhɔlik] *a.* 乙醇的，酒精的

She drank an occasional alcoholic beverage but did not smoke and took no drugs during pregnancy.

她偶尔饮用含酒精的饮料，但不吸烟，孕期亦无服药史。

As a rule, alcoholic drinkers do not care much for sugar.

一般地说，嗜酒的人不很喜欢吃糖。

n. 嗜酒者

Alcoholics are often hypertensive.

嗜酒者常患高血压。

Alcoholics may have a low blood sugar, and his comatose condition may be due to hypoglycemia.

酗酒者可能有低血糖，其昏迷即可能由低血糖造成。

alcoholism [ˈælkəhɔlizəm] *n.* 醇中毒，酒精中毒

Chronic alcoholism is the most common cause of fatty liver.

慢性酒精中毒是脂肪肝的最常见原因。

The differences may indicate a predisposition to alcoholism.

这些差异可能显示导致酗酒的诱发因素。

aldactone [ælˈdæktəun] *n.* 螺内酯

Aldactone is used to diagnose or treat a condition in which you have too much aldosterone in your body.

螺内酯被用来诊断及治疗醛固酮增多症。

Aldactone tablets contain the active ingredient spironolactone, which is a type of medicine called a potassium-sparing diuretic.

螺内酯片剂含有安体舒通活性成分，是一种保钾利尿剂。

aldehyde [ˈældihaid] *n.* 醛

Aldosterone is unique among naturally occurring steroids in having an aldehyde group in position 18.

醛固酮是惟一的一组在碳 18 位点上有一个醛基的自然生成的类固醇。

However, if the aldehyde dehydrogenase is inhibited, the level of acetaldehyde rises.

然而，如果醛脱氢酶受抑制，乙醛水平就会升高。

aldolase [ˈældəleis] *n.* 醛缩酶

The classic example of severe reactive hypoglycemia without hyperinsulinism is hereditary fructose intolerance (HFI). These children lack normal liver aldolase, which split fructose 1-phosphate.

有严重反应性低血糖而没有高胰岛素分泌的典型例子是遗传性果糖不耐症（HFI），这些儿童缺乏正常肝脏中能分解果糖 1 磷酸的醛缩酶。

aldosterone [ælˈdɔstərəun] *n.* 醛固酮

Renin acts on serum globulin to produce angiotensin which stimulates the adrenal cortex to produce aldosterone.

肾素作用于血清球蛋白产生血管紧张素，后者刺激肾上腺皮质产生醛固酮。

Aldosterone stimulates active absorption of sodium ion.

醛固酮促进钠离子的主动吸收。

In patients with heart failure, not only is aldosterone secretion elevated but the biologic half-life of aldosterone is prolonged.

在心衰病人，不仅体内醛固酮的分泌增加，而且醛固酮的生物半衰期也延长。

aldosteronism [ælˈdɔstərəunizəm] *n.* 醛固酮过多症

Aldosteronism is characterized by excessive production and excretion of aldosterone and typically by loss of body potassium, muscular weakness and elevated blood pressure.

醛固酮过多症的特征是患者过多地产生和分泌醛固酮、典型的体内钾排出增加、肌肉乏力和血压升高。

alert [əˈləːt] *a.* 留心的，警觉的

On physical examination the infant is alert and in moderate respiratory distress.

体检时小儿表现敏感，呈中度呼吸窘迫。

v. 使警觉

The appearance of proteinuria, even in the absence of excessive hypertension, should alert the clinician to the possibility of preeclampsia.

蛋白尿的出现，即使血压不过度升高，也应使临床医生警惕有子痫前期发生的可能。

alertness [əˈləːtnis] *n.* 警觉，苏醒

The prerequisite to the diagnosis of myocarditis is the awareness of its existence and alertness to its manifestations.

诊断心肌炎的先决条件是想到这一疾病的存在并对其临床表现有所警觉。

Return to alertness is usually slow after a seizure, prompt with syncope.

癫痫发作停止后病人的意识恢复较慢，而晕厥的病人其苏醒的恢复较快。

alga [ˈælgə] *n.*（常用 *pl.* algae [ˈældʒiː]）藻类，藻

Some algae have a plant's characteristic photosynthetic capabilities.

有些藻类具有植物特有的光合作用能力。

algal [ˈælgəl] *a.* 藻的

Algal blooms may occur in freshwater as well as marine environments.

淡水和海水中均可发生藻类的大量繁殖。

Algal toxins are a group of strongly toxic substances occurring in the cells of a number of Cyanophyceae (blue-green microalgae).

藻毒素是存在于蓝藻（铜绿微囊藻）细胞膜的一类高毒性物质。

alginate [ˈældʒineit] *n.* 海藻酸盐

Alginates are extracted from brown seaweed and are available in sodium, ammonium and potassium derivatives.

海藻酸盐可从褐藻中提取,并以钠、铵、钾衍生物的形式存在。

The freely permeable sodium alginate gel prevented the aggregation of islet cells that could lead to a loss of function.

具有自由渗透性的海藻酸钠凝胶阻止了可导致功能丧失的胰岛细胞聚集。

algorithm ['ælgəriðəm] *n.* 运算规则; 演示

This type of approach is used by drug regulatory agencies, such as in Australia, and has been used previously in an FDA algorithm.

这类方法被一些药品管理部门(如澳大利亚)所应用,以前亦一直在 FDA(美国食品及药物管理局)的运算规则中应用。

Predictive algorithms have been developed to identify potentially deleterious amino acid substitutions.

已开发出用于鉴别潜在有害氨基酸置换的预测算法。

alienate ['eiljəneit] *v.* 疏远,离间

Not gossiping is a sign that something is wrong and that you feel socially alienated or indifferent.

不聊天表明话不投机,在社交方面感到冷漠和疏远。

align [ə'lain] *v.* 排列,使成一直线

The polypeptide segments in a β-structure are aligned either in a parallel or antiparallel direction to its neighboring chains.

β-结构的多肽节段与毗邻链既可顺向平行排列,亦可反向平行排列。

Specific anatomical reference points on the patient's face are aligned to corresponding points on the three dimensional image.

患者面部特定解剖部位的参考点与三维影像中的对应点进行校正。

alimentary [ˌæli'mentəri] *a.* (关于)营养的,消化的

The alimentary canal is made up of the oral cavity, the pharynx, the esophagus, the stomach, the small intestines, large intestines and rectum.

消化道由口腔、咽、食管、胃、小肠、大肠和直肠组成。

The alimentary tract has a particularly varied flora which can be modified by dietetic change.

消化道有一种特别多样化的菌丛,它能随饮食而变。

alive [ə'laiv] *a.* 活着的

A cell is alive—as alive as you are.

细胞是活着的,就和你一样。

Of all the people who have ever lived to age 65, more than half are now alive.

在所有年龄超过 65 岁的人群中,有超过半数的人仍然活着。

alkali ['ælkəlai] *n.* 碱,强碱

Strong acids and alkalis, as well as very concentrated salts and amines, also denature proteins.

强酸和强碱,就像高浓度盐和胺一样,也可使蛋白质变性。

Acidosis is often intensified by infusion of abundent saline without alkali.

缺乏碱的生理盐水输注过多常会加重酸中毒。

alkaline ['ælkəlain] *a.* (强)碱的,碱性的

Acidic compounds are excreted more favorably if the urine is alkaline.

尿液为碱性时,更有利于酸性药物的排泄。

Investigation shows a high alkaline phosphatase and usually a high bilirubin.

检查可发现碱性磷酸酶升高,而且通常血胆红素也很高。

alkalinity [ˌælkə'liniti] *n.* 碱度,碱性

The pH scale is a measure of the relative acidity or alkalinity of the blood.

pH 标度是血液的相对酸碱度的测定方法。

alkaloid ['ælkəlɔid] *n.* 生物碱

Many alkaloids are important drugs, including morphine, quinine, atropine, and codeine.

很多生物碱是重要的药物，包括吗啡、奎宁、阿托品和可待因。
The new agent is obtained through methylation of an alkaloid extracted from the herbal medicine stephania tetrandra.
这种新药是对从草药千斤藤粉防己中提取的生物碱通过甲基化而得来的。

alkaloidal [ˌælkəˈlɔidəl] *a.* 生物碱的
Enzymes may be coagulated by heat, alcohol, strong acids, and alkaloidal reagents.
热、醇、强酸和生物碱试剂能使酶凝结。

alkalosis [ˌælkəˈləusis] *n.* 碱中毒
When the hydrogen ion concentration is less than normal, the person is said to have alkalosis.
当氢离子浓度低于正常时，我们说该患者有碱中毒。

alkalotic [ˌælkəˈlɔtik] *a.* 碱中毒的
These patients may vomit profusely and become dehydrated and alkalotic.
这些病人可因大量呕吐以致失水和碱中毒。

alkylate [ˈælkileit] *v.* 烷基化，用烷化剂处理
Pilot studies have not proved that alkylating agents or imunosuppressive drugs are beneficial.
小型实验性研究尚未证明烷化剂或免疫抑制药物是否有用。

alkylation [ˌælkiˈleiʃən] *n.* 烷基化
Alkylation of the bases in DNA can introduce gaps in the strand.
DNA 中碱基的烷基化能使该 DNA 链中产生缝隙。

allege [əˈledʒ] *v.* 断言，宣称，辩解
Many factors have been alleged to influence wound healing.
许多因素被断定会影响伤口愈合。
In the 404 cases of quadriceps myofibrosis that we have reviewed, 311 were alleged to have been caused by injections.
在我们研究过的 404 例四头肌肌纤维变性病例中，311 例归因于注射。

allele [əˈliːl] *n.* 等位基因（遗传学上指在同源染色体上占同一位点的基因）
Alleles are alternative forms of a gene at a given locus.
等位基因是一个基因在某一位点的不同形式。
Alleles govern chemical reactions that determine specific traits.
等位基因控制着决定特定性状的化学反应。
If the allele is X-linked dominant, the affected daughters must receive the gene from one of their parents.
如果对等位基因是显性 X-染色体基因，那么受影响的女儿必然会从父亲或母亲那里继承这种基因。

allelotaxis [əˌleləˈtæksis] *n.* 器官发育；异源发生
The neonate birthed at this time is called preterm infant; the birth weight is 1000-2499g, with allelotaxis still immature.
此时娩出的新生儿称早产儿，出生体重为 1000 ~ 2499g，各器官发育尚不够成熟。
Two birds of each replicate were slaughtered in 14, 35 and 49-day-old respectively to study the allelotaxis and enzyme activity in digestive tract.
分别在 14、35 和 49 日龄时各处死同组 2 只试验的鸟，以研究消化器官发育和消化酶活性。

allergen [ˈælədʒən] *n.* 变应原
Attempts to identify the allergen by history and skin testing then may be worthwhile.
病史和皮肤试验可能有助于找出变应原。
Skin tests can be used to test for sensitivity to allergens.
皮试可用于检测对过敏原的敏感性。

allergic [əˈləːdʒik] *a.* 过敏性的

Allergic reactions, as manifested by urticaria, are relatively common.
表现为荨麻疹的过敏反应是比较常见的。
Care should be exercised in the immunization of children with a family history of an allergic diathesis.
对具有过敏素质家族史的儿童,在进行免疫时应备加小心。
If the patient is allergic to penicillin and the infection is not responding to tetracycline, chloramphenicol can be used.
如果患者对青霉素过敏,而感染用四环素无效时,可使用氯霉素。

allergy [ˈælədʒi] *n.* 变态反应,过敏反应
Allergy is another condition that results from an abnormality of the immunity system.
变态反应是由于免疫系统异常所产生的另一种情况。
The child requires an allergy workup which includes a careful history, physical exam, and a few selective skin tests.
该患儿需要作变态反应检查,包括详细的病史、体格检查和几种选择性皮肤试验。
Allergy to drugs, septic pelvic vein thrombosis, and intra-abdominal abscesses are some causes of fever.
药物过敏、脓毒性盆腔静脉血栓形成以及腹腔内脓肿等,是引起发热的某些原因。

allesthesia [ˌælesˈθiːziə] *n.* 异位感觉
Visual allesthesia, along with palinopsia, differs from epileptic visual illusions and hallucinations from occipital and temporal lesions.
错位视觉以及视觉重复与枕叶和颞叶病变导致的癫痫性视错觉和幻觉不同。
At this low dose, naltrexone alone produced a strong potentiation of glucose-induced allesthesia.
低剂量的纳曲酮本身就对葡萄糖诱导的异位感觉产生了明显的增强作用。

alleviate [əˈlivieit] *v.* 减轻,缓和
Administration of vitamin C will alleviate the symptoms of scurvy.
给予维生素 C 可以减轻坏血病的症状。
During respiratory obstruction the cause must quickly be removed or alleviated.
当呼吸道堵塞时,必须迅速除去病因或使其缓解。

alliance [əˈlaiəns] *n.* 同盟,联合,良好合作
The importance of a good therapeutic alliance with the patient has assumed greater importance.
在治疗时取得病人的良好合作变得更为重要。

allied [əˈlaid, ˈælaid] *a.* 同类的,类似的
Furthermore, advances in toxicology and allied sciences will necessitate periodic review and revision of the protocol.
此外,毒理学及相关科学的进展将迫使人们对草案进行定期的审查和修正。

alloantigen [ˌæləuˈæntidʒən] *n.* 同种抗原
Antigenic differences between members of a species are called alloantigens.
同种抗原就是一个物种的不同个体之间的抗原性的差异。
The cells of the allograft will express alloantigens which are recognized as foreign by the recipient.
同种移植的细胞将表达同种抗原,它可被接受者作为外来抗原而识别。

allocate [ˈæləukeit] *v.* 分配,分派,拨(款)给
The director of the department allocates duties to all doctors and nurses.
科主任给所有的医生和护士分配任务。
Half of the medical supplies have already been allocated to the victims of the earthquake.
一半的医疗用品已经分配给了地震的受害者。
The municipal government has allocated five million yuan for building a new hospital.
市政府拨了 500 万元修建一个新医院。

allocation [ˌæləuˈkeiʃən] *n.* 分配，配给

Allocation of medical resources fairly and according to medical need is the basis for this principle.

实施此原则的基础是根据医学需要来公平地分配卫生资源。

allogeneic [ˌæləudʒiˈniːik] *a.* 同种（异体）的，同种基因的

In this case the graft is allogeneic(i. e. between members of the same species, having allelic variety of certain genes.)

在这种情况下，移植物是同种异体的（即同一物种不同的个体有不同的等位基因）。

allograft [ˈæləugrɑːft] *n.* 同种异体移植（物）

The course of an allograft reflects the result of a complex balance.

同种异体移植的过程反映出复杂平衡的结果。

Clinically, allograft rejection falls into three major categories: ①hyperacute rejection, ②acute rejection and ③chronic rejection.

临床上，同种异体移植排异反应分为三种主要类型：①超急性排异反应；②急性排异反应；③慢性排异反应。

Allografts that are commonly used clinically include blood, heart, kidney and liver.

常用于临床上的同种异体移植包括血液、心脏、肾脏和肝脏。

alloimmunization [ˌæləuiˌmjuːnaiˈzeiʃən] *n.* 同种免疫

Prophylactic transfusions result only in the development of alloimmunization in 80% of the patients.

预防性输血仅在 80% 患者中产生同种免疫作用。

allolalia [ˌæləuˈleiliə] *n.* 反常言语，言语障碍

Muscular strength and allolalia of hemiplegia were obviously recovered.

偏瘫引起的肢体肌力及语言障碍明显恢复。

Allolalia refers to any speech defect, especially one caused by a cerebral disorder.

反常言语指语言障碍，特别是由脑部疾病导致的语言障碍。

allopurinol [ˌæləuˈpjuərinɔl] *n.* 别嘌呤醇（治痛风药）

Allopurinol should be used before treatment of rapidly proliferating tumors.

在对增生迅速的肿瘤进行治疗之前应先给予别嘌呤醇。

Allopurinol may be required for hyperuricemia and dietary control for Type Ⅳ hyperlipdemia.

高尿酸血症时可能需用别嘌呤醇，如有Ⅳ型高脂血症时则需控制饮食。

alloreactivity [ˌæləuˌriækˈtiviti] *n.* 同种异体反应性

Alloreactivity describes the simulation of T cells by MHC molecules other than self; it marks the recognition of allogeneic MHC molecules.

同种异体反应性指的是非自身 MHC 分子对 T 细胞的刺激作用；它标志着同种异体 MHC 分子识别。

These findings about the basis of alloreactivity expand our understanding of this process.

有关同种异体反应性基础的发现拓宽了我们对于该过程的理解。

allorecognition [ˌæləuˌrekəgˈniʃən] *n.* 同种（异体）识别

Indirect allorecognition of a grafted tissue involves uptake of allogeneic proteins by the recipient's antigen-presenting cells and their presentation to T cells by self-MHC molecules.

对移植物的间接同种识别包括受者抗原提呈细胞摄取同种异体蛋白及其通过自身 MHC 分子提呈给 T 细胞等过程。

Protochordate allorecognition is controlled by a MHC-like gene system.

原索动物的同种异体识别受 MHC 样基因系统调控。

allosteric [ˌæləˈsterik] *a.* 变构的

Proteins which have two separate but interacting sites are called allosteric proteins.

具有两个不同而又相互作用部位的蛋白质称为变构蛋白。

Allosteric regulation is the regulation of an enzyme or other protein by binding an effector molecule at the protein's allosteric site.
变构调控是指一种酶或其他蛋白通过该蛋白的变构位点结合效应分子的调控。

allotransplantation [ˌæləuˌtræsplɑːn'teiʃən] *n.* 同种异体移植(术)
Allotransplantation usually results in rejection, unless histocompatible tissue and immunosuppression are used.
除非应用相容性的组织和免疫抑制,否则同种异体移植通常会导致排斥。
Cyclosporine is a compound that is becoming important for immunosuppression during allotransplantation.
在同种异体移植时,环孢霉素因其具有免疫抑制作用而变成一种重要的化合物。

allotropy [ə'lɔtrəpi] *n.* 同素异构,同素异形
Polymorphism in elements is called allotropy.
元素中的多晶型现象被称为同素异构性。
A structurally differentiated form of an element often exhibits allotropy.
一种化学元素的结构分化形式常表现为同素异形现象。

allotype ['ælətaip] *n.* (同种)异型
Allotypes occur mostly as variants of heavy chain constant regions.
同种异型的变化多数发生在重链的恒定区。

allowance [ə'lauəns] *n.* 供应量,许可量
The recommended daily allowance of copper in humans is 2 mg.
人的铜推荐日供应量为2mg。

alloy ['ælɔi] *n.* 合金
Lead is fairly reactive chemically and thus forms alloys with other metals, such as antimony, arsenic, copper and tin.
铅的化学性质相当活泼,因此能与其他金属(如锑、砷、铜和锡)形成合金。

almond ['ɑːmənd] *n.* 杏仁
The best prescription of the beverage was 5% almond, 4% lily bulb, and 6% sugar.
该饮料的最佳配方为杏仁5%,百合4%,白砂糖6%。
The skin of bitter almond can be easily removed with 0.8% boiling NaOH solution for 2 minutes.
用0.8% NaOH溶液煮沸两分钟能很容易去掉苦杏仁的皮。

aloesin ['æləusin] *n.* 芦荟苦素
Aloesin was isolated from the leaves of Aloe vera var. chinensis.
芦荟苦素是从芦荟叶子中分离出来的。

alopecia [ˌæləu'piːʃiə] *n.* 脱发,秃
Alopecia may be due to infection as well as to a number of other factors.
脱发可能是由于感染,也可能起因于多种其他因素。
A chronic fungous infection which involves the oil glands and hair follicles may result in alopecia.
累及皮脂腺和毛囊的慢性真菌性的感染都会引起脱发。
Many other cases of human Zn deficiency have been reported, with findings of poor growth, anorexia, alopecia and gonadal dysfunction.
人类锌缺乏的其他许多病例已有报道,表现为生长不良、厌食、脱发和生殖功能不良。

alpha ['ælfə] *n.* 阿尔法,希腊字母 α (第一个字母)
The researches are concerned with alpha rays.
这些研究均与阿尔法射线有关。
The particles expelled when the atom explodes are protons, alpha rays or neutrons.
原子爆炸时排出的粒子是质子、α 射线或中子。

alpha-fetoprotein (AFP) *n.* 甲胎蛋白

The level of AFP can be detected by a maternal blood test performed between the 16th and 18th weeks of pregnancy.
甲胎蛋白水平可于妊娠 16 至 18 周之间通过母体血液试验测定。
When AFP levels are unexpectedly high or low, further investigations (for example ultra-sound scanning) are indicated.
甲胎蛋白水平异常升高或降低时,应作进一步的检查(如超声波扫描)。

alphainterferon [ˌælfəˌintəˈfiərɔn] *n.* α 干扰素
Monitoring of alphainterferon therapy in chronic delta hepatitis is best accomplished by sequential testing for HDV RNA in serum.
慢性丁型肝炎最好连续检测血清中的 HDV RNA 来监测 α 干扰素治疗效果。

alpha-methyldopa [ˌælfəˌmeθilˈdəupə] *n.* α 甲基多巴
Alpha-methyldopa is used in the treatment of mild to moderate hypertension.
α 甲基多巴可用于治疗轻度到中度的高血压。

alpinetin [ˈælˌpaintin] *n.* 山姜素
We are making progress in the study of alpinetin.
我们在对山姜素的研究上有一定进展。
We use HPLC method to analyze the content of alpinetin in Alpinia katsumadai.
我们用 HPLC 法测定草豆蔻中山姜素的含量。

alter [ˈɔːltə] *v.* 改变
Ventricular hypertrophy and digitalis can alter the electrocardiogram considerably.
心室肥厚和洋地黄可使心电图发生较大的改变。
A number of other factors may alter the cytology.
很多其他因素可以改变其细胞学状态。

alterable [ˈɔːltərəbl] *a.* 可变的
The nature of the illness being treated sharply influences outcome by virtue of only partially alterable secondary effects.
所治疗的疾病种类单凭部分可变的次要因素,也可能对结局有重大影响。

alteration [ˌɔːltəˈreiʃən] *n.* 改变,变更,变化
Histamine synthesis probably explains capillary alterations.
组织胺的合成也许能解释毛细血管的变化。
The alterations in handling of a drug may be attributed to abnormalities at anatomic or at molecular levels.
药物处置上的改变可能是由于解剖水平或分子水平的异常所致。

alternate [ɔːlˈtənit] *a.* 交替的,轮流的
Fats have an alternate method of reaching the blood stream.
脂肪用另一种方法到达血流。
v. [ˈɔːtəneit] 交替,轮流
Diarrhoea or constipation may alternate in the same patient with amoebic dysentery.
患有阿米巴痢疾的同一个病人可以有腹泻或便秘交替出现。

alternating [ˈɔːltəneitiŋ] *a.* 更迭的,交替的
The pulse is rapid, of small volume, and rarely alternating.
脉搏快而弱,极少发生交替脉。
Some IBS(irritable bowel syndrome) patients have periods of constipation alternating with periods of diarrhea.
有些刺激性肠症候群患者的便秘期与腹泻期交替出现。

alternative [ɔːlˈtəːnətiv] *a.* 可选择的,替代的
In patients known to be truly allergic to penicillin, chloramphenicol is the alternative drug of choice.

对青霉素确有过敏的病人可改换氯霉素。

A lack of glucagon secretion has also been suggested as an alternative cause of hypoglycemia.

高血糖素分泌缺乏亦被提出为低血糖症的可能原因。

Thought should have been given to alternative ways of providing effective primary care.

应该考虑到能提供有效基本保健的其他可用方法。

n. 选择对象;替代方法;两者之一

Erythromycin, as a penicillin alternative, is a medium to broad spectrum antibiotic.

红霉素作为青霉素的替代药,是一种中谱到广谱的抗生素。

altretamine [ɔːltreˈtæmiːn] *n.* 六甲密胺

The main toxicities of altretamine are myelosuppression and neurotoxicity.

六甲密胺的主要毒性是骨髓抑制和神经毒性。

altruism [ˈæltruizəm] *n.* 利他主义;无私

The newest studies show a sharp rise in people's altruism at midlife, a key sign of new priorities.

最新的研究显示人们在中年时利他主义明显增长,这是优先考虑新问题的主要标志。

alum [ˈæləm] *n.* 明矾

You can clarify the water by adding a little alum.

你在水里加一点明矾就能使水净化。

But chemical mordants such as alum are popular today.

但是像明矾这样的化学腐蚀剂现今很普遍。

aluminum [əˈljuːminəm] *n.* 铝(=aluminium [ˌæljuˈminjəm])

Aluminum is the third most common element found on earth and is often used to purify drinking water.

铝是地球上第三大常见元素,常用于净化饮用水。

Aluminium has been blamed for the development of Alzheimer's.

铝一直被认为可引起早老性痴呆症的发生。

alveolar [ælˈviələ, ˌælviˈəulə] *a.* 肺泡的,小泡的

There is another rare type alveolar cell carcinoma (3%) which appears in many sites.

还有一种罕见的肺泡细胞癌(占3%),出现在许多不同的位置。

The fresh alveolar air has an oxygen tension of 100mm of mercury and virtually no carbon dioxide.

新鲜的肺泡内空气其氧分压为100毫米汞柱,几乎没有二氧化碳。

alveolitis [ˌælviəˈlaitis] *n.* 肺泡炎

Both types of alveolitis may progress slowly to a state of fibrosis, and both types usually respond to corticosteroid therapy.

两类肺泡炎均可缓慢发展成纤维变性状态,亦均可用皮质类固醇来治疗。

Cryptogenic fibrosing alveolitis is a cause of chronic interstitial lung disease.

原发性纤维化肺泡炎是引起慢性间质性肺病的一个原因。

alveolus [ælˈviələs] (*pl.* alveoli [ælˈviəlai]) *n.* 肺泡

The lungs are made up of clusters of small air sacs known as alveoli.

肺由一串串称为肺泡的小气囊所构成。

Air flows into the alveoli of the lungs because the pressure in the lungs becomes less than that of the atmosphere.

因为肺内压变得比大气压小,气流随之进入肺泡。

Alzheimer's disease [ˈæltshaimə] *n.* 阿尔茨海默病(早老性痴呆)

In the future there may be treatments for diseases such as Alzheimer's disease, which would encourage people to seek an early diagnosis.

未来可能会出现治疗诸如早老性痴呆疾病的方法,这将鼓励人们去寻求早期诊断。

A genetic locus on chromosome 21 has been found for some inherited forms of Alzheimer's disease.

现已发现某些遗传型阿尔茨海默病是由于在第 21 对染色体上的一个基因位点的异常所致。

amaranth [ˈæmərænθ] *n.* 苋菜红

Amaranth seeds are considered as an excellent complementary source of food protein due to their balanced amino acid composition.

苋菜红种子因其含有均衡的氨基酸成分,被认为是一种极好的食物蛋白补充剂。

We examined the degradation of amaranth, a representative azo dye, by Bjerkandera adusta Dec 1.

我们用烟管菌 Dec 1 检测苋菜红(一种典型的偶氮燃料)的降解。

amazing [əˈmeiziŋ] *a.* 令人惊异的

Much of the credit for this amazing progress can be given to modern drugs and improvements in medical care.

这种令人惊异的进步其荣誉应归于现代药品和医疗保健的提高。

amber [ˈæmbə] *n.* 琥珀;琥珀色

More than a century later, amber became sexy again with the advent of gene sequencing and cloning.

一个多世纪之后,随着基因序列和克隆技术的出现,琥珀再次变得有吸引力起来。

A new amber CRT display material was found.

人们发现了一种新型琥珀色 CRT 显示荧光材料。

amblyopia [ˌæmbliˈəupiə] *n.* 弱视

When one eye develops good vision while the other does not, the eye with poorer vision is called amblyopia. Usually, only one eye is affected by amblyopia.

当一个眼形成好的视力,而另一个眼没有好视力时,此视力不好的眼称作弱视,通常弱视只影响一个眼。

For example, in toxic amblyopia caused by tobacco, alcohol, certain other drugs, and vitamin deficiency, there is a disorder of the optic nerve.

例如,因烟草、酒精、某些其他药物及维生素缺乏引起中毒性弱视时便会有视神经障碍。

ambulance [ˈæmbjuləns] *n.* 救护车

The person who calls the physician or ambulance should tell the location of the injured person.

打电话叫医生或救护车的人应讲明受伤者的地点。

The injured man had died before the ambulance arrived here.

在救护车到达这里之前,伤者已经死亡。

ambulant [ˈæmbjulənt] *a.* 不必卧床的,可走动的

The doctor told the family that the patient was ambulant.

医生告诉病人家属,病人无需卧床。

ambulation [æmbjuˈleiʃən] *n.* 下床走动

Early ambulation is of benefit in a variety of medical conditions.

较早地起床活动,对多种内科疾病都有好处。

ambulatory [ˈæmbjulətəri] *a.* 非卧床的,流动的

The convalescent care provided to the ambulatory patient outside the hospital will not be reviewed here.

院外非卧床病人的恢复期护理将不在此讨论。

The EEG in association with video monitoring and ambulatory recording greatly increases the precision of EEG diagnosis.

配有电视图像监测和能走动记录的脑电图大大提高了脑电图诊断的精确性。

Ambulatory treatment is rarely indicated in the management of preeclampsia.

子痫前期患者一般不宜在门诊治疗。

ameba [əˈmiːbə] (*pl.* amebae [əˈmiːbiː] 或 **amebas** [əˈmiːbəs]) *n.* 阿米巴

The amebas invade the blood stream and are carried to the lungs, the liver, etc.

阿米巴侵入血液后，被带至肺、肝等处。

One of the main groups of protozoa is that consisting of the amebae.

阿米巴群是主要原虫群种之一。

amebiasis [ˌæmiˈbaiəsis] *n.* 阿米巴病

Amebiasis can be prevented by careful hygiene.

注意卫生能够预防阿米巴病。

Some cases of amebiasis begin with a very acute onset.

有些阿米巴病病例，发病很急剧。

The treatment of amebiasis remains unsatisfactory, because different forms of the infection require different treatment regimens.

阿米巴病的治疗仍不能令人满意，因为不同型的感染需要不同的治疗方案。

amebic [əˈmiːbik] *a.* 阿米巴的

Amebic dysentery bears some resemblance to the bacillary type.

阿米巴痢疾与杆菌痢疾有些相似。

Amebic hepatitis is common on a world basis and usually presents as a hepatic abscess.

阿米巴肝炎是世界范围内的常见病，一般表现为阿米巴肝脓肿。

ameboid [əˈmiːbɔid] *a.* 阿米巴样的

Besides degrading ECM, tumor cells can take a second mode of invasion, termed ameboid migration.

除了降解细胞外基质，肿瘤细胞还能采用第二种浸润方式，即阿米巴样迁移。

In ameboid migration the cell squeezes through spaces in the matrix instead of cutting through.

在阿米巴样迁移中，细胞在基质间隙中穿行，而不切断基质。

ameliorate [əˈmiːljəreit] *v.* 改善，改良

Antacids and diet often ameliorate symptoms but do not hasten healing.

抗酸剂和饮食常可使症状缓解，但不能加速痊愈。

Any factors that ameliorate or aggravate the discomfort should be noted.

任何使疼痛缓解或加重的因素都应注意。

amelioration [əˌmiːljəˈreiʃən] *n.* 改善，转佳

Controlling food intake by F344 rats results in amelioration of a number of these spontaneously manifested lesions.

控制 F344 大鼠的食物摄入量使那些自发的明显损伤得到改善。

Migraineurs often report amelioration of their headaches with prednisone.

偏头痛患者经常反映在服用强的松之后可以缓解头痛。

amenable (to) [əˈmiːnəbl] *a.* 有义务的，顺从的

The disease is amenable to treatment but rather prone to recurrence.

本病可以治好，但是比较容易复发。

Many aspects of mucocutaneous and visceral HSV infections are amenable to treatment with antiviral chemotherapy. (HSV = herpes simplex virus)

许多黏膜皮肤及内脏单纯疱疹病毒感染可接受抗病毒化疗。

The patients must be cooperative and amenable to careful follow-up.

患者必须合作并密切配合随访。

amendment [əˈmendmənt] *n.* 增补和修订，修正

With the passing of the FDA Amendments Act (FDAAA) in September 2007, registries increasingly continue to be used to fulfill safety-related objectives.

随着 2007 年 9 月《美国食品药品管理修正法案》的通过，注册登记系统被越来越多地用以实现安全相关的目的。

amenorrh(o)ea [eiˌmenə'riə] *n.* 经闭,无月经

The classic triad of amenorrhea, vaginal bleeding, and pain occur in only 25% of cases.

仅 25% 的病例出现停经、阴道出血和疼痛的典型三联征。

The cerebral cortex can exert a profound influence, exemplified by amenorrhea due to emotional disturbance.

大脑皮质能产生很大的影响,由于情绪纷乱引起闭经为一例证。

amensalism [ə'mensəlizəm] *n.* 偏害共栖

Amensalism is the type of symbiotic relationship that exists where one species is inhibited or completely obliterated and another one is unaffected.

偏害共栖是生物间存在的一类共生关系,即一种生物被抑制或完全被除掉,另一种却不受影响。

amentia [ə'menʃiə] *n.* 精神错乱,智力缺陷;痴呆

The handicapped also include deaf-mutes and some brain paralysis amentia patients.

残疾人还包括聋哑人及部分脑瘫智障患者。

Individualized care service can reduce agitated behavior of senile amentia patients during hospitalization.

个性化服务能减少老年痴呆病人住院期间激越行为。

amidase ['æmideis] *n.* 酰胺酶,脱酰胺酶

Mammalian tissues, including the plasma, contain a large number of nonspecific esterases and amidases.

哺乳动物组织,包括血浆,含有大量非特异性的酯酶和酰胺酶。

amikacin [ə'mikəsin] *n.* 丁胺卡那霉素,氨基羟丁基卡那霉素 A

Amikacin is active against tuberculosis and several of the nontuberculous species.

丁胺卡那霉素对结核病和其他一些非结核性的细菌感染有效。

Streptomycin, amikacin and neomycin have similar chemical structures and adverse effects.

链霉素、丁胺卡那霉素和新霉素的化学结构和副作用都相似。

amination [ˌæmi'neiʃən] *n.* 氨化

When the amine is used as an electrophile, the reaction is called electrophilic amination.

把胺用作亲电物质时,其反应被称作亲电氨化。

It was proposed that the catalytic amination of metyl t-butyl ether by solid acid was a promising green process.

有人提出,用固体酸催化甲基叔丁基醚的氨化是值得开发的绿色化工技术。

amine ['æmiːn] *n.* 胺

Aromatic amines produce papillomas and bladder cancer.

芳胺易引致乳头瘤和膀胱癌。

amino acid ['æminəu] *n.* 氨基酸

Some 40 different amino acids have been isolated from various proteins.

已经从各种蛋白质中分离出约 40 种不同的氨基酸。

Altered amino acid and trace element responses may have usefulness for detecting incubating infections.

异常的氨基酸和痕量元素反应可能对发觉潜伏的感染有用处。

aminoacid ['æminəu'æsid] *n.* 氨基酸

Glucagon infusion in patients with viral hepatitis did not induce a fall in free aminoacids.

病毒性肝炎患者输注高血糖素不曾诱发游离氨基酸下降的现象。

aminoacidopathy [ˌæminəuˌæsi'dɔpəθi] *n.* 氨基酸(缺陷)病

When blood ammonia, pH, and bicarbonate are normal, other aminoacidopathies should be considered.

当血液中氨、pH 和碳酸氢盐正常时,应考虑有其他氨基酸缺陷病。

All patients exhibit an unusual aminoacidopathy evident both in fasting plasma and in CSF.
所有病人在空腹血浆和脑脊液中均显示有异常氨基酸病的证据。

aminoglutethimide [ˌæminəuglu:ˈteθimaid] *n.* 氨基导眠能，氨鲁米特

Aminoglutethimide is an inhibitor of cholesterol metabolism, thereby reducing adrenocortical steroid synthesis, used in the treatment of Cushing's syndrome.
氨基导眠能是一种胆固醇代谢抑制剂，因而减少肾上腺皮质激素的合成，用于治疗库欣氏综合征。

Aromatase inhibitors, such as aminoglutethimide and anastrozole, work in a different way to lower estrogen levels.
芳香酶抑制剂，如氨鲁米特和阿那曲唑，降低雌激素水平的作用方式不同。

aminoglycoside [ˌæminəuˈglaikəusaid] *n.* 氨基苷

Aminoglycosides are bactericidal and inhibit protein synthesis in susceptible microorganisms.
氨基苷对敏感微生物具有杀菌作用，并抑制其蛋白质的合成。

The effectiveness of other aminoglycosides has not been evaluated in controlled studies.
对照研究(显示)其他氨基苷类的有效性尚未作评价。

aminophylline [ˌæminəuˈfilin] *n.* 氨茶碱

Aminophylline is an important drug for treating bronchial asthma.
氨茶碱是治疗支气管哮喘的一种重要药物。

Aminophylline, preferably given intravenously, is also beneficial but an overdose can lead to vomiting, convulsions and collapse.
氨茶碱也有效，最好采用静脉注射；但用药过量可引起呕吐、抽搐及虚脱。

aminopterin [ˌæmiˈnɔptərin] *n.* 氨蝶呤

Antimetabolites such as aminopterin and methotrexate may be incorporated into DNA and RNA.
抗代谢药物如氨蝶呤和甲氨蝶呤可渗入到 DNA 和 RNA 中。

aminopyrine [ˌæminəuˈpaiəri:n] *n.* 氨基比林

The assays for aminopyrine as the substrate is conducted as follows.
以氨基比林作底物的测定法可按下列(步骤)进行。

Male rats demethylate aminopyrine faster than females.
雄性大鼠比雌性大鼠的氨基比林脱甲基的速度快。

aminotransferase [æminəuˈtrænsfəreis] *n.* 转氨酶

Liver function tests frequently show elevated aminotransferases and bilirubin concentrations.
肝功能试验往往显示转氨酶及胆红素计量升高。

This kind of aciduria is caused by a defect in the peroxisomal enzyme—alanine glyoxylate aminotransferase.
这种酸尿是源于过氧化物酶——丙氨酸乙醛酸转氨酶的缺陷。

ammonia [əˈməuniə] *n.* 氨

Urea-splitting bacteria produce ammonia, which on combination with hydrogen ions forms ammonium.
分解尿素的细菌产生氨，后者与氢离子结合形成铵。

Among the toxic gases are sulfur dioxide, methane, the oxides of nitrogen, ammonia, hydrogen sulfide, and hydrogen cyanide.
常见的有毒气体有二氧化硫、甲烷、氧化氮、氨、硫化氢以及氰化氢。

ammonification [ə,mɔnifiˈkeiʃən] *n.* 氨化作用

The condensation and ammonification tests proceed by using pyrrolidone as the start material.
缩合和氨化试验是以吡咯烷酮为起始原料进行的。

Terrestrial microorganisms participate in important ecological processes such as nitrogen fixation, ammonification, nitrification and denitrification.
土壤微生物参与固氮作用、氨化作用、硝化作用和反硝化作用等重要生态过程。

ammonium [ə'məuniəm] *n.* 铵

Ammonium sulfate is the salt most frequently used.

硫酸铵是最常用的盐。

amnesia [æm'niːzjə] *n.* 遗忘(症),记忆缺失

Scopolamine depresses the CNS and in therapeutic doses causes fatigue, hypnosis, and amnesia.

东莨菪碱可抑制中枢神经系统,其治疗量可引起疲倦、催眠和遗忘。

Freud attributed this childhood amnesia to the repression of infantile sexuality.

弗洛伊德把这种童年记忆缺失归因于幼儿期性压抑。

amnestic [æm'nestik] *a.* (引起)遗忘的

If clouding of consciousness is present, a diagnosis of amnestic syndrome cannot be made.

若有意识模糊存在,就不能作出遗忘综合征的诊断。

However, prolonged untreated vitamin B_1 deficiency can result in an irreversible amnestic syndrome or even death.

然而,长期未经治疗的维生素 B_1 缺乏可导致患者产生不可逆的失忆症或甚至死亡。

amniocentesis [ˌæmniəusen'tiːsis] *n.* 羊膜穿刺术

Amniocentesis should be performed and an estimation of fetal maturity obtained starting at 33-34 weeks.

从 33 ~ 34 孕周开始可行羊膜穿刺术以估计胎儿成熟度。

amnion ['æmniən] *n.* 羊膜

The progress of human amnion on nervous system diseases based on related data was summarized.

(本文)就有关资料报道人羊膜在神经系统疾病中应用的进展进行了总结。

Human amnion, a new transplantation material for myringoplasty, is worthy to be popularized for it is easy to obtain and operate and regain great success.

人羊膜作为一种新的鼓膜成形术移植材料,因其易获得、易操作且成功率高,值得推广。

amnioscopy [ˌæmni'ɔskəpi] *n.* 羊膜镜检

Amnioscopy has been used for monitoring high risk pregnancy in our hospital.

我院用羊膜镜监护高危妊娠。

Five joint monitoring ways are used to monitor high risk pregnancy, i. e. , amnioscopy, measuring amniotic fluid volume by ultrasound B, nonstress testing (NST), determining E/C with urinoscopy and recording fetal movements.

采用羊膜镜检、B 超测羊水量、无负荷试验、测尿 E/C 值及记录胎动 5 项联合监测评分监护高危妊娠。

amniotic [ˌæmni'ɔtik] *a.* 羊膜的

Bilirubin is present in normal amniotic fluid in trace amounts.

在正常羊水中有微量胆红素存在。

As most of the amniotic fluid is fetal urine, diminished renal blood flow causes reduced amniotic fluid.

由于羊水主要是胎儿的尿液,所以肾血流减少时会导致羊水减少。

amniotomy [ˌæmni'ɔtəmi] *n.* 羊膜穿破术

Labour may be induced in cases of postmaturity by amniotomy in the usual way, followed if necessary by an oxytocin infusion.

过期妊娠病例可按常用方法给予人工破膜引产,必要时加用催产素滴注。

amodiaquine [ˌæmə'daiəkwin] *n.* 阿莫地喹,氨酚喹

The drugs of choice for the acute attack of malaria are the 4-aminoquinolines, chloroquine or amodiaquine.

疟疾急性发作选用的药物是 4-氨基喹啉类,氯喹或氨酚喹。

amorphous [ə'mɔːfəs] *a.* 不定形的

We have partially isolated the amorphous matrix densities.

我们已部分地分离出不定形基质致密物。

These amorphous matrix densities are found in irreversibly injured cells in other systems.

这些不定形的基质致密物，也见于其他系统的不可逆性损害的细胞内。

amoxicillin [ˌæmɔksiˈsilin] *n.* 羟氨苄青霉素，阿莫西林

Other effective regimens for sensitive strains include amoxicillin 4 ~ 4.5g/d for 2 weeks.

其他对敏感菌株的有效治疗还有每日服用 4 到 4.5g 阿莫西林，连服两周。

She was evaluated and found to have bilateral otitis media and treated with im ampicillin and oral amoxicillin.

检查时发现她患有双侧中耳炎，给予肌注氨苄青霉素和口服羟氨苄青霉素治疗。

amphetamine [æmˈfetəmiːn] *n.* 苯丙胺（中枢兴奋药），安非他明

Drug psychoses are due to consumption of drugs (notably amphetamines and barbiturates) and solvents.

药物性精神病由药物（主要为苯丙胺类、巴比妥酸盐类）和溶剂的滥用所引起。

At high altitudes, the toxicity of digitalis is decreased whereas that of amphetamine is increased.

在海拔高处，毛地黄的毒性降低而苯丙胺的毒性却增大。

The demand for amphetamines is particularly high in Scandinavia and Britain.

斯堪的纳维亚和不列颠对安非他明的需求量特别大。

amphipathic [ˌæmfiˈpæθik] *a.* 两亲（性）的

Molecules with both hydrophilic and hydrophobic groups are called amphipathic or amphiphilic.

分子兼有亲水的和疏水的两个基团，叫做两亲的分子或两性的分子。

Cell membranes containing a wide diversity of lipids are amphipathic; that is, they contain both hydrophilic and hydrophobic regions.

含有多种类型脂质的细胞膜是两性的，兼有亲水和疏水两个区域。

amphiphilic [æmfiˈfilik] *a.* 两性分子的；两亲性的

Being amphiphilic, the drug interacts with the polymers similar to the interaction of surfactants and polymers.

因为具有两亲性，该药物与聚合物的相互作用类似于表面活化剂与聚合物的相互作用。

An amphiphilic PAMAM dendron with aspartic acids on the periphery and an aliphatic chain at the focal point was synthesized.

合成了一种外周有天门冬氨酸，内含一条脂肪链的两亲性聚酰胺-胺树枝型大分子。

amphitheater [ˌæmfiˈθiətə] *n.* 手术示范教室，看台式教室

As soon as the operation was over, the doctors and students left the amphitheater.

当手术结束后，医生们和学生们都离开了观看手术的教室。

amphotericin [ˌæmfəˈterisin] *n.* 两性霉素

Amphotericin B bladder irrigation appeared to be the most effective treatment of uncomplicated funguria.

两性霉素 B 膀胱冲洗似乎是对无并发症霉菌尿最有效的治疗（方法）。

ampicillin [ˌæmpiˈsilin] *n.* 氨苄西林，氨苄青霉素

However, in protracted cases, antibiotic treatment with tetracycline or ampicillin may shorten the illness.

然而，对顽固性病例，四环素或氨苄西林等抗生素治疗可缩短病程。

Ampicillin is currently the drug of choice for sensitive strains in the United States.

在美国，对付敏感菌株，氨苄西林通常作为首选药物。

Resistance to ampicillin is now common, and resistance to TMP-SMX is increasing in frequency.

目前比较常见的是对氨苄青霉素耐药的问题，对 TMP-SMX 的耐药性问题也越来越多。

ample [ˈæmpl] *a.* 充分的，足够的

The animal study by Smith provides ample experimental support for this concept.

史密斯的动物实验，提供了支持这个观点的充分实验依据。

amplicon ['æmplikɔn] *n.* 扩增子

An amplicon is a piece of DNA formed as the product of natural or artificial amplification events.

一个扩增子是一段 DNA 序列，是天然或人工扩增的产物。

The males are distinguished as having two DNA amplicons present, while females have only a single amplicon.

男性有两个 DNA 扩增子，而女性只有一个，因而男女有别。

amplification [ˌæmplifi'keiʃən] *n.* 增强，扩大

Measurement and instrumentation are methods involving amplification of the examiner's senses.

检测和器械操作是增强检查者感官效能的方法。

amplifier ['æmplifaiə] *n.* 放大器

Cyclic AMP acts as a second messenger and amplifier by activating certain protein kinases.

环腺苷酸通过激活某些蛋白激酶而有第二信使和(生物)放大器的作用。

Conventional hearing aids have three components: a microphone, an amplifier and a speaker.

传统助听器有三个组成部分：一个麦克风，一个放大器和一个扬声器。

amplify ['æmplifai] *v.* 放大

The complex electrical potentials produced by the cardiac muscle at each beat are amplified and recorded.

对心肌每次搏动所产生的综合电位均加以放大并记录下来。

The steps involved in cell activation and the humoral factors elaborated by T cells that regulate and amplify cell-mediated immunity are shown in Fig 1.

这些步骤见图 1，包括有细胞活化以及可调节和放大细胞介导免疫的 T 细胞产生的体液因子。

amplitude ['æmplitjuːd] *n.* 范围，幅度，振幅

Tremor may be divided according to relationship to posture and amplitude.

震颤可以根据姿势和幅度的关系来进行分类。

After age 30, there is a progressive, almost linear decline in the amount of slow-wave sleep, and the amplitude of delta EEG activity comprising slow-wave sleep is reduced.

人在超过 30 岁之后，脑电图上慢波睡眠的数量有渐进性，甚至有线性的降低，同时脑电图(EEG)上可观察到由慢波睡眠组成的 δ 波的波幅也降低了。

ampoule ['æmpuːl] *n.* 安瓿

Closed ampoule isothermal microcalorimetry (IMC) is increasingly being used in medical and environmental sciences.

封闭安瓿等温微量热技术(IMC)正越来越多的应用于医学和环境科学。

The medication name on user-applied labels should be matched to that on the relevant ampoule.

用户应用标签上的药物名称应该与对应安瓿上的名称相一致。

ampullary [æm'pjuləri] *a.* 壶腹部的

Ampullary carcinoma presents early with obstructive jaundice and can be resected.

壶腹癌出现症状早，表现为阻塞性黄疸，可以切除。

amputate ['æmpjuteit] *v.* 切断，截(肢)

Manet agreed to have an operation to amputate his left foot.

马奈同意做手术截除他的左脚。

amputation [ˌæmpju'teiʃən] *n.* 切断术，截肢，切除术

The surgeon decided against amputation.

外科医生决定不做截肢。

The patient had an amputation of the left breast a year ago.

病人在一年以前做了左乳房切除。

amycolatopsis [ə'maikoulə'tɔpsis] *n.* 酸菌属，拟无枝酸菌

Amycolatopsis is a genus of high-GC content bacteria within the family Pseudonocardiaceae.
酸菌属是假诺卡菌科中富含 GC 的一个菌属。
Amycolatopsis can be isolated from soil, vegetable manner, and clinical specimens.
酸菌可从土壤、蔬菜和临床标本中分离出。

amygdala [ə'migdələ] *n.* 杏仁核
The amygdala is a key regulator of vigilance and heightens attention toward threat.
杏仁核是对威胁产生警觉性和提高注意力的关键调控部位。
It is unknown how corticosteroids affect the neural circuitry connected to the amygdala.
还不清楚类固醇是如何影响与杏仁核相连接的神经环路的。

amygdalase [ə'migdəˌleis] *n.* 苦杏仁酶
The experimental results showed that amygdalase was completely inactivated.
实验结果显示，苦杏仁酶的活性被完全抑制。

amygdale [ə'migdeil] *n.* 扁桃体
Co-distribution of the cannabinoid CB1 receptor and the 5-HT transporter in amygdale is an important topic for researchers.
扁桃体中大麻素受体 CB1 和 5-HT 转运蛋白的共分布是研究者们重要的研究课题。
There are many types of immunocytes in amygdale.
扁桃体中有多种免疫细胞。

amylase ['æmileis] *n.* 淀粉酶
Amylase is a starch-digesting enzyme, hydrolyzing starch to the sugar moltose.
淀粉酶是可以消化淀粉的一种酶，将淀粉水解成麦芽糖。
Another enzyme, amylase, acts on carbohydrates, and the third enzyme, lipase, acts on fats.
另一种酶—淀粉酶—作用于碳水化合物，第三种酶—脂肪酶—作用于脂肪。

amyloid ['æmilɔid] *n.* 淀粉样蛋白
The major sites of amyloid deposition are blood vessel walls and the mucous membranes.
淀粉样蛋白主要沉积在血管壁和黏膜上。
β-amyloid protein has been found in the brains of Alzheimer's patients but the significance of this is unclear.
β-淀粉样蛋白见于阿尔茨海默病患者的脑内，但其意义仍不清楚。

amyloidosis [ˌæmilɔi'dəusis] *n.* 淀粉样变性
Primary amyloidosis is characterized by accumulation of protein ground substance in many organs.
原发性淀粉样变性是以多脏器的蛋白基质的积累为特征的。
Secondary amyloidosis is uncommon but may follow prolonged chronic colitis.
继发性淀粉样变性并不常见，但可并发于迁延性慢性结肠炎。

amylopectinosis [ˌæmiləuˌpekti'nəusis] *n.* 支链淀粉病
Amylopectinosis can result from several mutations in the GBE1 gene, which result in a defective glycogen brancher enzyme.
支链淀粉病可以起因于 GBE1 基因的几个突变所致的糖原支链酶缺陷。

amyotrophy [əˌmai'ɔtrəfi] *n.* 肌萎缩（=amyotrophia [əˌmaiə'trəufiə]）
Diabetic amyotrophy usually occurs in middle-aged diabetics.
糖尿病性肌萎缩通常发生于中年糖尿病患者。

anabolic [ˌænə'bɔlik] *a.* 合成代谢的
The use of anabolic steroids has been suggested to be a factor in the increased incidence of cardiovascular risks.
已有人提出合成代谢类固醇的应用可能是引起心血管疾病发病率增高的一个危险因素。

anabolism [ə'næbəlizəm] *n.* 合成代谢
Biosynthetic reactions together make up anabolism.

生物的合成反应统称为合成代谢。

The term anabolism is used to describe that part of metabolism involving the building up of substances.

合成代谢这一术语被用来描述物质合成的那部分新陈代谢。

anaerobe [ə'neiərəub] *n.* 厌氧菌

Microbes that cannot grow in an atmosphere of oxygen are called anaerobes.

在大气的氧环境中不能生长的细菌被称为厌氧菌。

Anaerobes are present in 39 percent of animal bites and in 50 percent of human bites.

在被动物咬伤的伤口上有 39% 存在有厌氧菌，而在被人咬伤的伤口上则有 50% 存在厌氧菌。

anaerobic [əˌneə'rɔbik] *a.* 厌氧的

The tetanus bacillus is an anaerobic bacterium.

破伤风菌是一种厌氧菌。

The aerobic Bacillus and the anaerobic Clostridium are both gram-positive rods.

需氧芽孢杆菌属和厌氧梭状芽孢杆菌属均为革兰阳性杆菌。

anal ['einəl] *a.* 肛门的

The anal canal is the terminal portion of the digestive tract.

肛门是消化道的终末部分。

Surgery sometimes results in anal incontinence or stricture, especially in cases of complex fistulas.

外科手术治疗有时可以导致肛门失禁或造成狭窄不通，特别是在具有复合瘘管的病例。

analgesia [ˌænæl'dʒiːzjə] *n.* 痛觉缺失，止痛法

This dose is sufficient to produce analgesia in 70 percent of patients having moderate to severe pain.

这个剂量对 70% 具有中度或重度疼痛的患者足以产生镇痛作用。

Complete analgesia can be obtained for 12-24 hours with no interference with autonomic or motor function.

可获 12 ~ 24 小时的完全无痛而又不影响自主功能或运动功能。

The acute inflammation usually settles with bed rest, analgesia (pethidine) and antibiotics.

经卧床休息、止痛（哌替啶）和抗生素治疗，急性炎症一般可以平息下来。

analgesic [ˌænæl'dʒesik] *a.* 止痛的

Tolerance is developed to the narcotic and analgesic actions of morphine.

人体对吗啡的麻醉作用和镇痛作用可产生耐受性。

n. 止痛药

Analgesics are substances that lessen the perception of pain without the loss of consciousness.

镇痛药是在清醒的状态下减轻痛觉的物质。

analgin [ə'nældʒin] *n.* 安乃近

Analgin has brought about a drop in her temperature.

安乃近使她体温下降。

analog(ue) ['ænəlɔg] *n.* 类似物

Some enzymes have broader specificity and will accept several different analogs of a specific substrate.

一些酶有较宽的特异性，可接受一种特异性底物的几种不同类似物。

Tocainide, an analogue of lidocaine, is effective in suppressing chronic ventricular ectopy.

氨酰甲苯胺是利多卡因的类似物，能有效地抑制慢性室性异位节律。

analogous (to) [ə'næləgəs] *a.* 类似的，类同于

Heterozygous alpha thalassemia is analogous to thalassemia minor.

杂合子的 α 地中海贫血类似于轻型地中海贫血。

The tumour is analogous to a sebaceous cyst developing on the eyelids.
肿瘤类似长在眼睑上的皮脂腺囊肿。

analogy [əˈnælədʒi] *n.* 相似
No analogy exists between these two.
他们两个之间没有相似之处。
These fossils bear a close analogy to those described in the book.
这些化石的特征与那本书上所描述的化石有极其相似之处。

analyse [ˈænəlaiz] *v.* 分析
The pain has been fully analysed and a tentative diagnosis can often be made.
疼痛经充分的分析之后，常可作出初步的诊断。
The blood is sometimes analysed to determine the amount of sugar dissolved in the plasma.
有时进行血液分析是为了要测定溶解于血浆中的血糖含量。

analysis [əˈnæləsis] *n.* 分析
In common English usage "urinalysis" refers to the chemical analysis of urine.
通常英语中"尿液分析"一词指的是对尿液进行化学分析。
Upon analysis gastric juice is found to be a watery secretion containing some protein, some mucin and inorganic salts.
根据分析，发现胃液是一种含有一些蛋白质、黏蛋白和无机盐的水样分泌物。

anamnestic [ˌænæmˈnestik] *a.* 回忆的；抗体再生的
The producing rate of antibodies of anamnestic response goes up faster than that of the primary, but the dropping rate is slower.
与初次应答相比，回忆应答抗体产生的速度较快，而消失的速度较慢。
The secondary anamnestic response peaks last only 1-3 days
二次回忆应答峰值仅 1 ~ 3 天。

anaphase [ˈænəfeiz] *n.* 后期（细胞分裂的一个时期）
The centromere of each chromosome separates into two centromeres in the third stage, or anaphase, of mitosis.
有丝分裂的第三个时期即后期，每条染色体的着丝粒一分为二。
Anaphase is characterized by separation of the chromatids of each chromosome.
每条染色体的姐妹染色单体分离是（细胞分裂）后期的特征。

anaphylactic [ˌænəfiˈlæktik] *a.* 过敏性的，过敏反应的
Adrenaline must be available in case of acute anaphylactic reactions.
在遇到急性过敏反应的病例时，必须准备好肾上腺素。
Among which, 82 cases had anaphylactic shocks, which accounted for 2.12% of the total.
所有病例中发生过敏性休克者 82 例，发生率为 2.12%。
Fosfomycin may induce anaphylactic shock, which should arouse more attention in clinic.
磷霉素可致过敏性休克，应引起临床高度重视。

anaphylactogen [ˌænəfiˈlæktədʒən] *n.* 过敏原
This article explains the detection methods of anaphylactogen.
这篇文献阐述过敏原的检测方法。
As a very powerful anaphylactogen, house dust mite can induce mite asthma, anaphylactic asthma, allergic dermatitis.
屋尘螨作为一种非常强烈的过敏原，可引起尘螨性哮喘、过敏性哮喘、过敏性皮炎。

anaphylatoxin [ˌænəˌfiləˈtɔksin] *n.* 过敏毒素
Systemic complement activation generates large amounts of anaphylatoxin.
补体系统的激活产生大量的过敏毒素。
Elevated plasma levels of the anaphylatoxins C3a and C4a are associated with a fatal outcome in sepsis.

血浆中过敏毒素 C3a 和 C4a 水平升高与败血症的致命后果有关。

anaphylaxis [ˌænəfiˈlæksis] *n.* 过敏性,过敏反应

Anaphylaxis from penicillin affects not only the skin, but can affect the mucous membranes and tissues of any organ.

青霉素过敏反应不仅影响皮肤,而且能影响任何器官的黏膜和组织。

anaplasia [ˌænəˈpleisiə] *n.* 间变

The morphologic changes of anaplasia are often shown as pleomorphism, abnormal nuclear morphology and mitoses.

间变的形态学改变常表现为细胞的多形性、异常的核形态和核分裂象。

The expression of HLA-D/Dr antigen on tumor cells ran parallel to the degree of cellular anaplasia.

HLA-D/Dr 抗原在肿瘤细胞上的表达与细胞的退行性变化的程度是平行的。

anaplasmosis [ˌænəplæsˈməusis] *n.* 无浆体病

There will be a report tomorrow on research advances in the diagnostic techniques for bovine anaplasmosis.

明天将有一个关于牛无浆体病诊断方法的研究进展的报告。

Their research topic is detection of dairy cattle anaplasmosis and its application by PCR.

他们的研究题目是奶牛无浆体病 PCR 诊断方法的建立及应用。

anaplastic [ˌænəˈplæstik] *a.* 间变的,退行发育的

Anaplastic meningioma is a highly aggressive tumor and considered to be WHO grade Ⅲ/Ⅳ tumor.

间变性脑膜瘤是一种高侵袭性肿瘤,被认为是 WHO Ⅲ ~ Ⅳ级的肿瘤。

Neoplasms with no differentiation are said to be anaplastic.

未分化肿瘤被认为是退行发育。

anapnotherapy [əˌnæpnəuˈθerəpi] *n.* 吸入疗法

We have observed 68 cases of combined therapy of anapnotherapy and sinapisfango compressing chest on childhood asthma.

我们已经观察了 68 例以吸入疗法为主配合芥末泥敷胸来治疗儿童哮喘的综合治疗效果。

A good effect takes place also in topical administration via the oral mucosa, in nasal administration, and anapnotherapy.

通过口腔黏膜局部用药,鼻部用药和吸入疗法都有较好的疗效。

anastomose [əˈnæstəməuz] *v.* (使)吻合

The main veins and arteries should be anastomosed as early as possible, so that sufficient arterial blood supply and adequate vein return are ensured.

应尽早吻合主要静脉和动脉,从而保证足够的动脉血供应和适量的静脉血回流。

The inferior pulmonary vein, the superior pulmonary vein, the pulmonary artery, and the bronchus were anastomosed in that order.

按照肺下静脉、肺上静脉、肺动脉以及支气管的顺序进行(手术)吻合。

anastomosis [əˌnæstəˈməusis] *n.* 吻合,吻合术

A communication between two arteries is called an anastomosis.

两条动脉之间的沟通称为吻合。

These anastomoses are very important clinically.

这些吻合具有重要的临床意义。

This paper reports the procedures and therapeutic effects of fallopin tubal anastomosis without support after female sterilization.

本文介绍了女性绝育术后无支架输卵管复通术的操作方法和治疗结果。

anastomotic [ˌænəstəˈmɔtik] *a.* 吻合的

All cases were cured and discharged without anastomotic leakage and death during perioperative period.

所有的患者均治愈出院,无吻合口漏和围手术期的死亡。

Improved continuous suture is a kind of ideal suture mode which can reduce the incidence of anastomotic biliary strictures.

经改进的连续缝合法是一种理想的缝合方式,可降低吻合口胆管狭窄的发生率。

anatomic(al) [ˌænəˈtɔmik(əl)] *a.* 解剖学的,构造上的

Anatomic or histologic lesions in tissue may bear an obvious relation to the symptoms.

组织内解剖学或组织学上的病变可能与症状有明显的联系。

The hormones vary widely in composition and anatomical location.

各种激素的结构及解剖学的定位差异极大。

An important part of the physical examination is the evaluation of function of the part or organ as well as examination for anatomical change.

体检的一个重要部分是评估器官的功能,以及检查结构上的变化。

anatomist [əˈnætəmist] *n.* 解剖学家

Anatomists often compare the heart to a pump.

解剖学家常把心脏比喻为泵。

anatomy [əˈnætəmi] *n.* 解剖学

The first two years are devoted to the study of basic medical sciences, such as anatomy, physiology, biochemistry and others.

开头两年要学习基础医学课程,如解剖学、生理学、生物化学等。

In medicine, anatomy refers to the study of the form and gross structure of the various parts of the human body.

在医学上,解剖学指对人体各部分的形状和肉眼可见结构的研究。

anatoxin [ˌænəˈtɔksin] *n.* 类毒素

Anatoxin A can block acetylcholine receptors.

类毒素 A 能封闭乙酰胆碱受体。

ancestor [ˈænsistə] *n.* 祖宗,祖先

Of remoter ancestors I can only discover one who did not live to a great age.

至于较远的祖辈,我仅发现只有一位没活到高年。

ancestral [ænˈsestrəl] *a.* 祖先的,祖传的

These cells may be ancestral to the ordinary bone marrow stem cells and thus possess greater versatility.

这些细胞可能来源于普通的骨髓干细胞,因而具有更大的多面作用。

ancylostomiasis [ˌænsiˌlɔstəˈmaiəsis] *n.* 钩(口线)虫病

Ancylostomiasis is one of the main causes of anemia in the tropics.

钩虫病是热带地区引起贫血的主要原因之一。

Heavy ancylostomiasis may cause considerable damage to the wall of the intestine, leading to a serious loss of blood; this, in conjunction with malnutrition, can provoke severe anemia.

重症钩虫病可引起肠壁严重损伤,导致严重失血;失血和营养不良共同引起严重贫血。

androgen [ˈændrədʒən] *n.* 雄激素

Androgens have been used to stimulate erythropoiesis.

雄性激素已被用以促使红细胞的生成。

ACTH (adrenocorticotropic hormone) stimulates both adrenal androgens and adrenal corticosteroids.

ACTH 既兴奋肾上腺雄性激素又兴奋肾上腺皮质激素。

andrographolide [ˈændrəˈgræfəˌlaid] *n.* 穿心莲内酯

Gradient elution method was used to determine the content of andrographolide and dehydro-andrographolide in Qinghuo Zhimai tablets.

用梯度洗脱法测定清火栀麦片中穿心莲内酯和脱水穿心莲内酯的含量。

To control the quality of Qinghuo Zhimai tablets, we determine the content of andrographolide and dehydro-andrographolide.

我们通过测定穿心莲内酯和脱水穿心莲内酯的含量来控制清火栀麦片的质量。

andrology [æn'drɔlədʒi] *n.* 男科学

The article evaluates the ability of information collection and the characteristics of literatures requested by the scientists of andrology.

本文评估了信息收集能力以及男科学研究人员所需的文献的特征。

androstenedione [ˌændrə'stiːndiəun] *n.* 雄烯二酮

Androstenedione is a supplement made from a naturally occurring steroid hormone.

雄烯二酮是一种天然类固醇激素的衍生物。

Some androstenedione is also secreted into the plasma, and may be converted in peripheral tissues to testosterone and estrogens.

一些雄烯二酮也被分泌入血浆，可以在外周组织中转化为睾酮和雌激素。

anecdotal [ˌænik'dəutəl] *a.* 轶话的，轶事的

More recently anecdotal evidence has emerged that this new method may be associated with an improvement in renal outcome.

最近出现了有趣的现象，证明这种新方法可能会改善肾脏病的预后。

anemarrhena [ˌæni'mærinə] *n.* 知母

This method was simple, quick and accurate for the extraction of total flavonoid of anemarrhena.

该方法作为知母中总黄酮提取的方法具有简便、快速、准确的特点。

I am going to set up the HPLC fingerprint of anemarrhena.

我准备建立知母高效液相色谱指纹图谱。

an(a)emia [ə'niːmiə] *n.* 贫血

The overall clinical picture was compatible with pernicious anemia.

总的临床表现与恶性贫血相符。

Anaemia should be investigated and treated if it is suspected.

如怀疑有贫血，则应进行检查和治疗。

an(a)emic [ə'niːmik] *a.* 贫血的

Deleterious effects of chloramphenicol are seen in anemic patients.

在贫血病人中可见到氯霉素的有害作用。

The U. S. CDC (Center for Disease Control) estimates that 1 in 10 pre-menopausal women are anemic.

美国疾病控制中心估计绝经前的妇女 10 个人中就有一人贫血。

anemonin [ə'nemənin] *n.* 白头翁素

The purity of anemonin was 99% and yield rate was 0. 72‰. Its quality was controlled.

白头翁素纯度达 99%，收益率达 0 72‰，质量可控。

Protoanemonin and anemonin which exist in Ranunculaceae were extracted from Pulsatilla Chinesis.

从白头翁(Pulsatilla Chinesis)植物中提取的毛茛科植物含有的原白头翁素和白头翁素。

anencephalus [ˌænen'sefələs] *n.* 无脑儿

HPV-DNA was positive in 5 samples of neonatal cord blood or placenta, including 3 cases of fetal distress, 1 case of neonatal hyperbilirubinemia and 1 case of anencephalus.

有 5 例脐血或胎盘组织中的 HPV 呈阳性，其中包括 3 例胎儿窘迫、1 例新生儿高胆红素血症及 1 例无脑儿。

anergia [æ'nəːdʒiə] *n.* 能力缺失，无变应性，无力

Both under activity (anergia) and over activity (hyperergia) of the immune system have been reported as a result of mycoplasma infections.

支原体感染已被报道既可导致免疫系统的功能低下，又可导致免疫系统的功能亢进。

The initial symptoms, in the descending order of their frequencies, included fever, headache, anergia and dyskinesia.

最初症状，按发生频率递减排序，包括发热、头痛、无力和运动障碍。

anergic [æ'nəːdʒik] *adj.* 无反应的，无活动力的

Anergy is a state of nonresponsiveness to antigen. T cells and B cells are said to be anergic when they cannot respond to their specific antigen under optimal conditions of stimulation.

无反应性是一种对抗原刺激的不应答状态。当 T 细胞和 B 细胞在最佳条件下对特异性抗原刺激不能应答就被认为是无反应的。

By examining CD71 surface expression, we are able to distinguish and differentially isolate anergic and activated T cells.

通过检测细胞膜表面 CD71 分子的表达，我们能够鉴别并分离出无能的和活化的 T 细胞。

anergy ['ænədʒi] *n.* 无变应性

Anergy is defined as the lack of inflammatory response to skin test antigens.

无反应性的定义为对皮试抗原无炎性反应。

an(a)esthesia [ˌænis'θiːzjə] *n.* 感觉缺失，麻木，麻醉(法)

Anesthesia is a frequent symptom of lumbar intervertebral disc protrusion.

麻木是腰椎间盘突出症的常见症状。

Anesthesia is loss of feeling or sensation.

麻醉是指感觉或知觉的丧失。

Negative pressure pulmonary edema (NPPE) is a potentially life-threatening complication of laryngospasm that occurs during or after general anesthesia.

负压性肺水肿是在全身麻醉过程中或之后出现喉痉挛所致威胁生命的潜在并发症。

The development of anesthesia represents one of the most interesting aspects of US medical history.

麻醉学的发展是美国医学史上最引人入胜的篇章之一。

an(a)esthesiologist [ˌænisˌθiːzi'ɔlədʒist] *n.* 麻醉学家，麻醉师

It is essential that the anesthesiologist continuously assess the depth of anesthesia.

麻醉师必须不断地评估麻醉深度。

an(a)esthetic [ˌænis'θetik] *a.* 麻醉的

This is done to minimize the discomfort of wearing the anesthetic mask.

这样做能最大限度地减少带麻醉面罩的不适感。

n. 麻醉剂

Thiopental is an intravenous anesthetic.

硫喷妥是一种静脉麻醉药。

Anesthetics and analgesics readily cross both the blood brain and the placental barriers.

麻醉剂和镇痛剂易透过血脑和胎盘这两个屏障。

an(a)esthetist [æ'niːsθətist] *n.* 麻醉师

A surgical team usually consists of surgeons, anesthetists and operating room nurses.

手术组通常由外科医生、麻醉师以及手术室护士组成。

an(a)esthetization [æˌniːsθitai'zeiʃən] *n.* 麻醉(法)

Anaesthetization by acupuncture does not need any complicated apparatus; it can be applied regardless of equipment and other conditions.

针刺麻醉不需要任何复杂的仪器；不管设备和其他条件如何都能进行。

an(a)esthetize [æ'niːsθitaiz] *v.* 使麻醉

Central venous and arterial catheterization can usually by deferred until the patient is anesthetized.

中心静脉和动脉插管通常可以延迟到病人麻醉后进行。

aneuploid [ˌænjuˈplɔid] *n.* 非整倍体

Aneuploid often results in the death of the embryo at an early stage.

非整倍体通常导致胚胎在发育早期死亡。

Many forms of aneuploid result from nondisjunction during meiosis in the mother.

多种非整倍体是由于母方减数分裂期间染色体不分离造成的。

aneurysm [ˈænjuərizm] *n.* 动脉瘤

This patient may suffer from myocardial aneurysm.

此病人可能患心肌动脉瘤。

The mycotic aneurysms most commonly occur in the brain and they may rupture.

霉菌性动脉瘤最常发生于大脑,并可破裂。

aneurysmectomy [ˌænjurizˈmektəmi] *n.* 动脉瘤切除术

The treatment of aneurysmectomy may result in prolongation of life.

动脉瘤切除术的治疗方法可能会延长生命。

angelica [ænˈdʒelikə] *n.* 当归

Orange blossom, angelica, wheat germ, lavender, sage and sandalwood are just some of the natural essences.

橙花、当归、麦芽、薰衣草、鼠尾草和檀香只是部分天然香料。

To ensure the safety and utility in clinical medication, we predicted the stability of compound angelica powder for injection.

我们预测了复方当归粉注射的稳定性,以保证临床用药安全有效。

angiitis [ˌændʒiˈaitis] *n.* 血管炎,脉管炎

The treatment for primary angiitis of the central nervous system may be influenced by the clinical subset.

中枢神经系统原发性血管炎的治疗可能受临床亚型的影响。

Isolated angiitis of the CNS occasionally causes a chronic encephalopathy associated with confusion and disorientation.

中枢神经系统(CNS)单发的脉管炎有时可引起表现为意识模糊和定向力障碍的慢性脑病。

angina [ænˈdʒainə] *n.* 心绞痛;咽峡炎

Relief within 5 minutes by sublingual or buccal glyceryl trinitrate makes angina more likely.

舌下或口含硝酸甘油片使疼痛在 5 分钟内缓解者,更支持心绞痛诊断。

angina pectoris [ænˈdʒainəˈpektəris] *n.* 心绞痛

Surgery for angina pectoris performed in the United States during the 1950's turned out to be a mere placebo.

五十年代在美国流行的治疗心绞痛的手术后来证明只是一种安慰术。

anginal [ænˈdʒainəl] *a.* 心绞痛的

The use of nitroglycerin may give relief to the anginal pain at the time of its occurrence.

症状发生时,使用硝酸甘油可以缓解心绞痛。

angiocardiogram [ˌændʒiəuˈkɑːdiəgræm] *n.* 心血管造影

Postoperative angiocardiograms disclosed good perfusion of both lungs.

术后心血管的造影显示两肺的灌注良好。

angiocardiography [ˌændʒiːəuˌkɑːdiˈɔgrəfi] *n.* 心血管造影术

The lateral view of angiocardiography showed two adjacent chambers in the region of left atrium.

心血管造影侧位相显示左房区域有两个相邻的腔。

Rest equilibrium radionuclide angiocardiography (ERNA) will be performed on the patient after one week.

这位患者 1 周后将行静息平衡法核素心血管造影。

angioedema [ˌændʒiəui'diːmə] *n.* 血管水肿，血管神经性水肿

The respiratory stridor may indicate that there is angioedema of the epiglottis, and respiratory embarassment can possibly occur.

呼吸喘鸣这一事实可能表示有会厌处血管性水肿，并可能发生呼吸窘迫。

angiofibroma [ˌændʒiəufai'brəumə] *n.* 血管纤维瘤

Nasopharyngeal angiofibroma, a tumor most commonly found in adolescent males, may be manifested by epistaxis and nasal obstruction.

鼻咽血管纤维瘤好发于青少年男性，表现为鼻出血和鼻塞。

angiogenesis [ˌændʒiəu'dʒenisis] *n.* 血管生成，血管发生

Angiogenesis is necessary at the beginning and at the end of the metastatic cascade.

肿瘤转移的起始和终止都需要有血管生成。

Angiogenesis factor stimulates the growth of blood vessels after injury.

血管生成因子可在人体受到损伤后促进血管的生长。

angiogram ['ændʒiəugræm] *n.* 血管造影片

The left ventricular angiogram confirmed the presence of a membranous ventricular septal defect.

左心室造影证实有室间隔膜缺损。

angiography [ˌændʒi'ɔgræfi] *n.* 血管造影术

Selective angiography may show the site of active bleeding if not previously determined.

如果此前未能确定出血部位，则选择性血管造影检查可显示其出血部位。

Prof. Li has made a systematic study of recent advances in angiography.

李教授对血管造影术的新进展做了系统研究。

Hepatic angiography would be helpful if a hepatic neoplasm or abscess is suspected.

如果疑为肝肿瘤或肝脓肿，肝脏血管造影可有助于诊断。

angioma [ˌændʒi'əumə] *n.* 血管瘤

Angiomas are rarely seen on the lower trunk or extremities.

血管瘤很少见于躯干下部或下肢。

As with angiomas in the upper gastrointestinal tract, they may be associated with chronic renal failure or valvular heart disease.

如果血管瘤发生于上消化道，则可能伴有慢性肾功能衰竭或心脏瓣膜疾病。

angiomyolipoma [ˌændʒiɔmaiəuli'pəumə] *n.* 血管平滑肌脂肪瘤

Angiomyolipoma is a benign tumor consisting of vessels, smooth muscle, and fat.

血管平滑肌脂肪瘤是一种由血管、平滑肌和脂肪组织构成的良性肿瘤。

Fat density or fat signal can usually be found by angiomyolipoma imaging.

血管平滑肌脂肪瘤影像通常能发现脂肪密度或脂肪信号。

angioneurotic ['ændʒiəu, nju'rɔtik] *a.* 血管神经性的

Hereditary angioneurotic edema is the clinical name for a genetic deficiency of the C1 inhibitor of the complement system.

遗传性血管神经性水肿是一种由于补体系统中 C1 抑制因子遗传缺陷所引起的临床疾病。

The angioneurotic oedema resolved in all 3 patients within hours of discontinuing treatment with the agent.

在终止该药剂治疗后数小时内，所有 3 例患者的血管神经性水肿都得到恢复。

angioplasty [ˌændʒiəu'plæsti] *n.* 血管成形术

Angioplasty has already cut substantially into the heart-bypass business.

血管成形术实际上已进入心脏旁路手术领域。

50 patients have undergone percutaneous transluminal coronary angioplasty.

50 名患者进行了经皮透腔性冠状动脉成形术。

angiostatin [ˌændʒiəu'stætin] *n.* 血管生成抑制因子；血管抑素

Angiostatins contain four kringle domains which are associated with their potent angiostatic activity.

血管生成抑制因子含有四个与其有效的血管生成抑制活性相关的三环域。

The discovery of angiostatin provides a new way to restrain neoplasm metastasis.

血管抑素的发现为抑制肿瘤转移提供了新的思路。

angiotensin [ˌændʒiəu'tensin] *n.* 血管紧张素

Angiotensin has a powerful vasoconstrictor effect on the blood vessels generally.

通常血管紧张素对全身血管具有强有力的血管收缩作用。

Angiotensin Ⅰ is converted to angiotensin Ⅱ in the lung.

血管紧张素Ⅰ在肺部转变为血管紧张素Ⅱ。

anhidrosis [ˌænhai'drəusis] *n.* 无汗症

This drug can be applied clinically to cure several diseases such as cold, fever, asthma, anhidrosis, acute nephritis, and allergic rhinitis, and get good effect.

此药：临床可用于感冒、高热、哮喘、无汗症、急性肾炎、过敏性鼻炎等多科疾病，且取得了良好治疗效果。

The typical clinical manifestations are hypohidrosis/anhidrosis, sparse/scanty hair and absent teeth/teeth that are malformed.

该病典型的临床表现为少汗或无汗、毛发稀疏或全秃、少牙或牙齿形态异常等三联征。

anhydrase [æn'haidreis] *n.* 脱水酶

In patients with refractory heart failure, the action of loop diuretics may be potentiated by intravenous administration and the addition of other diuretics, i. e. , thiazides and carbonic anhydrase inhibitors.

对于顽固性心衰的病人，袢利尿剂的作用可通过静脉给药及加用其他利尿剂（如噻嗪类利尿剂和碳酸酐酶抑制剂）而得以加强。

anicteric [ænik'terik] *a.* 无黄疸的

Mild anicteric hepatitis is more common among infants than the icteric form.

轻症无黄疸型肝炎在婴儿中较黄疸型肝炎更为常见。

animal ['æniməl] *n.* 动物

The Laboratory Animal Resource Center of the University of California, San Francisco is administratively part of the Office of Research Services in the Research unit of the University.

美国旧金山加州大学试验动物资源中心隶属于该大学的科研机构的科研服务部。

In this Guide, laboratory animals include any vertebrate animal (e. g. , traditional laboratory animals, farm animals, wildlife, and aquatic animals) used in research, teaching, or testing.

在本指南中，实验动物包括用于科研、教学或测试的任何一类脊椎动物，如传统的实验动物、家畜、野生动物以及水生动物。

animate ['ænimit] *a.* 有生命的

Do you think animate beings exist on the Mars?

你认为火星上有生命之物存在吗？

These belong to the lowest orders of animate things.

它们属于有生命的物质中的最低等种类。

animation [æni'meiʃən] *n.* 动画片，动画片制作

The animation of China has made a great progress.

中国的动画片制作取得很大发展。

The animation is awesome and gets better and better every year.

动画片尤其精采，而且一年比一年好看。

anion ['ænaiən] *n.* 阴离子，负离子

Lactic and other organic acids are responsible for the increased anion gap.

乳酸和其他有机酸的增加使阴离子的间隙增大。

In acidic dyes, the color is carried by the anion (negative ion).

在酸性染料中,颜色是由阴离子着色的。

anisocytosis [æˌnaisəsaiˈtəusis] *n.* 红细胞(大小)不均

In addition to variations in size (anisocytosis), variations in shape may be seen.

红细胞不均除大小的变异之外,还可出现形态的变化。

ankle [ˈæŋkl] *n.* 踝

The patient has edema of the ankles.

病人踝部浮肿。

The usual sites of suicidal incisions are the neck, wrists, and ankles.

自杀切口的常见部位是颈部、腕部和踝部。

ankylosing [ˈæŋkiləuzing] *a.* 关节强硬的

Rheumatoid factor is usually negative in ankylosing spondylitis.

类风湿因子在强直性脊柱炎时常显示为阴性。

It has been found that 90% of patients with the clinical diagnosis of ankylosing spondylitis have HLA-B27 in their phenotype.

已发现在临床诊断患有强直性脊柱炎的病人中90%伴有HLA-B27.

annals [ˈænəlz] (*pl.*) *n.* 学会(或学科等)的年刊,年鉴

The findings of their study have been reported in the Annals of Internal Medicine.

他们研究的结果已在《内科学年刊》上作了报道。

anneal [əˈniːl] *vt.* 退火

Formation of double-stranded molecules is processed from two single strands of nucleic acid by base pairing of complementary sequence is called annealing.

两条单链核酸通过互补序列的碱基配对形成双链分子,这就称之退火。

annihilation [əˌnaiəˈleiʃən] *n.* (电子对)湮没

The radiation of positron annihilation in two aluminum samples from different origins was measured with the Ge(Li) detector.

用Ge(Li)探测器测量正电子在两种不同来源的铝样品中的湮没辐射。

The relative positions of the annihilation peak centers were repetitively determined.

湮没峰的相对位置被重复测定。

announce [əˈnauns] *v.* 宣布,宣告,发表

Only an initial dragging pain in the inguinal region announces a commencing epididymitis.

仅在腹股沟部分初现牵涉性痛就表示有了附睾炎症。

The discovery of another powerful killer of bacteria, the sulfas, was announced in 1935.

1935年公开宣布另一种强效杀灭细菌的磺胺药物被发现。

annual [ˈæŋjuəl] *a.* 每年的,年度的

The annual meeting of internal medicine is a week away.

内科学年会1周后举行。

Since 1972 the average annual incidence of M. audouinii at Cook County Hospital in Chicago has been 1.5 cases per year.

自1972年以来芝加哥库克县医院每年奥杜安小孢子菌的发病平均为1.5例。

n. 年刊,年鉴

Last week I received a copy of the annual of Immunogenetics Association in which you can find Dr. Baker's thesis.

上周我收到一份免疫遗传学学会的年刊,从中你可找到贝克博士的论文。

annually [ˈæŋnjuəli] *ad.* 全年地

In 1985 it was estimated that there were at least 24 million cases of diarrh(o)ea caused by food-borne microorganisms annually in the USA.

据 1985 年估计，一年中美国由于食物携带微生物而造成至少 2 400 万腹泻病例。

anomalous [ə'nɔːmələs] *a.* 不规则的，异常的

Regeneration of this nerve with misdirection of peripheral fibers results in anomalous movements.
具有周围纤维导向错乱的神经的再生会引起异常运动。

Pain can also result from damage to or anomalous activation of pain-sensitive pathways of the peripheral or central nervous system.
疼痛也可由对痛觉敏感的周围神经或中枢神经系统通路的损伤或异常刺激所致。

anomaly [ə'nɔməli] *n.* 异常，畸形

In most cases the anomaly consists in trisomy of a chromosome of the G group.
大多数病例的异常在 G 组染色体的 3 倍体上。

A plan for early surgical correction of predisposing anomalies must be developed.
对诱发性异常应制订早期手术矫正计划。

Serious adverse events(SAEs) include events that result in a congenital anomaly.
严重不良事件(SAEs)包括导致先天畸形的事件。

anorchia [æ'nɔːkiə] *n.* 无睾症

Anorchia (or anorchism, sometimes spelled anarchism) is a medical condition where both testes are absent at birth.
无睾症是指出生时双侧睾丸缺如的一种医学病症。

The presence of isolated micropenis in almost half of the patients with bilateral anorchia strongly suggests that the testicular alteration occurred during late gestation after male sex differentiation.
在将近一半的双侧无睾症患者中存在孤立的小阴茎，表明这种睾丸改变发生在妊娠后期男性性别分化之后。

anorexia [ˌænəu'reksiə] *n.* 厌食

Anorexia Nervosa is a disorder in which the main features are persistent active refusal to eat and marked loss of weight.
神经性厌食是一种主要特点为持续性地主动拒食和体重明显减轻的疾病。

It may be insidious with non-specific symptoms of anorexia and tiredness.
它可呈隐袭性，伴有一些非特异性症状如厌食和疲倦。

anovulation [ˌænɔvju'leiʃən] *n.* 排卵停止，无排卵

Episode of bleeding occurring at less than 21-day intervals is frequently due to anovulation.
月经的(出血)间隔短于 21 天常由于无排卵引起。

anovulatory [æ'nɔvjulətəri] *a.* 无排卵的

The treatment of anovulatory bleeding should have as its first aim the transformation of proliferative into secretory endometrium.
治疗无排卵型子宫出血的首要目标是将增生型的子宫内膜转化为分泌型的子宫内膜。

anoxia [æ'nɔksiə] *n.* 缺氧(症)

Anoxia may conduce to circulatory failure.
缺氧可导致循环衰竭。

Signs of tissue anoxia appear only after several hours of bacteremia.
组织缺氧体征仅在患细菌血症几小时后便可出现。

anoxic [æ'nɔksik] *a.* 缺氧的

A very early indication of anoxic damage is the disappearance of the dense granules.
缺氧损伤最早期的表现是致密颗粒消失。

After the severe anoxic episode the child was not able to maintain adequate oxygenation.
在严重缺氧发生后，患儿不能维持适当的氧化状态。

anoxygenic [æˌnɔksi'ʒenik] *a.* 不产氧的

A strain of the aerobic anoxygenic photosynthetic bacteria was isolated from a deep-ocean hydro-

thermal vent plume environment.
从深海热液喷口羽流环境中分离出一株需氧但不产氧的光合细菌菌株。
Anoxygenic photosynthesis is the phototropic process where light energy is captured and stored as ATP, without the production of oxygen.
不产氧光合作用是一个在无氧产生时,捕获光能并以 ATP 形式储存的趋光过程。

antacid [æn'tæsid] *n.* 抗酸剂,解酸药
All patients with liver injuries should be given antacids after operation.
所有肝外伤病人术后均需给抗酸药物。
The epigastric pain is managed by antacids and by other medications.
上腹部疼痛可用抗酸药和其他药物治疗。

antagonism [æn'tægənizəm] *n.* 对抗作用,拮抗作用
In physiologic antagonism, the drugs do not bind to the same receptor sites but produce functionally opposite results.
在生理性拮抗作用中,药物并未与相同受体结合,但产生功能上相反的结果。

antagonist [æn'tægənist] *n.* 拮抗剂,对抗剂
Drugs that interact with receptors preventing the action of agonists are referred to as antagonists.
凡与受体相结合后使激动剂不起作用的药物称为拮抗剂。
Many of the above mentioned factors already have their agonists and antagonists.
上面所提到的许多因素已经有它们相应的激动剂和拮抗剂。

antagonistic [ænˌtægə'nistik] *a.* 对抗(性)的
If two or more drugs antagonistic to each other are used, the effect may prove fatal.
如果两种或多种对抗药物同时使用,可能产生致命的结果。

antagonize [æn'tægənaiz] *v.* 中和,抵消,对抗
Neostigmine antagonizes the action of d-tubocurarine and curariform drugs.
新斯的明可拮抗右旋筒箭毒和箭毒样药物的作用。
The use of monoclonal antibodies to antagonize transmembrane receptors has met with tremendous clinical and commercial success over the course of the past decade.
在过去的十年,使用单克隆抗体来中和跨膜受体已经取得了巨大的临床和商业上的成功。

antecedent [ænti'siːdənt] *n.* 前例,前事
The characteristic antecedent of sudden death caused by infectious myocarditis is an upper respiratory tract infection.
传染性心肌炎引起的突然死亡特有的前驱表现是上呼吸道感染。

antegrade ['æntigreid] *a.* 前向的
Reentry requires that antegrade activation be slowed but spread in the normal direction.
折返需要前向传导的激活延缓但(传导的)方向不变。

antemortem [ˌænti'mɔːtəm] *a.* [拉] 死前的
The presence of diseases that might have induced antemortem fever must be taken into consideration.
必须考虑可能诱发死前高烧的疾病的出现。

antenatal [ˌænti'neitəl] *a.* 出生前的,产前的
In a few cases, the patients have not had any antenatal supervision, in that case complete examination will be necessary.
少数情况下,患者可能从未作产前检查,故全面检查是必要的。
Postpartum haemorrhage rate was 43.47%, antenatal diagnosis rate was 47.83%, and ultrasonography diagnosis rate was 23.81%.
产后大出血发生率为 43.47%,产前诊断率为 47.83%,超声诊断率为 23.81%。
Early diagnosis, especially antenatal diagnosis, can improve the cure rate of congenital intestinal

atresia.
早期诊断，尤其是产前诊断，可以提高先天性肠闭锁的治愈率。

antepartum [ˌænti'pɑːtəm] *a.* [拉] 产前的
Acute placental failure may result from accidental antepartum haemorrhage.
急性胎盘功能衰竭可因突发性产前出血所引起。

anterior (to) [æn'tiəriə] *a.* 前面的，在…之前的
Gastric ulcer pain may be epigastric or occur anywhere in the anterior upper abdomen.
胃溃疡疼痛可发生在上腹部，也可在上腹前部的任何部位。
The heart is anterior to the esophagus.
心脏在食管的前面。

anteriorly [æn'tiəriəli] *ad.* 在前部
When the foreign body is lodged anteriorly, it is obviously in the larynx.
如异物停留在前部则它显然是在喉部。

anteroposterior [ˌæntərəupɔs'tiəriə] *a.* 前后(位)的
Anteroposterior packing is a traditional technique for control of severe nose and ear emergency.
前后位包扎法是一种控制严重鼻子和耳朵急症的传统方法。
For critically ill patients or patients lying in bed, the anteroposterior radiography is needed.
对于危重病人或卧床患者，放射摄影需要采用前后位。

anterosuperior [ˌæntərəusju'piəriə] *a.* 前上方的
The stomach is anterosuperior to the transverse colon.
胃位于横结肠的前上方。

anterosuperiorly [ˌæntərəusju'piəriəli] *ad.* 在前上方
The transverse colon is related anterosuperiorly to the liver.
横结肠的前上方与肝脏相接触。

anthelmintic [ˌænθel'mintik] (=anthelminthic [ˌænθel'minθik]) *a.* 抗蠕虫的，驱肠虫的
Therapy of this disease includes anthelminthic drugs and correction of anemia.
此病的治疗包括使用驱肠虫药和矫正贫血。
n. 驱肠虫药
The pharmacology of most often used anthelminthics is summarized as follows.
最常用驱肠虫药的药理摘要如下。

anthrax ['ænθræks] *n.* 炭疽
Sometimes anthrax enters the body by way of the lungs through inhalation of the anthrax spores.
有时因为吸入炭疽芽孢，炭疽经肺侵入人体。
Anthrax often affects people who constantly come into contact with animals.
炭疽病常感染经常接触动物的人。

antiandrogen [ˌænti'ændrədʒin] *n.* 抗雄激素
An antiandrogen is a substance that inhibits the biological effects of androgenic hormones.
抗雄激素是一种具有抑制雄激素生物效应的物质。
The most common side effects from all antiandrogens are due to the decreased levels of hormones.
所有抗雄激素最主要的副作用是降低激素水平。

antiantibody [ˌænti'æntiˌbɔdi] *n.* 抗抗体
Antiantibody is an immunoglobulin formed in the body after administration of antibody acting as immunogen.
抗抗体是抗体作为免疫原给予后机体形成的一种免疫球蛋白。
Xolair is an antiantibody that reduces the level of IgE in the blood, which might increase the amount of peanut the patient can tolerate.
Xolair 是一种抗抗体，能减少血液中的 IgE 水平，从而增加病人对花生的耐受量。

antiarrhythmic [ˌæntiəˈriθmik] *a.* 抗心律失常的

Most of the major antiarrhythmic drugs are used to treat abnormally fast heart rates.

主要的抗心律失常药大多用于治疗异常快速心律。

Sudden cardiac death can be prevented by long-term administration of antiarrhythmic drugs.

心脏病引起的猝死可以通过长期服用抗心律失常药物来预防。

antiatherosclerotic [ˌæntiˌæθərəuskliəˈrɔtik] *a.* 抗动脉粥样硬化的

Noninvasive methods eventually may be expected to allow evaluation of the efficacy of antiatherosclerotic medical therapy.

将来可用非侵害性方法对抗动脉粥样硬化内科治疗的功效进行评估。

antibacterial [ˌæntibækˈtiəriəl] *n.* 抗菌剂,抗菌物

Both sulfonamides and penicillins are commonly used antibacterials.

磺胺类和青霉素类药物均为常用的抗菌剂。

a. 抗细菌的

Acidification of urine enhances the antibacterial action of methenamine.

酸化尿液能增强乌洛托品的抗菌作用。

antibiotic [ˌæntibaiˈɔtik] *n.* 抗生素 *a.* 抗菌的

If secondary infection is present, the steroid should be combined with an antibiotic.

如果出现继发性感染,类固醇就应与抗生素结合使用。

The selection of antibiotics is mostly based on the pattern of sensitivity of the infecting organism(s).

抗生素的选择大都依据所感染细菌的敏感性而定。

antibody [ˈæntiˌbɔdi] *n.* 抗体

Antibody appears at the onset of the illness and a rising titre indicates recent infection.

疾病开始时即有抗体生成,抗体的滴定度升高表明近期有感染。

Antibodies fight the viruses and bacteria that cause disease.

抗体能战胜引起疾病的某些病毒和细菌。

Antibodies are classified according to their mode of action as agglutinins, bacteriolysins, hemolysins, opsonins, precipitins, etc.

抗体可根据其作用方式分为凝集素、溶菌素、溶血素、调理素、沉淀素等等。

anticholinergic [ˌæntiˌkəuliˈnəːdʒik] *n.* 抗胆碱能药

Like other anticholinergics elorine reduces the flow of gastric juice, saliva and pancreatic juice.

像其他抗胆碱能药物一样,开马君也可减少胃液、唾液和胰液的分泌。

a. 抗胆碱能的

In addition to blocking H1 receptors, some of these agents have anticholinergic properties.

除阻断 H1 受体外,其中某些药物还有抗胆碱能作用。

anticholinesterase [ˌæntikəuliˈnestəreis] *n.* 抗胆碱酯酶

Anticholinesterase inhibitors can increase muscle weakness when given in excessive doses.

抗胆碱酯酶抑制剂使用过量时会加重肌无力。

Anticholinesterase tests are used in diagnosis of disorders of neuromuscular transmission.

抗胆碱酯酶试验被用于神经肌肉接头处传递障碍的诊断中。

anticipate [ænˈtisipeit] *v.* 预想

Emergencies must be anticipated and appropriate action taken before the physician arrives.

在医生到来之前,应预先想到将采用的急救方法并采取适当的配合措施。

Thus degeneration is an anticipated result of aging.

因此退行性病变是年老所带来的预料之中的结果。

anticipation [ænˌtisiˈpeiʃən] *n.* 预测

Fetal death and perinatal morbidity can be reduced with careful anticipation and vigilant monitoring of the fetus.

认真做出预先评估及密切监测能降低胎儿死亡及围产期发病率。

anticoagulant [ˌæntikəuˈægjulənt] *n.* 抗凝(血)剂

The pharmacologic properties of oral anticoagulants are identical qualitatively.

各种口服抗凝剂的药理特性在性质上是相同的。

a. 抗凝(血)的

With anticoagulant therapy, the danger of pulmonary embolism is greatly reduced.

由于抗凝疗法,肺栓塞症的危险显著减少。

anticoagulation [ˈæntikəuˌægjuˈleiʃən] *n.* 抗凝

Anticoagulation is indicated when atrial fibrillation develops or following systemic embolism.

当发生房颤时或体循环栓塞后适用抗凝。

Anticoagulation is not always feasible after major surgery.

在大手术后给予抗凝治疗并非都适宜。

anticoden [ˌæntiˈkəudən] *n.* 反密码子

On the tRNA molecule lies the anticoden.

在 tRNA 分子上有反密码子。

Each type of anticoden can bind only to a specific, complementary coden on an mRNA molecule.

每种反密码子只能与一个 mRNA 分子上的特异的互补密码子相结合。

anticomplement [ˌæntiˈkɔmplimənt] *n.* 抗补体

Gamimune can be safely given in large amounts and is free of spontaneous (nonspecific) anti-complement activity.

免疫球蛋白制剂可大剂量安全使用,且无自发性(非特异性)抗补体活性。

anticonceptive [ˌæntikənˈseptɪv] *n.* 避孕药 *a.* 避孕的

Taking anticonceptive pills is one of the safe and effective contraceptive ways.

口服避孕药片是安全有效的避孕措施之一。

anticongestive [ˌæntikənˈdʒestiv] *a.* 抗充血性的

Diuretic therapy in the form of furosemide was added to the patient's anticongestive regimen with considerable clinical improvement.

在抗充血性心力衰竭的治疗方法中加用了速尿作为利尿方法,临床上得到十分显著的改善。

anticonvulsant [ˌæntikənˈvʌlsənt] *n.* 抗惊厥药

Certain anticonvulsants can, after long periods, produce macrocytic anemia by interfering with folic acid metabolism.

某些抗惊厥药长期应用后,由于它可以干扰叶酸代谢,所以能产生巨细胞性贫血。

It is unwise to make frequent changes in the anticonvulsants if the attacks are not responding.

如果发作经治疗无效,频繁更换抗抽搐药物是不明智的。

antidepressant [ˌæntidiˈpresənt] *a.* 抗抑郁的

Extreme care must be taken when prescribing antidepressant drugs.

给病人开抗抑郁症药的处方时必须非常小心。

n. 抗抑郁药

Antidepressants seem specific for the panic attacks in agoraphobia.

抗抑郁剂似乎对旷野恐惧症的恐慌发作有特效。

antidiarrheal [ˌæntiˌdaiəˈriəl] *a.* 止泻的

The antitussive and antidiarrheal effects of meperidine are minimum.

哌替啶镇咳和止泻作用极微。

n. 止泻药

In older children with diarrhea, antidiarrheals may be used, but it is also very important that a sufficient amount of liquids be given to replace the fluid lost by the body.

较大年龄的腹泻患儿可使用止泻药,但必须给予足量的液体补充身体丧失的水分,这一点也很重要。

antidiuretic [ˌæntiˌdaijuə'retik] *a.* 抗利尿的 n. 抗利尿剂

Water is reabsorbed under the influence of antidiuretic hormone (ADH).

水是在抗利尿激素(ADH)的作用下被重吸收的。

Antidiuretic hormone or vasopressin from the posterior lobe regulates urine flow and the tone of smooth muscle in blood vessels.

后叶的抗利尿激素即后叶的加压素可以调节尿量和血管平滑肌的紧张度。

antidote ['æntidəut] *n.* 解毒药

An antidote is a substance that neutralizes the effects of a poison.

解毒剂是能将毒物的作用进行中和的物质。

Unfortunately there are no known specific antidotes for the large majority of poisons.

遗憾的是大多数毒物现在均无已知的特效解毒剂。

antidysrhythmic [ˌæntidis'riðmik] *a.* 抗心律失常的

Antidysrhythmic agents, electrical defibrillators, and pacers are able to reverse cardiac dysrhythmias effectively.

抗心律失常药、电除颤器和起搏器能有效地反转心律失常。

antiemetic [ˌæntii'metik] *a.* 止吐的 *n.* 止吐药

In case of the patient vomiting again, antiemetic should be given.

如果病人再呕吐,应该给他吃止吐剂。

antiendotoxin [ˌæntiˌendəu'tɔksin] *n.* 抗内毒素

The infusion of an antiendotoxin antiserum may be beneficial in patients in the early stage of septic shock.

在败血症患者休克的早期如给予抗内毒素抗血清可能是有效的。

antiepileptic [ˌæntiˌepi'leptik] *a.* 抗癫痫的

Use of antiepileptic drugs can produce smaller babies.

抗癫痫药物的应用能导致小样婴儿。

antiestrogen [ˌænti'estrədʒən] *n.* 抗雌激素药

An antiestrogen is a substance that blocks the production or utilization of estrogens, or inhibits their effects.

抗雌激素药是一种能阻止雌激素的产生、利用或抑制其效应的物质。

Clomiphene, an antiestrogen clinically used for ovulation induction, kills leukemic cells ex vivo via apoptosis.

克罗米芬,一种临床用来促排卵的抗雌激素药,在体内通过细胞凋亡杀死白血病细胞。

While antiestrogens have been available since the early 1970s, we still do not fully understand their mechanisms of action and resistance.

尽管抗雌激素类物质自20世纪70年代初已开始被应用,但我们还不能完全明白它们的作用和拮抗机制。

antifungal [ˌænti'fʌŋgəl] *a.* 抗真菌的

We evaluated the use of antifungal agents in the treatment of uncomplicated funguria.

我们评价了抗真菌制剂在无并发症的真菌尿症治疗中的应用。

n. 抗真菌药

With reference to specific groups of organisms such terms as antibacterial or antifungal are frequently employed.

对微生物的特定种群,像抗菌剂或抗真菌剂这样的术语经常被使用。

The administration of antifungals may prevent and treat infections with susceptible organisms but cause a concomitant increase in infections due to resistant fungi.

抗真菌药可以预防和治疗由敏感菌引起的感染,但如果该真菌有耐药性就会使感染加重。

antigen ['æntidʒən] *n.* 抗原

Hepatitis B has a surface antigen (HBsAg) and a core antigen (HBcAg).

乙型肝炎有一表面抗原(HBsAg)和一核心抗原(HBcAg)。

The skin tests used to diagnose anergy are those said to test recall antigens and delayed hypersensitivity.

用作无反应性诊断的皮试是要试验回忆性抗原和迟发性过敏反应。

antigenic [ˈæntiˈdʒenik] *a.* 抗原性的

Sensitized cells tend to elect domicile in the antigenic target.

敏感细胞容易在抗原靶中选择藏身处。

antigenicity [ˌæntidʒəˈnisiti] *n.* 抗原性

In some cell lines there is a similar periodicity in changes of cell surface antigenicity or response to wheat germ agglutinin.

在某些细胞系中,细胞表面抗原性或对麦胚凝集素的反应有相似的周期性变化。

This conformational change should alter the antigenicity of the determinant.

这种构象变化可能会影响抗原决定簇的抗原性。

antihistamine [ˌæntiˈhistəmin] *n.* 抗组胺药

For follow-up therapy, the patient should receive an antihistamine.

患者应接受抗组胺药以继续治疗。

Vitamin C can have an antihistamine effect, opening stuffy breathing passages.

维生素 C 具有抗组胺效果,打开不通气的呼吸道。

antihistaminic [ˌæntihistəˈminik] *n.* 抗组胺药 a. 抗组胺的

These effects are blocked by classic antihistaminics such as pyrilamine.

典型的抗组胺药如吡拉明(新安特甘)可阻断这些作用。

antihypertensive [ˌæntiˌhaipəˈtensiv] *a.* 抗高血压的

Neither of the agents is antihypertensive.

两种药都不能降压。

The headache associated with malignant hypertension is managed by antihypertensive agents.

恶性高血压引起的头痛用抗高血压药治疗。

Antihypertensive therapy if applied rapidly and effectively can often yield life-saving results.

降压治疗如果应用得迅速而有效,常能产生保命的效果。

n. 抗高血压药

The drugs used in this case are diuretics, sedatives, antihypertensives and others.

这种情况使用的药物为利尿剂、镇静剂、降压药及其他。

anti-idiotype (antiidiotypic) [ˌæntiˈidiətaip] *n.* 抗独特型

Anti-idiotype antibodies are antibodies raised against antigenic determinants unique to the variable region of a single antibody.

抗独特性抗体是指针对单一抗体可变区的抗原决定簇所产生的抗体。

Anti-idiotype antibodies can be used to monitor B-cell tumors and to investigate the biology of these tumors.

抗独特性抗体可用于监测 B 细胞瘤和研究这些肿瘤的生物学特性。

Antiidiotypic [ˌæntiˌidiəˈtipik] *a.* 抗特异基因型的

Antiidiotypic antibodies may prove to be a key mechanism for this type of manipulation of the recipient response.

抗特异基因型抗体可证明是这种受体反应操作类型的关键机制。

antiinflammatory [ˌæntiinˈflæmətəri] *n.* 消炎药 a. 消炎的

Acute rheumatic fever is treated with antiinflammatory agents such as aspirin.

急性风湿热可用抗炎药如阿司匹林治疗。

antimalarial [ˌæntiməˈlɛəriəl] *a.* 抗疟疾的

Antimalarial agents are used as therapy for several skin deseases but they also can induce cutaneous reactions.

抗疟疾药能用于治疗多种皮肤病，但是这些药也可诱发皮肤反应。

n. 抗疟疾药

This family of drugs is completely separate in structure from all other antimalarials.

这一族药物在结构上与所有其他抗疟疾药物完全不同。

antimetabolite [ˌæntiməˈtæbəlait] *n.* 抗代谢产物

Studies have shown beneficial effects of a single dose intraoperative mitomycin C, an antimetabolite, in inhibiting fibroblast proliferation.

研究证实，手术中单独一次应用抗代谢药丝裂霉素 C 能在抑制成纤维细胞增殖产生功效。

Pemetrexed is a multitargeted antimetabolite that has shown activity in malignant pleural mesothelioma and NSCLC.

培美曲塞是一种多靶点的抗代谢类药物，用于恶性胸膜间皮瘤和非小细胞肺癌治疗有效。

antimicrobial [ˌæntimaiˈkrəubiəl] *a.* 抗菌的，抗微生物的

Among aminoglycosides, amikacin has the broadest antimicrobial spectrum.

在氨基苷类中，丁胺卡那霉素的抗菌谱最广。

Antimicrobial agents should not be used during the acute phase of viral respiratory disease.

在病毒性上呼吸道疾病的急性阶段不能使用抗菌剂。

n. 抗菌剂

Symptoms of infection can be successfully removed by an appropriate antimicrobial.

感染症状可用一种适宜的抗菌药物有效地消除。

antimicrobic [ˌæntimaiˈkrɔbik] *a.* 抗微生物的

Antimicrobic susceptibility test of 13 antimicrobic agents in 76 clinical isolates of Klebsiella pneumoniae was studied.

通过 13 种抗微生物药物敏感试验对 76 株肺炎克雷伯菌临床分离株进行了研究。

antimony [ˈæntiməni] *n.* 锑

The earliest human was well aware of the toxic effects of the toxic mineral substances arsenic, lead and antimony.

最初的人类就已熟知有毒矿物质如砷、铅和锑的毒性。

The metabolism of antimony resembles that of arsenic.

锑的代谢与砷相似。

antimutagen [ˌæntiˈmjuːtədʒən] *n.* 抗诱变剂

Antimutagen is any substance that reduces the rate of spontaneous mutations or counteracts or reverses the action of a mutagen.

抗诱变剂是指可使自发突变率降低或抵消或逆转诱变剂作用的任何物质。

Chlorophyllin, an antimutagen, acts as a tumor promoter in the rat-dimethylhydrazine colon carcinogenesis model.

叶绿素是一种抗诱变剂，它在二甲肼诱发大鼠结肠癌模型中起促癌作用。

antineoplastic [ˌæntiˌniəuˈplæstik] *a.* 抗肿瘤的

Antineoplastic agents may be teratogenic, carcinogenic, and immunosuppressant.

抗肿瘤药可能致畸、致癌和抑制免疫。

n. 抗肿瘤药

Liposomal cytarabine belongs to the group of medicines known as antineoplastics.

脂质体阿糖胞苷属于抗肿瘤药一类。

antineutrino [æntiːnjuːˈtriːnəu] *n.* 反中微子

Antineutrinos are the antiparticles of neutrinos.

反中微子是中微子的反粒子。

Antineutrinos are neutral particles produced in nuclear beta decay.

反中微子是在核 β 衰变时产生的中性粒子。

antioncogene [ˌænti'ɔŋkədʒiːn] *n.* 抗癌基因,抑癌基因

The inactivation of antioncogene by methylation has become one of important pathogenesis mechanisms of leukemia.

抑癌基因甲基化失活已成为白血病的一个重要发病机制。

Antioncogenes are genes which prevent cells from transforming into cancerous cells, and loss of one or more antioncogenes is often found in cancer cells.

抑癌基因是能阻止细胞转变成癌细胞的基因,癌细胞常常出现一个或多个抑癌基因的缺失。

antioxidant [ˌænti'ɔksidənt] *n.* 抗氧化剂 (= antioxygen [ˌænti'ɔksidʒən])

Vitamins E and C and beta carotene, known as antioxidants, are considered powerful disease-fighters.

可称作是抗氧化剂的维生素 E、C 和 β-胡萝卜素也被认为是强有力的抗病药物。

Work from Cambridge University this year shows that heart disease patients have fewer heart attacks if they take high doses of antioxidant vitamins A, C and E.

今年剑桥大学的研究工作显示:心脏病患者如果服用大剂量抗氧化维生素 A、C 和 E,其心脏病发病的次数就会少得多。

The research indicates that a high dietary intake of various antioxidants is associated with lower rates of vascular disease.

这项研究显示从饮食中大量摄入多种抗氧化物质可使血管系统疾病的发病率降低。

antioxidation ['æntiɔksi'deiʃən] *n.* 抗氧化作用

Chocolate is antioxidation food, which has certain effect to delaying a senility.

巧克力是一种对延缓衰老有一定作用的抗氧化食物。

It was found in experiments that many protein extracts from animals and plants show antioxidation activity to some extent.

实验研究发现,很多来自于动植物的蛋白提取物具有一定的抗氧化活性。

antiproliferative [ˌæntiprəu'lifərətiv] *adj.* 抗增殖的

Rapamycin has antiproliferative actions on the arterial duct.

雷帕霉素对动脉导管具有抗增殖的作用。

These stents are often coated with antiproliferative drugs such as paclitaxel.

这些支架通常披覆抗增殖药物,诸如紫杉醇。

antiprostaglandin [ˌæntiˌprɔstə'glændin] *n.* 抗前列腺素

Antiprostaglandin agents may be the analgesics of first choice.

抗前列腺素制剂可为首选止痛剂。

The use of other anti-inflammatory drugs such as the antiprostaglandins is under active investigation.

其他抗炎药如抗前列腺素类药物的应用正在积极的研究之中。

antipruritic [ˌæntipruə'ritik] *n.* 止痒药,止痒剂

Histamine (H_2) blockers have been used as antipruritics and offer a nonsedating advantage.

组胺(H_2)阻断剂可被用做止痒药,其优点是无镇静作用。

Antipruritic is an agent that relieves itching (pruritus). Examples are calamine and crotamiton, applied in creams or lotions, and some antihistamine drugs (e. g. trimeprazine), used if the itching is due to an allergy.

止痒剂是减轻瘙痒的药物,例如以乳剂或洗剂形式使用的炉甘石和克罗米通,以及由变态反应所致的瘙痒而使用的一些抗组胺药(如阿利马嗪)。

antipsychotic [ˌæntisai'kɔtik] *a.* 抗精神病的

Clozapine ia an antipsychotic drug.

氯氮平是一种抗精神病药。

n. 精神病抑制药(如安定药)

Despite increasing use of antipsychotics, prescribing antipsychotics to children remains controversial.

尽管抗精神病药的使用日益增多,但给儿童开抗精神病药尚存争议。

An antipsychotic is a kind of medication primarily used to manage psychosis.

抗精神病药物是一类主要用于治疗精神病的药物。

antipyresis [ˌæntipaiˈriːsis] *n.* 退热(疗)法

Aspirin induces antipyresis.

阿司匹林产生解热作用。

antipyretic [ˌæntipaiˈretik] *a.* 退热的

The local application of the antipyretic drugs causes a fall in body temperature.

退热药的局部应用可使体温下降。

Several analgesic drugs have antipyretic activity, including aspirin, paracetamol, phenylbutazone, and mefenamic acid.

有几种止痛剂如阿司匹林、对乙酰氨基酚、保泰松和甲芬那酸等都具有退热作用。

n. 退热药

Table 1 lists some of the most commonly used antipyretics.

表 1 列举了一些最常用的退热药。

High fever(≥41℃) should be managed with antipyretics and physical cooling.

当发烧温度高(≥41℃)时必须服用退热药并进行物理降温。

antipyrine [ˌæntiˈpaiərin] *n.* 安替比林(解热镇痛药)

Antipyrine doesn't bind to plasma protein.

安替比林不与血浆蛋白结合。

antirachitic [ˌæntiræˈkaitik] *a.* 抗佝偻病的

Sunlight which has passed through ordinary window glass is deprived of its antirachitic potency.

阳光在透过一般玻璃窗后丧失其抗佝偻病的效能。

antiretroviral [ˌæntiˌretrəuˈvaiərəl] *a.* 抗逆转录病毒的

Antiretroviral therapy is to treat and prevent AIDS in developing countries.

抗逆转录病毒治疗将用于发展中国家艾滋病的治疗和预防。

antirheumatic [ˌæntiruˈmætik] *a.* 抗风湿(病)的

Phenylbutazone itself has both uricosuric and antirheumatic effects.

保泰松本身同时具有促尿酸排泄和抗风湿作用。

n. 抗风湿药

Aspirin, as one of the antirheumatics, is very effective in the treatment of rheumatoid arthritis.

作为一种抗风湿药,阿司匹林治疗类风湿性关节炎效果良好。

antiscorbutic [ˌæntiskɔːbˈjuːtik] *a.* 抗坏血酸病的

The antiscorbutic vitamin is a carbohydrate with strong acidic properties.

抗坏血病维生素是一种强酸性碳水化合物。

antisense [ˈæntisens] *a.* 反义的

Antisense oligodeoxyribonucleotides are described as "antisense" because they are complementary to the target mRNA.

反义寡脱氧核苷酸之所以被称为"反义",是因为它们与靶 mRNA 互补。

antisepsis [ˌæntiˈsepsis] *n.* 抗菌(法)

Prevention of wound infection involves application of techniques of antisepsis and asepsis in the hospital at large.

伤口感染的预防涉及在医院中充分应用抗菌和无菌的技术操作。

antiseptic [ˌæntiˈseptik] *a.* 防腐的,抗菌的

Joseph Lister has been considered the "father of antiseptic surgery".

约瑟夫·李斯特被称为是"无菌外科之父"。

n. 防腐剂,抗菌剂

A substance that prevents growth of bacteria in or on the body is called an antiseptic.

能防止细菌在体内或体表生长的物质叫做抗菌剂。

Neomycin has been used orally as an intestinal antiseptic to prepare the bowel for surgery.

口服新霉素作为肠道消毒剂,可用于肠道术前准备。

antiserum [ˌænti'siərəm] (*pl.* antisera [ˌænti'siərə]) *n.* 抗血清

Some specific immunizations appeared, such as diphtheria antitoxin and pneumococcic antisera.

出现了一些特别的免疫方法,如白喉抗毒素和肺炎球菌抗血清。

antisterility [ˌæntiste'riləti] *n.* 抗不育

The vitamin E substances have been shown to act as antisterility substances for white rats.

维生素 E 类物质作为抗不育类物质对大白鼠有效。

antistreptolysin [ˌæntiˌstreptə'laisin] *n.* 抗链球菌溶血素

Antistreptolysin O antibodies will be raised after infection with streptococci.

链球菌感染后抗链球菌溶血素 O 抗体将会升高。

Antistreptolysin O, commonly called ASO, is an antibody found in human blood produced upon an infection by Group A Streptococcus bacteria.

抗链球菌溶血素 O,俗称 ASO,是人血液中发现的一种抗体,系由 A 组链球菌感染引起。

antithrombin [ˌænti'θrɔmbin] *n.* 抗凝血酶

Another recent finding is that, unlike heparin, estrogen decreases the inhibition of Xa by antithrombin Ⅲ.

另一新发现是,同肝素不一样,雌激素减少凝血酶Ⅲ对Xa的抑制作用。

antithyroid [ˌænti'θairɔid] *a.* 抗甲状腺的 *n.* 抗甲状腺药剂

Although the use of antithyroid medications is a kind of standard therapy, it definitely has risk.

尽管应用抗甲状腺药物是一种标准治疗方法,但仍有一定的风险。

Some Chinese traditional herbs and compounds have shown their antithyroid functions including inhibition of the process of myocardial hypertrophy.

已发现有些中药和中药复方具有拮抗甲状腺素的作用,其中包括抑制心肌肥厚进程。

antitoxin [ˌænti'tɔksin] *n.* 抗毒素

Antitoxin is a substance in the blood that neutralizes the toxin or poison produced by bacteria.

血液里能中和细菌所产生的毒素的物质叫做抗毒素。

The prompt administration of diphtheria antitoxin in adequade amounts is the first and most important step.

及时地给予适量白喉抗毒素是首要的也是最重要的步骤。

antituberculous [ˌæntitju(:)'bə:kjuləs] *a.* 抗结核的,抗痨的

Response to standard antituberculous therapy is generally good.

常用的抗结核药物在治疗上一般均有良好效果。

If the clinical suspicion for tuberculosis is high, antituberculosis therapy should be initiated while awaiting cultural results.

如果临床上高度怀疑某病人患有结核病,便应在培养结果出来之前先给予抗结核药物治疗。

antitussive [ˌænti'tʌsiv] *a.* 镇咳的

Dextromethorphan is used as an antitussive preparation.

右甲吗喃被用作镇咳药。

n. 镇咳药

Nausea or vomiting may occur after taking a narcotic antitussive.

服用麻醉性镇咳药后可发生恶心呕吐。

antiulcer [ˌænti'ʌlsə] *a.* 治溃疡的，抗溃疡的

Bismuth potassium glycyrrhizate had antiulcer effect.

甘草酸铋钾有抗溃疡作用。

Synthesis methods, principle and technology of omeprazole (a new drug of peptic antiulcer) were reviewed. Their advantages and disadvantages were described in the paper.

该文综述了抗胃溃疡新药奥美拉唑的合成方法、原理及技术并评价了其优缺点。

antiviral [ˌænti'vaiərəl] *a.* 抗病毒的

There are no specific antiviral drugs available that are effective in treating viral upper respiratory disease.

尚无特效的抗病毒药物能有效地治疗病毒性上呼吸道疾病。

US researchers have shown for the first time that antiviral gene therapy can prolong the life of T cells in HIV infected individuals.

美国的研究者首次指出：抗病毒基因治疗可以延长受人类免疫缺陷病毒（HIV）感染者的T细胞寿命。

antral ['æntrəl] *a.* 窦的

Small antral follicle counts by ultrasound are one of the best ovarian reserve tests that we currently have available.

超声检测小窦卵泡数是目前可用的最好的卵巢储备检测方式之一。

Our study aims at exploring the value of predicting ovarian response using the antral follicle count in vitro fertilization (IVF) cycle.

我们的研究目的是探讨体外受精周期中窦卵泡数目对预测卵巢反应的价值。

antrectomy [æn'trektəmi] *n.* 窦切除术（如幽门窦切除术）

The most effective operation for treatment of gastric ulcers is simple antrectomy.

最能有效治疗胃溃疡的手术是单纯胃窦切除术。

antrophose ['æntrəfəus] *n.* 中枢性光幻觉

Antrophose is an optical illusion of motion produced by viewing a rapid succession of still pictures of a moving object.

中枢性光幻觉是一种由于看连续快速运动物体上的静止图片造成的运动性光幻觉。

Antrophose is a subjective sensation of light or color originating in the visual centers of the brain.

中枢性光幻觉是一种产生自大脑视觉中枢的对于光和颜色的主观感受。

antrum ['æntrəm] (*pl.* antrums or antra ['æntrə]) *n.* 窦，房

As the waves of contraction move toward the pylorus, they pinch off quantities of food and the wall of the antrum is stretched as this food is pressed onward.

收缩波在向幽门移动时推挤大量的食物，当食物被挤压向前时，胃窦壁就被牵张。

anucleate [ei'njuːkliːeit] *a.* 无核的

There has been a report about birth of infant after transfer of anucleate donor oocyte cytoplasm into recipient eggs.

已有一例无核供体卵细胞浆移植入受体卵细胞的胎儿出生的报道。

anuria [ə'njuəriə] *n.* 无尿（症）

Anuria is defined as less than 100ml urine daily.

当每日尿量少于100毫升时称为无尿症。

Renal failure with oliguria or anuria supervenes without the warning of persistent hypotension.

随着少尿或无尿的发生，肾功能衰竭可在无前兆的持续低血压情况下出现。

anus ['einəs] *n.* 肛门

The alimentary canal extends from mouth to anus.

消化道起始于口腔，延伸至肛门。

anxiety [æŋ'zaiəti] *n.* 焦虑，不安

Anxiety state is a condition in which anxiety dominates the patient's life; neuroses are now usually called anxiety disorders.

焦虑状态为患者生活处于焦虑为主导的状态；神经官能症现通常称作焦虑症。

The study will evaluate and compare the effectiveness of the therapy in reducing anxiety and depression.

此研究将评估和比较这种减轻焦虑和抑郁症的治疗方法的效果。

Anxiety disorders are currently divided into 12 separate categories.

焦虑症目前已被分为 12 种不同的类型。

The patient should strive to avoid anxiety and worry, never working to the point of fatigue.

病人应努力消除和避免焦躁与忧虑，决不要工作到已经疲劳的程度。

anxious [ˈæŋkʃəs] *a.* 担忧的，渴望的

The patient is anxious and perspires freely, and the sputum is frothy and blood-tinged.

病人显得焦虑，并有大量出汗，痰呈泡沫状，带有血。

The right suggestions may help the patient to stop being anxious.

正确的建议有助于患者解除忧虑。

aorta [eiˈɔːtə] (*pl.* aortae [eiˈɔːtiː]) *n.* 主动脉

Large arteries extend from the arc of the aorta and carry blood to the head and to the upper extremities.

大动脉从主动脉弓延伸，输送血液到头部和上肢。

The main artery carrying blood from the left ventricle of the heart to all parts of the body excepting the lungs is called aorta.

主动脉将左心室输出的血液输送至除了肺之外的身体的所有部位，故称作主动脉。

aortic [eiˈɔːtik] *a.* 主动脉的

Echocardiography will demonstrate dilatation of the aortic root and the separation of the cusps.

超声心动图检查可见主动脉根部扩张，瓣叶分开。

When any new heart murmur develops, it is usually due to aortic regurgitation.

如出现新的心脏杂音，通常是由于主动脉瓣关闭不全引起。

aortitis [ˌeiɔːˈtaitis] *n.* 主动脉炎

In the aorta, aortitis progesses to the point of producing an aneurysm.

在主动脉，主动脉炎已发展到了形成主动脉瘤的程度。

Aortitis principally affects the ascending thoracic aorta and may result in the formation of an aneurysm and obstruction to the coronary blood flow.

主动脉炎主要侵犯升主动脉，并可导致主动脉瘤形成使冠状动脉血流受阻。

aortoprosia [eiˌɔːtəuˈprəusiə] *n.* 主动脉下垂

Aortoprosia is defined as downward displacement of the aorta.

主动脉下垂是指主动脉的向下移位。

Patients with mitral valve regurgitation are subject to increase the risk for aortoprosia.

患二尖瓣逆流的病人患主动脉下垂的风险增加。

apathetic [ˌæpəˈθitik] *a.* 无情感的，情感淡漠的

I saw how electroshock therapy helped one apathetic and mute 76-year-old woman.

我见过电休克疗法是如何帮助一位情感淡漠、沉默不语的 76 岁妇女的。

apathy [ˈæpəθi] *n.* 无感情，感情淡漠

The patient has an apathy to food.

病人对于食物冷淡。

Later, there is central nervous depression with apathy, stupor and insensitivity to pain.

后来，中枢神经受抑制，伴有淡漠、迟钝及对疼痛反应麻木。

apelin [əˈpelin] *n.* 心血管活性多肽

A preliminary observation will be established for insulin up-regulates expression of apelin gene in 3T3-L1 cells.

将开展胰岛素上调 3T3-L1 细胞心血管活性肽基因表达的初步研究。

We want to know the progress of biological function of apelin.

我们想要了解心血管活性肽生物学功能的研究进展。

aperture [ˈæpətjuə] *n.* 口,孔

The spleen dominates muscles, and the mouth is the aperture of the spleen.

脾主肌肉,开窍于口。

The pulp cavity is continuous with a canal traversing the center of each root and opening by a small aperture at its extremity.

牙髓腔是一个连续不断的管道,经过每个牙根的中心,开口于其末端的一个小孔。

apex [ˈeipeks] (*pl.* apices [ˈeipisiːz]) *n.* 尖,尖端

The doctor found a shadow at the apex of the right lung.

医生在右肺肺尖上发现了一个阴影。

A loud friction rub was heard at the mid and lower left sternal border and the apex of the heart.

在胸骨左缘中部和偏下方以及心尖部可闻及响亮的摩擦音。

aphagia [əˈfeidʒiə] *n.* 吞咽不能

Aphagia signifies complete esophageal obstruction, which is usually due to bolus impaction and represents a medical emergency.

不能吞咽意味着食管完全阻塞,这通常是由于异物完全阻塞所致,属于急诊情况。

aphanizomenon [ˌəfæniˈzɔminɔn] *n.* 丝藻属

Aphanizomenon is a class of aquatic plants that may yield health benefits when used medicinally.

丝藻是一类水生植物,可制作药物用于保健。

aphasia [əˈfeizjə] *n.* 语言不能,失语症(=dysphasia)

Aphasia is the disorder of language with impairment of speaking and/or understanding speech.

失语症是语言能力性的疾患,伴有讲话和(或)理解能力的损伤。

If loss of speech is due to a defect in the cerebral hemispheres, the disorder is aphasia.

若为大脑半球缺陷所引起的语言能力的丧失,则称为失语症。

There are several different kinds of aphasia, depending on what part of the brain is affected.

由于脑受影响的部位不同,失语症也有多种不同的类型。

aphasic [əˈfeizik] *a.* 失语症的,患失语症的;*n.* 失语症患者

In the emergency room I found him aphasic, able to understand perfectly but unable to get a single word out.

在急诊室里我发现他患上了失语症,他的理解没有障碍,却完全无法通过言语来表达。

aphonia [əˈfəuniə] *n.* 失音症,失声症

Aphonia, absence or loss of the voice, is caused by disease of the larynx or mouth or by disease of the nerves and muscles involved in the generation and articulation of speech.

失音症是由喉或口腔疾病导致的发音能力的缺失或丧失,亦可因与语言生成或发音有关的神经或肌肉的病变所致。

Paralysis of both vocal cords causes complete aphonia, with no voice, and the patient only able to speak in whispers.

双侧声带麻痹导致完全失声,病人不能发音,只能用耳语声讲话。

apical [ˈæpikəl] *a.* 顶的,尖的

Abnormalities of the apical impulse and their indicated conditions are as follows.

心尖搏动的异常及其意义如下。

An acute apical abscess of a tooth is extremely painful, causing swelling of the jaw and sometimes also the face.

急性牙根尖脓肿非常疼痛,可引起颌部并有时包括面部的肿胀。

apicostomy [ˌæpiˈkɔstəmi] *n.* 牙根尖造口术

Apicostomy is a descriptive term applied to an operation in which a sterile channel is created to obtain cultures from the apical end of a tooth.

牙根尖造口术是一种形象的表达，指通过制造一条无菌引导在牙根尖提取培养物的手术。

Apicostomy has this limitation: one cannot always be sure of having reached the periapical tissue unless the operator feels the instrument drop into the rarefied area of destroyed bone.

牙根尖造口术有其局限性：操作者在感觉到器械触到受损骨质的稀疏区之前，无法确定是否已到达牙根尖组织。

aplasia [ə'pleisiə] *n.* 发育不全

Due to an organ total or partial failure of its development in the embryo, aplasia of total or partial failure of development of an organ may occur.

由于某器官有整个或部分器官在胚胎时期存在发育障碍，可出现某器官缺失或部分发育障碍等发育不全。

Erythroid aplasia may occur transiently during various infections and hemolitic disorders, and in association with tumors of the thymus.

红细胞系发育不良在各种感染和溶血性疾病时可暂时发生，也可能在有胸腺肿瘤时发生。

aplastic [ə'plæstik] *a.* 再生障碍的，发育不全的

Aplastic crises are the most serious complications which occur during childhood.

发育不全危象是发生在儿童时期的最严重的并发症。

Chloramphenicol is the drug most frequently associated with aplastic anemia.

氯霉素是产生再生障碍性贫血机会最多的一种药物。

apnea [æp'niːə] *n.* 呼吸暂停，窒息

Some insomnia sufferers have serious sleep disorders, such as sleep apnea.

有些失眠症患者常发生严重的睡眠紊乱，如睡眠窒息等。

The hallmark of medullary compression is respiratory failure: slow and irregular breathing followed by apnea.

延髓受压的标志是呼吸衰竭：呼吸缓慢而不规则，继而呼吸暂停。

apoenzyme [ˌæpəu'enzaim] *n.* 脱辅基酶蛋白

Apoenzyme enriching in mast cell can offer material basis for mast cell taking part in allergic reaction of I type.

肥大细胞中丰富的脱辅基酶蛋白可为肥大细胞参与 I 型变态反应提供物质基础。

Apoenzyme is an inactive enzyme that must associate with a specific cofactor molecule or ion.

脱辅基酶蛋白是一种无活性的酶，只有与特异辅助因子的分子或离子结合才能发挥作用。

apolipoprotein [ˌæpəˌlipə'prəutiːn] *n.* 载脂蛋白

The gene transcription of apolipoprotein is controlled by several factors.

载脂蛋白的基因转录受到多种因素的调控。

The apolipoprotein genes constitute a large family of genes encoding various binding proteins for plasma lipid transport.

载脂蛋白基因构成了一个复杂的多基因家族，为血浆脂质转运对不同绑定蛋白进行编码。

apomorphine [ˌæpəu'mɔːfiːn] *n.* 阿朴吗啡，脱水吗啡

Apomorphine, another dopamine 2-receptor agonist, is used to induce emesis.

阿朴吗啡，是另外一种多巴胺 2 受体激动剂，常用来催吐。

In nonemetic (lower) dosage, apomorphine has sedative, hypnotic, and expectorant action.

以不致呕吐（较低）的剂量使用时，阿朴吗啡具有镇静、催眠和祛痰作用。

aponecrosis [ˌæpəne'krəusis] *n.* 凋亡样坏死

Aponecrosis is a hybrid term derived from necrosis and apoptosis.

凋亡样坏死是由“坏死”和“凋亡”两个词组合而来的术语。

Aponecrosis has been described initially as the most common cell death in cultured rat fibroblasts.

凋亡样坏死起初被描述为培养的大鼠成纤维细胞最常见的细胞死亡。

aponeurosis [ˌæpənju'rəusis] *n.* 腱膜

Different in vitro mechanical tests were developed on eleven samples taken from the plantar aponeurosis of human cadaver by researchers.

研究者利用从人尸体获得的 11 个足底腱膜标本在体外做了不同的力学实验。

apophysis [ə'pɔfisis] (*pl.* apophyses[-siːz]) *n.* 骨突;骨棘

The endosternites are typically formed of a pair apophyses.

腹内骨是由一对骨突构成。

An experimental research is designed on the growth rate of acetabular ring apophysis.

设计一个实验来研究髋臼环状骨突的生长速度。

apoplexy ['æpəpleksi] *n.* 卒中,中风

The patient had an attack of apoplexy.

病人患了一次脑卒中。

Apoplexy is characterized by sudden loss of consciousness, followed by paralysis.

脑卒中的特征是突然失去知觉,随之全身麻痹。

apoprotein [ˌæpəu'prəutiːn] *n.* 脱辅基蛋白

A protein without its normal or characteristic prosthetic group is referred to as the apoprotein.

没有其正常或特征性辅基的蛋白质称为脱辅基蛋白。

apoptosis [ˌæpə'təusis] *n.* (细胞)凋亡

Programed cell death is often referred to as apoptosis.

程序性细胞死亡常称为凋亡。

Apoptosis represents physiological as opposed to pathological (necrotic) cell death.

和病理性的细胞死亡(坏死)相反,细胞凋亡代表了生理性的死亡。

The term apoptosis is used to define the type of individual cell death which is related to growth and morphogenesis.

凋亡一词用来解释与每个个别细胞的生长与形态形成有关的细胞死亡的形式。

Morphologically, apoptosis is recognised as death of scattered single cells which form rounded, membranebound bodies; these are eventually phagocytosed (ingested) and broken down by adjacent unaffected cells.

从形态上说,凋亡被认为是散在的单个细胞的死亡,它形成圆形的、有被膜包绕的小体,最终被毗邻未受影响的细胞吞噬(消化)和分解。

apoptotic [ˌæpə'təutik] *a.* 凋亡的

Apoptotic bodies are membrane-bound and composed of cytoplasm, organelles and nuclear fragments.

凋亡小体是有膜包裹的,由胞质、细胞器和核碎片组成。

The apoptotic bodies are rapidly ingested by macrophages.

凋亡小体很快被巨噬细胞吞噬。

apparatus [ˌæpə'reitəs] (*pl.* apparatus 或 apparatuses [ˌæpə'reitəsiːz]) *n.* 装置

Damage to the genetic apparatus more gross than that described above can sometimes be seen microscopically.

比上述更显著的遗传结构的损伤有时在显微镜下可见。

apparent [ə'pærənt] *a.* 明显的

One reason for the apparent increase in the number of red blood cells is that the capillaries are no longer normally intact.

红细胞数量明显增加的原因之一是毛细血管不再是正常完整的。

appeal [ə'piːl] *n.* 吸引力,感染力

Although appeals to logic and practicality have often appeared in the literature, a sound basis is

lacking.
虽然这些文献具有逻辑性和实践性的感染力，但缺乏充实的基础。

appealing [ə'piːliŋ] *a.* 有感染力的，吸引人的

The idea that a laboratory test could confirm a diagnosis is appealing.
实验室检验可证实一种诊断的想法是很吸引人的。

appear [ə'piə] *v.* 出现，显露

When the blood appears on the surface of any part of the body, the bleeding is called external.
当血液出现在身体某一部分的表面时，这种出血叫做外出血。

The authors of this study say the approach appeared to kill off tumors in mice infected with human ovarian cancer cells.
该项研究的作者们说，这种方法显示出能够杀灭感染人卵巢癌细胞的小鼠肿瘤。

appearance [ə'piərəns] *n.* 出现；外观，外貌；表象

The leukocytes are very different from the erythrocytes in appearance, quantity and function.
白细胞在外形、数量和功能上都和红细胞非常不同。

These three pairs of columns of gray matter give this cross section an H-shaped appearance.
这三对灰质脊髓柱使其横切面的外观呈现 H 型。

In the branched tubular glands the deep part of the tube becomes branched having a more complex appearance.
在分支管状腺内，管的深部变成分支状，外观较复杂。

The histopathology of the lesion can be studied in relation to the clinical appearance more directly in the skin than elsewhere.
研究损害的组织病理学与临床表现的关系，皮肤要比其他器官更为直接。

Good public relations are similar to good manners. They are developed from the appearance, behavior, and ability of the agency, collectively and individually.
好的公共关系类似好的举止。他们建立在仪表、行为及办事能力上，包括集体的和个人的。

appendage [ə'pendidʒ] *n.* 附件，附属物

We will approach the cell from the outside, starting with the external appendages.
我们将由外向内逐步对细胞进行剖析，先从外部附件开始。

Next, the surgeon will find out the condition of the uterine appendages.
下一步外科医生将要探查子宫附件的状况。

appendectomy [ˌæpən'dektəmi] *n.* 阑尾切除术

In this case appendectomy will be required later.
此病人以后还需做阑尾切除手术。

That is the way to do an appendectomy.
这就是做阑尾切除术的方法。

appendicitis [əˌpendi'saitis] *n.* 阑尾炎

Thus inflammation of the appendix is appendicitis, of the liver hepatitis and so on.
因此，阑尾的炎症称为阑尾炎，肝脏的炎症称为肝炎，以此类推。

If food gets into the appendix, a condition known as appendicitis will result.
如果食物进入阑尾，一种叫做阑尾炎的病就会发生。

appendix [ə'pendiks] *n.* 附录，附件；阑尾

Appendix 2 introduces abbreviations that are commonly used in medical literature.
附录二介绍医学文献中常用的缩略语。

Large thrombus masses may fill an auricular appendix in cases of cardiac disease with gross distention of the atria.
伴有心房显著扩张的心脏病病人可能有大血栓块充填心耳的现象。

The position of the appendix is variable.

阑尾位置变异颇多。

appetite ['æpitait] *n.* 欲望,强烈欲望,食欲

The patient's appetite has come back.

病人的食欲已经恢复。

He was a person of gross sexual appetites.

他是个性欲旺盛的人。

Case-control studies have demonstrated an association between long-term use of certain appetite suppressants and cardiac valve abnormalities.

病例对照研究证明,长期使用某些食欲抑制药和心脏瓣膜异常有关。

appetizer ['æpitaizə] *n.* 开胃剂

Small savoury biscuits provide a simple appetizer.

美味可口的小饼干可作简单的开胃品。

appetizing ['æpitaiziŋ] *a.* 开胃的

The list of ingredients sounds very appetizing.

这张配菜单听起来很能引起人的食欲。

appliance [ə'plaiəns] *n.* 器具,器械,设备

In Britain there is no need for registration because the product (skin tissue) is not classified as a drug or a medical appliance.

在英国不需要注册,因为这种产品(皮肤组织)没有归于药品或医疗器械之类。

applicability [ˌæplikə'biliti] *n.* 适用性

This section describes the specific applicability of the Common Rule to the creation and use of health information registries.

本节描述了卫生信息注册系统创建与使用通则的特殊适用性。

applicable (to) ['æplikəbl] *a.* 能应用的,适用于…的

This criterion is not applicable to children since personality disorders are not diagnosed before the age of 16.

这个标准不适用于儿童,因为在 16 岁之前不能做人格障碍的诊断。

The agent must document receipt and comply with regulatory requirements regarding adverse drug reaction reporting, to assure compliance with applicable drug and device regulations.

该代理人必须记录签收,并遵循药物不良反应报告的监管要求,以确保符合实用的药品和器械法规。

The term *human subject* is used throughout this chapter for consistency with applicable Federal law.

在本章节中使用的术语"人类受试者"可与适用的联邦法相一致。

applicant ['æplikənt] *n.* 申请者

Approximately half of all applicants are offered a position at one of the nation's accredited medical schools.

大约有一半的申请者可在国家认可的医学院谋得职位。

application [ˌæpli'keiʃən] *n.* 应用;敷用,敷剂;申请,申请表格

The mAbs have become standard research reagents and have extensive diagnostic and clinical application.

单克隆抗体已成为标准的研究试剂,并广泛应用于临床和诊断。(注:mAbs = monoclonal antibodies)

The potential long-term applications of this research are simply staggering.

这一研究成果潜在的长期用途将会是大得惊人的。

The topical application of Castellani paint is an effective but messy method of treatment.

局部敷用卡氏品红涂剂是一种有效但较脏的治疗方法。

This application will soothe the sore area.

这种敷料会减轻患部的疼痛。
The Sociaty of Microcirculation has approved his application for membership.
微循环学会已批准他入会的申请。
You must fill in an application for a passport within three days.
你必须在三天之内填写好护照申请表。

applicator ['æplikeitə] *n.* 敷贴器;涂药器
The effect of type of applicator is insignificant.
敷贴器的类型的影响不显著。
Remove applicator tip from the tube and wash with hot, soapy water.
取下与药管相连的涂药器头端,用肥皂热水冲洗。

applied [ə'plaid] *a.* 应用的,实用的
The Center for Food Safety and Applied Nutrition has a number of important reasons for interest in the area of dietary restriction as applied to toxicity and carcinogenicity testing.
食品安全与膳食营养中心有许多重要的理由来说明膳食限制(研究)领域的重要性,例如对于毒性和致癌性物质的检测等(就是最重要的理由)。

apply [ə'plai] *v.* 使用,应用于
When the suction is applied, the drainage is made to flow from the patient's respiratory tract into the bottle.
当进行抽吸时,抽取物从病人的呼吸道内被抽进瓶中。
When a stimulus is applied to a nerve cell, thus changing its environment, an electric impulse travels along its fibers.
如果刺激一个神经细胞,由此改变其环境,一个电冲动就会沿着其纤维前进。

appraisal [ə'preizəl] *n.* 估计,估价,评价
Evaluation of the status of the patient must include an appraisal of bowel function.
对病人状况的估计必须包括对肠功能的估计在内。

appraise [ə'preiz] *v.* 评价
The centenary of Koch's discovery should be dedicated to appraising our TB control strategies.
作为对柯霍的发现 1 百年的纪念,我们应该着眼于对结核防治战略的评价上。

appreciate [ə'priːʃieit] *v.* 赞赏;感激;理解;鉴别
His great achievement in cancer therapy was universally appreciated.
他在癌症治疗方面的重大成就获得普遍赞赏。
Any constructive criticism and suggestion will be greatly appreciated by the author.
任何积极的批评和建议都会受到作者衷心的感谢。
I fully appreciate her anxiety about her husband's illness.
我充分理解她对丈夫病情的忧虑。
The primary focus in the lung parenchyma and the involvement of the regional lymph glands are too small to be appreciated on the chest roentgenogram.
在肺实质的原发灶及局部受累淋巴结因太小而在胸片上无法识别。
Fetal heart tones were appreciated with the fetoscope at 19 weeks.
在 19 孕周用胎心听筒听到了胎心音。

appreciation [əpriːʃi'eiʃən] *n.* 感谢;正确评价;赏识
My colleagues join me in expressing deep appreciation to each of our guests.
我和我的同事们对各位客人表示由衷的感谢。
Proper appreciation of the nature of surgical shock is essential to proper treatment.
正确了解外科休克的性质对恰当的治疗是非常重要的。

apprehension [ˌæpri'henʃən] *n.* 了解,理解;恐惧,忧虑
Most of the students are quick of apprehension.
大多数学生头脑敏捷。

If each patient is told in simple language what to expect in each stage much of the apprehension can be removed before labour begins.

以简明的语言告诉每位患者各产程的正常状况，就可在分娩前消除许多顾虑。

apprehensive [ˌæpriˈhensiv] *a.* 忧虑的，担心的

The child appeared alert，shy，and apprehensive.

患儿呈现警惕、胆怯和忧虑不安的状态。

approach [əˈprəutʃ] *n.* 方法；探讨；接近

This approach overcomes the problem of disease complications which might occur with modified live vaccines.

该方法可克服由于改良的活疫苗所导致的疾病并发症的问题。

The diagnostic approach to epigastric pain should commence by first determining the character of the symptom.

对上腹部疼痛的诊断方法首先是要判定疼痛的性质。

Radiotherapy may form a combined approach together with surgery and chemotherapy.

放疗与手术和化疗一起组成联合治疗方法。

With the approach of the 21st century，various long-range plans of scientific research have been made.

随着 21 世纪的来临，科学研究的各种远景规划被制订出来。

appropriate [əˈprəupriit] *a.* 适当的，恰如其分的

Human milk is the most appropriate of all available milks for the human infant.

人乳对婴儿来说是所有可用的乳中最适当的一种。

Recently it has been appropriate to talk of molecular disease.

近来谈论分子疾病是很合时宜的。

The primary aim in treatment of all patients with diarrhea is to provide appropriate fluid and electrolyte replacement until the acute illness has spontaneously subsided.

治疗所有腹泻病人的首要目标是补充适宜的液体和电解质，直到急性病症自发地减退。

appropriateness [əˈprəuprieitnis] *n.* 合适程度

To assess the appropriateness of the target population in a medical study，one must ask the question：is this really the population that we need to know about?

要评价一项医学研究目标人群的合适程度，人们必须询问：这真是我们想了解的人群吗？

approval [əˈpruːvəl] *n.* 批准，认可

In 1992，they reviewed pharmaceutical products that received Food and Drug Administration approval between 1988 and 1991.

1992 年，他们回顾了 1988 ~ 1991 年间获得食品药品管理局批准的药品。

approve [əˈpruːv] *v.* 同意，赞成，认可

Dr. Zhang does not approve the therapeutic scheme afforded by Dr. Li.

张医生不同意李医生提供的治疗方案。

The Dean's Office approved the teaching programme of pathology.

教务处批准了病理学教学大纲。

approximate [əˈprɔksimit] *a.* 大概的

The physician made an approximate analysis of the case.

医生对病例做了大概的分析。

v. 近似，使接近

The average weight of the new born brain approximates 350gm.

新生儿脑的平均重量约 350 克。

Release of adrenaline produces bodily effects approximating generalized sympathetic nervous system activity.

肾上腺素对身体的作用如同交感神经系统活动一样。

approximately [ə'prɔksimitli] *ad.* 近似,大约

Every human cell contains approximately 30 000 genes.

人体每个细胞含有约 3 万个基因。

Expected time to clinical recovery of Chlamydia pneumonia is approximately 4 days.

衣原体肺炎临床恢复预期的时间约为 4 天。

Approximately 30% of patients undergoing laparoscopy for infertility have endometriosis.

因不孕症做腹腔镜检查的病例中,约 30% 为子宫内膜异位症。

apraxia [ə'præksiə] *n.* 失用症;失用

Apraxia, one of the most important and least understood major neurology syndromes, robs patients of the ability to use tools.

失用症是最重要并且了解得最少的神经病学综合征之一,它让病人丧失了使用工具的能力。

The dysfunction in the left inferior parietal lobule, the frontal lobes, or the corpus callosum is responsible for apraxia, a neurologic disorder.

左侧顶叶下部、额叶或胼胝体的功能失调是失用症这一神经障碍的主要原因。

aprotinin [ə'prəutinin] *n.* 抑肽酶

In patients undergoing CABG procedure, low dose aprotinin is effective in attenuating post bypass coagulopathy and decreasing blood product use.

在患者进行冠状动脉搭桥术中,低剂量的抑肽酶可以有效降低旁路后凝血障碍,减少血液制品的使用。

Recent studies suggest adverse events associated with aprotinin in adults may not occur in children.

近期研究表明成人中与抑肽酶有关的不良事件并不发生在儿童。

apt [æpt] *a.* 易于…的,有…倾向的

These side effects are most apt to occur and to be serious in the elderly.

在老年人身上这些副作用最容易出现并很严重。

aptitude ['æptitju:d] *n.* 智能

Moreover, practically all schools require a standard aptitude test and some type of personal interview.

而且所有学校都要求进行一次标准智能测验和某种类型的个别谈话。

aquacoat ['ækwəˌkəut] *n.* 乙基纤维素水分散体

Aquacoat ECD has been widely used in pharmaceutical coating applications.

乙基纤维素水分散体 ECD 已经广泛应用于药物包衣涂层。

The major advantage using Aquacoat ECD over polymer solvent solution is its low viscosity and non-tacky features.

相对聚合物溶剂溶液而言,乙基纤维素水分散体 ECD 的主要优点在于低黏度和无黏性。

aquatic [ə'kwætik] *a.* 水生的

The two main types of aquatic ecosystems are marine ecosystems and freshwater ecosystems.

水生生态系统的两个主要类型是海洋生态系统和淡水生态系统。

Aquatic Toxicology is an international journal on mechanisms of and responses to toxic agents in the aquatic environment.

《水生毒物学》是国际性期刊,主要刊登关于毒物在水生环境中的作用及机制的文章。

aqueous ['eikwiəs] *a.* 水的,水性的

The high acidity limits the aqueous solubility of the aspirin.

高酸性限制了阿司匹林的水溶性。

arachidonate [ə'rækiˌdɔneit] *n.* 花生四烯酸

Arachidonic acid (arachidonate) occurs in animal fats and is also formed by biosynthesis from dietary linoleic acid.

动物脂肪中有花生四烯酸存在，它也可由饮食中的亚油酸生物合成。

arachnoidcyst [ə'ræknɔidsist] *n.* 蛛网膜囊肿

Arachnoidcyst is a congenital intracranial lesion, which usually does not cause symptoms.

蛛网膜囊肿是一种先天性的颅内病变，通常不引起症状。

Arachnoidcysts occur in the temporal or occipital part, their CT appears as a circular low density lesion.

蛛网膜囊肿发生在颞部或枕部，CT 上表现为圆形低密度灶。

arachnoiditis [əˌræknɔi'daitis] *n.* 蛛网膜炎

We were originally not aware of the possible association between disc lesion and arachnoiditis.

我们原先未曾察觉到椎间盘的损伤与蛛网膜炎之间可能的联系。

arbitrarily ['ɑːbitrərili] *ad.* 任意，独断地

Arbitrarily, penicillin reactions are designated as acute, accelerated, and delayed.

青霉素反应被人为地划分为急性反应、加速反应和延迟反应。

arbitrary ['ɑːbitrəri] *a.* 任意的，简要的

Arbitrary etiologic divisions are employed for purposes of clarity.

为了明了起见，采用人为的病因学分类。

This section presents a somewhat arbitrary listing of the major groups of bacteria of medical importance.

本节简略地列出了医学上重要的主要细菌类别。

arbitrator ['ɑːbitreitə] *n.* 仲裁人

The institutional review board is the final arbitrator of the activities that constitute human subjects research.

伦理委员会是各种人体试验研究的最终裁决者。

arborization [ˌɑːbərai'zeiʃən] *n.* 树枝状；分支

Most of the external carotid artery branches were shown to be of arborization.

颈外动脉分支的形状大多为树枝状。

Postsynaptic currents and dendritic arborization in the rat hippocampal CA1 pyramidal neurons were postnatally developed.

大鼠海马 CA1 区椎体神经元的突触后电流和树突分支是产后才发育的。

arbovirus [ˌɑːbə'vaiərəs] *n.* 虫媒病毒

Sera of 402 healthy persons from Guizhou Province were tested for antibodies against arbovirus by the method of hemagglutination inhibition test.

用血凝抑制试验检测了贵州省 402 份健康人血清抗虫媒病毒抗体。

Group A arbovirus antibody positive rate was 31.68%, which included antibodies against MAY or related virus.

A 组虫媒病毒抗体阳性率为 31.68%，包括 MAY 或相关病毒抗体。

arbutin ['ɑːbjutin] *n.* 熊果苷；熊果酚苷

Determining the concentration of arbutin in cosmetics by RP-HPLC is a new program.

反相 HPLC 法测定化妆品中熊果苷的含量是一个新项目。

Natural herbage whiten essence contains arbutin, pearl powder and collagen protein.

天然本草美白精华含有熊果苷、珍珠粉和胶原蛋白。

arc [ɑːk] *n.* 弧，弓

Branchings issuing from the aorta below the arc, pass to the muscles of the trunk of the body and to the abdominal viscera.

从主动脉弓以下伸出的(血管)分支通向身体躯干(部分)的肌肉和腹腔的脏器。

arch [ɑːtʃ] *n.* 弓，弓形

The foot forms an arch which the leg bones rest on.

脚形成足弓，腿骨位于足弓上。

The vertebral arch protects the spinal cord and nerves from injury.
椎弓可保护脊髓和神经不受损伤。
After crossing the aortic arch the trachea divides into the right and left main bronchi.
越过主动脉弓以后，气管分成右和左主支气管。

archaea [ɑːˈkiːə] *n.* 古生菌，古细菌
Among 75 clones of archaea, 95% of which is MB, including 53% methanobacterium.
古细菌 75 个克隆中 95% 属于产甲烷菌群，包括 53% 甲烷细菌属。
Scientists believe that all three groups of living things, bacteria, archaea and eukaryota arose separately from some unknown ancestor.
科学家们相信细菌、古细菌和真核生物这三种生物都是分别来自不同的某未知祖先。

architecture [ˈɑːkitektʃə] *n.* 结构
The lobular architecture is preserved and there is little or no necrosis or fibrosis.
小叶结构仍保持完整，没有坏死和纤维化。

archive [ˈɑːkaiv] *n.* 档案馆；档案文件
The archive lets the public upload or download digital material for free.
这个档案馆允许公众免费上传和下载数字材料。
The archive showed that the product had high viscosity, constant viscosity, water-absorption capacity and good anti-synaeresis.
这些档案显示了这个产品的高黏度、常黏性、吸水性以及很好抗脱水收缩性能。
v. 把…存档
Archive or save everything important because you will have to get something from your archives at some point.
将重要的东西存档或保存下来，因为有时候你需要从你的档案里获取某些东西。

arctiin [ˈɑːktiin] *n.* 牛蒡子苷
HPLC method for determination of the content of arctiin in Yinqiao Jiedu tablets was established.
已建立 HPLC 法测定银翘解毒片中牛蒡子苷的含量。
We will study about pharmacokinetics and distribution of arctiin in rats.
我们将研究大鼠的牛蒡子苷的药物代谢动力学与分布情况。

arctinal [ˈɑːktinəl] *n.* 牛蒡子醛
Arctinal is a new anti-oxidation active compound.
牛蒡子醛是一种新型的活性抗氧化剂。
19 compounds were identified from roots of Rhapouticum uniflorum, and one of them was arctinal.
漏芦根中分离出了 19 种化合物，其中之一是牛蒡子醛

areca [əˈriːkə] *n.* 槟榔；槟榔树
The areca nuts were soaked in a solution with some flavors, and then dried.
用香料配制一种浸液，将槟榔浸泡其中，入味后，烘干就成为成品。
The formula of the functional beverage of Areca Catechu was studied through orthogonal design in this paper.
本文通过正交试验，对槟榔保健饮料的配方进行了研究。

areflexia [ˌeiriˈfleksiə] *n.* 反射消失
Patients with vestibular areflexia (VA) can be diagnosed by evaluating optokinetic nystagmus (OKN) responses.
前庭反射消失的病人可以通过评估视动性震颤反应进行诊断。

arenavirus [əˌrinəˈvaiərəs] *n.* 沙粒病毒属；沙粒病毒
Arenavirus infections are relatively common in humans in some areas of the world and can cause severe illnesses.
世界上某些地区沙粒病毒对人类的感染相对常见，并可引起严重疾病。

Arenavirus particles are roughly spherical and have an average diameter of 90-140nm.
沙粒病毒基本呈球形，直径平均为 90 ~ 140 纳米。

areola [əˈriːələ] *n.* 乳晕

Areola is most commonly used to describe the pigmented area around the human nipple.
通常情况下乳晕是指围绕在人体乳头周围的色素沉着区域。
Why is the areola darker than the rest of your breast tissue?
为什么乳晕区的颜色要比乳房其他区域颜色深？

arginine [ˈɑːdʒini(ː)n] *n.* 精氨酸

Following oral zinc therapy, their growth rate and their growth hormone response to arginine infusion improved.
经口服锌治疗后，他们的生长速率和生长激素对精氨酸输注的反应得到改善。
The diagnosis is determined by assessing the response to exogenous arginine vasopressin.
在给予外源性精氨酸加压素后再观察机体的反应可以帮助诊断。

argininemia [ˌɑːdʒiniˈniːmiə] *n.* 精氨酸血症

Arginase Ⅰ deficiency who exhibit argininemia is a rare autosomal recessive disorder.
精氨酸酶 I 缺乏症表现为精氨酸血症，是一种少见的常染色体隐性遗传病。
Argininemia is caused by a deficiency of arginase 1.
精氨酸血症是由于精氨酸酶 1 缺乏所导致的。

argininosuccinic acid [ˌɑːdʒiˌninəusʌkˈsinikˈæsid] *n.* 精氨(基)琥珀酸

Deficiency of argininosuccinate lyase results in an accumulation of argininosuccinic acid in tissues.
精氨基琥珀酸裂解酶缺乏症导致精氨(基)琥珀酸在组织中堆积。
Excretion of argininosuccinic acid in the urine leads to the condition of argininosuccinic aciduria.
精氨基琥珀酸在尿中排泄导致精氨基琥珀酸尿症。

argon [ˈɑːgɔn] *n.* 氩

The researchers used a special form of argon gas to eat away at the virus's outer shell.
研究工作者用一种特殊形式的氩气侵蚀病毒的外壳。

aristogenesis [əˌristəˈdʒenisis] *n.* 优生，适应突变

Aristogenesis and environment are closely related.
优生和环境是紧密联系的。
A new, rapid and clinically practical molecular cytogenetic method has been established for diagnosing the chromosomal subtelomeric deletion as well as for guiding aristogenesis and prenatal diagnosis.
建立了一个新的，快速的和临床实用的分子细胞遗传学方法诊断染色体亚端粒缺失以及指导优生与产前诊断。

aristogenics [əˌristəˈdʒeniks] *n.* 优生学

Aristogenics was practiced around the world and was promoted by governments, and influential individuals and institutions.
优生学在世界各地实行，各国政府和有影响力的个人和机构促进了它的发展。
Research on consanguineous mating and its genetic effects on generation is one of the research contents of human genetics and aristogenics.
对近亲婚配及其后代遗传效应的研究是人类遗传学和优生学的研究内容之一。

armamentarium [ˌɑːməmenˈtɛəriəm] *n.* 医疗设备

Definition of armamentarium is the equipment, pharmaceuticals, and methods used in medicine.
医疗设备的定义是医学所用的器材、药品和方法。

armpit [ˈɑːmpit] *n.* 腋窝

Skin temperature as obtained in the armpit is lower than mouth temperature.
自腋窝测得的皮肤温度较口腔温度低。

The usual places to take the temperature are the mouth, the armpit or the rectum.
测体温的部位通常是口腔、腋窝或直肠(等部位)。

aromatherapy [əˌrəumə'θerəpi] *n.* 芳香疗法

Aromatherapy, which uses herbal oils either massaged into the skin or inhaled, is the fastest-growing complementary therapy.
芳香疗法使用草药油剂无论通过按摩使之浸入皮肤或者采取吸入方式,这是发展最快的补充疗法。

aromatic [ˌærəu'mætik] *n.* 芳香的,有香味的

Normal urine has a characteristic faintly aromatic ordor.
正常尿液有一种特征性的轻微的香味。
Phenylbutazone undergoes aromatic hydroxylation to produce a metabolite.
保泰松是经芳香羟化后产生的一种代谢产物。

aromatization [əˌrəumətai'zeiʃən] *n.* 芳香化

Estrogen can derived by peripheral aromatization of androgen.
雄激素在外周经芳香化后能衍生出雌激素。

arousal [ə'rauzəl] *n.* 唤醒,激起

Catecholamines and adrenal corticosteroids are released during emotional arousal.
儿茶酚胺和肾上腺皮质类固醇在情绪激动状态下被释放出来。

arouse [ə'rauz] *v.* 唤醒,激起,引起

Patient should be aroused, if possible, and questioned regarding use of insulin, narcotics, recent trauma and headache.
如果病人可被叫醒的话,应仔细询问是否使用过胰岛素、麻醉药、近期有无外伤和头痛等情况。
Memory incorporation is inhibited at the onset of this stage, and subjects aroused from that stage frequently deny having been asleep.
处在这个阶段,记忆的融合受到抑制,在这个阶段被唤醒的研究对象通常否认曾经睡觉。

arrangement [ə'reindʒmənt] *n.* 安排,布置,排列

The arrangement quite fit in with our requirements of treatment.
这种安排与我们的治疗要求相符。
The heart changes its shape and size during each beat and friction damage is prevented by the arrangement of pericardium and its serous fluid.
每次心跳时心脏都改变其形状及大小,而心包膜及其中的浆液则防止了摩擦损伤。
Hair "form", or cross-sectional shape of the hair, depends upon the arrangement of cells in the bulb.
毛发的形态(即毛发横切面的形状)取决于毛球内细胞的排列。

arrest [ə'rest] *v.* 阻止,抑制

A Large thrombus may cause almost instantaneous death by arresting the circulation.
大血栓如阻断血循环,几乎可使患者立即死亡。
Some cancers can be arrested for long periods of time, others not.
有的癌症可以长期被抑制住,而另一些却不能。
n. 阻止,抑制
The patient developed bradycardia and then had cardiorespiratory arrest and could not be resuscitated.
患者出现心动过缓,接着呼吸心跳停止,复苏无效。
For a patient with severe burns, respiration and heart arrest might occur at any moment.
对于严重烧伤的病人来说,呼吸和心搏骤停随时都可能发生。

arrhythmia [ə'riθmiə] *n.* 心律不齐

Arrhythmias occur most commonly soon after symptoms are present.

心律不齐大多出现在症状出现时。

Atrial distension may provoke a variety of supraventricular arrhythmias.

心房的扩张可能引起各种室上性心律不齐。

arrhythmogenic [əˌriðmə'dʒenik] *a.* 致心律不齐的

The patient was suffering from a condition known as arrhythmogenic right ventricular dysplasia.

这病人患有一种称为致心律不齐的右心室发育异常的病。

arseniasis [ɑːsi'naiəsis] *n.* 砷中毒

It is demonstrated that arseniasis is an environmental phenomenon, which is affected by human activity.

已证实砷中毒是一种受人为活动影响的环境现象。

Characteristic features of arseniasis include skin manifestations, such as hyperpigmentation, hypopigmentation, and hyperkeratosis on the palms and soles, and skin cancer at later stages.

砷中毒的特征包括皮肤变化，如手掌和脚掌皮肤色素沉着、脱色素和过度角化，晚期还表现为皮肤癌。

arsenic [ɑː'senik] *n.* 砷

Arsenic is a chemical element whose compounds are extremely poisonous.

砷是一种化学元素，其化合物的毒性极强。

The cause of aplastic anemia can be a chemical agent (eg, benzene, inorganic arsenic), radiation, or drug (eg, antineoplastics).

再生障碍性贫血的病因可能是化学因子（如苯、无机砷）、辐射或药物（如抗肿瘤药）。

a. 砷的，含砷的

Bronze hyperpigmentation is seen in hemochromatosis and arsenic intoxication.

青铜色的过度色素沉着见于血色素沉着症和砷剂中毒者。

arsenism ['ɑːsinizəm] *n.* 砷中毒，慢性砷中毒

Skin changes of arsenism begin from hyperkeratosis, next affected by depigmentation and hyperpigmentation.

砷中毒的皮肤改变开始是过度角化，随后出现脱色和色素过度沉着。

Endemic arsenism caused by ingestion of arsenic-bearing drinking water has been an important public health problem in China.

由于摄入含砷的饮水而引起的地方性砷中毒已成为中国重要的公共卫生问题。

arterial [ɑː'tiəriəl] *a.* 动脉的

Arterial disease is clinically silent until far advanced.

动脉疾病不到晚期，临床上不显症状。

arteriography [ˌɑːtiəri'ɔgrəfi] *n.* 动脉造影术

After all other investigations, arteriography may be necessary.

如果用所有其他检查不能确诊，有时需要动脉造影检查。

arteriolar [ɑːtiəri'əulə] *a.* 小动脉的

BP may at first rise slightly because of reflex arteriolar constraction.

血压开始由于小动脉的反射性收缩而略有升高。

The information allows the brain to adjust heart rate and arteriolar tone so as to maintain an appropriate blood pressure.

此信息可使脑调节心率和小动脉的紧张度，以便维持适度的血压。

arteriole [ɑː'tiəriəul] *n.* 小动脉

The arterioles are extremely narrow tubes.

小动脉是极端窄小的管道。

Hypertrophy of arteriole is a well documented feature of prolonged hypertension.

小动脉肥厚是具有可靠记载的长期高血压的特征。

arteriolosclerosis [ɑːˌtiəriəuˌləuskliə'rəusis] *n.* 小动脉硬化，细动脉硬化

Hyaline arteriolosclerosis usually occurs in benign hypertension affected arterioles.
玻璃样细动脉硬化常发生于良性高血压，累及细动脉。
Hyperplastic arteriolosclerosis usually occurs in malignant hypertension, characterized by onion-skin lesions.
增生性细动脉硬化常发生于恶性高血压，以葱皮样病变为特征。

arteriosclerosis [ɑːˌtiəriəuˌskliəˈrəusis] *n.* 动脉硬化
Arteriosclerosis is usually the end result of atherosclerosis.
动脉硬化通常是由动脉粥样硬化造成。
In proper amounts, cholesterol is essential to health, but too much may cause arteriosclerosis.
适量的胆固醇为健康所必需，但过量的胆固醇会造成动脉硬化。

arteriosclerotic [ɑːˌtiəriəuskliəˈrɔtik] *a.* 动脉硬化的
This person has died suddenly of arteriosclerotic heart disease.
这个人突然死于动脉硬化性心脏病。

arteriovenous [ɑːˌtiəriəuˈviːnəs] *a.* 动静脉的
In addition, arteriovenous or arterial fistulas also predispose to endocarditis.
此外，动静脉瘘或动脉瘘也易发生心内膜炎。

arteritis [ˌɑːtəˈraitis] (*pl.* arteritides [ˌɑːtəˈritidiːz]) *n.* 动脉炎
Necrotizing arteritis may affect large vessels and give rise to digital gangrene, infarcted bowel or stroke.
坏死性动脉炎可发生在大动脉血管，引起手指坏疽、肠梗死或卒中。
Takayasu's arteritis affects primarily the aorta and its major branches, particularly those of the aortic arch.
Takayasu 动脉炎主要侵犯主动脉及其主要分支，尤其是主动脉弓处的分支。

artery [ˈɑːtəri] *n.* 动脉
Rapid sequence films may demonstrate unilateral renal artery stenosis.
快速顺序摄片可证实单侧肾动脉狭窄。
The arteries carry blood away from and the veins carry blood back to the heart.
动脉把血运出心脏，静脉把血运回心脏。

arthralgia [ɑːˈθrældʒiə] *n.* 关节痛
Arthralgia is also frequent in leukemia and can be migratory in nature.
关节痛也常见于白血病，可呈游走性。
Fewer patients complain of arthralgias, cough, testicular pain, dysuria, ocular pain, or visual blurring.
少数病人主诉患有关节痛、咳嗽、睾丸痛、排尿困难、眼痛或视力模糊(等症状)。

arthritic [ɑːˈθritik] *n.* 关节炎患者
It causes minimal stress across the joint, and hence it is often used for arthritics.
这种方法对关节压力很小，因此常用于关节炎患者。

arthritis [ɑːˈθraitis] *n.* 关节炎
Almost 49 percent of adults 65 and older suffered from arthritis.
大约有 49% 的年龄在 65 岁或 65 岁以上的老人患关节炎。
The next patient remembers grandpa grumbling about the damned arthritis as he got up from his chair.
第二位病人记起当祖父从椅子上起身时总是抱怨那该死的关节炎的情形。

arthrodesis [ˌɑːθrəuˈdiːsis] (*pl.* arthrodeses [ˌɑːθrəuˈdiːsiz]) *n.* 关节固定术，关节融合术
Arthrodesis is still used in cases in which total joint replacement is contraindicated or has failed.
如果采用全关节置换术属于禁忌证或者全关节置换术失败，仍然可以采用关节固定术。
Arthroscopic ankle arthrodesis is gaining in popularity.
关节镜下踝关节融合术正在逐步普及。

arthrogram [ˈɑːθrəɡræm] *n.* 关节造影片

We declared the importance of hip arthrogram in the diagnosis of Legg-Calvé-Perthes disease.

我们声明了髋关节 X 线片在 Perthes 病诊断中的重要性。

arthrography [ɑːˈθrɔɡrəfi] *n.* 关节照相术

An arthrography is an X-ray technique for examining joints. A contrast medium (either air or a liquid opaque to X-ray) is injected into the joint space, allowing its outline and contents to be traced accurately.

关节照相术是一种检查关节的 X 线照相术。将造影剂(采用空气或不透 X 线的液体)注入关节间隙,以准确显示其轮廓与内容物。

arthrogryposis [ˌɑːθrəuɡriˈpəusis] *n.* 关节挛缩

Arthrogryposis multiplex congenita is a rare disease, characterized by non-progressive, multiple joint contractures since birth.

先天性多关节挛缩是一种以先天性非进行性多关节挛缩为特点的罕见疾病。

These results show that the Pediatric Outcomes Data Collection Instrument is useful in evaluating functional outcomes of children with arthrogryposis.

这些结果提示 PODCI 系统对评估关节挛缩患儿的功能结局有用。

arthropathy [ɑːˈθrɔpəθi] *n.* 关节病

Neuropathic arthropathy, also known as Charcot's joint, represents the mechanical failure of a joint in a patient whose sensory input is impaired.

神经病理性关节病,也称 Charcot 关节,是由于病人感觉受损引起的关节运动障碍。

arthroplasty [ˈɑːθrəuˌplæsti] *n.* 关节成形术

The physician calls surgical repair of a joint an arthroplasty.

医生把"关节的外科修复"称为关节成形术。

Joint arthroplasty has revolutionized the management of severe and disabling osteoarthritis.

关节成形术使严重和可致残的骨关节炎的处理明显改善。

Our research tries to evaluate cardiac and thromboembolic complications and mortality in patients undergoing total hip and total knee arthroplasty.

我们的研究试图评估全髋和全膝关节成形术后患者的心脏和血栓栓塞并发症和死亡率。

arthropod [ˈɑːθrəpɔd] *n.* 节肢动物;*a.* 节肢动物的

Arthropods are animals with segmented bodies and six or more jointed legs.

节肢动物是身体分成节段并有 6 个或 6 个以上节足的动物。

The arthropods constitute over 90% of the animal kingdom and are classified in the phylum arthropoda.

节肢动物在动物界占 90% 以上,归属为节肢动物门。

The Japanese spider crab is the world's largest crustacean and arthropod.

日本蜘蛛蟹是世界上最大的甲壳动物和节肢动物。

This method is not only suitable to the arachnids, but also has certain model function to other arthropod genome DNA extraction.

盐析法不仅适用于蜘蛛类,对其他节肢动物基因组 DNA 提取也有一定的借鉴作用。

arthroscope [ˈɑːθrəskəup] *n.* 关节(内窥)镜

With the arthroscope, surgeon can look directly into your knee to diagnose your injury and decide on the best treatment for you.

外科医生用关节镜直接窥视你的膝关节,来诊断你的损伤,并为你设计最好的治疗方案。

Surgery for such injuries has become much simpler with the invention of the arthroscope.

对这类受伤的手术因为发明了关节内镜而变得简单多了。

arthrospore [ˈɑːθrəuspɔː] *n.* 节孢子

The arthrospore formed before conidium.

节孢子形成先于分生孢子。

Plant oil added to the culture medium highly stimulated swollen hyphal fragments into arthrospore.

植物油加入到培养基后，促进了高度膨胀的菌丝体断片形成节孢子。

article [ˈɑːtikl] *n.* 论文，文章

This medical article is out of date and not valuable.

这篇医学论文已经过时，无甚价值。

articular [ɑːˈtikjulə] *a.* 关节的

Each vertebra has seven processes: four articular, two to connect with the bone above, two to connect with the bone below; two transverse; and one spinous process.

每个脊椎骨都有七个突：四个关节突（两个与上脊椎骨连接，两个与下脊椎骨连接）、两个横突、一个棘突。

articulate [ɑːˈtikjulit] *v.* 连接，接合

The injured bone did not articulate well.

受伤的骨骼没有连接好。

articulation [ɑːˌtikjuˈleiʃən] *n.* 分节发音，发音清晰度；连接；关节

Articulation consists of contractions of the tongue, lips, pharynx and palate.

分节发音是由于舌、唇、咽和腭的收缩而产生的。

In addition, the articulation and resonance of speech are influenced by the structure of the nasopharynx.

此外，说话时发音的清晰度和共鸣也受鼻咽结构的影响。

The three main classes of articulation are diarthrosis (freely movable), amphiarthrosis (slightly movable), and synarthrosis (unmovable).

关节的三种主要类型为动关节（可自由活动的）、微动关节（可轻微活动的）及不动关节（不能活动的）。

artifact [ˈɑːtifækt] *n.* 人工制品；手工艺品；伪影

Many reasons can cause image imperfections or artifacts observed in CT systems.

很多因素可以导致 CT 系统中观察到的图像伪影。

The new technique can reduce significantly artifacts in images.

这项新技术能明显减少显像中伪影的产生。

The polychromatic spectrum leads to cup or streak beam hardening artifacts and reduces the image quality in X-CT.

在 X 射线断层成像技术中，X 射线束能谱的多色性将导致重建图像出现杯状或条状等射束硬化伪迹，降低成像质量。

Artificeial [ˌɑːtiˈfiʃəl] *a.* 人工的

After about ten minutes of artificial respiration, the patient came back to life.

在进行十分钟人工呼吸以后，病人复苏。

The distinction between synthetic compounds and those derived from living organisms is somewhat artificial.

合成化合物与生物衍生化合物，其区别有些是人为划分的。

artificially [ˌɑːtiˈfiʃəli] *ad.* 人工地，人造地

The membranes may be ruptured artificially to initiate labor or accelerate it.

可行人工破膜发动分娩或加速产程。

arundina [əˈrʌndinə] *n.* 竹叶兰属

Studies on chemical constituents of arundina graminifolia of Dai Medicine were established.

我们确立了傣药竹叶兰化学成分的研究课题。

All compounds were isolated from the genus of arundina for the first time.

首次从竹叶兰属植物中分离得到所有化合物。

arylhydrocarbon [æriləhaidrəu'kɑːbən] *n.* 芳香烃

The arylhydrocarbon receptor (AhR) is a member of the family of basic helix-loop-helix transcription factors.

芳香烃受体是碱性螺旋-环-螺旋转录因子家族中的一员。

Copper and zinc ions possess significant inhibiting effect on microsomal arylhydrocarbon hydroxylase.

铜和锌离子对微粒体芳烃羟化酶具有显著地抑制效应。

asbestos [æz'bestɔs] *n.* 石棉

Higher rates for gastrointestinal cancer are observed in asbestos workers.

已观察到在石棉工人中胃肠道癌肿的发病率较高。

asbestosis [ˌæsbes'təusis] *n.* 石棉肺,石棉沉着病

Asbestosis leaves the victim short of breath,often gasping for air.

石棉肺导致患者呼吸困难,经常喘息不已。

Asbestosis is caused by fibres of asbestos inhaled by those who are exposed to the mineral.

石棉沉着病是因接触矿物吸入石棉纤维所致。

ascariasis [ˌæskə'raiəsis] *n.* 蛔虫病

Discovery of ascariasis may be made by a routine stool examination.

蛔虫病可通过大便常规检查而发现。

The diagnosis of ascariasis is made by finding adult worms,larvae,or eggs.

发现成虫、幼虫或卵才可诊断蛔虫病。

ascaris ['æskəris] *a.* 蛔虫的

Ascaris eggs develop into the infective stage outside the human body and transmit disease when they are swallowed.

当人们吞入了已在人体外发育到有传染性阶段的蛔虫卵时便被传染了疾病。

The ascaris adults may perforate a suture line or cause a bile or pancreatic duct obstruction.

蛔虫的成虫可穿破缝线或引起胆管或胰腺管阻塞。

ascend [ə'send] *v.* 上升

In young children the eustachian tube is relatively short and straight and hence easily allows infection to ascend from the nose and throat into the middle ear.

幼儿咽鼓管相对地短且直,故容易使感染由鼻咽部上行至中耳。

ascendancy [ə'sendənsi] *n.* 优势,支配地位

Man's ascendancy over his environment and other species is related to the size of his cerebrum.

人支配其周围环境和其他种属的能力与人的大脑的大小有关。

The growth of world population and the ascendancy of multinational corporations have increased the necessity for concern for protecting nature resources and the environment.

世界人口的增长和多个国家的合作已经增加了关怀和保护自然资源和环境的迫切需要。

ascending [ə'sendiŋ] *a.* 上行的;向上的;上升的

The ascending colon is located on the right side of the body and is the first part of the large intestine.

升结肠位于人体右(下)侧,是大肠的起始部分。

The ascending aorta is near the heart and inside the pericardial sac.

升主动脉紧靠心脏,处于心包之内。

Transitory endometritis is consequently the precondition for ascending gonorrhea.

因此短暂的子宫内膜炎是逆行性淋病的必要前提。

Hyperkalemia may also cause an ascending muscle weakness.

高钾血症引起自下而上的肌无力。

ascertain [ˌæsə'tein] *v.* 查明,确定

An X-ray film of the abdomen should be taken to ascertain kidney size.

确定肾脏的大小,应当拍摄腹部 X 线片。

The kidneys are visible in the roentgenogram, and their size and position can be ascertained.

X 线片上可以看到肾脏,从而可以确定其位置和大小。

ascites [ə'saitiːz] *n.* 腹水

Ascites may be due to congestive heart failure, cirrhosis of liver and tuberculous peritonitis, etc.

腹水可以由充血性心力衰竭、肝硬化、结核性腹膜炎等病引起。

Patients with ascites are at risk of leaking ascites through the wound.

伴有腹水的患者,有经伤口溢漏腹水的危险。

ascitic [ə'sitik] *a.* 腹水的

Left untreated, ascitic leaks increase the incidence of wound infection.

如不予处理,腹水漏可增加伤口的感染率。

When ascitic fluid shows a lymphocytosis and a protein is excess of 3gm/100ml, tuberculous peritonitis should be considered.

当腹水液显示有很多淋巴细胞和蛋白质超过 3 克/100 毫升时,应当考虑是结核性腹膜炎。

ascorbic [əs'kɔːbik] *a.* 抗坏血的

Ascorbic acid is a moderately strong reducing agent.

抗坏血酸是一种中等强度的还原剂。

Ascorbic acid, or vitamin C, prevents the development of scurvy.

抗坏血酸,或称维生素 C,可以预防坏血病的发展。

ascospore ['æskəspɔː] *n.* 子囊孢子

The optimum temperatures for ascospore germination are 25℃ to 30℃ and for mycelium growth are 15℃ to 25℃.

子囊孢子发芽最适温度为 25 ~30℃,而菌丝体生长最适温度是 15 ~25℃。

At sexual stage, physalospora persicae produces the ascus and ascospore, with the size of 14. 5-23. 2×10. 1-14. 5μm.

桃疣皮病菌有性阶段产生子囊壳及子囊孢子,子囊孢子大小为 14. 5-23. 2×10. 1-14. 5 微米。

ascribe (to) [əs'kraib] *v.* 把…归于

The patient's death was ascribed to internal bleeding.

病人因内出血死亡。

Many of the deaths ascribed to infantile diarrhea are, in reality, caused by dysentery.

许多被认为由婴儿腹泻引起的死亡,其实是由于痢疾所致。

ascus ['æskəs] *n.* 子囊

An ascus is the sexual spore-bearing cell produced in ascomycete fungi.

子囊是产于子囊真菌含有孢子有性的细胞。

The surface of pink colony was smooth, without hypha, no ascus and ascospore produced on the colony.

粉红色菌落表面光滑无菌丝,不形成子囊和子囊孢子。

asepsis [æ'sepsis] *n.* 无菌

Basic principle of asepsis, antisepsis, and surgical technique should be implemented.

应当实施无菌术、抗菌术和手术操作技术的基本原则。

Medical asepsis involves the use of various methods of disinfection.

医学无菌包括使用各种不同的消毒方法。

aseptic [æi'septik] *a.* 无菌的

Meningitis with a clear fluid is likely to be either tuberculous or acute aseptic.

脑脊液清澈的脑膜炎既可为结核性的,也可为急性无菌的。

The nurse will encounter many situations on the clinical unit that require aseptic technique such

as catheterization or changing surgical dressings.
护士在病区遇到许多情况都需要无菌操作,如插入导管或更换外科敷料。

asexual [ei'seksjuəl] *a.* 无性(别)的

Cloning is also called asexual reproduction.
克隆也被称为无性生殖。

Asexual reproduction is often more rapid than sexual reproduction.
无性生殖通常比有性生殖更迅速。

aspartame [ə'spɑːteim] *n.* 甜味素,天冬甜素

Aspartame is an artificial, non-saccharide sweetener used as a sugar substitute in some foods and beverages.
甜味素是一种用在食品和饮料中替代糖的人造非糖甜味剂。

Aspartame is a methyl ester of the dipeptide of the natural amino acids L-aspartic acid and L-phenylalanine.
甜味素是由天然氨基酸 L-天冬氨酸和 L-苯丙氨酸形成二肽的甲酯。

aspartate [æs'pɑːteit] *n.* 天冬氨酸

The enzyme aspartate transcarbamylase has a quaternary structure comprised of 12 polypeptide subunits.
天冬氨酸转氨甲酰酶有由 12 个多肽亚基组成的四级结构。

aspect ['æspekt] *n.* 方面,外表,方位

Most physicians are now cognizant of the frequency and importance of psychologic aspects of disease.
许多医生现在都认识到了疾病心理方面的重要性和作用的经常性。

General aspects of hemolitic anemias will be discussed below, followed by a description of specific disorders.
下面讨论溶血性贫血的一般情况,接着讨论特殊的疾病。

The inner aspects of the thighs may also be irritated by inflammatory discharge.
股内侧也可由于炎症性排脓引起不适。

aspergillosis [ˌæspədʒi'ləusis] (=aspergillomycosis [ˌæspəˌdʒiləumai'kəusis]) *n.* 曲霉病

When there is asthma, allergic bronchopulmonary aspergillosis is the commonest cause.
如果有哮喘,最常见的原因是过敏性支气管肺曲霉病。

aspergillus [ˌæspə'dʒiləs] *n.* 曲霉菌属

Aspergillus is a genus of fungi (molds), several species of which are parasitic and opportunistic pathogens.
曲霉菌属是真菌的一个属,其中某些种属为寄生病菌或机会致病菌。

As a mold aspergillus can be found within indoor environments.
作为一种霉菌,曲霉菌可存在于户内环境中。

asphalt/bitumen ['æsˌfɔːlt] *n.* 沥青,柏油

Asphalt is a thick brown or black byproduct of crude oil.
沥青为黑褐色黏稠物,是一种原油副产物。

Asphalt is a sticky, black and highly viscous liquid or semi-solid that is present in most crude petroleums and in some natural deposits.
沥青是一种黑色的高黏性液体或半固体,存在于大多数原油和某些自然沉淀物中。

In asphalt workers there is an increased risk of respiratory symptoms, lung function decline, and COPD compared to other construction workers.
沥青作业工人出现呼吸系统症状、肺功能下降和慢性阻塞性肺疾病的危险较其他建筑工人高。

asphyxia [æs'fiksiə] *n.* 窒息

Accidental drowning is the most common form of fatal mechanical asphyxia.

意外性溺水是致命的机械性窒息的最常见形式。

The baby was believed to have experienced fetal and neonatal asphyxia.

这个婴儿被认为曾发生过胎儿和新生儿窒息。

aspirate [ˈæspərit] *v.* 抽吸

In addition the aspirated fluid should be examined for malignant cells.

此外,应检查吸出的液体有无恶性细胞。

n. 吸出物

In this case the aspirate will contain an unusually high bacterial content.

在这种情况下,吸出物通常含细菌量极高。

Aspirate from peritoneal cavity may be useful in confirming the clinical diagnosis of peritonitis.

腹膜腔的吸出物在证实腹膜炎的临床诊断中很有用。

aspiration [ˌæspəˈreiʃən] *n.* 吸入,抽吸(术)

Aspiration of bacteria from the oropharynx may follow dental anaesthesia.

自口咽中吸入细菌可在牙科麻醉时发生。

Aspiration of infectious material into the lung is the most common cause of lung abscess.

感染物吸入肺是肺脓肿的最常见病因。

In conclusion, we have found testicular fine needle aspiration (TEFNA) to be efficient, easy to learn, safe and well tolerated by all patients.

总之,我们发现睾丸精子细针抽吸术高效,简单易学,安全且患者耐受性较好。

aspirin [ˈæspərin] *n.* 阿司匹林,乙酰水杨酸

Aspirin is a weak or mild analgesic.

阿司匹林是一种弱的或中等程度的镇痛药。

Aspirin can increase the temporary hearing loss or damage from loud noise.

阿司匹林可以加剧巨大噪声造成的听觉暂时丧失或损伤。

assay [əˈsei] *n.* 测定(法),鉴定

Peripheral renin assays were done but were all within normal limits.

做过周围血肾素测定,但全在正常范围内。

Assays that could accurately measure the plasma levels of tricyclic antidepressants were introduced.

采用了能够准确测量血浆中三环类抗抑郁剂水平的测定法。

v. 测定,鉴定

Fetal hemoglobin was assayed by counter immunoelectrophoresis.

胎儿血红蛋白是通过对流免疫电泳测定的。

assemble [əˈsembl] *v.* 汇集

It is only after all the data have been assembled that the medical detective is in a position to begin his analysis.

只有在全部资料集中以后医学侦探才能开始他的分析。

Proteins fold and assemble in the endoplasmic reticulum.

蛋白质在内质网中进行折叠和组装。

assembly [əˈsembli] *n.* 组装体,装配

Membranes are lipid-protein assemblies.

膜是脂类蛋白质的组装体。

assess [əˈses] *v.* 评价,估计

As mentioned earlier, the patient should be assessed for side effects.

正如前面所述,应检查病人是否发生副作用。

The clinician must first assess the severity of the disorder.

临床医师必须首先评估病情严重程度。

The frequency of chromosomal breakage has been used to assess exposure to radiation.

染色体破损率已用于评估接触放射线情况。

assessment [ə'sesmənt] *n.* 检查,评定,估计

In the initial patient assessment arterial blood gases are crucial.

在对病人的最初检查中,动脉血气情况至关重要。

Clinical assessment of well being of mother and baby must never be omitted or disregarded.

对母婴健康情况的临床评估也不能忽视。

assign [ə'sain] *v.* 分派

Nurses assigned to each unit will be highly trained as clinical specialists in their particular area.

指派到各专科监护室工作的护士要接受高级培训,以便成为各自领域的临床专家。

Twenty students were randomly assigned to the experimental group and the control group.

二十名学生被随机分配到实验组和对照组。

assimilate [ə'simileit] *v.* 吸收

Vitamin is not digested but is assimilated into the tissues of the body in the form in which it is taken in.

维生素不是被消化,而是以其被摄取时的形式为人体所吸收。

Animal proteins can be assimilated up to 98 or 99 percent.

动物蛋白质的吸收率可达98%或99%。

assist [ə'sist] *v.* 援助,帮助

The function and fate of lymphocytes are unknown, perhaps they assist in the formation of antitoxins.

淋巴细胞的功能和存活期尚未弄清楚,也许它们有助于抗毒素的形成。

assistance [ə'sistəns] *n.* 帮助

The nurse may also set up and record an electrocardiogram, carry out closed chest massage, and use a respirator when respiratory assistance is needed.

护士还要操作心电图机,记录心电图,进行胸外按摩,在需要协助病人呼吸时使用呼吸器。

assistant [ə'sistənt] *a.* 助理的,辅助的

Dr. Li is an assistant research fellow in this organ transplantation center.

李医生是这个器官移植中心的助理研究员。

I would like to see the assistant manager of this medical and pharmaceutical company.

我想见见这家医药公司的副经理。

The assistant nurses have carried out a part of the service work for the patients.

卫生员承担了为病人服务的部分工作。

n. 助理,助教

He is an assistant to the general manager of this company.

他是这家公司的总经理助理。

His elder brother is a teaching assistant in this medical college.

他哥哥是这所医学院的一名助教。

associate [ə'səuʃieit] *v.* 使发生联系,使联合,关联

Sebaceous glands are normally associated with hair follicles.

皮脂腺通常与毛囊相关。

The presence of an associated skin rash supports the likelihood of RSV infection.

如同时出现皮疹,则支持呼吸道合胞病毒感染。

Bacterial endocarditis is the most common associated infection.

细菌性心内膜炎是最常见的并发感染。

Acute effects have been associated with impairments in attention, concentration, and reaction time.

急性效应涉及注意力、思想集中和反应时间的下降。

n. [ə'səuʃiət] 伙伴,同事;相关的事物

The physician found valuable most of the information he received from patients and their associates.

这位内科医生发觉他从病人及其陪伴人那里获得的信息大多数都是有价值的。

According to the interrelation between two associates different forms of symbiosis may be distinguished.

根据两个相关动物之间的相互关系，可以区分出不同的共生形式。

association [əˌsəusiˈeiʃən] *n.* 联合，联系，协会

Dr. John Smith is a member of the American Geriatrics Association.

约翰·史密斯博士是美国老年病学协会会员。

But there was significant association between dry eye syndrome and duration of diabetes (P = 0.01).

但是干眼症和糖尿病的病程有显著关联(P=0.01)。

No association was observed between age and alcohol consumption.

没有观察到年龄和酒精摄入之间的关联性。

assortative [əˈsɔːtətiv] *a.* 相称的；相配的

Assortative mating is the choice of a mate who possesses some particular traits.

选型婚配是指选择具有一些特定特质的配偶。

A clinically important aspect of assortative mating is the tendency to choose partners with similar medical problems, such as congenital deafness or blindness.

选型婚配的一个重要的临床问题是一些人往往选择具有相似医学问题如先天性耳聋或失明的人作为对象。

assortment [əˈsɔːtmənt] *n.* 分类；基因分配

The phenomenon of independent assortment has the consequence of increased variation among the gametes formed.

独立分配现象增加了配子形成过程中发生变异的机会。

assume [əˈsjuːm] *v.* 假定，设想；承担；采取；呈(某种形式、面貌)

The amoeba assumes various shapes.

阿米巴呈现各种形态。

These contiguous, undifferentiated cells subsequently assume the characteristics of keratinocytes.

这些毗邻的未分化的细胞随后显示出角质形成细胞的特征。

For all women, cancer is the second leading cause of death, although in certain population AIDS has assumed first place.

对女性而言，癌症居死因第二位，而在某些人群中，艾滋病已被认为居死因首位。

It is assumed that high levels of glucose are responsible and good diabetic control is therefore important before pregnancy.

有人认为高血糖是病因而且在妊娠前控制好糖尿病是很重要的。

She will assume the new duties of a head nurse tomorrow.

明天她就要开始执行护士长的新任务了。

Assuming the patient goes into shock, what shall we do?

假定病人休克了，我们怎么办?

assumption [əˈsʌmpʃən] *n.* 假定，设想

This assumption has never been subjected to a properly controlled clinical trial.

这一假定从未经过具有适当对照的临床试验。

The assumption was borne out by the course of the disease.

这一设想为病程所证实。

assurance [əˈʃuərəns] *n.* 保证；把握；信念

I have full assurance of the effect of this drug.

我充分相信这药的效力。

There is no assurance that the candidate who has fulfilled all the requirements for admission will be accepted.
符合一切入学条件者也不能保证一定被接受入学。

astereognosis [əˌsteriəugˈnəusis] *n.* 实体觉缺失

In a simple test for astereognosis, the doctor has her patient close his eyes, places a key in his hand, and asks him to identify the object.
在实体觉缺失的一个简单测试中，医生让患者闭眼，把一个钥匙放在他的手里，然后让他辨认手中的物品。

It is likely that a lesion of the nucleus itself or its related sensory tracts may cause astereognosis.
很可能是核团本身或其相关传导通路的损伤引起实体觉缺失。

asterixis [ˌæstəˈriksis] *n.* 扑翼样震颤

Asterixis occurs when a group of contracted muscles suddenly and temporarily go limp.
当一组收缩肌肉突发短暂的无力时出现扑翼样震颤。

Asterixis commonly results from liver failure and so has been called liver flap.
扑翼样震颤通常由于肝功能衰竭所致，所以又称作肝病性扑动。

asthenic [æsˈθenik] *a.* 虚弱的，衰弱的

The body build is asthenic with evidence of weight loss.
体型无力并伴有体重减轻。

Asthenic personality disorder is characterized by passivity and a weak or inadequate response to the demands of daily life.
衰弱性人格障碍是以具有对日常生活需求呈消极状态和冷漠反应为特征的人格障碍。

asthenopia [ˌæsθiˈnəupiə] *n.* 眼疲劳

Asthenopia is a sense of fatigue brought on by use of the eyes for prolonged close work.
眼疲劳是长时间用眼进行精细工作引起的视力疲劳感觉。

asthenozoospermia [əsˈθenəˌzəuəˈspəːmiə] *n.* 弱精症

Asthenozoospermia is the medical term for poor sperm movement, or poor sperm motility。
弱精症这一医学术语是指精子活力或运动能力很差。

Some men are infertile because of asthenozoospermia, i. e. , the poor sperm motility.
有些男士不育是因为弱精症，即：精子活力低下。

asthma [ˈæsmə, ˈæzmə] *n.* 气喘，哮喘

Bronchial asthma, especially in adult life, is often associated with chronic bronchitis.
支气管哮喘，特别在成年人中常与慢性支气管炎有关。

Many conditions, such as asthma and hay fever, are now being treated successfully.
像哮喘和枯草热等许多疾病现在都能有效地治疗了。

asthmatic [æsˈmætik] *a.* 哮喘性的

The patient with chronic asthmatic bronchitis has a long history of cough and sputum production with a later onset of wheezing.
此慢性哮喘性支气管炎患者有长期咳嗽及咯痰史，后来肺部出现哮鸣音。

Many who were asthmatic as children have turned out to be outstanding athletes.
许多儿童时期患过哮喘的人，后来成了优秀的运动员。

astigmatism [æsˈtigmətizm] *n.* 散光

Astigmatism occurs when the lens system becomes ovoid (egg-shaped) rather than spherical.
散光发生于透镜系统变成卵圆形（蛋形）而不是球形时。

An intrastromal corneal ring can correct long-sightedness, short-sightedness and astigmatism.
一种基质内角膜环可用来校正远视、近视和散光。

astringent [əˈstrindʒənt] *a.* 收敛的 *n.* 收敛药

Alcohol is an astringent.
酒精是一种收敛剂。

As an astringent, tea can cause temporary contraction of the blood vessels.
作为收敛剂,茶叶能引起血管暂时性收缩。

astrocyte [ˈæstrəsait] *n.* 星形(胶质)细胞

Astrocyte foot processes are closely associated with the blood vessels to form the blood-brain barrier.
星形胶质细胞的足突与其周围的血管紧密结合在一起形成血脑屏障。

The astrocytes have been ascribed the function of providing nutrients for neurones and possibly of taking part in information storage processes.
据认为星形细胞具有营养神经元的功能,并可能参与信息的存贮处理。

astrocytoma [ˌæstrəsaiˈtəumə] *n.* 星形细胞瘤

In glioma, astrocytoma is the most common, followed by glioblastoma.
在胶质瘤中,星型细胞瘤最多见,其次为胶质母细胞瘤。

Study of astrocytoma CT enhancement scanning characteristics and its relationship to the malignant degree, has high value for diagnosis and differential diagnosis.
研究脑星形细胞瘤 CT 增强扫描特征及其与恶性程度的关系,对诊断和鉴别诊断有很高的价值。

asymmetrical [ˌæsiˈmetrikəl] *a.* 不对称的,偏位的

More often the enlargement of the uterus is asymmetrical; the tumour does not occupy a median position.
不对称子宫增大更为常见,肿瘤并不在正中位置。

asymmetry [əˈsimitri] *n.* 不对称

Asymmetry is induced in the substrate by the asymmetric binding surface of the enzyme.
酶的不对称结合表面诱发底物分子的不对称性。

asymptomatic [əˌsimptəˈmætik] *a.* 无症状的

He remained asymptomatic after his initial infection.
他在初次感染后一直无症状。

Over one-third of postoperative myocardial infarctions are asymptomatic.
术后心肌梗死无症状者超过三分之一。

asynchronous [əˈsiŋkrənəs] *a.* 非同步的

With asynchronous respiration expiratory abdominal expansion can exceed inspiratory abdominal expansion.
由于呼吸不同步,呼气时腹部扩张可能超过吸气时的腹部扩张。

asystole [əˈsistəli] *n.* 心脏停止

Our study shows that the third-degree-burn to one side of the neck can induce bradycardia and asystole.
我们的研究显示半边颈部三度烧伤能诱发心动过缓和心搏停止。

ataxia [əˈtæksiə] *n.* 运动失调,共济失调,协调不能

He began to feel the symptoms of a nerve disease called ataxia which interfered with his movements.
他开始感到具有干扰活动称作运动性共济失调的神经性疾病症状。

Numerous drugs in toxic doses produce ataxia and slurred speech.
许多药物在中毒量时产生共济失调和吐词不清。

atelectasis [ˌætiˈlektəsis] *n.* 肺不张,肺萎陷

Atelectasis is more common in patients who are elderly or overweight and in those who smoke.
肺不张较常见于老年、超重或抽烟的病人。

The tube then blocks ventilation of the other main bronchus, and atelectasis may ensue.
此时管道阻塞了另一侧主支气管的通气而产生肺不张。

atelectatic [ˌætilekˈtætik] *a.* 肺不张的,(肺)膨胀不全的

The perfused but atelectatic left lung was acting as afunctional shunt.
灌注后仍膨胀不全的左肺在功能上只起短路的作用。

atherogenic [ˌæθərəuˈdʒenik] *a.* 致动脉粥样硬化的

Decreased adiponectin levels in familial hyperlipidemia patients promote the formation of the atherogenic lipid profile.
家族性高脂血症患者脂联素水平下降促进了致动脉粥样硬化脂质谱形成。

The diagnostic criteria for metabolic syndrome definition are abdominal obesity, atherogenic dyslipidemia, elevated blood pressure and elevated blood glucose.
代谢综合征定义的诊断标准为腹部肥胖、致动脉粥样硬化性血脂异常、血压升高和血糖升高。

atherogenicity [ˌæθərəudʒeˈnisiti] *n.* 致动脉粥样硬化

Low-dose testosterone is a safe therapy for atherogenicity.
低剂量睾丸酮对预防动脉粥样硬化是安全的。

atheroma [ˌæθiˈrəumə] *n.* 动脉粥样化

Atheroma tends to be particularly severe in individuals with chronic hypertension.
动脉粥样化在慢性高血压患者身上往往特别严重。

atheromatous [ˌæθiˈrəumətəs] *a.* 动脉粥样化的

The arterial walls were moderately dilated and showed scattered atheromatous plaques.
动脉壁中度扩张，并有散在的粥样斑块。

atheroprotective [ˌæθərəuprəˈtektiv] *a.* 抗动脉粥样硬化的

High-density lipoproteins possess many atheroprotective functions, including reverse cholesterol transport, antioxidant, anti-inflammatory, and antithrombotic effects.
高密度脂蛋白具有多种抗动脉粥样硬化功能，其中包括胆固醇逆转运、抗氧化、抗炎和抗血栓形成。

atherosclerosis [ˌæθərəuskliəˈrəusis] *n.* 动脉粥样硬化

This paper discusses mainly the pathogenesis of atherosclerosis.
本文主要讨论动脉粥样硬化的发病机制。

Coronary atherosclerosis is the most common cause of sudden death of adults.
冠状动脉粥样硬化是成人突然死亡最常见的原因。

atherosclerotic [ˌæθərəuskliəˈrɔtik] *a.* 动脉粥样硬化的

An infarct may occur without thrombosis and the lumen of the coronary artery is greatly narrowed by atherosclerotic thickening of the inner coat.
梗塞可能不带血栓，冠状动脉腔由于内层的动脉粥样硬化增厚而显著变窄。

The doctor successfully dilated an atherosclerotic obstruction in a peripheral artery by means of an intraluminal catheter.
这位医生用腔内插管的方法成功地扩张了周围动脉粥样硬化梗阻。

athetosis [ˌæθəˈtəusis] *n.* 手足徐动症

Athetosis is a movement disorder that afflicts numerous persons with cerebral palsy.
手足徐动症是一种困扰大量脑瘫病人的运动障碍。

athlete [ˈæθliːt] *n.* 运动员

Sinus bradycardia is often found in healthy individuals, especially athletes.
窦性心动过缓在健康人尤其是运动员中较为常见。

atlas [ˈætləs] *n.* 图谱，图表集；寰椎(第一颈椎)

The National Library of Medicine has published the first electronic atlas of the entire human body.
国家医学图书馆最近出版了第一本人的整体电子图谱。

It is especially important to consider atlas fractures in any patient with a severe closed head injury.

对于任何有严重头部闭合性损伤的患者，都应考虑到是否有寰椎的骨折，这一点尤其重要。

atmosphere [ˈætməsfiə] *n.* 大气；空气

The atmosphere causes rain.

Watery vapour in the atmosphere causes rain.

大气中的水蒸气导致下雨。

The atmosphere is a carrier of microorganisms.

空气是微生物的携带者。

Nitrogen and oxygen are the gases present in the atmosphere.

氮气和氧气是大气中的气体。

Respiratory paralysis may be caused in any confined space where the atmosphere has been stagnant for long periods of time.

在任何长时间空气不流通的空间都可能引起呼吸麻痹。

atom [ˈætəm] *n.* 原子

The particles in an atom are infinitely small.

原子里的粒子极小。

The atom is a basic unit of matter.

原子是物质的基本单位。

atomic [əˈtɔmik] *a.* 原子的，原子能的；微粒子的

The atomic reactor generates enormous amounts of thermal energy.

原子反应堆能产生巨量的热能。

The atomic particles resist being accelerated past the velocity of light.

这些原子粒子无法被加快到超过光速。

Atomic force microscopy can be used to reveal the chemical identity of individual atoms on a surface.

原子力显微镜能够用于显示表面单个原子的化学特性。

atomize [ˈætəmaiz] *v.* 使雾化，喷雾

The solution of a drug can be atomized into an aerosol for inhalation therapy.

一种药物的溶液可以雾化成气雾剂用于吸入疗法。

atonic [æˈtɔnik] *a.* 张力缺乏的，弛缓的

The spastic type of constipation is probably much more common than the atonic lazy kind.

痉挛型便秘可能比弛缓性无张力型的便秘更常见。

atopic [əˈtɔpik] *a.* 特(异反)应性的

A response to sodium cromoglycate occurs in about 40% of all atopic asthmatics.

色甘酸钠对40%的特异反应性哮喘患者有效。

atopy [ˈætəpi] *n.* 特(异反)应性，特异性变态反应

Atopy is a term used to describe IgE-mediated anaphylactic responses in humans.

特应性是用来描述人的免疫球蛋白 E 介导的过敏反应。

Reaction to this may be mild(as in urticaria or atopy) or life-threatening(as in anaphylaxis).

此反应可能较轻微(如荨麻疹或特异性反应)或者严重到危及生命(如过敏症)。

atoxic [əˈtɔksik] *a.* 无毒的

Curcumin is an atoxic antioxidant.

姜黄是一种无毒的抗氧化剂。

An atoxic immunogenic product, adaptable to injection, was prepared by the method of Claim 1.

根据要求 1 的方法制备了一种可用于注射的无毒免疫药品。

Curcumin is a natural and atoxic antioxidant.

姜黄素是一种天然的、没有毒性的抗氧化剂。

atractylodes [ətrækˈtailədis] *n.* 苍术属，苍术

An analysis of nuclear types in chromosome of atractylodes was made.
对苍术的染色体核型进行了分析。
Doctors of traditional Chinese medicine usually use atractylodes in the treatment of gastroptosis.
中医经常运用苍术治疗胃下垂。

atractylone [ə'træktailəun] *n.* 苍术酮
Methodological studies were set up on quantitative determination of atractylone in atractylodes by HPLC.
我们启动了用高效液相色谱法(HPLC)测定苍术中苍术酮含量的方法学研究。
A method to keep atractylone stable was established.
确立了一种能使苍术酮保持稳定的方法。

atractyloside [ətræk'tailəsaid] *n.* 苍术苷
Atractyloside can inhibit mitochondrial energy transduction.
苍术苷能够抑制线粒体的能量转换。
The sensitive heat production of atractyloside was abolished in anoxic solution.
苍术苷的敏感的产热效果在缺氧的溶液中被消除了。

atransferrinemia [eiˌtrænsfəri'niːmiə] *n.* 缺转铁蛋白血症,缺载铁蛋白性贫血
Atransferrinemia appears when Fe cannot move from storage sites to the erythron.
缺转铁蛋白血症发生在铁不能从贮存部位运往红细胞系时。

atraumatic [ətrɔː'mætik] *a.* 无外伤的
A steady but remarkable increase has occurred in the availability and usefulness of atraumatic noninvasive methods in diagnosing diseases.
在疾病诊断上的无创伤非侵害性方法的有效性和可用性,已出现稳定而显著的进展。

atresia [ə'triziə] *n.* 闭锁(畸形),不通
Extrahepatic biliary atresia continues to account for 30%-60% of all cases of prolonged "obstructive" jaundice in neonates.
肝外胆道闭锁仍占全部新生儿持续性“阻塞性”黄疸病例的30% ~60%。
Sometimes menstruation is concealed because the vagina is occluded by a congenital septum or atresia.
有时月经是隐蔽的,这是因为阴道被先天性隔膜所闭塞或阴道闭锁所致。

atretic [ə'tretik] *n.* 闭锁;萎缩
Atretic follicles was gone in the periodic process in which immature ovarian follicles degenerate and are subsequently re-absorbed during the follicular phase of the menstrual cycle.
闭锁卵泡是在不成熟的卵泡退化和随后在月经周期卵泡期重新吸收的周期过程中消失。
The formation of atretic follicle is a hormonally controlled apoptotic process.
闭锁卵泡形成是一个受到激素控制的凋亡过程。

atrial ['ɑːtriəl] *a.* 心房的
Ventricular rate in atrial fibrillation is controlled by digitalisation.
房颤时的心室率可用洋地黄化控制。

atrioventricular ['ɑːtriəven'trikjulə] *a.* 房室的
The primary indication of permanent artificial pacing has been for the treatment of complete atrioventricular (AV) block.
长期性人工起搏的首要适应证是治疗完全的房室传导阻滞。

atrium ['ɑːtriəm] (*pl.* atria ['ɑːtriə]) *n.* 心房
The systemic circulation begins at the aorta and ends in the right atrium.
体循环始于主动脉,止于右心房。

atrophic [æ'trɔfik] *a.* 萎缩的,衰退的
The muscles are weak, thin, and atrophic, but there may be an excess of subcutaneous fat.
肌肉瘦弱和萎缩,但皮下脂肪可能过多。

atrophy [ˈætrəfi] *n.* 萎缩

Cell numbers are reduced in various forms of pathological atrophy.

在发生各种类型的病理性萎缩时细胞数目减少。

Addison' s disease results primarily from atrophy of cortices and tuberculosis of adrenal gland.

艾迪生病主要是由于皮质萎缩和肾上腺结核所致。

v. 萎缩

After the menopause the tumour ceases to grow, and may atrophy, sometimes becoming calcified.

绝经后肿瘤停止生长，可发生萎缩，有时形成钙化。

atropine [ˈætrəpin] *n.* 阿托品，颠茄碱

Atropine is able to oppose these muscarinic effects.

阿托品可对抗这些毒蕈碱样作用。

atropinization [æˌtrəupinaiˈzeiʃən] *n.* 阿托品化，阿托品处理(法)

Atropine 0.5-2mg is given iv every 15min until complete atropinization is achieved (dry mouth).

阿托品每 15 分钟静脉推注 0.5 ~2 毫克，直到达到完全阿托品化(表现为口干)为止。

attach [əˈtætʃ] *v.* 缚，系，贴；使附属；使附着

Thrombi are usually attached in one or more places to the vessel wall.

血栓通常在一处或多处黏着于血管壁。

The first four cranial nerves are located near the front of the brain and are attached to the undersurface.

前四对脑神经靠近脑前部，与底面相连接。

Drugs such as penicillin can attach to erythrocytes and cause IgG-mediated damage to erythrocytes.

青霉素类的药物可吸附在红细胞上使其产生 IgG 介导的损伤。

This hospital is attached to the medical college of Peking University.

这所医院附属于北京大学医学院。

attachment [əˈtætʃmənt] *n.* 附着，接合

The attachment of a muscle to a bone occurs by means of a fibrous structure known as a tendon.

肌肉借助一种称为键的纤维结构附着在骨上。

The interaction between drug and protein is not a chemical one but a reversible attachment.

药物和蛋白之间的相互作用不是一种化学作用，而是一种可逆性接合。

attack [əˈtæk] *n.* 攻击；(疾病)发作

One attack of measles confers high degree of immunity.

麻疹发病一次可使人产生高度免疫力。

The attack rate for disease due to Hemophilus influenza type B is about 1%.

由 B 型流感嗜血杆菌所致疾病的发病率约为 1%。

v. 攻击，(疾病)侵袭

Children are commonly attacked with measles.

儿童易患麻疹。

attain [əˈtein] *v.* 达到，完成，获得

The blood in the veins of the liver may attain a temperature of 39.7℃.

肝静脉内血液的温度可达到 39.7℃。

Some lesions quickly attain complete formation without any intermediate stage (macules).

有些损害可以不经任何中间阶段(发斑疹)便会很快形成。

attainable (to) [əˈteinəbl] *a.* 可达到的

This is the quality of health that is attainable to people with positive attitudes.

这是持积极态度的人们所能达到的健康质量。

attainment [əˈteinmənt] *n.* 成就

Albert Einstein was noted for his scientific attainments in various fields.
阿伯特·爱因斯坦凭他在许多科学领域的成就而闻名。

It would be premature to attempt to ascertain at this early stage what progress has been made towards the attainment of these targets.
目前阶段试图确定为实现这些目标已取得多少进展尚为时过早。

attempt [ə'tempt] *v.* 试图,企图

Wheezing is most marked as the child attempts to force air out.
当患儿企图用力呼气时喘鸣最为明显。

Arterioles may be tightly constricted, as they usually are in shock, attempting to preserve arterial pressure.
处于休克时,小动脉强烈收缩以维持动脉压。

A topical chemical provocation test can be attempted in questionable cases.
对可疑的病例可尝试用局部化学刺激试验。

Resuscitation attempts failed in the patient.
该病人经抢救无效。

Owing to anoxia, the alpinists failed in all their attempts at climbing the mountain.
由于缺氧,登山运动员登顶失败。

attend [ə'tend] *v.* 参加;照顾,护理

The attending doctor insists that a blood-sugar determination be made once a month.
主治医生坚持要求每月测定血糖一次。

The young researchers will be strongly encouraged to attend this conference and present their own research.
强烈鼓励年轻的研究人员参加这次会议并展示他们自己的研究工作。

attendance [ə'tendəns] *n.* 出席;照顾,护理

It is very encouraging indeed to find such a large attendance of delegates.
这么多的代表出席确实令人鼓舞。

Friendly attendance is provided at the out patient department of this hospital.
这家医院的门诊部提供良好的服务。

In case of pneumonia as complication patients should be given a careful attendance.
对合并肺炎的病人应给予细心的护理。

Have you a good doctor in attendance?
有一个好医生给你治疗吗?

attenuate [ə'tenjueit] *v.* (使)减毒,减弱

It seems that the pathogenicity may be attenuated.
看来致病力可被减弱。

The primary infection was caused by an attenuated strain of bacillus.
原发性感染是一种毒性减弱的菌株引起的。

attenuation [əˌtenju'eiʃən] *n.* 减毒,减弱

Gamma globulin is administered for the prevention or attenuation of measles.
可给予丙种球蛋白来预防或减轻麻疹。

Moreover, a chemical or genetic marker for attenuation remains to be identified.
而且,减毒的化学和遗传标志仍有待鉴定。

attenuator [ə'tenjueitə] *n.* 衰减子,衰减器

Attenuator DNA sequence lies between the operator and the structural genes for trp biosynthesis. (trp = tryptophan 色氨酸)
衰减子的 DNA 序列位于合成色氨酸的操纵基因和结构基因之间。

The Variable Optical Attenuator is an important optical communication device without source.
可调光衰减器是一种重要的无源光通信器件。

attest [ə'test] *v.* 证实,表明

The inpatient and the outpatient services of most institutions will attest to the continuing problem.

大多数医院的住院和门诊服务表明问题继续存在。

attitude ['ætitjuːd] *n.* 姿式;态度

The leg gestures often reflect one's attitude towards something or someone that person is with.

腿的姿势常常反映出一个人对某事或某人的态度。

Science seeks to be pure, while the application of a scientific discovery are social, governed by the attitudes of people.

科学偏向纯理论,而一项科学发现的应用则是社会性的,要受到人民意愿的制约。

attractant [ə'træktənt] *n.* 诱引剂,吸引剂

The attractant has been identified and is cyclic AMP.

诱引剂已被鉴定是环腺苷酸。

attributable (**to**) [ə'tribjutəbl] *a.* 可归因的,可归属的

The symptoms are attributable largely to hypoxia.

这些症状主要归因于缺氧。

The disease has characteristics usually attributable to acute hepatitis.

本病具有一般属于急性肝炎的特征。

attribute (**to**) [ə'tribjuːt] *v.* 把…归因于

Some attributed their fatigue to overwork, although many said they could think of no reason for their exhaustion.

有些人把疲劳归于过度的工作,尽管许多人说他们对自己的疲惫找不出什么理由来。

The clinical and electrocardiographic abnormalities are attributed to degenerative changes.

临床与心电图异常被归因于退行性变化。

n. ['ætribjuːt] 属性,特征

Cellular proliferation is a characteristic feature of tumor tissue, though not necessarily an essential attribute of the individual tumor cell.

细胞的增殖是肿瘤组织的一种特征,虽然不一定是单个肿瘤细胞的基本特征。

atypical [ə'tipikəl] *a.* 非典型的,不标准的

Atypical measles can develop in patients who received killed measles vaccine and can present with a variety of rashes.

非典型性麻疹常出现在已接种过灭活麻疹病毒疫苗的患者,而且表现为皮疹的多样化。

An atypical pneumonia is one of a group of community-acquired pneumonias that do not respond to penicillin but do respond to such antibiotics as tetracycline and erythromycin.

非典型性肺炎是一种用青霉素无效而用四环素和红霉素类抗生素有效的社区性肺炎。

In the case of an atypical growth and questionable identification the culture is examined under the microscope for characteristic morphologic forms.

遇有不典型的生长和在鉴定上有疑问时,可将此培养物置于显微镜下检查其特殊的形态。

audible ['ɔːdəbl] *a.* 听得见的

In asthma wheezing is distinctly audible.

哮喘时可清楚地听到喘鸣。

audiometer [ˌɔːdi'ɔmitə] *n.* 测听器

Quantification of hearing loss is obtained with an audiometer.

利用测听器量化听力丧失的程度。

audiometric [ˌɔːdiəu'metrik] *a.* 听力测验的

Ophthalmologic examination was normal but audiometric evaluation showed a moderate hearing loss at high frequencies.

视力检查正常,然而听力测定显示在高频率时有中度听力丧失。

audit ['ɔːdit] *n.* (卫生)审计

Its success is measured by a process of medical audit.

其成功率由医学审计的方法来衡量。

auditory ['ɔːditəri] *a.* 听的,听觉的

Responses to auditory and sometimes to visual stimuli are abnormal.

(病人)对听觉,有时也对视觉的刺激反应异常。

auger ['ɔːgə] *n.* 俄歇

A Monte-Carlo Method is proposed for quantitative Auger analysis.

本文提出了一种用 Monte Carlo 模拟进行俄歇定量分析的方法。

Raman, Auger Electron Spectroscopy (AES) and X ray Photoelectron Spectroscopy (XPS) were used to analyze the samples.

(我们)用拉曼谱(Raman)、俄歇电子能谱(AES)以及 X 射线光电子能谱(XPS)等方法对样品进行了分析研究。

augment [ɔːg'ment] *v.* 增长,增加,加强

The action of oxytocin is augmented by estrogen and inhibited by progesterone.

催产素的作用可被雌激素增强,而被孕激素抑制。

It is not clear whether the response rate or longevity of serum conversion can be augmented by more frequent or higher dosing of the vaccine.

反应速率或血清转化的时间长短,是否随着疫苗剂量的增高和使用次数的增加而增长尚不清楚。

augmentation [ˌɔːgmen'teiʃən] *n.* 扩大,增加

Augmentation of the uterine action by administration of an oxytocic infusion is to be considered.

可考虑点滴催产素加强宫缩。

aura ['ɔːrə] *n.* 先兆

Approximately 20% of migraineurs experience aura.

大约有 20% 的偏头痛患者伴有先兆症状。

Migraine with aura seems to be a risk factor for cardiovascular events.

伴有先兆的偏头痛可能是心血管事件的一个危险因素。

auricle ['ɔːrikl] *n.* 心耳,心房(过去曾用作此义)

The pressure of blood in the auricle is great enough to force the valves apart.

心房血液压力之大,足以把瓣膜挤开。

(注:left auricle of heart 左心耳,right auricle of heart 右心耳)

auricular [ɔː'rikjulə] *a.* 耳的

Large thrombus masses may fill an auricular appendix in cases of cardiac disease with gross distention of the atria.

伴有心房显著扩张的心脏病的病例,可能有大的血栓块充填心耳的现象。

aurum ['ɔːrəm] *n.* 金

Aurum(Au) and Platinum(Pt) doping techniques are widely used to fabricate the fast recovery diodes(FRD), and both of them have merits and demerits.

掺金和掺铂技术被广泛地应用于制造快恢复二极管中,这两种技术各具优缺点。

Experiments need to be carried out to set proper conditions of spraying tin and plating aurum.

需进行实验以设定喷锡和镀金的适宜条件。

auscultate ['ɔːskəlteit] *v.* 听诊

In this case the fetal heart should be auscultated twice daily.

对这种病例,每天应听两次胎心。

auscultation [ɔːskəl'teiʃən] *n.* 听诊

The four classical techniques of the physical examination are inspection, palpation, percussion and auscultation.

体检的四项传统技能是望诊、触诊、叩诊和听诊。
The rest of the chest is clear to auscultation.
胸部其余部分听诊清晰。

autacoid ['ɔːtəkɔid] *n.* 内分泌物
The biological half-life of the very lipophilic endothelium-derived nitric oxide is only 3-5 sec and this allows it to function locally as an autacoid.
内皮细胞源性一氧化氮生物半衰期仅为 3 ~5 秒,因此可作为一种在局部发挥作用的内分泌物质。
Nitric oxide can function as an intracellular messenger, an autacoid, a paracrine substance, a neurotransmitter, or as a hormone that can be carried to distant sites for effects.
一氧化氮可作为细胞内信使、内分泌物质、旁分泌物质、神经递质或作为激素被转运到远处发挥作用。

authoritative [ɔː'θɔrətətiv] *a.* 权威的
In 1947, one authoritative clinician reviewed 200 cases of IDDM that he had personally treated over many years.
1947 年一位权威的临床医生对已经自己治疗过多年的 200 名 IDDM 病例进行了总结。
(注:IDDM = insulin-dependent diabetes mellitus 胰岛素依赖性糖尿病)

authority [ɔː'θɔriti] *n.* 权力,权威 (*pl.*);当局
It is believed that insufficient attention to foodborne disease is paid by health authorities in many parts of the world.
人们认为世界上许多国家的卫生当局对食物传播性疾病重视不够。

autism ['ɔːtizəm] *n.* 孤僻症
Atypical childhood psychosis may show some, but not all of the features of infantile autism.
非典型性童年精神病可显示婴儿孤僻症的某些而不是全部特点。

autistic [ɔː'tistik] *a.* 孤独的,内向的
Autistic children have been extensively studied over the past 30 years.
在过去 30 年中对孤独症患儿进行了广泛的研究。

autoantibody [ˌɔːtəu'æntiˌbɔdi] *n.* 自身抗体,自体抗体
Autoantibodies to erythrocytes result in autoimmune hemolytic anemias.
红细胞产生自身抗体可导致自身免疫溶血性贫血。

autoantigen [ˌɔːtəu'æntidʒən] *n.* 自身抗原,自体抗原
The antigens leading to this type of hypersensitivity can be microbial antigens, autoantigens and foreign serum components.
引起此型过敏反应的抗原可以是微生物抗原、自身抗原和外来血清成分。

autoclave ['ɔːtəukleiv] *n.* 高压消毒器,压热器
The laboratory apparatus designed to use steam under regulated pressure is called an autoclave.
实验室内所使用的可调节蒸汽压力的仪器称为高压消毒器。
v. 用压热器消毒
Sterilization by autoclaving is necessary.
用压热器消毒的灭菌方法是必不可少的。

autocrine [ˌɔːtəu'krain] *n.* 自分泌
These so-called autocrine and paracrine systems are used commonly during development and by most growth factors.
由大多数生长因子促进的发育(过程),多采用所谓自分泌和旁分泌系统发挥作用。

autograft ['ɔːtəgraːft] *n.* 自身移植物 *v.* 自体移植
Autograft is that tissues/organs are transplanted from one part of the body to another.
自体移植是将组织或器官从身体的某个部位移植至另一部位。
An autograft creates a wound at the donor site almost as serious as the one it is supposed to heal.

移植自己的皮肤在供体部位所造成的伤口几乎和打算治疗的伤口一样严重。

Thanks to the tiny skin grafts and the two dozen major and minor operations, skin autografts finally spread all over the body.

由于进行了微小皮肤的移植和24次大小手术，自体移植的皮肤终于扩布了全身。

autohemolysis [ˌɔːtəuhiˈmɔlisis] *n.* 自体溶血

The autohemolysis test is useful in diagnosing hereditary spherocytosis.

自体溶血试验对于诊断遗传性球形红细胞症是有用的。

autoimmune [ˌɔːtəuiˈmjuːn] *a.* 自体免疫的，自身免疫的

Type Ⅱ diabetes is not autoimmune related or HLA (human leucocyte antigen) associated.

Ⅱ型糖尿病与自身免疫和人类白细胞抗原无关。

Considerable difficulty, however, has been encountered in assessing the exact significance of observed autoimmune phenomena.

然而，在评价已观察到的自身免疫现象的真正意义时却遇到了很大的困难。

autoimmunity [ˌɔːtəuiˈmjuːniti] *n.* 自体免疫性

Autoimmunity is an acquired immune reactivity to self antigens.

自身免疫性是一种对自身抗原的获得性免疫反应。

Interest has centered in particular on the challenging question of autoimmunity and its possible pathogenic role.

自体免疫性及其可能具有的病理作用这一挑战性的问题，引起了人们的特别兴趣。

autointoxication [ˈɔːtəuinˌtɔksiˈkeiʃən] *n.* 自体中毒

In the 19th century, studies in biochemistry and microbiology seemed to support the autointoxication hypothesis, and mainstream physicians promoted the idea.

在19世纪，自体中毒的假说似乎获得了生物化学与微生物学研究的支持和多数临床医生的推崇。

Other factors we should consider in autointoxication are the stresses put on society today.

必须考虑自体中毒的其他因素：给予当今社会的种种压力。

autologous [ɔːˈtɔləgəs] *a.* 自身固有的

Burn victims and others who need new skin have always received autologous grafts.

烧伤患者及其他需要新皮肤的人往往只能接受从自身取得的移植物。

autolysate [ˌɔːtəuˈlaiseit] *n.* 自溶物，自溶产物

Autolysates are produced similar to the yeast extracts but the cell walls are not removed in the process.

自溶物产生与酵母抽提相似，但该过程并不清除细胞壁。

The autolysate of yeast cells is a valuable source of various substances which can be used as ingredients in foods, feeds and fermentation.

酵母细胞的自溶产物是多种物质的一个重要来源，这些物质可用作食物、饲料和发酵的组分

autolysis [ɔːˈtɔlisis] *n.* 自溶

The histological features of necrosis attributable to autolysis do not develop.

由自溶引起的坏死的组织学表现不会发生。

I should note that severe permanent ischemia found in the posterior papillary muscle infarct is essentially equivalent to total ischemia or autolysis.

我应当指出，在后乳头肌梗死时出现的严重的持久性缺血，在本质上与完全缺血和自溶相等。

automate [ˈɔːtəmeit] *v.* 使自动化

An engineer is designing how to automate the production of this new drug.

一位工程师正在设计如何使这种新药的生产自动化。

With the development of automated technology, such concerns have been largely resolved, and it is now feasible to raise a large relatively reasonable cost.

随着自动化技术的发展,那些人们关心的事项已大多解决了,而且在大范围内推行较为合理的成本,目前已有可能。

automatic [ɔːtə'mætik] *a.* 自动的,机械的

By conscious effort, you may hold your breath for a while, but eventually unconscious automatic breathing starts again.

你可以有意识地屏住呼吸一会儿,但最后不自主的呼吸又自动开始了。

The automatic nervous system is subdivided into sympathetic and parasympathetic nervous system.

自主神经系统又被分为交感神经系统和副交感神经系统。

automatically [ˌɔːtə'mætikəli] *ad.* 自动地,自主地

Independent of its nerve supply cardiac muscle can contract automatically and rhythmically at a slow rate.

在不受其神经支配的情况下,心肌能够自主和有节奏地缓慢收缩。

automaticity [ɔːˌtəmə'tisiti] *n.* 自动性,自律性

Disopyramide depresses automaticity primarily in the ventricular conducting system.

双异丙吡胺主要抑制心室传导系统的自律性。

automation [ˌɔːtə'meiʃən] *n.* 自动化

The amount of work required from clinical laboratories has led to the introduction of automation.

对临床实验室大量工作的需要导致了自动化的应用。

Automation is realized by means of computers.

借助计算机而实现自动化。

Electronic automation equipment is very expensive.

电子自动化设备非常昂贵。

automatism [ɔ'tɔmətizəm] *n.* 自动症;自动(作用)

Sleep-walking is a state of automatism occurring in the course of normal sleep, most commonly in childhood.

梦游症是在正常睡眠过程中发生的一种自动症状态,多见于童年。

autonomic [ˌɔːtəu'nɔmik] *a.* 自主的

The sinus node is richly supplied with autonomic nerves, both sympathetic and parasympathetic.

窦房结分布有丰富的自主神经,包括交感的和副交感的。

autonomous [ɔː'tɔnəməs] *a.* 自主的,自律的;自治的

All living organisms are capable of autonomous movement, although in some forms it is slight.

一切生物都能自主地运动,虽然某些生物的运动是微不足道的。

Benign and malignant neoplasmas of the skin reflect autonomous proliferation of a specific cell type.

皮肤的良性和恶性肿瘤反映出一种特异的细胞类型的自主性增生。

autonomy [ɔː'tɔnəmi] *n.* 自主性,自律性

Furthermore, his definition does not stress the autonomy of tumors as much as some of the older definitions did.

再者,他的定义对肿瘤的自主性不像有些旧定义那样强调。

A significant number of physicians in the United States have either a poor or no understanding of the laws of states regarding the principle of autonomy.

在美国有许多医生对联邦法律中的自主原则不了解或知之甚少。

autophage ['ɔːtəufeidʒ] *n.* 自噬,自身消耗;自身消瘦,自食己肉(精神病患者)

The hemiterpene matters used by the invention are all excretive by the autophage process of the plants, thus having no toxic hazard。

本发明所使用的半松油精物质均是植物自身代谢过程中分泌的物质,所以没有毒害。

Phenomena of autophage in pancreatic acinar cells of acute pancreatitis rat was studied in this paper.

本文研究了急性胰腺炎大鼠胰腺腺泡细胞的自噬现象。

autophagosome [ˌɔːtəu'fægəsəum] *n.* 自噬体

Autophagosome is a secondary lysosome in which elements of a cell's own cytoplasm are digested.

自噬体是一种可以消化细胞质中细胞器的次级溶酶体。

The membrane origin of autophagosomes remains unclear.

自噬体膜结构的起源仍不是很清楚。

autophagy [ɔː'tɔfədʒi] *n.* 自我吞噬，自食症

we focus on susceptibility genes related to autophagy.

我们重点关注自食症的敏感基因。

According to the author, autophagy is the only known process that gets rid of abnormal proteins within cells.

作者认为，自我吞噬是清除细胞内异常蛋白质的唯一途径。

Autophagy occurs in all types of eukaryotic cells, which has a rigid connection with the normal or abnormal development of cells and is associated with many diseases.

自噬存在于所有类型的真核细胞，它与细胞的正常或异常发育以及多种疾病密切联系。

Remarkably, autophagy may also play a role in determining the human life span.

显然，自噬在决定人类寿命方面可能也发挥作用。

Autophagy, present in almost all cells that have mitochondria, is a highly conserved homeostasis process.

自噬存在于几乎所有的含线粒体的细胞中，它是细胞中一种高度保守的自稳机制。

Our study tries to explore the role of autophagy in COPD.

我们的实验试图探寻自噬在慢性阻塞性肺疾病中的作用。

autopsy ['ɔːtəpsi] *n.* 验尸，尸检

The autopsy findings revealed hemorrhagic necrosis in the cerebral cortex.

尸检所见为大脑皮层出血性坏死。

One mystery is why some autopsies have found such a striking disparity.

难以理解的是为什么有些尸检的分析全然不同。

autoradiography [ˌɔːtəuˌreidi'ɔgrəfi] *n.* 放射自显影术，自动射线照相术

The distribution of radioactively labelled substances taken up by the cell is followed by autoradiography.

细胞吸收的放射性标记物的分布情况由自动射线照相术追踪显示出来。

autoreactive [ˌɔːtəuri'æktiv] *a.* 自身反应的

The pathogenesis of autoimmune disease includes production of autoantibodies or autoreactive T cells, infiltration of target tissues by destructive inflammatory cells, and deposition of immune complexes in vascular sites.

自身免疫性疾病的发病机制包括：自身抗体或自身反应性 T 细胞的产生、靶组织遭受破坏性炎细胞的浸润、以及免疫复合物在血管部位的沉积。

autoreactivity [ˌɔːtəuˌriæk'tiviti] *n.* 自身反应性

Autoreactivity describes immune responses directed at self antigens.

自身反应性是指针对自身抗原的免疫反应。

$CD4^{+}CD7^{-}CD28^{-}$ T cells are expanded in rheumatoid arthritis and are characterized by autoreactivity.

$CD4^{+}CD7^{-}CD28^{-}$ T 细胞在类风湿性关节炎中增殖，以自身反应性为特征。

autosomal [ˌɔːtə'səuməl] *a.* 常染色体的

Genes located on the autosomes are termed autosomal genes.

位于常染色体的基因称为常染色体基因。

Most patients with autosomal dominant polycystic kidney disease have a gene defect linked to markers on chromosome 16.

患常染色体显性遗传的多囊肾的病人大多数存在基因缺陷,这种基因缺陷与链接在 16 号染色体上的标记物有关。

autosome [ˈɔːtəsəum] *n.* 常染色体

Autosomes are chromosomes other than the sex chromosomes.

除性染色体之外,其他染色体均为常染色体。

In humans the gene for albinism has its locus on autosome.

人类白化病基因位于常染色体上。

autosuggestion [ˌɔːtəusəˈdʒestʃən] *n.* 自我暗示

Autosuggestion is used primarily in autogenic training, a technique used to help patients control their anxiety or their habits.

自我暗示主要是应用自律训练来帮助患者控制他们的焦虑或习惯的一种技术。

autotransplant [ˌɔːtəuˈtrænsplɑːnt] *v.* 自体移植

Large defects in the cervical esophagus are being replaced by autotransplanted segments of bowel.

食道颈段大面积缺损正在由自体肠段移植所代替。

autotransplantation [ˈɔːtəuˌtrænsplɑːnˈteiʃən] *n.* 自体移植

Surgery such as free skin flap transfer and autotransplantation of the testicle to the scrotum are now being performed routinely.

游离皮瓣移植和将自体睾丸回纳到阴囊之类的手术,现在正成为常规手术。

autotroph [ˈɔːtətrɔf] *n.* 自养生物

Autotrophs can manufacture their own energy-rich organic compounds.

自养生物能生产自身需要的高能有机化合物。

The more than 400 000 plant species on earth are autotrophs.

地球上有 40 多万种植物是自养生物。

autoxidation [ɔːˌtɔksiˈdeiʃən] *n.* 自然氧化(作用)

Autoxidation of cholesterol can occur through reactions initiated by free radical species.

胆固醇的自氧化作用可以通过自由基引发的反应而发生。

The peak areas of oxidation products were at least five times higher as compared with autoxidation.

氧化产物的峰面积比自氧化作用至少高了五倍以上。

auxiliary [ɔːgˈziljəri] *a.* 辅助的,附属的

Auxiliary cells, including mast cells, basophils and platelets, are important sources of the vasoactive mediators histamine and 5-hydroxytryptamine.

辅助细胞,包括肥大细胞、嗜碱性粒细胞和血小板,是缩血管介质组胺和 5-羟色胺的重要来源。

availability [əˌveiləˈbiliti] *n.* 可用性,有效性

The availability of choline regulates the synthesis of acetylcholine.

胆碱的可利用度调节乙酰胆碱的合成。

Still drug experts say that availability alone is the answer.

药物专家依然认为药物的有效性是第一位的。

available [əˈveiləbl] *a.* 可利用的,可获得的

Vitamin B_{12} is available in meat, animal protein foods, and legumes.

维生素 B_{12} 可以从肉类、动物蛋白类食物和豆类食物获得。

Tests that use hair samples to detect drugs are available but may not be as accurate.

可以用头发来检查药品,但精确度较低。

There are a number of drugs available that suppress the immune reaction.
有许多可抑制免疫反应的药物。
A scientist must make full use of all information available.
科学家应充分运用可得到的信息。

avenue [ˈævinjuː] *n.* 途径
To the basic researchers, microsurgical expertise will also provide new avenues for experimentations.
对于基础研究人员来说,显微外科专门技术也将为实验提供新的途径。

average [ˈævəridʒ] *a.* 平均的
The average life span of a red blood cell is 120 days.
红细胞的平均寿命是 120 天。
The average follow-up was 8.4 months for the women treated with placebo and 9.1 months for women treated with melphalan.
用安慰剂的妇女,治疗后随访时间平均是 8.4 个月,而用米尔法兰的是平均 9.1 个月。
n. 平均(数)
On average, alcoholic women drink less than alcoholic men.
一般来说,酗酒的女性的饮酒量小于酗酒的男性。
v. 平均为
The contractions of the heart average about 72 per minute and are carried on increasingly for the whole of a lifetime.
心脏每分钟收缩平均为 72 次,一生中从不间断。
The incubation period of this type of hepatitis is relatively short, averaging between two to four weeks.
此型肝炎的潜伏期较短,平均 2 ~4 周。

avert [əˈvəːt] *v.* 转移;防止,避免
Complete loss of consciousness may be averted if subject can promptly lie down.
如果病人马上躺下就可避免出现完全的意识丧失。
Contact sports should be avoided for 6-8 weeks to avert splenic rupture.
6 ~8 周不能做触及身体的运动以避免发生脾破裂。

avidity [əˈviditi] *n.* 亲和力
Avidity is the sum total of the strength of binding of two molecules or cells to one another at multiple sites. It is distinct from affinity, which is the strength of binding of one site on a molecule to its ligand.
Avidity 是两个分子和两个细胞之间在多个位点结合强度的总和,它不同于 affinity,后者是一个分子和其配体在一个位点的结合强度。
These findings support a differential avidity model of T cell selection.
这些结果支持 T 细胞选择的差异性亲和力模型。

avirulent [æˈvirjulənt] *a.* 无毒力的
Several properties of virulent, avirulent, and interferon-resistant Rickettsia prowazekii strains were compared.
已对有毒、无毒和干扰素耐性普氏立克次体株的几种特性进行了比较。
Experimental infection of mice with avirulent Semliki Forest virus (SFV) has been used as a model of demyelinating disease in humans.
用无毒力的西门利克森林病毒实验性感染小鼠已被用作人类脱髓鞘疾病的一种模型。

avitaminosis [eiˌvaitəmiˈnəusis] *n.* 维生素缺乏(病),营养缺乏病
The role of malnutrition and avitaminosis is difficult to separate from the direct effects of alcohol.
营养不良和维生素缺乏病的作用很难与酒精的直接作用分开。

avoid [əˈvɔid] *v.* 避免,回避

An enteric coated preparation may avoid gastric side effects.
肠溶片可用来避免对胃的副作用。
The best way to avoid DNA amplification during qPCR is to design primers on 2 different exons of your gene.
定量 PCR 中避免 DNA 扩增的最好方法是在目的基因的 2 个不同外显子上设计引物。

avulsion [əˈvʌlʃən] *n.* 撕裂
The anal fissure may be due to avulsion of an anal valve.
此例肛裂可能由肛瓣的撕裂所致。

await [əˈweit] *v.* 等候,期待
These agents await evaluation by controlled trials.
这些试剂有待用对照试验来估价。
The patient is trained to use his or her existing potential and abilities, while awaiting any recovery that may occur.
应当训练病人发挥自身的能力和潜能,而不是等待康复。

awake [əˈweik] *v.* 唤醒,醒
The patient began to awake, with some delirium, 6 hours after the operation.
手术后 6 小时病人开始苏醒过来,但仍处于谵妄状态。
a. 醒的,警觉的
It is also common to find patients awake and alert but most uncomfortable, shivering on a cooling blanket.
通常也可以发现病人非常警醒,但非常不舒服,在冰冷的毯子上发抖。

aware [əˈwɛə] *a.* 意识到的
An alert clinician must be aware of the possibility of myocarditis complicating any acute viral infection.
有警觉的医生应当知道任何急性病毒感染都可能并发(于)心肌炎。
We are all now aware that some new scientific or technological advance, though useful, may have unpleasant side effects.
我们现在都意识到一些新科技的进展,尽管有用,也可能产生令人不愉快的副作用。
Following infection, some have no signs and symptoms, often such individuals are not aware that they have been exposed to infection.
感染后有些人可以没有任何症状和体征,这些人通常没意识到他们已被感染。

awareness [əˈwɛənis] *n.* 察觉,意识
Awareness of an irregularity suggests fibrillation.
如察觉其节律不规则,则可能为纤维性颤动。
Public awareness of dangers of drugs has greatly increased.
人们对药物危险性的了解已大大增加。

awkward [ˈɔːkwəd] *a.* 笨拙的
Nerve impulses to muscles may be affected, making the person slow and awkward.
传至肌肉的神经冲动可能受到影响,使人的动作变得缓慢而笨拙。

axial [ˈæksiəl] *a.* 轴的
The shape of a spirochete is maintained in part by an axial filament.
螺旋体的形态在部分程度上是由轴丝维持着的。

axilla [ækˈsilə] (*pl.* axillae [ækˈsiliː]) *n.* 腋,腋窝
The axilla is a roughly pyramidal fossa between the arm and the upper part of the thorax.
腋窝大体上为一锥形窝,位于臂与胸上部之间。
The axilla contains large important nerves which are branches of the brachial plexus.
腋窝内有大的重要神经,这些神经是臂丛的分支。

axillary [ækˈsiləri] *a.* 腋下的

The rectal temperature is about half a degree higher and the axillary about half a degree lower than the mouth temperature.
直肠温度比口腔温度约高半度,腋下温度比口腔温度约低半度。
Axillary nerve arises from the posterior cord of the brachial plexus and supplies the teres minor and deltoid muscles.
腋神经起于臂丛后索,分布于小圆肌和三角肌。

axis [ˈæksis] *n.* 轴
Many outside influences play upon the hypothalamic-pituitary-ovarian axis.
很多外界影响对下丘脑-垂体-卵巢轴起作用。
Hinge joints permit movement in one axis at right angles to the bones involved.
屈戌关节,可使骨在一个轴上作直角运动。

axon [ˈæksɔn] *n.* 轴突,轴索
This axon reflex was described more than 50 years ago.
这种轴索反射 50 多年前就被描述过。

axonopathy [æksəˈnɔpəθi] *n.* 轴突病变
The current study supports the hypothesis that microtubule mechanisms are disrupted during episodes of lysosome stress or dysfunction, leading to axonopathy.
本研究支持这一假说:在发生溶酶体应激或功能障碍时,微管机制被破坏,从而引起轴突病变。

axonotmesis [ˌæksɔnɔtˈmiːsis] *n.* 轴索断裂
Electrical stimulation in the acute phase of axonotmesis promotes nerve regeneration and functional recovery.
轴索断裂急性期使用电刺激可促进神经再生和功能恢复。
We present here a lesion with complete axonotmesis of the axillary nerve.
这里我们提供了一个完全性腋神经轴索断裂的病例。

azathioprine [ˌeizəˈθaiəpriːn] *n.* 硫唑嘌呤
Azathioprine has been used to treat various autoimmune disorders.
硫唑嘌呤已被用于治疗各种自身免疫性疾病。
Azathioprine has also been used in the treatment of acute and chronic leukaemias and inflammatory bowel disease (e. g. ulcerative colitis).
硫唑嘌呤亦用于治疗急性和慢性白血病和炎症性肠病(如溃疡性结肠炎)。

azide [ˈæzaid] *n.* 叠氮化合物,叠氮
Reduction of azides is an important method to introduce amino group to organic molecules.
叠氮还原是向有机分子中引入氨基的重要方法。
Zinc metal in near-critical water (250℃) reduces azides to amines.
在近临界水中(250℃),锌可将叠氮化合物还原为胺。

azidothymidine (AZT) [ˌæzidəˈθaimidiːn] *n.* 叠氮胸苷
The most prominent initial success has been achieved with azidothymidine, which is an inhibitor of HIV reverse transcriptase.
获得的最突出初步成就是叠氮胸苷(AZT)的应用,本品为 HIV 反转录酶抑制剂。

azo [ˈæzəu] *n.* 偶氮,*a.* 含氮的
Bacterial azo reduction is a process that azo compound are decomposed into aromatic amines by the azo reductase from bacteria.
细菌偶氮还原是在细菌偶氮还原酶作用下偶氮化合物分解为芳香胺的过程。
Azo compounds are compounds bearing the functional group R—N ═N—R′, in which R and R′ can be either aryl or alkyl.
偶氮化合物含有功能团 R—N ═N—R′,其中 R 和 R′可以是芳基或烷基。

azole [ˈæzəul] *n.* 唑类

Vaginal yeast infections can reoccur over time so these medicines like azole are recommended.
随着时间的推移,阴道酵母菌感染会再发,因此建议使用这些唑类药物。

The susceptibility rates of 161 strains of yeastlike fungi to azole antifungals, such as fluconazole, were 95.7%.
161 株酵母样真菌对唑类抗真菌药(如氟康唑)的敏感率为 95.7%。

azone [eiˈzəun] *n.* 氮酮

Moreover, using azone together with propylene glycol, the permeation effect of elemene was even better.
另外,同时使用氮酮和丙二醇后,榄香烯的渗透作用实际上更好。

The transdermal absorption reached peak when the ratio of azone to propylene glycol was 1.6% : 2.0%.
当氮酮和丙二醇的比例为 1.6% :2.0% 时透皮吸收达到了高峰。

azoospermia [əˌzəuəˈspəːmiə] *n.* 精子缺乏,无精症

A biopsy of the testis is necessary in order to differentiate these two causes of azoospermia; if a blockage is present it may be possible to relieve it surgically.
需作睾丸活组织检查以辨别精子缺乏的这两种原因;若有阻塞,可用手术排除。

Obstructive azoospermia is because of an absent vas deferens.
梗阻性无精症是因为输精管道的缺失。

Obstructive azoospermia refers to no sperm in a man's semen, as a result from problems with sperm delivery.
梗阻性无精症指没有精子,由输精障碍产生。

azotemia [æzəˈtiːmiə] *n.* 氮血症

Aggravating factors are azotemia, prolonged endotracheal intubation, and severe associated infection.
加重因素有氮血症、延长气管内置插管的置放时间以及严重的复合感染。

Patients with long-term severe hypertension may develop renal failure and azotemia.
长期患严重高血压的病人可发生肾功能衰竭和氮血症。

B

bacillary [bəˈsiləri] *a.* 杆菌的，杆菌性的；杆状的

Gram-negative bacillary meningitis occurs mostly in patients whose anatomic defense against CNS infection has been compromised.

革兰氏阴性杆菌性脑膜炎大多发生于(那些)抗 CNS 感染的解剖屏障受到损害的患者。

Blood and pus are grossly apparent in severe bacillary dysentery.

患严重细菌性痢疾的病人粪便中肉眼便可见到脓和血。

bacillin [bəˈsilin] *n.* 杆菌素

Bacillin is highly active against gram-positive and gram-negative bacteria.

杆菌素具有很高的抗革兰氏阳性和革兰氏阴性细菌的活性。

bacillus [bəˈsiləs] (*pl.* bacilli [bəˈsilai]) *n.* 杆菌

Bacilli are cylindrical or rod-shaped cells.

杆菌是呈柱状或杆状的细胞。

Many diseases are referred to the action of bacilli.

许多疾病归因于杆菌的作用。

bacitracin [ˌbæsiˈtreisin] *n.* 杆菌肽

There is bacitracin, which was discovered by two scientists at Columbia University's College of Physicians and Surgeons.

杆菌肽是由哥伦比亚大学医学院的两位科学家发现的。

backache [ˈbækeik] *n.* 背痛

Involvement of the pancreas may produce backache which can mistakenly be attributed to an orthopaedic lesion.

涉及胰脏后会发生背痛，这可能被误认为矫形损伤所致。

backbone [ˈbækbəun] *n.* 主链；脊柱，脊椎

The backbone of nucleic acids consists of alternating phosphates and pentoses.

核酸的主链由交替出现的磷酸和五碳糖组成。

Only a few animals with backbones are able to produce light.

只有少数几种脊椎动物能发光。

backflow [ˈbækfləu] *n.* 回流，反流

These valves prevent backflow in the same way as those which are found in some veins.

这些瓣膜如同某些静脉中的瓣膜那样，起着防止回流的作用。

background [ˈbækgraund] *n.* 本底；背景；基底

The unwanted radiation is referred to as background radiation.

这种有害辐射称为背景辐射。

Many instruments are equipped to carry out this background correction on an automatic basis.

许多仪器具有进行这种自动本底校正的功能。

baclofen [bækˈləufən] *n.* 巴氯芬

Baclofen is a derivative of gamma-aminobutyric acid (GABA).

巴氯芬是一种 γ-氨基丁酸(GABA)的衍生物。

Baclofen is primarily used to treat spasticity and is under investigation for the treatment of alcoholism.

巴氯芬主要用来治疗痉挛性疾病，是否能够治疗酒精中毒还在研究中。

Becquerel [bekə'rel] *n.* 贝可(放射性活度单位)

According to the legal metrological units, the Becquerel (Bq) is taken as activity unit.

根据法定计量单位选用了贝克(Bq)作为放射性活度单位。

One Becquerel corresponds to the transformation (disintegration) of one atomic nucleus per second.

1 贝可相当于每秒转换(分解)1 个原子核。

bacteremia [ˌbæktə'riːmiə] *n.* 菌血症

Signs of tissue anoxia appear only after several hours of bacteremia.

组织缺氧的体征仅在菌血症几小时后便可出现。

The diagnosis is established by the demonstration of persistant bacteremia.

诊断是根据有持久菌血症的表现而确定的。

bacteria [bæk'tiəriə] (bacterium [bæk'tiəriəm] 的复数) *n.* 细菌

In the uncomplicated case, bacteria are not present in the vegetations.

在无并发症的病例中,疣赘物内无细菌存在。

(另见 bacterium)

bacterial [bæk'tiəriəl] *a.* 细菌的

Not all food poisoning has a bacterial cause.

并不是所有食物中毒都是由细菌引起的。

Macrophages may thus help to control some bacterial and viral infections.

这样巨噬细胞可有助于控制某些细菌性和病毒性感染。

Successful treatment of bacterial meningitis depends on early diagnosis.

细菌性脑膜炎的有效治疗依赖于早期诊断。

Ascitic fluid should be examined for bacterial and malignant cells.

腹水应送去检查菌细胞和恶性肿瘤细胞。

bactericidal [bækˌtiəri'saidl] *a.* 杀菌的

Nalidixic acid is bactericidal in nature.

萘啶酸具有杀菌性。

Isoniazid moves freely into caseous tissues and has bactericidal and bacteriostatic actions.

异烟肼可自由进入干酪化组织中,并有杀菌和抑菌作用。

bactericide [bæk'tiərisaid] *n.* 杀(细)菌剂

A bactericide is similar to a germicide, but it is restricted to bacteria and does not affect their spores.

杀细菌剂与杀病菌剂类似,但只作用于细菌,对菌孢无影响。

bactericidin [ˌbæktəri'saidin] *n.* 杀菌素

A bactericidin for Bacillus Subtilis has been found in amniotic fluid and intervillous space blood.

在羊水和绒毛间隙血中已经发现有枯草杆菌杀菌素。

Bactericidin is an antibody that kills bacteria in the presence of complement.

杀菌素是一种抗体,在有补体存在时可以杀死细菌。

bacterin ['bæktərin] *n.* 菌苗

Bacterin means bacterial vaccine.

菌苗就是细菌的疫苗。

bacteriocin [bæk'tiəriəsin] *n.* 细菌素

Specific bacteriocins attach to specific receptors on cell walls and induce specific metabolic block, e. g. , cessation of nucleic acid or protein synthesis of oxidative phosphorylation.

特异的细菌素附着于细胞壁上的特异受体,可诱发特异性的代谢阻滞,例如可使核酸或蛋白质合成的氧化磷酸化活动停止。

bacteriological [bækˌtiəriə'lɔdʒikəl] *a.* 细菌学的

The lack of efficient bacteriological laboratories contributes to the unwise use of antibiotics.

缺乏有效的细菌实验室必然会导致抗生素的滥用。

bacteriologist [bækˌtiəriˈɔlədʒist] *n.* 细菌学家

Bacteriologists have methods of differentiating between these two types of germs.

细菌学家有办法鉴别这两种细菌。

An English bacteriologist, Fred Griffith, ultimately revealed the answer.

英国细菌学家 Fred Griffith 最终揭示了这个问题的答案。

bacteriology [bækˌtiəriˈɔlədʒi] *n.* 细菌学

Nevertheless, men developed the science of bacteriology from the speculations of these philosphers.

然而,人们根据这些哲学家的预测发展了细菌学。

The bacteriology of acute upper respiratory infections has been well defined.

急性上呼吸道感染的细菌学已有可靠的解释。

bacteriolysin [bækˌtiəriˈɔlisin] *n.* 溶菌素

Bacteriolysins are antibodies that dissolve the specific microorganisms which stimulate the development of the antibodies.

溶菌素是一种抗体,它能溶解特异的能刺激抗体生成的微生物。

bacteriophage [bækˈtiəriəfeidʒ] *n.* 噬菌体

Bacteria may be infected with viruses called bacteriophages.

细菌可以感染上称为噬菌体的病毒。

One is the use of naturally occurring bacteriophages capable of destroying the bacterial cell both in vitro and in vivo.

一种情况是使用能在体内和体外杀死细菌细胞的自然产生的噬菌体。

bacteriosis [ˌbæktiəriˈəusis] *n.* 菌群失调;细菌性疾病

Abuse of antibiotics may cause bacteriosis.

滥用抗生素可引起菌群失调。

Vaginal bacteriosis is an alteration and imbalance of the normal and healthy bacterial make-up of the vagina.

阴道菌群失调是指阴道中有益健康的正常菌群比例的改变和失去平衡。

bacteriostasis [bækˌtiəriəˈsteisis] *n.* 抑菌作用

Bacteriostasis is the process of inhibiting the growth of bacteria.

抑菌作用是抑制细菌生长的过程。

bacteriostatic [bæktiəriəˈstætik] *a.* 抑制细菌的

Practically all strains of meningococci are susceptible to the bacteriostatic action of the sulfonamide drugs.

几乎所有脑膜炎双球菌菌株对磺胺药物的制菌作用都是很敏感的。

bacteriotherapy [bækˌtiəriəuˈθerəpi] *n.* 细菌疗法

Bacteriotherapy using harmless bacteria to displace pathogenic organisms is an alternative and promising way of combating infections.

用无害的细菌替代致病微生物进行的细菌治疗,是一种可供选择的、具有发展前景的抗感染方法。

Bacteriotherapy has already long been used in animals—for example, to prevent salmonellosis in chickens.

细菌疗法已经在动物身上应用很久了,例如预防鸡沙门菌病。

bacteriotropic [bæktiəriəˈtrɔpik] *a.* 亲细菌的

The agglutinin titres and the bactericidal and bacteriotropic properties of the sera from these rabbits were also investigated.

对这些兔血清的凝集素效价、杀菌和亲菌特性也进行了研究。

Bacteriotropic substance is an opsonin or other substance that alters bacterial cells in such a manner that they are more susceptible to phagocytic action.

亲菌素是一种能改变细菌细胞的调理素或其他物质,从而使其更容易遭受吞噬作用。

bacterium [bæk'tiəriəm] (*pl.* bacteria [bæk'tiəriə]) *n.* 细菌

The morphologic, biochemical, immunologic and genetic characteristics of a bacterium are used for its identification.

细菌的形态学、生物化学、免疫学和遗传学的特性均可用于其鉴定。

None of these staining procedures are used routinely in the identification of a bacterium.

这些染色法中没有一项用于常规的细菌鉴定。

bacteriuria [bækˌtiəri'juəriə] *n.* 细菌尿

However, significant bacteriuria may be absent in some circumstances when true urinary infection exists.

然而,在某些情况下确有泌尿道感染却无明显的菌尿。

This study did not correlate the level of bateriuria with other clinical and laboratory parameters that indicate infection.

这项研究没有将菌尿水平与表示感染的其他临床与实验室指标联系起来。

bacteroides [ˌbæktə'rɔidiːz] *n.* 拟杆菌属,类杆菌属

The bacteria, apart from bacteroides, are nearly all penicillin sensitive.

除了类杆菌属,细菌几乎都对青霉素敏感。

baicalin ['baikəlin] *n.* 黄芩苷

Methods established were simple and reliable, and were suitable for the quality control of baicalin.

建立的各项方法简便、可靠,可用于黄芩苷原料生产的质量控制。

We should investigate the relation between the quality of baicalin production and the pyrogen.

我们应该研究黄芩苷产品质量与致热原的关系。

balance ['bæləns] *v.* 权衡,使平衡

The normal production of red cells balances their continuous destruction.

红细胞的正常生成与不断的破坏相平衡。

n. 平衡

Cytokines act as key communicators for immune cells and maintaining a delicate balance in the level of these communicators is vital for health— in many chronic diseases, this balance is disrupted.

细胞因子是免疫细胞的关键信息分子,保持这些信息分子水平的精细平衡对健康至关重要,在很多慢性疾病,这种平衡被破坏。

balanitis [ˌbælə'naitis] *n.* 龟头炎

Balanitis is sometimes accompanied by a purulent exudate, depending on the causative agent.

由于致病微生物不同,龟头炎有时可伴有脓性分泌物。

balanoposthitis [ˌbælənəupɔs'θaitis] *n.* 龟头包皮炎,阴茎头包皮炎

In order to prevent recurrence, the parts with vaginitis, genital inflammation and dermatitis should also be coated with iodine glycerin, and meanwhile her husband's balanoposthitis should be cured.

为了预防女性生殖道炎症复发,应将碘甘油同时涂在患者的阴道炎、外阴炎和周边有炎症的皮肤上,并应将其丈夫的龟头包皮炎一并治愈。

Balanoposthitis should not be confused with balanitis, which is inflammation of the glans penis or the clitoris.

不应混淆龟头包皮炎与龟头炎,后者指龟头或阴蒂的炎症。

Balanoposthitis is sometimes accompanied by a purulent exudate, depending on the causative agents.

阴茎头包皮炎有时伴有脓性分泌物,这取决于是什么致病微生物引起的。

ballooning [beˈluːniŋ] *a.* 气球样的

Hepatocytes undergo diffuse swelling called ballooning degeneration in acute hepatitis.

急性肝炎时，肝细胞发生广泛肿胀，称气球样变。

Ballooning degeneration is a kind of severe hydropic change.

气球样变是一种严重的水变性。

ban [bæn] *v.* 禁止

Smoking in the public places is banned.

禁止在公共场所吸烟。

bandage [ˈbændidʒ] *n.* 绷带

Bandages are used to hold dressings in place, apply pressure to a part, immobilize a part, and aid in checking hemorrhages.

绷带用于固定敷料、局部加压、局部固定及帮助止血。

In most cases pressure with a clean bandage directly on the wound will stop the bleeding effectively.

在多数情况下，用清洁的绷带直接压迫伤口即可有效地制止出血。

bandwidth [ˈbændwitθ] *n.* 频带宽度，通带宽度

The bandwidth was reduced by two-thirds.

频带宽度减少了三分之二。

This wastes bandwidth and makes the network unusable.

这会浪费网路频宽并造成网路无法使用。

bank [bæŋk] *n.* 库

Although blood can be transferred directly, the usual practice for hospitals is to use blood that has been collected earlier and stored in so-called blood banks.

尽管可以直接输血，但医院的常规作法是使用早先收集并储存在血库中的血。

barbiturate [bɑːˈbitjurit] *n.* 巴比妥酸盐

Barbiturates do not raise the pain threshold and have no analgesic property.

巴比妥类不提高痛阈，也无镇痛作用。

The barbiturates apparently reduced brain metabolism and the swelling caused by lack of oxygen.

巴比妥酸盐明显地降低了脑代谢，减轻了由于缺氧引起的脑水肿。

bariatrics [ˌbæriˈætriks] *n.* 肥胖病学，肥胖治疗学

Bariatric surgery provides substantial, sustained weight loss.

减肥手术提供了大量的、持续的体重下降。

Spend some time for online reading about bariatrics abroad.

建议你花些时间在网上浏览国外的减肥治疗情况。

barium [ˈbɛəriəm] *n.* 钡

Many rectal lesions can be demonstrated by barium enema.

许多直肠疾病可由钡灌肠检出。

Sigmoidoscopy and barium enema may cause endocarditis.

乙状结肠镜检查与钡灌肠可引起心内膜炎。

bariumism [ˈbɛəriəmizm] *n.* 钡中毒

The arrhythmias in acute bariumism are due to secondary hypokalemia, direct effect of barium on myocardium, and toxic myocarditis.

急性钡中毒引起的心律失常是由于继发性低血钾、钡剂直接作用于心肌以及中毒性心肌炎所致。

Barium meal examination rarely leads to bariumism.

钡餐检查很少会导致钡中毒。

baroreceptor [ˌbærəuriˈseptə] *n.* 压力感受器

One of the most important nervous reflexes is the baroreceptor reflex.

最重要的神经反射之一为压力感受器反射。

barotrauma [ˌbærəˈtrɔːmə] *n.* 气压伤

Barotrauma is physical damage to body tissues caused by a difference in pressure between the body and the surrounding fluid.

气压伤是由于身体和外界气流压力差导致的物理性组织损伤。

Barotrauma typically occurs in air spaces within a body when that body moves to or from a higher pressure environment.

当人体移动到气压高的环境或从气压高区移动出时,气压伤通常会发生在人体气腔。

barrier [ˈbæriə] *n.* 屏障

The placental barrier differs anatomically among various animal species.

不同动物物种的胎盘屏障在解剖学上存在差异。

The body's first line of defence against pathogenic bacteria consists of simple barriers to the entry or establishment of the infection.

机体抵抗病原菌的第一道防线由可以阻挡细菌进入或感染的简单屏障组成。

bartholin [ˈbɑːθəlin] *n.* 前庭大腺(囊肿)

The clinical effects of Bartholin cyst and abscess drainage with insertion of flap were observed.

观察了前庭大腺囊肿或脓肿皮片对穿引流术的临床效果。

bartholinitis [ˌbɑːθəliˈnaitis] *n.* 前庭大腺炎

An 18-month-old infant suffered from the acute bartholinitis caused by Pseudomonas aeruginosa.

1 例 18 月龄婴儿患急性绿脓杆菌性前庭大腺炎。

Bartonella [ˌbɑːtəˈnelə] *n.* 巴通体属

Bartonella, a gram-negative bacterium, has the ability to cause human disease in many different ways.

巴通体属是一类革兰阴性细菌,能以多种不同的方式引起人类疾病。

Bartonellosis is an infectious disease produced by bacteria of the genus Bartonella.

巴通体病是一种由巴通体属细菌引起的传染病。

bartonellosis [ˌbɑːtəneˈləusis] *n.* 巴通体病

This human disease caused by the gram-negative bacterium in many different ways is called Bartonellosis.

这种革兰阴性菌以多种方式引起的人类疾病称为巴通体病。

Bartonellosis is geographic-specific, meaning they all don't occur everywhere.

巴通体病具有地区特异性,也就是说并非所有地方都发生这种病。

barylalia [ˌbæriˈleiliə] *n.* 言语不清

He had barylalia and could only say some simple words.

他言语不清并且仅能说些简单的词。

She developed barylalia about three months ago, had excessive salivation from the left side of her mouth, and experienced a burning sensation on her skin.

她大约 3 个月前发生言语不清,有过度唾液分泌从左侧口角流出,以及皮肤有烧灼感。

basal [ˈbeisəl] 基底的

Basal cell carcinoma usually occurs at sun-exposed sites in aged persons.

基底细胞癌常发生于老年人的阳光暴晒部位。

Basal cell carcinomas are slow-growing and local invasive tumors that rarely metastasize.

基底细胞癌生长缓慢,局部浸润,很少转移。

basaloid [ˈbeisəlɔid] *a.* 基底样的

In cervical carcinoma in situ, the normal epithelium is replaced by atypical basaloid cells.

在宫颈原位癌中,正常上皮被异型的基底样细胞取代。

In basaloid carcinoma, the infiltrating tumor nests are composed of atypical squamous cells that resemble immature cells from the basal layer of the normal epithelium.

在基底样癌，浸润的癌巢由异型的鳞状细胞构成，癌细胞类似正常上皮基底层的不成熟细胞。

base [beis] *n.* 碱

Generally, drugs that are bases are excreted when the urine is acid.

通常当尿液为酸性时，碱性药物被排泄。

baseline ['beislain] *n.* 基线

The baseline assessment included measurements of demographic and health information, smoking behaviors, and psychosocial variables.

基线调查包括人口与健康信息、吸烟行为以及社会心理变量的测试。

Although blinded assessments were conducted at baseline, blinded follow-up evaluations were not possible for two reasons.

尽管在基线时我们使用了盲评，但是因为两个原因不可能在随访中进行盲评。

basement ['beismənt] *n.* 地下室

It is rather damp in the basement.

地下室里很潮湿。

basic ['beisik] *a.* 碱的，盐基的

Most drugs, whether acidic, basic, or neutral in character, are absorbed mainly from the small intestine.

无论是酸性、碱性还是中性，多数药物主要是从小肠吸收的。

basidiomycota [bəˌsidiəu'maikəutɑː] *n.* 担子菌门

Russula subnigricans Hongo is a kind of toxic mushroom, which belongs to Basidiomycota, Agaricales, Russulaceae, Russula.

亚稀褶黑菇是一种毒蘑菇，属担子菌亚门，伞菌目，红菇科，红菇属。

Many species from Basidiomycota and Ascomycota are valuable edible and medicative fungi which deserve to be developed and utilized.

担子菌门和子囊菌门的许多种是可食用和药用真菌，具有开发利用价值。

basidiospore [bə'sidiəuspɔː] *n.* 担孢子

The optimal germinating temperatures were 17 ~ 20℃ for teliospore, 15 ~ 23℃ for basidiospore, and 10 ~ 25℃ for aeciospore.

孢子发芽的最适温度为：冬孢子 17 ~ 20℃，担孢子 15 ~ 23℃，锈孢子 10 ~ 25℃。

Single teliospore or basidiospore has no resistance to dry condition in which the single spore died completely within 1 ~ 2 days.

单个冬孢子及担孢子不耐干燥，1 ~ 2 天便全部死亡。

basophilia [ˌbeisə'filiə] *n.* 嗜碱性，嗜碱粒细胞增多

At high power, the reason for the basophilia is clear: the thymus is packed with lymphocytes with darkly stained nuclei.

在高倍镜下，其嗜碱性的原因很明显，是因为胸腺内充满了核深染的淋巴细胞。

Note that excessive basophilia in chronic myeloid leukaemia may indicate the transformation into an accelerated or blastic phase.

需注意在慢性髓细胞性白血病时过度的嗜碱性粒细胞增多可能提示疾病向加速期或急变期转化。

bathe [beið] *v.* 沐浴，冲洗；把…沉浸在液体中

Children should bathe regularly in order to keep the body clean.

儿童应经常洗澡以便保持身体清洁。

The plasma exudes through the thin capillary walls and bathes the surrounding tissues.

血浆通过毛细血管的薄壁渗出并浸泡周围的组织。

The doctor told him to bathe his eyes with the lotion twice a day.

医生叫他用洗液每天冲洗眼睛两次。

battery [ˈbætəri] *n.* 电池;一组,一套,一副;一系列,一连串;一群,一批

The artificial cardiac pacemaker functions in initiating the electrical impulses generated by small batteries.

人工心脏起搏器是由小电池所发动的电冲动激发的。

When these drug safety programs include registries, which often prospectively collect a battery of information using standardized instruments.

当这些药品安全规划中包含注册登记时,后者往往会用标准化手段前瞻性收集一系列相关信息。

Bdellovibrio [ˌdeləˈvibriəu] *n.* 蛭弧菌

The four Bdellovibrio strains broke down 15 out of 16 pathogens, amounting to 93. 8% lysis ability.

4 株蛭弧菌可裂解 16 株病原菌中的 15 株,裂解率达 93. 8% 。

Researchers in China mostly study the Bdellovibrio for applying in aquatic products.

中国的研究人员大多研究蛭弧菌应用于水产品。

beam [biːm] *n.* (光)束

Lasers are devices which produce pure, intensive beams of light or radiation.

激光是能产生纯而密度极大的光束或辐射的装置。

Ultravidet of 365nm wavelength is obtained by passing the beam through a Wood' s Filter composed of nickel oxide-containing glass.

365nm 波长的紫外线光束是通过含氧化镍玻璃的伍氏滤器得来的。

bear [bɛə] *v.* 承担;具有;忍受

The head nurse of a ward bears a heavy load of responsibility at all times.

病房护士长总是承担着重大的责任。

beargall [ˈbɛəgɔːl] *n.* 熊胆

We use FDMS to control the quality of beargall.

我们用场解吸质谱(FDMS)的方法来控制熊胆的质量。

We study the quality control and fingerprint of beargall pill.

我们研究了熊胆丸的质量控制及指纹图谱。

bearing [ˈbɛəriŋ] *n.* 忍耐;关系,联系

All past illnesses may have an important bearing on the present illness.

所有既往的疾病与现在的病都可能有重要的联系。

beclomethasone [ˌbekləuˈmeθəsəun] *n.* 丙酸倍氯米松

50 cases were treated with beclomethasone dipropionate aerosol.

50 例用二丙酸倍氯米松气雾剂治疗。

becquerel [bekəˈrel] *n.* 贝克(勒尔)(放射性强度的国际制单位)

The becquerel is named after Henri Becquerel, who shared a Nobel Prize with Pierre and Marie Curie in 1903 for their work in discovering radioactivity.

贝克勒尔以亨利・贝克勒尔的名字命名,亨利・贝克勒尔与皮埃尔和玛丽・居里因为发现放射现象而在 1903 年共享诺贝尔奖。

One becquerel is defined as the activity of a quantity of radioactive material in which one nucleus decays per second.

1 贝克勒耳被定义为一些放射性物质每秒发生一个核衰变时的(放射性)活度。

bedpan [ˈbedpæn] *n.* 便盆

Patients who are recovering from myocardial infraction and others should not be forced to use a bedpan if it is possible to move them from bed to bedside toilet.

心肌损害和其他正处于恢复期的病人,如能起床去床边厕所,就不应强迫他们使用便盆。

bedsore [ˈbedsɔː] *n.* 褥疮

The nurse should have the patients changing their recumbent positions frequently so as to prevent

bedsore.
护士应让病人不断地改变躺卧的体位以预防褥疮。

beeswax [ˈbiːzwæks] *n.* 蜂蜡

Beeswax is a tough wax formed from a mixture of several compounds.
蜂蜡是由几种化合物混合形成一种硬蜡。

Beeswax is used commercially to make fine candles.
蜂蜡的商业用途是制造精致的蜡烛。

beforehand [biˈfɔːhænd] *ad.* 预先

Please accept our thanks beforehand for the favor of an early reply.
请预先接受我们对早日赐复的谢意。

Glucose is also detected in most insulin assays and must be either removed beforehand or measured independently in the sample.
在大多数检测胰岛素的方法中也可测到葡萄糖，必须先去除或单独测定标本中的葡萄糖。

behavio(u)r [biˈheivjə] *n.* 行为，举止

This was the first hint that chromosomal abnormality could affect behaviour.
这是染色体异常可能影响行为的第一个暗示。

The term disturbance of conduct should be used for abnormal behaviour in individuals of any age.
行为障碍这一术语应当用于不论有多大年岁者的人的异常行为。

Studies reveal that a physician's advice alone can substantially influence smoking behaviour.
有研究表明仅仅是医生的建议就能使有吸烟行为的人受到重要影响。

behavioral [biˈheivjərəl] *a.* 行为的

From behavioral quirks to brain cancer, researchers have looked for any health risks associated with cellphone radiation for years.
从行为怪癖到脑癌，数年来研究人员一直在寻找与手机辐射有关的健康风险。

Research has shown that physical abuse during childhood is associated with various mental and behavioral problems in adolescence.
研究显示童年时期的身体虐待与青少年时期的多种精神和行为问题有关。

belch [beltʃ] *v.* 打嗝；喷出

The doctor explained to the patient how to treat ceaseless belch.
医生向病人解释如何治疗不停的打嗝。

Belching (also known as burping, ructus, or eructation) is the release of gas from the digestive tract (mainly esophagus and stomach) through the mouth.
打嗝是消化道（主要是食管和胃）通过嘴释放气体。

belching [ˈbeltʃiŋ] *n.* 嗳气

In patients with a complaint of chronic belching, each belch can often be observed to be preceded by a swallow of air.
长期嗳气的病人，在每次嗳气前常可见到吞咽空气的动作。

belladonna [ˌbeləˈdɔnə] *n.* 颠茄

Belladonna usually gives relief in such cases.
在这种病例中，服用颠茄往往可以缓解病情。

belly [ˈbeli] *n.* 肚，腹部，胃

It was thought that only the brain produced this hormone, but no, your belly fat can make it too.
这种荷尔蒙被认为产生于大脑，但是不，你的肚子脂肪也可以产生它。

One technique is belly breathing, which fills the lungs completely and speeds vital oxygen to the brain.

其中一个技巧为“腹部呼吸”，它使肺部吸满空气并加速将维持生命必需的氧气输送到大脑。

benadryl [ˈbenədril] *n.* 苯海拉明(商品名，抗组胺药)

IM(intramuscularly) benadryl is satisfactory to prevent further reactions, but does not reverse on-going inflammation.

肌肉注射苯海拉明对于防止反应进一步发展是令人满意的，但却不能使正在进展中的炎症逆转。

benchmark [ˈbentʃˌmɑːk] *n.* 基准

The benchmark dose method has been proposed as an alternative to the no-observed-adverse-effect level (NOAEL) approach for assessing noncancer risks associated with hazardous compounds.

基准剂量方法被建议替代无明显有害作用水平(NOAEL)方法来评价有害物的非致癌危险度。

In the United States the U. S. Environmental Protection Agency (EPA) already uses the benchmark dose in health risk assessment.

美国环境保护局已使用基准剂量作健康风险评价。

This absorbed dose is used in conjunction with a soil exposure scenario to derive the benchmark soil concentration of hydrogen cyanide.

吸收剂量结合土壤暴露情况得出氰化氢的土壤基准浓度。

beneficence [biˈnefisəns] *n.* 善行，有利

These principles are respect for persons, beneficence, and justice.

这些原则是尊重人、善行和公正。

beneficial [ˌbeniˈfiʃəl] *a.* 有利的，有益的

Athletic sports are beneficial to the health.

体育运动有益于健康。

The activation of complement by immune complexes is normally beneficial.

免疫复合物激活补体通常有利于机体。

Splenectomy is beneficial when the RBC defect is associated with selective splenic sequestration.

如红细胞缺陷与选择性脾潴留有关则宜行脾切除术。

The antiinflammatory effects of the corticosteroids are markedly beneficial.

皮质类固醇的抗炎效果明显。

benign [biˈnain] *a.* 良性的

Duodenal ulcers are virtually always benign.

十二指肠溃疡通常是良性的。

Such a close resemblance is especially true in benign tumours.

这种相似性尤其多见于良性肿瘤。

bentonite [ˈbentənait] *n.* 硅皂土，膨润土

Bentonite was investigated to remove Ni(Ⅱ) from aqueous solutions because of its strong sorption ability.

膨润土因其强大的吸附功能而被研究用于去除水溶液中的镍(Ⅱ)。

On bentonite, calcium carbonate and humic acid no significant sorption was observed.

膨润土对碳酸钙和腐殖酸没有显著的吸附作用。

benzene [ˈbenziːn, benˈziːn] *n.* 苯

On the contrary, benzene hexachloride and several related compounds frequently produce illness in which a convulsion is the first sign of injury.

相反，六氯苯和几种有关化合物致病时，惊厥往往是损伤的第一个体征。

benzidine [ˈbenziˌdiːn] *n.* 联苯胺

In the present study, the expression of nuclear mitotic apparatus protein 22 (NMP22) in workers

occupationally exposed to benzidine was investigated.
本文研究了联苯胺职业接触人群中核有丝分裂器蛋白22(NMP22)的表达情况。
Benzidine has been linked to bladder and pancreatic cancer.
联苯胺与膀胱癌和胰腺癌的发生有关。

benzoate [ˈbenzəeit] *n.* 苯甲酸盐
Treatment with intravenous caffeine sodium benzoate given over a few minutes as a 500mg dose will terminate headache in 75 percent of patients.
每隔数分钟静脉给予500mg苯甲酸钠咖啡因可以使75%的病人终止头痛。

benzodiazepine [ˌbenzəudaiˈæzəpiːn] *n.* 苯二氮䓬类,地西泮
Benzodiazepine is a psychoactive drug whose core chemical structure is the fusion of a benzene ring and a diazepine ring.
苯二氮䓬类是一类精神科药物,其核心化学结构是融合了的苯环和氮的杂合环。
Benzodiazepines enhance the effect of the neurotransmitter gamma-aminobutyric acid (GABA).
苯二氮䓬类药物能够增强抑制性神经递质γ-氨基丁酸的作用。

benzofuran [ˌbenzəuˈfjurən] *n.* 苯并呋喃
Benzofuran is the heterocyclic compound consisting of fused benzene and furan rings.
苯并呋喃是由稠苯环和呋喃环组成的杂环化合物。
Dronedarone is a benzofuran derivative of amiodarone that has been developed for the treatment of atrial fibrillation and atrial flutter.
决奈达隆作为胺碘酮的一种苯并呋喃衍生物已经用于治疗心房纤维性颤动和心房扑动。

benzoic [benˈzəuik] *a.* 苯甲酸的
Benzoic acid and cobalt chloride are reported to be causes of type 1 allergic responses.
苯甲酸和氯化钴已被报道是引起Ⅰ型超敏反应的原因。

benzoin [ˈbenzəuin] *n.* 安息香
The pain of acute tracheitis usually responds to the inhalations of steam medicated with benzoin.
急性气管炎引起的胸痛,通常吸入安息香药物蒸气即可缓解。
Other fixatives which may be used include the oleoresins such as benzoin, or styrax.
其他可用的固定剂包括安息香或苏合香等含油树脂。
We study the synthesis and properties of siloxane containing benzoin ether group.
我们研究含有安息香醚的硅氧烷的合成及性能。

benzopyrene [ˌbenzəuˈpairiːn] *n.* 苯并芘
A vast number of studies have documented links between benzo [a] pyrene and cancers.
大量研究表明苯并芘和癌症之间存在着联系。
Properly speaking, benzopyrene is a procarcinogen.
确切地说,苯并芘是一种前致癌物。

berberine [ˈbəːbəriːn] *n.* 黄连素,小檗碱
Determine the content of berberine hydrochloride tablets.
请测定盐酸小檗碱片的含量。
We get to study the hypoglycemic action of the berberine and its clinical efficacy.
我们要研究小檗碱(黄连素)的降血糖作用及临床疗效。

bereave [biˈriːv] *v.* 使丧失(亲人等)
Usually, bereaved persons feel that the depressed mood is normal.
通常,沮丧的人觉得忧郁情绪是正常的。

bereavement [biˈriːvmənt] *n.* (亲人等的)丧失
Bereavement means deprivation, leaving a sad or lonely state due to loss or death.
丧亲意为丧失,因丧失或死亡而使人处于悲伤或孤独状态。

beriberi [ˌberiˈberi] *n.* 脚气(病)
Among such deficiency diseases are rickets, beriberi, scurvy, anemia, to mention just a few.

在这类缺乏症中有佝偻病、脚气病、坏血病、贫血，仅列举这几种。

beryllium [bə'riljəm] *n.* 铍

Beryllium is used primarily as a hardening agent in alloys, notably beryllium copper.

铍主要用来作为合金硬化剂，特别是铜铍合金。

The high thermal conductivity of beryllium and beryllium oxide has led to their widely use in heat transport and heat sinking applications.

铍及铍氧化物的高导热性使其已广泛应用于热传输和散热。

beta ['beitə] *n.* 贝塔，希腊字母第二个字母 β

Each emission of an alpha or beta ray accompanies the transmutation of an atom; because the energy communicated to these rays comes from inside the atom.

每一次 α 射线或 β 射线的放射都伴随着原子的蜕变，因为赋予给这些射线的能量来自于原子的内部。

Beta cells make and release insulin, a hormone that controls the level of glucose in the blood.

β 细胞生成和释放胰岛素，后者是一种控制血液中葡萄糖水平的激素。

beverage ['bevəridʒ] *n.* 饮料

Some individuals gulp air excessively because of chronic anxiety, rapid eating and drinking carbonated beverages.

有些人因为长期焦虑不安、快速进食以及饮用碳酸饮料而大口吞咽空气。

beware(of) [bi'wɛə] *v.* 谨防，当心

Hypertensive persons must beware of constipation.

高血压病人必须预防便秘。

Beware of cosmetics that purportedly aid the skin in breathing.

要小心那些据称帮助皮肤呼吸的化妆品。

bezoar ['biːzɔː] *n.* 牛黄(解毒剂)

Where would you look for it if I asked you to find bezoar?

如果我要你拿一块牛黄，你要到哪找？

The free and total cholesterol contents in three kinds of bezoar are between 0.072% to 0.214% and 0.546% to 0.608% respectively.

三批天然牛黄的测定结果为：游离胆固醇含量 0.072% ~ 0.214%，总胆固醇含量 0.546% ~ 0.608%。

bias ['baiəs] *n.* 偏见，偏向；偏移

Girls exceed boys in language abilities, and this early linguistic bias often prevails throughout life.

女孩的语言能力超过男孩，这种早期的语言偏向常常在一生中都占优势。

Dr. Li discusses some strategies for detecting bias: analysis of variance, Chi square and so on.

李博士论述为检测偏倚所用的某些对策，如方差分析、卡方检测等。

Inverted funnel plots and the Egger's test were used to examine the influence of publication bias.

倒漏斗图以及 Egger 检验用来检测发表性偏倚的影响。

Zhang et al. considered the possibility that selection bias may have led them to overestimate the strength of the association between cannabis smoking and this cancer.

Zhang 等人认为选择性偏移可能使得他们高估了吸食大麻和该肿瘤之间的关联强度。

v. 使有偏见

Some doctors were biased against essential medicines.

某些医生曾对基本药物有偏见。

biatrial [ˌbai'eitriəl] *a.* 两心房的

Electrocardiography reveals evidence of biatrial and biventricular enlargement.

心电图显示(心脏的)两房和两室扩大。

biaxial [bai'æksiəl] *a.* 二轴的

Condyloid joints are biaxial joints which allow movement in two directions.

髁状关节为双轴性关节,可容许骨向两个方向运动。

bicarbonate [bai'kɑːbənit] *n.* 重碳酸盐

Many medicines for the relief of pain, indigestion and constipation contain bicarbonates that neutralize the acid in the stomach.

许多可以缓解疼痛、消化不良和便秘的药物(几乎)都含有中和胃酸的重碳酸盐。

An alkali such as sodium bicarbonate may relieve the pain to an even greater degree.

碱性物质如重碳酸钠可更有效地减轻疼痛。

bicuspid [bai'kʌspid] *a.* 二尖的 *n.* 二尖瓣;双尖牙

The left atrium now contracts and forces the blood over the open bicuspid valve into the left ventricle, as is described for the right side of the heart.

左心房收缩迫使血液经过开着的二尖瓣进入左心室,就如同对心脏右边所描述的一样。

bidirectional [ˌbaidi'rekʃənəl] *a.* 两个方向的,双向的

This is a bidirectional model of DNA replication in eukaryotes.

这是真核生物的 DNA 双向复制的模型。

bidirectionally [ˌbaidi'rekʃənəli] *ad.* 两个方向地,双向地

DNA duplication proceeds bidirectionally starting from a fixed origin of replication.

DNA 的复制是从一个固定的复制起点开始向两个方向进行的。

bifendate [ˌbai'fendeit] *n.* 联苯双酯

The method of emulsification-evaporation was appropriate for the preparation of bifendate-loaded solid lipid nanoparticles.

乳化蒸发法适用于带有联苯双酯固体脂质纳米粒的制备。

Bifendate pills are indicated for the treatment of chronic persistent hepatitis with increased ALT.

联苯双酯片可用于治疗谷丙转氨酶升高的慢性持续性肝炎。

bifunctional [bai'fʌŋkʃənəl] *a.* 双功能的

All antibodies are bifunctional.

所有的抗体都具有双重功能。

Each immunoglobulin molecule is bifunctional.

每一个免疫球蛋白分子都具有双重功能。

One mRNA may synthesize two kinds of protein, this mRNA is called bifunctional.

一个信使核糖核酸(mRNA)可以合成两种蛋白质,此 mRNA 则被称为双功能的(核糖核酸)。

bilateral [bai'lætərəl] *a.* 两侧的,双侧的

This pathologic process may be unilateral or bilateral, and generally begins in the deep calf veins.

这种病理过程可以是单侧的或双侧的,通常开始于深部腓肠静脉。

Proliferation of lymphocytes in lacrimal and salivary glands may cause bilateral painless enlargement.

泪腺和唾液腺内淋巴细胞增生可引起两侧腺体无痛性肿大。

bilaterally [bai'lætərəli] *ad.* 两侧,双向地

Neck was supple with absence of cervical lymph nodes bilaterally.

颈软且两侧颈淋巴结无肿大。

bilayer ['baileiə] *n.* 双 [分子] 层

Phospholipids dispersed in water tend to interact to form bilayers.

分散在水中的磷脂具有相互作用形成双[分子]层的倾向。

bile [bail] *n.* 胆汁

Long-continued cholestasis can lead to cirrhosis from the harmful effect of retained bile upon the

hepatocytes.
长期持续性胆汁郁积,可因潴留的胆汁对肝细胞的损害作用而引起肝硬化。
Liver secretion contains large amounts of bile salts.
肝分泌液含有大量胆盐。

biliary ['biljəri] *a.* 胆的,胆管的,胆囊的
The onset after a heavy meal is one of the distinguishing features in biliary colic.
饱餐后发病是胆绞痛的显著特征之一。

bilioenteric [ˌbiljəen'terik] *a.* 胆肠的
Myofibroblast is the main cause to result in scar contracture of bilioenteric anastomosis.
肌成纤维细胞是导致胆肠吻合口瘢痕性挛缩的主要原因。
In the research, they observed histological changes of healing process after bilioenteric anastomosis.
在该研究中,他们观察了胆肠吻合术后愈合过程的组织学变化。

bilious ['biljəs] *a.* 胆汁的
Fatty food makes some people bilious.
多脂肪食物可使某些人患胆汁病。
The most common symptoms are abdominal distension and bilious vomiting.
常见的症状有腹胀和胆汁性呕吐。

bilirubin [ˌbili'ru:bin] *n.* 胆红素
There are three main constituents in gall stones: cholesterol, bilirubin and calcium.
胆石有三种主要成分:胆固醇、胆红素和钙质。
Investigation of blood of jaundice patient shows a high alkaline phosphatase and a high bilirubin.
检查黄疸病人血液显示碱性磷酸酶和胆红素很高。

bilirubinuria [ˌbiliru:bi'njuəriə] *n.* 胆红素尿
Bilirubinuria often precedes a noticeable yellow tint and may be the only indication of mild jaundice.
胆红素尿往往发生在显著黄染之前,并且可能是轻度黄疸的惟一指征。

billion ['biljən] *n.* ,*a.* (美)10 亿; 大量,无数
China has a population of more than 1. 3 billion.
中国有 13 亿多人口。
The human body is composed of thousands of billions of cells.
人体是由无数细胞组成的。

bimolecular [ˌbaimə'lekjulə] *a.* 双分子的
Recent research has confirmed the bimolecular structure of the lipid part of the plasma membrane.
近来的研究证实,质膜由双分子层脂质构成。

binder ['baində] *n.* 结合剂
In the one-site assay, the excess antibody that is not bound to the sample is removed by addition of a precipitating binder.
采用一位点测定法时,未与样品结合的剩余的抗体可用加入沉淀结合剂(的方法)来除去。

binding ['baindiŋ] *n.* 结合
The binding of drug to plasma protein is not usually a disadvantage.
药物与血浆蛋白相结合并不一定是缺点。
Some drugs may alter the protein binding of other agents.
有些药物可以改变另一些药物与蛋白质的结合。

binomial [bai'nəumjəl] *n.* 双名法;二项式 a. 双名的;二项式的
Biologists have adopted the binomial system of nomenclature.

生物学家已经接受了(生物)命名的双名法系统。

binucleate [bai'nju:kliit;-eit] *a.* 双核的

Regenerative hepatocytes are usually binucleate with prominent nucleoli.

再生的肝细胞往往是双核,核仁突出。

Mirror image cells are binucleate Reed-Sternberg cells that are specific and diagnostic in Hodgkin lymphoma.

镜影细胞是双核的 R-S 细胞,是霍奇金淋巴瘤特异的和诊断性的肿瘤细胞。

bioaccumulation [ˌbaiəuəkju:mju'leiʃən] *n.* 生物累积,生物浓缩

Bioaccumulation occurs when an organism absorbs a toxic substance at a rate greater than that at which the substance is lost.

单个有机体吸收的某有毒物质的速率大于失去该物质的速率称为生物累积。

Coastal fish and seabirds are often monitored for heavy metal bioaccumulation.

海鱼和海鸟体内常可监测到重金属的生物累积。

Bioaccumulation occurs within a trophic level, and is the increase in concentration of a substance in certain tissues of organisms' bodies due to absorption from food and the environment.

生物浓缩存在某个营养级别范围,指的是在生物体内某组织中由食物和环境中摄取的物质浓度的增加。

bioactivation [ˌbaiəuˌækti'veiʃen] *n.* 生物活化(作用)

Genotoxic carcinogens usually require bioactivation to reactive intermediates before eventually producing DNA adducts in target cells.

遗传毒性致癌物,在靶细胞最终产生 DNA 加合物之前,通常需要生物活化成反应性中间产物。

bioaerosol [baiəu'eərəˌsɔ:l] *n.* 生物气溶胶

A bioaerosol is a suspension of airborne particles that contain living organisms.

生物气溶胶是含有活的有机物的空气颗粒物的悬浮物。

Bioaerosols can be a source of microbial pathogens, endotoxins, and other allergens.

生物气溶胶可以作为病原微生物,内毒素和其他过敏原的来源。

bioaminergic [ˌbaiəuˌæmi'nə:dʒik] *a.* 生物胺能的

The neurons that secrete biogenic amines is bioaminergic.

可以分泌生物源性胺的神经细胞被称为生物胺能的(细胞)。

bioamplification [ˌbaiəuˌæmplifi'keiʃən] *n.* 生物扩增,生物放大

After bioamplification for 5 times, 24 positive clones were obtained from 60 clones screened randomly.

经过 5 次生物扩增,从随机筛选的 60 个克隆中获得了 24 个阳性克隆。

Bioaccumulation and bioamplification of mercury compounds occurred in a second level consumer.

汞化合物的生物蓄积和生物扩增过去发生于二手物品消费者中。

Bioamplification, or biomagnification, is the process that results in the increase in concentration of a pollutant from one trophic level in a food chain to another.

生物放大是指污染物在食物链中从一个营养级别到另一个营养级别其浓度增加的过程。

The present study quantified polychlorinated biphenyl (PCB) bioamplification in male and female mayflies at three sites.

本文在三个地点对多氯联苯(PCB)在雄性和雌性蜉蝣中的生物放大进行了定量研究。

bioassay [ˌbaiəuə'sei] *n.* 生物测定,生物测试

Within this project, all the six gasoline oxygenated additives, alone or blended with gasoline, have been submitted to long-term carcinogenicity bioassays.

在这个科研项目中,全部六种汽油氧化添加剂(单一或与汽油混和在一起)都已提交了长期致癌性的生物检测报告。

Bioassay typically were of 2 years duration and utilized B6C3F1 mice or Sprague-Dawley or Fisher 344 rats, although other strains were also used.
典型的生物测试期为两年,使用 B6C3F1 小鼠,或 Sprague-Dawley 或 Fisher 344 大鼠,尽管也有使用其他种属的。

bioavailability [ˌbaiəuəˌveilə'biliti] *n.* 生物利用度
The oral bioavailability of numerous drugs has been increased by a reduction in particle size.
药物的颗粒减小,可使许多药物的口服生物利用度提高。

biochemical [ˌbaiəu'kemikəl] *a.* 生物化学的,生化的
Vitamins are a class of biochemical compounds essential for normal growth and development.
维生素是正常生长和发育所必需的一类生化化合物。
The classification system used here is based on major morphological and biochemical properties.
此处采用的分类系统依据的是细菌的主要形态和生化性质。

biochemistry [ˌbaiəu'kemistri] *n.* 生物化学
The aspect of the biochemistry of this hormone is developing rapidly.
这种激素的生物化学方面的发展是迅速的。
They completed doctoral thesis in biochemistry on different topics under the same supervisor.
他们在同一个导师指导下完成了在生物化学方面不同题目的博士论文

biocompatibility [ˌbaiəukəmˌpæti'biliti] *n.* 生物适应性
All these factors are then subject to the overriding requirements of medical safety, biocompatibility of absorbent and so on.
所有这些因素应服从于医疗安全、吸附剂的生物相容性等压倒一切的需要。

bioconcentration [ˌbaiəukɔnsən'treiʃən] *n.* 生物浓缩
Bioconcentration is defined as occurring when uptake from the water is greater than excretion.
生物浓缩的定义是从水中的摄取量大于排泄量。
Thus bioconcentration and bioaccumulation occur within an organism, and biomagnification occurs across trophic (food chain) levels.
生物浓缩和生物累积发生在单个有机体内,生物放大则是发生在食物链的整个营养级别。

biodefense [ˌbaiəudi'fens] *n.* 生物防护
Starting this month, the US Food and Drug Administration(FDA) has lowered the bar for biodefense drugs.
从这个月开始,美国食品和药物管理局(FDA)降低了生物防护药物的标准。

biodegradable [ˌbaiəudi'greidəbl] *a.* 生物可降解的
The dermal matter is grown in a sterile plastic bag that contains a biodegradable mesh.
皮肤代用物是在盛有生物降解作用的网状物的无菌塑料袋中培育的。
The engineering process involves making a mesh of biodegradable suture material similar to that used by surgeons in operations.
工程设计的过程包括设计一种网状的可生物降解的缝线材料,类似外科医生在外科手术中使用的缝线材料。

biodegradation ['baiəuˌdegrə'deiʃən] *n.* 生物降解(作用)
Microorganisms play important roles in biodegradation.
微生物在生物降解方面起着重要作用。
Is biodegradation the same as biotransformation?
生物降解与生物转化是相同的吗?
Biodegradation or biotic degradation or biotic decomposition is the chemical dissolution of materials by bacteria or other biological means.
生物降解是指物质借助细菌或其他生物学方法发生的化学分解。
To be able to work effectively, most microorganisms that assist the biodegradation need light, water and oxygen.

为了能够有效发挥作用，大多数促使生物降解的微生物需要光，水和氧气。

biodiversity [ˌbaiəudaiˈvəːsəti] *n.* 生物多样性

Biologists most often define biodiversity as the "totality of genes, species, and ecosystems of a region".

生物学家常将生物多样性定义为"一个地区的基因、物种和生态系统的整体"。

Biodiversity is the result of 3.5 billion years of evolution.

生物多样性是 35 亿年生物进化的结果。

biodynamics [ˌbaiəudaiˈnæmiks] *n.* 生物动力学

The science that study the nature and determinants of all organismic behavior is Biodynamics.

研究有机体行为的本质和决定因素的科学被称作生物动力学。

bioelectricity [ˌbaiəuilekˈtrisiti] *n.* 生物电

Bioelectricity may appear in muscle and nerve tissue.

生物电现象可以出现于肌肉或神经组织。

bioencapsulation [ˌbaiəuinˌkæpsjuˈleiʃən] *n.* 生物包裹

Bioencapsulation has provided a range of promising therapeutic treatments for diabetes, cancer and renal failure.

生物包裹技术为糖尿病、癌症和肾功能衰竭提供了一系列有效的治疗方法。

bioenergetics [ˌbaiəuˌenəˈdʒetiks] *n.* 生物能学

This paper introduced the measurement of revolution, bioenergetics and the dynamics.

该论文介绍了转速测量、生物能学以及动力学。

Bioenergetics is the subject of a field of biochemistry that concerns energy flow through living systems.

生物能学是生物化学领域中的一个学科，研究通过生物体系的能量流。

bioengineer [ˈbaiəuˌendʒiˈniə] *n.* 生物工程师

A useful contribution can be made by bioengineers to the overall problem of liver disease.

生物工程学者对肝脏疾患的全盘问题能作出有益的贡献。

bioengineering [ˈbaiəuˌendʒiˈniəriŋ] *n.* 生物工程学

Despite the many recent advances in bioengineering, much remains to be done.

尽管生物工程学已获得了许多新进展，但还有许多工作有待去做。

bioenrichment [ˌbaiəuinˈritʃmənt] *n.* 生物富集，生物浓缩

Because rice is a staple food in China, selenium-enriched rice obtained by bioenrichment of selenium to increase the Se content of rice could be a good selenium source for the population in selenium-deficient regions.

大米是中国的主食，富硒大米由于硒的生物富集而使大米中的含硒量增加，可以作为缺硒地区人群补硒的理想来源。

We study the important factor and resolution methods which influence quality during the process of bioenrichment selenium tea beverage.

我们研究了在富硒茶饮料生产过程中影响其品质的重要因素和解决方法。

bioequivalence [ˌbaiəuiˈkwivələns] *n.* 生物等效性

This research group investigates the bioequivalence of loratadine tablets in healthy volunteers.

该研究小组研究氯雷他定在健康志愿者中的生物等效性。

During development of generic product, similar safety and efficacy as reference product is usually proven in bioequivalence study.

在一般产品研制过程中，生物等效性试验常可确证其与对照品相似的安全性和有效性。

Interchangeability of drugs is determined by bioequivalence studies.

药物的可替换性取决于其生物等效性研究。

bioethics [ˈbaiəueθiks] *n.* 生命伦理学；生物伦理学

Activities include the development of standards for patient rights, admission, discharge practices, management of conflict of interest, clinical decision making, and bioethics education and services.

这些活动包括针对下列项目制定一些标准:患者权利、入院、出院手续、利益冲突处理、临床决策的制定、以及生命伦理学教育和服务。

The committee decided to broaden education in bioethics.

委员会决定拓展生物伦理学的教育。

We read it in a recent report on bioethics.

我们在最近的一篇生物伦理学报道中读到它。

biofeedback [ˌbaiəuˈfiːdbæk] *n.* 生物反馈

Information as "reinforcement" plays a significant role in biofeedback.

信息增强在生物反馈中起重要作用。

biofilm [ˌbaiəuˈfilm] *n.* 生物膜

The isolation rate of ESBLs producing strains in klebsiella biofilm were 42. 5%.

超光谱 β-内酰胺酶在具有生物膜的肺炎克雷伯菌中检出率为 42. 5%。

The challenge is that bioburden and biofilm often go unchecked, leading to an unrecognized infection.

我们所面临的挑战是,对生物负荷和生物膜往往不做检查,导致无法识别的感染。

A biofilm is an aggregate of microorganisms in which cells adhere to each other on the surface.

生物膜是附着在表面的细胞黏合在一起的一种微生物群落。

Biofilms may form on living or non-living surfaces and can be prevalent in natural, industrial and hospital settings.

活性和非活性的附着面都可以形成生物膜,它在自然界、工业和医疗设施中都广泛存在。

biogas [ˈbaiəugæs] *n.* 沼气

Biogas typically refers to a gas produced by the biological breakdown of organic matter in the absence of oxygen.

沼气是在缺氧条件下由有机物生物分解而产生的气体。

The methane contained within biogas is 20 times more potent as a greenhouse gas than is carbon dioxide.

沼气中含有的甲烷,与温室效应气体一样,比二氧化碳强 20 倍以上。

bioinformatics [ˌbaiəuˌinfəˈmætiks] *n.* 生物信息学

Bioinformatics is the application of computer science and information technology to the field of biology and medicine.

生物信息学是计算机科学与信息技术在生物学和医学上的应用。

The primary goal of bioinformatics is to increase the understanding of biological processes.

生物信息学的主要目的是加深对生物过程的理解。

Bioinformatics is fundamental to the modern day study of biology and essential to 21st century biomedical research.

生物信息学是当今生物学研究的基础,也是 21 世纪生物医学研究的基础。

The leading journal in its field, *bioinformatics* publishes the highest quality scientific papers.

作为该领域一流的杂志,《生物信息学》发表最高质量的科学研究论文。

Assembly of the human genome is one of the greatest achievements of bioinformatics.

人类基因组拼接是生物信息学的最大成就之一。

The topology prediction of transmembrane protein is a hot in bioinformatics.

跨膜蛋白拓扑结构预测是生物信息学的研究热点之一。

The European Bioinformatics Institute (EBI) is a centre for research and services in bioinformatics, and is part of European Molecular Biology Laboratory (EMBL).

欧洲生物信息学中心(EBI)是一个信息学研究和服务中心,是欧洲分子生物学实验室(EMBL)的一部分。

biological [ˌbaiəˈlɔdʒikəl] *a.* 生物学的

Numerous biological studies have been carried out using the radioisotope technique.

已采用放射性同位素技术进行了大量的生物学研究。

It is quite interesting that these one-cell animals carry on complex biological functions.

非常有趣的是这些单细胞动物执行着复杂的生物学功能。

Scientists have discovered some very interesting facts about biological clock.

科学家们已经发现了有关生物钟的一些有趣事实。

biologist [baiˈɔlədʒist] *n.* 生物学家

Mr. Blom is a noted biologist in the world.

布洛姆先生是一位世界知名的生物学家。

biology [baiˈɔlədʒi] *n.* 生物学

The era of transplantation produced the most fantastic change in the history of biology and medicine.

(器官)移植的时代使生物学和医学的历史产生了极大的变化。

biomacromolecule [ˌbaiəuˌmækrəuˈmɔlikjuːl] *n.* 生物大分子

Some carcinogens react with nucleophilic biomacromolecules to form adducts.

一些致癌物与亲核的生物大分子反应形成加合物。

biomagnification [ˈbaiəuˌmægnifiˈkeiʃən] *n.* 生物放大

Suedel et al. (1994) concluded that although biomagnification is probably more limited in occurrence than previously thought, there is good evidence that DDT, DDE, PCBs, toxaphene, and the organic forms of mercury and arsenic do biomagnify in nature.

1994 年 Suedel 等人指出,尽管生物放大的发生远较预期的少,但已有证据表明,DDT、DDE、多氯联苯、毒杀芬、有机汞和砷的确在自然界中发生了生物放大。

The success of top predatory-bird recovery (bald eagles, peregrine falcons) in North America following the ban on DDT use in agriculture is testament to the importance of biomagnification.

在北美,农业上禁止使用 DDT 后,顶端肉食鸟(白头鹰,游隼)数量的恢复证明了生物放大作用的重要性。

biomarker [ˌbaiəuˈmɑːkə] *n.* 生物标志物

The National Academy of Sciences defines a biomarker as a xenobiotically induced alteration in cellular or biochemical components that is measurable in a biological system or sample.

国家科学院定义"生物标志物"为外源化合物所诱导的可在生物系统或样品中测量到的细胞成分或生化成分的改变。

biomedical [ˌbaiəuˈmedikəl] *a.* 生物医学的

It is indeed a pleasure to welcome you to the fifth in the series of Biomedical Research Symposia held in Groton.

我怀着极其愉快的心情欢迎您们出席在格洛顿举行的生物医学系列研讨会的第五次会议。

biomethylation [ˈbaiəumeθilˈleiʃən] *n.* 生物甲基化作用

Methylcobalamin (methyl-B12) has been implicated in the biomethylation of the heavy metals (mercury, tin, platinum, gold, and thallium) as well as the metalloids (arsenic, selenium, tellurium and sulfur).

甲钴胺参与了重金属(汞、锡、铂、金、铊)和类金属(砷、硒、碲、硫)的生物甲基化作用。

Biomethylation of mercury is reportedly increased by lower pH.

据报道,在低 pH 条件下汞的生物甲基化作用是增加的。

biomimetic [ˈbaiəumiˈmetik] *a.* 仿生的

The high performance inorganic materials synthesized in the biomimetic ways have established the focus of biomimetic synthesis technology in the material chemistry field.

以仿生方式合成无机材料的高性能使得仿生合成技术成为材料化学领域的热点。

biomimetics [ˈbaiəumiˈmetiks] *n.* 生体模仿学

Biomimetics is the study of the structure and function of biological systems as models for the design and engineering of materials and machines.

生体模仿学是一门以生物系统的结构与功能作为模型对材料和机器设计和工程进行研究的学科。

biomonitoring [ˈbaiəuˈmɔnitəriŋ] *n.* 生物监测

The US Forest Service administers a long-term, nationwide ozone biomonitoring program in partnership with other state and federal agencies to address national concerns about ozone impacts on forest health.

由美国国家林务局协同其他州和联邦机构执行一项全国范围内的长期臭氧生物监测计划，旨在设法解决全国有关臭氧对森林健康产生影响的问题。

We performed a retrospective human biomonitoring study by investigating the metabolites of the five most prominent phthalates in urine.

我们通过调查尿液中五种最常见的邻苯二甲酸酯的代谢产物，开展了人群生物监测的回顾性研究。

bionic [baiˈɔnik] *a.* 仿生的

Prostheses replace body parts and may be a plastic eye or nose or a bionic substitute for a demaged organ.

假体代替身体的某个部分，可以是塑料的眼、鼻或者是一个受损器官的仿生代替物。

biopharmaceutical [ˌbaiəuˌfɑːməˈsjuːtikəl] *a.* 生物制药的

Medical product registries include patients who have been exposed to biopharmaceutical products or medical devices.

医药产品注册包括已使用（已暴露于）生物制药产品或医疗器械的病人。

biopsy [baiˈɔpsi] *n.* 活（组织）检（查）

Biopsy is an absolute necessity in the differential diagnosis of breast cancer and fat necrosis.

活检在乳腺癌和脂肪坏死的鉴别诊断中是绝对必要的。

The diagnosis is based on serial biopsy in patients with biochemical evidence of hepatitis.

诊断是基于对有生化变化证据的肝炎病人的连续活检。

biopsychology [ˌbaiəsaiˈkɔlədʒi] *n.* 生物心理学，精神生物学

This is a nonlinear analysis toolbox of biopsychology.

这是一个生物心理学的非线性分析工具箱。

This biopsychology documentation is available freely.

这份生物心理学文件是可以免费得到的。

biopsychosocial [ˌbaiəuˌsaikəuˈsəuʃəl] *a.* 生物心理社会的

A biopsychosocial approach is commonly used to treat affective disorders in children.

生物心理社会的方法经常用于治疗儿童情感性障碍。

Drug therapy in the older adult population is a complex phenomenon influenced by numerous biopsychosocial factors.

老年人群的药物治疗是一个受诸多生理、心理和社会因素影响的复杂问题。

biosphere [ˈbaiəsfiə] *n.* 生物圈，生物界

Mitochondrial genomes are, with the exception of viruses, the most economically packed forms of DNA in the whole biosphere.

线粒体基因组是除病毒基因组外生物圈中最经济的 DNA 包装形式。

Selective mechanisms exist in organism and biosphere, which select the cells with less DNA injury and reproduces them.

生物界和生物圈中存在筛选机制，它将 DNA 损伤较小的细胞筛选出来并进行增殖。

The biosphere is the global sum of all ecosystems.

生物圈是地球上所有生态系统的总和。

The actual thickness of the biosphere on earth is difficult to measure.
地球上生物圈的实际厚度难以测量。

biostatistics [ˌbaiəustəˈtistiks] *n.* 生物统计学

The regression model for contaminated data is a useful model in biostatistics.
在生物统计学中，污染数据回归模型是常用的模型。

He is a professor of biostatistics at the University of Pittsburgh.
他是美国匹兹堡大学的一名生物统计学教授。

biosynthetic [ˌbaiəusinˈθetik] *a.* 生物合成的

The bacterial cellulose is widely applied to food, medicine, textile and chemical industry as a new biosynthetic material.
细菌纤维素是一种新型微生物合成材料，在食品、医药、纺织、化工等方面有着巨大的应用潜力。

NADPH is required for many biosynthetic pathways and particularly for synthesis of fatty acid and steroids.
NADPH 对许多生物合成途径都是需要的，特别是对脂肪酸和甾体的合成。

biotechnology [ˌbaiəutekˈnɔlədʒi] *n.* 生物技术

Application of scientific and technical advances in life science to develop commercial products is biotechnology.
运用生命科学中科学技术的进展成就来开发商业产品就是生物技术。

Modern biological sciences are intimately entwined and dependent on the methods developed through biotechnology.
各种现代生物科学相互密切渗透并依赖利用生物技术开发的各种方法。

"Application of scientific and technical advances in life science to develop commercial products" is biotechnology.
生物技术即在生命科学领域里应用科学和技术的进步来开发商业产品。

Green biotechnology is biotechnology applied to agricultural processes.
绿色生物技术指的是应用于农业生产过程的生物技术。

bioterrorism [ˌbaiəuˈterərizm] *n.* 生物恐怖主义

Smallpox as a possible agent for bioterrorism is much in the news of late, but there is no evidence of use so far.
最近常有消息称天花可能用于生物恐怖主义，但至今仍无证据。

biotic [baiˈɔtik] *a.* 生命的，来自生物的

Biotic pesticides H-14 was sprayed.
已经喷洒了生物杀虫剂 H-14。

biotin [ˈbaiətin] *n.* 生物素

Biotin is identical with vitamin H and coenzyme R.
生物素和维生素 H 以及辅酶 R 是相同的（东西）。

Strategies include inducing the bacteria to excrete glutamate by excluding biotin from the nutrient medium.
（科研设计的）策略是在营养环境中去除生物素，迫使细菌分泌谷氨酸。

Deficiency of biotin is known as egg-white injury.
生物素的缺乏称为蛋清性损害。

biotransformation [ˌbaiəuˌtrænsfəˈmeiʃən] *n.* 生物转化

Biotransformation may be defined as enzyme catalyzed alteration of drugs by the living organism.
生物转化（一词）可定义为药物在生物体内被酶催化所引起的改变。

In general, biotransformation may be divided into hepatic and nonhepatic metabolism.
通常生物转化可分为肝内和肝外代谢。

biotype [ˈbaiətaip] *n.* 生物类型

The current cholera vaccines composed of classic or biotype Eltor strains are of limited value.
内含有经典的或生物型 Eltor 菌株的现行霍乱疫苗(应用)价值有限。

biparietal [ˌbaipəˈraiətəl] *a.* 二顶的;二顶骨的

B-mode ultrasound scans were applied to measure the biparietal diameter, gestational sac, femur length and abdominal circumference of fetuses in 380 cases of pregnant women at the different pregnant week.
应用 B 型超声检查,对 380 例孕妇的胎儿根据不同孕周分别测量了胎头双顶径、妊娠囊、股骨长度、腹围等有关数值。

bipartite [baiˈpɑːtait] *a.* 双边的,由两部分构成的,双方的

Bipartite genome means that the genome is segmented into two segments.
双基因组是指基因组被分割为两段。
Bipartite uterus is a type of uterus found in deer and moose.
对分子宫是子宫形状中的一种,可见于鹿和驼鹿中。

biphasic [baiˈfeizik] *a.* 两相的

Clinically, such a biphasic illness suggests that the causative organism of the disease is viral.
临床上这种两相性疾患可提示此病的病原体是病毒。

biphenyl [baiˈfenl] *n.* 联苯

Biphenyl is an intermediate for the production of a host of other organic compounds such as emulsifiers, crop protection products and plastics.
联苯是可供生产许多其它有机化合物(如乳化剂、作物保护产品和塑料制品)的中间体。
The results show that the glass transition temperature of the copolymer increases obviously as a result of the introduction of biphenyl units.
结果表明,联苯的引入明显提高了聚合物的玻璃化转变温度。

bipolar [baiˈpəulə] *a.* 有两极的,双极的

Genetic factors are most important in schizophrenia and bipolar disorders.
遗传因素在精神分裂症和双相情感障碍症中是最重要的。
Patients were excluded from the study if they had a current or past history of bipolar disorder.
在这个研究中,如果病人现在或曾有双向情感障碍者将被排出在外。

birth [bəːθ] *n.* 出生

In early times, both the birth rates and death rates were high.
过去,出生率和死亡率都很高。

bisphosphonate [bisˈfɔsfəuneit] *n.* 二膦酸盐

Bisphosphonates are a class of drugs used to treat osteoporosis and similar diseases.
二膦酸盐类是一种用于治疗骨质疏松和类似疾病的药物。
Evidence shows that bisphosphonates reduce the risk of osteoporotic fracture in those who have had previous fractures.
有证据表明,二膦酸盐类药物可以减少曾有骨折史的病人发生骨质疏松性骨折的风险。

bitter [ˈbitə] *a.* 苦的,痛苦的

Four classes of taste are recognized: sweet, salt, sour, and bitter.
人能辨别四种味道:甜、咸、酸和苦。
Black coffee leaves a bitter taste in the mouth.
黑咖啡(清咖啡)喝着有点苦味。
Failing the exam was a bitter disappointment to him.
没有通过考试使他失望伤心。

bivalent [baiˈveilənt, ˈbivə-] *a.* 二价的

Synapsis is complete, and each pair of homologues appears as a bivalent.
联会完成时,每一对同源染色体显示为二价体。
The new formulation is known as B. O. P. V., or bivalent oral polio vaccine.

该新剂型被称为 B. O. P. V. ,或二价口服脊髓灰质炎疫苗。

bladder [ˈblædə] *n.* 囊;膀胱

The gall bladder is removed 2-3 months later after the inflammation has settled.

在炎症控制后 2 ~ 3 个月施行了胆囊切除。

The bladder acts as a reservoir for urine, it is a pear-shaped organ.

膀胱作为尿液的储存器,是一个梨形器官。

blade [bleid] *n.* 刀口;板

Direct viewing of the pharynx by use of a tongue blade should not be attempted.

不应该试图利用压舌板直接观察咽部。

Shelley's method of shaving the nail, with half of a flexible Gillette Super Blue razor blade, is an excellent one.

Shelley 氏法削刮指甲是一种很好的方法:取可弯可曲可变的吉利剃须刀片的半片,按指甲形状来削刮指甲。

blame [bleim] *v.* 责备,把…归于;应负责

He blamed the assistant for his failure.

他把失败归于他的助手。

If you fail the exam you'll only have yourself to blame.

如果你考不好,只能怪自己。

Influenza C has been blamed for only minor epidemics in closed communities.

丙型流感已造成在不开放团体内仅小范围的流行。

blank [blæŋk] *a.* 空白的

Write on one side of the page and leave the other side blank.

在纸的一面写字,另一面空着。

n. 空白

I have filled in this form incorrectly. Can I have another blank?

我把这份表填错了,能再给我一张空白的吗?

blast [blɑːst] *n.* 爆炸;冲击波;气浪

Primary blast injury is responsible for most early deaths and may exist without other evidence of external injury.

大多数早期死亡都由原有的爆炸伤引起,但爆炸引起的伤害可以在没有任何外在损伤时存在。

blastoconidium [ˌblæstəukəˈnidiəm] *n.* 芽分生孢子

Blastoconidium is produced singly or in chains, and detached at maturity leaving a bud scar, as in the budding of a yeast cell.

芽分生孢子以单个或链状产生,在成熟时脱离开,并留下一个芽痕,像酵母细胞出芽一样。

These medical condition or symptom topics may be relevant to medical information for blastoconidium.

这些临床状况的议题均与芽分生孢子的医学信息有关。

blastocyst [ˈblæstə(u)sist] *n.* 囊胚,胚泡

The blastocyst is a sphere of about 150 cells, composed of the trophoblast, the blastocoel, and the inner cell mass.

胚泡是一个由滋养层、囊胚腔、内细胞团组成的约 150 个细胞的球体。

Blastocyst culture of the in-vitro-fertilization-embryo-transfer for 5 days allows selection of the best quality embryos for transfer.

体外受精胚胎移植囊胚培养的第 5 天,可以选择最好的优质胚胎进行移植。

blastomere [ˈblæstə(u)miə] *n.* 卵裂球

A blastomere is a type of cell produced by division of the egg after fertilization.

卵裂球是卵子受精后分裂产生的一种细胞类型。

Preimplantation genetic diagnosis can be performed separately on the removed cell(s) from blastomere biopsy.

植入前遗传学诊断可以从卵裂球活检中分别取得的单个或多个细胞上进行。

blastomycosis [ˌblæstəumaiˈkəusis] *n.* 酵母菌病

Blastomycosis is a fungal infection caused by the organism *Blastomyces dermatitidis*.

酵母菌病是由皮炎芽生菌感染引起的真菌性疾病。

Blastomycosis can present in many ways.

酵母菌病可以多种方式表现。

blastulation [ˌblæstjuˈleiʃən] *n.* 囊胚形成

Blastulation is the formation of a blastula from a morula.

囊胚形成是从桑葚胚形成囊胚。

During blastulation, cells continue to divide and begin to differentiate.

在囊胚形成过程中,细胞继续分裂并开始分化。

bleed [bliːd] *v.* 流血

Were it not for the blood clotting mechanism, one would bleed to death even in the case of a slight injury.

如果没有凝血机制,一个人即使是轻伤,也会流血致死。

bleeding [ˈbliːdiŋ] *n.* 出血

The slight bleeding commonly occurs from small vessels in the wall of a cavity.

空洞壁小血管经常发生轻度出血。

They at last successfully stopped the bleeding and got the patient out of danger.

他们终于成功地把血止住,使病人脱离了危险。

blemish [ˈblemiʃ] *n.* 损伤,瑕疵;瘢痕

Skin blemishes can also be removed by means of lasers.

皮肤上的瘢痕与瑕疵也能通过激光清除。

In burns of the first and second degree, healing occurs rapidly with little or no permanent blemish.

对于第一、二度烧伤,痊愈迅速,几乎没有或完全没有永久的瘢痕。

bleomycin [bliəˈmaisin] *n.* 博来霉素

The doctor may suggest to inject bleomycin to treat the skin cancer.

医生会建议注射博来霉素治疗皮肤癌。

bletilla [bliˈtilə] *n.* 白芨

We did a research to identify the influencing factors on the extraction of bletilla.

我们做了一个研究来确认对白芨提取的影响因素。

Bletilla glucomannan (Bg) was used as the preservation material.

白芨葡甘露聚糖被用作保鲜材料。

blindness [ˈblaindnis] *n.* 盲,视觉缺失

In some developing countries, vitamin A deficiency is a major cause of blindness in the young.

在一些发展中国家,维生素 A 缺乏是年轻人致盲的主要原因。

Marked pallor occurs in complete optic atrophy, when there is blindness or severe visual impairment.

在完全性视神经萎缩时,视盘呈明显的苍白色,此时失明或有严重的视力障碍。

Color blindness is the one most common genetic disease in human race.

色盲是人类最普通的遗传病之一。

blister [ˈblistə] *n.* 水疱,疱

The patient also developed a "fever blister" on his lip.

患者还患有唇部单纯疱疹。

In a severe burn there is a copious loss of fluid at the burnt surface, into the blisters and in the oedematous tissues deep to the burn.
在严重烧伤时,烧伤表面有大量的液体流失,并流入水疱和烧伤深部的水肿组织之中。

block [blɔk] *n.* 大块,块料;阻滞,阻断
Sections from serial blocks did not show a great degree of atherosclerosis.
在连续的组织块切片上,未见明显的动脉粥样硬化病变。
Hypertension may occur also in certain chronic diseases as well as in heart block.
有些慢性疾病和心脏传导阻滞患者也可有高血压。
v. 阻断
Doctors say the operation extends the life of persons whose arteries are partly blocked.
医生说这种手术能延长动脉部分受阻的病人的生命。
Spinal anesthesia blocks the spinal nerve roots and dorsal root ganglia and probably also blocks the periphery of the spinal cord.
脊髓麻醉阻断脊神经根和背根神经节,也可能阻滞脊髓的外周部分。

blockade [blɔ'keid] *n.* 阻断,阻塞,阻滞
Prazosin causes alpha-adrenergic receptor blockade and direct vasodilatation.
哌唑嗪可阻断 α 肾上腺素能受体和直接扩张血管。
H_2 blockade relieves symptoms and favours healing of duodenal ulcer.
阻滞 H_2 受体可以缓解症状,并有利于十二指肠溃疡的愈合。

blockage ['blɔkidʒ] *n.* 阻碍物,阻塞
A year later the blockage in his artery had been reduced to 59 percent, while blood flow through the artery had nearly tripled.
一年后,动脉阻塞减少到59%,而且经过该动脉的血流量几乎增加到 3 倍。

blocker ['blɔkə] *n.* 阻断剂
Phenoxybenzamine is a noncompetitive alpha-adrenergic receptor blocker.
酚苄明为非竞争性 α 肾上腺素能受体阻断药。

bloodstained ['blʌdsteind] *a.* 沾染血的
In pyloric growths pain resembles that of duodenal ulcer, but ultimately the pain becomes constant with vomiting which may be bloodstained.
在幽门癌时,疼痛与十二指肠溃疡相似,但最终变成持续性的并伴有呕吐,吐物可能带血。

bloodstream ['blʌdstriːm] *n.* 血流
Accumulation of bilirubin in the bloodstream causes yellow pigmentation of the plasma.
胆红素在血流中蓄积使血浆呈黄色。
Electrolytes are the charged particles found in the bloodstream within and around body cells.
电解质是围绕人体细胞内外血流中的带电颗粒。
The bloodstream may carry a carcinoma to other parts of the body.
血流可把癌变带到身体的其他部位。

bloody ['blʌdi] *a.* 带血的
Bloody sputum is caused by the opening of a tumor in the bronchus into a blood vessel.
痰中带血是由于支气管肿瘤侵入血管所致。
During acute glomerulonephritis the urine is usually frankly bloody.
患急性肾小球性肾炎时,通常有明显血尿。

blot [blɔt] *n.* 污点,污迹;印迹
Our Western blot results revealed that there were no statistically significant ($p>0.05$) differences for NGF in any of the experimental groups when compared to sham operated controls.
我们的免疫印迹结果显示,任一实验组的 NGF 与假手术对照组比,都没有统计学差异($p>0.05$)。
[注] Western blot (蛋白)免疫印迹

blotting ['blɔtiŋ] *n.* 印迹

Generally, Southern blotting can successfully identify chromosomal rearrangements and small deletions.

通常情况下,Southern 印迹能有效地鉴定染色体重排和小的缺失。

blueprint ['bluːprint] *n.* 蓝图

Each person has a unique set of chemical blueprints that determines how his or her body looks and functions.

每个人都有一套独一无二的、决定他(或她)的身体结构和功能的化学蓝图。

bluish ['blu(ː)iʃ] *a.* 带蓝色的

This lack of oxygenation causes a bluish color in the child suffering a severe attack of asthma.

缺乏氧合作用使得患有严重哮喘的儿童肤色发青。

blunt [blʌnt] *a.* 钝的,迟钝的

A detailed discussion of blunt injury of the brain and spinal cord will be found in chapter 7.

关于大脑和脊髓钝挫伤的详细讨论见第七章。

In some respects, the circumstance has the pattern of an "internal" Fe deficiency to which the normal compensatory responses are blunted.

在某些方面,所谓内在性缺铁是由于正常铁代偿性反应较差的缘故。

blur [bləː] *v.* 变模糊

Distinctions between these groups are often blurred by the existence of transitional forms.

这些分组之间的区别往往因存有过渡形态而模糊不清。

Visual blurring accompanies papilledema in some patients with intracranial tumor.

某些有颅内肿瘤病人的视神经乳头水肿常伴有视力模糊。

blurred [bləːd] *a.* 模糊的

However, the distinction between exogenous and endogenous pyrogens is sometimes blurred.

然而,外源性和内源性致热原物质的区别有时很模糊。

The line between food and medicine will become increasingly blurred.

食品和药品之间的界线将变得越来越模糊。

boil [bɔil] *n.* 疖

Boil is an inflamed swelling arising from a hair follicle caused by bacterial infection.

疖是细菌感染引起的毛囊炎性肿大。

bolus ['bəuləs] *n.* 团,块(如药丸,食团)

After being prepared, the Chinese medicine comes in the forms of bolus, powder, plaster, pellet, tablet and oral liquid.

中药在经过制备后,会以丸、散、膏、丹、片和口服液等形式出现。

What effect does carsick bolus have?

晕车丸有什么作用?

Small bolus doses of fentanyl were repeated to maintain reasonable levels of anesthesia.

重复给小剂量丸药芬太尼以便使麻醉维持在适当的水平。

bombard [bɔm'bɑːd] *v.* 炮击,撞击,照射

Malignant tumors(cancers) are bombarded with the rays of radioactive materials.

恶性肿瘤(癌)受到放射性物质发射的射线照射。

bombardment [bɔm'bɑːdmənt] *n.* 轰击,撞击

Even nonmotile bacteria bounce back and forth because of bombardment from water molecules.

即使无动力的细菌也可因水分子的撞击而前后弹动。

bony ['bəuni] 骨的

In the healing of a fracture, bony callus is composed of woven bone.

在骨折愈合中,骨性骨痂由编织骨构成。

The bony callus remodeling is accomplished by coordination of osteoclasts and osteoblasts.

骨性骨痂的改建是在破骨细胞和骨母细胞协调作用下完成的。

boost [buːst] *v.* 增强

"Messages" from the brain may boost or impair the immune system.

来自大脑的"信息"可以增强或削弱免疫系统。

Using human stem cells, scientists have developed methods to boost the production of red blood cells, according to a new study.

根据一项新的研究,科学家们通过使用人干细胞已经研究出了促进红细胞生成的方法。

booster [ˈbuːstə] *n.* 加强剂量

For contaminated or severe wounds, a booster is given if more than 5 years have elapsed since immunization.

对于污染伤口或重伤,在免疫接种 5 年以后要给予加强剂量。

Booster injections are given one, three, and five years after completion of the initial course.

完成了初始疗程后,以后过一、三、五年再给予加强注射。

bootstrap [ˈbuːtstræp] *n.* 引导程序,自展

Using a bootstrap procedure, we design a mechanism to extract significant factors from the support vector approach.

本研究中,我们利用引导程序设计出一种机制可从支持矢量途径获取显著因子。

One of the most dependably accurate methods for deriving 95% confidence intervals for cost-effectiveness ratios is the nonparametric bootstrap method.

非参数自展法是最可靠精确的方法之一,用此法可获得成本-效果比值 95% 可信区间。

borax [ˈbɔːræks] *n.* 硼砂

Borax is a compound of boron, used in making glass, enamels and detergents.

硼砂是硼的化合物,多用于制造玻璃、瓷釉或清洁剂。

You have to identify all the constituents and determine the contents of Borax in Xingqi Tannikaer capsule.

你必须鉴别行气坦尼卡尔胶囊中的全部成分并且测定硼砂的含量。

The running buffer was composed of 30mmol/L borax.

运行缓冲液由 30mmol/L 硼砂缓冲溶液组成

border [ˈbɔːdə] *v.* 边缘,接近

The vessels enter and leave the spleen at the concave medial border.

血管在凹陷的内侧缘中心出入脾。

The spleen is a spongy organ with the lateral border in contact with the diaphragm.

脾为一海绵状的器官,以其外缘与膈相接。

In the study of microbiology, we encounter "organisms" which may represent the border line of life.

在微生物的研究中,我们遇到处于生命边缘的"有机体"。

v. 镶边

It is not unusual to find the bronchiolar and alveolar walls bordered by a homogeneous acidophilic hyaline membrane.

常可见在细支气管壁和肺泡壁上形成同质的嗜酸性透明膜边。

Favus is also prevalent in the Middle East, Southeastern Europe, and the countries bordering the Mediterranean Sea.

黄癣也在中东、东南欧和地中海沿岸的国家内流行。

Her condition borders on insanity.

她的病情接近于精神错乱。

borderline [ˈbɔːdəlain] *n.* ,a. 边界(上的),边缘(的)

Borderline states may be made worse by antidepressants.

抗抑郁剂可加重边缘状态。

Borderline state is a poorly defined term employed with reference to three groups of mental aberration.

临界状态是一种定义不明确的术语,指的是三种精神迷乱状态。

boredom ['bɔːdəm] *n.* 厌烦,无聊

As a result of boredom and mental apathy the patient neglects his personal toilet and loses all self-respect.

由于厌倦和情感淡漠,病人忽视个人梳洗,失去自尊心。

Besides getting rid of boredom, daydreaming can make truly grim situations a little easier to endure.

除了排除厌倦情绪外,白日梦还可使残酷的现实易于被人忍受。

boric ['bɔːrik] *a.* 硼的

Don't use boric acid soaks in treating large burns, enough boric acid could be absorbed to be dangerous.

不要使用含硼酸的溶剂治疗大面积烧伤,因为硼酸可被大量吸收造成危险。

Borax and boric acid are used in mouth and nasal washes, gargles, eye lotions and contact-lens solutions, and in dusting powder.

硼砂和硼酸可用于口腔和鼻腔的冲洗,或用于含漱、洗眼液、浸泡隐形眼镜以及扑撒患部。

borneol ['bɔːniɔl] *n.* [中医] 冰片;龙脑

The solid water is like the borneol taken out of the fridge.

冰晶看起来像是从冰箱里拿出的冰片。

The product is a yellowish and transparent liquid with the fragrance of borneol.

本品为微黄色澄明的液体,具有冰片香味。

borrelia [bə'reliə] *n.* 疏螺旋体属

Some species of borrelia cause Lyme disease or borreliosis and are transmitted by ticks.

疏螺旋体属中的某些菌种引起莱姆病或莱姆疏螺旋体病,该病由扁虱传播。

Lyme disease caused by borrelia is considered to be one of the fastest growing illnesses in the world.

疏螺旋体引起的莱姆病被认为是全球增长最快的疾病之一。

botanical [bə'tænikəl] *a.* 植物的

The experience enforced his passionate interest in botanical drugs.

这些经验增强了他对植物药物浓厚的兴趣。

botulin ['bɔtjulin] *n.* 肉毒毒素

The control effects of D type botulin at these 3 concentrations were equal to that of 0. 1% C type botulin.

这 3 个不同浓度的 D 型肉毒毒素的控制效果与 0. 1% 的 C 型肉毒毒素相当。

Botulin is a protein produced by the bacterium Clostridium botulinum and is the most powerful neurotoxin yet discovered.

肉毒毒素是一种由肉毒梭菌产生的蛋白质,是迄今发现的毒性最强的神经毒素。

botulinum [ˌbɔtju'lainəm] *n.* 肉毒杆菌

Botulinum toxin causes the complete inhibition of release of Ach evoked by nerve impulses.

肉毒杆菌毒素能够完全抑制由神经冲动诱导的乙酰胆碱的释放。

Clostridium botulinum grows freely in badly preserved canned foods, producing a toxin causing serious food poisoning(botulism).

肉毒梭状芽孢杆菌能在保存不好的罐头食品中迅速生长,产生的毒素引起严重的食物中毒(肉毒中毒)。

botulism ['bɔtjulizəm] *n.* 肉毒中毒

The neurologic symptoms noted with botulism help differentiate it from staphylococcal food poisoning.

具有明显肉毒中毒的神经系统症状，有助于将其与葡萄球菌性食物中毒相区别。

boundary [ˈbaundəri] *n.* 界线，边界

Yet the boundaries between injury and inflammation, and between inflammation and healing, are indistinct.

然而损伤与炎症之间，以及炎症与愈合之间，界线是不清楚的。

bout [baut] *n.* 一回，一次，一阵发作

Like a bad bout of winter flu, she couldn't shake the virus.

就像得了一次极重的冬季流行性感冒一样，她对病毒毫无办法。

The sick child was coughing and occasionally had bouts of sneezing this morning.

患儿今天早晨不断地咳嗽，偶尔阵发性打喷嚏。

boutonniere [ˌbuːtəˈnjεə] *n.* 纽孔，钮孔状切开术

The boutonniere deformity (BD) is a well-described condition in hand surgery.

钮孔状变形是一种在手外科中有明确描述的疾病。

bovine [ˈbəuvain] *a.* 牛的

The bovine bacillus is more liable to cause tuberculosis of the tonsils and alimentary tract.

牛型结核菌比较容易引起扁桃体和消化道的结核病。

bowel [ˈbauəl] *n.* 肠

Hepatic amoebiasis is a common complication of the bowel infection.

肝阿米巴病是肠道感染的一种常见并发症。

During intestinal obstruction, on auscultation excessive bowel sounds may be heard.

当肠梗阻发生时进行听诊可以听到肠鸣音亢进。

You must move the bowels every day so as not to cause constipation.

你必须每日进行排便以免产生便秘。

bow-legs [ˈbəu-legz] *n.* 弓形腿

Bow-legs is a physical deformity marked by outward bowing of the leg in relation to the thigh, giving the appearance of an archer's bow.

弓形腿是指双下肢向外侧呈弧形凸出的畸形病变，像弓箭手的弓而由此得名。

Children until the age of 3 to 4 have certain degree of bow-legs.

3 到 4 岁前的幼儿都有一定程度的膝内翻。

brace [breis] *n.* 支架

Gait training is practiced with the assistance of canes, crutches, walkers, braces, and artificial limbs.

步法的训练可借助于手杖、拐杖、扶车、支架或是假肢进行。

brachial [ˈbreikjəl] *a.* 臂的，肱的

Femoral and brachial pulses are moderately strong and equal.

股动脉和肱动脉的搏动强度适中，且两者近似。

Radial nerve is an important mixed sensory and motor nerve of the arm, forming the largest branch of the brachial plexus.

桡神经是臂部重要的感觉和运动混合神经，是臂丛的最大分支。

brachytherapy [ˌbrækiˈθerəpi] *n.* 近距离放射治疗

Brachytherapy for prostate cancer indicates to the cases with prostate cancer in low-risk group.

近距离放射治疗适合治疗低危组的前列腺癌患者。

Brachytherapy is becoming a useful tool to control cancers.

近距离放射疗法正在成为控制各种癌症的有效工具。

bradycardia [brædiˈkɑːdiə] *n.* 心动过缓

Bradycardia occurs commonly during the early phases of acute myocardial infarction.

心动过缓通常发生在急性心肌梗死早期。

Tachycardia is usual, although in certain infectious diseases a relative bradycardia may be seen.

尽管在某些传染病中可以见到相对的心动过缓，但心动过速则是常见的。

bradykinesia ['brædiki'niːziə] *n.* 运动过慢，身心反应迟钝

Bradykinesia describes a slowness of movement and slow reaction times.

运动过慢用来表示动作缓慢且反应迟钝(的现象)。

bradykinin ['brædi'kainin] *n.* 缓激肽(血管舒张药)

Subsequently, kinin system activation results in the production of bradykinin, a powerful vasodilator.

接着激肽系统激活因而产生了强有力的血管扩张物——缓激肽。

Bradykinin is a potent vasodilator, it increases vascular permeability and causes contraction of extravascular smooth muscles.

缓激肽是一种强力血管扩张剂，它可增加血管的通透性，并可引起血管以外的平滑肌收缩。

bradyphrenia [ˌbrædi'friːniə] *n.* 思维迟钝；智力迟钝

A 27-year-old man only showed symptoms of slight bradyphrenia after the first seizure.

一个27岁的男性患者在首次癫痫发作后，仅表现为轻微的思维迟钝。

Bradyphrenia in Parkinson's disease may reflect advancing age or slower movement.

帕金森病的思维迟钝可能反映了高龄或运动缓慢。

brain [brein] *n.* 脑

Because of the development of industry, the incidence of traumatic brain injury is increasing every year.

由于工业的发展，创伤性脑损伤的发病率正在逐年增长。

Try your best to protect brain when you subject to a traffic accident.

当你遭遇车祸的时候，请设法保护你的脑。

brainstem ['breinstem] *n.* 脑干

Brainstem plays an important role in the control of respiratory system.

脑干在呼吸系统的控制中起重要作用。

branch [brɑːntʃ] *n.* 分支

When reaching the coronary sulcus, the left coronary artery divideds into an anterior interventricular branch and a circumflex branch.

左冠状动脉到达冠状沟后分为前室间支和旋支。

The International Life Sciences Institute accomplishes its work through its branches and institutes.

国际生命科学研究院通过其分支机构和下属研究所完成它的工作。

breach [briːtʃ] *v.* 攻破，突破

Natural boundaries can be breached; e. g. , intestinal cutaneous fistulas may form, or blood vessel walls may be penetrated.

自然的边界可被突破，如肠壁瘘管的形成、或血管壁的穿透。

Metastatic spinal tumors seldom breach the dura.

转移性脊柱肿瘤很少会突破硬脊膜。

breakdown ['breikdaun] *n.* 分解；衰竭

Cortisol promotes the breakdown of proteins and inhibits protein synthesis.

氢化可的松促进蛋白质的分解，抑制蛋白质的合成。

The energy requirements are fulfilled by the breakdown of glucose to lactic acid.

能量的需要是由葡萄糖分解为乳酸获得的。

breakthrough ['breikθruː] *n.* 突破；成就

The discovery of insulin was considered to be a breakthrough in medicine.

胰岛素的发现被认为是医学上的一个突破。

breast-fed ['brest'fed] *a.* 人乳喂养的

The stool of the breast-fed infants is naturally softer than that of the infant fed cow's milk.
人乳喂养的婴儿粪便要比牛乳喂养的婴儿粪便软些。

breathe [briːð] *v.* 呼吸

Throughout the operation the patient was fully conscious and breathed easily.
整个手术过程中，病人完全清醒，且呼吸通畅。

breathing ['briːðiŋ] *n.* 呼吸

Breathing is a unique human function in that it can be fully voluntary or involuntary.
呼吸是一种独特的人体功能，既可完全随意，又可非随意进行。

Proper breathing nourishes the central nervous system.
适宜的呼吸对中枢神经系统具有营养作用。

breech [briːtʃ] *n.* 臀

The head is recognized because it is rounder and harder than the breech.
可识别头部是因头部比臀部圆而且硬。

Indications of cesarean section are as follows: hypamnion, breech presentation, premature rupture of fetal membranes, prolonged pregnancy, giant baby and fetal distress.
剖宫产指征如下：羊水过少、臀位、胎膜早破、过期妊娠、巨大儿和胎儿窘迫。

breed [briːd] *v.* 繁殖，饲养；培养；滋生 n. 品种

This discovery is likely to be of great significance in breeding new strains of animals.
这一发现可能在繁殖新种动物方面具有重大意义。

The heart valves present an especially appropriate breeding place for the bacteria.
心瓣膜为细菌提供了非常适合繁殖的场所。

bremsstrahlung ['bremˌʃtrɑːləŋ] *n.* 韧致辐射

The ratio of the microwave radiation to the X-ray bremsstrahlung radiation is dependent on the density in the emitting region.
微波辐射与 X 射线韧致辐射的比值与发射区的密度有关。

The nonlinear inverse bremsstrahlung absorption is a main mechanism in the plasma heating at laser-plasma interaction.
非线性逆韧致吸收是激光-等离子体相互作用中对等离子体的加热起重要作用的机制。

brevibacterium [ˌbrevibæk'tiəriəm] *n.* 短杆菌属

Some species of brevibacterium is ubiquitously present on the human skin where it causes foot odor.
有些短杆菌属广泛存在于人的皮肤，引起脚臭。

Brevibacterium is a genus of bacteria, gram-positive soil organisms, of the order Actinomycetales.
短杆菌属归属放线菌目，为革兰阳性土壤微生物。

brevity ['brevəti] *n.* 简洁，简短

In preparing this book, attempts were made to maintain brevity.
在编写本书的过程中，我们力求保持简洁。

bridging ['bridʒiŋ] *adj.* 桥接的

Bridging necrosis is confluent necrosis of hepatocytes usually occurred in chronic hepatitis.
桥接坏死是肝细胞的融合性坏死，常发生于慢性肝炎。

Bridging necrosis may span adjacent lobules in portal-to-portal, central-to-central, or portal-to-central fashions.
桥接坏死可跨越相邻小叶，形成门管区-门管区、中央-中央区或门管区-中央区之间的坏死带。

brittle ['britl] *a.* 易碎的，脆弱的

When the nails are affected they become brittle, irregularly thickened, and crusted under the free margins.
当指甲受感染时，指甲变脆，有不规则增厚，并在指甲的游离缘下结痂。

broad-spectrum [ˈbrɔːdˈspektrəm] *a.* 广谱的

Amoxicillin and ampicillin are broad-spectrum penicillins.

羟氨苄青霉素和氨苄青霉素都是广谱青霉素。

Some antibiotic drugs are called broad-spectrum antibiotics because they are effective against both gram-positive and gram-negative bacteria.

有些抗生素被称为广谱抗生素，因为它们既对革兰氏阳性菌有效，也对革兰氏阴性菌有效。

bromate [ˈbrəumeit] *n.* 溴酸盐

In this paper the formation and danger of bromate and its analytical methods are introduced.

本文介绍了溴酸盐的形成、危害以及分析方法。

Therefore, it is necessary to investigate ozone's bactericidal mechanism and the control technologies for bromate in order to realize the balance between ozone, pathogens and bromate.

因此，要实现臭氧、致病菌与溴酸盐三者的平衡就必须研究臭氧的灭菌机制及溴酸盐的控制技术。

bromocriptine [ˌbrəuməˈkriptiːn] *n.* 溴隐亭

Bromocriptine is used to treat symptoms of hyperprolactinemia including lack of menstrual periods, discharge from the nipples, infertility and hypogonadism.

溴隐亭用于治疗高泌乳素血症的症状，包括闭经、溢乳、不孕和性腺功能减退。

Bromocriptine QR is an effective and safe antidiabetic drug which can be employed as monotherapy or with metformin to achieve and maintain optimal glycemic control.

溴隐亭四射体是一种安全有效的抗糖尿病药物，它可以单用或者与二甲双胍合用以达到并维持良好的血糖控制。

bronchial [ˈbrɔŋkjəl] *a.* 支气管的

Bronchial asthma, especially in adult life, is often associated with chronic bronchitis.

支气管哮喘，特别在成年人中常与慢性支气管炎有关。

The operation on the patient ill with bronchial carcinoma has successfully been brought to an end.

对患支气管癌的病人所施行的手术已成功地结束了。

bronchiectasis [ˌbrɔŋkiˈektəsis] *n.* 支气管扩张

Lung abscess and bronchiectasis are common complications.

肺脓肿和支气管扩张是常见的合并症。

Bronchiectasis differs from chronic bronchitis in that the former is more of a localized disease.

支气管扩张与慢性支气管炎的区别，在于前者是一种更加局限性的疾患。

bronchiolar [ˌbrɔŋkiˈəulə] *a.* 细支气管的

It is not unusual to find the bronchiolar and alveolar walls bordered by a homogeneous acidophilic hyaline membrane.

常可见到在细支气管壁和肺泡壁上形成同质透明膜边。

bronchiole [ˈbrɔnkiəul] *n.* 细支气管

In most instances the cause of atelectasis is not obstruction but closure of the bronchioles.

在大多数情况下，肺不张的原因不是梗阻，而是细支气管的关闭。

Small bronchioles are prone to close when lung volume reaches a critical point (closing volume).

当肺容量达到一临界点（闭合容量）时毛细支气管趋于关闭。

bronchiolitis [ˌbrɔŋkiəuˈlaitis] *n.* 细支气管炎，毛细支气管炎

Viral pneumonia may be indistinguishable from acute bacterial bronchitis or bronchiolitis in children and infants.

在婴儿及儿童患者，患有病毒性肺炎者不易与急性细菌性支气管炎或细支气管炎相区别。

bronchitis [brɔŋˈkaitis] *n.* 支气管炎

The history is initially often of acute bronchitis.

病史上常以急性支气管炎发病。

He has had acute bronchitis twice since January.

自从一月份以来他已经患过了两次急性支气管炎。

bronchoconstriction [ˌbrɔŋkəukən'strikʃən] *n.* 支气管狭窄，支气管收缩

How airway cooling or drying produces bronchoconstriction is also unclear.

目前还不清楚为何气道干燥或受冷会引起支气管收缩。

Exercise induced bronchoconstriction may be an isolated disorder in a child who is otherwise free from asthmatic attacks.

对于那些没有其他哮喘发作的儿童，由运动诱发的支气管缩小可能是一种单独的疾病。

bronchodilatation [ˌbrɔŋkəuˌdailei'teiʃən] *n.* 支气管扩张

There are enough evidences that can prove the relationship between bronchodilatation and pulmonary infection.

有足够的证据证明支气管扩张与肺部感染有关。

Positive reaction in bronchodilatation test was found in 15. 2% of COPD patients and in 93. 3% of asthmatic patients.

15. 2% 的 COPD 患者和 93. 3% 的哮喘患者呈支气管舒张试验阳性反应。

bronchodilator [ˌbrɔŋkəudai'leitə] *n.* 支气管扩张器；支气管扩张药

There was no significant improvement after bronchodilator administration.

应用支气管扩张剂后，无明显改善。

bronchogenic [ˌbrɔŋkəu'dʒenik] *a.* 支气管源性的

The most common mistake in diagnosis is the confusion of bronchogenic carcinoma and primary lung abscess.

最常见的误诊是把支气管癌和原发性肺脓肿相混淆。

bronchography [brɔŋ'kɔgrəfi] *n.* 支气管造影术

Bronchography is a radiographic examination of the tracheobronchial tree following the injection of a radiopaque material.

支气管造影术是通过注射一种不透射线的造影剂来显影支气管树的一种射线检查。

As a result of improved computerized tomography (CT scan) and bronchoscopy technology, bronchography is performed on an infrequent basis.

随着 CT 和支气管镜技术的发展，支气管造影术的应用减少了。

bronchopneumonia [ˌbrɔŋkəunjuː'məunjə] *n.* 支气管肺炎

Most patients with staphylococcal pheumonia will have radiographic evidence of bronchopneumonia early in the illness.

大多数葡萄球菌肺炎患者，在疾病早期可有支气管肺炎的 X 线征象。

bronchopulmonary [brɔŋkəu'pʌlmənəri] *a.* 支气管肺的

Bronchopulmonary drainage should be maintained in patient with hypersecretion.

痰多的病人应持续做支气管肺引流。

bronchoscope ['brɔŋkəskəup] *n.* 支气管镜

The lung cancer is often readily seen by means of the bronchoscope.

肺癌通常容易通过支气管镜检查发现。

bronchoscopy [brɔŋ'kɔskəpi] *n.* 支气管镜检法

Bronchoscopy may be required to remove solid matter.

支气管镜检法可用以取出固体物质。

Chest X-ray was carried out together with bronchoscopy.

胸部 X 线检查与支气管镜检查同时进行。

bronchospasm ['brɔŋkəuˌspæzm] *n.* 支气管痉挛

Signs of pulmonary congestion are difficult to interpret, since they may be indistinguishable from those produced by bronchospasm.

肺充血的体征很难解释,因为不易与支气管痉挛产生的体征相区别。

bronchus ['brɔŋkəs] (*pl.* bronchi ['brɔŋkai]) *n.* 支气管

The persistent cough is due to irritation of the bronchus by the growth.

持续的咳嗽是生长物(肿瘤)对支气管的刺激所致。

Branches of the trachea or windpipe are called bronchi.

气管的分支叫做支气管。

broth [brɔ(ː)θ] *n.* 肉汤

Cola beverages, fruit juices, and broths are also beneficial.

可乐饮料、水果汁和肉汤也是有益的。

On subsequent examination Needham found that the broth was swarming with the animalcules.

随后检查时,尼达姆发现肉汤(培养基)充满了微生物。

browser ['brauzə] *n.* 浏览者;【电脑】浏览器

Load the Web page again in a browser.

在浏览器中再次加载该网页。

It is now time to start building your Web browser.

现在是开始生成 Web 浏览器的时候了。

brucella [bru'selə] (*pl.* brucellae [bru'seli]) *n.* 布鲁(杆)菌

Brucellae are small, nonmotile aerobic gram-negative coccobacilli.

布鲁菌是一类形态较小的、无动力的革兰阴性需氧球杆菌。

Brucella is associated with a history of contact with goats or cattle and often affects the aortic valve.

布鲁菌病与牛羊接触史有关,常侵及主动脉瓣。

Humoral factors may be important in the host defence against Brucella.

体液因素对宿主抵抗布鲁(杆)菌感染是重要的。

brucellosis [ˌbruse'ləusis] *n.* 布鲁菌病

Brucellosis remains a significant health and economic burden in many countries.

在许多国家布鲁菌病仍是重大的健康及经济负担。

A vital role for mononuclear phagocytes and cell-mediated immunity in brucellosis has been demonstrated.

现已证实布鲁菌病中单核吞噬细胞及细胞介导的免疫功能起重要作用。

bruise [bruːz] *n.* 青肿,挫伤

Examination of the extremities revealed numerous bruises over the lower ones.

检查肢体发现两下肢有许多挫伤。

bruit [bruːt] *n.* [法] 杂音

The abdomen should be palpated for renal enlargement, and auscultated for bruits.

应触诊腹部是否有肾增大,听诊以判断有无杂音。

The presence of bruit over the carotid is a possible clue to the presence of atherosclerotic disease of the internal carotid arteries.

颈动脉杂音的存在很可能提示存在有颈内动脉的粥样硬化病。

bubo ['bjuːbəu] *n.* 腹股沟淋巴结炎

When inguinal nodes become enlarged, they are often referred to as buboes.

腹股沟淋巴结肿大常称为腹股沟淋巴结炎。

bubonic [bju(ː)'bɔnik] *a.* 腹股沟淋巴结炎的

Bubonic plague must be suspected in any febrile patient with painful adenopathy.

凡是发热病人并伴有淋巴结肿大和疼痛时,应怀疑该病人患有鼠疫引起的腹股沟淋巴结炎。

buccal ['bʌkəl] *a.* 口的,口腔的

Relief within 5 minutes by sublingual or buccal glyceryl trinitrate makes angina more likely.

舌下或含服硝酸甘油片使疼痛在 5 分钟内缓解者,更支持心绞痛诊断。

buccally [ˈbʌkəli] *ad.* 向颊地,由(口腔)颊内面地

Nifedipine is absorbed orally or buccally.

硝苯吡啶口服或含服用药均可吸收。

bucking [ˈbʌkiŋ] *n.* 呛咳

Please don't swallow the saliva to prevent bucking, let it flow out naturally.

请不要吞咽口水以免呛咳,让它自然流出来。

The bucking incidence was 8% (2/25) in Group A; whereas it was 60% (15/25) in Group B, having significant difference between the two groups (P<0.01).

A 组呛咳发生率为 8% (2/25),而 B 组为 60% (15/25),这两组有显著差异(P<0.01)。

bud [bʌd] *n.* 芽,蕾

The taste buds on your tongue have nerve receptors in them.

在你舌头的味蕾上都有神经感受器。

budding [ˈbʌdiŋ] *n.* 芽殖

In budding yeast, cohesin at least includes Scc1, Scc3, Smc1 and Smc3 four subunits in mitosis.

在芽殖酵母的有丝分裂中,黏合素至少包括 SCC1、SCC3、SMC1 和 SMC3 四个亚基。

Budding could be easily seen on the cytoplasmic membrane of the host cells.

在宿主细胞的细胞质膜上可以很容易地看到芽殖。

budesonide [bjuˈdesənaid] *n.* 布地奈德

Among these patients, the clinical remission rate was 66% in the budesonide group and 49% in the mesalazine group.

在这些患者中,布地奈德和美沙拉嗪组的临床缓解率分别为 66% 和 49%。

Smokers and non-smokers with asthma gain similar benefits from budesonide therapy in terms of limiting their lung function decline, research shows.

研究显示,在限制肺功能下降方面,患有哮喘的吸烟者和非吸烟者会从布地奈德疗法中获得相似的益处。

buffer [ˈbʌfə] *n.* 缓冲剂,缓冲器

A fresh blood smear is briefly fixed and then exposed to a phosphate buffer of specific pH.

取新鲜血液涂片,迅速固定,然后放入特定 pH 的磷酸盐缓冲液。

The baroreceptor system is sometimes called a moderator system or a buffer system.

压力感受器系统有时称为调节系统或缓冲系统。

v. 缓冲

In such cases, the excess acid is neutralized or buffered by bicarbonates in the blood.

在这种情况下,过量的酸可能被血中的重碳酸盐所中和或缓冲。

building [ˈbildiŋ] *n.* 建筑物,建筑

The term "sick building syndrome" (SBS) is used to describe situations in which building occupants experience acute health and comfort effects that appear to be linked to time spent in a building, but no specific illness or cause can be identified.

"病态建筑物综合征"是对在建筑物中居住的人出现的急性不良健康情况的描述,与在建筑物中停留的时间长短有关,但不能确定特定疾病或病因。

The term "building related illness" (BRI) is used when symptoms of diagnosable illness are identified and can be attributed directly to airborne building contaminants.

"建筑物相关疾病"(BRI)指的是症状可确诊、并可直接归因于空气中的建设污染物的疾病。

bulbogastrone [ˌbʌlbəuˈgæstrəun] *n.* (十二指肠)球抑胃素

The existence of a specific inhibitory agent named bulbogastrone in the upper duodenum has been extensively documented in a series of physiological studies.

球抑胃素是一种存在于十二指肠上半部的特定抑制剂,目前有一系列生理学研究对其进

行了广泛报道。

The inhibitory effect of antral distension on gastric acid secretion in healthy subjects does not seem to be mediated by secretin, cholecystokinin or bulbogastrone.

健康人的胃窦扩张对胃酸的分泌的抑制作用似乎不是由肠促胰液素、胆囊收缩素或球抑胃素所介导的。

bulge [bʌldʒ] *v.* 肿胀,隆起

The abdomen was distended and the flanks were bulging.

腹部膨胀并向两侧隆起。

The endothelial cell nuclei bulge prominently into the lumen, but no subendothelial tissue is visible.

内皮细胞的细胞核向管腔内明显凸出,但看不到内皮下组织。

bulimia [bjuːˈlimiə] *n.* 贪食症,食欲亢进

Bulimia means eating a lot of food.

贪食症是指吃太多的食物。

Eating disorders include anorexia and bulimia.

饮食失调包括厌食和贪食症。

bulk [bʌlk] *n.* 大体积纤维性物质(不为肠所吸收,但可促进肠蠕动);大批,大量

To lose weight quickly, she went on a fad diet, high in fiber and bulk, but low in protein.

为快速减肥,她采用了一种一时风行的食谱:高纤维素、低蛋白质。

The bulk of lymphoid tissue that is found in association with mucosal surfaces is called the mucosa-associated lymphoid tissue(MALT).

在黏膜表面出现大量的淋巴组织被称为黏膜相关的淋巴组织。

bulla [ˈbulə, ˈbʌlə] *n.* 大疱,肺大泡(*pl.* bullae)

Bulla is a fluid-filled raised lesion greater than 5 mm in skin diseases.

大疱在皮肤病中指大于5mm的含液体的隆起性病变。

Both chest radiography and CT could depict the size, location and morphology of the giant bulla.

胸片和CT均能清晰显示巨型肺大泡的大小、位置和形态。

bullet [ˈbulit] *n.* 子弹;弹丸

The bullet went clean through his shoulder。

子弹穿透他的肩膀。

There is no magic bullet against cancer.

没有抗癌灵药。

bullous [ˈbuləs] *a.* 囊泡性

In bullous emphysema, rupture of the bullae may give rise to pneumothorax.

患囊泡性肺气肿时,大泡破裂会导致气胸。

Bullous emphysema sometimes is associated with old tuberculous scarring.

囊泡性肺气肿有时与陈旧性结核瘢痕有关。

bump [bʌmp] *v.* 碰到;撞倒

Air currents flow and bump into each other, carrying the water vapor from place to place.

气流移动并相互撞击,将水蒸气从一地携带到另一地。

Environmental factors such as winds, bumps in the road, and hills require continual small adjustments of the steering wheel and the accelerator.

环境因素如风、路面不平、坡面等需要对方向盘和加速器不断进行小的调整。

bunion [ˈbʌnjən] *n.* 踇囊炎;踇趾囊肿

A bunion is a deformity characterized by lateral deviation of the great toe.

踇囊炎是脚大踇趾侧偏(向第二趾)畸形。

The symptoms of bunions include irritated skin around the bunion, pain when walking, joint redness and pain.

䟹囊炎的症状有踇趾周围皮肤炎症、走路时疼痛及关节红肿疼痛等。

bupleurum [bʌ'pluərəm] *n.* 柴胡,柴胡属

Bupleurum Chinense Emulsion has a marked suppressive effect on inflammation.

北柴胡乳剂具有显著的抑制炎症的作用。

I am interested in the classification and distribution of Bupleurum L. (Umbelliferae Juss.) in Mongolia.

我对蒙古柴胡属 L.(伞形科)植物的分类和分布很感兴趣。

burden ['bəːdən] *n.* 负担,负荷

Four different methods have been applied to estimate the burden of disease due to indoor air pollution from household solid fuel use in developing countries.

采用了四种不同的方法评估发展中国家由于家用固体燃料的使用造成室内空气污染引起的疾病负担。

The economic burden of cancer is the economic cost to the nation associated with expenditures on cancer preventive, screening and treatment services.

肿瘤的经济负担是指国家在肿瘤预防、筛查和治疗上的开支。

burdock ['bəːdɔk] *n.* 牛蒡,牛蒡子

Burdock is a powerful blood purifier.

牛蒡子为强力的净血剂。

Studies on antimutagenicity of burdock are important.

牛蒡子对抗基因突变作用的研究很重要。

burn [bəːn] *n.* 烧伤

Severe burns are among the most difficult of all medical problems to bandle.

严重烧伤是所有医疗课题中最难处理的问题之一。

Modern burn treatment has been eminently successful in saving the lives of many people.

现代的烧伤治疗(方法)已在拯救众多病人生命上取得了突出的成就。

burning ['bəːniŋ] *a.* 燃烧的;高热的; *n.* 灼热,烧灼感

Herpes simplex begins with grouped vesicles, often accompanied by burning pain.

生殖器疱疹开始时多为成群水疱,常伴有烧灼样疼痛。

bursa ['bəːsə] *n.* 滑囊,黏液囊 (*pl.* bursae ['bəːsiː])

A bursa is a small fluid-filled sac lined with synovial membrane.

滑囊是一个内衬有滑膜并充满滑液的小囊。

Bursae function as cushions between bones and tendons and/or muscles around a joint.

滑囊主要功能为缓冲骨骼与肌腱或/和关节周围肌肉的相互作用。

bursitis [bə'saitis] *n.* 黏液囊炎 滑囊炎

There were 11 cases of subcutaneous bursitis with pain on the tip of the Kirschner pins (65%).

其中克氏针尖端皮下痛性滑囊炎 11 例,占全部并发症的 65%。

Diathermy may be prescribed for arthritis, bursitis, and other conditions requiring heat treatment.

对关节炎、黏液囊炎还有其他需要热医疗的病症,都可用透热疗法治疗。

butazone ['bjuːtəzəun] *n.* 保泰松,苯丁唑啉

Butazone should be discontinued at the first signs of the above side effects.

一旦出现上述副作用,应立即停止使用保泰松。

buttock ['bʌtək] *n.* 半边臀部, [*pl.*] 臀部

Pain referred to the low back or buttocks is often associated with diseases of the cervix, urethra, or lower portions of the bladder and rectum.

涉及腰骶部或臀部的疼痛往往与宫颈、尿道、膀胱下部或直肠下段的疾病有关。

Male human buttocks are different from female human buttocks.

男性的臀部和女性的不一样。

The buttocks are formed by the masses of the gluteal muscles superimposed by a layer of fat.

臀部是由大量的臀肌和一层叠加的脂肪组成。

bypass [ˈbaipɑːs] *n.* 分流，旁路

Coronary bypass surgery has been attempted, but the results are poor.

已试行冠状动脉旁路术，但效果不佳。

The patient has a history of coronary artery bypass graft.

该病人有冠状动脉搭桥史。

v. 绕过；忽视；回避

And for people with spinal-cord injuries, we could bypass the injury to a certain extent.

对于那些脊髓受伤的人，我们可以在一定程度上绕过受伤部位。

by-product [ˈbaiˌprɔdʌkt] *n.* 副产品

Heat is an important by-product of the many chemical activities constantly going on in the tissues all over the body.

热量是在全身所有组织中不断进行着的众多的化学活动中产生的一种重要的副产品。

Useful drugs are made from inorganic substances or are plant and animal by-products.

有用的药物是由无机物制造的或者是植物和动物的副产品。

Ammonia, coal tar, and coke are all by-products obtained in the manufacture of coal gas.

氨、煤焦油和焦炭都是生产煤气时产生的副产品。

byssinosis [ˌbisiˈnəusis] *n.* 棉尘病，棉屑沉着病

Byssinosis is an occupational lung disease caused by exposure to cotton dust in inadequately ventilated working environments.

棉尘病是一种在通风不畅的工作场所接触棉尘而引发的职业性肺病。

Byssinosis commonly occurs in workers who are employed in yarn and fabric manufacture industries.

棉尘病通常发生在纱线和织物制造业的从业工人中。

C

cable [ˈkeibəl] *n.* 电缆，有线

They are building a submarine cable tunnel.

他们正在建设一条海底电缆隧道。

It can even transmit shows, via a cable or wirelessly, to big TV screens if you like.

如果你愿意的话，它甚至还可以通过有线或无线方式将节目传输到更大的电视屏幕上。

v. 发电报

Don't forget to cable us as soon as you arrive.

别忘了一到就给我们打个电报。

cache [kæʃ] *n.* [计] 高速缓冲存储器；缓存

The data needed are found in the cache.

在高速缓冲存储器中找到所需数据。

The battery is no longer powering the cache.

电池将不再给高速缓存供电。

A cache is typically used for quick data access.

缓存通常用于快速数据访问。

cachectin [kəˈkektin] *n.* 恶病质素

Cachectin plays a central role in mediating the toxic effects of endotoxin and other microbial products.

恶病质素在介导内毒素及其他微生物产物的毒性作用中起主导作用。

cachexia [kəˈkeksiə] *n.* 恶病质

In addition, tumor necrosis factor induces catabolic responses of chronic inflammation which contribute to the profound wasting(cachexia) associated with many chronic diseases.

此外，肿瘤坏死因子诱发慢性炎症的分解代谢，因而使许多有慢性病的患者机体过度消耗（恶病质）。

cadaver [kəˈdeivə] *n.* 尸体

Cadaver kidneys are removed as soon as possible after the donor's death, preferably within an hour.

尸体的肾在捐献者死亡后最好是在一小时内尽快取出。

The Visible Human Male consists of 1871 images showing cross-sections of a normal male cadaver.

《男性可视人体》电子书内有 1871 幅影像，显示一个正常男性尸体的各种横断面。

cadence [ˈkeidəns] *n.* 步调

Cadence may refer to the number of steps per minute.

步调可解释为每分钟的步数。

Cadence may have other meanings.

步调可能还有其他的含义。

cadherin [kædˈhiərin] *n.* 钙黏素，钙黏着蛋白

The cadherins are a large family of glycoproteins.

钙黏素是一个糖蛋白大家族。

cadmium [ˈkædmiəm] *n.* 镉

Arsenic compounds are by-products of the mining and the smelting of cadmium, cooper, lead,

nickel and zinc.
砷化合物是镉、铜、铅、镍和锌等采矿和熔炼的副产品。

caffeine [kæ'fiːn,'kæfˌiːn] *n.* 咖啡因
In humans' body, caffeine also acts as a central nervous system stimulant.
在人体内,咖啡因也能起到中枢神经系统兴奋剂的作用。
I like energy drinks that just have herbs and vitamins in them, but no caffeine.
我喜欢那种只含有药草和维生素的能量饮料,但不含咖啡因。

calamine ['kæləmain] *n.* [中医] 炉甘石
Please establish a method to determine the content of chloramphenicol in calamine chloramphenicol lotion compound.
请建立一个复方炉甘石氯霉素洗剂中氯霉素的含量测定方法。
Their product is a kind of calamine lotion.
他们的产品是一种炉甘石洗剂。

calamus ['kæləməs] *n.* 菖蒲
The thesis mainly introduces calamus, a traditional Chinese medicine.
本论文主要介绍了一种中药——菖蒲。
We should know about extraction and separation of insecticidal constituents from calamus.
我们需要了解菖蒲的杀虫活性成分的提取与分离。

calcaneocuboid [kælˌkeiniəu''kjuːbɔid] *a.* 跟骰的
In this study, clinical and radiological results after lateral column lengthening by calcaneocuboid traction arthrodesis and calcaneus osteotomy were compared.
在本研究中比较了用跟骰牵引关节融合术与跟骨截骨术进行侧柱延长术之后的临床效果与放射学结果。

calcaneum [kæl'keiniəm] *n.* 跟骨
For the human, the calcaneus is a bone of the tarsus of the foot which constitutes the heel.
在人类,跟骨是脚骨中跗骨的一块,它构成脚跟。
In the human body, the calcaneus is the largest of the tarsal bones and the largest bone of the foot.
在人类,跟骨是跗骨中最大一块同时也是足骨中最大一个。

calcicosilicosis ['kælsikəuˌsili'kəusis] *n.* 钙矽肺
Calcicosilicosis is a type of mixed dust pneumoconiosis due to the inhalation of mineral dust containing silica and calcium-containing minerals.
钙矽肺是一种混合性粉尘的尘肺,由吸入含硅的矿物性粉尘和含钙的矿尘所致。
Pneumoconiosis is caused by more than one type of dust, such as anthracosilicosis, calcicosilicosis, or silicosiderosis.
尘肺病由多种粉尘导致,例如煤矽肺、钙矽肺、矽铁尘肺。

calcific [kæl'sifik] *a.* 钙化的
Idiopathic, calcific aortic stenosis is a degenerative disorder common in the elderly and usually mild.
特发性的由于主动脉钙化引起的主动脉瓣狭窄是一种退行性病变,多见于老年人并且病变程度较轻。

calcification [ˌkælsifi'keiʃən] *n.* 钙化,沉钙(作用)
Pericardial calcification as a result of chronic constrictive pericarditis is rare in children.
由患慢性缩窄性心包炎所致的心包钙化在儿童中较少见。
The mass showed some fine calcification and appeared to be in the area of the lower pole of the kidney.
该肿块有细小的钙化点,似乎位于肾的较下端区域。

calcify ['kælsifai] *v.* 钙化

The primary complex heals with fibrosis and frequently, calcifies without therapy.
原发性综合病变愈合并纤维化,常常未经治疗就钙化。
The necrotic mass may become calcified.
坏死区可发生钙化。

calcineurin [ˌkælsiˈnjuərin] *n.* 神经钙蛋白,钙神经素,钙调磷酸酶
The cytosolic serine/threonine phosphatase calcineurin has a crucial role in signaling via the T-cell receptor.
细胞浆中丝氨酸/苏氨酸磷酸酶钙神经素在 T 细胞受体的信号转导中起重要作用。
The protein calcineurin (CaN) regulates transcriptional programs that control synapse formation and function.
神经钙蛋白(CaN)调节控制突触形成与功能的转录程序。
The research was carried out in 22 pediatric heart transplant recipients who have had a long-term treatment with calcineurin inhibitors.
对长期接受钙调磷酸酶抑制剂治疗的 22 例儿科心脏移植受体进行了研究。

calcinosis [kælsiˈnəusis] *n.* 钙质沉着
Scleroderma is complicated by atrophy, ulceration, calcinosis, and(or) pain.
硬皮病的并发症为萎缩、溃疡、钙质沉积和(或)疼痛。

calcite [ˈkælsait] *n.* [矿物]方解石;南寒水石
Natural calcium carbonate is the chief component of calcite.
天然碳酸钙是方解石中的最主要的成分。
Calcite is used to treat patients with strong fever, extreme thirst and excessive perspiration.
南寒水石可用于治疗壮热、烦渴、大汗的病人。

calcitonin [ˌkælsiˈtəunin] *n.* 降钙素
Calcitonin can promote osteoclast apoptosis.
降钙素能促进破骨细胞凋亡。
High serum calcium levels cause production of the hormone calcitonin.
血清内高钙水平可引起降钙激素的产生。

calcitriol [kælˈsitriɔl] *n.* 骨化三醇
Calcitriol is effective on bone mineral density in the treatment of corticosteroid-induced osteoporosis.
骨化三醇在治疗皮质类固醇诱导的骨质疏松症中可改善骨密度。
The effect of calcitriol plus alendronate is s uperior to calcitriol alone for senile osteoporosis.
对老年性骨质疏松的治疗,阿仑膦酸钠和骨化三醇联合治疗的效果优于单用骨化三醇。

calcium [ˈkælsiəm] *n.* 钙
Vitamin D increases the amount of calcium in our blood.
维生素 D 能增加血中钙的含量。
Finally, parathyroid hormone inhibits calcium excretion in the kidney.
最后,甲状旁腺激素可抑制肾内钙的排泄。

calculate [ˈkælkjuleit] *v.* 计算;预测
Science teaches us that all energy of whatever type can be measured or calculated in terms of heat units.
科学教给我们不论任何类型的能量都能以热单位来测量或计量。
Scientists have calculated that the world's population will double by the end of the century.
科学家预测在本世纪末世界人口将翻一番。
Brown et al calculated curves which describe the progressive decrease in VDRL titer after treatment.
布劳恩等制订了反映治疗后 VDRL 滴定度逐渐下降的曲线。

calculous [ˈkælkjuləs] *a.* 结石的

The patients in this ward all suffer from calculous cholecystitis.
这个病室的病人均患结石性胆囊炎。

calculus [ˈkælkjuləs] (*pl.* calculi [ˈkælkjulai]) *n.* 结石

Decubitus ulcers and mobilization of calcium stores with formation of renal calculi may also be seen.
褥疮性溃疡和伴随肾结石形成的钙堆积活动均可见到。

Calculi in the urinary tract are commonly composed of calcium oxalate and are usually visible on X-ray examination.
泌尿道结石通常由草酸钙组成,经 X 线检查便可发现。

calf [kɑːf] *n.* 腓肠肌(俗名小腿肚)

Inspection of the calves and intravenous cannula dressings may reveal thrombophlebitis.
观察腓肠肌和静脉插管敷料能发现血栓性静脉炎。

When standing, the venous return from the legs depends largely on the muscular activity of the calf muscles.
站立时小腿的静脉回流主要靠小腿肌的活动。

caliber [ˈkælibə] *n.* 管径,口径

It is chiefly the caliber of the arterioles that controls the systemic vascular resistance.
全身性血管阻力主要由小动脉的管径决定。

calibrate [ˈkælibreit] *v.* 校准,校正

You do not need to calibrate the motion sensor.
你无需校准运动传感器。

A direct means is required to calibrate the indirect method.
要求用直接测定法校正间接测定法。

calibration [ˌkæliˈbreiʃən] *n.* 校准;刻度;标度

Insufficient calibration of detector sensitivity may cause system artifact.
探测器灵敏度校准不充分可以导致系统伪影的产生。

The standards used for calibrating an instrument are simply referred to as calibration standards.
用于校准仪器的标准称作校准标准。

We can increase the accuracy by constructing a calibration curve.
我们可以通过建立标准曲线来提高精确度。

calibrator [ˈkæliˌbreitə] *n.* 校准仪

Transformer calibrator is widely used by the electric power department and the measure department.
互感器校验仪是电力和计量部门广泛使用的检测仪器。

A novel comparator-type instrument transformer calibrator with electric zero adjustment is presented in this paper.
该论文介绍了一种带有电子调零线路的新型比较仪式互感器校验仪。

Caliciviridae [kəˌlisiˈviridiː] *n.* 杯状病毒科

Viruses in three of the four established genera of the family Caliciviridae have been detected in pigs.
杯状病毒科中已确立的 4 个病毒属中有 3 个属的病毒已在猪身上检测到。

Research on porcine caliciviruses has yielded new insights into the mechanisms of pathogenesis, replication, and evolution of the family Caliciviridae.
通过猪杯状病毒的研究,对杯状病毒科的致病机制、复制和进化有了新的理解。

callosity [kəˈlɔsiti] *n.* 皮肤硬结;老茧

Callosity is a symptom that appears in many diseases.
许多疾病有皮肤硬结的症状。

A callosity is a piece of skin that has become thickened as a result of repeated contact and friction.

皮肤硬结是指一片皮肤反复的接触和摩擦而导致的皮肤增厚。

callostasis [ˌkæləˈsteisis] *n.* 骨痂

Callostasis is the sign of gradual healing of a fracture

骨痂是骨折逐渐愈合的标志。

The formation of callostasis is the fourth stage of fracture healing.

骨痂的形成属于骨折愈合的第四阶段。

callous [ˈkæləs] *a.* ,无情的;麻木的;硬结的

His behaviour was notably aberrant and showed a callous disregard for others.

他的行为明显异常,并表现为对他人无情的冷漠。

His muscles became hard as iron and grew callous to ordinary pain.

它的肌肉变得如钢铁般坚硬,对一般的疼痛已经麻木。

callus [ˈkæləs] *n.* 胼胝;骨痂

Tackle calluses and hard skin with a foot file or pumice.

用足锉或浮石修整双足的胼胝和硬茧。

calm [kɑːm] *a.* 镇静的

It is important to keep calm in an emergency.

在紧急情况下保持镇静是重要的。

v. 使平静,使镇静

Heavy sedation should be avoided, but small doses of tranquilizers may be helpful in calming the emotionally disturbed patient during the first few days.

应避免使用大剂量镇静剂,但在最初的几天内使用小剂量的镇静剂可能有助于使情绪失常的病人平静下来。

calmodulin [ˈkælməˌdjulin] *n.* 钙调蛋白,钙调素

Calmodulin (CaM) is a protein that binds calcium and it is expressed in all complex structures.

钙调节蛋白是一种和钙结合的蛋白,机体所有复杂结构中都有表达。

Amino acid sequence of yeast calmodulin shares 60% identity with other calmodulins.

酵母钙调节蛋白的氨基酸序列和其他钙调节蛋白有 60% 的同源性。

calnexin [ˈkælneksin] *n.* 钙连接蛋白(内质网的一种磷酸化的钙结合蛋白)

The protein calnexin binds to partly folded members of the immunoglobulin superfamily of proteins and retains them in the endoplasmic reticulum until folding is completed.

钙联接蛋白结合那些部分折叠的免疫球蛋白超家族成员,并将它们滞留在内质网内直到折叠完毕。

calomel [ˈkæləmel] *n.* [中医] 轻粉

The hospitals were worrying about the scarcity of calomel.

各个医院因为轻粉的缺乏而发愁。

Calomel contains the powder of mercury..

轻粉中含有水银的粉末。

calorie [ˈkæləri] *n.* 卡(热量单位)

By definition a calorie is the amount of heat required to raise the temperature of 1 kilogram of water 1 degree C.

按定义来说,一卡就是 1000g 水升高 1℃ 所需要的热量。

One world-renowned gerontologist claims that sticking to 1800 calories a day will keep us all younger.

一位世界闻名的老年病学家声称,固定每天摄入 1800 卡路里的热量,将使我们永保年轻。

For most people excessive calorie intake beyond daily energy requirements leads to weight gain in the form of fat.

对大多数人来说,摄入超过日需的热量就会以脂肪积累的形式导致体重增加。

calorimetry [ˌkæləˈrimitri] *n.* 测热法

The amount of heat given off in the breakdown of food can be measured by either direct or indirect calorimetry.

食物分解所释放的热量可以用直接或间接测热法测量。

calreticulin [ˌkælriˈtikjulin] *n.* 钙网蛋白

Calreticulin is the molecular chaperone that binds initially to MHC class Ⅰ, MHC class Ⅱ, and other proteins that contain immunoglobulin-like domains, such as the T-cell and B-cell antigen receptors.

钙网蛋白是一种分子伴侣，最初结合到 MHC Ⅰ类、MHC Ⅱ类分子以及其他含有免疫球蛋白样结构域的蛋白，如 T 细胞和 B 细胞抗原受体。

calsequestrin [ˌkælsiˈkwestrin] *n.* 贮钙蛋白

Calsequestrin occurs on the inner membrane surface of the sarcoplasmic reticulum, it is a calcium binding protein, it serves to chelate and store calcium ions.

贮钙蛋白存在于肌浆网内膜表面，它是一种能结合钙的蛋白，其作用是螯合和贮存钙离子。

camera [ˈkæmərə] *n.* 照相机，摄影机

The department of pediatrics has bought two digital cameras.

小儿科买了两台数字照相机。

There is a very close functional relationship between the eye and the camera.

人的眼睛和摄影机之间有着十分密切的功能关系。

camphor [ˈkæmfə] *n.* 莰酮，樟脑

These clothes have smell of camphor.

这些衣服闻起来有樟脑的气味。

Camphor oil has recently been evaluated for its effectiveness in treating demodicoses that often occur with rosacea.

樟脑油对常出现于酒糟鼻中的蠕形螨病有治疗效果。

camphorwood [ˈkæmfəwud] *n.* 樟木；龙脑香木

This research is about extracting camphorwood oil from camphor tree seeds.

这个实验是关于从樟树籽中提取樟木油的。

The step is made out of a complete piece of camphorwood.

这个台阶是由一块完整的樟木做成的。

camptodactyly [ˌkæmptəuˈdæktili] *n.* 屈曲指，先天性屈指畸形

Camptodactyly is a medical condition involving fixed flexion deformity of the interphalangeal joints of the little finger.

先天性屈指畸形是指累及小指指间关节的固定屈曲畸形。

A number of congenital syndromes may cause camptodactyly.

许多先天性的综合征可以引起屈曲指。

camptomelic [kæmptəuˈmelik] *a.* 肢弯曲的

Camptomelic dysplasia is due to mutations in the SOX9 gene on chromosome 17q.

肢弯曲发育异常是由于染色体 17q 上的 SOX9 基因突变造成的。

Camptomelic dysplasia is an autosomal dominant disorder with usually lethal skeletal malformations.

肢弯曲发育异常为常染色体显性遗传病，常造成致命的骨骼畸形。

campylobacter [ˌkæmpiləuˈbæktə] *n.* 弯曲菌属

Campylobacter is gram-negative, spiral, and microaerophilic, causing opportunistic infection in humans.

弯曲菌为革兰阴性、螺旋状的微需氧细菌，可引起人类机会感染。

At least a dozen species of campylobacter have been implicated in human disease.

弯曲菌属中至少有十多个菌种与人类疾病有关。

campylobacteriosis [ˈkæmpiləuˌbæktiəriˈəusis] *n.* 弯曲菌病

Campylobacteriosis is an infection by the campylobacter bacterium, most commonly *C. jejuni*.

弯曲菌病是一种弯曲菌引起的感染，其中空肠弯曲菌感染最常见。

Campylobacteriosis produces an inflammatory diarrhea or dysentery syndrome, mostly including cramps, fever and pain.

弯曲菌病表现为炎症性腹泻或痢疾样综合征，多数有肠痉挛、发热和腹痛。

canal [kəˈnæl] *n.* 管，道；沟渠

The spinal cord is contained entirely within the vertebral canal.

脊髓充满在椎管内。

The mouth cavity is the beginning of the alimentary canal.

消化道起始于口腔。

canalicular [ˌkænəˈlikjulə] *a.* 小管的

Additional findings include bile stasis (intracellular and canalicular) and portal and perilobular fibrosis.

其他发现包括胆汁淤滞（细胞内的和小管的）以及门静脉和小叶周围的纤维化。

canaliculus [ˌkænəˈlikjuləs] *n.* 小管；小沟

In an early embryo, a bile canaliculus has been found.

胆小管在胚胎早期已经形成。

The objective of our study is to estimate the curative effect of anastomosed laceration canaliculus.

本研究的目的是评估吻合外伤性泪小管断离的临床疗效。

cancer [ˈkænsə] *n.* 癌，恶性肿瘤

The risk of breast cancer increases with age.

患乳腺癌的危险随着年龄的增长而增加。

In 60 seconds, the tumor became an ice ball, all cancer cells were killed.

60 秒后，肿瘤变成了一冰块，所有的癌细胞都被杀死。

The therapy is a breakthrough in cancer treatment.

这种治疗方法是在癌症治疗上的一个突破。

cancerous [ˈkænsərəs] *a.* 癌的

The X-ray revealed a cancerous growth in the breast of this middle-aged woman.

X 线显示这位中年妇女的乳房部位有癌性生长物。

If there are multiple cancerous nodules in an organ, they are probably metastatic.

如果一个器官有多个恶性瘤结节，则可能为转移瘤。

cancrum [ˈkæŋkrəm] *n.* 坏疽性溃疡

Cancrum oris is now rarely seen in the industrial world, but in many developing countries it is not uncommon.

坏疽性口炎在发达国家已经几乎绝迹，但在一些发展中国家却时有发生。

Noma also known as cancrum, is gangrenous disease leading to tissue destruction of the face, especially the mouth and cheek.

坏疽性口炎（坏疽性溃疡）是一种坏疽疾病，它能破坏脸部组织，特别是嘴部和面颊。

Candida [ˈkændidə] *n.* 念珠菌属

The commonest causes of vaginitis in adult women are infection with Trichomonas vaginalis or with Candida albicans.

成年妇女阴道炎的最常见原因是阴道滴虫感染或白色念珠菌属感染。

candidate [ˈkændidit] *n.* 候选人；报考者

Patients for research must be candidates for operation and must have accepted surgery as alternative therapy.

供研究的患者必须是手术预选对象，并且必须已同意手术可作为替换疗法。

Because pathways involved in drug response are often known or at least partially known, pharmacogenetic studies are highly amenable to candidate gene association studies.

因为参与药物反应的通路常常是清楚的或至少部分是清楚的，遗传药理学的研究是全然经得起候选基因关联性研究的检验的。

candidiasis [kændiˈdaiəsis] *n.* 念珠菌病

In patients at risk for AIDS, oral candidiasis is strongly indicative of subsequent development of overt AIDS.

艾滋病高危患者若患口腔念珠菌病，则强烈提示其日后定将患艾滋病。

The presence of candidiasis in the upper urinary tract is more commonly secondary to hematogenous spread.

上尿路念珠菌病的发生更多地继发于血源性感染。

candidosis [ˌkændiˈdəusis] *n.* 念珠菌病

Candidiasis is a fungal infection (mycosis) of any of the Candida species, of which Candida albicans is the most common.

念珠菌病是念珠菌属真菌感染性疾病，其中白色念珠菌最常见。

Superficial infections of skin and mucosal membranes by Candida causing local inflammation and discomfort are very common in the people.

由念珠菌引起的皮肤表浅或黏膜感染导致的局部炎症和不适在人群中是十分常见的。

candiduria [ˌkændiˈdjuəriə] *n.* 念珠菌尿

Wise et al observed an increased incidence of candiduria from 1% to 8% over a 10-year period.

Wise 等观察到念珠菌尿发病率在 10 年内由 1% 升至 8%。

The investigation concluded that candiduria is benign and self-limiting and rarely requires specific treatment.

这项研究的结论是，念珠菌尿是良性的与自限性的，很少需要特殊治疗。

canid [ˈkænid] *n.* 犬科动物

Canid is the biological family of carnivorous and omnivorous mammals.

犬科动物在生物学上属肉食和肉草兼食性哺乳动物家族成员。

cannabinoid [ˈkænəbiˌnɔid] *n.* 大麻的化学成分；大麻素

Blocking these cannabinoid receptors can reduce the sense of hunger and help people lose weight.

阻断这些大麻素受体可以减少饥饿感，从而帮助人们减肥。

The cardiac cannabinoid receptors have the effect of regulating the cardiac rhythm and myocardial contractility.

心肌大麻素受体具有调节心律和心肌收缩力的作用。

cannabis [ˈkænəbis] *n.* 大麻

Hallucinogens, cannabis, and amphetamines may produce a delusional disorder.

致幻剂、大麻和苯丙胺可能造成妄想症。

cannula [ˈkænjulə] (*pl.* cannulae [ˈkænjuliː] 或 cannulas) *n.* 套管，插管

It is well known to the surgical world for the low cost and hard-wearing cannulas and artificial vessels that can be made from polyester.

外科界都知道，聚酯制成的导管和人造血管既便宜又耐用。

A cannula is a hollow tube designed for insertion into a body cavity, such as the bladder, or a blood vessel.

套管是用以插入体腔如膀胱或血管的中空插管。

cantharides [ˌkænˈθæridiːz] *n.* 斑蝥

Cantharides are a kind of pharmaceutical insects.

斑蝥是一种重要的药用昆虫。

Pharmaceutical research and resource development on cantharides were important.

斑蝥的药用研究及资源开发很重要。

capability [keipə'biliti] *n.* 能力,才能

The patient with a long-term disability tends to suffer a decline in their functional capabilities in the ordinary hospital.

长期伤残者在普通医院里容易造成身体功能衰退。

capable ['keipəbəl] *a.* 有能力的

The outer hair cells are capable of slow and fast motility.

外毛细胞有缓慢和快速的(两种)活动能力。

Malignant tumors are composed of cells which are capable of invading adjacent tissues.

恶性肿瘤由能够侵袭邻近组织的细胞组成。

capacity [kə'pæsiti] *n.* 能力;容量

Energy is defined as the ability or capacity to do work.

“能”就是做功的能力。

Air pollution reduces the capacity of the lung to combat viruses and possibly bacteria.

空气污染降低了肺部对抗病毒和某些细菌的能力。

All cells have a capacity to repair some damage by radiation, but this seems to be greatest in normal tissue.

所有的细胞都有能力修复某些放射线所致的损伤,但在正常组织中最为明显。

Early shock is usually due to a decrease in blood volume, or an increase in the capacity of the vascular space, or both.

早期休克通常是由于血量减少,或血管腔的容量增大,或二者并存。

capillarisin [kə'pilərisin] *n.* 茵陈色原酮

Capillarisin was isolated from Herba Artemisiae Capillaris.

茵陈色原酮已从茵陈中分离出来。

The antioxidant bioactivity of Capillarisin (Cap) was studied.

我们研究了茵陈色原酮的抗氧化生物活性。

capillarization [kəˌpilərai'zeiʃən] *n.* 毛细血管化

In liver cirrhosis, the deposition of collagen in the space of Disse leads to capillarization of sinusoids.

肝硬化时,狄氏腔内胶原的沉积导致肝窦毛细血管化。

Capillarization of sinusoids impairs the function of sinusoids and blocks the exchange of solutes between hepatocytes and plasma.

肝窦毛细血管化会损伤肝窦功能,阻碍肝细胞和血浆之间的物质交换。

capillary [kə'piləri] *n.* 毛细血管

Capillaries are one of the fine, thin walled blood vessels connecting arteries and veins.

毛细血管是连接动脉和静脉的一种很细和薄壁的血管。

In the lungs, the exceedingly minute arteries branch out and form capillaries.

在肺里,极微小的动脉分支形成毛细血管。

capital ['kæpitəl] *a.* 股骨头的;重要的

Slipped capital femoral epiphysis can result in posterior and inferior displacement of the epiphysis on the femoral neck.

股骨头骨骺滑脱症能导致股骨颈上骨骺向后向下移位。

capitellum [ˌkæpə'teləm] *n.* 肱骨小头

In human anatomy of the arm, the lateral portion of the articular surface of the humerus consists of a smooth, rounded eminence, named the capitellum.

在人类的臂骨中,肱骨近端关节的侧面包含一个光滑的,圆形的小突起,叫做肱骨小头。

The role of capitellum is to adhere tendons to the bones and then to form the joints.

肱骨小头的作用是附着肌腱和形成关节。

capping [ˈkæpiŋ] *n.* 顶裂，帽化

The capping was stable at proper environmental pH and salt concentration.

在适宜的 pH 值和盐浓度环境中这种帽化作用是稳定的。

G-quadruplex-interactive compounds have been shown to inhibit telomerase access as well as telomere capping.

研究显示 G 四链体化合物可抑制端粒末端转移酶的靠近和端粒加帽。

capsid [ˈkæpsid] *n.* 衣壳，外壳

The capsid protects the nucleic acid from enzymes or physical agents.

衣壳保护核酸免受酶或物理因素的破坏。

capsule [ˈkæpsjuːl] *n.* 囊；包膜，荚膜；胶囊（剂）

Fibromyomata receive their blood supply from the vessels in the surrounding capsule.

纤维肌瘤血供来自周围包膜中的血管。

Some capsules even appear to be toxic for phagocytes.

有些荚膜甚至对吞噬细胞具有毒性。

Drugs are often made in the forms of tablets，capsules or liquids.

药品常被制成片剂、胶囊剂或液体剂型。

capture [ˈkæptʃə] *v.* 捕获；夺取

The pseudopodia permit the organism to move and to capture food by encircling food particles.

伪足使生物体移动，并且用包围食物颗粒的方法来获取食物。

This captures the specific cytokine released in a spot around the active T cell.

这可捕获在激活的 T 细胞周围某一位点上释放的特异细胞因子。

Caralluma [kærəˈlumə] *n.* 水牛角属

They are going to establish a method to identify illegally added Caralluma in Lingyangganmao Capsules.

他们打算设计一个检测方法来测量在羚羊感冒胶囊中非法添加的水牛角属。

The medicinal value of caralluma is extraordinarily different from that of chamoishorn.

水牛角属的药用价值与羚羊角非常不同。

caramel [ˈkærəmel] *n.* 焦糖

The method proved to be useful for the analysis of 4MeI in other foods such as caramel colors，drinks，and Worcestershire sauce.

这种方法在分析其他食物例如焦糖色素、饮料、辣酱油中的 4-甲基咪唑时被证实是有用的。

Early researches have detected caramel color contains 5-hydroxymethyl-2-furaldehyde which is toxic and should be removed from caramel color as much as possible.

早期研究已经检测到焦糖色素中含有 5-羟甲基-2-呋喃甲醛，后者是有毒的，应该尽可能的从焦糖色素中去除。

carbachol [ˈkɑːbəkɔl] *n.* 卡巴可，氯化氨甲酰胆碱

Carbachol may be used chronically for therapy of noncongestive，wide-angle glaucoma.

氯化氨甲酰胆碱可长期用于非充血性、开角型青光眼病人。

carbamazepine [ˌkɑːbəˈmæzəpiːn] *n.* 卡马西平，酰胺咪嗪（抗惊厥药）

If further attacks occur it is best to start with either carbamazepine or phenytoin，200mg at night for an adult.

如果出现进一步发作，最好先启用卡马西平或苯妥英，成人在晚上服用 200mg。

carbenicillin [kɑːbeniˈsilin] *n.* 羧苄青霉素（用于尿路感染）

This organism，however，is only moderately sensitive to carbenicillin.

这种微生物仅对羧苄青霉素有中度敏感性。

Carbenicillin is poorly absorbed from the gastrointestinal tract and must be given by intramuscular injection.

羧苄青霉素胃肠道吸收不佳,必须肌注。

carbide [ˈkɑːbaid] *n.* 碳化物

The orifices of this nozzle are almost chocked up with carbide.

这个油嘴的喷孔几乎被碳化物堵死。

This important carbide precipitates both inter and intragranularly.

这种重要的碳化物向晶体内和晶体间沉淀。

carbodiimide [ˌkɑːbədaiˈimaid] *n.* 碳二亚胺

Chitosan was thiolated by carbodiimide method and thiolation was confirmed qualitatively and quantitatively.

壳聚糖用碳二亚胺法作了硫醇化,并且对硫醇化进行了定性和定量上的证实。

In this study, densified collagen films were fabricated by a plastic compression technique and cross-linked using carbodiimide.

在该研究中,致密的胶原蛋白薄膜是用一种塑料压缩技术制造,并通过碳二亚胺交联。

carbohydrase [ˌkɑːbəuˈhaidreis] *n.* 糖酶,碳水化物酶

Carbohydrase is an enzyme that breaks down (cleaves) carbohydrates into simple sugars.

糖酶是一种可将糖类分解成单糖的酶。

We hypothesized that this decrease in carbohydrase activity might be due to a decrease in the carbohydrate.

我们猜测这种糖酶活性的下降可能是由于碳水化合物的下降。

carbohydrate [ˌkɑːbəuˈhaidreit] *n.* 碳水化合物,糖类

For an adequate diet, the emphasis on carbohydrates is beneficial.

为了使饭食能够满足需要,强调一下碳水化合物的含量是有益处的。

carbomer [ˈkɑːbəumə] *n.* 卡波姆

In organic chemistry, a carbomer is an expanded molecule obtained by insertion of a C_2 unit in a given molecule.

在有机化学中,卡波姆是在一种给定分子中插入一个 C_2 单元而获得的扩展性分子。

Carbomer is also a generic name for synthetic high molecular weight polymers of acrylic acid used as thickening, dispersing, suspending and emulsifying agents in pharmaceuticals and cosmetics.

卡波姆也是丙烯酸合成高分子聚合物的通用名,其在药学和化妆品领域可作为增稠剂、分散剂、悬浮剂和乳化剂使用。

carbon [ˈkɑːbən] *n.* 碳

Proteins consist of carbon, hydrogen, oxygen, nitrogen, sulphur and phophorus.

蛋白质是由碳、氢、氧、氮、硫和磷构成的。

By means of the respiratory system the body takes in oxygen and eliminates carbon dioxide.

机体通过呼吸系统吸入氧气而排出二氧化碳。

The amount of carbon monoxide per cigarette may vary with the type of filter but 12 to 19mg per cigarette.

由于过滤嘴不同,每支香烟吸入人体的一氧化碳总量也不同,但是大约为 12 ~ 19mg/支。

carbon dioxide [ˈkɑːbən-daiˈɔksaid] *n.* 二氧化碳

When you exercise, your metabolism is faster, you produce more carbon dioxide (CO_2)

当你运动时,你的代谢增加,可以产生更多的二氧化碳。

carbonic [kɑːˈbɔnik] *a.* 碳的

In the plasma, some of dissolved carbon dioxide reacts with water to produce carbonic acid.

在血浆中,有些溶解的二氧化碳会和水发生反应而生成碳酸。

carboplatin [ˌkɑːbəuˈplætin] *n.* 卡铂

The thrombocytopenia caused by carboplatin was a direct function of AUC, which in turn was determined by renal clearance of the parent drug.

卡铂所致血小板减少与其药时曲线下面积直接相关，而后者则取决于其原药的肾清除率。

carbopol [ˈkɑːbəpɔl] *n.* 聚羧乙烯

Different types of carbopols are frequently applied excipients of various dosage forms.

不同类型的聚羧乙烯是各种剂型常用的赋形剂。

The formulation containing gellan gum showed better sustained release compared to carbopol based gels.

含结冷胶的配方比含聚羧乙烯凝胶的配方有着更好的缓释作用。

carboxyhaemoglobin（COHb） [kɑːˈbɔksiˌhiːməuˈgləubin] *n.* 碳氧血红蛋白

They found that tobacco smoking was the most important factor in producing elevated COHb.

他们发现，吸烟是导致碳氧血红蛋白含量升高的最重要因素。

The effects are dependent upon the combination of carbon monoxide with hemoglobin to form carboxyhemoglobin.

这些后果取决于一氧化碳同血红蛋白结合生成的碳氧血红蛋白。

carboxylase [kɑːˈbɔksileis] *n.* 羧基酶，羧化酶

Pyruvate carboxylase deficiency is an inherited disorder that causes lactic acid and other potentially toxic compounds to accumulate in the blood.

丙酮酸羧化酶缺乏症是一种遗传性疾病，可导致血中乳酸和其他可能有毒物质的积累。

Carboxylase is an enzyme that catalyzes the incorporation of carbon dioxide into a substrate molecule.

羧化酶是一种酶，可以催化二氧化碳结合到底物分子中。

carboxylation [kɑːˌbɔksəˈleiʃən] *n.* 羧化作用

Carboxylation in chemistry is a chemical reaction in which a carboxylic acid group is introduced in a substrate.

化学中，羧化作用就是在底物中引入羧酸的化学反应。

The key chemical step in which carbon dioxide is "fixed" is called a carboxylation.

固定一个二氧化碳分子的主要化学过程称为羧化。

carboxypolymethylene [kɑːˌbɔksiˌpɔliˈmeθiliːn] *n.* 羧聚乙烯，聚丙烯酸

An antiseptic composition containing a peroxide, glycerol, and a carboxypolymethylene polymer.

防腐剂组成成分里含有过氧化物、甘油和聚丙烯酸聚合体。

It has been disclosed that carboxypolymethylene polymers are effective agents for thickening glycerol.

已经证实聚丙烯酸聚合物是浓缩甘油的有效物质。

carbuncle [ˈkɑːbʌŋkl] *n.* 痈

The bacteria that cause carbuncles grow in a cluster like a bunch of grapes.

引起痈的细菌像成串葡萄一样成群生长。

Carbuncles produce fever, leukocytosis, extreme pain, and prostration.

痈会使患者发热、白细胞增多、剧烈疼痛和乏力。

carcinoembryonic [ˌkɑːsinəuembriˈɔnik] *a.* 癌胚的

Carcinoembryonic antigen (CEA) found primarily in serum of patients with cancers of the gastrointestinal tract, especially cancer of the colon.

癌胚抗原（CEA）主要存在于有消化道癌肿病人的血清中，特别结肠癌的病人。

carcinofetal [ˌkɑːsinəuˈfitəl] *a.* 癌胚的

In liver injury or in association with some neoplasms where the ferritins may be linked to a carcinofetal antigen, serum ferritin levels are elevated also.

当肝脏受损时，或与某些肿瘤有关联时，其铁蛋白可能与癌胚抗原有关，血清铁蛋白质水平也会升高。

carcinogen [kɑːˈsinədʒən] *n.* 致癌物质

Some carcinogens can occur in the environment.

某些致癌物质可能存在于周围环境中。

Besides job-related carcinogens, most people are exposed to several potent cancerous agents.

除了与工作有关的致癌物质外，大多数人还会接触到几种强有力的致癌物质。

carcinogenesis [ˌkɑːsinəuˈdʒenisis] *n.* 致癌作用

There is not sufficient epidemiological, biochemical or genetic data to demonstrate a causal relationship between manganese exposure and carcinogenesis.

没有充分的流行病学、生物化学或遗传学的数据来证明接触锰与其致癌作用之间具有因果关系。

carcinogenic [ˌkɑːsinəuˈdʒenik] *a.* 致癌的

Several cancer producing or carcinogenic agents exist in our environment, naturally or artificially.

在我们生活的环境中有若干种致癌因子，包括天然的和人造的。

carcinogenicity [ˌkɑːsinəudʒiˈnisiti] *n.* 致癌性

As a result of these limitations, most studies of refinery populations provide limited information to directly assess the carcinogenicity of gasoline.

由于这些局限性，大多数对炼油人群的研究资料，用于直接评价汽油的致癌性时，只能提供有限的信息。

carcinoid [ˈkɑːsinɔid] *n.* 类癌瘤

Typically, carcinoid presents with cough, with or without hemoptysis, in young adults.

年轻人患类癌瘤病，通常伴有咳嗽，伴有或不伴有咯血。

Carcinoid syndrome means that hepatic metastases are present.

患类癌瘤综合征（时）表明出现了肝脏转移。

carcinoma [ˌkɑːsiˈnəumə] (*pl.* carcinomas 或 carcinomata [ˌkɑːsiˈnəumətə]) *n.* 癌

The presence of an epigastric mass suggests a carcinoma.

上腹部如有包块提示为癌肿。

In general, carcinomas tend to metastasize through the lymphatic vessels.

通常癌倾向于通过淋巴管转移。

carcinomatosis [ˌkɑːsiˌnəuməˈtəusis] *n.* 癌扩散，癌症

How long will the person with rectum carcinomatosis live after operation?

直肠癌扩散的人术后的寿命有多长？

Pulmonary lymphangitic carcinomatosis (PLC) is a term that refers to tumor growth in the lymphatic system of the lungs.

肺部淋巴管转移癌（PLC）是指在肺部淋巴系统生长的肿瘤。

carcinomectomy [ˌkɑːsinəuˈmektəmi] *n.* 癌切除术

218 patients have received carcinomectomy of esophagus and cardia in the past 10 years in this hospital.

在过去的十年中，218 名患者在该医院接受了食管和贲门的癌切除术。

carcinosarcoma [ˌkɑːsinəusɑːˈkəumə] *n.* 癌肉瘤

Carcinosarcoma is a mixed tumor with carcinoma and sarcoma.

癌肉瘤是含有癌和肉瘤两种成分的混合性肿瘤。

Endometrial carcinosarcomas consist of adenocarcinoma mixed with the malignant mesenchymal elements.

子宫内膜癌肉瘤包括腺癌和恶性间叶成分。

cardia [ˈkɑːdiə] *n.* 贲门

The cardia is the anatomical term for the part of the stomach attached to the esophagus.

贲门是解剖学术语，指连接胃和食管的部位。

Just proximal to the cardia at the gastroesophageal (GE) junction is the lower esophageal sphincter (LES) that is anatomically indistinct but physiologically demonstrable.

紧邻贲门的胃食管交界处是食管下括约肌，这一结构在解剖学上是模糊的但在生理学上

已被证明存在。

cardiac [ˈkɑːdiæk] *a.* 心(脏)的,贲门的

Cardiac massage was tried but all in vain.

试行了心脏按摩,但毫无结果。

There is an opening at the upper part of the stomach called cardiac orifice which allows food in.

胃的上部有一个叫做贲门的开口可让食物入内。

cardinal [ˈkɑːdinəl] *a.* 主要的,基本的

The cardinal clinical features of aseptic meningitis include fever, headache, and a stiff neck.

无菌性脑膜炎的主要临床特征包括发热、头痛及颈部僵直。

The neuroleptic drugs reduce the cardinal signs of the hyperactive syndrome in children.

精神抑制药可减轻儿童多动症的主要体征。

cardioaccelerator [ˌkɑːdiəuækˈseləreitə] *a.* 心动加速的 *n.* 心动加速药

At the same time the cardioaccelerator center of this cardioregulatory center is inhibited by the impulses from the pressure receptors.

同时,心脏调节中枢内的心加速中枢接受了压力感受器来的冲动而产生抑制。

cardiogenic [ˌkɑːdiəuˈdʒenik] *a.* 心源的

Severe cardiogenic shock may occur during the course of diphtheria.

在白喉病程中可能发生严重的心源性休克。

cardioinhibitory [ˌkɑːdiəuinˈhibitəri] *a.* 心(动)抑制的

The cardioinhibitory center of the cardioregulatory center is stimulated to increased activity.

心脏调节中枢内的心抑制中枢被刺激因而增加了活动。

cardiology [ˌkɑːdiˈɔlədʒi] *n.* 心脏病学

Professor Smith has published his second book "Fundamental Theory and Practice of Cardiology".

史密斯教授出版了他的第二本著作《心脏病学基本原理与实践》。

cardiomegaly [ˌkɑːdiəuˈmegəli] *n.* 心肥大

Cardiomegaly and venous congestion are seen in the chest X-ray.

胸部 X 线可见心脏肥大和静脉充血。

Dyspnea and hepatomegaly are nearly always manifest, and cardiomegaly is invariably present.

呼吸困难和肝大几乎总是明显存在,心肥大则是必有的体征。

cardiomyopathy [ˌkɑːdiəumaiˈɔpəθi] *n.* 心肌病

The patient was wrongly thought to have idiopathic cardiomyopathy.

这病人被错误地认为患有特发性心肌病。

cardioneurosis [ˌkɑːdiəunjuəˈrəusis] *n.* 心脏神经症

The diagnosis of cardioneurosis should rule out the organic heart disease.

心脏神经症的诊断应排除器质性心脏病。

The symptoms of cardioneurosis can be similar to angina pectoris.

心脏神经症的症状可与心绞痛相似。

cardioplegia [ˌkɑːdiəuˈpliːdʒiə] *n.* 心麻痹;心脏停搏(法)

Cardioplegia is intentional and temporary cessation of cardiac activity, primarily for cardiac surgery.

心脏停搏是人为的暂时的停止心脏搏动,主要为了进行心脏手术。

The objective of our study is to investigate the effects of clod plasma cardioplegia on the function and structure of immature myocardium.

本研究的目的是评价冷血浆停搏液对未成熟心肌结构及功能的影响。

cardiopulmonary [ˌkɑːdiəuˈpʌlmənəri] *a.* 心肺的

If anemia produces cardiopulmonary symptoms, packed RBC transfusions may be necessary.

如贫血产生了心肺症状,可能需要(给患者)输注纯红细胞。

The recent development of cardiopulmonary resuscitation methodology is changing the pattern of survival from acute infarction.
最新研究出的一种心肺复苏方法正在改变着急性梗死的生存模式。

cardioregulatory [ˌkɑːdiəu'regjulətəri] *a.* 心脏调节的
These areas are therefore called the vasomotor center and the cardioregulatory center.
因此这些区域被称为血管舒缩中心和心脏调节中心。

cardiorespiratory [ˌkɑːdiəuˌris'paiərətəri] *a.* 心肺的，呼吸循环的
The fundamental purpose of the cardiorespiratory system is to deliver oxygen to the cells and to remove carbon dioxide from them.
呼吸循环系统的基本任务是为细胞输送氧气和清除细胞产生的二氧化碳。

cardiotonic [ˌkɑːdiəu'tɔnik] *a.* 强心的
In addition to bronchodilatation, methylxanthine stimulates respiration and has cardionotic and diuretic properties.
除了有扩张支气管的作用外，甲基黄嘌呤药可以兴奋呼吸，并有强心和利尿的作用。

cardiotoxicity ['kɑːdiəˌtɔk'sɪsɪtiː] *n.* 心脏毒性
Anthracyclines remain a mainstay of chemotherapy in spite of their well-recognized cardiotoxicity.
尽管公认蒽环类具有心脏毒性作用，但其仍然是化疗的主体。
Cardiotoxicity was observed in 90-days exposure to bis(2-chloroethoxy)methane in rats.
双-(2-氯乙氧基)甲烷染毒 90 天观察到对大鼠的心脏毒性。

cardiovascular [ˌkɑːdiəu'væskjulə] *a.* 心血管的
Prof. Wang is a specialist in cardiovascular diseases.
王教授是心血管疾病专家。
Hypertension is second only to coronary arteriosclerosis as a cause of cardiovascular disease.
高血压作为心血管疾病的病因，仅次于冠状动脉硬化。
In hospital deaths from acute fibrillation used to account for 30% of cardiovascular deaths.
因急性纤维性颤动而死于医院的病人过去占心血管疾病死亡率的 30%。

cardioversion ['kɑːdiəˌvəːʃən] *n.* 电复律
The restoration of normal rhythm of the heart by electrical shock is called cardioversion.
用电击恢复心脏的正常节律被称为电复律。

carditis [kɑː'daitis] *n.* 心脏炎
The acute rheumatic fever is of limited duration, but the carditis may lead to permanent valvular damage.
急性风湿热持续期有限，但心脏炎却会导致永久性瓣膜损害。

caries ['kɛəriiːz] *n.* 龋
Deficiency in vitamins C and D has a direct influence upon caries of the teeth.
维生素 C 和维生素 D 缺乏，对龋齿形成有直接的影响。

carina [kə'rainə] *n.* 隆凸
Carina is an important mark for judgment of the bifurcation of trachea.
隆凸是判断气管分叉的重要标志。
The mucous membrane of the carina is the most sensitive area of the trachea and larynx for triggering a cough reflex.
隆凸部位的黏膜是气管和喉部引发咳嗽反射最敏感的区域。

carminative ['kɑːminətiv] *a.* 驱风的，排气的 *n.* 驱风剂
Alcohol is a carminative and facilitates the expulsion of gas from the stomach.
酒精是驱风剂，使胃部气体容易排除。

carnitine ['kɑːnitiːn] *n.* 肉毒碱
Carnitine also increases the level of isovaleric acid in plasma.

肉毒碱也增加血浆中异戊酸的水平。

Carnitine appears to decrease muscle soreness.

肉毒碱似可减少肌肉酸痛。

carotene [ˈkærətiːn] *n.* 胡萝卜素

Vitamin A and carotenes are subject to oxidation.

维生素 A 和胡萝卜素易被氧化。

carotid [kəˈrɔtid] *n.* 颈动脉

A second common indication for testing is the evaluation of the asymptomatic carotid bruit.

进行试验第二个常见的指征是对无症状颈动脉杂音的评估。

carotin [ˈkærətin] *n.* 胡萝卜素

Carotin is readily transformed in the cell of the intestinal wall into vitamin A.

胡萝卜素在肠道壁的细胞内很容易转变成维生素 A。

In the experiment, crystalline carotin was fed to the rat.

在这次实验中,用晶体胡萝卜素喂大鼠。

carpus [ˈkɑːpəs] *n.* 腕骨 carpal [ˈkɑːpəl] *a.* 腕骨的,腕的

The carpus is the sole cluster of bones in the wrist between the radius and ulna and the metacarpus.

腕骨是位于腕部在尺骨和桡骨与掌骨之间的骨的集群。

The main role of the carpus is to facilitate effective positioning of the hand and powerful use of the extensors and flexors of the forearm.

腕骨的主要作用是方便手的有效定位并且加强前臂屈肌和伸肌的运用。

carrier [ˈkɛəriə] *n.* 载体,媒介物,带菌者

Iron is an essential component of hemoglobin, the oxygen carrier of the blood.

铁是血红蛋白(即血中氧的运载者)的基本组成要素。

Other carrier proteins may also be defective.

其他的载体蛋白也可发生缺陷。

A person who has the germs of some disease in his body but is not affected by them is called a carrier.

体内藏有某种疾病的病菌但未发病的人称为带菌者。

cartilage [ˈkɑːtilidʒ] *n.* 软骨

A few cartilages are also included in the skeletal system.

有少数软骨也包括在骨骼系统中。

The lining for joints contains cartilage.

关节的内衬含有软骨。

carvedilol [ˈkɑːvəˌdilɔl] *n.* 卡维地洛

Another study is underway to monitor the introduction of carvedilol for the treatment of cardiac failure.

另一项监测卡维地洛治疗心力衰竭的研究正在进行中。

cascade [kæsˈkeid] *n.* 串联,级联,链锁

There might then be a cascade effect as more and more proteins change shape.

随着愈来愈多的蛋白质构形的改变,有可能发生级联效应。

It has provided important paradigms for how receptors activate intracellular signalling cascade.

这为细胞受体如何激活细胞内信号级联反应提供了重要的范例。

casein [ˈkeisiin] *n.* 酪蛋白

Casein is a milk protein commonly used in processed foods.

酪蛋白是加工食品中常用的一种牛奶蛋白。

Casein mRNA activity was assayed by immunoprecipitation.

酪蛋白 mRNA 活性已用免疫沉淀反应进行了测定。

caseous [ˈkeisiəs] *a.* 干酪(似)的

There is no evidence that caseous tissue is reduced by corticosteroids.

尚无证据说明皮质类固醇能减少干酪组织。

Caseous necrosis is a form of cell death in which the tissue takes on a cheese-like appearance.

干酪性坏死是细胞死亡的一种形式,在这种形式中组织呈现奶酪样外观。

Frequently,caseous necrosis is encountered in the foci of tuberculous infections.

干酪性坏死多见于结核性感染病灶内。

caspase [ˈkæspeis] *n.* 胱天蛋白酶,凋亡蛋白酶

They have managed to introduce a human suicidal protein,called caspase-3,in infected cells.

在受感染的细胞中他们已经引入一种人类细胞自杀性蛋白称为凋亡蛋白酶3。

cast [kɑːst] *n.* 管型;模型

The basic structure of the cast is a protein matrix.

管型的基本结构是一种蛋白质。

During acute glomerulonephritis the urine is usually frankly bloody but certainly contains protein and red blood cells,white blood cells and red cell casts.

急性肾小球肾炎时,尿液通常带血,但一定含蛋白、红细胞、白细胞及红细胞管型。

A plaster cast is designed to protect a broken bone and prevent movement of the aligned bone ends until healing has progressed.

石膏模型是用来保护断骨,防止骨折断端活动,直至充分愈合。

castorbean [ˈkɑːstəbiːn] *n.* 蓖麻子

The deadliest plant seed in the world is the castorbean.

世界上最致命的植物的种子是蓖麻子。

Purification and effect against pests of ricin from castorbeans were studied.

研究了蓖麻子中蓖麻毒蛋白的提纯及杀虫效果。

castration [kæsˈtreiʃən] *n.* 阉,阉割,性腺切除术

Furthermore,castration in experimental animals has been shown to reduce the zinc concentration in different tissues.

而且,实验表明实验性切除性腺后的动物在不同组织中的锌浓度降低。

casual [ˈkæʒuəl] *a.* 临时的,随便的,偶然的

Doctors should not wear casual dress when visiting the ward.

医生们查房不应穿便服。

That medical student has saved a lot of casual expenses this term.

那位医学生这一学期节省了不少临时费用。

catabolism [kəˈtæbəlizəm] *n.* 分解代谢

Corticosteroids cause an elevation in the BUN because of their positive effect on protein catabolism.

皮质类固醇可引起 BUN 升高,这是因为它们可以促进蛋白质分解。(BUN=blood urea nitrogen 血液尿素氮)

Low density lipoprotein is probably,perhaps totally,a product of VLDL(very low density lipoprotein)catabolism.

低密度脂蛋白可能(也许全部)是极低密度脂蛋白分解代谢的产物。

catabolize [kəˈtæbəlaiz] *v.* (使)发生分解代谢

Nitroglycerin is catabolized very rapidly in the liver if it is given orally.

硝酸甘油若口服会迅速在肝脏代谢。

One of the most characteristic phenotypes of rapidly growing cancer cells is their propensity to catabolize glucose at high rates.

快速生长的癌细胞最具特征性的一种表型是其葡萄糖的分解代谢速率通常很快。

catalase [ˈkætəleis] *n.* 过氧化氢酶

Numerous enzymes, including alcohol dehydrogenase, alkaline phosphatase, catalase, cytochrome C oxidase, and so on, require copper for activity.
许多酶的作用都需要铜,包括乙醇脱氢酶、碱性磷酸酶、过氧化氢酶、细胞色素 C 氧化酶,等等。

In the liver homogenates, we measured the activities of superoxide dismutase and catalase.
我们检测了肝脏匀浆中的超氧化物歧化酶和过氧化氢酶的活性。

Hydrogen peroxide increased in catalase-deficient cells.
在过氧化氢酶缺乏的细胞中,过氧化氢增加了。

catalyse [ˈkætəlaiz] *v.* 催化

Chemical reactions in cells, collectively known as metabolism, are catalysed by the class of proteins called enzymes.
细胞内的化学反应总称为物质代谢,是由一类称为酶的蛋白质催化的。

catalysis [kəˈtælisis] *n.* 催化(作用)

The separate reactions of metabolism are feasible in the absence of enzymic catalysis.
物质代谢的各个反应在没有酶催化时是可以进行的。

catalyst [ˈkætəlist] *n.* 催化剂

A catalyst is a substance which can hasten the reaction speed.
催化剂是一种能加快反应速度的物质。

Enzymes, like inorganic catalysts, accelerate progress towards equilibrium.
像无机催化剂一样,酶可加速反应达到平衡的进程。

catalytic [ˌkætəˈlitik] *a.* 催化的

Enzymes are complex proteins which act as catalytic agents.
酶是具有催化剂作用的复杂的蛋白质。

Among the phase 1 biotransforming enzymes, the cytochrome P450 system ranks first in terms of catalytic versatility.
在 1 相生物转化酶类中,细胞色素 P450 在催化的多样性方面首屈一指。

cataplexy [ˈkætəpleksi] *n.* 猝倒,昏倒

To quantify structural brain changes associated with cataplexy, we used high-resolution T1-weighted magnetic resonance imaging (MRI).
为量化昏厥相关的大脑结构变化,我们使用了高分辨率的 T_1-加权磁共振成像。

Cataplexy is a pathognomonic symptom of narcolepsy.
昏倒是发作性嗜睡病的一个确诊性症状。

cataract [ˈkætərækt] *n.* 白内障

Cataract may result from long standing diabetes.
长期的糖尿病可能引起白内障。

catarrh [kəˈtɑː] *n.* 黏膜炎,卡他

Based on the animal model, we observed the therapeutic effect of seabuckthorn seed oil on acute radioactive catarrh.
本文在沙棘籽油动物实验研究基础上,观察其对急性放射性黏膜炎的治疗作用。

The combined use of corticosteroid drugs has a very good effect in the treatment of spring catarrh conjunctivitis.
皮质类固醇类药物的联合使用在春季卡他性结膜炎的治疗中有很好的作用。

catarrhal [kəˈtɑːrəl] *a.* 卡他性的

The disease is highly infectious during the catarrhal stage.
在卡他期此病传染力很强。

Acute laryngitis may be defined as an acute catarrhal inflammation of laryngeal mucosa.
急性喉炎可以解释为喉黏膜急性卡他性炎症。

catecholamine [ˌkætikəˈlæmin] *n.* 儿茶酚胺

Dopamine, norepinephrine, and epinephrine are classified as catecholamines.
多巴胺、去甲肾上腺素和肾上腺素均为儿茶酚胺类。

catechu [ˈkætitʃuː] *n.* 儿茶

The dyewood is known to have the suppression action of catechu phenol-O-methyl shift enzyme.
染料木素有抑制儿茶酚-O-甲基转移酶的作用。

The aim is to explore clinical responses of oral lichen planus of erosive type to catechu.
目的是研究儿茶对糜烂型口腔扁平苔藓的临床治疗效果。

categorically [ˌkætiˈgɔrikəli] *ad.* 绝对地

Some physicians misuse laceration as a synonym for cut; this is categorically incorrect.
有些内科医生把 laceration（撕裂，裂伤）误用为 cut（切伤）的同义词，这是绝对错误的。

categorize [ˈkætigəraiz] *v.* 把…分类

All maternal deaths are carefully investigated, analyzed and categorized.
所有母体死亡病例都经过了慎重的研究、分析和分类。

The host defence mechanism may be categorized as either nonspecific or specific.
宿主的防御机制可分为非特异性的或特异性的。

category [ˈkætigəri] *n.* 种类，类型，范畴

There are six major categories of nutrients: carbohydrates, fats, proteins, vitamins, minerals and water.
有六种主要营养素：碳水化合物、脂肪、蛋白质、维生素、矿物质和水。

In general, asepsis is divided into two categories: A. medical asepsis and, B. surgical asepsis.
一般说来，无菌分为两类：A. 内科无菌；B. 外科无菌。

Treatment of the poisoned patient can be divided into four general categories.
中毒病人的治疗可以分为四大类型。

catenin [ˈkætinin] *n.* 连环蛋白

The operation samples of patients with renal cell carcinoma are studied for β-catenin expression by means of immunohistochemistry.
采用免疫组织化学方法对肾细胞癌患者手术标本的 β-连环蛋白表达进行研究。

cathartic [kəˈθɑːtik] *n.* 泻药

The patient has a sense of being constipated and may feel the need for a cathartic or an enema.
患者有便秘感，似乎需用泻剂或灌肠。

Lubricant cathartic acts by softening the feces reducing friction between them and the intestinal wall.
润滑泻剂使粪便变软，减少粪便和肠壁之间的摩擦。

Cathartics may sometimes be helpful, but they can also be dangerous.
泻药有时可能是有益的，但也可能是危险的。

cathepsin [kəˈθepsin] *n.* 组织蛋白酶

DNase treatment does not increase the activities of protease 3 and cathepsin G, indicating their different distribution in sputum.
用脱氧核糖核酸酶处理没有增加蛋白酶 3 和组织蛋白酶 G 的活性，显示出它们在痰液中的不同分布。

Several new approaches are being explored, including cathepsin K inhibitors, and drugs that act on calcium sensing receptors.
正在探索几种新的方法，包括组织蛋白酶 k 抑制剂和对钙敏感受体起作用的药物。

catheter [ˈkæθitə] *n.* 导（液）管

If bladder distention will interfere with exposure in the pelvis, a catheter should be placed preoperatively.
如果膀胱膨胀会妨碍盆腔内脏器的暴露，在术前应放置导尿管。

The catheter was left in place for a minimum of 7 postoperative days.

术后导尿管至少在原处留置 7 天。

catheterization [ˌkæθitərai'zeiʃən] *n.* 导管插入(术)

Catheterization can be done on the nursing unit just before the patient leaves for the operating room.

可以在病人离开护理病房去手术室前进行插管。

In case the patient fails to urinate in another hour, catheterization should be attempted.

如果病人在 1 小时后仍不排尿,则应该导尿。

Cardiac catheterization is used for determination of intracardiac pressure and detection of cardiac anomalies.

心导管插入术用来测定心内压力和检测心脏异常。

catheterize ['kæθitəraiz] *v.* 插管

The patient is placed in the lithotomy position and the bladder is catheterized.

病人处于切石术的位置,然后进行膀胱插管(术)。

caudal ['kɔːd(ə)l] *a.* 近尾部的,[解剖][动] 尾部的

Rats in model group were fed with AOAC-modified low-dosage iron feeds to establish IDA models by blooding at caudal vein.

模型组采用 AOAC 改良的低铁饲料配方辅以尾静脉放血建立缺铁性贫血模型。

Of them, 2 rats received lateral cord transection at caudal injection region.

对其中 2 只大鼠在尾侧注射区作脊髓外侧索横断。

causal ['kɔːzəl] *a.* 原因的;因果关系的

The prognosis of epilepsy is obviously correlated with that of the causal condition.

癫痫的预后显然与导致癫痫病变的病因有关。

causalgia [kɔː'zældʒiə] *n.* 灼性神经痛

The presented cases demonstrate that the use of mirror therapy in patients with causalgia related to neuroma is worthy of further exploration as a potential treatment modality.

提供的病例证明镜子疗法对于神经瘤引起的灼性神经痛是一个潜在的值得深入研究的治疗法。

causally ['kɔːzəli] *ad.* 原因(地),在因果关系上

It has been suggested that the schizophrenia and epilepsy are in some way causally related.

有人提出精神分裂症和癫痫有某些因果关系。

causation [kɔː'zeiʃən] *n.* 引起,因果关系

A toxic blood concentration of a drug is one that has been associated with causation of serious toxic effects.

一种药物的中毒血浓度是指能引起严重中毒作用的血浓度。

In children, there is evidence that biological and genetic causation is important.

在儿童身上,证据表明生物的和遗传的原因是重要的。

causative ['kɔːzətiv] *a.* 成为原因的,引起…的

When the causative bacteria is highly virulent, a normal heart may be affected by endocarditis.

当病原菌毒力强时,正常的心脏也可受到心内膜炎的影响。

Ingestion of asbestos in food or in drinking water could also be a causative factor for gastrointestinal cancer.

摄入食物或饮水中的石棉,可能也是引起胃肠癌的一个原因。

cause [kɔːz] *v.* 引起

Itai-itai disease was caused by cadmium poisoning due to mining in Toyama Prefecture.

痛痛病是由于在富山县采矿致镉中毒引起的。

Minamata disease is an encephalopathy and peripheral neuropathy caused by daily intake of fish and shellfish highly contaminated by methylmercury.

水俣病是因每天摄入被甲基汞高度污染的鱼贝类所引起的脑病和周围神经病。

cauterization [ˌkɔːtəraiˈzeiʃən] *n.* 腐蚀;烧灼;烧烙术

All of these cases received a simple cauterization of the ear drum under the microscope.

所有病例均在显微镜下接受了简单的鼓膜烧烙术。

Cauterization means using heat to burn tissue to stem bleeding or destroy diseased tissue.

烧灼术是指使用高温烧灼组织从而阻止出血或破坏病变组织。

caution [ˈkɔːʃn] *n.* 警告;小心,谨慎

Caution must be taken not to traumatize the inflamed joint.

务必保持谨慎,避免使发炎的关节受到损伤。

The prognosis of the spontaneously developing posterior urethritis must be made with caution.

必须谨慎提出有关自发发生的后尿道炎的预后。

cautious [ˈkɔːʃəs] *a.* 谨慎的,细心的

Physicians should be cautious about assessing pain intensity by visually inspecting a patient.

医生在通过视诊评估疼痛的程度时应慎重。

It is advisable to be cautious before substituting them for established and safe ones.

用新药取代已知的和安全的药物时以小心为宜。

Oxygen, low sodium intake, diuretics, and cautious digitalization are the essential features of treatment.

治疗要点是输氧、摄入低钠、使用利尿药和谨慎地服用洋地黄。

cautiously [ˈkɔːʃəsli] *ad.* 谨慎地

Blood pressure must be reduced cautiously.

血压必须慎重地降低。

caveolin [ˈkæviəulin] *n.* 窖蛋白,小窝蛋白

Regulatory effect of caveolin-1 on endothelial cell proliferation is strong.

窖蛋白-1 抑制内皮细胞增殖的调控效应很强。

Our study suggests that caveolin-1/AKT could be a candidate target of gene therapy in the future.

我们的研究提示窖蛋白-1/AKT 可以作为今后基因治疗的方向之一。

cavernitis [ˌkævəˈnaitis] *n.* [泌尿]海绵体炎

The viewpoint that the disease of cavernitis is caused by trauma has been universally accepted.

创伤引起海绵体炎的观点已被普遍接受。

Middle-aged people are more susceptible to cavernitis.

中年人更易得海绵体炎。

cavernosogram [ˌkævəˈnəuzəgræm] *n.* 海绵体造影片

The latter was categorized into 5 groups according to the findings on cavernosogram.

根据海绵体造影片的结果,后者被分成了 5 类。

Cavernosogram techniques were used in 3 cases.

海绵体造影片技术被用于三个病案中。

cavernous [ˈkævənəs] *a.* 海绵状的

Cavernous hemangioma is composed of large, cavernous blood-filled and thin-walled vascular spaces.

海绵状血管瘤由大的海绵状含血的薄壁的血腔组成。

Cavernous hemangiomas are the most common benign liver tumors.

海绵状血管瘤是最常见的肝脏良性肿瘤。

cavitate [ˈkæviteit] *v.* 形成空洞,形成腔

The miliary lesions do not cavitate.

粟粒性病变不形成空洞。

cavitation [ˌkæviˈteiʃən] *n.* 成洞,成腔

In lung infection, cavitation is uncommon, and most patients do not have underlying pulmonary

disease.
发生肺部感染时很少会形成空洞，并且大多数病人也不会留下肺部的潜在疾病。

cavity [ˈkæviti] *n.* 腔，(空)洞

In the thoracic cavity the pleura surrounds the lungs and the pericardium the heart.
在胸腔里，胸膜包被着肺，而心包则包被着心脏。
Cigarette smoking is believed to be related to cancer of the bladder and the oral cavity.
据说膀胱癌和口腔癌与吸烟有关。
Cavity formation, when observed, is often in an immunocompromised patient.
如有空洞形成，则常出现在有免疫缺陷的病人。
The dentist filled the cavity in the patient's tooth.
牙医填塞了病人牙中的空洞。

cavus [ˈkævəs] *n.* 弓形足

Some people with cavus foot may also experience foot drop.
一些弓形足患者常伴有足下垂。
Pes cavus is a descriptive term that covers a spectrum of deformity.
弓形足是涵盖了一系列畸形的一个描述性术语。

cease [siːs] *v.*, *n.* 停止，停息；结束

With this, uterine contractions cease with transient relief of pain.
随之而来的是子宫收缩停止和短暂的疼痛缓解。
In contrast to the rapid proliferation of embryonic cells, some cells in adult animals cease division altogether (e.g., nerve cells) and many other cells divide only occasionally.
与胚胎细胞的快速增殖相反，成年动物中的一些细胞完全停止分裂(如神经细胞)，很多其他细胞则只是偶尔分裂。

cecum [ˈsiːkəm] (*pl.* ceca [ˈsiːkə]) *n.* 盲肠；盲端

This syndrome is most common among patients with carcinoma, especially of the sigmoid and cecum.
在癌症病人中这种综合征很常见，尤其在乙状结肠癌和盲肠癌的病人。
The colonoscope can be passed to the cecum within 30 minutes in over 90% of patients.
(用结肠镜进行检查)在90%以上的患者中，30分钟以内结肠镜就可到达盲肠。
In the adult cecum and transverse colon, there are 10^8-10^{10} bacteria/gm of contents.
在成年人的盲肠和横结肠内，每克内容物含有10^8～10^{10}个细菌。

cefazolin [siˈfæzəlin] *n.* 头孢唑林，唑啉头孢菌素

For all other patients, gentamicin plus cefazolin is the combination of choice.
对所有其他病人宜选用庆大霉素联合头孢唑啉。

cefotaxime [siˈfɔtæksaim] *n.* 头孢噻肟

The interference of cefotaxime sodium for injection to the determination of bacterial endotoxin can be excluded when it was diluted 100 times.
将注射用头孢噻肟钠稀释100倍，可排除其对细菌内毒素测定的干扰作用。

ceftazidine [sefˈtæzidiːn] *n.* 头孢他啶

Bacillus pyocyaneus showed 100% sensitivity to ceftazidine. The low infective rate of the patients proved that our anti-infective measures were effective.
绿脓杆菌对头孢他啶显示出100%敏感。病人的低感染率证实我们的抗感染措施是有效的。

cefuroxime [ˌsefjuˈrɔksiːm] *n.* 头孢呋辛

Cefuroxime is generally well tolerated and side effects are usually transient.
大部分人对头孢呋辛耐受良好，其副作用通常很短暂。
Sodium cefuroxime solution is usually conditioned in pre-filled syringes then frozen for storage.
头孢呋辛钠溶液一般用载药注射器保存，冷冻后储存。

Celastrol [si'læstrəl] *n.* 雷公藤红素

We want to know whether celastrol can inhibit neovascularization.

我们想知道是否雷公藤红素能够抑制血管生成。

The production of IL-1 and IL-2 can be affected by celastrol.

IL-1 和 IL-2 的产生可能受到雷公藤红素的影响。

cell [sel] *n.* 细胞

The central role of cells in living systems was not recognized until the cell theory was put forward around 1840.

直到 1840 年前后有人提出细胞理论,人们才认识到细胞在生物体内的中心作用。

Any precursor cell may be called stem cell.

任何前体细胞可称作干细胞。

cellular ['seljulə] *a.* 细胞的

Scientists claim to have found the "cellular foundain of youth".

科学家们宣称已找到了"青春细胞的源泉"。

Heat is constantly produced by the body as a result of muscular and cellular activity.

由于肌肉和细胞活动的结果,身体就不断地产生热。

cellularity [ˌselju'læriti] *n.* 细胞构成

This astrocytoma demonstrates increased cellularity and pleomorphism, as compared to normal brain.

与正常大脑相比,星形细胞瘤显示出细胞构成丰富和明显多形性。

During 24-28 weeks, the epithelial layer increased to 4-10 layers, the cellularity was clear, with more gap junction and less intermediate junction.

在 24 ~ 28 周时,上皮增至 4 ~ 10 层,细胞结构清晰,细胞间连接以缝隙连接为主,而中间连接较少。

cellulitis [ˌselju'laitis] *n.* 蜂窝织炎

The expanding diffuse infection of the skin and subcutaneous tissue is known as cellulitis.

皮肤和皮下组织的弥漫性感染被称为蜂窝织炎。

In contrast to spreading cellulitis, gas gangrene begins with sudden pain in the region of the wound.

与蜂窝织炎不同,气性坏疽的发病是以来自伤口区域的突发疼痛开始的。

cellulose ['seljuləus] *n.* 纤维素

Dietary fibre falls into four groups: cellulose, hemicelluloses, lignins, and pectins.

食物纤维分为四类:纤维素、半纤维素、木质素和果胶。

The plant cell is bounded by a comparatively thick wall made of cellulose.

每个植物细胞外面有一层由较厚的纤维素构成的(细胞)壁。

The bacteria produce enzymes that can digest some of the food material not previously broken down (for example, cellulose).

细菌产生酶,能消化一些先前没有被分解的食物(如纤维素)。

cement [si'ment] *n.* 牙骨质;粘固粉(牙科用);水泥

The dentin of the root is covered by cement.

牙根部的牙质被牙骨质覆盖着。

census ['sensəs] *n.* 人口调(普)查

The current census will provide important information on which a sound long-term care policy can be based-measuring the numbers and living environments of elders and their families.

这次人口普查将查清老年人及其家庭成员的数目及其生活条件,为制定一种合理的长期照顾老年人的政策提供重要依据。

Centella ['sentelə] *n.* 雷公藤,积雪草

Our purpose is to evaluate the efficacy of centella cream in the treatment of burn wounds.

我们的目的是评估雷公藤霜对治疗烧伤创面的疗效。

Centella is a kind of antirheumatic drugs.

雷公藤是一种抗风湿药。

centenarian [senti'nɛəriən] *n.* 百岁以上老人

Recent research shows there are plenty more ideas for improving life expectancy and forming would be centenarians.

近代研究表明对于提高预期寿命和造就未来百岁老人的问题有很多见解。

Many centenarians have intact memory function and no evidence of clinically significant dementia.

许多百岁老人拥有完整的记忆功能,未出现临床上明显的痴呆。

centenary [sen'tiːnəri] *n.* 一百周年纪念

The hospital will celebrate its centenary next year.

该医院明年将庆祝它的一百周年。

centigrade ['seitigreid] (also Celsius) *a.* 百分度的,摄氏温度计的

The formula for converting from centigrade(C) to Fahrenheit(F) is:F=(C+32)9/5

摄氏度(C)换算成华氏度(F)的公式是:华氏度=(摄氏度+32)9/5

On the centigrade thermometer, the freezing point of water is zero degree.

在摄氏温度计上水的冰点定为零度。

centimeter ['senti,miːtə] *n.* 厘米

The individual lesions, which begin as small nodules, slowly enlarge to several centimeters.

开始时单个的损害呈小结节状,缓慢增大后可达数厘米。

centimorgan ['sentimɔːgən] *n.* 厘摩(基因交换单位)

The map distance between two loci is measured in units called centimorgans.

两个基因座之间的图距单位称为厘摩。

A centimorgan (cM) is a unit that describes a recombination frequency of 1 percent.

一个厘摩代表百分之一的重组频率。

centrally ['sentrəli] *ad.* 中心地

The pain in acute intestinal obstruction is visceral and is therefore felt centrally and usually in the umbilical area.

急性肠梗阻的疼痛是内脏性的,因此感觉在腹部中心部位痛,通常在肚脐周围。

centrifuge ['sentrifjuːdʒ] *n.* 离心机

The liquid can be forced more quickly to pass through the filter by means of a centrifuge.

用离心机可以迫使这液体更快地通过过滤器。

v. 离心

A rubber cap is placed over the end of the tube, and the tube is centrifuged at 2000r. p. m. for five minutes.

在试管一端加上橡皮盖后,将试管在每分钟 2000 次的转速下离心 5 分钟。

The Hct is measured by centrifuging a volume of blood and determining the percentage of RBCs. (Hct=hematocrit)

血细胞压积的测定就是将一定容积的血液经离心沉淀后测定其红细胞所占的百分比。

centrilobular [,sentri'lɔbjulə] *a.* 小叶中央的

Centrilobular necrosis is ischemic coagulative necrosis of hepatocytes in the central region of the lobule.

小叶中央性坏死是小叶中央区域肝细胞的缺血性的凝固性坏死。

In chronic liver congestion, fatty change of the hepatocytes initially occurs in the centrilobular regions.

慢性肝淤血时,肝细胞脂肪变性首先发生于小叶中央区。

centroblast ['sentrəublæst] *n.* 生发中心母细胞

Centroblasts are large, rapidly dividing cells found in germinal centers. Antibody-secreting and

memory B cells derive from these cells.
生发中心母细胞就是(淋巴结)生发中心体积大、分裂快的细胞,分泌抗体的和记忆性 B 细胞来源于这些细胞。
Distinct role of follicular dendritic cells and T cells in the proliferation, differentiation, and apoptosis of a centroblast cell line, L3055.
滤泡树突状细胞和 T 细胞在生发中心母细胞系 L3055 的增殖、分化和凋亡过程中的作用是不同的。

centrocyte [ˈsentrəusait] *n.* 中心细胞,中央细胞
Centrocytes are the small B cells in germinal centers that derive from centroblasts.
中心细胞是(淋巴结)生发中心里来源于生发母细胞的小 B 细胞。
Somatic mutation leads to efficient affinity maturation when centrocytes recycle back to centroblasts。
当中心细胞再循环回到生发中心母细胞时,体细胞突变将导致有效的亲和力成熟。

centromere [ˈsentrəmiə] *n.* 着丝点,着丝粒
The two identical chromatids which compose each chromosome are joined at the centromere.
组成每条染色体的两条相同染色单体在着丝粒处相连。
In the anaphase of mitosis, the centromere of each chromosome separates into two centromeres.
在有丝分裂后期,每条染色体的着丝粒一分为二。

centrosome [ˈsentrəsəum] *n.* 中心体
The centrosome is involved in cell division.
中心体参与细胞分裂。

cephalad [ˈsefəlæd] *adv.* 向头部地,头向,向头侧
Management of bezoars is usually surgical with fragmentation and milking it cephalad or cauda depending on its location and level of obstruction.
处理胃肠结石通常以手术将其碎裂,然后根据其位置和阻塞的水平向头端或尾端挤出。
At a more cephalad level, patchy consolidation and ground-glass opacity are visible.
在近头侧层面,可见斑片状实变和毛玻璃样影。

cephalic [siˈfælik] *a.* 头的
The patients with gestational age more than 37 weeks presented with cephalic presentation.
这位怀孕超过 37 周的孕妇的胎儿为头先露。
The left cephalic vein was developed.
左侧的头静脉显影了。

cephalohematoma [ˌsefələuˌhiːməˈtəumə] *n.* 头颅血肿
A cephalohematoma in an older baby or child is evidence of some recent injury to the head; occasionally an unsuspected fracture is revealed on X-ray.
稍大的婴儿或儿童的头颅血肿是近期头部外伤引起,在 X 线下偶尔可发现意外骨折。

cephalosporin [ˌsefələuˈspɔːrin] *n.* 先锋霉素,头孢菌素
Cephalosporins are structurally related to penicillins.
头孢菌素结构与青霉素相似。

ceramide [ˈserəmaid] *n.* 神经酰胺
Environmental stress and chronic inflammation can stimulate p38MAPK and ceramide signaling and induce cellular senescence.
环境压力和慢性炎症可以刺激 p38MAPK 和神经酰胺信号,并且引起细胞衰老。
At the onset of transferrin internalization both ceramide level and acid sphingomyelinase activity returned to their basic levels.
在转铁蛋白内化开始时,神经酰胺水平和酸性鞘磷脂酶活性都回到了基本水平。

cercaria [səːˈkɛəriə] (*pl.* cercariae [səːˈkɛəriiː]) *n.* 尾蚴
Infection occurs during immersion in fresh water containing schistosome cercariae.

当浸入带有血吸虫尾蚴的淡水中时，人体常产生感染。

cereal [ˈsiəriəl] *n.* (*pl.*)谷物，粮食

Riboflavin is found in meats, milk, cereals, and leafy vegetable, but no food is particularly rich in this vitamin.

核黄素存在于肉类、牛奶、粮食及叶状蔬菜中，但是没有哪种食物特别富含这种维生素。

a. 谷类的

Soybeans are handled differently from cereal grains.

大豆的加工处理与谷类的加工处理不同。

cerebellum [ˌseriˈbeləm] *n.* 小脑

The part of the brain underneath the back part of the cerebrum is the cerebellum.

大脑后部的下方是小脑。

cerebral [ˈseribrəl] *a.* 大脑的

Cerebral abscess is a rare complication.

脑脓肿是较少见的合并症。

About one-fourth of all leukemia patients die of cerebral hemorrhage.

大约 1/4 的白血病患者死于大脑出血。

cerebritis [seriˈbraitis] *n.* 大脑炎

TLDH of cerebral spinal fluid in virogenetic cerebritis was significantly lower than that of the control group (P<0. 01).

病毒性脑炎与对照组比较，脑脊液总乳酸脱氢酶（TLDH）明显降低（P<0. 01）

These two types of MR imaging manifestations correspond in the main with the etiologic and pathologic classifications of the sporadic cerebritis.

磁共振影像的这两类表现与散发性脑炎的病因及病理分类基本相符。

cerebroside [ˈseribrəsaid] *n.* 脑苷脂

Cerebroside is also called cerebrogalactoside, it is abundant in membranes of nervous tissue, especially the myelin sheath.

脑苷脂也称脑半乳糖苷，在神经组织膜内，特别是在髓鞘中很丰富。

cerebrospinal [ˌseribrəuˈspainəl] *a.* 脑脊髓的

Normal cerebrospinal fluid is colorless and clear.

正常的脑脊液是无色透明的。

Send cerebrospinal fluid samples for cell count and for a serologic test for syphilis.

请送脑脊液标本作细胞计数和梅毒的血清学检查。

These are generally found in special locations such as cerebrospinal fluid or intraocular fluid.

这些液体通常被发现处于一些特定部位，如脑脊液、眼内液等。

cerebrovascular [ˌseribrəuˈvæskjulə] *a.* 脑血管的

Stroke is the acute onset of a neurologic deficit due to cerebrovascular disease.

脑卒中是由于脑血管病而突发的神经障碍。

cerebrum [ˈseribrəm] (*pl.* cerebra [ˈseribrə]) *n.* 大脑

The largest part of the brain is the forebrain or cerebrum.

脑的最大部分是前脑或称大脑。

The cerebrum is the part of the brain in which thought occurs.

大脑是脑的一部分，它能产生思想。

Man has a better-developed cerebrum than animals.

人有一个比动物进化得更好的大脑。

ceresin [ˈserisin] *n.* 地蜡，微晶蜡

Ceresin is a waxy mineral that is a mixture of hydrocarbons and occurs in association with petroleum.

地蜡是由碳氢化合物混合而成的一种蜡质矿物，常与石油伴生。

Ceresin is commonly used in the production of semisolid lubricants.
地蜡常用来生产半固态的润滑油。

certainty [ˈsəːtənti] *n.* 确实，肯定

A diagnosis of this condition may be made with a fair degree of certainty.
这个病的诊断可以有较大程度的可靠性。

About 20 naturelly-accurring amino acids have been identified with certainty.
约有 20 种天然氨基酸已肯定被识别。

The viral etiology of myocarditis in a given patient is not easy to establish with certainty.
对某一患有心肌炎病人来说，很难有把握地确定其病原就是病毒。

certificate [səˈtifikeit] *n.* 证件，证书

He has a certificate that he is a member of medical education committee.
他持有证件，证明他是医学教育委员会的委员。

That practitioner has got a certificate from the Municipal Bureau of Health.
那位开业医生已从市卫生局领到证书。

She has obtained a certificate for passing the College English Test, Band 4.
她已获得大学英语四级考试通过的证书。

certification [ˌsəːtifiˈkeiʃən] *n.* 证明，证明书

Hospital privileges and academic posts now tend to be given on the basis of completion of graduate medical education and board certification.
现在的倾向是，研究生毕业和委员会的证明是获得医院工作权利和学术地位的基础。

certify [ˈsəːtifai] *v.* 证明

There are special boards that review and certify the qualifications of doctors in a specialized area.
设有专门委员会审查和证明各个专科医生的合法资格。

This is to certify that Miss Wu Ming is a registered nurse in the pediatric department of our hospital.
兹证明吴明小姐是我院小儿科的一名注册护士。

ceruloplasmin [siˌruːləuˈplæzmin] *n.* 血浆铜蓝蛋白

Ceruloplamin is an alpha$_2$-globulin that transports copper.
血浆铜蓝蛋白是一种转运铜的 α_2-球蛋白。

cervical [ˈsəːvikəl] *a.* 颈的；子宫颈的

The cervical vertebrae are located at the top end of the vertebral column.
颈椎位于脊柱的顶端。

Cervical polyps are frequently seen in association with chronic cervicitis.
子宫颈息肉常与慢性子宫颈炎同时存在。

cervicitis [səːviˈsaitis] *n.* 子宫颈炎

Chronic cervicitis may be clinically indistinguishable from cervical cancer.
临床上慢性子宫颈炎与子宫颈癌难以区别。

In the tissues of cervicitis, cervical intraepithelial neoplasia, and cervical cancer, the P53 positive expression rate was 9.0% ,31.6% and 40.0% respectively.
子宫颈炎、宫颈上皮内瘤变和子宫颈癌组织的 P53 阳性表达率分别为 9.0%、31.6%、40.0%。

cervix [ˈsəːviks] *n.* 颈；子宫颈

Before removal of the speculum, the color of the cervix is noted.
窥阴器取出前要注意宫颈的颜色。

This is particularly true of carcinoma of the cervix.
对宫颈癌来说尤其如此。

cesarean [siːˈzεəriən] *a.* 剖腹的，剖宫的

Incision through the abdominal and uterine wall for delivery of a fetus is called cesarean section.

切开腹壁和子宫壁取出胎儿称为剖宫产。

In a patient with a very premature infant and a very unfavorable cervix, a cesarean delivery without a trial of labor may be indicated.

对于不成熟胎儿及宫颈条件极差者,应作剖宫产,无须试产。

Cesarean section is poorly tolerated by the patient with this condition.

有这种情况的病人,对剖宫产是不能耐受的。

cessation [se'seiʃən] *n.* 停止,休止

Secondary amenorrhoea refers to cessation of the periods after menstruation has been established.

继发性闭经系指月经建立后又停止者。

This change develops within a few minutes of cessation of the circulation.

这种变化在血循环停止数分钟内发生。

cetirizine [seti'riziːn] *n.* 西替利嗪,仙特明(商品名:zyrtec)

Cetirizine, an antihistamine, is used to relieve hay fever and seasonal allergy symptoms。

仙特明系抗组胺药,用于缓解干草热和季节性过敏症状。

chain [tʃein] *n.* 链

A protein chain can fold into its correct conformation without outside help.

蛋白链无需外界帮助就能折叠成其正确构象。

The most characteristic histologic lesion of light chain deposition disease (LCDD) is nodular glomerulosclerosis.

轻链沉积病最具特征的组织学损害是结节性肾小球硬化。

chalazion [kə'leiziɔn] (*pl.* chalazia [kə'leiziə] 或 chalazions) *n.* 睑板腺囊肿,霰粒肿

Treatment of the chalazion includes local steroid injection or incision and curettage for elimination.

霰粒肿的治疗包括局部注射类固醇或局部切开刮除。

challenge ['tʃælindʒ] *v.* 向…挑战,对…怀疑

Some drug manufacturers challenged the justice of New Drug Law.

有些药品生产厂家对新药法的公正性表示怀疑。

n. 挑战

The government will have to meet the challenge of rising prices.

政府将面临价格上涨的挑战。

chamber ['tʃeimbə] *n.* 腔

The heart has four chambers, an apex, three surfaces and four borders.

心脏有四腔、一尖、三面和四缘。

Neisseria gonorrhoeae can be grown only in a moist chamber, at 35 ~ 37℃, at a pH of 7.2, with CO_2 enrichment.

奈瑟淋球菌只能在室温 35 ~ 37℃、pH 7.2 和 CO_2 丰富的湿润的房间内生长。

chamoishorn ['ʃæmihɔːn] *n.* 羚羊角

Chamoishorn is a kind of Chinese herbs which are widely used.

羚羊角是一种常用中药。

Chamoishorn has high medicinal value, and is very expensive.

羚羊角药用价值高,价格昂贵。

chancre ['ʃæŋkə] *n.* 下疳

The chancre is most common on cervix, but it may occur on the labia.

下疳最常见于宫颈,但可能发生于阴唇。

chancroid ['ʃæŋkrɔid] *n.* 软下疳

Chancroid, also called soft chancre, is an acute, sexually transmitted disease.

软下疳又称软性下疳,是一种急性的性传播性疾病。

The ulcer of chancroid is not indurated, irregular and painful.

软下疳的溃疡没有硬结，不规则而且疼痛。

changeability [ˌtʃeindʒəˈbiliti] *n.* 可变性

The changeability and sociality of the legal action is the key of theoretical basis of legal act education, and various kinds of education should be applied to the medical students' legal action.

法律行为的可变性和社会性是法律行为教育理论依据的关键，应采取多种方式加强对医学生法律行为的教育。

channel [ˈtʃænəl] *n.* 系统；途径；管

Nifedipine is thought to be more selective toward blocking the Ca^{2+} channels.

应考虑硝苯吡啶对钙通道的阻断作用具有更大的可选用性。

Endoplasmic reticulum is a system of deep channels that winds throughout the cytoplasm.

内质网是一个弯弯曲曲地分布于整个细胞质中具有深沟状的体系。

chapter [ˈtʃæptə] *n.* 章，回

The etiologic agents of respiratory viral disease are discussed in detail in Chapter 57.

呼吸道病毒性疾病的病原因子将在第 57 章详细讨论。

characteristic [ˌkæriktəˈristik] *a.* 特异的，特有的，表示特性的

The characteristic neuronal necrosis can occur in the absence of raised intracranial pressure.

在颅内压不升高的情况下，特有的神经元坏死也能发生。

The expression of the face is characteristic of certain diseases.

（特异的）面部表情是某些病所特有的。

The symptoms and signs of pneumococcal pneumonia are so characteristic as to make the diagnosis relatively easy.

肺炎球菌性肺炎的症状和体征是如此典型以致使诊断比较容易。

n. 特性，特征

They developed a doublelumen dilation catheter with unique expansive characteristics.

他们创制了具有极为良好扩张性能的双腔扩张插管。

characteristically [ˌkæriktəˈristikəli] *ad.* 特有地

Suicidal incised wounds are characteristically on the neck, wrists, or ankles.

自杀性切伤特有的部位是颈部、腕部或踝部。

An impact at high velocity and over a small contact area characteristically produces a local fracture.

与小面积接触的高速碰撞必然产生局部骨折。

characterize [ˈkæriktəraiz] *v.* 表示…的特性，成为…的特性

Bronchial asthma is characterized by respiratory distress, apnea, wheezing, flushing and cyanosis.

支气管哮喘的特征为呼吸困难、窒息、喘息、面红和发绀。

Nephrotic syndromes are characterized by edema, albuminuria, and renal failure.

肾病综合征以水肿、蛋白尿和肾功能衰竭为特征。

check [tʃek] *v.* 制止，控制；核对，检查

The principal use of ergonovine is to prevent or check postpartum hemorrhage.

麦角新碱的主要用途是用于预防和控制产后出血。

The haemoglobin level is checked and blood transfusion given if necessary.

检查血红蛋白水平，如有必要需进行输血。

checklist [ˈtʃeklist] *n.* 清单，检查表，备忘录，目录册

Dr. Pronovost and his colleagues compared hospital deaths in the state of Michigan, where the checklist program was in use, with nearby states that weren't in the program.

普罗诺沃斯特医生和他的同僚们将使用这个工作清单的密西根州医院的死亡率，与邻近还没有使用这种方法的州进行比较。

Through the use of a checklist, we will help you decide which method is best suited for you and your application.

通过使用清单，我们将帮助您确定哪种方法最适合您和您的应用程序。

checkpoint [ˈtʃekpɔint] *n.* 关键点，检查点

In nondividing cells, DNA damage activates a checkpoint that depends on the presence of a normal p53 gene.

在非分裂细胞中，DNA 损伤对一个检查点的激活取决于正常 p53 基因的存在。

Cell cycle checkpoints are control mechanisms that ensure the fidelity of cell division in eukaryotic cells.

细胞周期检查点是确保真核细胞中细胞分裂保真性的调控机制。

When DNA damage is found, the checkpoint uses a signal mechanism either to stall the cell cycle until repairs are made or, if repairs cannot be made, to target the cell for destruction via apoptosis.

当发现 DNA 损害时，检查点通过信号机制要么暂停细胞周期直到损害被修复，要么在不能修复时通过凋亡靶向破坏该细胞。

chelation [kiːˈleiʃən] *n.* 螯合（作用）

These exogenous conditioning dietary factors, with the exception of alcohol, probably influence zinc nutrition by chelation.

除酒精外，这些外源性饮食因素可能通过螯合作用来影响锌的营养（吸收）。

Because of the already significant Fe burden such transfusions hasten the advent of clinical symptoms secondary to hemosiderosis, and Fe-chelation therapy should be considered.

由于已有明显的铁负荷，这种输血促使继发于含铁血黄素沉积症的临床症状出现，必须考虑铁螯合疗法。

chemerin [ˈkemərin] *n.* 趋化素

Chemerin is a potent chemoattractant for cells expressing the GPCR CMKLR1.

趋化素是细胞表达 G 蛋白偶联受体 CMKLR1 的一种有效的化学引诱物。

Chemerin is thought to play important roles in cell migration and recruitment to sites of tissue damage and inflammation.

趋化素被认为在细胞迁移以及组织损伤和炎症的发生中起到重要作用。

chemobiodynamics [ˌkiməuˌbaiədaiˈnemiks] *n.* 化学生物动力学

The basic knowledge about chemobiodynamics has been reviewed in this paper in detail.

有关化学生物动力学的基本知识已经在该文章中做了详细的阐述。

After graduating from university, he entered the chemobiodynamics laboratory for further study.

大学毕业后，他进入到化学生物动力学实验室继续深造。

chemokine [ˌkeməuˈkain] *n.* 化学趋化因子

The chemokines are a group of at least 25 small cytokines.

化学趋化因子是一群小细胞因子，至少有 25 个。

chemokinesis [ˌkeməukaiˈniːsis] *n.* 趋化作用

In chemokinesis, mediators such as histamine enhance the overall motility of cells.

在趋化作用中，像组胺这样的介质可以增强细胞的运动。

chemolysis [keˈmɔləsis] *n.* 化学分解

Some recycling technologies are based on chemolysis, including alcoholysis, glycolysis and hydrolysis.

一些回收技术是基于化学分解，包括醇解，糖酵解和水解。

For chemolysis of polyurethanes, it is preferable to process feedstock of known composition in order to obtain consistent and predictable regenerated products.

对于聚氨酯的化学分解，最好对已知组成的原料加工，以获得相符的且可预测的再生产品。

chemonucleolysis [ˌkeməuˌnjuːkliəˈlaisis] *n.* 髓核化学溶解术

The surgical findings in a series of 50 patients who had previously undergone lumbar chemonucleolysis without success were analyzed with the aim of finding signs that would permit us to predict (and thus avoid) failures of chemonucleolysis.

对一系列曾有过腰椎髓核化学溶解术失败经历的 50 名患者外科结果进行了分析，目的在于找到迹象可预测(因而避免)髓核化学溶解术的失败。

Analysis of this series emphasizes the need for meticulous screening of patients by careful clinical examination and extensive x-ray and computed tomography studies prior to chemonucleolysis.

这组分析结果强调在髓核化学溶解术之前应通过仔细的临床检查、广泛的 X 线和 CT 扫描来精细筛选患者。

chemoprophylaxis [ˌkeməuˌprɔfiˈlæksis] *n.* (化学)药物预防

The treatment of tuberculosis is subdivided into chemoprophylaxis and active treatment.

结核病治疗可细分为化学药物预防和积极治疗。

Chemoprophylaxis has also been shown to be effective in preventing certain nosocomial infection.

业已表明药物预防对防止医院内的某些感染确实有效。

chemosis [keˈməusis] *n.* 球结膜水肿

Ophthalmological check-up revealed a firm mass palpable over the lateral portion of left upper eyelid and chemosis of adjacent conjunctiva.

眼部检查显示在左上眼睑的侧部可摸到一个质硬的肿块和邻近的球结膜水肿。

External examination revealed erythema, warmth, eyelid edema, marked proptosis, conjunctival chemosis and complete ophthalmoplegia in the right eye.

外眼检查显示右眼红、热、眼睑浮肿、明显凸眼、球结膜水肿以及完全眼肌麻痹。

chemotactic [ˌkeməuˈtæktik] *a.* 趋化性的

Chemotactic stimuli result in neutrophil margination and diapedesis.

趋化性刺激导致中性粒细胞的迁移和渗出。

Chemotactic substances are related by infected tissues, and these substances cause white blood cells to migrate into the infected area.

感染组织释放趋化物质，而这些物质使白细胞向感染区移动。

chemotaxis [ˌkeməuˈtæksis] *n.* 趋化性

Some cells exhibit chemotaxis.

有些细胞具有趋化性。

Once in the tissues, cells migrate towards the site of infection by a process of chemical attraction known as chemotaxis.

在组织中细胞受到化学物质的吸引向已有炎症的部位迁移的过程称为趋化性。

chemotherapeutic [ˌkeməuθerəˈpjuːtik] *a.* 化学疗法的

The administration of antibiotics or chemotherapeutic agents is not always necessary.

抗生素或化学药物的应用并非总是必需的。

chemotherapy [ˌkeməuˈθerəpi] *n.* 化学疗法

Chemotherapy means the treatment of disease with chemical drugs.

化疗就是用化学药品治疗疾病。

The sensitivity of the organism to chemotherapy and the response of the patient to it should be known.

应该了解细菌对化疗的敏感性以及病人对化疗的反应。

Chernobyl [tʃiəˈnɔːbil] *n.* 切尔诺贝利(乌克兰北部城市)

The Chernobyl disaster was a nuclear accident that occurred on 26 April 1986 at the Chernobyl Nuclear Power Plant in Ukraine.

切尔诺贝利灾难是指 1986 年 4 月 26 日在乌克兰的切尔诺贝利核电厂发生的一起核事故。

The United Nations Scientific Committee of the Effects of Atomic Radiation (UNSCEAR) has conducted 20 years of detailed scientific and epidemiological research on the effects of the

Chernobyl accident.

联合国原子辐射效应科学委员会(UNSCEAR)对切尔诺贝利事故的影响进行了为期20年的详细的科学研究和流行病学调查。

chest [tʃest] *n.* 胸,胸廓;箱,盒

Acute chest pain is associated with a fractured rib, a fibrinous pleurisy secondary to pneumonia or a pulmonary infarct.

急性的胸痛与肋骨骨折、继发于肺炎的纤维蛋白性胸膜炎或肺梗死有关。

chew [tʃuː] *v.* 咀嚼

Chew your food well before you swallow it.

在吞咽食物之前要细细咀嚼。

The purpose of saliva is to dissolve the food and to facilitate the processes of chewing and swallowing.

唾液的作用是使食物分解,以利于咀嚼和吞咽。

In older people with dentures, it is often very hard for them to chew properly.

镶有假牙的老人常常很难咀嚼。

chiasma [kaiˈæzmə] *n.* (染色体的)交叉,(视神经的)交叉,交叉融合

The average number of chiasma seen in human spermatocytes is about 50, that is, several per bivalent.

人类精母细胞的平均交叉数约为50,也就是每个二价染色体上有数个。

Genetic recombination can occur without the formation of a chiasma.

基因重组在没有形成交叉的情况下,也可以发生。

chicken-pox [ˈtʃikin-pɔks] *n.* 水痘

Influenza, chicken-pox and some kinds of sore throats are all virus infections.

流行性感冒、水痘和某些种类的咽喉炎都是病毒性感染。

Two children with liver transplants died of the common children's disease, chicken-pox.

两个做了肝脏移植的儿童死于普通小儿疾病——水痘。

childbearing [ˈtʃaildˌbɛəriŋ] *n.* 分娩,生产

In the childbearing age the most important causes of uterine bleeding are associated with disorders of reproduction.

生育年龄的妇女出现子宫出血的原因主要与生育引起的病症有关。

chill [tʃil] *n.* 寒冷;寒战

There is quite a chill in the air this morning.

今天早晨的空气颇有寒意。

Chills are often associated with fever.

寒战常伴有发热。

Acute severe hemolysis may be accompanied by chills, fever, pain in the back and abdomen, prostration, and shock.

急性而又严重的溶血可能伴有寒战、发烧、背部和腹部疼痛、虚脱以及休克。

But the influenza may, with almost typical chills, act like malaria, or may, when the fever is continuous, act like typhoid fever.

当流感伴有几乎典型的寒战时可能像疟疾,当发烧持续时又可能像伤寒。

chimera [kaiˈmiərə] *n.* 嵌合体

Plant expression plasmid pROSB carrying the gene encoding chimera SBR-CT and bar gene was transferred into Agrobacterium tumefaciens LBA4404.

携带编码嵌合体 SBR-CT 和 bar 基因片段的植物表达质粒 pROSB 被转移入农杆菌 LBA4404。

Many patients with heart transplant of a pig or cow valve, they are dissimilar chimera.

许多心脏病患者移植了猪或牛的瓣膜,他们都是异种嵌合体。

chimeric [kaiˈmiərik] *a.* 嵌合的

The human organ chimeric animals may be used for organ transplants.

人器官嵌合体动物有可能被应用于器官移植。

Then they harvested these chimeric fetal livers for transplant into lethally irradiated hosts.

然后他们采集嵌合体胚胎肝脏移植至受致命性辐射照射的受体。

chimerism [kaiˈmerizəm] *n.* 嵌合体,嵌合现象,嵌合性,嵌合状态

Mixed hematopoietic chimerism is a state in which bone marrow hematopoietic stem cells from two genetically different individuals coexist.

造血干细胞混合嵌合体是指两个不同基因型个体的骨髓造血干细胞共存的一种状态。

Chinonin [ˈkainənin] *n.* 知母宁

The results suggest that Chinonin has preventive effects against apoptotic and necrotic cell death.

结果显示知母宁具有防止细胞凋亡和坏死的作用。

The possible mechanisms of Chinonin for scavenging reactive oxygen species are related to genes bcl-2 and p53.

知母宁清除活性氧的机制可能与 bcl-2 和 p53 基因相关。

chipping [ˈtʃipiŋ] *n.* 裂片,破片

This may be due to the rough stem surface chipping away bone fragments, rather than the bone being cut away precisely as is done with a rasp.

这可能是由于粗糙茎杆表面刮除骨碎片,而不是被锉刀准确地切掉骨头。

A transition from chipping to splitting occurs at higher loads for contacts near the central axis of the tooth.

当牙齿中央轴附近接触到更高负荷时,就会发生由裂片到分裂的转换。

chitin [ˈkaitin] *n.* 几丁质,壳质,壳多糖,角质素

Both radiation heating and an irradiation without heating intensify chitin and cellulose decomposition and distillation.

辐射加热和不产热的照射都会增强角质素和纤维素的分解和蒸馏。

Chitin and chitosan are the most widely accepted biodegradable and biocompatible materials subsequent to cellulose.

壳多糖和壳聚糖是仅次于纤维素的最广为接受的可生物降解和生物相容性材料。

chitosan [ˈkaitəsæn] *n.* 壳聚糖

Chitosan coating followed by cold storage delayed anthocyanin degradation and prevented colour deterioration in the pomegranate arils.

冷藏壳聚糖包衣可以延缓花青素的分解,并防止石榴种皮的褪色。

Lecithin-chitosan nanoparticles are a promising carrier for topical delivery of quercetin.

卵磷脂-壳聚糖纳米粒是一种有前景的槲皮素局部转运载体。

chlamydia [kləˈmidiə] (*pl.* chlamydiae [kləˈmidiiː]) *n.* 衣原体

Chlamydiae cause conjunctival, genital and respiratory infections.

衣原体常会引起结膜、生殖道和呼吸道的感染。

The chlamydiae are smaller than the rickettsiae.

衣原体比立克次体更小。

Chlamydia is the best-studied organism of those that cause the afebrile pneumonitis syndrome.

衣原体是引起无热肺炎综合征的病原体中研究得最好的一个。

chlamydial [kləˈmidiəl] *a.* 衣原体的

In women with chlamydial infection, tetracycline should be used.

对衣原体感染的女性患者应该用四环素治疗。

chlamydiosis [kləˈmidiəusis] *n.* 衣原体病

268 serum samples collected from Tibetan sheep in Chengduo country were used to detect the antibody of chlamydiosis by indirect hemagglutination.

应用间接血凝试验,对采集的 268 份治多县藏系羊血清进行了衣原体病的血清学抗体定性检测。

chloralose [ˈklɔːrələus] *n.* [化] 氯醛糖,氯醛缩葡萄糖(用作安眠剂)

The experiments were performed on New Zealand rabbits anaesthetized with urethane and chloralose.

实验是在氨基甲酸乙酯和氯醛糖麻醉下的新西兰兔身上进行。

chloramphenicol [ˌklɔːræmˈfenikɔl] *n.* 氯霉素

Chloramphenicol(chloromycetin) has a broad spectrum of bacteriostatic activity.

氯霉素具有广谱的抑菌作用。

The hematologic reactions to chloramphenicol may be severe.

氯霉素的血液反应可能很严重。

chlordiazepoxide [ˌklɔːdaiˌeiziˈpɔksaid] *n.* 甲氯二氮,利眠宁

Chlordiazepoxide works fastest when administered orally.

口服时利眠宁发挥作用最快。

Chlordiazepoxide is a sedative and tranquillizing drug with muscle relaxant properties.

甲氯二氮(利眠宁)为镇痛安定药,具有肌肉松弛的作用。

chloride [ˈklɔːraid] *n.* 氯化物

The two minerals which occur in the extracellular fluid and regulate water balance are sodium and chloride.

细胞外液中存在的两种可以调节水平衡的矿物质是钠和氯。

This may be due in part to reduced delivery of chloride to the collecting tubules.

这部分原因可能是由于传送至集合管的氯化物减少。

In amphetamine toxicity, acidification of urine with ammonium chloride will be required.

在苯丙胺中毒时,需要采用氯化铵来酸化尿液。

chlorinate [ˈklɔːrineit] *v.* 用氯处理,使氯化

Philadelphia chlorinates its water.

费城使用氯气对水进行处理。

chlorination [ˌklɔːriˈneiʃən] *n.* 氯化

Chlorination does not kill everything.

氯化处理并不能杀死所有的病菌。

chlorine [ˈklɔːriːn] *n.* 氯

Chlorine is widely used to sterilize drinking water and purify swimming baths.

氯气被广泛用于消毒饮水与清洁游泳池水。

In high concentrations chlorine is toxic; it was used in World War I as a poison gas in the trenches.

高浓度氯气有毒性,第一次世界大战中曾用作战壕阵地毒气。

Chlorine(Cl) is a reactive gas that is intermidiate in water solubility, denser than air, and yellow in color.

氯气(Cl)是一种反应性气体,中度溶于水,密度比空气大,呈黄色。

chlorobutanol [ˌklɔːrəˈbjuːtənɔl] *n.* 三氯叔丁醇

Chlorobutanol is a short acting depressant drug.

三氯叔丁醇是一种短效镇静药。

Chlorobutanol is made into chloral hydrate when it passes through the body.

三氯叔丁醇进入体内后转变为水合氯醛。

Chlorobutanol is a medicine available in a number of countries worldwide.

三氯叔丁醇是一种在全球许多国家使用的药品。

chlorocresol [ˌklɔːrəˈkresəl] *n.* 氯甲酚

Chlorocresol is a medicine available in a number of countries worldwide.

氯甲酚是一种在全世界许多国家使用的药物。

Chlorocresol is an activator of ryanodine receptor-mediated Ca^{2+} release.

氯甲酚是兰尼碱受体介导的钙离子释放的活化剂。

chloroethylnitrosourea [ˌkləurəˈeθilnaiˌtrəusəuˈjuəriə] *n.* 氯乙基亚硝基脲类

Chloroethylnitrosoureas cause delayed and prolonged suppression of both platelets and granulocytes.

氯乙基亚硝基脲类引发血小板和粒细胞滞后而持久的抑制。

chlorofluorocarbon（CFCs） [ˌklɔːrəuˌfluərəuˈkɑːbən] *n.* 含氯氟烃，氟利昂

Many CFCs have been widely used as refrigerants, propellants and solvents.

许多含氯氟烃被广泛用做制冷剂，推进剂和溶剂。

Chlorofluorocarbons（CFCs）are nontoxic, nonflammable chemicals containing atoms of carbon, chlorine, and fluorine.

含氯氟烃是含有碳原子、氯原子和氟原子的无毒、不燃化学品。

chloroform [ˈklɔrəfɔːm] *n.* 氯仿

Chloroform has a multitude of natural sources, both biogenic and abiotic.

自然界通过多种生物性和非生物性渠道生成氯仿。

It is estimated that greater than 90% of atmospheric chloroform is of natural origin.

据估计，大气中超过90%的氯仿来源于自然界。

chloroma [kləˈrəumə] *n.* 绿色瘤

The clinical features, pathology, diagnosis, treatment and prognosis of orbital chloroma were also reviewed.

本篇还综述了眼窝绿色瘤的临床特征、病理学、诊断、治疗与预后。

There was a tendency of chloroma formation in acute myeloblastic leukemia（AML）.

患急性髓细胞性白血病时往往有形成绿色瘤的倾向。

chloromycetin [ˌklɔːrəumaiˈsiːtin] *n.* 氯霉素

Chloromycetin has no demonstrable effects on the central nervous system.

氯霉素对中枢神经系统无明显作用。

chlorophyll [ˈklɔrəfil] *n.* 叶绿素

Chlorophyll, the green pigment in plants, is almost always found in plastids known as chloroplasts.

叶绿素——植物的绿色色素，几乎总是存在于叫做叶绿体的成形粒中。

chloroplast [ˈklɔːrəplæst] *n.* 叶绿体

The ribosomes in mitochondria and chloroplasts are also 70s.

在线粒体和叶绿体中核糖体也都是70s。（注：s表示沉降系数）

chloroquine [ˈklɔːrəkwin] *n.* 氯奎

Chloroquine phosphate is absorbed rapidly and completely by the intestinal tract.

磷酸氯奎迅速而彻底地为肠道吸收。

chlorpromazine [klɔːˈprəuməziːn] *n.* 氯普马嗪，氯丙嗪，冬眠宁

One of the side effects of chlorpromazine is mild to severe agranulocytosis.

氯丙嗪的不良反应之一是轻度到重度粒细胞缺乏症。

chlortetracycline [ˌklɔːtetrəˈsaikliːn] *n.* 氯四环素

Some of the sulfonamides, and antibiotics like chlortetracycline, are bacteriostatic rather than bactericidal in their action.

有些磺胺类药物和抗生素（如氯四环素）具有抑菌而无杀菌的作用。

chocolate [ˈtʃɔkəlit] *n.* 巧克力

Chocolate cysts of ovary are often found with endometriosis or other hemorrhagic conditions within the ovary.

卵巢巧克力囊肿常在子宫内膜异位症或者其他卵巢内出血性疾病中出现。

The stale hemorrhage resembles chocolate, and thus it is called a chocolate cyst of ovary.
因陈旧性出血看来似巧克力，故被称为卵巢巧克力囊肿。

choke [tʃəuk] *v.* 哽住；阻塞；窒息

Anger choked his words.
他气得话也说不出来。

An acute episode of dyspnea often occurs in patients with mitral stenosis at night when they wake up from sleep with a choking sensation.
二尖瓣狭窄时病人常在夜晚发作严重呼吸困难，使他们在睡梦中惊醒时感到窒息感。

cholangiocarcinoma [kəuˌlændʒiəuˌkɑːsiˈnəumə] *n.* 胆管癌

Cholangiocarcinoma is a late complication of chronic clonorchiasis.
胆管癌是慢性华支睾吸虫病的晚期并发症。

cholangiography [kəˌlændʒiˈɔgrəfi] *n.* 胆管造影术

Cholangiography is the imaging of the bile duct by x-rays. There are at least two kinds of cholangiography: percutaneous transhepatic cholangiography and endoscopic retrograde choledochography.
胆道造影术是通过 X 线进行胆道成像。至少有两种胆管造影术：经皮肝穿胆管造影术和内镜下逆行胆总管造影术。

Cholangiography is an examination that uses X-rays and contrast medium (dye) to view your bile ducts.
胆管造影术是一种检查方法，通过使用 X 线和造影剂来查看你的胆管。

A retrospective review was made of the records of 152 patients undergoing cholangiography at the time of cholecyctectomy.
本文对 152 名在胆囊切除术时做过胆管造影术的患者的病历进行了回顾性复习。

cholangiopancreatography [kəuˌlændʒiəˌpænkriəˈtɔgrəfi] *n.* 胰胆管造影术

Endoscopic retrograde cholangiopancreatography (ERCP) is a technique that combines the use of endoscopy and fluoroscopy to diagnose and treat certain problems of the biliary or pancreatic ductal systems.
内镜逆行胰胆管造影(ERCP)是结合使用内镜和 X 线透视来诊断和治疗胆或胰导管系统某些疾病的一种技术。

Magnetic resonance cholangiopancreatography (MRCP) is a medical imaging technique that uses magnetic resonance imaging to visualise the biliary and pancreatic ducts in a non-invasive manner.
磁共振胰胆管造影是一种医学成像技术，它使用磁共振成像以无创方式来显示胆胰管。

cholangitis [kɔlænˈdʒaitis] *n.* 胆管炎

Obstruction of the bile duct is associated with cholangitis, and eggs may be deposited in the liver.
胆管梗阻可并发胆管炎，而且虫卵会沉积于肝内。

With recurrent pyogenic cholangitis cirrhosis may eventually develop.
复发型化脓性胆管炎最终可发展成肝硬化。

cholecalciferol [kɔlikælˈsifərɔl] *n.* 胆钙化醇

Both cholecalciferol and ergocalciferol are metabolized identically.
胆钙化醇和麦角钙化醇(两者的)代谢途径相同。

cholecystectomy [ˌkɔlisisˈtektəmi] *n.* 胆囊切除术

Cholecystitis may require treatment by cholecystectomy.
胆管炎患者常需要做胆囊切除术。

Most surgeons prefer to perform definitive cholecystectomy on the next available operating day during regular working hour and after the patient has been stabilized medically.
在病人的病情稳定之后，大多数外科医生多倾向于择期给病人进行胆囊切除术。

cholecystis [ˈkɔlisistis] *n.* 胆囊

There is no significant disparation in the percentage of polypoid lesions of gallbladder, cholesterol crystallization in cholecystis between the test group and the control group.

测试组和对照组相比,胆囊息肉样病变和胆囊内胆固醇结晶的百分率无显著性差异。

cholecystitis [ˌkəulisisˈtaitis] *n.* 胆囊炎

The patient told the doctor that he had a previous history of cholecystitis.

病人告诉医生他有胆囊炎的既往史。

As a rule, acute cholecystitis calls for immediate operation.

一般地说,急性胆囊炎需要立即进行手术。

The positive rate of FasL in carcinoma was significantly higher than that in chronic cholecystitis.

FasL 在癌中的阳性率显著高于慢性胆囊炎。

cholecystography [ˌkɔlisisˈtɔgrəfi] *n.* 胆囊造影术

Cholecystography is a procedure that helps to diagnose gallstones using X-rays and contrast medium to show up the gallbladder and bile duct.

胆囊造影术是通过使用 X 线和造影剂来显示胆囊和胆管从而有助诊断胆结石的一种操作。

Cholecystography may be performed when signs and symptoms of gallbladder disease, such as right upper quadrant abdominal pain, jaundice and intolerance of fat in the diet, are present.

胆囊造影术可以在胆囊疾病的症状和体征出现时进行,如右上腹疼痛、黄疸和在饮食上不耐受脂肪。

cholecystokinin [ˌkəulisistəˈkinin] *n.* 胆囊收缩素

There are a range of peptides that regulate appetite——including central cholecystokinin, an anorectic agent, and neuropeptide-Y, a potent appetite stimulant.

有一系列可以调节食欲的肽类,包括中枢性胆囊收缩素(一种食欲抑制剂)和神经肽 Y(一种强效的食欲刺激剂)。

cholecystostomy [ˌkəulisisˈtɔstəmi] *n.* 胆囊造口术(引流)

Cholecystostomy, the surgical placement of a drainage tube in the gallbladder, on occasion may be appropriate.

偶尔也可采用胆囊造口术,即用手术方法在胆囊内安置引流管引出胆汁。

cholecystotomy [ˌkɔlisisˈtɔtəmi] *n.* 胆囊切开术

Cholecystotomy is performed only when cholecystectomy would be impracticable or dangerous.

胆囊切开术仅在采用胆囊切除术无法施行时或有危险时才采用。

choledocholithiasis [ˌkɔlidəuˌkɔliθiˈæsis] *n.* 胆总管结石病

Juxtapapillary duodenal diverticulum might be one of the causes for choledocholithiasis and recurrent stones.

十二指肠乳头旁憩室可能是胆总管结石和复发结石的病因之一。

Choledocholithiasis is the presence of at least one gallstone in the common bile duct.

胆总管结石病是指在胆总管至少出现一个胆结石。

cholelithiasis [ˌkəuliliˈðaiəsis] *n.* 胆囊结石,胆石病

Cholecystitis and cholelithiasis occur more commonly in females than in males.

胆囊炎和胆石症两者发生于女性均较男性为常见。

The precise mechanism by which cholecystitis and cholelithiasis occur is not fully understood.

产生胆囊炎和胆囊结石的确切机制还没有完全被认识。

cholera [ˈkɔlərə] *n.* 霍乱

Koch also discovered the bacillus which causes cholera.

郭霍还发现了引起霍乱的杆菌。

Cholera can be eliminated only by improved standards of living, public health, and sanitation.

惟有改善生活条件、公共卫生和环境卫生才能消灭霍乱。

choleretic [ˌkəuləˈretik] *n.* 利胆剂

Bile salts are choleretics which stimulate the flow of bile and increase the efficiency of its production.

胆盐是利胆剂,它可刺激胆汁流出并有增加胆汁产生的功效。

Some type of choleretic is usually used thereafter as well as broad-spectrum antibiotics for a minimum of 1-2 weeks.

随后通常使用某些利胆剂以及广谱抗生素至少 1 ~2 周。

cholestasis [ˌkɔliˈsteisis] *n.* 胆汁淤积

The intrahepatic cholestasis results in jaundice, pale stools, dark urine and steatorrhoea.

肝内胆汁淤积引起黄疸,大便色白而小便色深,同时可有脂肪下痢。

Hepatitis with predominant cholestasis is uncommon in children.

儿童患有胆汁淤积性肝炎者,并不多见。

cholesterol [kəˈlestərəl] *n.* 胆固醇

A high cholesterol level in the blood can cause heart disease.

血液中胆固醇含量高能引起心脏病。

Cholesterol is synthesized in the body from acetate, mainly in the liver.

胆固醇在体内(主要在肝脏)由乙酸盐合成。

He cut his dietary cholesterol to 300mg a day and started exercising.

他把一天饮食中的胆固醇含量减少到 300mg,并且开始锻炼身体。

cholesteryl [kəˈlestəˌril] *n.* 胆甾烯醇

ACAT is present in a variety of tissues and is responsible for catalyzing the conversion of free cholesterol to the more readily stored cholesteryl esters.

胆固醇乙酰转移酶(ACAT)存在于不同的组织中,可催化游离胆固醇向更易储存的胆固醇酯转化。

Cholesteryl ester transfer protein CETP is a key member of bactericidal gene family and plays an important role in reverse transportation of cholesterol from the peripheral tissues to the liver.

胆固醇酯转运蛋白(CETP)是杀菌蛋白基因家族的重要成员,其主要功能是将血浆中的胆固醇逆向从外周组织转运至肝脏中。

cholinergic [ˌkəuliˈnəːdʒik] *a.* 胆碱能的

Atropine will counteract the muscarinic side effect of the cholinergic drugs.

阿托品对胆碱能药物的毒蕈碱性副作用有拮抗作用。

cholinesterase [ˌkəuliˈnestəreis] *n.* 胆碱酯酶

A decrease in cholinesterase activity≥50% in plasma or red cells is diagnostic.

血浆或红细胞内的胆碱酯酶活性下降≥50%可诊断(有机磷中毒)。

chondral [ˈkɔndrəl] *a.* 软骨的

Physicians have taken a greater interest in treating chondral defects recently partly because of our better understanding of cartilage biology and pathology and partly because of advances in imaging and arthroscopy.

内科医生最近在治疗软骨疾病方面显示出巨大的兴趣,部分是因为我们对软骨的生物学和病理学了解更多了,部分是因为图像技术和关节内镜技术的进步。

Patients with acute chondral injuries of the patellofemoral joint often complain of pain and catching in the knee.

患有急性髌股关节软骨损伤的患者经常主诉膝部疼痛和僵硬感。

chondroblastoma [ˌkɔndrəuˌblæsˈtəumə] *n.* 软骨母细胞瘤,成软骨细胞瘤

Chondroblastoma is rare, accounting for less than 1% of primary bone tumors.

软骨母细胞瘤罕见,占原发性骨肿瘤不到 1%。

In chondroblastoma, the tumor cells have well-defined cytoplasmic borders, moderate amounts of pink cytoplasm, and nuclei with longitudinal grooves.

在软骨母细胞瘤，肿瘤细胞界限清楚，胞质粉染、中等量，核有纵沟。

Because chondroblastoma may extend upto subchondral bone, it is difficult to perform marginal excision or complete curettage.

因为软骨母细胞瘤可能会累及软骨下骨，所以很难找到肿瘤的边缘并完整切除肿瘤。

chondrocyte [ˈkɔndrəsait] *n.* 软骨细胞

The progenitors of chondrocytes arise in the bone marrow, in a form of stem cell.

软骨细胞的前体以一种干细胞的形式产生于骨髓中。

chondrodysplasia [ˌkɔndrəudiˈspleiziə] *n.* 软骨发育不全

A number of chondrodysplasias are caused by mutations in the gene for collagen Ⅱ.

许多软骨发育不全是由于胶原基因 2 的突变引起的。

This model will be useful for the study of FGFR3 function of cartilage and the future therapeutic approaches of chondrodysplasias.

此模型有助于对软骨 EGFR3 基因的功能研究，并有助于未来对软骨发育不全的治疗方法的研究。

chondrolysis [kɔnˈdrɔlisis] *n.* 软骨溶解

Chondrolysis is the disappearance of articular cartilage as the result of the disintegration or dissolution of the cartilage matrix and cells.

软骨溶解是由于软骨基质和细胞的裂解或溶解造成的关节软骨消失。

This systematic review provides a synthesis of existing clinical evidence that helps identify factors associated with the development of glenohumeral chondrolysis after arthroscopy.

这个系统性回顾提供了综合现有临床证据的情况，有助于确定与关节镜检查后出现盂肱软骨溶解的有关因素。

chondroma [kɔnˈdrəumə] *n.* 软骨瘤

Chondromas are benign tumors of hyaline cartilage that usually occur in small tubular bones.

软骨瘤是透明软骨的良性肿瘤，常发生于短的管状骨。

Characteristic features of chondroma include the vascular axes within the tumor, which make the distinction with normal hyaline cartilage.

软骨瘤与一般的透明软骨不同的显著特征是在肿瘤内部有血管轴。

chondrosarcoma [ˌkɔndrəusɑːˈkəumə] *n.* 软骨肉瘤

Chondrosarcoma is the third most common primary malignant neoplasm of bone, producing neoplastic cartilage.

软骨肉瘤是第三最常见的骨原发的恶性肿瘤，可产生肿瘤性软骨。

The most common sites for chondrosarcoma to grow are the pelvis and shoulder, along with the superior metaphysial and diaphysial regions of the arms and legs.

软骨肉瘤好发部位是骨盆和肩部，以及四肢干骺端及骨干上方的区域。

chordoma [kɔːˈdəumə] *n.* 脊索瘤

Chordoma is a rare slow-growing malignant neoplasm thought to arise from cellular remnants of the notochord.

脊索瘤是一种罕见的生长缓慢恶性肿瘤，被认为源于胚胎期脊索细胞残留物。

chorea [kɔˈriə] *n.* 舞蹈病

Chorea may be generalized or limited to one side of the body.

舞蹈病可表现为全身性发作或仅局限于半侧肢体。

In Huntington's chorea the involuntary movements are accompanied by a progressive dementia.

在亨廷顿氏舞蹈病中不自主运动伴有进行性痴呆。

choreiform [kɔˈriːifɔːm] *a.* 舞蹈病样的

A patient with chronic hepatitis C showed an increase in choreiform movements associated with Huntington's disease.

一例慢性丙型肝炎病人表现为与亨廷顿病相关的舞蹈病样运动。

She had a history of minor choreiform limb movements for the past few years, but no cognitive impairment was observed.

在过去几年里她有轻微的舞蹈样肢体运动的病史，但是没有认知障碍。

choreoathetoid [ˌkɔriəˈæθəˌtɔid] *n.* 舞蹈病；手足徐动症

Different from spastic cerebral palsy, persons with choreoathetoid cerebral palsy have variable muscle tone often with decreased muscle tone.

不同于痉挛性大脑性麻痹，舞蹈病患者的大脑性麻痹肌紧张程度可变并伴有肌紧张程度下降。

chorioamnionitis [ˌkɔːriəuˌæmniəˈnaitis] *n.* 绒毛膜羊膜炎

Chorioamnionitis is inflammation of the placental membranes.

绒毛膜羊膜炎是胎膜的炎症。

Chorioamnionitis indicates intrauterine infection, is one of the major risk factors for prematurity.

绒毛膜羊膜炎提示宫内感染，是引起早产的主要危险因素之一。

choriocarcinoma [ˌkɔːriəuˌkɑːsiˈnəumə] *n.* 绒(毛)膜癌

Invasive mole and choriocarcinoma are treated with great success by chemotherapy.

化疗治疗侵蚀性葡萄胎及绒毛膜癌已取得了巨大成就。

A high proportion of patients with certain cancers such as choriocarcinoma, testicular cancer, and a number of childhood neoplasms can now expect to be cured.

相当多的患有绒膜癌、睾丸癌和一些儿童肿瘤的患者有治愈的希望。

chorio-epithelioma [ˌkɔːriɔepiˌθiːliˈəumə] *n.* 绒(毛)膜上皮癌

Chorio-epithelioma, which rapidly invades and causes secondary deposits, is highly malignant; it may occur after hydatidiform mole, pregnancy, or abortion.

绒毛膜上皮癌的生长极为迅速并易转移，其恶性程度极高，多发生于葡萄胎、妊娠或流产之后。

chorion [ˈkɔːriɔn] *n.* [胚] 绒毛膜；浆膜

It also, when possible, noted whether fetuses were surrounded by their own chorionic membrane, or whether that chorion was shared.

这个资料也可能记载了胎儿是否各自拥有一个绒毛膜，还是与孪生同胞共享。

He thinks the harm is done if the blood supply is shared between the two individuals, something more common in twins who share a chorion.

他认为当血液同时要供给两个胎儿的时候，危害就产生了，这在共用一个绒毛膜的双胞胎妊娠中是很常见的。

chorionic [ˌkɔːriˈɔnik] *a.* 绒毛膜的

Dynamic monitoring of serum human chorionic gonadotropin levels for early diagnosis of ectopic pregnancy is helpful.

动态监测血清人绒毛膜促性腺激素水平对异位妊娠早期诊断是有帮助的。

Chorionic villus sampling is a form of prenatal diagnosis to determine chromosomal or genetic disorders in the fetus.

绒毛膜绒毛取样是对胎儿进行染色体和遗传缺陷检查的一种产前诊断方法。

chorioretinitis [ˌkɔːriəuˌretiˈnaitis] *n.* 脉络膜视网膜炎

Chorioretinitis can occur with all of the above infections.

脉络膜视网膜炎可见于所有上述感染。

choroid [ˈkɔːrɔɪd] *n.* 脉络膜

The brain contains pockets or spaces called ventricles with a spongy layer of cells and blood vessels called the choroid plexus.

脑内包含一些袋子或间隙，称作脑室，脑室内含有细胞海绵层和称作脉络膜丛的血管。

Choroid plexus cysts are cysts that occur within choroid plexus of the brain.

脉络膜丛囊肿是发生在脑内脉络丛内的囊肿。

chromatic [krəu'mætik] *a.* 染色质的;彩色的

The irregular agglomerate of chromatic pycnosis and periphery distribution of nucleus and crescent moon of the cell, were observed.

已观察到染色质固缩不规则团块、核边缘化分布以及细胞呈新月形。

chromatid ['krəumətid] *n.* 染色单体

In prophase, each chromosome appears as a double strand of identical chromatids.

在有丝分裂前期,每条染色体含有两条相同的染色单体。

In mitosis the sister chromatids and the centromere become clearly visible and line up along the plane of eventual cleavage.

在有丝分裂过程中姐妹染色单体和着丝粒变得清晰可见并且排列在最终的分裂面上。

chromatin ['krəumətin] *n.* 染色质

In chromatolysis or karyolysis, the nuclear chromatin appears to be dissolved and the nucleus gradually fades from sight.

在染色质溶解或核溶解时,核染色质呈现溶解状态,而且核也逐渐消失。

chromatogram [krəu'mætəgræm] *n.* 色谱图

We have the instruments such as gas chromatogram, surface aperture, etc.

我们拥有气相色谱仪和表面孔径测定仪等设备。

Ion-exchange pillar is used in ion-exchange chromatogram.

离子交换柱用于离子交换色谱。

chromatography [ˌkrəumə'tɔgrəfi] *n.* 色层分析,色谱分析法

The inclusion bodies were purified by ion-exchange chromatography.

这些包涵体是用离子交换色谱法进行纯化的。

Plasma was fractionated by chromatography.

血浆用色谱法进行了分离。

chromatolysis [ˌkrəumə'tɔlisis] *n.* 染色质溶解,尼氏体溶解

Chromatolysis is the dissolution of the Nissl bodies in the cell body of a neuron.

尼氏体溶解是指神经元胞体内的尼氏体崩解。

The event of chromatolysis is characterized by a prominent migration of the nucleus towards the periphery of the cell and an increase in the size of the nucleolus, nucleus, and cell body.

染色质溶解的特点是细胞核向细胞周边的显著迁移,以及核仁、细胞核与细胞体的体积变大。

chromium ['krəumjəm] *n.* 铬

Dermal exposure to chromium may result in the development of allergic contact dermatitis.

皮肤接触铬可引发变态反应性接触性皮炎。

Chromium is used for the production of alloys, in paint pigment and in the tanning industry.

铬常用于生产合金,并用于油漆颜料和电镀工业中。

chromoblastomycosis [ˌkrəuməˌblæstɔmai'kəusis] *n.* 着色芽生菌病

Chromoblastomycosis is a chronic fungal infection of the skin and the subcutaneous tissue.

着色芽生菌病是一种慢性皮肤和皮下组织的真菌感染。

Chromoblastomycosis is caused by traumatic inoculation of a specific group of dematiaceous fungi.

着色芽生菌病是通过创伤而带入某特异着色真菌引起的。

chromogenic [ˌkrəumə'dʒenik] *a.* 显色的

Chromogenic or precipitating substrates have been used widely for many years and offer the simplest and most cost-effective method of detection.

显色或沉淀底物已经被广泛使用了很多年,它们提供了最简单和最经济有效的检测方法。

Unlike chemiluminescent or fluorescent blotting applications, chromogenic substrates do not re-

quire special equipment for visualization of the assay results.
与化学发光或荧光印迹应用不同,显色底物不需要特殊设备来显示分析结果。

chromomycin [ˌkrəuməˈmaisin] *n.* 色霉素

Sperm chromatin status was evaluated by Chromomycin A3 (CMA3), Aniline Blue (AB) and Toluidine Blue (TB).
精子染色质状态通过色霉素 A3、苯胺蓝和甲苯胺蓝作了评价。

Chromomycin SA3 and chromomycin SA2 are the first naturally occurring chromomycin analogs with truncated side-chains.
色霉素 SA3 和色霉素 SA2 是人类最先发现的侧链缩短的天然色霉素类似物。

chromophore [ˈkrəuməfɔː] *n.* 生色团,色基

Four kinds of azo chromophore compounds containing oxygen were synthesized.
合成了 4 种含氧偶氮生色团化合物。

The activity lost after the chromophore was rearranged.
生色团重排后,活性丢失。

chromophoric [krəuməˈfɔrik] *a.* 发色团的,载色体的

The results showed that the chromophoric group of the fluorescent monomer tagged with FC-POCA wasn't changed much.
这些结果显示:标记了 FC-POCA 的荧光单体发色基团并没有发生很大变化。

Chromophoric dissolved organic matter (CDOM) is a major component of the total dissolved organic matter in seawater.
有色可溶解有机物是海水中总溶解有机物的主要组成部分。

chromoprotein [ˌkrəuməˈprəutiːn] *n.* 色蛋白

The colored chromoproteins, such as hemoglobin, contain an organic prosthetic group that is linked to some metal ion.
有颜色的色蛋白,如血红蛋白,含有连接某些金属离子的有机辅基。

chromosomal [ˌkrəuməˈsɔməl] *a.* 染色体的

The gross chromosomal abnormalities described above lead to complex abnormalities since many genes must be involved.
上述显著的染色体异常可引起复杂的变化,因为要涉及许多基因。

The degree of chromosomal damage seems to be associated with disease progression and poorer prognosis.
染色体损伤的程度似乎与疾病的进展和不良的预后有联系。

chromosome [ˈkrəuməsəum] *n.* 染色体

Chromosomes are strings or beads of genetic material.
染色体是线状或串珠状的遗传物质。

There are 46 chromosomes present in somatic cell of man, including the two (xx or xy) which determine the sex of the organism.
人体细胞内有 46 条染色体,包括两条(xx 或 xy)决定机体性别的染色体。

Each chromosome has already divided into two chromatid, which are held together by a centromere.
每一个染色体有分开的两条染色单体被一个着丝点连在一起。

In 1960 an international conference was held in Denver to establish a standard numbering-system for human chromosomes.
1960 年在丹佛举行的国际会议上,制订了一套标准的人类染色体标记系统。

chronic [ˈkrɔnik] *a.* 慢性的

Just because you're older doesn't mean you have to have these chronic diseases.
只是因为年老,并不意味着你就得染上这些慢性病。

Amoebic dysentery usually runs a chronic course with pains in the abdomen.

阿米巴痢疾通常是伴有腹痛的一种慢性病程。

chronically [ˈkrɔnikəli] *ad.* 慢性地，长期地

There is little doubt that a chronically inflamed appendix can be responsible for symptoms of dyspepsia.

阑尾慢性炎症可引起消化不良症状，这一点几乎是不容怀疑的。

Numerous drugs when taken in large doses and chronically may alter receptor functions.

许多药物如果长期大剂量使用，可改变受体的功能。

chronobiology [ˌkrɔnəbaiˈɔlədʒi] *n.* 生物钟学

Chronobiology is the study of the biological mechanism that governs the rhythmic activities of organisms.

生物钟学研究支配生物节奏性活动的生物机制。

chronology [krəˈnɔlədʒi] *n.* 年代学，年代；（按事物发生）顺序的排列

You can find the date for discovery of blood circulation from the Medical Advances Chronology.

你可从《医学进展年表》中查到发现血液循环的日期。

Painstaking attention must be paid to the chronology of symptoms in relation to the use of drugs or treatments.

应特别注意与药物或治疗的使用相关的症状出现的时间顺序。

chronopharmacokinetics [ˌkrɔnəˌfɑːməkəukiˈnetiks, -kai-] *n.* 时辰药物动力学，时间药物动力学

Chronopharmacokinetics is the study of the absorption, distribution, metabolism, and elimination of medicines according to the time of day, menstrual cycle, or year.

时辰药物动力学是研究日、月或年周期内药物的吸收、分布、代谢和消除。

The pig represents a useful model for the study of chronopharmacokinetics of drugs given intravenously in human.

猪是研究人静脉内给药时辰药物动力学的一种有用模型。

chrysomonad [kriˈsɔmənæd] *n.* 金滴虫目

Chrysomonads are usually small flagellates.

金滴虫目通常是小鞭毛虫。

chyle [kail] *n.* 乳糜

Chyle is the milky-appearing fluid formed by the combination of fat globules and lymph.

乳糜液是由脂肪球和淋巴液组成的乳状液。

The milky fluid draining away into the lymphatics is the chyle.

流入淋巴管的乳样液就是乳糜。

chylomicron [ˌkailəuˈmaikrɔn] *n.* 乳糜微粒

Impaired clearance of chylomicron remnants is associated with increased risk of atherosclerosis and cardiovascular disease.

乳糜微粒残留物清除受损与动脉粥样硬化及心血管疾病的风险增加相关。

chylothorax [ˌkailəuˈθɔːræks] *n.* 乳糜胸

Chylothorax is an infrequent but serious complication after thoracic surgery.

乳糜胸是胸外科手术后罕见的但十分严重的并发症。

Ligation of thoracic duct can effectively prevent patients with middle or upper carcinoma of esophagus undergoing esophagectomy from suffering chylothorax.

中上段食管癌行食管切除术时，胸导管结扎能有效防止乳糜胸的发生。

chylous [ˈkailəs] *a.* 乳糜的

Chylous ascites is still more uncommon; it is usually related to traumatic lymphatic injury.

乳糜性腹水则更加少见，其通常和淋巴损伤相关。

The clinical manifestation of chylous ascites may mimic retroperitoneal cystic lymphangioma.

乳糜腹水的临床表现和后腹腔的囊状淋巴瘤十分类似。

chyluria [kaiˈljuəriə] *n.* 乳糜尿;乳糜尿检验

What is the role of radionuclide lymphoscintigraphy in chyluria?

放射性核素淋巴闪烁显像在乳糜尿检验中的作用是什么?

This article summarizes our experience in retroperitoneoscopic ligation of renal lymphatic vessels for the treatment of chyluria.

本文总结了我们用后腹腔镜进行肾蒂淋巴管结扎术治疗乳糜尿的经验。

chymotrypsin [kaiməˈtripsin] *n.* 糜蛋白酶,胰凝乳蛋白酶

Although chymotrypsin contains three polypeptide chains, it is not considered to have a quaternary structure.

尽管胰凝乳蛋白酶有三条多肽链,但并不被认为具有四级结构。

cicatricial [ˌsikəˈtriʃəl] *a.* 瘢痕的

The oesophageal stenosis may be caused by cicatricial tissue or by compression.

食道狭窄可由瘢痕组织或压迫所引起。

The purpose of the study is to investigate the use of micro grafts and minigrfts for the treatment of cicatricial alopecia.

这项研究的目的是调查使用微、小头发移植体治疗瘢痕性秃发的应用情况。

cigarette [ˌsigəˈret] *n.* 香烟

These two people have reacted to cigarette smoke differently.

这两个人对于吸烟有着不同的生理反应。

Cigarette smoke causes oral cancer, gum diseases and tooth loss.

香烟烟气导致口腔癌、牙龈炎和牙齿脱落。

ciliary [ˈsiliəri] *a.* 睫状的,纤毛的

Ciliary defects are not always inherited.

纤毛的功能缺陷并非皆由遗传所致。

ciliat [ˈsilieit] *a.* 纤毛的

Nasal secretions are normally swept backward to the pharynx by ciliat action, and one is usually unaware of this.

鼻分泌物在正常情况下被纤毛作用向后清除到咽部,但是人们通常没有意识到这一点。

ciliated [ˈsilieitid] *a.* 纤毛的

The ciliary activity of ciliated tracheobronchial epithelium is influenced by numerous agents, it is stimulated by acetylcholine, weak acid and is inhibited by low humidity, cigarette smoke.

有纤毛的气管支气管上皮的纤毛活动受很多因素影响,乙酰胆碱、弱酸可刺激它;湿度低、香烟的烟可抑制它。

cilium [ˈsiliəm] (*pl.* cilia [ˈsiliə]) *n.* 纤毛;睫

Cilia are shorter than flagella.

纤毛比鞭毛短。

In land vertebrates, thousands of cilia occur on the epithelial cells.

陆生脊椎动物的上皮细胞上有无数的纤毛。

Cilia normally are present in many organs, and their absence or abnormality may cause clinical problems.

正常情况下许多脏器都具有纤毛,若纤毛缺失或异常时,常能引起疾病。

cimetidine [saiˈmetiˌdiːn] *n.* 西咪替丁,甲氰咪胍(抗消化性溃疡药)

Recently, clinical studies showed that cimetidine had antitumor effects.

近年来,临床研究显示西咪替丁具有抗肿瘤作用。

The article reviews the clinical application of cimetidine in this field.

文章综述了西咪替丁在这一领域的临床应用。

cinnamaldehyde [ˈsinəˈmældihaid] *n.* 肉桂醛;桂皮醛

GC method for the determination of cinnamaldehyde in cassia bark capsules has been developed.

采用气相色谱测定中成药桂皮胶囊中桂皮醛含量的方法已制定出来。

This young technician has quickly mastered the method for the determination of cinnamaldehyde content in cassia.

这位年轻技术员很快掌握了测定桂皮中桂皮醛含量的方法。

cinnamicalcohol [siˌnæmik'ælkəhɔl] *n.* 肉桂醇

The cinnamicalcohol content among them was highest.

肉桂醇的含量在它们中是最高的。

Data from these patients showed that the top allergen was cinnamicalcohol.

患者的数据显示最常见的致敏原是肉桂醇。

cinnamon ['sinəmɔn] *n.* 肉桂;肉桂色;肉桂皮

Someone once said that cinnamon has no synonym.

有人曾说肉桂没有同义词。

These smells included cinnamon, black pepper, chocolate, paint thinner, and smoke.

这些气味包括肉桂、黑胡椒粉、巧克力、油漆稀释剂和烟味。

ciprofloxacin [ˌsiprəu'flɔksəsin] *n.* 环丙沙星

The treatment of acute bacterial pneumonia with high-dose parenteral ciprofloxacin appears to be efficacious and well tolerated.

注射大剂量羟嗪环丙沙星治疗急性细菌性肺炎似乎是有效的和耐受良好的。

One hundred and fifty three hospitalized patients were enrolled in an open, prospective, multi-center study on the efficacy and safety of intravenous ciprofloxacin (400mg i. v., b. i. d.) for acute bacterial pneumonia.

153 位住院病人加入了一项开放的前瞻性多中心研究,研究的是使用静脉注射环丙沙星(400 毫克 2 次/天)治疗急性细菌性肺炎的有效性和安全性。

circadian [sə'keidiən] *a.* 以 24 小时为周期的,生理周期的

The normal 24h circadian temperature rhythm is associated with temperatures varying by 0. 5℃.

正常体温 24 小时周期性变化表现为体温波动在 0. 5℃。

Sleep deprivation or disruption of the circadian timing system can lead to serious impairment of daytime functioning.

失眠或昼夜节律的失衡可导致白日机体功能的严重紊乱。

Fever is an elevation of body temperature above the normal circadian range.

发热是指体温高于正常生理变化范围。

circulate ['səːkjuleit] *v.* 循环,传播

Lymph is a watery fluid that circulates throughout the body.

淋巴是一种循环于全身的水状液。

Blood is the fluid which circulates around the cardio-vascular system by the contractions of the two ventricles.

血液是一种液体,由两个心室的收缩使其周而复始的沿着心血管系统(不断的)循环。

circulation [səːkju'leiʃən] *n.* 循环

The period of a complete circulation of the blood throughout the body is short.

血液流经全身的完整循环的周期时间很短。

Blood from the left ventricle may pass through the coronary circulation to nourish the heart itself.

左心室的血液可以通过冠状动脉循环来滋养心脏自身。

circulatory ['səːkjulətəri] *a.* 循环的

For instance, circulatory shock may cause weakness of the heart.

例如,循环休克可引起心脏衰弱。

Severe peripheral circulatory failure is combined with severe pulmonary congestion.

严重的周围循环衰竭和严重的肺充血是相互联系着的。

circumcise ['səːkəmsaiz] *v.* 割除包皮;对…进行环切术

The bank was set up by using discarded tissue from circumcised new-born babies.
该细胞库系利用从新生儿包皮环切下来的废弃组织建立起来。

circumcision [ˌsəːkəm'siʒən] *n.* 包皮环切术

Otherwise, some people could develop a false sense of security and engage in high-risk behaviors that could undermine the partial protection provided by male circumcision, the agencies said.
另外，该机构认为有些人可能产生错误的安全感，并进行高危的（性）行为习惯，结果是削弱了包皮环切所产生的部分保护作用。

Public health leaders think circumcision may be a powerful way to reduce HIV infection in Africa, the continent hardest hit by AIDS.
公共卫生系统的官员认为包皮环切术可有效减少非洲（遭艾滋病最严重肆掠的大陆）HIV 感染。

circumduction [ˌsəːkəm'dʌkʃən] *n.* 环转

Flexion and extension, abduction and adduction, medical and lateral rotation, and circumduction can occur at ball and socket joints.
联结球窝关节（的肢体）可作屈伸、收展、旋内旋外和环转运动。

circumference [sə'kʌmfərəns] *n.* 圆周，周围

His height, weight and chest circumference are 165cm, 56kg and 80cm respectively.
他的身高、体重和胸围分别为 165 厘米、56 公斤和 80 厘米。

circumscribe ['səːkəmkraib] *v.* 限制；使外接，使外切

All living cells are circumscribed by limiting membranes or cell walls; and all contain nuclei or an equivalent nuclear substance.
所有生活的细胞都受限于界膜或细胞壁，并都含有细胞核或相当于核的物质。

circumstance ['səːkəmstəns] *n.* 情况，环境

Each case of suspected postmaturity should be dealt with according to its special circumstances.
每例怀疑过期妊娠患者都应根据具体情况来处理。

Culture shock can occur also when life circumstances change radically with a society.
文化冲击在一个社会生活环境发生根本改变时也可发生。

cirrhosis [si'rəusis] *n.* 肝硬化，肝硬变

Cirrhosis is a condition involving the entire liver.
肝硬化是整个肝脏受累的一种疾病。

Cirrhosis is a pathological diagnosis and therefore implies liver biopsy in all suspected cases.
肝硬化是一病理诊断，这就表明需对所有的拟诊病例进行肝活体组织检查。

cisplatin [sis'plætən] *n.* 铂化合物，顺铂；顺氯氨铂

Cisplatin plus gemcitabine is an appropriate option for the treatment of patients with advanced biliary cancer.
顺铂加吉西他滨是治疗晚期胆道癌病人的一种合适的抉择。

The inorganic drug of the metal complexes has been a new anticancer drug of chemical therapy, since cisplatin was used in clinic as an anticancer drug.
自从顺铂作为抗肿瘤药物被临床应用以来，金属络合物类无机药物已成为一类新的抗癌化疗药物。

cis-platinum [sis'plætinəm] *n.* 顺铂

Cis-platinum is a chemotherapy drug. It is used to treat various types of cancer, including sarcoma, some carcinoma (e. g. small cell lung cancer, and ovarian cancer), lymphoma, and germ cell tumors.
顺铂是一种化学治疗药物，通常用来治疗不同类型的恶性肿瘤，包括肉瘤，癌（如小细胞肺癌，卵巢癌），淋巴瘤，和生殖细胞瘤。

Cis-platinum crosslinks DNA in several different ways, interfering with cell division by mitosis.
顺铂用不同方法交链 DNA 来干扰细胞的有丝分裂。

cisterna [si'stəːnə] *n.* 池;内胞浆网槽

In fact, surgeons seldom see the cisterna chyle during upper lumbar spinal surgeries.

事实上,外科医师在行上腰椎手术时很少会看到乳糜池。

Leakage of lymph from below the cisterna chili can cause a retroperitoneal lymphocele, which is an accumulation of clear fluid.

乳糜池以下的淋巴漏则可以引起腹膜后淋巴管囊肿,它是由清亮的液体聚集而成。

cistron ['sistrɔn] *n.* 顺反子

Cistron is a segment of DNA that is involved in producing a polypeptide chain.

顺反子是一个参与产生一条多肽链的 DNA 片段。

The study of genes involves the study of the individual genetic units called cistrons.

基因的研究涉及称为"顺反子"的单个遗传单位的研究。

cite [sait] *v.* 引证,引用

According to Smith, who cites 10 authors, the incidence ranges from 10 to 15 per cent.

根据史密斯引用的 10 个作者的资料,其发病率为 10% ~15% 。

In a medical review the writer cited quotations from many original articles or other literatures.

在医学综述中,作者从许多原始论文或其他文献中引用了一些资料。

Several studies could be cited in support of this view.

有好几项研究成果可引用来支持这个论点。

citrate ['sitrit] *n.* 枸橼酸盐,柠檬酸盐

Citrate binds calcium, which is essential for the coagulation cascade and thus serves as an anticoagulant.

枸橼酸盐与钙结合是凝血过程的基础,因此枸橼酸盐可作为一种抗凝剂。

In order to keep the blood from clotting, sodium citrate in solution is added.

为了防止血液的凝固,可以加入枸橼酸钠溶液。

citrobacter [ˌsitrə'bæktə] *n.* 柠檬酸杆菌属

Citrobacter can be found almost everywhere in soil, water, wastewater, as well as in the human intestine.

柠檬酸杆菌存在于土壤、水、废水以及人体肠道的几乎任何地方。

Citrobacter is a genus of gram-negative coliform bacteria in the enterobacteriaceae family.

柠檬酸杆菌属是肠杆菌科中的一类革兰阴性大肠型细菌。

citrullinemia [siˌtrʌli'niːmiə] *n.* 瓜氨酸血症,精氨基琥珀酸合成酶缺乏症

Adult-onset type Ⅱ citrullinemia is a disorder caused by an inborn error of metabolism affecting the liver.

成年起病的Ⅱ型瓜氨酸血症是由影响肝脏的先天性代谢性疾病引起的。

This is the first description for a patient with adult onset type Ⅱ citrullinemia in Korea.

这是韩国对成年起病的Ⅱ型瓜氨酸血症的第一次描述。

civilization [ˌsivilai'zeiʃən] *n.* 文明,文化

Historical records show that ancient civilization conducted breeding experiments to improve stocks of plants and animals.

历史记载表明古文明进行大量繁殖试验以改进动植物品种。

cladothrix ['klædəθriks] *n.* 分枝丝菌属

Cladothrix is a thread-like form in which false branching may be recognized.

分枝丝菌呈丝状,其中可以辨认出假分枝。

In 1873 Ferdinand Cohn discovered, and in 1875 he described, a new type of a microorganism that he called Cladothrix dichotoma.

费迪南德·科恩在 1873 年发现,并于 1875 年描述了一种新型微生物,他称之为岐分枝丝菌。

claim [kleim] *v.* 要求,声称;主张

Many users claim that this drug is less potent than the others.
许多使用者都认为这种药物的(疗效)不及其他药物的效力强。

clamp [klæmp] *v.* 夹紧,夹住

All bleeding points are clamped and tied.
(手术时)所有出血点被夹紧和系牢。

These babies had blood volumes 32% higher than babies whose cords were clamped immediately after birth.
这些婴儿的血容量比出生后立即夹紧脐带的婴儿高 32%。

clarify [ˈklærifai] *v.* 阐明;(使)易懂

Further research is needed to clarify the relationship of seasonal factors to depression in children.
需进一步研究以弄清季节因素与儿童抑郁症的关系。

A period of observation may be necessary to clarify the diagnosis.
为了弄清诊断,还需观察一段时间。

clarithromycin [klæˌriθrəˈmaisin] *n.* 甲红霉素,克红霉素(商品名:klacid 克拉仙)

Clarithromycin, an antibiotic belonging to the group of macrolides, has different dosage forms.
甲红霉素属大环内酯类抗生素,具有多种剂型。

Clarithromycin is used to treat bacterial infections in many different parts of the body.
甲红霉素可用于治疗身体许多不同部位的细菌感染。

Clarithromycin is available only with a doctor's prescription in the dosage forms of oral suspension, tablets or extended-release tablets.
甲红霉素需经医生处方才能获得,其剂型有口服悬液、片剂和缓释片剂。

clarity [ˈklæriti] *n.* 清楚,透明

This lack of clarity has compounded difficulties in identifying effective interventions for colic.
缺乏透明度使确定急腹痛的有效干预措施更加困难。

Stability was assessed from turbidity measurement, size analysis and clarity of dispersion on standing.
稳定性从浊度测量、大小分析和静置分散澄清度上进行了评估。

classical [ˈklæsikəl] *a.* 典型的,标准的

Glomerulonephritis is the classical nephritis.
肾小球性肾炎是典型的肾炎。

The salivary glands are classical examples of compound racemose glands.
唾液腺就是复合泡状腺的典型例子。

classification [ˌklæsifiˈkeiʃən] *n.* 分类(法);类别;等级

There are so many different types of bacteria that their classification is very complicated.
细菌种类繁多,因此它们的分类是很复杂的。

Another more generally used classification of heart disease is based on causative and age factors.
另一种常用的心脏病的分类法是以造成疾病的原因和病人的年龄因素为基础的。

Risk factors for surgical wound infection include classification of wound, presence of a drain, length of surgery and surgeon.
发生手术伤口感染的危险因素有:伤口的等级、是否有引流、手术时间的长短和医生等。

classify [ˈklæsifai] *v.* 把…分类

Proteins are classified as complete or incomplete on the basis of the amount and the number of essential amino acids they contain.
基于蛋白质所含必需氨基酸的数量可以将蛋白质分为完全的和不完全的两种。

There are many ways of classifying heart disease.
心脏病的分类有多种。

The classified list comprises four broad interlinked categories.
分类名单包括有相互关联的 4 大类。

As there are five types of white cells it is necessary to classify them separately in the white cell count.

由于有五种类型的白细胞，因此在白细胞分类计数时有必要将它们分别归类。

clastogen [ˈklæstəudʒən] *n.* 断裂剂

A clastogen is a material that can cause breaks in chromosomes, leading to sections of the chromosome being deleted, added, or rearranged.

断裂剂可导致染色体断裂，并引发染色体缺失、扩增或重组。

Known clastogens include acridine yellow, benzene, ethylene oxide, arsenic, phosphine and mimosine.

公认的断裂剂包括吖啶黄、苯、环氧乙烷、砷、磷和含羞草碱。

clastogenesis [ˈklæstəuˈdʒenəsəs] *n.* 断裂作用

Clastogenesis is any process that leads to breaks in chromosomal material, or rearrangement, gain or loss of pieces of chromosome.

染色体断裂作用是指导致染色体断裂或重组、染色体片段的扩增或缺失的过程。

Pre-treatment of mice with quercetin significantly reduced cisplatin-induced clastogenesis and apoptosis in the bone marrow cells and these effects were dose and time dependent.

以槲皮素预处理小鼠可显著性降低顺铂引起的骨髓细胞染色体断裂和凋亡，其结果取决于剂量大小和时间的长短。

claudication [ˌklɔːdiˈkeiʃən] *n.* 跛行

When atherosclerosis involves the arteries of the lower extremities, patients may present with intermittent claudication.

当动脉粥样硬化累及下肢远端血管时，患者可以出现间歇性跛行。

claustrophobia [ˌklɔːstrəuˈfəubjə] *n.* 幽闭恐惧症

Claustrophobia can involve intense fear or even panic as a result of being in a small space.

幽闭恐惧症是指患者因为处在一个狭小空间内而产生强烈的恐惧感甚至恐慌。

The criterion variance predicted was impressive, clearly sufficient to legitimize both the research preparation and the conceptualization of claustrophobia that was evaluated.

预计的诊断标准的差异令人印象深刻，无疑足以使评价幽闭恐惧症的研究准备和概念确定下来。

clavicle [ˈklævikəl] *n.* 锁骨

In human anatomy, the clavicle or collarbones is a long bone with short length that serves as a strut between the scapula and the sternum.

在人体解剖学中，锁骨是用来连接肩胛骨和胸骨的一段短的长骨。

Clavicle fractures are common in adults and children.

锁骨骨折在成人和孩童均常见。

cleanse [klenz] *v.* 使清洁，净化

The site of injection should be cleansed with a suitable antiseptic.

注射部位必须用适当的消毒剂使之清洁。

For abdominal operations the skin should be cleansed with a suitable anticeptic such as chlorhexidine one percent in spirit.

对于腹部手术，应该使用合适的抗菌剂，如：1% 的氯己定酒精溶液，进行皮肤清洗消毒。

cleanser [ˈklenzə] *n.* 清洁剂

Skin cleansers containing mild detergents may be used in place of soap.

应以含有温和去垢剂的洁肤剂来代替肥皂。

clearance [ˈkliərəns] *n.* 清除率，廓清率

The patient was noted to have a creatinine clearance of 5. 8mg/dl.

已注意到患者的肌酸酐廓清率为 5. 8mg/dl。

cleavage [ˈkliːvidʒ] *n.* 劈开；分裂；卵裂

The quantity of yolk affects cleavage.
卵黄量影响卵裂。
Cleavage patterns depend on several factors.
卵裂方式有赖于几个因素。
Cotton developed the chemical cleavage of mismatch method.
科顿发展了错配化学切割法。

cleft [kleft] *n.* 裂,沟

In basal cell carcinoma, the stroma retracts away from the carcinoma and produces clefts or separation artifacts.
在基底细胞癌中,间质回缩使其与癌巢之间产生裂隙或人为的间隔。
Cleft lip is compatible with life when it occurs as an isolated anomaly.
唇裂(兔唇)单独发生时对生命并无大碍。

client ['klaiənt] *n.* 客户;【计算机】客户端

The client only has to know the server name.
客户端只需要知道服务器名称即可。

climacteric [klai'mækterik] *n.* 更年期 *a.* 更年期的

The doctor diagnosed his illness as climacteric arthritis.
医生诊断他的疾病为更年期关节炎。

climate ['klaimit] *n.* 气候

Britain has a temperate climate.
英国气候属于温带气候。
She moved to a warmer climate.
她移居到气候较温和的地区。
Bejel and pinta are endemic only in tropical climates.
非性病性梅毒和品他病只限于热带区域。

clindamycin [ˌklində'maisin] *n.* 氯林可霉素

Clindamycin is an alternative to penicillin.
氯林可霉素是青霉素的一种替代药。

clindodactyly [ˌklindəu'dæktili] *n.* 先天性指内屈

Clinodactyly is a medical term describing a bend or curvature of the fifth finger toward the adjacent fourth finger.
先天性指内屈这一医学术语是指第五指向相邻的第四指弯曲的状况。

clinical ['klinikəl] *a.* 临床的

Investigation are used to confirm or deny a doubtful or difficult clinical diagnosis.
以实验室检查方法来确定或否定疑似的或困难的临床诊断。
A clinical depression is by far the most common cause of memory loss and intellectual deterioration.
临床抑郁症是记忆力丧失和智力衰退最常见的原因。

clinically ['klinikəli] *ad.* 临床上

In most cases, the emboli were small and were often unsuspected clinically.
在大多数情况下,栓子小通常不引起临床上怀疑。
The usual age at which the disease appears clinically is between sixteen and thirty.
这病具有临床特征的通常年龄是在 16 ~30 岁之间。

clinician [kli'niʃən] *n.* 临床医生

There is no agreement among clinicians as to the amount of antitoxin that should be administered.
临床医生对给多少量的抗毒素尚无一致意见。
An alert clinician must be aware of the possibility of myocardities complicating any acute viral in-

fection.
有警觉的医生都应当知道任何急性的病毒感染都可能并发心肌炎。

clinicopathologic [ˌklinikəuˌpæθəˈlɔdʒik] *a.* 临床病理(学)的
Clinicopathologic observation in humans and results of numerous experiments in animals indicate that arterial injury may favor lipid deposition in the injured arterial wall.
对人的临床病理观察和许多动物实验结果表明动脉的损伤可能有利于脂肪沉积在损伤的动脉壁上。

clitoris [ˈklitəris] *n.* 阴蒂
The size of the clitoris should be noted.
应该注意阴蒂的大小。

cloaca [kləuˈeikə] (*pl.* cloacae [kləuˈeisiː] *n.* 瘘,孔
A retrospective review of 411 patients diagnosed with cloaca was performed to identify the ones with a posterior cloaca.
对 411 名被诊断为肛瘘的患者进行了回顾性调查,以确认其中患直肠后位肛瘘的患者。

clofibrate [kləˈfaibreit] *n.* 安妥明
Clofibrate does have a rather potent activity as an inhibitor of cholesterol synthesis.
安妥明作为一种胆固醇合成的抑制剂确实相当有效。
Clofibrate reduces VLDL, triglyceride, and cholesterol.
安妥明可能降低极低密度脂蛋白、甘油三酯和胆固醇。

clog [klɔg] *v.* (使)阻塞,塞满
In this type of case, neurologist may prescribe anticlotting medication or advise surgical opening of a clogged blood vessel.
出现这一类症状时,神经科医生会开出抗凝类药物或劝患者动手术切开阻塞的血管。

clomiphene [ˈklɔmifiːn] *n.* 克罗米酚
Ovulation and menstruation may often be induced with clomiphene.
使用克罗米酚常可诱导排卵及月经。

clonal [ˈkləunəl] *a.* 克隆的,无性(繁殖)系的,细胞系的,纯系的
According to the account, the clonal offspring, now two years old, is living with his "father" in California.
根据报道,该克隆后代现年两岁,随其"父"住在加利福尼亚州。

clone [kləun] *v.* 无性繁殖,复制,克隆
He and others cloned three goats last April.
去年四月他和其他人一起克隆了三只山羊。
Cloned sheep may age prematurely.
克隆的羊可能会早衰。
The team tested the theory by isolating and cloning NK cells from two individuals.
研究小组验证这一学说采用的方法是从两个个体分离出天然杀伤细胞进行克隆。
Clone is a group of genetically identical cells or organisms derived by asexual reproduction from a single parent.
通过无性繁殖,从单一亲代派生出在遗传上完全相同细胞群或生物体(的过程)称作克隆。
The progeny of such a lymphocyte all share the same specific receptor for a given antigen and are termed clones.
这个淋巴细胞的后代都有针对指定抗原的相同的特异性受体,称之为克隆。

clonidine [ˈkləunidiːn] *n.* 氯压定,可乐定(降压药)
Sudden discontinuation of clonidine may induce rebound hypertension.
可乐定的突然停药会引起高血压(症状)反跳。

cloning [ˈkləuniŋ] *n.* 克隆形成,克隆(化),无性繁殖

If so, adult human cloning may never be possible.
果真如此,那么成年人的无性繁殖将永远无法实现。
Using cloning techniques it is possible to obtain portions of a genome that are specific for a given genus, species, or subspecies.
采用克隆技术有可能获得对一定属、种或亚种有特异性的基因组片段。

clonorchiasis [ˌkləunɔːkaiəsis] *n.* 华支睾吸虫病
Clonorchiasis occurs in all parts of the world where there are Asian immigrants from endemic areas.
世界上凡有来自流行疫区的亚洲移民的地方都可能发生华支睾吸虫病。

clonotypic [ˌkləunə'tipik] *n.* 克隆型
A feature unique to individual cells or members of a clone is said to be clonotypic.
单个细胞或一个克隆中成员所具有的独有特征被称为克隆型。

clonus ['kləunəs] *n.* 阵挛,抽筋
Tissue viscoelasticity appeared to have a strong effect on the emergence and persistence of clonus.
组织的黏弹性好像对阵挛的出现和持续时间有强烈的影响。
Lack of calcium in women, especially pregnant women, would cause quadriplegia, ache, clonus etc.
妇女,特别是怀孕妇女缺钙会引起手足麻木、腰酸背痛、抽筋等。
Deep-tendon hyperreflexia and clonus may signal impending seizures.
深部腱反射亢进和阵挛是即将抽搐的信号。

closed-circuit ['kləuzd-'səːkit] *a.* 闭路式的
During X-ray therapy, observation is maintained by closed-circuit television.
在病人接受 X 线治疗时,通过闭路电视对其进行持续观察。

clostridial [klɔ'stridiəl] *a.* 梭状芽孢杆菌的
Clostridial poisoning typically occurs in fairly large outbreaks.
梭状芽孢杆菌食物中毒的典型情况为大面积的暴发。
Clostridial gas gangrene is a highly lethal necrotizing soft tissue infection of skeletal muscle caused by toxin-and gas-producing species.
梭状芽孢杆菌性气性坏疽是一种由产毒素和产气的菌种引起的骨骼肌软组织高度致命的坏死性感染。

clostridium [klɔs'tridiəm] *n.* 肉毒杆菌,梭状芽孢杆菌属(*pl.* clostridia)
Spores of clostridium botulinum are killed in 4 to 20 minutes by moist heat at 120℃.
肉毒杆菌的芽孢在 120℃湿热下 4 ~20 分钟即可被杀死。
The clostridia (sulfite-reducing bacteria) are a class of firmicutes, including clostridium and other similar genera.
梭状芽胞杆菌(还原亚硫酸盐细菌)是一类硬壁菌门中的细菌,包括梭状芽胞杆菌属和其他相近的菌属。
The toxins produced by certain members of the clostridia are among the most dangerous known to man.
梭状芽胞杆菌中某些菌产生的毒素是已知对人最危险的毒素之一。

clot [klɔt] *n.* (血)凝块
Clot is a semisolid mass, as of blood or lymph.
凝块是一种半固体团块,如血凝块或淋巴凝块。
The upper(usually anterior) part of the clot is yellow and gelatinous.
血凝块上部(通常是前面)呈黄色和胶冻状。
v. (使):凝结
Four substances are essential for the clotting of the blood.

有四种物质为血液凝结作用所必需。

clotrimazole [kləu'triməzɔl] *n.* 克霉唑,氯三苯甲咪唑

Clotrimazole is used for the topical therapy of superficial fungal infections.

克霉唑是用于表皮真菌感染的外用药。

Clotrimazole is an inhibitor of Cyp3A, the most abundant P450 enzymes in the human liver.

克霉唑是人类肝脏中最丰富的 P450 酶类中 Cyp3A 的一种抑制剂。

cloud [klaud] *v.* 使混浊,使模糊

The term "clouded consciousness" refers to a reduction in the clarity of awareness of the environment.

"意识模糊"这个术语指的是对环境认识的清晰度下降。

cloudy ['klaudi] *a.* 浑浊的

The osmotic swelling gives the cell cytoplasm a swollen, cloudy and granular appearance.

这种渗透性肿胀使细胞浆呈肿胀、混浊和颗粒状。

clubbing ['klʌbiŋ] *n.* 杵状变(指、趾)

Clubbing is the selective enlargement of the distal segments of fingers and toes.

杵状变是手指和脚趾的远端选择性的变粗。

clue [kluː] *n.* 线索,暗示

This particular symptom has provided an important clue to our making of the diagnosis.

这一特殊的症状为我们做出诊断提供了重要线索。

clump [klʌmp] *n.* 丛;凝块

In such cases the Gram stains may still show clumps of gram-positive cocci.

在这类病例中,革兰氏染色仍可发现革兰氏阳性球菌凝块。

Clumps of cancer cells which are reproducing break off from the original growth and get into the blood or lymph.

不断繁殖的癌细胞块从原先生长的肿瘤上脱落,并进入血液或淋巴。

cluster ['klʌstə] *v.* 成群,丛生,群集

The clustering of two or more nonpolar side chain groups may occur in small regions of the protein surface.

蛋白质表面较小的区域也可有两个或更多的非极性侧链基团集簇。

These studies found affective disorders clustered in families.

这些研究发现情感性障碍在家族中成群出现。

Clusters of these neurons are supplied by a rich and permeable vascular network.

这些神经元群有丰富的和具有通透性的血管网供给能量。

coadministration [kəuəd,minis'treiʃən] *n.* 同时服用

The coadministration of pyridoxine prevents these side effects.

同时服用吡哆醇可防止这些副作用。

coaggregation [kəu,ægri'geiʃən] *n.* 共凝作用

Erythrocytes can be rapidly and effectively separated by coaggregation from negatively charged colloidal magnetic particles.

红细胞通过共凝可迅速且有效地与带负电荷的胶体磁性颗粒分离。

There is an initial study of coaggregation between oral Actinomycetes and Streptococci.

对口腔放线菌和链球菌之间的共凝作用已做了初步研究。

coagulability [kəu,ægjulə'biliti] *n.* 凝固性

Coartisol, like epinephrine, enhances the coagulability of blood.

氢化可的松像肾上腺素一样可增加血液的凝固性。

coagulase [kəu'ægjuː,leis] *n.* 凝固酶

The coagulase negative staphylococci accounted for 57.0%, which was the most common among the Gram positive cocci.

凝固酶阴性葡萄球菌占57.0%,在革兰阳性球菌中最常见。

Oxacillin resistance was identified in 17.6% of staphylococcus aureus and 69.9% of coagulase negative staphylococcus.

17.6%的金黄色葡萄球菌和69.9%的凝固酶阴性葡萄球菌被确认对苯唑西林耐受。

coagulate [kəu'ægjuleit] *v.* (使)凝结

Protein may also coagulate in the tubular lumen.

蛋白质也可在肾小管腔内凝结。

A deficiency of vitamin K in the food results in the inability of the blood to coagulate.

食物中缺乏维生素K可引起血液凝固能力的降低。

coagulation [kəuˌægju'leiʃən] *n.* 凝结

Occasionally the red cells settle before coagulation occurs.

偶尔在血液凝固前,红细胞发生沉降。

Soon after the blood escapes, coagulation occurs in and around the opening in the vessel.

当血液流出(血管)之后,在血管切口内及其周围(血液)会立即凝固。

coagulative [kəu'ægjuleitiv] *a.* 凝结的

This type of necrosis is appropriately described as coagulative necrosis.

这种类型的坏死恰如其分地被称为凝固性坏死。

coagulin [kəu'ægjulin] *n.*

A protease-sensitive antibacterial substance produced by Bacillus coagulans I4 strain, isolated from cattle faeces, was classified as a bacteriocin-like inhibitory substance and named coagulin.

凝结芽孢杆菌I4株产生的一种对蛋白酶敏感的抗菌物质,从牛粪中分离出来,被归类为细菌素样抑制物质,并被命名为凝固素。

Coagulin and pediocin differed only by a single amino acid at their C terminus.

凝固素和片球菌素只在C末端的一个氨基酸上存在差异。

coagulopathy [kəuˌægju'lɔpəθi] *n.* 凝血病

The platelet count, thrombin time, and protamine test are useful in defining consumptive coagulopathy.

血小板计数、凝血时间和鱼精蛋白试验可用于诊断消耗性凝血病。

coagulum [kəu'ægjuləm] (*pl.* coagula [kəu'ægjulə]) *n.* 凝块,血块,凝结物

A longitudinal section taken through the attached head of a thrombus shows a framework of pale granular material partly surrounded by a fibrin coagulum containing red cells and leucocyte.

从血栓附着头的纵切面上可看到其框架为苍白颗粒物质,部分被含有红细胞和白细胞的纤维蛋白凝块包绕。

coal [kəul] *n.* 煤

Coal workers' pneumoconiosis (CWP), colloquially referred to as black lung disease, is caused by long exposure to coal dust.

煤工尘肺通俗称为黑肺病,是由于长期接触煤尘引起。

Researcher tries to find link between coal pollution and disease.

研究人员试图找到煤污染和疾病之间的联系。

coalesce [ˌkəuə'les] *v.* 合并,融合,连合

The rheumatoid nodules may calcify, cavitate or coalesce and may produce clinical arthritis.

这些类风湿结节可以钙化、形成空洞或融合,甚至在临床上出现关节炎。

The cysts may be multiple in the early stages but subsequently coalesce into a single large cyst.

囊肿在发病的早期阶段可为多发性,但随后就会融合为单个的大囊肿。

coarctation [ˌkəuɑːk'teiʃən] *n.* 缩窄

Coarctation of the aorta can lead to secondary hypertension.

主动脉狭窄能导致继发性高血压。

coat [kəut] *n.* 外衣，表层，膜

Rarely the amoebic ulcers penetrate through the muscular coat of the colon.

阿米巴溃疡极少穿透结肠肌膜引起穿孔。

The poliovirus protein coat contains 60 polypeptide subunits.

脊髓灰质炎病毒蛋白包膜含 60 个多肽亚基。

v. 在…上涂

Saliva also coats the food with mucus, allowing it to "go down" more easily.

唾液还使食物外面包上一层黏液，使之易于"下行"。

The tablet is coated with a substance, which does not dissolve until it reaches the intestines.

药片上涂上一层物质，到肠后才溶解。

coating ['kəutiŋ] *n.* 外膜，表皮

Many protozoa can secrete a thick coating around themselves to protect them from an adverse environment.

许多原虫能分泌一层厚的外膜包于其外，以便在逆境中保护其自身。

cobalamin [kəu'bɔləmin] *n.* 钴胺素，维生素 B_{12}，氰钴胺

Cobalamin is always tightly bound to proteins and undergoes a series of transfers during its absorption.

维生素 B_{12} 与蛋白质紧密结合，通过一系列转运机制吸收入体内。

cobalt [kəu'bɔːlt] *n.* 钴

Cobalt is an essential element found in vitamin B_{12}.

钴是一种存在于维生素 B_{12} 中的基本元素。

Cobalt itself forms part of the vitamin B_{12} molecule.

钴是维生素 B_{12} 的组成成分。

The artificial radioisotope cobalt-60, or radiocobalt, is a powerful emitter of gamma radiation and is used in the radiation treatment of cancer.

人工放射性同位素钴-60（放射性钴）能发射强大的 γ 射线，用于治疗癌症。

cocaine [kə'kein, 'kəukein] *n.* 可卡因，古柯碱

Unfortunately cocaine experimentation and use went up dramatically from 1982 to 1985.

不幸的是，从 1982 年到 1985 年，可卡因的实验和使用都大幅度增加。

In this unusual experiment scientists were looking inside a man's head to see what cocaine does.

在这次不寻常的实验中，科学家们正窥视人脑内部试图了解可卡因起什么作用。

co-carcinogen ['kəukɑː'sinədʒən] *n.* 辅癌物

A co-carcinogen is a chemical that promotes the effects of a carcinogen in the production of cancer.

辅癌物是指在癌症发生发展过程中起促进作用的化学物质。

A chemical may both have anti-carcinogenic properties and yet still be a co-carcinogen in combination with some carcinogens.

某化学物在与某些致癌物联合作用时可同时扮演抗癌物和辅癌物的角色。

co-carcinogenesis ['kəukɑːsinə'dʒenəsəs] *n.* 辅癌作用

Acetaldehyde seems to be involved in ethanol-associated co-carcinogenesis.

乙醛似乎参与了乙醇的辅癌作用。

Metronidazole reduces its tumor-promoting effect, suggesting that fecal anaerobes are important in bile acid co-carcinogenesis.

甲硝唑肿瘤促进作用的下降提示粪便中厌氧菌对胆汁酸发挥辅癌作用十分重要。

coccobacillus [ˌkɔkəubə'siləs] *n.* 球杆菌

Bartonella is a group of Gram-negative pleomorphic coccobacillus, widely parasitizing in a diverse array of mammals.

巴尔通体是一群广泛寄生在多种哺乳动物体内的革兰阴性多形性球杆菌。

There were kinds of bacteria on the clue cells such as coccobacillus and microbacterium.
索细胞上有几种细菌,例如球杆菌和微小杆菌。

coccus [ˈkɔkəs] (*pl.* cocci [ˈkɔksai]) *n.* 球菌
Cocci are spherical cells.
球菌是球形细胞。

coccyx [ˈkɔksiks] (*pl.* coccyxes 或 coccyges [kɔkˈsaidʒiːz]) *n.* 尾骨
In the same way the coccygeal vertebrae are firmly united to form the coccyx.
同样,尾椎牢固地连接起来形成尾骨。
The vertebral column is formed by twenty-four bones called vertebrae and by the sacrum and coccyx.
脊柱是由叫做脊椎的 24 块骨骼加上骶骨和尾骨构成的。

cochlea [ˈkɔkliə] *n.* 耳蜗
The cochlea is where the hearing nerve cells are located.
耳蜗内排列有听觉神经细胞。

cocktail [ˈkɔkteil] *n.* 鸡尾酒;混合剂
The doctors tried to treat these patients with a cocktail of powerful antiviral drug and steroids.
医生们试图用强效抗病毒药和类固醇的混合剂治疗这些病人。

code [kəud] *v.* 编码,把…译成电码
There are also probably errors in genes coding for proteins which regulate the activities of other genes.
在为调节其他基因活动的蛋白质编码的基因中也可能有错误。
Diseases and operations can be coded according to standard nomenclature.
疾病和手术均可按标准的命名法编码。

codeine [ˈkəudiːn] *n.* 可待因
Codeine(methylmorphine) is a naturally occurring analgesic.
可待因(甲基吗啡)是一种天然生成的镇痛药。

codominant [ˌkəuˈdɔminənt] *a.* 共显性的,等显性的
The phenotype expressed depends on whether alleles are dominant, recessive or codominant.
表达的表现型取决于等位基因是显性的、隐性的、还是共显性的。
As a codominant genetic marker, restriction fragment length polymorphisms, referred as RFLPs, has been widely applied to the prenatal diagnosis of some genetic diseases.
限制性酶切片段长度多态性(被称为 RFLP)作为共显性的遗传标记,已广泛应用于一些遗传病的产前诊断。

codon [ˈkəudən] *n.* 密码子
Each three RNA nucleotides is called a codon, serving to insert a single amino acid into the protein molecule.
每三个 RNA 的核苷酸称为一个密码子,用来将一个氨基酸插入到蛋白质分子中。

coefficient [ˌkəuiˈfiʃənt] *n.* 系数
The absorption coefficient is often strongly wavelength-dependent.
吸收系数往往与波长密切相关。
Engel's coefficient on urban and rural households has dropped by more than 20 percentage points.
城乡居民恩格尔系数已经下降了 20 个以上的百分点。

coenzyme [kəuˈenzaim] *n.* 辅酶
Thiamine functions biologically as a coenzyme in some enzymatic reactions.
硫胺素的生物学功能是在某些酶反应中起辅酶作用。
Drugs may produce their actions or side effects by interacting with coenzymes.
药物可通过与辅酶之间的相互影响而产生作用或副作用。

coexist [kəuig'zist] *v.* 同时存在，共存

Malignancy may coexist and this necessitates a more radical therapeutic approach.

恶性肿瘤可能同时存在，这就需要更彻底的治疗手段。

This condition may coexist with invasive cancer.

这种病状可能与浸润癌同时存在。

cofactor [kəu'fæktə] *n.* 辅助因子

Most cofactors are coenzymes.

绝大部分辅助因子是辅酶。

In some enzymes, cofactors take part in the catalyzed reactions.

在一些酶中，辅助因子参与催化反应。

coferment [kəu'fəːmənt] *n.* 辅酶

They called the unidentified factor responsible for this effect a coferment.

他们将产生这种效应、尚未被确定的因子称之为辅酶。

v. 辅助发酵

Our results indicated that C. beijerinckii SA-1 was able to coferment hexose/pentose sugar mixtures in the absence of a glucose repression effect.

我们的结果显示当缺乏葡萄糖抑制作用时，拜氏梭菌 SA-1 能够辅助己糖/戊糖混合物的发酵。

coffee ['kɔfi] *n.* 咖啡

In addition, information on smoking history, coffee consumption, and obesity were obtained.

另外，有关吸烟史、咖啡消费量和肥胖的资料也得到了。

cognitive ['kɔgnitiv] *a.* 认识的，认知的

In delirium and dementia, there is global cognitive impairment.

在谵妄和痴呆中，存在着总的认知能力损伤。

Developmental dyslexia is attributable to a constitutional cognitive disability.

发育中的阅读困难可归因于体质上的认知能力的丧失。

cognizant ['kɔgnizənt] *a.* 认识的，认知的；知晓的，觉察到的

Registry developers should become cognizant of the patient privacy considerations confronting their likely data sources.

注册登记开发者应该认识到患者在面对其可能资料来源时的隐私考虑。

cohesion [kəu'hiːʒən] *n.* 结合，凝聚，内聚力

The cohesion of chains in the tense form is due largely to ionic or salt bonds.

紧密型链的结合主要是由离子键或盐键维持。

The force that causes various particles to unite is called cohesion.

使各种颗粒联合的力称为内聚力。

cohesive [kəu'hiːsiv] *a.* 有附着力的，有内聚力的

The stratum corneum consists of several layers of thin, cohesive, dead cells.

角质层由几层薄的有内聚力的死细胞构成。

cohesiveness [kəu'hiːsivnis] *n.* 黏着性

The concentration of lubricants did not significantly change the cohesiveness of the granules.

润滑剂的浓度并没有显著改变颗粒剂的黏着性。

Some texture parameters such as cohesiveness and resilience were altered in berries of infected plants.

在受感染植物的浆果中，一些结构参数例如黏着性和弹性发生了改变。

cohort ['kəuhɔt] *n.* 同期组群，队列

Also, the authors reported that they were unable to obtain a complete work history for approximately 50% of the cohort, and in some instances only the last job classification was available.

再者，作者们报告，约有 50% 的队列人员，无法获得他们完整的职业史，而且有些只能获

得最后的职业分类。

In addition, the follow-up period was relatively short, and the cohort under study was relatively young, as is reflected in the small number of overall observed deaths.

另外,由于随访时间比较短,接受研究的队列人员比较年轻,因而观察到的死亡总数少。

coil [kɔil] *v.* 盘绕

The chromosomes in affected individuals are longer and less tightly coiled than normal.

受累个体的染色体比正常的长,但不像正常的盘绕得那样紧。

coin [kɔin] *v.* 创造(新词等)

Hooke coined the word "cell".

虎克创造了"细胞"一词。

coincide [ˌkəuin'said] *v.* 恰好相同,相符

In pleurisy, the chest pain usually coincides with the appearance of a friction rub.

胸膜炎时,胸痛常和摩擦音同时出现。

coincidence [kəu'insidəns] *n.* 巧合,一致

It's rather a coincidence that a new drug received just a few days ago can be used in his treatment.

颇为凑巧,几天前刚收到的新药正好可用于他的治疗。

coincident [kəu'insidənt] *a.* 同时发生的,一致的

If there is a coincident chronic urinary infection, the clinical picture will be different.

如果同时发生慢性尿道感染,临床表现将会有所不同。

coincidental [kəuˌinsi'dentl] *a.* 巧合的,同时发生的

It is not clear whether the occurrence of these lesions is coincidental.

还不清楚,这些损害是否同时发生。

These two cases are believed to be coincidental.

这两个病例被认为是巧合。

coitus ['kəuitəs] *n.* 性交,交媾

In the description of vaginal discharge, the relation to the menses and coitus should be noted.

在描述阴道分泌物时应记录它与月经及性交的关系。

By age 15, 26 percent of white females and males, and 69 percent of black males experience coitus.

15 岁时,26% 的白人男性和女性以及 69% 的黑人男性有过性经验。

coke [kəuk] *n.* 焦炭

Exposure to coke oven emissions may occur for workers in the aluminum, steel, graphite, electrical, and construction industries.

在铝、钢、石墨、电子和建筑企业工作的工人可能接触焦炉排放物。

Coke-oven emissions are known to be human carcinogens based on sufficient evidence of lung cancer in humans exposed to coke-oven emissions.

根据接触焦炉排放物人群罹患肺癌的充分证据,焦炉逸散物被认为是人类致癌物。

cokeromyces [ˌkɔkərə'maisiːz] *n.* 科克霉科

Some species of Cokeromyces are opportunistic agents, and most cases involve some degree of immunosuppression.

科克霉科中的某些毛霉菌是机会致病菌,其引起的疾病多与一定程度的免疫抑制有关。

Described as a new species in 1950, Cokeromyces was isolated from rabbit dung collected in Illinois.

科克霉科是在 1950 年从美国伊利若斯州的兔粪便分离到并报道的一个新种。

colchicine ['kɔltʃisiːn] *n.* 秋水仙素,秋水仙碱(治痛风药)

Because of severe gastrointestinal side effects, high-dose oral colchicine is rarely used for an acute attack.

因为有严重的胃肠道的副作用,所以大剂量口服秋水仙碱很少用于治疗急性发作。

colectomy [kəu'lektəmi] *n.* 结肠切除术

Total colectomy with ileostomy is the elective operation performed in most centers.

在大多数治疗中心以全结肠切除和回肠造口术作为选择性手术。

colibacillosis [ˌkəulibæsi'ləusis] *n.* 大肠杆菌病,大肠杆菌感染

Colibacillosis occurs in all species, especially in the very young less than one week old.

所有大肠杆菌菌种可引起大肠杆菌感染,对不足一周龄的极幼婴儿尤其易于发生。

The form of colibacillosis is characterized by varying degrees of diarrhea.

大肠杆菌感染的特点是腹泻的程度轻重不一。

colic ['kɔlik] *a.* 绞痛的;结肠的

The patient suffered from a colic pain every now and then.

病人时时发作绞痛。

n. 绞痛

The old man began to suffer from biliary colic last week.

这位老人上周开始患胆绞痛。

The causes of chest or/and abdomen colic within one week after prostatectomy and transurethral resection of the prostate (TURP).

对前列腺切除术和经尿道前列腺切除术后 1 周内患者出现胸部或(和)腹部绞痛的原因进行了分析。

colicky ['kɔliki] *a.* 绞痛的

Colicky pain is usually promptly alleviated by analgesics.

绞痛通常可用止痛剂迅速缓解。

In chronic intestinal obstruction there may be recurrent colicky pain accompanied by visible peristalsis.

慢性肠梗阻时,可有反复的绞痛,伴有明显的肠蠕动波。

coliform ['kɔləˌfɔːm] *n.* 大肠杆菌类,大肠菌群

Coliform bacteria are a commonly used bacterial indicator of sanitary quality of foods and water.

大肠杆菌常用作反映食物和水卫生质量的细菌指标。

The presence of fecal coliform in aquatic environments may indicate that the water has been contaminated with the fecal material of humans or other animals.

水环境中出现粪大肠菌意味着水受到了人和动物粪便的污染。

colitis [kə'laitis] *n.* 结肠炎

Secondary amyloidosis is uncommon but may follow prolonged chronic colitis.

继发性淀粉样变并不常见,但可继发于迁延性慢性结肠炎。

collaborate [kə'læbəreit] *v.* 合作

A network of occupational health institutions will collaborate with WHO in the international exchange of information.

在信息的国际交流方面,职业卫生机构的网站将与世界卫生组织合作。

collaboration [kəˌlæbə'reiʃən] *n.* 合作

Collaboration in evaluating and adapting these technologies will be accomplished through a network of collaborating centres.

可通过合作中心的网络来完成对这些技术进行评价和修改的合作。

collaborative [kə'læbəreitiv] *a.* 合作的

Countries will be encouraged to establish collaborative activities and training schemes on a technical cooperation among developing countries basis.

在发展中国家技术合作的基础上,鼓励各国进行合作活动并建立培训规划。

collagen ['kɔləˌdʒən] *n.* 胶原

Among the albuminoids are the collagen, elastins, and keratins.

类白蛋白中有胶原、弹性蛋白和角蛋白。

Lack of vitamin C causes defective collagen fiber formation.

缺乏维生素 C 会引起胶原纤维形成不全。

collagenase [kəˈlædʒineis] *n.* 胶原酶

Different families of tumor-derived collagenases degrade the interstitial collagen (Ⅰ ~ Ⅲ) and type Ⅳ basement membrane collagen.

不同种类的肿瘤衍生的胶原酶能降解 Ⅰ ~ Ⅲ 型的间质胶原和 Ⅳ型基底膜胶原。

collagenous [kɔˈlædʒinəs] (=collagenic [ˌkɔləˈdʒenik]) *a.* 胶原的；产生胶原的

The passage of the hormones into the vascular stream is facilitated by the replacement of thick collagenous connective tissue fibers by fine reticular fibers.

由细小的网状纤维代替厚的胶原结缔组织纤维，使激素容易进入血管内血流。

collapse [kəˈlæps] *n.* 萎陷；虚脱

Chest X-ray initially shows only collapse or consolidation.

胸部 X 线检查最初仅见萎缩与实变。

Too rapid infusion may cause circulatory collapse.

注射过速可引起循环虚脱。

v. 塌陷

The neck veins may be distended during expiration, yet they collapse quickly with inspiration.

在呼气时可见颈静脉扩张，在吸气时迅速塌陷。

collateral [kəˈlætərəl] *a.* 侧的，副的

If the heart survives the shock as is frequently the case, a collateral circulation is in time established.

如果心脏像通常那样度过了休克期，此时会形成侧支循环。

colleague [ˈkɔliːg] *n.* 同事

The Lancet contains the revolutionary results of a yearlong experiment conducted by Ornish and his colleagues.

近期出版的医学杂志《柳叶刀》上载有奥尼斯和他的同事们所做的历时一年的具有革命意义的试验成果。

collectin [kəˈlektin] *n.* 胶原凝集素

Mannose binding protein (MBP) is a member of C type collectin proteins in the plasma.

甘露糖结合蛋白(MBP)是血浆中 C 型胶原凝集素蛋白的一个成员。

Mannan-binding lectin is a member of collectin family and plays an important role in innate immune defense.

甘露聚糖结合凝集素是胶原凝集素家族的一个成员，在天然免疫防御中起重要作用。

colletotrichum [ˌkɔləˈtɔtrikəm] *n.* 炭疽菌属

This book focuses on the genus Colletotrichum and the development of new Colletotrichum species epidemics worldwide.

此书重点阐述炭疽菌属及其在世界范围流行的新种发生情况。

collimator [ˈkɔlimeitə] *n.* 瞄准仪，准直器

The width of collimator aperture, which can be adjusted with the scope of 1-10mm, decides the slice thickness.

准直器孔径的宽度范围能够调整 1 ~ 10 毫米，它决定层厚。

With a multileaf collimator, conformal radiotherapy can be realized by shaping the beam to target contour.

多叶准直器使射线束的截面形状与病灶的轮廓相吻合，可以实现适形放射治疗。

The collimator projects a reticle to infinity.

准直仪将十字线投射到无穷远。

colliquative [kəˈlikwətiv] *a.* 液化的

An infarct undergoes coagulative or colliquative necrosis.
梗塞可以继发凝固性或液化性坏死。

colloid [ˈkɔlɔid] *n.* 胶体,胶质;胶态
Some have advocated administration of colloid solutions to maintain intravascular volume.
有些人提倡用胶体补液来维持血容量。

colloidal [kəˈlɔidəl] *a.* 胶体的,胶态的
The plasma proteins, being large, colloidal molecules, are nondiffusible.
血浆蛋白是大的胶体分子,因而是非扩散性的。

colon [ˈkəulən] (*pl.* colons 或 cola [ˈkəulə]) *n.* 结肠
The small intestine extends from the stomach to the colon.
小肠从胃延伸到结肠。
Occult blood does not always mean colon cancer, and colon cancer can occur without bleeding.
有隐血不一定意味着直肠癌,而直肠癌也不一定会出血。

colonic [kɔˈlɔnik] *a.* 结肠的
Colonic obstruction is, except in the cases of volvulus, chronic.
结肠梗阻,除扭转的病例外,都是慢性的。

colonization [ˌkɔlənaiˈzeiʃən] *n.* 移生,定植
Antibiotics will suppress normal flora and increase the chance for colonization with gram negatives.
抗生素抑制正常菌群,增加革兰氏阴性细菌定植的机会。
Colonization of oropharynx with gram-negative bacteria occurs in only 20% of normal individuals.
仅有20%的正常人口咽部革兰氏阴性菌能移地发育。

colonize [ˈkɔlənaiz] *v.* 移生,移地发育
Approximately 30%-40% of family members of a child with hemophilus influenza disease are colonized.
流感嗜血杆菌病患儿的家庭成员中约30%~40%为此种细菌的带菌者。

colonoscopy [ˌkəuləˈnɔskəpi] *n.* 结肠镜检查
Most commonly, colonoscopy is used to evaluate abnormal barium enema findings.
钡灌肠检查结果异常的病人常进行结肠镜检查。

colony [ˈkɔləni] *n.* 集落,菌落,群体
This colony of rats has been employed for various experiments in the Bentivoglio laboratory for nearly 25 years.
在 Bentivoglio 实验室里,这一种系的大鼠用于各种试验已将近25年了。
Saprophytes turn the medium green; C. albicans does not cause color changes, but produces a typical yeast colony.
腐生菌使培养基变为绿色;而白色念珠菌不引起颜色的改变,但产生一种典型的酵母菌落。
In recent years, bone marrow colony-stimulating factors have been isolated and are now available for clinical use.
近年来,骨髓集落刺激因子已被分离出来,现在正应用于临床。

color [ˈkʌlə] *v.* 着色
Only the background will be colored, and the colorless cell bodies will stand out.
通过背景着色,可使无色的菌体显示出来。

colorblindness [ˈkʌləblaindnis] *n.* 色盲
Colorblindness is inherited as a sex-linked recessive.
色盲是性联(或伴性)隐性遗传的。
Colorblindness can be understood very readily on the basis of the above mentioned knowledge.

在上述知识的基础上可容易理解色盲。

colorectal [kɔlə'rektəl] *a.* 结肠直肠的

Aspirin may block colorectal cancer.

阿司匹林可以抑制结肠癌。

Approximately half of cases of early postoperative small bowel obstruction follow colorectal surgery.

在手术后早期肠梗阻的病例中约有半数发生于结肠直肠手术后。

coloring ['kʌləriŋ] *n.* 着色

The health effects of hair coloring are, to a certain extent, unknown.

染发对健康的影响在某种程度上还并不清楚。

Although the FDA says that adding food coloring to food is safe, some groups, including the Center for Science in the Public Interest (CSPI), insist that they aren't and want them banned.

尽管 FDA 宣称食品中添加食用色素是安全的,但某些团体包括公共利益科学中心(CSPI)坚持否认,并希望对其禁止使用。

colostomy [kə'lɔstəmi] *n.* 结肠造口术

A colostomy is a surgical procedure in which a stoma is formed by drawing the healthy end of the large intestine or colon through an incision in the anterior abdominal wall and suturing it into place.

结肠造口术这种手术是在健康的结肠的尾端置孔,并将此孔与前腹壁的切口缝合到位。

Timing of colostomy closure is a debatable issue among general surgeons.

普通外科的医生们对结肠造口术缝合的时机仍有争议。

colostrum [kə'lɔstrəm] *n.* 初乳

Adiponectin was presented abundantly in human milk and higher in colostrum compared to that in mature milk.

人乳中含有丰富的脂联素,初乳中脂联素水平明显高于成熟乳。

The applications of agar single/double immunodiffusion method in determination of immunoglobulin in bovine colostrum were analysed.

对琼脂单/双扩散免疫法在牛初乳免疫球蛋白测定的应用进行了分析。

Colostrum (also known as beestings or first milk) is a form of milk produced by the mammary glands in late pregnancy and the few days after giving birth.

初乳是在妊娠晚期或分娩初期由乳腺产生的乳汁。

colposcopy [kɔl'pɔskəpi] *n.* 阴道镜检查

Colposcopy is a medical diagnostic procedure to examine an illuminated, magnified view of the cervix and the tissues of the vagina and vulva.

阴道镜检是一种运用照亮和放大视野来检查子宫颈和阴道及外阴组织的一种医学诊断过程。

The main goal of colposcopy is to prevent cervical cancer by detecting precancerous lesions early and treating them.

阴道镜检查的目标是通过早期发现和治疗癌前病变来预防宫颈癌。

coltivirus [kɔlti'vaiərəs] *n.* 科罗拉多壁虱热病毒

Coltivirus is characterized by being the causative agent for Colorado Tick Fever.

科罗拉多壁虱热病毒是科罗拉多壁虱热的病原体。

In virology, the causative organism, coltivirus, is a member of the Reovirus family.

在病毒学中,环状病毒这种致病微生物归属于呼肠孤病毒科。

column ['kɔləm] *n.* 柱,圆柱

Slight to moderate degrees of lateral curvature of the spinal column are common.

脊柱轻度到中度侧弯是常见的。

coma [ˈkəumə] *n.* 昏迷

Hepatic coma is often seen in late stage of liver disease.

肝昏迷常见于肝脏疾病的晚期。

Coma is an advanced state of brain failure in which a person lies in a sleeplike state with eyes closed.

昏迷是人闭着眼睛处于睡眠状态的晚期脑衰竭病症。

comatose [ˈkəumətəus] *a.* 昏迷的

The management of comatose patient is to find the cause of the coma, according to the procedures already outlined and remove it.

处理昏迷病人要找出昏迷的原因，再根据规定的步骤将其消除。

These are necessary steps in the early management of comatose patients.

这些是昏迷病人早期处理的必要措施。

At first the condition is rather that of collapse than of true coma, though later the patient is completely comatose.

最初病情是虚脱而不是真正昏迷，可是后来病人完全昏迷了。

combat [ˈkɔmbət] *v.* 跟…战斗，搏斗

The inflammatory response is essential in combating most infections.

炎症反应在对抗大多数感染中是不可缺少的。

The doctors are concentrating their efforts on combating cancer.

医生们正在集中力量以战胜癌症。

combination [ˌkɔmbiˈneiʃən] *n.* 结合；化合；组合；配合

The color purple is a combination of red and blue.

紫色是由红色与蓝色合成的。

Most of the modern drugs come from chemical combinations worked out by research scientists.

大多数现代药物都是研究人员经过化学合成而得到的。

The ear is a combination sensory organ, related to both hearing and equilibrium.

耳是一个组合的感觉器官，与听觉和平衡觉都有关系。

Chinese herbal medicine is used alone or in combination with nonoperative procedures like gastro-intestinal decompression, intravenous infusions and antibiotics.

中草药可以单独使用或与非手术治疗结合使用，如胃肠减压、静脉输注和抗生素等。

combustion [kəmˈbʌstʃən] *n.* 燃烧

When oxygen unites with the food in the cells, combustion takes place.

在细胞内氧与食物结合的时候发生燃烧。

comedocarcinoma [ˌkɔmidəuˌkaːsiˈnəumə] *n.* 粉刺癌

Comedocarcinoma is ductal carcinoma in situ of high grade.

粉刺癌是高级别导管原位癌。

Comedocarcinoma is characterized by the presence of solid sheets of pleomorphic cells and central necrosis.

粉刺癌的特点是多形性肿瘤细胞实体片状排列并伴有中央坏死。

comet [ˈkɔmit] *n.* 彗星

The Single Cell Gel Electrophoresis assay (also known as comet assay) is an uncomplicated and sensitive technique for the detection of DNA damage at the level of the individual eukaryotic cell.

单细胞凝胶电泳试验（也称彗星试验）是一种简单而敏感的可在单个真核细胞水平上检测 DNA 损伤的技术。

The comet assay is an extremely sensitive DNA damage assay.

彗星试验是一种极为灵敏的检测 DNA 损伤的试验。

command [kəˈmaːnd] *n.* 命令，指挥，掌握，[计算机] DOS 命令

This command will halt the machine.
这个命令将停止计算机。
Double-clicking a control-menu box is the same as choosing the close command.
双击一个控制菜单框与选择关闭命令具有相同作用。

commence [kə'mens] *v.* 开始
Measles commences in much the same way as a common cold.
麻疹开始时和普通感冒的状况差不多。

commencement [kə'mensmənt] *n.* 开始
The cecum is the commencement of the large intestine and is almost entirely enveloped by peritoneum.
盲肠是大肠起始部,几乎全被腹膜包绕。

commend [kə'mend] *v.* 称赞;推荐
The patient commends the director on the efficiency of his hospital.
病人称赞院长说他的医院工作效率高。

commensal [kə'mensəl] *n.* 共生体
Most of the bacteria causing gram-negative sepsis are normal commensals in the gastrointestinal tract.
引起革兰氏阴性脓毒血症的大多数细菌是胃肠道中的正常共生体。

commensurate [kə'menʃərit] *a.* 同量的,相当的
Therefore, active immunization is begun as early as is commensurate with the production of a satisfactory immune response.
因此,为了获得相当满意的免疫反应,自动免疫应尽早开始。

commercial [kə'məːʃəl] *a.* 商业的
It was not until 1956 that commercial urine test strips resembling those used today were marketed.
直到 1956 年,与今天使用的相似的商业用尿检测试纸才投入市场。

commercially [kə'məːʃəli] *ad.* 商业上,商品上
The commercially prepared extract of the posterior lobe is known as pituitrin.
在商业上将已提取的(垂体)后叶浸膏称作垂体后叶素。

comminuted ['kɔminjuːtid] *a.* 粉碎的,捣碎的
When due to direct violence, the fracture occurs at the point of impact, and is generally transverse and often comminuted.
直接由暴力所致的骨折发生于撞击点时,(骨折)通常是横向的,且往往是粉碎性的。

comminution [ˌkɔmi'njuːʃən] *n.* 粉碎
Older patients tend to have acetabular fractures with medial displacement patterns and associated comminution.
老年病人易发生内侧移位粉碎性髋臼骨折。
Clinically, this may assist proximal humeral fracture fixation in osteoporotic bone with medial cortex comminution.
临床上,这可能有助于内侧皮层粉碎的骨质疏松症骨近端肱骨骨折的固定。

commissure ['kɔmisjuə] *n.* 连合,接缝处
Rheumatic endocarditis scars the mitral valve and commonly causes fusion of the commissures.
风湿性心内膜炎使二尖瓣瘢痕化,并使瓣膜结合处融合。

commissurotomy [ˌkɔmiʃə'rɔtəmi] *n.* 连合部切开术;交界分离术
Commissurotomy of cardiac valves is called valvulotomy.
心脏瓣膜的交界分离术叫做瓣膜切开术。
In neurosurgery, a commissurotomy may be performed to sever the corpus callosum.
在神经外科中,可以行交界分离术来分割胼胝体。

commit [kə'mit] *v.* 承诺;交托;犯(错误等)

The company has committed funds to an advertising campaign.

公司已承诺给广告宣传活动提供资金。

He has committed himself to support his brother's children.

他答应抚养他兄弟的子女。

He committed the papers to the care of the lawyer.

他把文件交托律师处理。

The nurse committed an error by oversight.

那位护士由于疏忽而犯了错误。

Being driven to despair, she committed suicide.

由于被逼得绝望,她自杀了。

commitment [kə'mitmənt] *n.* 许诺,承诺

We should make a new commitment to eliminate TB as a major health problem, at the latest by the year 2000.

我们应当承担新的义务:最迟到2000年以前消灭结核这一严重影响健康问题的疾病。

Developing red blood cells, with their almost total commitment to hemoglobin synthesis, are such a source.

发育中的红细胞,就是这样一种来源,其任务几乎完全是合成血红蛋白。

commonplace ['kɔmənpleis] *n.* 普通的事物,平凡的事情

The unusual of yesterday has become the commonplace of today.

昨天不寻常的事物今天成为普通的事物。

a. 平凡的,普通的

Sinus surgery using a fiber-optic endoscope inserted through the nostril to see inside the sinus has become commonplace.

现在使用光学纤维内镜由鼻孔插入以了解窦内病变的鼻窦手术已十分普遍。

communicable [kə'mjuːnikəbl] *a.* 有传染性的,传播的

A communicable disease is one which can be transmitted from one person to another.

传染病是指可以由一个人传给另一个人的疾病。

Fever is one of the symptoms of measles, influenza and other communicable diseases.

发烧是麻疹、流感和其他传染性疾病的症状之一。

More and better food, combined with medical advances such as the control of communicable diseases, greatly reduced the death rate.

更多更好的食物,加之对传染性疾病的控制这类医学的进展,大大地降低了死亡率。

communication [kəmjuːni'keiʃən] *n.* 交流,通讯

This area has not been covered by the communication net.

这个地区还不在通讯网的覆盖之内。

Telegraph communication was broken off.

电讯中断了。

community [kə'mjuːniti] *n.* 群体,社区(居民)

For years the AIDS community has rallied around the battle cry "Silence = Death".

多少年来,艾滋病族一直在竭力呐喊"沉默就是死亡"。

comorbid [kə'mɔːbid] *a.* 共存的;共病

Instead, the authors observed that age, race, comorbid conditions, and tumor stage were independent predictors of disease.

相反,作者观察到年龄、种族、伴发病、肿瘤分期是该病独立的预测指标。

Evidence is increasing that comorbid patients have more problems and higher functional losses and a higher mortality.

越来越多的证据显示存在伴发病的患者问题更严重,功能丧失更多且病死率更高。

comorbidity [kemɔːˈbiditi] *n.* 并发症,共病,伴随疾病

In medicine, comorbidity is either the presence of one or more disorders (or diseases) in addition to a primary disease or disorder, or the effect of such additional disorders or diseases.

并发症在医学上是指除了一种原发疾病之外,要么出现一种或一种以上其他疾病,要么出现这些其他疾病的效应。

Comorbidity refers to the presence of one or more disorders in addition to a primary disease.

共病是指与原发病并存的一种或多种疾病。

compact [kəmˈpækt] *a.* 紧密的,致密的,坚实的

The teeth consist principally of a compact tissue—dentin.

牙齿主要由致密组织——牙质组成。

comparable [ˈkɔmpərəbl] *a.* 可与相比的,比得上的

Mexiletine is comparable to procainamide.

慢心利与普鲁卡因类似。

The patients were observed under comparable controlled conditions on a clinical investigation unit.

病人是在一个临床研究单位的相似对照的条件下接受观察的。

compare [kəmˈpɛə] *v.* 比较

Our aim was to compare the survival rate of the patients with clear cell carcinoma (CC) with that of the patients with endometrioid carcinoma (EC).

我们的目的是比较透明细胞癌(CC)和子宫内膜样癌(EC)患者的生存率。

The demographic data was compared using t-test.

人口学数据的比较采用 t 检验。

compartment [kəmˈpɑːtmənt] *n.* 隔间

The thorax is divided into three compartments.

胸腔分为三个部分。

compatibility [kəmˌpætəˈbiliti] *n.* 相容(性),一致(性)

An absolute prerequisite before transplantation of any organ is the presence of ABO blood group compatibility.

任何器官移植前的绝对先决条件是 ABO 血型相容。

Those who donate blood to others must have it typed to determine compatibility.

向别人输血的人必须检验血型以测定是否适合。

compatible (with) [kəmˈpætəbl] *a.* 相容的,一致的

This infant's clinical picture is compatible with an intrauterine infection.

此婴儿的临床表现与宫内感染是相符合的。

The diagnosis of infectious hepatitis is compatible with the findings.

传染性肝炎的诊断与检查所见符合。

compel [kəmˈpel] *v.* 强迫,迫使

We cannot compel you to do it, but we think you should.

我们不能强迫你做这件事,可是我们认为你应该做。

Bad health compelled him to resign from his job.

身体虚弱迫使他辞去工作。

compensate [ˈkɔmpenseit] *v.* 代偿,补偿

When the respiratory system is unable to compensate adequately for the increased load, it fails to maintain normal arterial blood gas tension. This situation is termed respiratory failure.

当呼吸系统已不能随着增加负荷而适当地代偿时,便不足以保持正常的动脉血气张力,此种情况称为呼吸衰竭。

compensatory [kəmˈpensətəri] *a.* 代偿性的,补偿的

The specific symptoms and signs of anemia represent cardiovascular-pulmonary compensatory re-

sponses to the severity and duration of the hypoxia.
贫血特有的症状和体征是心血管和肺对这种缺氧的严重程度和持续时间的代偿性反应。

competence [ˈkɔmpitəns] *n.* 能力，胜任
There are special boards that review and certify the qualifications of doctors who claim competence as specialists.
设有专门委员会审查和证明申请专家资格的医生的合法资格。

competent [ˈkɔmpitənt] *a.* 有能力的，合格的
Every year people in the United States spend millions of dollars for drugs without the advice of a competent physician.
在美国，人们未请合格的医生看病，每年购买药物所花去的费用不计其数。
Competent physicians prescribe drugs only with full knowledge of a particular patient and his condition.
称职的医生是在完全了解了病人及病情的情况下才开处方的。

competition [kɔmpiˈtiʃən] *n.* 比赛，竞争
Intense competition for resources frequently results in wasteful duplication and ineffective use of the resources given.
人力和物力的激烈竞争，常常引起现有人力和物力的成倍的浪费以及无效使用。

competitive [kəmˈpetitiv] *a.* 比赛的，竞争的
Naloxone is a competitive antagonist of morphine at its receptor site.
在吗啡受体部位，纳洛酮是吗啡的竞争性拮抗剂。

compilation [ˌkɔmpiˈleiʃən] *n.* 收集
Consent may have two components: (1) consent to registry creation by the compilation of patient information; (2) consent to the initial research purpose and uses of registry data.
“同意”可以有两种含义：(1) 同意收集患者信息用于建立登记；(2) 同意初始研究目的和登记资料的使用。

compile [kəmˈpail] *v.* 汇编，编纂
This is a guidebook compiled from a variety of sources.
这是利用各种资料编辑的一本导游手册。
The police have compiled a list of suspects.
警察已编制了一份嫌疑犯的名单。
It takes years of hard work to compile a good dictionary.
编写一本好字典需要经多年的辛勤工作。

compiler [kəmˈpailə] *n.* [计算机] 编译器，编译程序
That's exactly what happens with a compiler.
这就是编译程序所要完成的。
Can you double check your compiler settings?
你能否再检查一次编译器的设置？

complain [kəmˈplein] *v.* 主诉
He complains of constipation over the past two months.
他主诉已有两个月的便秘。
The patient complained of a bad headache.
患者主诉有强烈头痛。
What did the patient complain of?
患者有何主诉？

complaint [kəmˈpleint] *n.* 主诉，病痛
Some patients with active duodenal ulcer have no gastrointestinal complaints.
某些病人有活动性十二指肠溃疡，却无胃肠道主诉。
The doctor carefully noted every complaint on the cards of his patients.

医生在病人的卡片上细心记录下病人的每一个陈诉。

Arthritis is a common complaint among the elderly.

关节炎是老年人的常见病。

complement [ˈkɔmplimənt] *n.* 补充物,补体

Complement is required for the cytolytic destruction of cellular antigens by specific antibodies.

特异性抗体作用于细胞抗原所致的细胞溶解需要补体参与。

After 6 weeks the gonococcal complement fixation test on the patient's serum may become positive.

6 周后病人血清中淋球菌补体结合试验可能变为阳性。

complementarity [ˌkɔmplimenˈtɛəriti] *n.* 互补性,补充,补足

The complementarity-determining regions (CDRs) of immunoglobulins and T-cell receptors are the parts of these molecules that determine their specificity and make contact with specific ligand.

免疫球蛋白和 T 细胞受体的互补决定区(CDRs)是这些分子决定其特异性和与特异性配体接触的部位。

complementary [ˌkɔmpliˈmentəri] *a.* 补偿的,互补的

Because of this property, given an order of bases on one chain, the other chain is exactly complementary.

由于这种特性,若一条链的碱基为某种顺序,另一条链上的碱基顺序准确的与之互补。

The T loop is thought to interact with a complementary region of 5s ribosomal RNA during protein synthesis.

在蛋白质合成的过程中,T 环与 5s 核糖体 RNA 上的互补区相互作用。

complex [ˈkɔmpleks] *n.* 复合物

Good medical care today is much more complex than it was in the past.

现代良好的医疗保健比过去要复杂得多。

There is evidence of circulating immune complexes in most cases.

在大多数病例中出现循环性免疫复合物。

Cholesterol and triglycerides are transported to the blood in the form of lipoprotein complexes.

胆固醇和甘油三酯以脂蛋白复合体形式转运到血内。

compliance [kəmˈplaiəns] *n.* 顺应性;遵循

Isolated systolic hypertension (systolic>160, diastolic<90) is most common in elderly patients, due to reduced vascular compliance.

单纯性的收缩性高血压(收缩压>160,舒张压<90)通常在老年患者中常见,原因是血管的顺应性已经下降了。

With careful planning and legal guidance, health registries can be designed and operated in compliance with applicable rules and regulations.

借助周密的规划和法律的指导,卫生注册能在遵循适用规章制度条件下进行设计与运作。

complicate [ˈkɔmplikeit] *v.* (使)变复杂,(使)并发

Unless endocrine abnormalities complicate the picture, its diagnosis is not difficult.

除非内分泌异常使病情复杂化,此病的诊断并不困难。

The pulmonary fat embolism is complicated by pulmonary oedema and haemorrhages.

肺动脉脂肪栓塞并发肺水肿和出血。

Scleroderma is complicated by atrophy, ulceration, calcinosis, and/or pain.

硬皮病的并发症为萎缩、溃疡、钙质沉积和(或)疼痛。

complication [kɔmpliˈkeiʃən] *n.* 合并症,并发症

Few complications are more common than the head pain.

几乎没有比头痛更常见的合并症。

Pelvic venous thrombosis is a complication of operations on the pelvic organs.

盆腔静脉血栓形成是盆腔器官手术的并发症。

compliment [ˈkɔmplimənt] *v.* 向…致意，祝贺

We complimented him on his scientific achievements.

我们祝贺他在科学上的成就。

comply [kəmˈplai] *v.* 遵守，依从

When a physician's medical decision is medically questionable, a nurse may refuse to comply with it.

当医生的治疗决定在医学上可疑时，护士可以不遵守。

component [kɔmˈpəunənt] *n.* 组成部分，成分

The components of this weight gain include the fetus, placenta, liquor, uterus, breasts and the fat store.

构成孕妇体重增加的成分包括胎儿、胎盘、体液、子宫、乳房和脂肪储备。

Apoptosis is an essential component of normal cell turnover.

凋亡是正常的细胞周期必不可少的组成部分。

The molecular structure and the macro molecular components of the calcium channels have not been established.

钙通道的分子结构和大分子成分尚未证实。

composite [ˈkɔmpəzit] *n.* 复合材料，合成物

Our topic is: Research and Prospect of Conductive Polyaniline/rubber Composites.

我们的题目是"导电聚苯胺/橡胶复合材料的研究进展"。

a. 复合的，合成的

And by building composite applications, you can get quick access to your business information in one view.

并且通过构建复合应用程序，您可以在一个视图中快速访问业务信息。

composition [ˌkɔmpəˈziʃən] *n.* 成分

The composition of thrombus are platelets, fibrin, and blood cellular.

血栓的成分是血小板、纤维蛋白和血细胞。

Each organism has its own distinctive genetic composition.

每个有机体都有其独特的基因组成。

compound [ˈkɔmpaund] *n.* 混合物，化合物，复合物

Medicine is usually a compound.

药品通常是一种化合物。

Water is a compound of hydrogen and oxygen.

水是氢和氧的化合物。

a. 混合的，化合的，复合的

I treated stab wounds of the belly, punctured lungs, compound fractures, etc.

我治疗过腹部刺伤、肺部穿孔和复合性骨折等病例。

comprehend [ˌkɔmpriˈhend] *v.* 了解，领悟

Most patients should be told "the truth" to the extent that they can comprehend it.

大多数病人只应在其能理解的限度内被告知其"真实情况"。

comprehension [ˌkɔmpriˈhenʃən] *n.* 理解，包含

A lack of comprehension of spoken words occurs in lesions of the first and second temporal convolutions.

（患者）当有脑的第一和第二颞回损伤时，就可能出现不能理解言语的症状。

Other mental faculties may also be affected such as attention, judgement, comprehension, learning, calculation, and behavior.

其他精神方面的功能也会受到影响，如注意力、判断力、理解力、学习能力、计算能力和行为。

comprehensive [ˌkɔmpriˈhensiv] *a.* 综合性的,综合的

The microsurgical problems in the different fields of surgery are sufficiently related that this comprehensive book was necessary.

外科学各个领域的显微外科问题都有充分的联系,因此需要这本综合性的论著。

compress [kəmˈpres] *v.* 压迫

Neck hematomas may expand rapidly and compress the trachea.

颈部血肿可迅速膨胀而压迫气管。

compressibility [kəmˌpresəˈbiliti] *n.* (可)压缩性,压缩系数

The ideal gas model can be improved by introducing the compressibility factor.

理想气体模型可通过引入压缩因子改进。

Compressibility is the fractional change in volume per unit increase in pressure.

压缩系数是压力单位体积增加的分数变化。

compression [kəmˈpreʃən] *n.* 压迫,加压

An assistant can control hemorrhage by aortic compression against the vertebral column either manually or using a "sponge-stick".

助手用手或海绵条将腹主动脉压在脊柱上以控制出血。

A hematoma discovered days after surgery may be evacuated by gentle compression of the wound edges.

术后数天出现血肿时,可通过轻压伤口边缘使其排出。

comprise [kəmˈpraiz] *v.* 包含;由…组成,构成

Adenocarcinoma of the cervix comprises about 5 percent of cervical cancer.

子宫颈腺癌约占子宫颈癌的5%。

compromise [ˈkɔmprəmaiz] *n.* 折衷办法; 遭致损害

Asepsis is absolute, there is no compromise or modification.

无菌是绝对的,不存在任何折衷或权宜之计。

Respirations become irregular and may suddenly cease, owing to compromise of the respiratory centers in the medulla.

由于延髓呼吸中枢受压,呼吸不规则并可突然停止。

v. 使遭到损害,危及

When fluid enters the alveoli, gas exchange is compromised.

当液体进入肺泡,气体交换就要受到损害。

In an immune deficient and compromised host, the prognosis of chemotherapy is uncertain.

对缺乏免疫能力和免疫功能受损的宿主来说,化疗的预后是难以肯定的。

compulsive [kəmˈpʌlsiv] *a.* 强迫的,强制的

The person might begin compulsive drinking or gambling, which further add to his/her problems.

患者可能开始强迫自己饮酒或赌博,这更增加了他/她的问题的严重性。

compulsory [kəmˈpʌlsəri] *a.* 规定的,强制的

Is "Immunology" a compulsory subject in a medical college?

"免疫学"在医学院里是必修课吗?

The incidence of smallpox has been greater in countries where vaccination is not nationally compulsory.

在不强制普遍接种牛痘的国家里,天花的发病率较高。

computer [kəmˈpjuːtə] *n.* 计算机,电脑

A computer can easily perform simple and complex calculations.

计算机做简单的和复杂的计算都很容易。

Is the information available on the computer?

在计算机里有可利用的资料吗?

These complex statistics were all processed by the computer.

这些复杂的统计都是用计算机来处理。

concavity [kɔn'kæviti] *n.* 凹,凹面,凹度

A method for describing and measuring the concavities of digital objects is developed.

已研发出一种用于描述和测量数字对象的凹度的方法。

conceal [kən'siːl] *v.* 隐瞒;隐蔽

Self medication is often concealed by the patient, for fear this may be disapproved of by his doctor.

病人怕医生责难,常常隐瞒自己用药。

Clever though she was, she could not conceal her eagerness for praise.

尽管她很聪明,但还是无法掩饰急于受到表扬的心情。

concede [kən'siːd] *v.* (退一步)承认;给予

Sinus node dysfunction is generally conceded to be the cause of the sick sinus syndrome.

一般认为,窦房结功能障碍是病窦综合征的原因。

conceivably [kən'siːvəbli] *ad.* 可以想象

It could conceivably speed the onset of inspiratory muscle fatigue.

可以想象,这种情况能够加速吸气肌肉疲劳的发生。

conceive [kən'siːv] *v.* 受孕,怀胎

Her first operation went well, and by late 1981 she was again trying to conceive.

她的第一次手术很成功,到 1981 年晚些时候,她决定再次试着怀孕。

concentrate ['kɔnsentreit] *v.* 集中,浓缩

These neurotransmitters concentrate in nerve ends and are released by nerve impulses.

这些神经递质集中于神经末梢,并由神经冲动所释放。

The impairment may be so severe that the gallbladder is no longer capable of receiving or concentrating bile.

损害可能非常严重,以致胆囊不能再容纳或浓缩胆汁。

Subsequently the larger bile ducts become dilated and filled with concentrated bile.

随后,大胆管也扩张并充满浓缩的胆汁。

concentrated ['kɔnsəntreitid] *a.* 浓缩的;聚集的;集中的

The blood filtrate moving along in the nephron becomes a more concentrated solution.

沿着肾单位流动的血液滤液变成了一种浓缩的溶液。

These changes are often concentrated in the macular region, where they appear to fan out from the disc.

这些变化常集中于黄斑处,并由视盘呈扇状排开。

concentration [ˌkɔnsən'treiʃən] *n.* 浓度,浓缩

High concentration of oxygen is given in pulmonary oedema or shock.

肺水肿或休克时应给以高浓度的氧气。

The sputum was examined by means of the concentration method.

通过浓缩方法检查痰液。

concentric [kən'sentrik] *a.* 向心性的,同心的

Raised systemic vascular resistance increases the work of the left ventricle and leads to the concentric hypertrophy of the heart.

全身血管阻力的增加使左心室负荷增加并导致心脏向心性肥厚。

conception [kən'sepʃən] *n.* 妊娠,受孕

The difficulty in making any definition is that the precise date of conception in any particular pregnancy is unknown.

下定义困难是因为不知道某一具体妊娠的准确受孕日期。

concern [kən'səːn] *n.* 关心;关系;忧虑

As a physician, that is not, and cannot be, my primary concern.

作为一名医生,这不是,而且不能是我的主要关注。

From the viewpoint of treatment, the prime concern is the location of the tumor and the malignant potential of invasion and metastasis rather than the presence of the carcinoid syndrome.

从治疗的观点来看,主要考虑的是肿瘤的位置、侵袭的恶性程度和转移,而不是出现类癌综合征。

concerted [kən'səːtid] *a.* 通力合作的,协调的

A medical study could evolve from a concerted effort to discover associations.

一项医学研究可由为了揭示相关内容的通力合作努力中发展而来。

conclude [kən'kluːd] *v.* 结束,得出结论

The doctor concluded his talk with an interesting case.

这位医生用一个有趣的病例结束了他的谈话。

The jury concluded, from the evidence, that she was guilty.

陪审团根据证据作出结论,判明她有罪。

The authors concluded that these modifications were not necessarily related to the cancer preventive activity of dietary restriction.

作者们的结论是,没有必要把这些修正与膳食限制的防癌活动联系起来。

conclusion [kən'kluːʒən] *n.* 结论

What conclusions do you draw from the evidence you have heard?

你从听到的证据中能得出什么结论?

The researchers came to the conclusion that smoking accelerates platelet activity.

研究人员已得出结论:抽烟可以促进血小板的活性。

Old age is not the necessary conclusion of human existence.

老年并不是人生的终结。

conclusive [kən'kluːsiv] *a.* 最后的,结论性的

Usually a number of skin tests are given, but the results of these are far from conclusive in most cases.

通常要做多种皮肤试验,但在多数情况下,试验结果还远不足以作出定论。

The evidence for the hypothesis will not be presented here, but it is certainly far from conclusive.

本文不拟讨论这种假说的证据,当然这还远非结论性的。

conclusively [kən'kluːsivli] *ad.* 最终,最后

The fact remains that we cannot prove conclusively how good or how bad the health care system in the United States really is.

事实仍然是我们不能最终证明,美国的卫生保健制度究竟是如何好还是如何不好。

concomitant [kən'kɔmitənt] *a.* 相伴的,伴随的

Concomitant measures are therefore required in all these areas so that human body can make the most of its own defence mechanisms.

因此,有必要在所有这些领域里采取相应的措施,使人体充分发挥自身防御机制。

Multiple biopsies should be performed to exclude concomitant malignant lesions.

要排除恶性病变的并存,必须做多种活组织检查。

Concomitant disinfections should be done to destroy all pathogenic microorganisms.

应进行随时消毒以杀灭所有致病微生物。

This unpleasant side effect is managed readily by the concomitant use of an antiemetic agent.

同时使用止吐剂,就容易处理这种不舒服的副作用。

n. 相伴物,伴随的情况

Neuralgic pains are frequent concomitants of pregnancy.

神经痛经常随着妊娠发生。

concomitantly [kən'kɔmitəntli] *ad.* 同时

Concomitantly, the haemoglobin acts as a buffer.

同时,血红蛋白还起着缓冲作用。

Fluid resuscitation should be carried out concomitantly.

要同时补充液体。

concrete [ˈkɔnkriːt] *a.* 具体的,确定的

Physics deals with the forces acting on concrete objects.

物理学研究作用于实际物体的力。

concurrently [kənˈkʌrəntli] *ad.* 并发地,同时发生地,并存

Loop diuretics should not be used concurrently with ototoxic aminoglycoside antibiotics.

襻利尿剂不能与具有耳毒性的氨基甙类抗生素合用。

concussion [kənˈkʌʃən] *n.* 震荡;脑震荡

Concussion, from the Latin concutere, is the most common type of traumatic brain injury.

脑震荡(源自拉丁语的"剧烈震动"一词)是一种最常见的创伤性脑损伤。

Treatment of concussion involves monitoring and rest.

脑震荡的治疗措施包括监测和休息。

condense [kənˈdens] *v.* 冷凝;浓缩

Steam condenses to water when it touches a cold surface.

水蒸气触及冷的表面即凝结成水。

condition [kənˈdiʃən] *n.* 情况,状态,条件;疾病

The labouring conditions for workers in the factories and mines have been greatly improved.

工厂和矿山工人的劳动条件已大大改善。

Fever is a condition in which the body temperature is higher than normal.

发热是体温高于正常的一种情况。

Arthritis is the most common chronic condition among the elderly.

关节炎是老年人最为常见的慢性病。

condom [ˈkɔndəm] *n.* 避孕套

The rate of condom-use adherence increased from 32.9% before interventions to 50.0%, 63.2% and 69.1% respectively in the different times after interventions.

安全套坚持使用率由干预前的 32.9% 逐步上升至干预后不同时间的 50.0%、63.2% 和 69.1%。

conduce(to) [kənˈdjuːs] *v.* 导致,有助于

Taking a walk after supper conduces to health.

晚饭后散步可以增进健康。

Dusty occupation and excessive smoking conduce to chronic bronchitis.

粉尘作业和吸烟过多常导致慢性支气管炎。

conducive(to) [kənˈdjuːsiv] *a.* 有助于…的,有益于…的

Cycling is a sport conducive to health, so in some countries children normally go to school on bikes.

骑自行车是一项有益健康的运动,所以许多国家的儿童常骑自行车上学。

As pathology is conducive to medical practice, so the latter makes the former more perfect.

正像病理学有助于医疗实践一样,医疗实践也会使病理学更加完善。

conduct [kənˈdʌkt] *v.* 实施,进行

An extensive testing of this patient's contacts at school and in the neighborhood was conducted.

对此患儿在学校及邻居中的接触者进行了广泛的检查。

conduction [kənˈdʌkʃən] *n.* 传导

Vasodilation and sweating dissipate heat through radiation and conduction from the skin.

血管舒张和出汗通过皮肤的辐射和传导散热。

condyle [ˈkɔndil;-dail] *n.* 骨节;踝

A condyle is the round prominence at the end of a bone, most often part of a joint-an articulation with another bone.

骨节是骨一端圆形突起，通常情况下是关节的一部分，与另一骨构成关节。

condyloma [ˌkɔndiˈləumə] (*pl.* condylomata [ˌkɔndiˈləumətə]) *n.* 湿疣，尖锐湿疣 (*pl.* condylomata)

The purpose of this study is to investigate the cellular immune function in patients with condyloma acuminata.

这项研究的目的是要了解尖锐湿疣患者细胞免疫功能的状况。

Condylomata are rarely seen in the urethra and most often situated in the distal part of the urethra.

尖锐湿疣在尿道少见，而最常出现在尿道远端。

confer [kənˈfəː] *v.* 授予(称号，学位等)，给予

The university conferred on him the title of Doctor of Medicine.

该大学授予他医学博士学位。

One attack of measles confers high degree of immunity.

麻疹发病一次可有高度免疫力。

A mother who has had measles confers passive immunity on her infant for the first six months of life.

曾患麻疹的母亲可使婴儿出生后头 6 个月内具有被动免疫力。

conference [ˈkɔnfərəns] *n.* 会议，讨论会

Nowadays many international conferences are held in China.

现在有很多国际会议在中国召开。

The hospital director is in conference now.

现在医院的院长正在开会。

confidential [ˌkɔnfiˈdenʃəl] *a.* 秘密的，获得信任的

The physician must provide assurance of the confidential nature of all information.

医生必须为所有信息保密。

confidentiality [ˌkɔnfiˌdenʃəˈæliti] *n.* 保密性；隐私

For clinical research, it is also essential to ensure that appropriate processes are in place to safeguard research participants and their confidentiality.

临床研究也应建立适当程序，以保护研究参与者及其隐私。

configuration [kənˌfigjuˈreiʃən] *n.* 外形，形状

The lesions preserve to some degree the wedge shaped configuration of infarcts.

病变保持一定程度的梗死的楔形外观。

Films of good quality will provide much information concerning the position and configuration of normal organs.

质量好的片子可以提供有关正常器官的位置和轮廓的许多情况。

confine [kənˈfain] *v.* 限制；禁闭；分娩

She confines her remarks to scientific management.

她所讲的仅限于科学管理问题。

He is confined to the house by illness.

他因病而不出门。

Today the majority of patients are confined in hospital.

目前大多数患者住院分娩。

confinement [kənˈfainmənt] *n.* 限制；分娩

His doctor recommended confinement to a vegetarian diet.

他的医生建议他限于素食。

Inadequate housing is a clear obstacle to home confinement.

住房条件不佳显然是家庭分娩的障碍。

Her confinement will come about in a week.
她大约在 1 周以后即可分娩。

confirm [kən'fəːm] *v.* 确认,证实;坚定

Chest radiography may be helpful in confirming the cause of the cough.
胸片可能有助于明确咳嗽的原因。
The diagnosis of viral pneumonia is confirmed by a rise in specific titre.
特异性抗体滴度升高可确定病毒性肺炎的诊断。
The diagnosis is confirmed if the enema is returned clear and no flatus is passed.
如果灌肠液转为清亮而且没有排气即可确诊。
Please telephone the passenger center to confirm your reservation.
请打电话给乘客中心确认你预定的座位。
This confirms me in the view that robotic operation is a new approach in the evolution of surgery.
这更坚定了我的看法:机器人手术是外科进展中的新方法。

confirmation [ˌkənfə'meiʃən] *n.* 确定,证实

Confirmation of the etiology is possible only by the virus isolation in the laboratory.
病因的确定只需在实验室做病毒分离便可。
Since the Papanicolaou's smear is only a screening procedure, histologic confirmation is required before any treatment is initiated.
由于帕氏涂片仅为一种筛选手段,因此在任何治疗开始前需经组织学证实。

confluence ['kənfluəns] *n.* 汇合;聚集

The severity of the disease is directly related to the extent and confluence of the rash.
本病的严重程度直接与皮疹的范围和融合的程度有关。

confluent ['kənfluənt] *a.* 融合的,连合的

In mild measles the rash tends not to be confluent.
在轻症麻疹患者,其皮疹往往不融合。
The lesions may become confluent in the lower parts of the lungs, where they are most numerous.
在病变最多的肺下部,病变可发生融合。

conform(to) [kən'fɔːm] *v.* 符合,与…一致

The results of the present study conformed to those reported previously.
目前研究的结果与以前所报道过的结果一致。
The drugs must conform in every way to the standards set up by the government.
药物必须完全符合政府规定的标准。

conformation [ˌkənfɔː'meiʃən] *n.* 构造,构象

The secondary structure refers to the conformation of the polypeptide chain in the protein.
二级结构系指蛋白质内的多肽链构象。

conformational [ˌkənfɔː'meiʃənəl] *a.* 构象的,结构的

The interaction of the substrate with the enzyme induces a conformational change in the enzyme.
底物与酶相互作用诱导酶发生构象改变。

confounder [kən'faundə] *n.* 混杂变量,混杂因素

We included the following confounders in the model: sex, duration of smoking, inhalation habits, and type of tobacco smoked.
我们将下列混杂因素纳入模型:性别、烟龄、吸入习惯,以及所用烟草的类型。
In most studies, age is viewed as a potential confounder.
在大多数研究中,年龄都被视为一个潜在的混杂因素。
Clinical confounders for such studies are preexisting viral diseases, certain prescription and over-the-counter medications, alcohol abuse, and preexisting HIV(human immunodeficiency virus) infection or AIDS.
对于这样的研究来说,临床混杂变量有事先存在的病毒性疾病(感染)、某些处方和非处

方用药、乙醇滥用、以及事先存在的 HIV(人类免疫缺陷病毒)感染或艾滋病。

confounding [kən'faundiŋ] *n.* 混杂;混乱

We will describe some important confounders in pharmacoepidemiology and we will show that it is sometimes difficult to distinguish between confounding and selection bias.

我们将介绍药物流行病学中几种重要混杂因素并将显示有时难以区分混杂和选择偏倚。

confront [kən'frʌnt] *v.* 使面对,使面临

Any practitioner may today be confronted by an unfamiliar imported disease.

今日任何一名医师都可能面临一种不熟悉的、自外传入的疾病。

Some people appreciate health only when they are seriously confronted with disease.

有些人只在严重面临疾病时,才感到健康之可贵。

confuse [kən'fjuːz] *v.* 混淆

Pain originating in the thoracic muscles is often confused with pleurisy, since it is generally aggravated by deep breathing.

由于胸膜炎在深呼吸时加重所以与起源于胸部肌肉的疼痛相混淆。

confusion [kən'fjuːʒən] *n.* 精神混乱;混淆;意识模糊

Reactive confusion is often accompanied by excessive activity and apparently provoked by emotional stress.

反应性精神混乱经常伴有过度活动并且显然是由情绪紧张所诱发。

Confusion is often the first feature of cognitive impairment noticed by relatives or the examiner.

病人家属或检查者常首先发现认知障碍的病人有精神错乱。

confusional [kən'fjuːʒənəl] *a.* 混乱的,意识模糊的

Acute confusional state is a short-lived transient psychotic condition, lasting hours or days.

急性精神混乱状态是持续数小时或数日的短暂的精神病症状。

congenital [kən'dʒenitəl] *a.* 先天的,天生的

The majority of these congenital abnormalities did involve the central nervous system.

大多数先天畸形确实累及中枢神经系统。

Some genetic disorders are congenital.

有些遗传病是先天性的。

congenitally [kən'dʒenitli] *ad.* 先天性地

Infants congenitally infected with cytomegalovirus may tend to be small-for-gestational age.

有巨细胞病毒先天感染的婴儿常小于胎龄儿。

congest [kən'dʒest] *v.* (使)充血

After early death, the brain and cord are congested at autopsy.

早期死亡的病例,在尸检时呈现脑和脊髓充血。

The patient has congested eyes.

病人眼睛充血。

The patient also tries very hard to cough up the congesting mucus in his chest, but usually cannot breathe in enough air to do this successfully.

病人(虽然)也想用力咳出淤积于胸中的痰液,但通常都是不能吸入足量的空气来达到此目的。

congestion [kən'dʒestʃən] *n.* 充血;(交通)拥挤

At first the infarcted tissue is dark red from congestion.

最先,梗死的组织由于充血呈暗红色。

He was delayed by the congestion of traffic in town.

他因城里的交通拥挤而耽搁。

congestive [kən'dʒestiv] *a.* 充血的

Congestive heart failure is classed according to functional capacity.

充血性心力衰竭根据心功能状况进行分级。

congression [kən'greʃən] *n.* 集会,聚会,会议

Such phosphorylation is essential for faithful chromosome congression in mitosis.

这种磷酸化对于有丝分裂时染色体准确的集合非常重要。

The chromosomes begin to move toward a point midway between the spindle poles, a process called congression.

染色体开始向介乎两个纺锤体极之间的一个位点移动,这个过程叫做染色体的中板集合。

conical ['kɔnikəl] *a.* 圆锥形的

The heart is conical in shape.

心脏呈圆锥形。

conidia [kəu'nidiə] *n.* 分生孢子

Conidia were hyaline, lunate to reniform.

分生孢子是透明的,呈新月形或肾形。

For conidia, its size was ranged by 32μm ~ 160μm×8 9μm ~ 141μm.

分生孢子,其大小为 32 微米 ~ 160 微米×8 9 微米 ~ 141 微米。

conidiophore [kəu'nidiəfɔː] *n.* 分生孢子柄

Conidiophore is an asexual reproductive structure that develops at the tip of a fungal hypha and produces conidia.

分生孢子柄是一种无性繁殖结构,长在真菌菌丝的顶端,产生分生孢子。

Mostly conidiophores develop a flat layer of relatively short ones which then produce masses of spores.

分生孢子柄多数先长成一个较短的扁平层,然后长出大量孢子。

conidium [kəu'nidiəm] *n.* 分生孢子;无性孢子 (*pl.* conidia)

The morphology of conidium is often distinctive of a specific species of fungi.

不同种的真菌分生孢子形态通常不同。

Conidia are also called mitospores due to the way they are generated through the cellular process of mitosis.

由于可通过细胞有丝分裂方式产生,分生孢子也称为有丝分裂孢子。

conjoined [kən'dʒɔind] *a.* 联体的;结合的;联合的

Four cases of conjoined twins underwent various imaging examinations and the imaging findings were compared with the results of the operation and pathology.

运用多种影像学检查手段对 4 例联体儿进行检查,并将检查结果与手术及病理结果进行了比较。

The preoperative materials of radiology, CT, MRI and sonography exactly showed the location, degree and cerrelative anatomy of the conjoined twins.

联体儿术前的 X 线、CT 和超声学检查结果准确地显示了患儿联体畸形的部位、程度和相关的解剖学信息。

conjugate ['kɔndʒugeit] *v.* 使结合

Proteins can be classified as simple or conjugated proteins.

蛋白质可分为简单蛋白和结合蛋白。

The conjugated product may appear in the bile and finally be excreted in the small intestine.

这种结合产物可出现在胆汁中,最后被排泄入小肠。

a. ['kɔndʒugit] 结合的;共轭的

Gaze movement are the normal conjugate movements of the two eyes moving to the same direction.

注视运动是双眼向同一方向运动的自然的联合运动。

conjugation [ˌkɔndʒu'geiʃən] *n.* 结合,结合作用

Conjugation of bilirubin to other sugars also occurs but only to a small extent.

只有小部分胆红素与其他糖类结合。

Methyl conjugation is an important pathway in the metabolism of many drugs, neurotransmitters, and xenobiotics.
甲基结合作用在药物、神经递质和外来化合物的代谢中是一条重要的路径。

conjugative [ˌkɔn'dʒugətiv] *a.* 接合性的
Elimination of 20 Shigella strains with conjugative drug resistance plasmids by norfloxacin and berberine in vitro was analyzed.
对试管内用诺氟沙星和黄连素来消除 20 株携带有接合性耐药质粒的志贺菌进行了分析。
Conjugative plasmid can be mediated by sex pilus and transferred from one cell to another cell of bacteria.
接合性质粒可通过性菌毛介导从一个菌细胞转移到另一个菌细胞。

conjunction [kən'dʒʌŋkʃən] *n.* 结合,联合
Reserpine may be used in conjunction with a diuretic in the treatment of mild to moderate hypertension.
利血平可与利尿剂合用治疗轻、中度高血压。

conjunctiva [ˌkəndʒʌŋk'taivə] *n.* 结膜
The conjunctiva on the right is slightly red but without discharge.
右眼结膜轻度发红但无分泌物。

conjunctivitis [kənˌdʒʌŋkti'vaitiə] *n.* 结膜炎
If significant conjunctivitis is also present, the most likely causative agent is an adenovirus.
如果还出现较重的结膜炎,其病因最大可能是腺病毒。

consanguineous [ˌkɔnsæŋ'gwiniəs] *a.* 血缘的;血亲的;同族的
Couples who have one or more ancestors in common are consanguineous.
有共同祖先的夫妇称为近亲。
The chief cause of high morbidity-rate of congenital defect in Qatar is consanguineous marriages, experts of the society said.
据学会的专家们说,导致卡塔尔先天性缺陷发病率居高的主要原因就是近亲婚姻。

consanguinity [ˌkɔnsæŋ'gwiniti] *n.* 近亲婚配
Consanguinity brings about an increase in the frequency of autosomal recessive disease.
近亲婚配导致常染色体隐性遗传病的发病率升高。
In each and all of these systems they are bound to each other in fact by consanguinity and affinity.
在所有这些系统中,他们实际上都是通过血缘和姻亲相互联系在一起的。

conscientious [ˌkɔnʃi'enʃəs] *a.* 认真的,谨慎的
The selection of a competent and conscientious physician is vitally important in the diagnosis and treatment of cancer.
选择一位合格而又认真的医生,对于诊断和治疗癌症是极为重要的。

conscientiousness [ˌkɔnʃi'enʃəsnis] *n.* 认真,谨慎
In people with frontal lobe syndrome, conscientiousness and powers of concentration are often diminished.
在出现额叶综合征的人们中,认真态度和集中注意的能力常常减弱。

conscious ['kɔnʃəs] *a.* 神志清醒的,有意识的,意识到的
Patients are fully conscious during operations when this kind of anaesthetization is used.
当采用这种麻醉方法时,病人在手术中神志完全清醒。
He is in a coma for days, but now he is fully conscious again.
他昏迷几天了,但现在已完全苏醒过来了。
His observations, his selections and his inference depend on conscious thought and on intuition.
他的观察、选择和结论取决于有意识的思维和直觉。
He is deeply conscious of his responsibility as a doctor.

他深刻意识到他作为一个医生的责任。

consciousness [ˈkɔnʃəsnis] *n.* (有)意识,知觉,清醒

Consciousness is the state of the awareness of self and the environment.

意识就是对自身和周围环境有认知的状态。

Severe cases of such poisoning may bring about convulsions, loss of consciousness and even death.

这种中毒的严重病例可引起惊厥、失去知觉甚至死亡。

The patient recovered his consciousness, but he could not eat or drink.

病人神志已经恢复,但既不能吃,又不能喝。

It has been found that even though the skin is anesthetized, there still is consciousness of pressure.

已发现,皮肤即使被麻醉之后也仍然具有压力感觉。

consecutive [kənˈsekjutiv] *a.* 连贯的,连续的

It is generally agreed that infants with two consecutive blood glucose levels of 30mg/dl or less should be treated.

通常认为对连续两次血糖水平为 30mg/dl 或其以下的婴儿应予治疗。

This drug was used for 5 consecutive cycles.

这药已连续用了 5 个周期。

consensus [kənˈsensəs] *n.* 一致;同感

The consensus is that the small size should be used for nulliparous women.

一致认为未经产妇女应该使用小号的。

The consensus is that weather does not affect the inflammatory diseases.

共同的看法是气候并不影响炎症性疾病。

consent [kənˈsent] *v.* 同意;答应

They consented to simple mastectomy and are presently free of disease.

她们已同意做单纯乳房切除术,目前没有其他疾病。

consequence [ˈkɔnsikwəns] *n.* 结果;影响;重要(性)

This complication can have very dangerous consequence.

这种并发症可以有非常危险的后果。

Several important practical consequences flow from the differences between microorganisms and viruses.

根据病毒和微生物之间的差异得出了几个重要的实际结论。

The failure of a TB control program has two consequences in term of drug resistance.

就抗药性而论控制结核病计划的失败有两方面的影响。

These molecules may protect microorganisms from the normal consequences of antibody and complement binding.

这些分子可以保护微生物使其免遭抗体与补体结合后通常发生的效应。

consequent [ˈkɔnsikwənt] *a.* 作为结果的

Occasionally rupture is consequent upon instrumentation of the bladder.

有时,破裂是因为对膀胱使用了器械的结果。

conservation [ˌkɔnsəˈveiʃən] *n.* 保存

Hysterectomy, with conservation of the ovaries, cures the condition but is obviously a final step.

切除子宫但保留卵巢用以治愈此病显然为最后一步。

conservative [kənˈsəːvətiv] *a.* 保守的,守旧的

This patient is under conservative treatment with propranolol.

此患者现在用心得安进行保守治疗。

Conservative measures should be adopted since operation carries a high mortality in such cases.

这类病例应该采用保守疗法治疗,因为手术的死亡率高。

conserve [kən'səːv] *v.* 保存

The spleen conserves the iron from red cell breakdown—which then goes to the liver.

脾保存被破坏的红细胞中的铁，这些铁以后进入肝脏。

In addition there is often a failure to conserve sodium while potassium accumulates together with phosphate and other acidic radicals.

此外，钠常不能保留，而钾则与磷酸盐及其他酸根一起蓄积。

The synthesized cAMP is conserved by theophylline.

茶碱减少了已合成的 cAMP 受到的破坏。

considerable [kən'sidərəbl] *a.* 相当(大，多)的，大量的

Considerable digestion of food takes place in the small intestine and some in the large intestine.

食物的大部分消化在小肠进行，部分则在大肠进行。

Considerable loss of heat occurs with the help of the sweat glands.

大量热借助于汗腺发散。

The site of formation of antibodies has evoked considerable dispute.

抗体形成的部位已经引起了许多的争论。

considerably [kən'sidərəbli] *ad.* 相当大地

The right bronchus differs considerably from the left bronchus.

右支气管与左支气管有很大的不同。

consideration [kɔnsidə'reiʃən] *n.* 考虑，思考

Admission of some patients to cardiac care units with the implied diagnosis of coronary disease may also be prejudicial to further diagnostic considerations.

将某些疑诊为冠心病的病人收入心脏病监护室，可能不利于进一步的诊断思考。

The correct approach to the problem of hospital treatment of the elderly must be based on a consideration of the desirability of rest.

正确探讨老年患者住院治疗问题必须从休息的需要出发来考虑。

consistency [kən'sistənsi] *n.* 一贯；坚实度

His actions lack consistency.

他的行动缺乏一贯性。

The size, mobility, consistency, position, and shape of the uterus should be recorded.

应记录子宫的大小、活动度、硬度、位置及形状。

consistent(with) [kən'sistənt] *a.* 一贯的，一致的

Ultrasonic examination at 18 weeks was consistent with her dates.

18 孕周超声波检查结果与孕龄相符。

The doctor has done everything consistent with the emergency treatment of a shock case.

医生已经做了符合抢救休克病人应急治疗的一切工作。

Several consistent abnormalities have been detected in MS(multiple sclerosis) body fluids.

在多发性硬化症的体液中发现了某些始终存在的异常。

consistently [kən'sistəntli] *ad.* 连贯地，始终如一地

The drug aspirin lowers fever and alleviates pain more consistently than it produces harmful side effects.

阿司匹林这种药可连续地用于退热并减轻疼痛，而不易引起有害的副作用。

consist of [kən'sist] *v.* 由…构成

A new study finds that older people who follow a diet that consists of greater amounts of fish show a better means of preserving bone density as compared to people who do not eat as much fish.

一个新的研究发现饮食中含大量鱼的老人比吃鱼少的老人更能维持骨密度。

Having a diet plan consisting of high protein and low carbohydrate meals may possibly cause your breath to bad.

含高蛋白低碳水化合物膳食可能会让你有口臭。

console [ˈkɔnsəul] *n.* 控制台，仪表板

Doctors sit several feet away from the patient at a console where they see inside the patient on a monitor.

医生们坐在离病人数英尺远的控制台旁，可以在监视器上看到病人体内的情况。

consolidate [kənˈsɔlideit] *v.* 巩固，加强；变硬

In the succeeding decade T. tonsurans has consolidated and extended its territory.

在以后的十年间，断发癣菌发生的地域将进一步巩固和扩展。

The transplanted lung was consolidated due to massive intraalveolar exudate.

植入的肺因肺泡内充满大量的渗出物而变硬。

consolidation [kənˌsɔliˈdeiʃən] *n.* 坚实，实变

Many patients develop hemorrhagic consolidation of the lung after transplantation.

许多病人移植后发生肺出血性实变。

Chest X-ray shows consolidation in lobar distribution.

胸部 X 线检查见有呈大叶性分布的实变阴影。

conspicuous [kənˈspikjuəs] *a.* 明显的，显著的

The episodes are not due to excessive consumption, and without conspicuous neurological signs of intoxication.

由于没有明显的中毒性神经系体征，所以其发作不是由于过量吸收引起的。

The reactions are most conspicuous in patients with bacteremia.

菌血症的病人反应也很明显。

In many patients, a heart murmur is the only or the most conspicuous finding on physical examination.

体检时有很多患者其心脏杂音是惟一的也是最显著的体征。

constancy [ˈkɔnstənsi] *n.* 坚定，恒定

Because of the constancy of the mother's internal environment the composition of the blood reaching the placenta is unlikely to vary much.

由于母体内环境的稳定，到达胎盘的血液成分不大可能有大的变化。

constant [ˈkɔnstənt] *a.* 经久不变的，恒定的

Children need constant encouragement from parents, teachers and elders.

孩子需要从父母、老师和长者那里不断地得到鼓励。

The amount of water lost in expired air and in the faeces is fairly constant.

经呼气及排出粪便失去的水分量相当恒定。

The mortality rate of 10% for severe upper gastrointestinal bleeding has remained constant over the past 30 years.

在过去 30 年中，严重的上消化道出血的死亡率仍然稳定在 10% 左右。

constantly [ˈkɔnstəntli] *ad.* 恒定地，不变地，经常地，不断地

Red blood cells do not live very long, so they constantly need to be replaced.

红细胞的寿命不很长，因此需要不断地更新。

constipation [ˌkɔnstiˈpeiʃən] *n.* 便秘

Constipation, if chronic, brings on numerous complications.

慢性便秘常引起许多并发症。

Anorexia, nausea and vomiting, constipation, or diarrhea often accompanies abdominal pain.

食欲不振、恶心和呕吐、便秘或腹泻常伴有腹痛。

constituent [kənˈstitjuənt] *n.* 成分，要素

When some basic dyes bind to highly negatively charged cellular constituents, they undergo a change in color.

当一些碱性染料结合到带强负电荷的细胞成分时，其颜色发生改变。

Cholesterol is far from (being) a minor constituent of the body.

胆固醇绝对不是人体内的次要成分。

constitute ['kɔnstitjuːt] *v.* 构成，组成

Early diagnosis and treatment constitute secondary prevention.
早期诊断和治疗构成第二级预防。

Shock and hemorrhage constitute the number one cause of maternal death.
休克和出血是构成母体死亡的首要原因。

constitution [ˌkɔnsti'tjuːʃən] *n.* 体质，结构

The alertness and liveliness show that the baby has an unusually sound constitution.
这小孩机灵、活泼，说明他有特别强健的体质。

The classical, or complete, hydatidiform mole has a 46, XX chromosomal constitution.
典型的或完全性葡萄胎具有 46，XX 染色体结构。

constitutional [ˌkɔnsti'tjuːʃənəl] *a.* 全身的，体质的

There is real constitutional peculiarity in this race.
这个种族确实有其体质上的特点。

We have recently shown that children with constitutional growth delay have reduced zinc concentration in hair and serum.
我们最近证明身体生长延迟儿童的头发和血清中的锌浓度下降。

constitutionally [ˌkɔnsti'tjuːʃənli] *ad.* 全身，体质性地

Some infants are constitutionally small by virtue of having small parents.
有些婴儿是体质性小样儿，这是由于其父母身材较矮小之故。

constitutively ['kɔnstitjuːtivli] *ad.* 组成性地，基本地

Resting T cells constitutively express the γ chain(CD134).
静息的 T 细胞组成性表达 γ 链(CD134)。

constrain [kən'strein] *v.* 强迫，强使；抑制

The state of each family member is constrained or stimulated by the state of the other members.
每个家庭成员的状态均受家庭其他成员状态的抑制或刺激。

constrict [kən'strikt] *v.* 收缩，压缩；使狭窄

The pupil of a blind eye will not constrict when its retina is exposed to light.
一只失明眼的视网膜受到光线照射时，其瞳孔不收缩。

During the process of swallowing, the muscles of the pharynx contract and so constrict the space.
在吞咽过程中咽部肌肉收缩而使(口腔)的空间缩小。

Arterioles may be tightly constricted, as they usually are in shock, attempting to preserve arterial pressure.
通常在休克时，小动脉收缩加强以维持动脉压。

The neck of a tooth is the constricted portion between the root and the crown.
牙颈是牙根和牙冠之间的狭窄部分。

constriction [kɔns'trikʃən] *n.* 收缩；狭窄

Constriction of the arterioles decreases the amount of leak, increasing arterial pressure.
小动脉的收缩使流出量减少，动脉压增加。

Shallow breathing raises levels of the body's stress hormones, leading to constriction of blood vessels and tension in the heart.
浅呼吸使体内应激激素升高，导致血管狭窄，心肌张力增加。

constrictive [kən'striktiv] *a.* 缩窄性的

Constrictive pericarditis never follows acute rheumatic fever.
急性风湿热决不会引起缩窄性心包炎。

consult [kən'sʌlt] *v.* 查阅；商量，咨询

I have consulted a number of pathological terms in a medical dictionary.
我已在一本医学词典里查阅了许多病理学术语。

He consulted a doctor about his health.
他找大夫进行了健康咨询。
Never discontinue a prescription drug on your own without consulting your physician.
如果没有同医生商量,不要擅自停止使用你处方上的药。

consultand [kən'sʌltənd] *n.* 询者
The person who brings the family to attention by consulting a geneticist is referred to as the consultand.
为了家庭成员的问题而来咨询遗传学家的人被称为咨询者。

consultant [kən'sʌltənt] *n.* 顾问医师,会诊医师
Hospital consultants and general practitioners cannot always agree on many clinical problems.
医院高级医师和全科医师对许多临床问题不能总是看法一致。

consume [kən'sjuːm] *v.* 消费,用尽
People aged 80 or more consume a greater proportion of health care and social services than any other age group.
80 岁或 80 岁以上的老年人,比任何其他年龄组在卫生保健和社会服务方面所需的消费都多。

consumption [kən'sʌmpʃən] *n.* 消费,消耗量
The annual consumption of gasoline has been estimated at over 600,000,000 tons throughout the world.
全世界汽油的年消耗量估计超过 6 亿吨。
Low birth weight, early consumption of cows' milk, and poor dietary iron intake are considered the main risk factors.
出生体重低,饮用牛奶过早,以及饮食摄入中铁质含量少被认为是主要的危险因素。
Intrauterine growth retardation is increased with alcohol consumption.
(孕妇)饮酒可使(胎儿)宫内生长迟缓率增加。

consumptive [kən'sʌmptiv] *a.* 消耗性的
The platelet count, thrombin time, and protamine test are useful in defining consumptive coagulopathy.
血小板计数、凝血时间和鱼精蛋白试验可用于诊断消耗性凝血病。

contact ['kɔntækt] *n.* 接触,联系
Scarlet fever is capable of being passed on by direct contact with a diseased individual.
猩红热可以通过直接接触病人而传染。
Contact radiotherapy is a form of radiotherapy in which a radioactive substance is brought into close contact with the part of the body being heated.
接触放射线疗法是放射线疗法的一种,此时放射性物质与机体受照射部位紧密接触。
The spleen is a spongy organ with the lateral border in contact with the diaphragm.
脾为一海绵状器官,其外缘与膈相接。
Contact lenses are more convenient than spectacles.
隐形眼镜较普通眼镜要方便些。
v. 接触,联系
His father was shocked and he contacted the doctor at once.
他的父亲休克了,他立即跟医生联系。

contactant [kən'tæktənt] *n.* 接触物
Contact dermatitis is the term used for inflamed skin resulting from external contactants.
接触性皮炎是指由外源性接触物引起的皮肤炎症。

contagious [kən'teidʒəs] *a.* 传染的,传染性的
Mumps is a contagious disease with painful swellings in the neck.
腮腺炎是一种颈部肿痛的传染病。

Measles is one of the most contagious of infections.
麻疹是传染病中传染性最强的一种疾病。

contagium [kən'teidʒiəm] *n.* 接触传染物

Contagium is a causative agent capable of causing a communicable disease.
接触传染物是一种能导致传染病的致病物。

The third notion was the germ theory, or infection was caused by a living organism, a contagium vivum.
第三个概念是病菌理论,或者感染是由活的微生物(活的接触传染物)引起。

container [kən'teinə] *n.* 容器

The radioactive material is stored in a special radiation-proof container.
放射性物质被储存在特制的防辐射容器内。

One may dissect these factors if one considers the arterial tree as an elasitic container.
若把动脉及其分支看作为一个弹性储库,就可能详细分析这些因素。

contaminant [kən'tæminənt] *n.* 沾污物,污染物

Such disease is caused by contaminants acquired during production, storage and distribution of food.
这种疾病是在食物的制作、储存和分配期间所接触的污染物引起的。

The microorganisms in a wound or sewage in a stream are common contaminants.
伤口内的微生物或河流中的脏东西都是常见的污染物。

contaminate [kən'tæmineit] *v.* 污染,弄污

Care must be taken during surgery not to contaminate the wound with cancer cells.
外科手术时必须小心,不要使癌细胞污染伤口。

Contaminated materials or objects exposed to boiling water cannot be sterilized with certainty.
污染的物品或物质,经煮沸并不一定能达到灭菌的目的。

contamination [kəntæmi'neiʃən] *n.* 污染,沾染

Upon completion of filtration, precautions must be taken to prevent contamination of the filtrated material.
过滤中,应特别注意防止被过滤物质的污染。

Water pollution is the contamination of water bodies (e. g. lakes, rivers, oceans and groundwater).
水污染是指水体(如湖泊、河流、海洋、地下水)受到了污染。

Analysis of groundwater contamination may focus on the soil characteristics and site geology, hydrogeology, hydrology, and the nature of the contaminants.
地下水污染的分析应该特别注意对土壤特性和现场地质、水文地质、水文以及污染物性质的分析。

contemplate ['kɔntempleit] *v.* 注视,仔细思考

If cholestasis is prominent, initiation of treatment with phenobarbital, 5-10mg/kg/day, should be contemplated.
如果胆汁淤积显著,应考虑采用苯巴比妥每天 5 ~ 10mg/kg 来治疗。

Provided that one fetal heart can be heard at a normal rate no interference should be contemplated for fetal distress.
倘若能听到一个正常胎心率,不应认为有胎儿窘迫而进行手术。

contempt [kən'tempt] *n.* 轻视,蔑视

The conversation of the old and young ends generally with contempt or pity on either side.
老年人与青年人之间谈话往往以双方相互瞧不起或遗憾而结束。

content ['kɔntent] *n.* 含量,容量;内容物,内容

When the content of oxygen in the plasma is increased, the hemoglobin begins drawing it to itself.

当血浆内氧的含量增加时，血红蛋白便开始与氧结合。

Each red blood cell is filled with red hemoglobin and has no other contents, not even nucleus.

每个红细胞只含有红色的血红蛋白而不含任何其他物质，甚至没有核。

The cavity of the stomach is always the size of its contents.

胃腔的大小与其内容物的多少一致。

contention [kən'tenʃən] *n.* 争论，争辩

Retention of normal ovaries in women after the menopause is still a matter of contention.

绝经期后妇女的正常卵巢是否保留仍然是个争论的问题。

context ['kɔntekst] *n.*（词、句的）上下文

Can't you guess the meaning of the word from the context?

你不能从上下文猜出词意吗？

In a medical context depression refers to a morbit mental state dominated by a lowering of mood, accompanied by a variety of associated symptoms.

在医学文献中，抑郁指的是一种病态的精神状态，以情绪低沉为主，伴有不同的有关症状。

contiguous [kən'tigjuəs] *a.* 接触的

Superficial infections may spread along skin not only by contiguous necrosis but also by metastasis.

表浅感染不仅通过接触性坏死，而且也通过转移而沿皮肤扩散。

continuation [kəntinju'eiʃ ən] *n.* 继续，持续；续篇

The May number of the magazine will contain an important continuation of the report.

本杂志五月号将刊载该报道的重要续篇。

continuity [kɔnti'njuiti] *n.* 连续性，连贯性

ATN is characterized by a loss of tubular epithelial continuity.

急性肾小管坏死（ATN）的特点是小管上皮的连续性中断。

continuously [kən'tinjuəsli] *ad.* 持续不断地

There is currently no technique available to monitor local arterial flow continuously.

目前尚无用以连续不断地测量局部动脉血流的技术。

continuum [kən'tinjuəm] *n.* 连续

Most cells are alive, and most can also reproduce and thereby sustain the continuum of life.

大多数细胞是活的，而且大多数还可以繁殖，从而维持生命的延续。

contour ['kɔntuə] *n.* 外形，轮廓

X-ray screening may show abnormal pulsation and an abnormal cardiac contour.

X 线透视可见到不正常的心脏搏动及不正常的心脏外形。

Asymmetry of the abdominal contour suggests an abnormal mass.

腹形不对称提示腹部肿块。

The crucial procedure of contour detection for corneal endothelium image is to segment cells from background.

为角膜内皮细胞图像而做的轮廓检测的关键步骤是把细胞与背景分隔开来。

contraception [ˌkɔntrə'sepʃən] *n.* 避孕，避孕药

The efficacy of progestational agents for oral contraception is an established fact.

口服孕酮类物质对避孕的效力为既定事实。

Women were excluded from the analysis if they were younger than 45 years and using oral contraception.

如果妇女年龄小于 45 岁并正在服用口服避孕药，她们就会被排除在分析之外。

contraceptive [ˌkɔntrə'septiv] *a.* 避孕的

Married couples may choose contraceptive methods according to age and health.

已婚夫妇可以根据年龄和健康状况选择节育方法。

n. 避孕药

These contraceptives are provided by the state free of charge.
这些避孕药是国家免费供应的。
It is important to counsel patients to discontinue oral contraceptives for several months prior to conception.
指导病人在怀孕之前停止口服避孕药数月是很重要的。

contract [kən'trækt] *v.* 得病,患病;收缩,感染
There is some danger of a patient's contracting pneumonia after the use of ether as an anesthetic.
当乙醚作为麻醉剂使用后,病人有患肺炎的危险性。
Arterial walls are able to expand and contract.
动脉壁能够扩张和收缩。
Babies can acquire bacteria from their mothers if the mother contracts listeriosis while pregnant.
如果母亲在妊娠时感染李斯特菌病,会导致母婴传播。

contractile [kən'træktail] *a.* 有收缩性的
Both skeletal and cardiac muscles are striated muscles, and they have similar contractile mechanisms.
骨骼肌和心肌都是横纹肌,而且它们的收缩机制类似。

contraction [kən'trækʃən] *n.* 收缩,缩短
Pituitrin has the effects of stimulating the contraction of the pregnant uterus.
垂体后叶素有刺激妊娠子宫使之收缩的作用。
Muscle tissue, whatever its kind, is designed to produce power by a forcible contraction.
肌肉组织,不论是哪一种,都旨在以强有力的收缩来产生力量。

contracture [kən'træktʃə] *n.* 挛缩
Fixed limitation of both active and passive assisted joint motion is termed contracture.
主动和被动辅助关节运动的固定受限称为挛缩。
Contracture of a muscle may be due to ischemia, as by a tight bandage or from injury or cold.
肌肉的挛缩可以因绷带太紧而局部缺血引起,也可因损伤或寒冷而引起。

contraindicate [kɔntrə'indikeit] *v.* 禁忌
Elevated intracranial pressure, especially when a posterior fossa mass is suspected, contraindicates lumbar puncture.
当颅内压增高,尤其怀疑为后颅凹肿块时,切忌作腰穿。
Sedation may depress respiration further and is contraindicated.
镇静剂可加重呼吸抑制,应禁用。
Sympathomimetic agents are contraindicated in hypertension and hyperthyroidism.
拟交感药为高血压和甲亢所禁用。

contraindication [ˌkɔntrəˌindi'keiʃən] *n.* 禁忌证
Contraindications to atropine and related drugs are glaucoma and prostatic hypertrophy.
青光眼和前列腺肥大禁用阿托品及其同类药。
If there are no contraindications, some patients may have a needle biopsy of the liver to confirm the diagnosis.
如果没有禁忌证,有些病人可用肝穿刺活检来确诊。
An attack of pneumonia in a patient would be a strong contraindication against the use of a general anaesthetic.
采用全身麻醉对肺炎患者是绝对危险和禁忌的。

contralateral [ˌkɔntrə'lætərəl] *a.* 对侧的
Each measurement was compared with those of the nasal cavity on the contralateral side and of normal control subjects.
每项测定结果都与对侧鼻腔的以及正常对照组的数值进行对比。

Basal ganglia infarction can cause contralateral limb motor or sensory disturbance.
基底节区的梗塞会引起对侧肢体运动或感觉障碍。

contrary [ˈkɔntrəri] *ad.* 相反地

The concept is described contrary to current understanding of renal physiology.
这一观点与现在流行的肾脏生理学的观点相反。

contrast [ˈkɔntræst] *n.* 对比,对照

Visual acuity and contrast sensitivity decrease rapidly after 60 years of age even in the absence of recognizable eye disease.
即使没有明显的眼部疾病,人的视力敏感性和对比感在 60 岁以后也会迅速下降。

Radio-opaque materials, many of them containing iodine, are used as contrast media.
许多含有碘的不透 X 线的物质可用作(放射照相术中的)对比剂(造影剂)。

In contrast, certain syndromes appear only after certain drugs have been given.
与此对比,某些综合征只是在给予某些药物后出现。

v. 和…成对照

The abrupt onset of weakness caused by an arterial obstruction contrasts with the steadily progressive weakness.
由动脉闭塞引起突然发生的肌无力和稳定的进行性无力形成对照。

The extreme susceptibility of some individuals must be contrasted with the great tolerance of others.
一些人(对药物)的极度感受性必须与另一些人的巨大耐受性进行对照。

The infected hair fluoresces bright green, like beads on the hairs contrasting strongly with the dark field.
感染的头发发出亮绿色的荧光,好像珠子在头发上,在暗淡视野中形成强烈的对照。

contribute [kənˈtribjut] *v.* 贡献出;起作用;有助于

The liver is a store-house of many vitamins, some of which in turn contribute to its own proper functioning.
肝脏是许多维生素的储存库,其中某些维生素又对肝脏发挥正常功能有所助益。

Many physicians are reluctant to use these agents because of the risk of inducing or contributing to hemorrhage.
许多医生不愿使用此药剂,因其有引起或促成出血的危险。

contribution [kəntriˈbjuːʃən] *n.* 贡献

Koch made an outstanding contribution to the understanding of the specific relationship between a microbiologic entity and a disease entity.
柯霍做出杰出贡献,使人们懂得一种微生物与一种疾病之间的特定关系。

Another contribution to the digestive mechanism furnished by the oral cavity is the production of saliva.
口腔在完成消化机制方面的另一贡献是分泌唾液。

contributor [kənˈtribjutə] *n.* 捐助者;撰稿人;起一份作用者

Prof. Smith is a regular contributor to this medical magazine.
史密斯教授是这个医学杂志的长期撰稿人。

Koch and Pasteur were celebrated contributors to the development of bacteriology.
柯霍和巴斯德是对细菌学发展做出卓越贡献的人。

Prolonged pregnancy remains a significant contributor to perinatal mortality.
过期妊娠仍对围产儿死亡率有重要影响。

control [kənˈtrəul] *n.* 控制,对照

Unfortunately none of these studies included normal controls for comparison.
遗憾的是这些研究中没有一项包含了供比较的正常对照受试者。

The present study includes 42 control cases and 40 carcinoma cases.

目前的研究包括 42 个对照病例和 48 个癌症病例。

v. 控制,对照

Two studies have used a double blind placebo controlled methodology.

两项研究使用了双盲安慰剂对照的方法。

Such therapy has recently been proved to be efficacious in the treatment of allergic asthma in a double-blind controlled study.

最近在一项双盲法对照的研究中,已证实这种疗法治疗变态反应性哮喘有效。

controllability [kənˌtrəuləˈbiliti] *n.* 可控性

The controllability and observability are of great importance in both theory and applications.

可控性和可观测性在理论和运用方面都很重要。

Controllability is an important property of a control system.

可控性是控制系统的一个重要特性。

controversial [ˌkɔntrəˈvəːʃəl] *a.* 有争论的

The use of respiratory stimulants in the treatment of acute respiratory failure is controversial.

使用呼吸中枢兴奋剂治疗急性呼吸衰竭尚有争论。

The aetiology of chronic active hepatitis is controversial.

慢性活动性肝炎的病因是有争论的。

controversy [ˈkɔntrəvəːsi] *n.* 论战,争论

Much of the controversy stems from difficulties in establishing an accurate diagnosis.

许多论战的缘由是难于做出一个准确的诊断。

Chronic tonsilitis is a condition on which there has been much controversy.

慢性扁桃腺炎是有不少争论的一种疾病。

The biggest controversy is over the so-called "irreversible" shock, or that shock which does not respond to apparently adequate blood replacement.

争论最大的是所谓"不可逆性"休克,即显然补足适当血量之后仍无反应的休克。

contuse [kənˈtjuːz] *vt.* 打伤,撞伤,挫伤

Of 48 cases with colonic injury, 71% were injured by stab, 25% by contusing, and 4% by firearm.

48 例结肠损伤中,刀刺伤占 71%,腹部钝性伤占 25%,火器伤 4%。

contusion [kənˈtjuːʒən] *n.* 挫伤

A contusion is a discoloration of tissue by blood that has extravasated into it as a result of damage.

挫伤是由于(小血管)受伤,血液渗入组织而使之变色。

The functional disturbances produced by contusion of internal tissue are variable.

内组织挫伤引起的功能紊乱是可变异的。

convalesce [ˌkɔnvəˈles] *v.* 恢复健康,渐愈

Would you consider going north to convalesce this summer?

今年夏天你考虑到北方去疗养吗?

How long do patients convalesce after inguinal herniorrhaphy?

病人在腹股沟疝修补术后需要多长时间康复?

convalescence [ˌkɔnvəˈlesns] *n.* 恢复(期),康复(期)

During convalescence from scarlet fever the patient may manifest all the signs and symptoms of acute tonsilitis.

在猩红热恢复期间,患者可出现急性扁桃体炎的全部体征和症状。

Fever is rare after the first week in patients who had a normal convalescence.

正常恢复的病人在第一周后极少发热。

convalescent [kɔnvəˈlesnt] *a.* 恢复健康的

Many children recover completely and resume full activity without this prolonged convalescent pe-

riod.
许多儿童不经此延长的恢复期,立即全部复原并开始正常活动。

convection [kən'vekʃən] *n.* (热的)对流

Conduction and convection normally make up only 10% to 15% of heat loss.
热量的散发仅有10%到15%是通过传导和对流的方式进行的。

convenience [kən'vinjəns] *n.* 便利

The gate of out-patient department is always open for the convenience of patients.
为了病人看病方便,门诊部的大门总是开着的。

convenient [kən'viːniənt] *a.* 方便的,适宜的

A convenient approach to most anemias that result from production defects is to examine cellular changes.
处理大多数由于生成不足所致的贫血的合适的方法是检查血细胞的变化。

conventional [kən'venʃənəl] *a.* 传统的,常规的

By the standard of conventional medicine, the impossible had happened.
按照传统医学的标准,不可能的事终于发生了。

Nor did the women with enlarged radical mastectomies do better than those who had conventional radical mastectomies.
做彻底根治性乳腺切除术的妇女并不比做一般根治性乳腺切除者情况好。

conventionally [kən'venʃənəli] *adv.* 按惯例,照传统

Amenorrhea is conventionally divided into primary and secondary amenorrhea. With primary amenorrhea, menstruation never takes place.
闭经惯常分为原发性闭经和继发性闭经,对于原发性闭经,就是从没来过月经。

Our review indicates that there is currently no evidence to support the selection of organically over conventionally produced foods on the basis of nutritional superiority.
我们的研究表明在营养价值的优越性上,当前没有证据支持挑选有机食品比传统生产的食品更好。

convergence [kən'vəːdʒəns] *n.* 会聚;集合

The response of pupil to convergence, although slow, is often extensive and its redilation is slow and steady.
瞳孔对会聚的反应虽然缓慢,但经常是持续较久,瞳孔的再扩大缓慢而平稳。

converse ['kɔnvəːs] *a.* 相反的

The converse is also true.
反之亦然。

Right ventricular hypertrophy causes converse changes with small R-waves in S_1, dominant R-waves in the leads over the right ventricle V_2-V_4 where the T-wave is inverted.
右心室肥厚可引起相反的变化,在S_1导联有小的R波,而在右心室胸前导联$V_2 \sim V_4$上则以R波占优势,T波倒置。

conversely [kɔn'vəːsli] *ad.* 反之,相反

Conversely, dilation of arterioles increases the leak and lowers arterial pressure.
反之,小动脉的舒张则增加其流出量,因而降低动脉血压。

conversion [kən'vəːʃən] *n.* 转化,转变

The conversion of the uterine mucosa into decidua occurs in pregnancy.
妊娠期子宫内膜转化为蜕膜。

The liver has been identified as the major site of conversion of progesterone to carbohydrates.
肝脏作为孕酮转化为碳水化合物的主要部位已被确认。

convert [kən'vəːt] *v.* 转变,转化

Sometimes the body converts a drug to several active metabolites with dissimilar pharmacologic properties.

有时机体将一种药物转化成几种具有不同药理性质的活性代谢物。

The popularity of these lenses is growing so fast that eyeglass wearers are converting to contacts at the rate of more than 2 million a year.

这些新式眼镜迅速受到人们的欢迎,因而每年换用隐形眼镜的超过 200 万人。

convertase [kən'vəːteis] *n.* 转化酶

Proprotein convertases activate a large number of protein precursors.

前蛋白转化酶可激活大量蛋白前体细胞。

The larger C2a fragment is the active protease component of the C3 convertase.

大片段 C2a 是 C3 转化酶的活性酶成分。

converter [kən'vəːtə] *n.* 转换器

The converter has 2 external timers.

这种转换器有两个外部定时器。

There is currently no converter available.

目前没有可用的转换器。

convertor [kən'vəːtə] *n.* 转炉;变流器;转化器;转换器

It is needed in the computerized control system to convert analog signal into digital signal, so A/D convertor is an essential component.

在计算机控制系统中,需将模拟量转换成数字量,因此,A/D 转换器是一个必需的部件。

A/D convertor and D/A convertor are two essential structures for CT scanner.

模数转换器和数模转换器是 CT 的两个必需构件。

convex [kɔn'veks] *a.* 凸面的,凸的

The inferior and lateral convex border of the stomach is the greater curvature.

胃的下方及侧面凸缘是胃大弯。

The lenses become more convex or concave, depending on whether the wearer is long-sighted or short-sighted.

镜片可以根据佩戴者的近视或远视情况变得更凸出或更凹陷。

n. ['kɔnveks] 凸面

Because there is no abrasion between the concave and convex, the nut is reusable.

因为凹面与凸面没有磨损,螺母可以重复使用。

convey [kən'vei] *v.* 传送,传播,传达

The secretions from the lobes are conveyed through lactiferous ducts, all of which converge at the nipple.

乳腺小叶的分泌物通过输乳管来输送,所有的输乳管(最后)都汇集于乳头。

This infection is often conveyed to man by animals.

这种传染病常由动物传染给人。

convoluted ['kɔnvəluːtid] *a.* 卷曲的

Microvilli abound in the lining of the convoluted tubules in the kidney.

肾曲小管的内膜有丰富的微绒毛。

convulsion [kən'vʌlʃən] *n.* 惊厥,抽搐

In children, alcohol may cause severe hypoglycemia and convulsions.

酒精可引起儿童严重低血糖和惊厥。

The patient suddenly fell into convulsions.

病人突然发生抽搐。

coolant ['kuːlənt] *n.* 冷冻剂

The atomic reactor used a gas coolant.

这个原子反应堆使用了一种气态冷冻剂。

A coolant, which may be liquid sodium, water or some other substances can carry away the heat produced in the reactor.

像液体钠、水或其他一些物质这样的冷却剂能吸走反应堆所产生的热。

cooperation [kəuˌɔpə'reiʃən] *n.* 合作,协作

WHO will provide technical support to intercountry cooperation for strengthening the training of technical and managerial staff.

世界卫生组织将对国家间的协作提供技术支援,以加强技术与管理人员的训练。

coordinate [kəu'ɔːdineit] *v.* (使)协调

That is why the activity of the whole nervous system is coordinated.

这就是整个神经系统能够协调的原因。

The shortage of human donor organs is highlighted in another report from the United Network for Organ Sharing which coordinates the use of donated organs in the US.

另一来自人体器官供应网的报道强调人类供体器官的短缺,该供应网是美国协调捐献器官使用的一个机构。

coordination [kəuˌɔːdi'neiʃən] *n.* 联合,协调

Good coordination of the eyes will come about in some children only at a later date.

某些儿童两只眼睛的完全协调,只在晚一些的时候才出现。

cope [kəup] *v.* 对付;处理;斗争(with)

A high temperature is a sign that the body is coping with some infection.

发热是一种标志,说明人体正在和感染进行着斗争。

copious ['kəupjəs] *a.* 富裕的,丰富的

Hemorrhage is a frequent sign, varying from a slight oozing of blood to a copious flooding that may prove fatal.

出血是一种常见体征,其程度从轻微渗血到可能导致死亡的大量流血。

Because of copious vomiting, there is often associated loss of weight and constipation.

因大量呕吐,故常伴有体重减轻和便秘。

copolymer [kəu'pɔlimə] *n.* 共聚物

Advanced development of block copolymer micelle has been mentioned.

嵌段共聚物胶束的研究进展已提及。

coprecipitate [kəupri'sipiteit] *n.* 共沉淀物

Chitosan-silica coprecipitate (C-S) has recently been proposed as a tablet disintegrant.

脱乙酰壳聚糖-二氧化硅共沉淀物(C-S)最近被推荐用作片剂崩解剂。

These cations diffuse away from their particulate mineral sources and coprecipitate with Al and Si in the soil clay matrix.

这些阳离子从它们的颗粒矿物源中扩散出来,并在黏土矩阵中与铝和硅形成共沉淀物。

coprolalia [ˌkɔprə'leiliə] *n.* 秽语症

Coprolalia is an occasional characteristic of Tourette syndrome.

秽语症是图雷特综合征的一个偶然特征。

Coprolalia is not unique to tic disorders.

秽语症不是抽搐性运动障碍所特有的。

copy ['kɔpi] *n.* 复制品 复份,副本

The painting is a copy of one in the museum.

这幅画是博物馆中的一幅画的复制品。

This is a mark that discriminates the original from the copy.

这是一个使原作与复制品有区别的标志。

He asked his secretary to make a copy of the document.

他叫秘书把文件复制一份。

v. 复制

You can't copy your file with this disk; it's full.

你不能用这张磁盘拷文件,这张盘已满。

copyright [ˈkɔpirait] *n.* 版权

No part of this material can be reproduced or utilized in any form without written permission from the copyright holder.

未经版权所有者书面允许,不得以任何形式复制或使用本材料中的任何部分。

v. 获得版权保护

This article is copyrighted but readers may reproduce it in part or in whole only with proper acknowlegement.

本文享有版权,但只要作出适当声明读者可部分或全部进行复制。

coracoid [ˈkɔrəkɔid] *n.* 喙突

The coracoids is a small hook-like structure on the lateral edge of the superior anterior portion of the scapula.

喙突是肩胛骨前上方横侧面的一个勾样结构。

Coracoid and acromial fractures were noted. Open reduction and internal fixation were performed.

放射学检查显示出右肩喙突与肩峰骨折,因而对其进行了开放性复位及内固定术。

cordotomy [kɔːˈdɔtəmi] *n.* 脊髓前侧柱切断术

Percutaneous cordotomy is presently the most common neurosurgical procedures for the relief of chronic cancer pain.

目前经皮脊髓前侧柱切断术最常用于缓解慢性癌痛。

core [kɔː] *n.* 核心

There is a tiny round-shaped core known as nucleus in the centre of a cell.

细胞的中央有一个称为细胞核的小圆核。

Other symptoms, not easily recognized but having their source in the core problem of depression, relate to daily living.

其他不容易认识到但源于抑郁症的核心问题的症状与日常生活有关。

In pemphigus foliaceus, the circulating antibodies bind specifically to desmoglein I, a desmosomal core glycoprotein.

在落叶性天疱疮中,循环抗体与桥粒芯蛋白 I(即一种桥粒的核心糖蛋白)发生特异性结合。

coreceptor [ˌkəuriˈseptə] *n.* 辅助受体,共同受体

Deletion of CD4 and CD8 coreceptors permits generation of αβT cells that recognize antigens independently of the MHC.

CD4 和 CD8 共受体缺失会允许 αβT 细胞产生,后者可以不依赖 MHC 分子而识别抗原。

MHC-independent αβT cells were indeed generated in mice deficient in both coreceptors as well as MHC。

在共受体和 MHC 分子缺陷的小鼠体内确实产生了 MHC 分子非依赖性 αβT 细胞。

corepressor [ˌkəuriˈpresə] *n.* 辅阻遏物

Corepressor in nuclei of hTC 4 is the important molecule of signaling pathway.

hTC 4 细胞核中的辅阻遏物是信号转导的重要分子。

This review focuses on a family of transcriptional corepressor proteins.

这篇综述重点介绍辅阻遏物蛋白转录家族。

corn [kɔːn] *n.* 鸡眼

Wearing high heels can cause long-term foot problems, such as blisters, corns and calluses, and also serious foot, knee and back pain and damaged joints.

穿高跟鞋可引发长期的足部疾病,比如水疱、鸡眼,老茧,以及严重的脚部、膝部和背部疼痛和关节损伤。

cornea [ˈkɔːniə] *n.* 角膜

Leukemic nodules are occasionally found in the cornea and sclera.

白血病小结有时可发现于角膜和巩膜内。

His corneas, the windows over the pupil, had turned thick, white and opaque.

他的角膜(瞳孔上的窗户)增厚、变白,也不透明。

The central part of cornea is the best site for measuring intraocular pressure.

角膜中心部分是测量眼内压的最佳位置。

corneal [ˈkɔːniəl] *a.* 角膜的

Corneal ulcerations are often found if checked up carefully.

如果仔细查看的话,经常可发现角膜溃疡。

cornerstone [ˈkɔːnəˌstəun] *n.* 基础,柱石,地基

In patients with functional heartburn, pain modulators are the cornerstone of therapy.

对那些有功能性胃灼热的病人,疼痛调节剂是治疗的基础。

Inefficient signal transduction represents the cornerstone in the pathogenesis of type 2 diabetes mellitus.

无效率的信号转导是 2 型糖尿病发病机制的基础。

coronary [ˈkɔrənəri] *a.* 冠状的

The incidence of death from coronary disease increases rapidly over 40 years of age.

冠心病的死亡发生率在 40 岁以上的人中增长很快。

Coronary arteriography has a small morbidity and mortality.

冠状动脉造影引起的并发症及死亡率甚小。

coronavirus [ˌkɔrənəˈvaiərəs] *n.* 冠状病毒

The present data suggest that coronaviruses cause about 10 percent of common colds.

现有的数据表明冠状病毒引起约 10% 的普通感冒。

In March 2003, a novel coronavirus(SARS-CoV) was discovered in association with cases of severe acute respiratory syndrome(SARS).

2003 年 3 月,科学家们发现了引起严重急性呼吸系统综合征的一种新型冠状病毒(SARS-CoV)。

Researchers have shown that the SARS coronavirus can undergo rapid evolution in our population.

研究人员指出 SARS 冠状病毒在人群中能迅速演变。

cor pulmonale [ˈkɔːpʌlməˈnɑːli] *n.* 肺心病,肺源性心脏病

A right ventricular hypertrophy, enlargement, or failure resulting from pulmonary arteral hypertension with no primary disease of the left heart is known as cor pulmonale.

肺心病(的发病)是由肺动脉高压引起右心室肥大、扩张并衰竭所致,左心室并无原发疾病。

corpus [ˈkɔːpəs] (*pl.* corpora [ˈkɔːpərə]) *n.* [拉] 体

A corpus luteum cyst develops from a mature Graafian follicle.

一个黄体囊由一个成熟的囊状卵泡发育而成。

Corpus luteum secretes the hormone progesterone, which prepares the womb for implantation.

黄体分泌孕酮以备子宫受精着床。

corpuscle [ˈkɔːpʌsl] *n.* 血细胞;粒子

Blood corpuscles are too small to be seen by the naked eye.

血细胞太小,肉眼看不见。

An electron is an extremely small corpuscle with negative charge which rounds about the nucleus of an atom.

电子是绕着原子核运行、带有负电荷的极其微小的粒子。

correct [kəˈrekt] *v.* 矫正,改正

Animal experiments some ten years ago convinced Dr. Smith that Protein C was a key in correcting the coagulation response.

大约十年前的动物实验使史密斯医生坚信 C 蛋白正是矫正凝血反应的关键所在。

correction [kəˈrekʃən] *n.* 校正

Am I suitable for laser vision correction?

我适合于激光矫正视力吗?

This lesion can be lessened by surgical correction.

这种损害可通过外科矫治减轻。

correlate(with) [ˈkɔrileit] *v.* (使)相互关联

An adequate medical history permits the physician to correlate the physical findings with the information previously acquired.

足够的病史可使医生将体检结果与以往获得的资料联系起来。

The structure and form of a cell is closely correlated with its function.

细胞的结构及形状和它的功能之间有着密切的相互关系。

correlation [ˌkɔriˈleiʃən] *n.* 相互关系,相关性,关联

Though the classification is based on pathology, there are fairly clear clinical correlation.

虽然该分类是建立在病理学基础上的,但是其临床上的相关性是很明显的。

There was a positive correlation between age and pulse wave velocity (r=+0.90).

年龄和脉搏波传播速度之间存在正关联(r=+0.90)。

correlative [kɔˈrelətiv] *a.* 相关的

Few roentgen pathologic correlative studies in bronchiectasis appear in the literature.

文献中发表的有关支气管扩张的 X 线病理学相关的研究为数很少。

correspond [kɔrisˈpɔnd] *v.* 符合,一致;相当

The location of the discomfort generally corresponds to the segmental level of nerves.

不适感的部位一般和神经节段水平相对应。

This functional difference between the anterior and posterior urethra does not correspond to the anatomical division.

这种在前后尿道之间的功能差别并不与解剖学分类一致。

It is likely that these bands correspond to genes or groups of genes.

这些带状物似乎就是基因或基因群。

corroborate [kəˈrɔbəreit] *v.* 确证,证实

The response to therapy corroborates the diagnosis.

对治疗的反应可使诊断得到确证。

corrosive [kəˈrəusiv] *a.* 腐蚀性的

Ingestion of corrosive agents such as strong alkalies or acids can lead to esophagitis and esophageal perforation.

食入腐蚀性物质如强碱或强酸可引起食管炎和食管穿孔。

The structure may be nonspecific, such as any tissue in direct contact with corrosive chemicals.

直接与腐蚀性化学物质接触的任何组织,其结构可以是非特异性的。

n. 腐蚀性物质

The intentional or accidental ingestion of corrosives causes a severe chemical gastritis.

有意或无意吃进腐蚀性东西可引起严重的化学性胃炎。

Liquid corrosives are more likely to cause serious esophageal damage than crystalline products, because liquids are more easily ingested.

因为液体比固体更易于吸收,所以液态腐蚀剂更易于引起严重的食管损伤。

cortex [ˈkɔːteks] (*pl.* cortices [ˈkɔːtisiːz]) *n.* 皮质,皮层

The scientists experimented with rats that had damaged part of the brain called the cortex.

科学家们用大脑皮质局部受到损伤的老鼠来做实验。

In most regions of the cortex six separate cell layers can be recognized under the microscope.

大部分皮层区在显微镜下可见六层分离的细胞层。

cortical [ˈkɔːtikəl] *a.* 外皮的，皮质的

At autopsy, a small 0.5cm papillary renal cortical adenoma with focal areas of calcification was identified.

在尸检中，发现一处有钙化集中点的 0.5cm 的小乳头状肾皮质腺瘤。

corticoid [ˈkɔːtikɔid] *n.* 皮质激素类

Adrenocorticoid therapy was first offered as ACTH (adrenocorticotropic hormone), and then synthetic corticoids gain more widespread use.

肾上腺皮质激素类治疗开始时用 ACTH，以后合成的皮质激素得到更为广泛的应用。

corticosteroid [ˌkɔːtikəuˈstiərɔid] *n.* 皮质醇，皮质激素

Almost all of these cases can be produced by large doses of corticosteroids.

以上所有这些表现，在使用大剂量皮质醇时，几乎都可出现。

Even a slight excess of corticosteroid given for prolonged periods will induce Cushing's syndrome.

长期应用即使稍过量的皮质激素，也会引起库欣综合征（肾上腺皮质功能亢进）。

corticosterone [ˌkɔːtikəuˈstiərəun] *n.* 皮质酮

Sabatino et al. (1991) found that dietary restriction results in daily afternoon peak concentrations of plasma free corticosterone in male F344 rats.

Sabatino 等人（1991）发现，限制饮食引起 F344 雄性大鼠的血浆游离的皮质酮的峰浓度在每天下午时出现。

corticotropin [ˌkɔːtikəuˈtrəupin] *n.* 促肾上腺皮质激素（= corticotrophin [ˌkɔːtikəuˈtrəufin]）

Corticotropin deficiency may be isolated or occur in association with other pituitary hormone deficiencies.

促肾上腺皮质激素的缺乏可以单独出现或与其他垂体激素的缺乏共同存在。

Corticotropin (ACTH) can increase aldosterone secretion, but its effect is short (<24 hours).

促肾上腺皮质激素能增加醛固酮的分泌，但它的作用时间比较短（小于 24 小时）。

Corticotrophin releasing factor is a peptide from the pituitary. Infusion of this peptide into the animal's brain induce anxiety-like behaviour.

促皮质素释放因子是来自脑下垂体的一种肽，将此种肽灌注于动物的脑内时可以诱发焦虑不安的活动。

cortisol [ˈkɔːtisɔl] *n.* 氢化可的松，可的索，皮质醇

Cortisol causes hypernatremia, hypokalemia, and hypercalciuria.

氢化可的松可引起高血钠、低血钾和尿钙增加。

Cortisol, like other 11-oxygenated corticosteroid, has the property of maintaining the glycogen stores of liver.

皮质醇与其他的 11 氧合的皮质类固醇一样有保持肝脏糖原储存的特性。

cortisone [ˈkɔːtisəun] *n.* 可的松，肾上腺皮质激素

That is why there is often pigmentation of the skin in adrenocortical insufficiency when cortisone is lacking.

这就是为什么肾上腺皮质功能低下缺乏可的松时，常有皮肤色素沉着的原因。

The patient showed marked improvement on cortisone therapy.

在可的松治疗下，患者病情显著改善。

coryza [kəˈraizə] *n.* 鼻卡他，鼻炎

Upper respiratory symptoms including sore throat, nasal congestion, and coryza are infrequently reported.

咽痛、鼻充血以及鼻炎等上呼吸道的症状很少报道。

Ordinarily, upper respiratory tract symptoms of several day's duration, including fever, coryza, hoarseness, sore throat and cough, precede the pulmonary illness.

通常，在肺部症状出现前，有若干天的上呼吸道症状，如发热、鼻炎、声音嘶哑、咽喉疼痛及咳嗽出现。

cosmesis [kɔz'mesis] *n.* 美容术

Long-term cosmesis from the patient's perspective is compared to the doctor's appraisal.

从病人的角度对长期美容的看法与医生对长期美容的评估做了比较。

Factors that determine judgment of cosmesis are analyzed.

分析了判断美观的决定性因素。

cosmetic [kɔz'metik] *n.* 化妆品

Cosmetics do not always cover up the deficiencies of nature.

化妆品并非总能遮盖天生的缺陷。

a. 整形的，整容的

Contact dermatitis may result from exposure to many cosmetic and personal hygiene products.

接触性皮炎可能会由接触许多化妆品和个人卫生用品而引起。

Cosmetic surgery deals with operations pertaining to correcting physical defects and beautifying the body.

整形外科是从事矫正身体缺陷和美容的手术。

cosmopolitan [ˌkɔzmə'pɔlitən] *a.* 全世界性的

Measles is a disease of cosmopolitan distribution, endemic in all but isolated populations.

麻疹分布于世界各地，除隔离的人群外，各地均可流行。

co-stimulation [kəu,stimju'leiʃən] *n.* 共刺激，共刺激作用

We have tested the role of ICOS co-stimulation in eliciting effector function from these memory T cells.

我们检测了 ICOS 共刺激作用在激发这些记忆性 T 细胞效应功能中的作用。

costimulator [ˌkəu'stimjuleitə] *n.* 共刺激分子

In vitro T cell activation requires both antigen presentation and a second stimulus provided by the lymphocyte costimulator.

在体外，T 细胞活化需要抗原呈递和由淋巴细胞共刺激分子提供的第二刺激。

An inducible costimulator (ICOS) is expressed on activated T cells.

可诱导的共刺激分子(ICOS)的表达部位在活化 T 细胞表面。

costotransversectomy [ˌkɔstəuˌtrænzvəː'sektəmi] *n.* 肋骨椎骨横突切除术

Fifteen patients with thoracic spinal cord compression from metastatic neoplastic processes were managed by spinal canal decompression via a modified costotransversectomy approach.

对十五位因肿瘤迁徙患有胸部脊髓受压的病人做了通过改良的肋骨椎骨横突切除术来进行椎管减压。

cough [kɔf] *n.* 咳嗽

During asthma, in many cases, there is a hard, tight cough.

哮喘时，往往会有难以忍受的胸部发紧并透不过气来的咳嗽。

v. 咳

The patient also tries very hard to cough up the congesting mucus in his chest, but usually cannot breathe in enough air to do this successfully.

病人也想使劲咳出淤积在胸中的痰液，但通常都是不能吸入足够量的空气来达到这一目的。

coulomb ['kuːlɔm] *n.* 库仑

The unit of electric quantity is coulomb.

物体的电量单位是库仑。

In quantum electrodynamics two electrons obeyed Coulomb's inverse square law.

在量子电动力学中两个电子遵从库仑反平方定律。

council ['kaunsəl] *n.* 理事会，委员会

Such boards or councils have the important duty of keeping the curriculum under constant review.

这样的委员会或理事会的职责是使课程设置置于经常的考核下。

counsel ['kaunsəl] *n.* 咨询;律师,法律顾问

They should consult legal counsel early in the registry planning process for the necessary assistance.

早在登记计划制订过程中他们就应该咨询法律顾问,以获得必要的帮助。

counseling ['kaunsəliŋ] *n.* 咨询

Training of involved physicians, nurses, and pharmacists can be undertaken with written instructions or via telephone and/or face-to-face counseling.

有关的医生、护士和药剂师的培训,可以通过书面指导、或通过电话和(或)面对面咨询来进行。

count [kaunt] *v.* 计数; *n.* 计数

We count the number of photos arriving at D1 without the mirror.

我们对没有放入镜子时达 D1 的光子进行计数。

The count showed that twenty thousand votes had been cast.

统计表明已投票两万张。

counter ['kauntə] *v.* 反对,反击

These effects are not countered by atropine.

阿托品不能对抗这些作用。

Certain fibers also help counter high cholesterol, protect against cancer and maintain a normal blood sugar level.

某些纤维还有助于抵制高胆固醇,防止癌症和维持正常血糖水平。

counteract [ˌkauntə'rækt] *v.* 对抗,中和

These agents do not counteract the effect of aldosterone on the distal tubule.

这些药物不能中和醛固酮对远曲小管的作用。

If we can understand how cancer works, we can counteract its action.

如果我们能了解癌细胞如何工作,我们就能设法抵消它的作用。

counterfeit ['kauntəfit] *a.* 伪造的 *n.* 伪造品,仿冒品

The influence of co-medication with traditional medicines, and the unexpected failure of efficacy because of substandard of counterfeit medicines, will have to be covered by the pharmacovigilance system.

同时服用传统药物的影响以及因使用假冒劣质药品所导致治疗意外失败,都必须接受药物警戒系统监督。

counterpulsation [ˌkauntəpʌl'seiʃən] *n.* 对抗搏动法,反搏术

Intra-aortic counterpulsation is a most promising technique.

主动脉内反搏术是一项非常有前途的技术。

countershock ['kauntəʃɔk] *n.* 对抗休克

Ventricular fibrillation was promptly terminated by direct current countershock.

用直流电对抗休克使心室纤颤立刻停止。

countertransference [ˌkauntətræs'fəːrəns] *n.* 反转移法,反移情作用

Countertransference is a key concept in psychodynamic therapies, but it occurs in all therapies.

反移情是精神动力治疗法的一个关键概念,但它也出现在所有治疗法中。

couple ['kʌpl] *v.* (使)连接,(使)结合

The release of insulin is closely coupled with the level of glucose.

胰岛素的释放与血糖的水平密切相关。

Glucose transport, no less than potassium, is coupled to sodium flux.

葡萄糖的转运和钾一样,也与钠流通偶联。

Immunotoxins are antibodies that are chemically coupled to toxic proteins usually derived from plants or microbes.
免疫毒素是与毒性蛋白化学偶联的抗体，这些毒性蛋白通常源自植物或微生物。

coupler [ˈkʌplə] *n.* 耦合器，联接器
This product is of secure type consisting of telephone set and coupler.
本产品为安全型，由电话机和耦合器两部分组成。
The relative equipment' s coupler adopts the casting-seal structure.
关联设备耦合器采用浇封结构。

court [kɔːt] *n.* 法庭
Court records show that many juvenile criminals are boys and girls who have become addicted to marijuana-cigarette smoking.
法庭记录表明许多幼稚无知的罪犯为大麻吸毒成瘾的男女青少年。

courtesy [ˈkəːtisi] *n.* 礼貌
Many sponsors report adverse events potentially associated with another manufacturer' s drug to that manufacturer' s safety department as a courtesy, rather than report events directly to FDA.
很多申办方按照礼节，将可能与其他制造商的药物有潜在关系的不良事件报告给该药品制造商的安全部门，而不是直接报告给 FDA。

covalent [kəuˈveilənt] *a.* 共价的
In covalent bonds, electrons are shared by different atoms.
在共价键中，电子为不同原子所共有。
Covalent bonds are stronger than hydrogen bonds.
共价键强于氢键。

covariable [kəˈvɛəriəbl] *n.* 协变量
These differences were also significant when we used female body size as a covariable.
当我们把女性体尺作为协变量时，这些差异也很显著。
Energy intake was a covariable in regression models.
在回归模型中，能量摄入是一个协变量。

covariate [kəuˈvɛərieit] *n.* 协变量
Significant covariates will be identified to allow refinement of dosing in the context of drug interactions and disease influences.
在药物相互作用和疾病影响的情况下，重要的协变量将被确定，以便较精确地调整用药剂量。

cowpox [ˈkaupɔks] *n.* 牛痘
Edward Jenner observed that people who had had cowpox were immune to smallpox.
爱德华·詹纳尔注意到得过牛痘的人对天花具有免疫力。

crack [kræk] *v.* 破裂，裂化 *n.* 破裂声；裂缝，裂开；皲裂
Pain often accompanies movement of the parts by opening or deepening the cracks or forming new ones.
由于裂缝裂开或裂口加深或新的裂隙形成的局部区域通常在运动时都会感觉疼痛。

cramp [kræmp] *n.*（肌肉）痉挛
Hypocalcemia and hypnatremia predispose to muscle cramp.
低血钙和低血钠容易发生肌肉痉挛。
The swimmer was seized with cramp and had to be helped out of water.
游泳者突然抽筋，只好由别人救助出水。
v. 使起痉挛
Cramping or colicky pain is characteristic of obstruction of a hollow viscus.
痉挛性疼痛或绞痛是空腔脏器梗阻所特有的。

cranial [ˈkreinjl] *a.* 颅的，颅侧的

Cranial arteritis is an inflammatory condition involving the cranial blood vessels.
颅动脉炎是一种累及脑血管的炎症。
Cranial nerves are those which carry impulses to and from the brain.
脑神经是那些将冲动传入和传出脑的神经。
In about 15 percent of strokes a weak wall of a cranial vessel bursts, causing bleeding into the brain.
在大约15%的中风病例中,脑血管壁因脆弱而迸裂,继而导致脑内出血。

craniocerebral [ˌkreiniəu'seribrəl] *a.* 颅脑的
Craniocerebral trauma is of particular interest from a forensic standpoint for several reasons.
由于多种原因颅脑损伤从法医学观点来看具有特殊意义。

cranioplasty ['kreiniəˌplæsti] *n.* 头颅成形术;颅骨成形术
Cranioplasty following decompressive craniectomy is reported to result in improved blood flow and cerebral metabolism.
报道称减压性颅骨切除术后的颅骨成形术能够改善脑部血供和脑代谢。

craniosynostosis ['kreiniəˌsinɔs'təusis] *n.* [胚] 颅缝早闭;颅缝骨接合
In certain of the craniosynostoses, the new mutations responsible are usually missense mutations that arise nearly always in the paternal germline.
在某种颅缝早闭中,致病的新突变通常由父本生殖细胞的错义突变造成。
If a baby has craniosynostosis, it is usually present at birth, but it is not always noticeable straight away.
如果一个婴儿颅缝早闭,通常在出生时即可显现,但它并不总是立刻能被发现。

craniotabes [kreiniə'teibiːz] *n.* 颅骨软化
One of the early signs of rickets is craniotabes.
佝偻病早期的症状之一是颅骨软化。

craniotomy [kreini'ɔtəmi] *n.* 颅骨切开术
Brain tumours are normally treated by surgery after a section of the skull has been removed—a drastic procedure known as craniotomy.
脑肿瘤通常是在切开部分颅骨后用外科手术治疗,这种剧烈而带损伤性的操作称为颅骨切开术。

cranium ['kreiniəm] *n.* 颅
The cranium consists of eight bones connected together by immovable joints.
颅骨由不动关节连接在一起的八块骨头组成。
The skull can be divided into the cranium, which enclosed the brain, and the face(including the lower jaw).
头颅可分为颅骨(包围大脑)和面骨(包括下颌骨)两大部分。

cream [kriːm] *n.* 乳(膏)剂,膏状物
Traditionally, topical estrogen cream application has been the choice of conservative treatment.
按传统的做法,局部应用雌激素乳剂是一种保守的治疗选择。
The disease is chronic, has exacerbations and remissions and can be managed with hot water treatments and capsaicin cream.
这种慢性疾病反复发作,可以用热水和辣椒素乳剂来治疗。

creaming ['kriːmiŋ] *n.* 乳析,乳状液分层
Emulsions were characterised with respect to droplet size, interfacial tension, creaming, surface load and electron microscopy.
乳状剂可根据微滴大小、界面张力、乳析、表面负荷和电子显微镜检查鉴定。
The resulting emulsions were stable against coalescence but were subject to creaming.
这种合成的乳状剂不易聚结但是易产生乳油化。

creatine ['triːətin] *n.* 肌酸(或作 creatin)

Diagnosis of myocardial infarction is substantiated by electrocardiographic changes and elevated serum creatine phosphokinase levels, especially the MB isoenzyme.
心电图改变和血清肌酸磷酸酶水平，尤其是 MB 同工酶等的增高可证实心肌梗死的诊断。

creatinine [kriˈætinin] *n.* 肌酸酐
There is an accumulation of the products of protein metabolism, urea, creatinine, uric acid and ammonia.
出现蛋白代谢产物（尿素、肌酸酐、尿酸、氨）的蓄积。
The serum creatinine is not increased unless renal disease is also present.
如果没有肾脏疾患，血清肌酸酐水平一般不升高。

credible [ˈkredəbl] *a.* 可信的，可靠的
His report of the success of the liver transplantation done by Prof. Smith is credible.
他撰写的关于史密斯教授所做肝脏移植手术成功的报道是可信的。

credit [ˈkredit] *n.* 名誉，名望，功劳
He is a physician in high credit.
他是一位有名望的内科医生。
The credit for discovering the new technique goes to two young doctors.
发明该项新技术的功劳，归于两个青年医生。
Credit is given to Li Shizhen for compiling the first book on medicinal herbs in a great volume.
编写第一部中草药巨著的功劳应归于李时珍。

creep [kriːp] *n.* 蠕变，爬行
The modelling of the creep phase was based on the creep recovery test.
蠕变阶段建模是基于蠕变回复试验。
Fluid creep may be influenced by practitioner error.
实际工作者的过失可能影响流体蠕变。

crepitant [ˈkrepitənt] *a.* 劈啪响的，捻发音
Crepitant rales are common in patients with heart failure.
捻发音常见于心衰病人。

crepitation [ˌkrepiˈteiʃən] *n.* 咿轧音，捻发音，水泡音
On examination, coarse crepitations are often heard in patients with bronchopneumonia.
在支气管肺炎病人体检时常可听到有粗的水泡音。

crescendo [kriˈʃendəu] *n.* 逐渐增强，恶化型
Crescendo angina is an intermediate state between stable angina and acute myocardial infarction.
恶化型心绞痛是介于稳定型心绞痛和急性心梗之间的一种临床状态。

crescent [ˈkresənt] *n.* 新月体
Crescents composed of proliferating epithelial cells are seen within the glomeruli.
在肾小球内可见由增生的上皮细胞组成的新月体。

crescentic [kreˈsəntik] *a.* . 新月体性的
Rapidly progressive glomerulonephritis is a syndrome associated with severe glomerular injury, also called crescentic glomerulonephritis.
快速进行性肾小球肾炎是一种与严重肾小球损伤相关的综合征，又称为新月体性肾小球肾炎。
The renal manifestations of crescentic glomerulonephritis include hematuria with red blood cell casts in the urine, moderate proteinuria, and variable hypertension and edema.
新月体性肾小球肾炎的肾脏表现包括：血尿、红细胞管型、中度蛋白尿以及程度不一的高血压和水肿。

cresol [ˈkriːsɔl] *n.* 甲酚，甲苯酚
We discussed the characteristics of adsorption and removal of cresol.
我们讨论了甲酚吸收和消除的特点。

Several animal studies suggest that cresols may act as tumor promotors.
一些动物研究表明甲酚可能是促癌物。

crest [krest] *n.* 嵴;波峰

Find the lumbar spinous processes and then the process at the level of the iliac crest.
查明腰椎各棘突,然后找出髂嵴水平的棘突。

cretinism [ˈkriːtinizm] *n.* 克汀病,呆小病

Cretinism is a syndrome of dwarfism, mental retardation, and coarseness of the skin and facial features due to lack of thyroid hormone from birth.
克汀病是表现为身材矮小、智力低下、皮肤粗糙和容貌特殊的一种综合征,系先天性缺乏甲状腺激素所致。

cricothyroidotomy [ˌkraikəuˌθairɔiˈdɔtəmi] *n.* 环甲膜切开术

A cricothyrotomy is an incision made through the skin and cricothyroid membrane to establish an airway during certain life-threatening situations.
环甲膜切开术是指在某些威胁生命的情况下通过皮肤和环甲韧带置切口来建立通气道。

Cricothyrotomy is easier and quicker to perform than tracheotomy, does not require manipulation of the cervical spine, and is associated with fewer complications.
环甲膜切开术比气管切口操作更容易也更迅速,不需要处理颈椎,而且并发症要少。

crime [kraim] *n.* 犯罪

Crime in Western Europe has increased along with the drug problem.
在西欧,犯罪随着吸毒问题在不断上升。

criminal [ˈkriminəl] *a.* 犯罪的,违法的

Criminal investigations are under state or federal government authority.
州或联邦政府人员才可进行犯罪的调查。

cripple [ˈkripl] *v.* 使残疾,使损伤

The crippled virus becomes harmless.
这种有缺陷的病毒变得对人无害。

crisis [ˈkraisis] (*pl.* crises [ˈkraisiːz]) *n.* 危机,危象;骤退

The fever may fall by crisis or lysis.
发热可以骤退或渐退。

The ICU(intensive care unit) is frequently the scene of crisis situations.
重症监护室是危象多发之地。

criterion [kraiˈtiəriən](*pl.* criteria [kraiˈtiəriə]) *n.* 标准,准则

One major criterion for classification is the morphology of bacteria, i. e. , their size and shape.
细菌的形态,即其大小和形状,是分类的一个主要标准。

The presence or absence of metastases is one of the most important criteria in determining the prognosis of an individual cancer case.
转移出现与否,在决定每个恶性瘤病例的预后上是最重要的标准之一。

critical [ˈkritikəl] *a.* 关键的;危急的,临界的

It is critical in management of a patient with placenta previa that no digital vaginal or rectal examination be performed.
处理前置胎盘患者,禁止做阴道指检或肛门检查是非常关键的。

Family members of a patient in a critical care unit may be restricted as to how long they may visit.
危重病房的病人,其家属探视的时间要受到限制。

The mechanical sensor arm enables the surgeon to see the exact relationship of the sinuses to critical nearby areas such as the eye socket and the brain.
这种机械臂可以使外科医生清楚地看到鼻窦与眼窝和大脑等紧邻结构间的确切关系。

cromoglycate [ˌkrəuməˈglaikeit] *n.* 色甘酸盐

Those who have symptoms which are troublesome despite adequate bronchodilator therapy should be tried on sodium cromoglycate.
在使用了充分的支气管扩张剂治疗后仍有不令人满意的症状时，应当试用色甘酸钠。

cromolyn [ˈkrəuməlin] *n.* 色甘酸

The aim of this study was to compare cromolyn sodium cream 4% with placebo for the treatment of renal pruritus.
本研究的目的是比较4%色甘酸钠奶油和安慰剂对肾脏疾病引起的瘙痒症的疗效。

Cromolyn sodium can be used by pregnant women and children.
色甘酸钠可以用于孕妇和儿童。

crospovidone [ˌkrɔsˈpəuvidəun] *n.* 交聚维酮

The results show that crospovidone Type B is more effective in enhancing the dissolution rate of poorly soluble drugs.
结果显示B型交聚维酮可以更有效地提高难溶性药物的溶解速率。

The superdisintegrant AC-Di-Sol and crospovidone were used for immediate release of drug from tablet.
表面崩解剂交联羧甲基纤维素钠和交聚维酮可用于促进片剂中药物的快速释放。

cross [krɔs] *n.* 十字形，交叉

The nervous system and the endocrine system demonstrate pharmacologic cross reactivities.
神经系统与内分泌系统在药理学上有交叉反应。

crossing-over [krɔsiŋˈəuvə] *n.* 交换，互换，交叉

Interchange of segments of homologous chromatids is termed crossing-over.
同源的染色单体间片段的交换称为互换。

Crossing-over occurs while the chromosomes are in synapsis.
互换发生在染色体联合时。

In cross-over trial the patients act as their own controls, new treatment and control treatment being applied in random order.
交叉试验中，病人自己起对照作用，新疗法与对照疗法被随机交替使用。

cross-linkage [ˈkrɔsˈliŋkidʒ] *n.* 交联键

The cross-linkages may be of several sorts: hydrogen bonds, salt links or sulphur bridges.
交联键可能有几种：氢键、盐键或硫桥。

The sulphur bridges are the strongest cross-linkages.
硫桥是最强的交联键。

cross-match [ˈkrɔs-ˈmætʃ] *v.* 交叉配血

Blood was drawn for hemoglobin and hematocrit as well as for type and cross-match.
采血是为了血液分型和交叉试验，也为了测血红蛋白和血细胞容量。

cross-presentation [krɔs, prezənˈteiʃən] *n.* 交叉递呈，交叉提呈

Phagosomes are competent organelles for antigen cross-presentation.
吞噬小体是胜任抗原交叉提呈的细胞器。

MHC Class Ⅰ-restricted cross-presentation is biased towards high dose antigens and those released during cellular destruction.
MHC-Ⅰ类分子限制性的交叉提呈偏向于高剂量抗原和那些细胞损伤时释放的抗原。

cross-reaction [ˈkrɔsriˈækʃən] *n.* 交叉反应

Cross-reaction tests were done with purified monoclonal antibody.
对纯化后的单克隆抗体进行交叉反应试验。

A similar cross-reaction explains the allergy to apple skin found in southern Europe.
类似的交叉反应解释了南欧人对苹果皮过敏的原因。

crossreactivity [ˌkrɔsri(ː)ækˈtiviti] *n.* 交叉反应性

Similarly steroids exhibit no physiologically significant crossreactivity among their receptors.

同样，类固醇激素对于相应受体不发生生理显著性的交叉反应性。

croton [ˈkrəutən] *n.* 巴豆

It is said that ten drops of croton oil, taken internally, will have fatal results.

据说摄入十滴巴豆油会致死。

We want to observe the inhibiting effect of croton oil on the growth of multi-drug-resistance mycobacterium tuberculosis in vitro.

我们想观察巴豆油体外对多重耐药结核杆菌的生长抑制作用。

crotonaldehyde [ˌkrəutəˈnældəhaid] *n.* 巴豆醛

The hydrogenation of crotonaldehyde has been studied.

已研究了巴豆醛的氢化作用。

Studies on selective catalytic hydrogenation of crotonaldehyde have aroused wide concern.

巴豆醛选择性催化加氢的研究引起广泛关注。

crown [kraun] *n.* 着冠

Once the fetal head is "crowned" the patient should be discouraged from bearing down by telling her to take rapid shallow breaths.

一旦胎头"着冠"，让患者作快速而浅的呼吸，勿再向下用力。

crucial [ˈkruːʃəl] *a.* 决定性的

Identifying both the etiology and pathophysiologic mechanisms of megaloblastic anemia is crucial.

弄清巨幼红细胞性贫血的病因和病理生理两种机制才是至关重要的。

The diagnosis is crucial to the problem.

诊断对解决这个问题是极其重要的。

cruciferous [krusiˈferəs] *a.* 十字花科的，有十字形的

Scientists hope to be able to tell consumers which cruciferous plants offer the greatest protection against cancer.

科学家们希望能够告诉消费者哪种十字花科植物抗癌能力最强。

crude [kruːd] *a.* 天然的，粗糙的

A simpler system, which provides a crude measure of complement activity is single-radial hemolysis.

一种提供天然补体活化测定的简单系统是单向辐射溶血。

Plain films of the kidneys provide a crude index of renal anatomy.

肾脏的平片显示肾脏大致的解剖学结构。

crumble [ˈkrʌmbl] *v.* 粉碎，崩溃，瓦解

The doctor keeps telling me that if I continue to drink a lot of carbonated drinks, my bones will crumble.

医生告诫我如果我再继续饮用大量的碳酸饮料我的骨骼系统会出严重问题。

Crumble the peanuts up so that the old woman can have some.

把花生米捣碎，老妇人才能吃点。

crust [krʌst] *n.* 外壳；痂

Copper is an abundant element making up approximately 0.1% of the earth's crust.

铜是一种丰富的元素，约占地壳组成的0.1%。

crutch [krʌtʃ] *n.* 拐杖

The patient will soon get used to walking on the crutches.

病人不久就会习惯于架拐走路了。

cryoglobulin [ˌkraiəuˈglɔbjulin] *n.* 冷球蛋白

Cryoglobulins are immunoglobulins that precipitate in the cold.

冷球蛋白是一种有遇冷沉淀现象的免疫球蛋白。

cryosurgery [ˈkraiəuˈsəːdʒəri] *n.* 冷冻手术

Cryosurgery has its proponents in the poor risk patient.

对手术耐受差的病人,有人尝试用冷冻治疗。

cryotherapy [ˌkraiəu'θerəpi] *n.* 冷冻疗法,冷凝疗法

If there are only a few lesions, cryotherapy with liquid nitrogen is the most rapid and satisfactory treatment.

如果病变少,那么最快和最令人满意的疗法是液氮冷冻治疗。

cryptdin ['kripdin] *n.* 隐窝素

Paneth cells in small intestine crypts secrete microbicidal alpha-defensins, termed cryptdins, as components of enteric innate immunity.

小肠隐窝潘氏细胞分泌杀菌的 α-防御素,即隐窝素,属小肠天然免疫的组成成分。

cryptic ['kriptik] *a.* 神秘的,含义模糊的; [动] 隐藏的

These alternative sites are termed cryptic splice sites because they are normally not used by the splicing apparatus when the correct site is available.

这些可选择的位点被称为隐藏性拼接位点,因为在通常情况下若有正确的位点可利用,那么这些位点并不会被使用。

They can be quite cryptic, but are worth learning because of the inherent power they give you for text processing.

它们可能十分神秘,但是值得您去学一学,因为它们给予您内在的能力去进行文本处理。

cryptococcal [ˌkriptəu'kɔkl] *a.* 隐球菌的

Diagnosis is greatly assisted by positive cryptococcal antigen response or possive culture results, or both.

隐球菌抗原反应或培养为阳性结果,或两者均为阳性者对诊断的帮助很大。

cryptogenic [ˌkriptəu'dʒenik] *a.* 隐源性的,病因不明的

In about 20% of cases the inciting cause of the cirrhosis cannot be determined, so labeled as cryptogenic cirrhosis.

肝硬化的激发原因约 20% 的病例难以确定,被认为是隐源性肝硬化。

Transfusion-transmitted virus (TTV) would be accounted for part of the reason in patients with cryptogenic hepatitis.

输血传播病毒可以解释病人患隐源性肝炎的部分病因。

cryptopatche ['kriptəpætʃi] *n.* 隐窝小结

Cryptopatches are aggregates of lymphoid tissue in the wall of the intestine.

隐窝小结就是肠壁淋巴组织的集合。

cryptospermia [ˌkriptəu'spəːmiə] *n.* 少精子症

After the operation, the sperm density increased by 62. 5% of the patients with varicocele, while the cases with azoospermia (cryptospermia) showed no significant improvement.

精索静脉曲张患者在手术后精子密度提高了 62. 5%,但少精症患者无明显改善。

cryptosporidiosis [ˌkriptəuspəˌridiː'əusis] *n.* 隐孢子虫病

Cryptosporidiosis is an important apicomplexan disease with medical and veterinary significance.

隐孢子虫病是一种重要的人兽共患的原虫病。

In this paper, cryptosporidium and the occurrence, epidemiological characteristics, symptoms and influence of cryptosporidiosis are reviewed.

本文对隐孢子虫及隐孢虫病的发生、流行病学特点、症状和影响进行了综合评述。

Polymerase chain reaction (PCR) is another way to diagnose cryptosporidiosis.

聚合酶链反应(PCR)是另一种对隐孢虫病作出诊断的方法。

cryptosporidium [ˌkriptəuspɔː'ridiəm] *n.* 隐孢子虫属

Another less common protozoa in AIDS patients is cryptosporidium.

艾滋病病人另一种少见的感染是隐孢子虫感染。

crystalline ['kristəlain] *a.* 结晶的,晶状的

Sanamycin is a reddish yellow crystalline substance which has a cytostatic action.

萨纳霉素(放线菌素 C)为带微红的黄色结晶物质,具有抑制细胞作用。

crystallize [ˈkristəlaiz] *v.* 使结晶,使成形

However, some viruses have been crystallized and these crystals are capable of infecting cells.

然而,有些病毒已形成晶体,这些晶体能使细胞感染。

They further crystallized these observations into a system of medicine.

他们进一步把这些观察提炼成为一个医学体系。

crystalluria [ˌkristəˈljuəriə] *n.* (结)晶尿症

Good urine flow should be maintained by adequate fluid intake to prevent crystalluria.

饮用足够的液体以便保持足够的尿量来防止晶尿症。

cubic [ˈkjuːbik] *a.* 立方的,立方体的,立方形的

There are about 7,500 white blood cells per cubic millimeter of blood.

在每立方毫米的血液中大约含有 7500 个白细胞。

The columnar epithelium is replaced by cubic or even flattened epithelium.

柱状上皮由立方形上皮或甚至由扁平上皮替代。

cuff [kʌf] *n.* 袖口(状构造);环带

The vest, developed by researchers at Johns Hopkins University, looks like an oversize blood pressure cuff.

约翰斯·霍普金斯大学研究人员研制的这种背心看起来就像一个特大号的量血压袖带。

culdocentesis [ˌkʌldəusenˈtiːsis] *n.* 后穹隆穿刺术

If ultrasonography is not available, you can use culdocentesis.

在不能得到超声探查时,可使用后穹隆穿刺术。

culminate [ˈkʌlmineit] *v.* 到绝顶,达到高潮;使结束

Endoplasmic reticulum (ER) stress triggers tissue-specific responses that culminate in either cellular adaptation or apoptosis。

内质网应激引发组织特异性反应,最终导致细胞适应性改变或者凋亡。

These data suggest that short-term hyperglycemia initiates compensatory mechanisms, which culminate in improvements in the ventricular response, infarcted area, and mortality rate in diabetic rats exposed to ischemic injury.

这些数据表明,在暴露于缺血损害的糖尿病大鼠,短期高血糖引发代偿机制,最终使心室反应、梗塞区域和死亡率得到改善。

culprit [ˈkʌlprit] *n.* 元凶,事故的原因

The new findings suggest the culprit causing rejection is a class of immune system cells called natural killer(NK) cells.

新近研究成果提示,排斥的根本原因在于一种免疫系统细胞,名为自然杀伤细胞。

cultivate [ˈkʌltiveit] *v.* 培养

Experimenters often cultivate living micro-organisms in artificial media.

实验人员常在人工培养基内培养活的微生物。

cultivation [ˌkʌltiˈveiʃən] *n.* 培养

Chlamydiae are bacteria which require living cells(cell culture) for cultivation.

衣原体是需要在活体细胞中培养的细菌(细胞培养)。

culture [ˈkʌltʃə] *n.* 培养

Thus, blood cultures must be obtained immediately when endocarditis is suspected clinically.

因此,临床上一旦怀疑为心内膜炎,须立即进行血液培养。

The method of making cultures of tissues is one of the greatest achievements of contemporary science.

组织培养法是当代科学上最大的成就之一。

v. 培养

The spinal fluid should be cultured for bacteria, mycobacteria, and fungi.

应对脑脊液做细菌、分枝杆菌和真菌培养。

cumulate [ˈkjuːmjuleit] *v.* 堆积，累积

Atheromatous substances cumulate in the arterial intima forming atherosclerosis.

粥样化物质堆积在动脉内膜内形成动脉粥样硬化。

cumulative [ˈkjuːmjulətiv] *a.* 累积的

The effects of exposure to X-rays are cumulative.

暴露于 X 线所造成的后果是累加的。

In polygenic inheritance, each gene contributes to the whole effect in cumulative fashion.

在多基因遗传中，每个基因的作用效果对整体是累积式的。

cupping [ˈkʌpiŋ] *n.* 拔火罐；拔罐疗法

Cupping is a therapeutic approach by attaching small jars in which a vaccum is created.

拔火罐通过负压吸住小的罐状器来产生治疗作用。

curable [ˈkjuərəbl] *a.* 可医好的

Colon cancer is highly curable in its early stages.

结肠癌在其发病早期阶段是很有可能治好的。

Treated early, skin cancer is highly curable.

只要及早治疗，皮肤癌是很有可能治好的。

curative [ˈkjuərətiv] *a.* 治疗的，医治的

For curative purpose of bronchitis or coughs, a reliable cough mixture should first be sought for.

治疗支气管炎或咳嗽首先需选用可靠的止咳合剂。

The other class includes the many conditions for which there is no specific curative treatment.

另外一类疾病包括那些没有特异治愈方法的病症。

curcumenol [kəːˈkjuːmenəl] *n.* 莪术醇，莪术烯醇

It provides the basis for purification and standardization of curcumenol reference substance.

它为莪术醇对照品的纯化和标准化提供了依据。

Our objective is to determine the difference of the effective constituents of curcumenol, curzerenone and germacrone in Rhizoma Curcumae from different areas.

我们的目的是测定不同产地莪术药材中莪术烯醇、莪术酮和吉马酮有效成分的差异。

curcumin [ˈkəːkjumin] *n.* 姜黄素，姜黄色素

But they wanted to pinpoint the exact components in curcumin, which is a kind of complex compound.

但他们想查明姜黄素中的确切成分，因为姜黄素是一类混合物。

We developed a reversed-phase HPLC method for the quantitative determination of curcumin.

我们制定了反相高效液相色谱法测定姜黄素含量的方法。

curd [kəːd] *n.* 凝乳

The curd time of Streptococcus thermophilus ferment milk was shortened from 12h to 4h.

嗜热链球菌发酵乳的凝乳时间从 12 小时缩短到 4 小时。

Curds are a dairy product obtained by curdling milk with rennet or an edible acidic substance such as lemon juice or vinegar.

凝乳是用柠檬汁或醋使牛奶凝化而成的乳制品。

curettage [ˌkjuriˈtɑːʒ, kjuəˈretidʒ] *n.* [法] 刮(除)术

Curettage may reveal that there is a local cause for the irregular bleeding.

刮宫可显示不规则出血的局部原因。

Hysteroscope and diagnostic curettage are important methods to diagnose the unusual bleeding.

宫腔镜和诊断性刮宫不失为异常出血的重要诊断手段。

Cervical curettage is the usual method of diagnosis.

子宫颈刮术是诊断的常用方法。

curie [ˈkjuəri] *n.* 居里

Millicurie is a unit of radioactivity, equal to one thousandth of a curie.
毫居里放射单位,等于千分之一居里。
The Curie temperature and saturation magnetization increase with the Fe content.
居里温度和饱和磁化强度都随着 Fe 含量的增加而增高。

curious [ˈkjuəriəs] *a.* 好奇的
A good medical worker is always curious.
优良的医学工作者总是好奇的。

currently [ˈkʌrəntli] *ad.* 当前
Many strains of bacteria and fungi are naturally resistant to all currently available antibiotics and other chemotherapeutic drugs.
许多细菌株和真菌株,能自然地抵抗所有现在使用的抗生素和其他化疗药物。
It is currently unknown whether the occurrence of these two lesions is coincidental.
目前还不清楚,这两种损害是否碰巧同时发生。

curriculum [kəˈrikjuləm] *n.* 课程
During the final two years, the curriculum consists of the clinical subjects.
最后两年的课程包括各种临床学科。

curvature [ˈkəːvətʃə] *n.* 弯曲
Deficiency of vitamin D is responsible for rickets in children, causing bones to become soft and liable to curvature.
缺乏维生素 D 可使儿童患佝偻病,造成骨骼变软并易于弯曲。

curve [kəːv] *n.* 弯曲;曲线,曲线图表
The spinal column of a human being has thoracic, lumber and sacral curves besides the cervical one.
人的脊柱除了颈曲之外还有胸曲、腰曲和骶曲。
When hypoxia occurs consequent to respiratory failure, $PaCO_2$ usually rises and the oxygen dissociation curve is displaced to the right.
当低氧血症由呼吸衰竭所致时,CO_2 分压通常增高,同时氧分离曲线向右侧偏移。

cusp [kʌsp] *n.* 瓣尖,瓣叶
Echocardiography will demonstrate dilatation of the aortic root and the separation of the cusps.
超声心动图检查可见主动脉根部扩张,瓣叶分开。

customary [ˈkʌstəməri] *a.* 通常的,习惯的
It is customary to use an appropriate safety factor or a mathematical model.
通常采用一种合适的安全因子或数学模型。
It is now customary to use the CD marker to indicate the molecule recognized by each group of monoclonal antibody.
现在常用 CD 标志来表示被每组单克隆抗体所识别的分子。

cutaneous [kju(ː)ˈteinjəs] *a.* 皮(肤)的
A large number of growth factors and cytokines are involved in cutaneous wound healing.
大量生长因子和细胞因子参与皮肤创伤的愈合过程。
In textbooks of medicine, there is a chapter describing in detail the major systemic disorders that can be identified by cutaneous signs.
医学教科书中有一章详细介绍了可通过皮肤的体征来进行诊断的主要的全身性疾病。

cyanide [ˈsaiənaid] *n.* 氰化物
Many toxicants produce immediate toxic effects, a notable example being cyanide poisoning.
许多毒物产生即发性毒性效应,其典型的例子是氰化物中毒。
Sodium or potassium cyanide taken by mouth may also cause death within minutes.
口服氰化钠或氰化钾在几分钟内亦可致死。

cyanobacteria [ˌsaiənəbækˈtiəriə] *n.* 蓝菌

Because these organisms possess a procaryotic cell strucure, they have been renamed the cyanobacteria.
因为该类生物具有原核生物的细胞结构,故被重新命名为蓝菌。

cyanobacterium [ˌsaiənəubæk'tiəriəm] *n.* 蓝细菌,蓝藻门
Cyanobacterium is a phylum of bacteria that obtain their energy through photosynthesis.
蓝细菌是一类通过光合作用获得能量的细菌。

cyanocobalamin [saiənəukə'bæləmin] *n.* 氰钴胺,维生素 B_{12}
Vitamin B_{12} or cyanocobalamin was isolated and crystallized from liver in 1948.
维生素 B_{12} 或氰钴胺素是在 1948 年从肝脏组织分离和结晶出来的。

cyanosis [saiə'nəusis] *n.* 发绀,青紫
Entry of the tube into the larynx may produce cyanosis.
管子插进喉部以后,可以出现发绀。
With right ventricular failure the cyanosis deepens and peripheral edema becomes prominent.
有右心室衰竭时,发绀加深,外周水肿更明显。

cyanotic [saiə'nɔtik] *a.* 发绀的,青紫的
The bluish color of a cyanotic patient is usually most marked in the lips, nail beds, ears, and malar eminences.
发绀病人的淡蓝色通常在嘴唇、指甲床、耳部和颧骨隆起部最明显。
The patient with predominant bronchitis is often overweight and cyanotic.
以支气管炎为主要病变的患者,常超重并有发绀。

cyclase ['saikleis] *n.* 环化酶
Adenylate cyclase is the enzyme that converts adenosine triphosphate(ATP) to cAMP.
腺苷酸环化酶是转变三磷酸腺苷为环腺苷酸的酶。

cyclodextrin [ˌsaikləu'dekstrin] *n.* 环糊精
Cyclodextrins are a group of structurally related natural products formed during bacterial digestion of cellulose.
环糊精是细菌消化纤维素时产生的一组结构相关的天然产物。
Cyclodextrins are produced from starch by means of enzymatic conversion.
环糊精是由淀粉经酶消化后产生的。

cyclophilin [saikləu'filin] *n.* 环孢亲和素,亲环蛋白,亲环素
Cyclophilin A could participate in the tumorigenesis, invasion, cell proliferation, vascular growth of oral squamous cell carcinoma.
环孢亲和素 A 可能参与口腔鳞状细胞癌的发生、侵袭、增殖、血管生长等过程。

cyclophosphamide [ˌsaikləu'fɔsfəmaid] *n.* 环磷酰胺
Cyclophosphamide is a powerful immunosuppressive drug that is more toxic for B than T lymphocytes.
环磷酰胺是一种强有力的免疫抑制剂,它对 B 淋巴细胞的毒性强于 T 细胞。
Immunosuppressive therapy(cyclophosphamide) is thought by some to decrease the frequency of attacks and stabilize progressive disease.
有些人认为采用免疫抑制治疗(环磷酰胺)可降低发作频率并稳定病情。
Cyclophosphamide is mainly used together with other chemotherapy agents in the treatment of lymphomas, some forms of leukemia and some solid tumors.
环磷酰胺主要是与其他化疗药物一起使用来治疗淋巴瘤、某些白血病和某些实体瘤。

cyclosporin [ˌsaikləu'spɔːrin] *n.* 环孢菌素
Cyclosporin A is a fungal metabolite.
环孢菌素 A 是一种真菌的代谢产物。
Cyclosporin, however, suppresses only part of the body's immune system.
然而,环孢菌素只能抑制人体的部分免疫系统。

Interferon and cyclosporin A are not used for this infection.
干扰素和环孢菌素 A 不能用于治疗这种感染。

cyclothymia [ˌsaikləu'θaimiə] *n.* 循环性情感气质

Cyclothymia is a term to designate the milder forms of depressive and elated mood-swings.
周期性情绪波动症是一个用来表明轻型的抑郁和兴奋情绪波动的术语。

cyclotron ['saikləˌtrɔn] *n.* 回旋加速器

Today many radioisotopes are produced using the particle accelerator called a cyclotron.
今天许多放射性同位素是用被称为回旋加速器的粒子加速器来制造的。

China's first atomic reactor and cyclotron were built in 1958.
中国的第一个原子反应堆和回旋加速器建于 1958 年。

cylinder ['silində] *n.* 圆柱,圆柱体

Some cells grow as elongated cylinders or produce long shoots or branches.
有些细胞长成长圆柱状或长出触角或长出分枝。

cylindrical [si'lindrikəl] *a.* 圆柱状的

The cylindrical bacteria are known as bacilli.
圆柱形细菌被称为杆菌。

cynamorlum [sinə'mɔːləm] *n.* 肉苁蓉

Where are the Cynamorlum listing and contents?
肉苁蓉的清单和目录在哪?

Do you want to show cynamorlum or other products of your own company?
你想展示自己公司的肉苁蓉或者其他产品吗?

Cynanchol ['sinəkəl] *n.* 白薇醇

Cynanchol is a crystalline substance obtained from the milky juice of Cynanchum Linn.
白薇醇是从白前的根的乳汁中提取的一种透明物质。

Cynanchol can lower fever and promote diuresis.
白薇醇能够降温和利尿。

cyperene ['saipərin] *n.* 香附烯

The efficacy of Aifunuangong Wan may have something to do with its element of cyperene.
艾附暖宫丸的功效与其含有的成分香附子烯有关。

However, there is no reported evidence for the antioxidative activity of cyperene.
然而,没有已报道的证据证明香附烯有抗氧化活性。

cyst [sist] *n.* 囊肿,(包)囊

When punctured, such cysts yield an exudate.
当穿刺时,这样的囊肿产生渗出液。

Hydatid cysts occur more frequently in the liver than in any other organ.
包虫囊在肝脏里比在任何其他器官更为多见。

cystadenoma [sistədi'nəumə] *n.* 囊腺瘤

With the formation of retained fluid such a structure becomes a papillary serous cystadenoma.
随着液体蓄积,这一结构就变成乳头状浆液性囊腺瘤。

An ovarian borderline mucinous cystadenoma is a sub type of ovarian mucinous tumors and as the name stands, it is intermediate between a mucinous cystadenoma and a mucinous cystadenocarcinoma.
卵巢交界性黏液性囊腺瘤是卵巢黏液性肿瘤的子类型,正如其名,是介于黏液性囊腺瘤和黏液性囊腺癌之间的一种类型。

cystathionine β-synthase [ˌsistə'θaiəniːn-'beitə-'sinθeis] *n.* 胱硫醚 β-合酶

Cystathionine β-synthase has a common 68 base pair insertion/deletion polymorphism that has been linked to folate levels.
胱硫醚 β-合酶基因中有一常见的 68 个碱基对的插入/缺失型多态性,被认为与体内叶酸

盐的水平有关。

cystectomy [sisˈtektətmi] *n.* 膀胱切除术

Cystectomy is necessary in the treatment of certain bladder conditions, notably cancer.

在治疗某些膀胱疾患,特别是膀胱癌时,必须施行膀胱切除术。

cysteine [ˈsisˌtiiːn] *n.* 半胱氨酸

Cysteine is an α-amino acid with the chemical formula HO_2CCH.

半胱氨酸是一种 α-氨基酸,分子式为 HO_2CCH。

Cysteine is an essential amino acid and plays an important role in cell functions.

半胱氨酸是一种基本氨基酸,在细胞功能中起着重要作用。

cystic [ˈsistik] *a.* 囊的;囊性的

On inspection alone, cystic tumours may be indistinguishable from ascites.

仅凭望诊不能将囊肿与腹水加以区别。

Respiratory failure is the most dangerous consequence of cystic fibrosis.

呼吸衰竭是囊性纤维化最危险的后果。

Disease registries are defined by patients having the same diagnosis, such as cystic fibrosis or heart failure.

疾病注册被定义为有相同诊断的病人,如囊性纤维化或心力衰竭。

cystine [ˈsistiːn] *n.* 胱氨酸

The first-limited amino acids are methionine and cystine in two kinds of milk.

两种牛奶中的第一限制氨基酸都是蛋氨酸和胱氨酸。

Suitable quantities of tryptophan, arginine, cystine, glycine and serine were used to supplement the medium.

给培养基补充适量的色氨酸、精氨酸、胱氨酸、甘氨酸和丝氨酸。

cystitis [sisˈtaitis] *n.* 膀胱炎

Cystitis and acute pyelonephritis may occur together or independently.

膀胱炎与急性肾盂肾炎可以同时或单独发生。

cystoma [sisˈtəumə] *n.* 囊瘤

A cystoma is a tumor containing cyst of neoplastic origin.

囊瘤是一种包含有瘤源性囊的肿瘤。

Its management is essentially the same as that described for simple serous cystoma.

其处理与对于单纯浆液性囊瘤所描述者,基本上是一样的。

cystoscope [ˈsistɔskəup] *n.* 膀胱镜

The cystoscope consists of a metal sheath surrounding a telescope and light-conducting bundles.

膀胱镜由望远镜与光导纤维束构成,其外罩有一层金属套管。

cystoscopy [sisˈtɔskəpi] *n.* 膀胱镜检查

Let' s proceed to cystoscopy and retrograde pyelography if necessary.

必要时我们可进行膀胱镜检查和逆行性肾盂造影。

cytochalasin [ˌsaitəukəˈlæsən] *n.* 细胞松弛素

Cytochalasins are fungal metabolites that have the ability to bind to actin filaments and block polymerization and the elongation of actin.

细胞松弛素是真菌代谢物,能与肌动蛋白丝结合并阻止肌动蛋白的聚合和伸长。

Cytochalasins can change cellular morphology, inhibit cellular processes such as cell division, and even cause cells to undergo apoptosis.

细胞松弛素能够改变细胞形态,抑制细胞过程如细胞分裂,甚至导致细胞遭受凋亡。

cytochrome [ˈsaitəkrəum] *n.* 细胞色素

Cytochromes act as electron transfer agents in biological oxidation-reduction reactions.

细胞色素是生物氧化-还原反应中的电子传递体。

Certain carrier molecules in electron transport chain are cytochromes.

电子传递链中的某些载体分子是细胞色素。

cytogenetics [ˌsaitəudʒiˈnetiks] *n.* 细胞遗传学

Clinical cytogenetics is the study of chromosomes, their structure and their inheritance, as applied to the practice of medical genetics.

临床细胞遗传学是研究染色体及其结构与遗传性,并将之应用于医学遗传学实践的一门学科。

We will discuss the general principles of cytogenetics and the various types of numerical and structural abnormalities observed in human karyotypes.

我们将讨论细胞遗传学的基本原理,以及人类核型中看到的不同类型的数目或者结构异常。

cytokine [saitəuˈkain] *n.* 细胞因子

Cytokine is the general term for a large group of molecules involved in signalling between cells during immune response.

细胞因子是在免疫应答中介导细胞间信息传递的一大类分子的总称。

All cytokines are proteins or peptides, some with sugar molecules attached(glycoproteins).

细胞因子均为蛋白质或多肽,有些与糖基连接(糖蛋白)。

cytokinesis [ˌsaitəukaiˈniːsis] *n.* 胞质分裂

In cell division, cytoplasmic division is referred to as cytokinesis.

在细胞分裂过程中,细胞质的分裂叫做胞质分裂。

The visible division processes in cell division are nuclear division and cytokinesis.

在细胞分裂过程中可以观察到的分裂为核分裂和胞质分裂。

cytology [saiˈtɔlədʒi] *n.* 细胞学

Clinical cytology can be a great assistance if properly understood and utilized.

如能正确地理解和利用临床细胞学,那是极其有帮助的。

Biopsy and exfoliative cytology can give histological confirmation.

活检和脱落上皮的细胞学检查可以提供组织学上的证据。

cytolysin [saiˈtɔlisin] *n.* 溶细胞素

Cholesterol-dependent cytolysins are secreted from various types of bacteria and are involved in various diseases.

胆固醇依赖的溶细胞素系由多种细菌分泌,许多疾病均受此影响。

Cytolysin is secreted by cells to dissolve other cells.

溶细胞素由细胞分泌,用于溶解其他细胞。

This microorganism secretes a few extracellular products including capsular polysaccharide (CPS), protease, cytolysin and phospholipase.

这种微生物能分泌多种细胞外产物,包括荚膜多醣体、蛋白酶、溶细胞素与磷脂酶等。

cytolysis [saiˈtɔlisis] *n.* 细胞溶解

Cytolysis is a cell death that occurs because of a rupture in the cell' s membrane.

细胞溶解是一种细胞死亡,它的发生是因为细胞的膜破裂。

The ultrastructure changes showed various degrees of degeneration and edema and focal cytolysis necrosis in liver, heart, lung and kidney.

超微结构变化显示肝、心、肺、肾出现不同程度的变性、水肿以及局灶性细胞溶解坏死。

cytomegalovirus [ˌsaitəuˌmegələuˈvaiərəs] *n.* 巨细胞病毒

Cytomegalovirus is a very frequent pathogen in patients with AIDS.

巨细胞病毒是艾滋病患者极常被感染的病原体。

Congenital cytomegalovirus appears to be the most common cause of chronic intrauterine infection.

先天性巨细胞病毒看来是慢性宫内感染最常见的原因。

cytometry [saiˈtɔmitri] *n.* 血细胞计数(仪)

Aneaphoid cells in mucosal epithelium of gastric antrum were detected by Flow cytometry.
胃窦黏膜上皮内的异倍体细胞可用流式细胞仪检出。

cytopathic [ˌsaitəˈpæθik] *a.* 细胞病变的

It produced obvious cytopathic effects in Marc145 cells.
它在 Marc145 细胞上产生明显的细胞病变。

Two strains of cytopathic rotavirus (AN1 and AN2) were isolated.
已分离出两株细胞病变的轮状病毒(AN1 和 AN2)。

cytopathology [ˌsaitəupəˈθɔlədʒi] *n.* 细胞病理学

5 to 10ml of subarachnoid fluid should be sent to the cytopathology laboratory to determine if there are malignant cells.
应送 5 ~ 10ml 脑脊液到细胞病理学实验室,以确定其是否有恶变细胞。

cytopenia [ˌsaitəuˈpiːniə] *n.* 血细胞减少(症)

Laboratory abnormalities include cytopenias and elevated alkaline phosphatase with liver involvement.
实验室检查的异常包括有血细胞减少和由于肝脏受损引起的碱性磷酸酶升高。

Increased destruction of the cellular elements is the fundamental mechanism of the cytopenia.
血细胞减少的根本原因是由于细胞的破坏增加。

cytoplasm [ˈsaitəplæzəm] *n.* 细胞浆

The cytoplasm is enclosed by the plasma membrane.
细胞浆由浆膜包裹。

cytoplasmic [ˌsaitəuˈplæzmik] *a.* 细胞质的,细胞浆的

Cytoplasmic division is termed cytokinesis; nuclear division is termed mitosis.
细胞质的分裂称为胞质分裂,细胞核的分裂称为有丝分裂。

Cytoplasmic division usually occurs during cell division.
细胞质分裂通常发生在细胞分裂的过程中。

cytoreduction [ˌsaitəuriˈdʌkʃən] *n.* 缩减细胞,细胞减少

Moreover, the expression of the gene has close relationship with tumor prognosis and cytoreduction mediated by adenoviruses.
此外,该基因的表达与肿瘤的预后和腺病毒介导的减瘤效应有密切的关系。

Surgery is necessary for diagnosis, accurate staging and optimal cytoreduction, and is crucial for the successful treatment of EOC (epithelial ovarian cancer).
手术对上皮性卵巢癌的诊断、精确分期和最理想的减瘤是必需的,并且对于成功的治疗也是关键。

cytoreductive [ˌsaitəuriˈdʌktiv] *a.* 减少细胞的

Since the leukemic transition may take up to 10yr and since early therapy(with currently available cytoreductive agents) of the pre-leukemic phase does not result in improved survival, no special therapy is indicated.
由于转变成白血病可能需时 10 年之久,而且白血病前期的早期治疗(用目前可用的减少细胞的药剂)并不能延长存活时间,因此没有特异疗法可推荐。

cytosine [ˈsaitəˌsiːn] *n.* 胞嘧啶

Four heterocyclic compounds were: maltol, allantoin, adenosine, cytosine.
四种杂环化合物分别是:麦芽酚、尿囊素、腺苷、胞嘧啶。

Cytosine is one of the four main bases found in DNA and RNA.
胞嘧啶是 DNA 和 RNA 中的四种主要碱基之一。

cytoskeletal [ˌsaitəuˈskelitəl] *n.* 细胞骨架的

Chemicals that bind to tubulin or actin impair the assembly and/or disassembly of these cytoskeletal proteins.
结合到微管蛋白或机动蛋白上的化学物质能损伤这些细胞骨架蛋白的组合和(或)分解。

cytoskeleton [ˌsaitəu'skelitən] *n.* 细胞支架，细胞骨架

These molecules traverse the membrane and are linked to the cell's cytoskeleton.

这些分子穿过胞膜并连接成细胞的支架。

The cytoskeleton enable eukaryotic cell to carry out activities impossible for prokaryotic organisms.

细胞骨架使真核细胞能够完成原核细胞不可能完成的活动。

cytotoxic [ˌsaitəu'tɔksik] *a.* 细胞毒素的

From our discussions, we will assume that high concentration of metal and metalloid ions are cytotoxic.

通过我们的讨论，我们愿设想那些高浓度的金属和类金属的离子都是具有细胞毒性的。

Cytotoxic chemotherapy has recently altered the dismal prognosis in some cases of ovarian cancer.

细胞毒素化疗近来改变了某些卵巢癌病例令人绝望的预后。

cytotoxicity [ˌsaitəutɔk'sisiti] *n.* 细胞毒性，细胞毒作用

The cytotoxicity of tobacco smoke can be tested with short-term predictive assays.

烟草烟雾的细胞毒性可通过短期预测分析来测定。

Cytotoxicity assays are widely used by the pharmaceutical industry to screen for cytotoxicity in compound libraries.

在制药业，细胞毒性试验广泛用于筛选化合物数据库中各种化合物的细胞毒性。

D

dacryoadenitis [ˌdækriəuˌædiˈnaitis] *n.* 泪腺炎

Diagnosis of chronic granulomatous dacryoadenitis often requires lacrimal gland biopsy.

慢性肉芽肿性泪腺炎通常需要做泪腺的活检。

daemon [ˈdiːmɔn] *n.* [计]守护程序

How do I get my program to act like a daemon?

我怎样使我的程序作为守护程序运行?

This file must contain suitable startup information for the meta-daemon.

此文件包含了超级守护程序所使用的适当的启动信息。

daily [ˈdeili] *a.* 每日的,日常的

The average daily intake of CO^{2+} in nonoccupational population is 5 to 45μg.

非职业人群 CO^{2+} 的每日平均摄入量为 5 ~ 45 微克。

dairy [ˈdɛəri] *n.* 乳制品

Dairy food like yogurt or milk helps your bones and teeth to develop.

像酸乳酪或牛奶这类乳制食品有助于骨骼和牙齿的发育。

damage [ˈdæmidʒ] *n.* 损伤,损害

Once inside, the bacteria may cause damage.

细菌一旦侵入体内就会造成损害。

Damage to the nerve fibres is considered elsewhere.

至于神经损伤在别处另有叙述。

v. 损害,毁坏

Pathological processes can damage the self-purification mechanisms of the vagina.

患病期间阴道自身的自我清洁机制可能遭到破坏。

damp [dæmp] *a.* 有湿气的,潮湿的

You should wipe the window with a damp cloth.

你应当用湿布擦窗子。

The sweat between the toes and on the soles has a high pH, and keratin damp with it is a good culture medium for the fungi.

趾间和跖部的汗液 pH 高,含有汗液而且湿润的角蛋白是真菌良好的培养基。

n. 瓦斯;湿气

Fire damp is distinguished from black damp (choke damp), which does not ignite.

沼气与矿内的窒息性气体不同,后者不能点燃。

darken [ˈdɑːkən] *v.* 变黑,(颜色)变深

The urine of children deprived of ascorbic acid darkens when exposed to air.

缺乏抗坏血酸的儿童尿液,暴露于空气时颜色变深。

database [ˈdeitəbeis] *n.* 数据库

I have database programming experience and network knowledge.

我有数据库编程经验并具有网络知识。

This database is only accessible by the authorized manager.

只有授权的管理员才可以访问此数据库。

Disease natural histories and drug-induced diseases are now being described in large population database.

疾病的自然史和药源性疾病目前在大的人群数据库中均有说明。

There are several databases that contain information on polymorphisms and mutations in human genes, which allow the investigator to search by gene for polymorphisms that have been reported.

有几个含有人类基因多态性和突变信息的数据库，这使研究者可通过已有的报道来查找基因的多态性。

dataset [ˈdeitəset] *n.* 数据集

The minimum dataset required to consider information as a reportable adverse event is indeed minimal.

报告不良事件信息所要求的最小数据集的确是很小的。

datum [ˈdeitəm] (*pl.* data [ˈdeitə]) *n.* 数据，资料

It is only after all the data have been assembled that the medical doctor is in a position to begin his analysis.

只有当全部的资料收集后，医生才能开始分析。

daunting [ˈdɔːntiŋ] *a.* 使人畏缩的

While the requirements for health rules may seem daunting, they are not insurmountable barriers to medical research.

这些卫生法规的要求可能令人望而生畏，但对医学研究并非不可逾越的障碍。

daydream [ˈdeidriːm] *n.* 白日梦

Singer sums up the advantage of daydreams to the average person.

辛格总结了白日梦对普通人的好处。

v. 白日做梦

The amount of time and the frequency that a person daydreams is what's important.

人的白日梦时间的长短与频率正是重要的东西。

deadly [ˈdedli] *a.* 致命的

Smallpox used to be a deadly disease.

天花过去是一种致命疾病。

AIDS is one of the deadliest illness of the human race.

艾滋病是人类最能致死的疾病之一。

deaf [def] *a.* 聋的

He is deaf in one ear.

他有一侧耳朵聋。

Hearing aid is an electronic device to enable a deaf person to hear.

助听器是一种能使聋人听到声音的电子仪器。

deafness [ˈdefnis] *n.* 耳聋

Deafness, either partial or complete, may be caused by a variety of conditions.

耳聋，不管是半聋或全聋，可由许多种原因引起。

There have been rapid advances in the molecular genetics of deafness in recent years.

近年来，耳聋的分子遗传学研究进展迅速。

deal [diːl] *v.* 处理；对待

I will recommend you how to deal with these difficult diseases.

我会建议你如何治疗(处理)这些疑难病症。

In dealing with toxicity of anticancer agents, the physician must provide vigorous supportive care, including platelet transfusions, antibiotics, and hematopoietic growth factors.

在处理抗癌药毒性时，医生必须给予有力的支持治疗，包括输注血小板、应用抗生素及造血生长因子。

deaminase [diːˈæmineis] *n.* 脱氨酶

A-D-A stands for adenosine deaminase, an important component of the human immune system.

A-D-A 表示腺苷脱氨酶，是人类免疫系统中一个很重要的成分。

debatable [di'beitəbl] *a.* 可争论的

The term senile emphysema is of debatable value.

老年性肺气肿这名称是否恰当，是有争议的。

debate [di'beit] *n.* 争论，辩论

The debate over the appropriate role of scientific technology in health care will continue for many years to come.

对于科学技术在卫生保健中的作用的争论仍将继续若干年。

debilitate [di'biliteit] *v.* 使衰弱

In a very debilitated elderly patient a gastrojejunostomy alone may be carried out.

对于一个极为虚弱的老年病人，只能进行胃空肠吻合术。

These serious complications are particularly liable to develop in very young, malnourished or debilitated children.

这些严重的并发症尤其易发生于很年幼的、营养不良的或身体衰弱的儿童。

debilitating [di'biliteitiŋ] *a.* 使人衰弱的

Manet was upset by the debilitating effect of the disease.

疾病的折磨导致马奈体质虚弱。

The factors that cause a person loss of strength, such as malnutrition and wasting disease, are called debilitating factors.

使人丧失力量的因素如营养不良和消耗性疾病称为使人衰弱的因素。

debility [di'biliti] *n.* 衰弱

Extensive tuberculous bronchopneumonia is associated with fever, severe debility and rapid weight loss.

广泛的结核性支气管肺炎伴有发热、极度衰弱和体重迅速减轻等症状。

debride [de'bri:d] *v.* 清创

All severe localized infections, especially with gas formation, should be widely debrided and drained.

所有严重的局部感染，特别有气体形成时，一定要广泛清创并引流。

debridement [debrid'mɔŋ] *n.* [法]清创术

Debridement should be considered if there is a poor response to therapy in the first 48h.

治疗在头 48 小时内无效就应考虑行清创术。

debris ['debri:] *n.* 碎屑，碎片，残骸

The menstrual flow consists of partially haemolysed blood, mucus and cellular debris.

月经血包括部分溶血的血液、黏液和细胞碎屑。

Undigested debris and water remain through the great length of the small intestine.

通过很长一段小肠之后，剩下的只有尚未消化的残渣和水分。

They evolve to become very dense, hard, pustular lesions, which are filled with what turns out to be tissue debris.

它们逐渐变成黏稠、发硬的脓疱性损害，脓疱内充满的实际上是组织残骸。

debrisoquine [de'brisəkwin] *n.* 异喹胍

Debrisoquine is a derivative of guanidine.

异喹胍是胍的衍生物。

debugger [di:'bʌgə] *n.* 调试器，调试程序

The debugger must be in break mode .

调试器必须处于中断模式。

Debugger did not perform a state change.

调试程序没有进行状态更改。

debulk [di'bʌlk] *v.* 去除主体

Debulking is the surgical removal of the greater part of a malignant tumor to enhance the effectiveness of radiation or chemotherapy.
去除主体是手术切除恶性肿瘤的大部分，以增强放疗或化疗的效率。
Ovarian carcinoma and some types of brain tumor are debulked prior to radio-chemotherapy.
卵巢癌和某些脑肿瘤在放化疗前要尽可能切除大部分肿瘤。

decade [ˈdekeid] *n.* 十年
During the past decade, considerable progress has been made in the reduction of cardiac death.
过去十年中，在减少心脏病患者死亡方面已取得了重大的进展。
These powerful drugs can save lives which would have been lost a few decades ago.
这些特效药可以挽救那些几十年前可能失去生命的人们。
For many decades, attempts were made to isolate the common cold virus.
几十年来，人们一直试图分离感冒病毒。

decay [diˈkei] *v.* 衰退，衰变，蜕变；腐烂
As we know, vast numbers of red blood cells decompose and die in the organism daily. Other cells of the body decay and die also.
我们知道，机体内每天有大量红细胞分解和死亡，体内其他细胞也同样衰退和死亡。
Such superheavy elements are usually very radioactive and decay away almost instantly.
这些超重元素通常是具有非常强的放射性，并且几乎立即会发生衰变。
n. 衰减，衰变
Alpha particles are positively charged helium nuclei obtained from natural radioactive decay.
α 粒子是从天然放射性衰变得到的带正电的氦核。

deceased [diˈsiːst] *a.* 已死的
Grief reaction proceeds from a phase of shock and bewilderment, via a depressive preoccupation with the deceased, to a gradual period of resolution.
忧伤反应病状的进展是从震惊和迷乱阶段，经过抑郁性全神贯注于死者，到症状逐渐消失。
However, kidneys from a deceased donor have also proved satisfactory in many cases.
然而，在不少例子中，用从已死的供肾者身上提供的肾脏，也得到了满意的结果。

deceleration [diːˌseləˈreiʃən] *n.* 减速(度)
Watch for a drop in the fetal heart rate, deep variable decelerations, and persistant bradycardia.
要观察是否有胎儿心率的下降、可变减速和持续的心动过缓。
Prolonged deceleration or loss of beat-to-beat variation may be sinister signs.
恢复期长的减速或者心跳间变异消失可能是危险的征兆。

deceptively [diˈseptivli] *ad.* 靠不住地，易使人上当的
During and immediately after hemorrhage, the RBC count, Hb, and Hct are deceptively high because of vasoconstriction.
在出血期间或刚出血后，由于血管收缩，红细胞计数、血红蛋白和血细胞压积反而显得高。

dechallenge [diˈtʃælindʒ] *n.* 去激发
This assessment of causality may be based on factors such as dechallenge (discontinuation of the product to determine if the adverse reaction resolves) and so on.
这种因果关系的评估可能建立在诸如去激发(停药以确定不良反应是否消失)等影响因素基础上。

decidua [diˈsidjuə] *n.* 蜕膜
Basal decidua is the maternal portion of the placenta.
底蜕膜是胎盘的母体成分。
If pregnancy is established the endometrium becomes the decidua, which is shed after birth.
一旦妊娠，子宫内膜将变成蜕膜，并在胎儿娩出后脱落。

decidual [diˈsidjuəl] *a.* 蜕膜的

Hypertrophy of the stroma cells continues until they resemble the decidual cells of pregnancy.
间质细胞继续肥大,直到它们增生至类似妊娠时的蜕膜细胞。

TGF-β_3 was mostly found in trophoblast and decidual cell.
TGF-β_3 主要表达于滋养细胞和蜕膜细胞。

decidualization [diˌsidjuəlaiˈzeiʃən] *n.* 蜕膜化

This study was undertaken to investigate the biological significance of transforming growth factor-α, which shares a significant sequence homology with epidermal growth factor EGF, in the regulation of decidualization.
这项研究探讨转化生长因子-α 在蜕膜化调节中的生物学意义,它与表皮生长因子有重要的序列同源性。

We previously reported the gene expression of epidermal growth factor in the process of decidualization in the human endometrium.
我们曾经报道过表皮生长因子在人类子宫内膜蜕膜化的过程中的基因表达。

deciliter, decilitre [ˈdesiˌliːtə] *n.* 分升

Scleral icterus may be detected at a serum bilirubin concentration as low as 2.0 to 2.5 mg per deciliter.
血清胆红素浓度降低至 2.0 至 2.5 毫克/分升时将会出现巩膜黄染。

decisive [diˈsaisiv] *a.* 决定性的

Their reform is a decided victory, but whether it is a decisive one only time can tell.
他们的改革取得了成功,但是否是决定性的胜利只能由时间来回答。

Because specific clinical and laboratory findings of Reiter's disease are unknown, the general clinical features are decisive.
由于尚不清楚莱特尔病的特殊临床表现及其实验室表现,所以一般的临床特征具有决定性的意义。

declare [diˈklɛə] *v.* 宣布,断言

In 1941, penicillin was declared safe for use on humans and made available to doctors.
1941 年,青霉素被宣称为可安全用于人体并可提供给医生们使用。

decline [diˈklain] *v.* 下降,减弱,衰退,拒绝

His health was declining after the illness.
病后他的健康逐渐衰退。

As one grows older one's memory declines.
一个人随着年龄的增长,记忆力便会逐渐衰退。

Those individuals decline use of their health information in a research project.
那些人拒绝在研究项目中使用他们的健康信息。

n. 下降,减少

This decline in risk is evident soon after giving up smoking and continues with time.
戒烟后不久就很明显地看到这种危险性降低,随着时间的推移将会更明显。

Complete cessation of RBC production results in a decline of about 10% wk of the control value.
红细胞的生成完全停止就会使其数值与对照相比每周下降 10% 左右。

decoction [diˈkɔkʃən] *n.* 汤剂

Joloo is a Nigerian herbal decoction used for managing breast tumor, ulcer, pain, fever and general malaise in southwestern Nigeria.
Joloo 是一种尼日利亚草药汤剂,在尼日利亚西南部用于乳腺肿瘤、溃疡、疼痛、发烧和全身不适的治疗。

Decoction of Sipunculus nudus has traditionally been used to remedy sternalgia in folk medicine.
在民间医药中,方格星虫汤剂常用于心绞痛的治疗。

decode [diːˈkəud] *n.* 解码,译码

No ribosome proteins are involved in decoding messages.

解码信息不涉及核糖体蛋白。

As such, this central domain of the 30s subunit serves as the decoding center.

这样,30s 亚基的中心结构域就作为解码中心。

decolorize [diˈkʌləraiz] *v.* 使脱色,漂白

Bacteria are stained with violet, decolorized with ethanol and counterstained with safranin. Those bacteria that retain violet stain are said to be gram-positive.

细菌用紫罗兰染色,用乙醇脱色,再用番红复染,那些保留有紫罗兰染料的细菌称为革兰氏阳性。

decompensation [diːkəmpenˈseiʃən] *n.* 代偿失调,代谢失常,呼吸困难

In such circumstances propranolol may be useful in alleviating the cardiac decompensation.

在这种情况下心得安可能减缓心脏的代偿失调。

Recurrent, life-threatening metabolic decompensations often occur in patients with methylmalonic aciduria.

周期性的威胁生命的代谢失常经常发生于甲基丙二酸尿症病人。

This is a rare cause of fatal right ventricular cardiac decompensation.

这是致命的右心室功能衰竭的一个少见原因。

decompose [diːkəmˈpəuz] *v.* 分解,解体

Methenamine decomposes in solution to generate formaldehyde.

乌洛托品在溶液中分解产生甲醛。

The speed at which RNA molecules decompose is a critical determinant of many biological processes.

RNA 分子的分解速度是很多生物学过程的重要决定因素。

decomposer [ˌdiːkəmˈpəuzə] *n.* 分解者；分解体

Millipede is an important decomposer in the forest ecosystem.

千足虫是森林生态系的重要分解者。

decomposition [ˌdiːkɔmpəˈziʃən] *n.* 分解,解体,腐败

Louis Pasteur demonstrated that such microorganisms could cause the decomposition of organic matter such as body tissue.

路易・巴斯德证明,这些微生物能分解有机物如机体组织。

decompress [ˌdiːkəmˈpres] *v.* 使减压

Emergency surgical intervention is sometimes necessary to decompress the intracranial contents.

有时需要立即手术以便使颅内压降低。

decompression [ˌdiːkəmˈpreʃən] *n.* 减压,降压

A decompression chamber is the chamber in which divers may return to normal pressure.

减压舱是潜水员能在其中返回至常压的箱室。

Recurrent symptoms usually respond to a second surgical decompression.

反复发生的症状通常可通过第二次外科减压手术改善。

decongestant [diːkənˈdʒestənt] *n.* 减充血剂

Many cough preparations containing expectorants and decongestants are shown to be more effective than an antitussive agent used alone.

许多含有祛痰剂和减充血剂的咳嗽制剂比单独使用镇咳药更有效。

decontamination [ˌdiːkəntæmiˈneiʃən] *n.* 去污染(法)

Prompt GI decontamination is followed by activated charcoal.

用活性炭及时去除胃肠道中的毒物。

decortication [ˌdikɔtiˈkeiʃən] *n.* 剥外皮;[外科]去皮质术

The exposure allows for decortication of the pars, facet joint, and transverse processes for bone-grafting and fusion.

暴露过程中可对峡部、关节突关节和横突皮质剥除以便进行植骨融合。

Clearance of blood clot and decortication of lung were adopted in 27 cases.
在 27 例患者中采用了血凝块清除和肺纤维板剥脱术。

decrease [diː'kriːs] *v.* 减小,减少

Anything that compromises the amount of oxygen coming to the brain will decrease brain function.
任何有损氧含量的东西进入大脑都将降低大脑的功能。

Normally, approximately 85 to 90 percent of all scalp hairs are in the anagen phase, a figure which decreases with age.
正常情况下约 85% ~90% 的头发处于生长期,此数字随年龄增长而减少。

n. 减少(量),减小

The destruction of melanocytes leads to decrease in their number.
黑色素细胞被破坏导致其数目减少。

But even a less severe blood-sugar decrease can alter brain function and cause memory problems.
但是,血糖下降即使不太严重,也能改变大脑的功能,产生记忆力问题。

decubitus [di'kjuːbitəs] *n.* 褥疮

Decubitus ulcers and mobilization of calcium stores with formation of renal calculi may also be seen.
褥疮性溃疡和随着肾结石形成的钙堆积活动均可见到。

dedifferentiated [diːdif'renʃieitid] *a.* 失分化的

Dedifferentiated liposarcoma is uncommon, and only a small number of cases have been documented.
失分化的脂肪肉瘤并不常见,仅仅少数病例记录在案。

Dedifferentiated chondrocytes reexpress the differentiated collagen phenotype when cultured in agarose gels.
失分化的软骨细胞在琼脂糖凝胶中培养时再表达分化的胶原表型。

deduce [di'djuːs] *v.* 推论,推断

To deduce is to figure something out based on what you already know.
推断是基于已知的东西来判定某事。

How do you deduce that a child has an ear infection?
你如何推断一个孩子有耳部感染?

deduction [di'dʌkʃən] *n.* 扣除,减除,推论,演绎

The two main methods of reasoning are called deduction and induction.
这两种主要的推理方法被称为演绎和归纳。

Your donation will result in a tax deduction in accordance with IRS rules.
依照美国国税局条例,捐款可以减税。

defecation [ˌdefi'keiʃən] *n.* 排便

Defecation is effected by relaxation of internal anal sphincter in response to rectal distention.
直肠扩张引起的肛门内括约肌松弛可影响排便。

Constipation is the decrease in frequency of stools or difficulty in defecation.
大便次数减少或排便困难称为便秘。

defect [di'fekt] *n.* 缺陷

The chromosome abnormality leads to the physical and mental defects found in this condition.
在这种疾病中发现染色体异常导致机体和智力缺陷。

defective [di'fektiv] *a.* 有缺陷的

He is defective in intelligence, manner and body.
他在智力、举止和身体上均有缺陷。

Deficient or defective heme or globin synthesis produces a hypochromic-microcytic RBC population.

血红素或球蛋白合成不足或有缺陷会产生低色素小红细胞性的红细胞群（低色素小红细胞贫血）。

defense [diˈfens] *n.* 防御，防护

Walking is a vital defense against the ravages of degenerative diseases and aging.

散步是一种对身体退行性疾病和衰老的重要防御（活动）。

defensin [diˈfensin] *n.* 防御素

β-defensins are antimicrobial peptides made by virtually all multicellular organisms.

β-防御素实际上是由多细胞生物所产生的抗菌多肽。

Plant defensins are the low molecular weight peptides, which have a broad spectrum of inhibiting the growth of plant pathogens.

植物防御素是广谱的抑制植物病原菌生长的低分子量多肽。

defer [diˈfəː] *v.* 推迟，使延期

The knowledge that some drugs are available gives her confidence and she may prefer to defer their use for a time.

知道可以得到这些药物后，她满怀信心，宁可暂时延缓这些药物的应用。

Can you defer menstruation while traveling abroad?

你是否能在出国旅游时推迟月经？

defervesce [ˌdiːfəˈves] *v.* 退热

Most patients defervesce within 12-36h of initiation of therapy, but some take up to 4d.

大多数病人在治疗开始后 12～36 小时内退热，但有些则需 4 天。

defervescence [ˌdiːfəˈvesəns] *n.* 退热（期）

Untreated, high fever and cough persist for 7-10d, followed by defervescence.

如果不治疗，高热和咳嗽持续了 7～10 天之后会自行退热。

Eradication was defined as a decrease in colony counts or improvement as indicated by defervescence and patients' increased well-being.

根治指的是集落计数减少或体温下降和病人一般状况的改善。

defibrillate [diːˈfaibriˌleit] *v.* 去纤颤

When one is faced with a patient in ventricular fibrillation, all attempts should be made to defibrillate the patient as soon as possible.

碰到室颤患者时应尽快采用各种可能的措施给病人除颤。

defibrillator [diːˌfaibriˈleitə] *n.* 除颤器

Long-term antiarrhythmic drug therapy, implantation of an automatic defibrillator, and/or cardiac surgery may be necessary.

病人需要服用长效抗心律失常药物、在体内植入自动除颤器和（或）接受心脏手术。

Defibrillators are often used in intensive care unit to save patients suffering from cardiac arrest.

在重症监护病房内，除颤器常被用来挽救心脏骤停病人的生命。

deficiency [diˈfiʃənsi] *n.* 缺乏，不足

Vitamin C deficiency can ultimately lead to scurvy.

缺乏维生素 C 最终能导致坏血病。

Iron deficiency anaemia is the most common form of anaemia.

缺铁性贫血是最常见的一种贫血。

Parenteral administration of folate will overcome these deficiencies.

肠道外给予叶酸治疗可纠正这些缺乏症。

deficient [diˈfiʃənt] *a.* 缺乏的，不足的

Drug metabolism is very deficient qualitatively and quantitatively in the newborn.

新生儿对药物的代谢，无论在质量上或数量上都非常不足。

A clinically important form of nuclear damage is encountered in patients deficient in vitamin B_{12} or folic acid.

一种具有临床重要性的核损伤类型常见于维生素 B_{12}或叶酸缺乏症的病人。

deficit ['defisit] *n.* 缺乏,缺陷

Acute infections and the chronic disturbances associated with deficits of calories, vitamins, minerals or proteins were studied intensively.

对各种急性传染病及与热量、维生素、矿物质或蛋白缺乏有关的慢性疾患,都在加强研究。

Cerebral hemorrhage typically causes abrupt coma with profound neurologic deficits.

脑溢血一般会引起突然昏迷并伴有明显的神经障碍。

define [di'fain] *v.* 给…下定义,解释,界限,限定

Shock may be defined as an inadequate capillary perfusion.

休克可以定义为毛细血管灌注不足。

Early latent syphilis is defined as that during the first year after infection.

早期潜伏梅毒是指感染梅毒后的第一年内的患病期。

Define cholesterol: state the functions, food sources, and health concerns associated with it.

请解释胆固醇:说明其功能、食品来源及其与健康的关系。

From the radiologic point of view, the infiltrates in viral pneumonia tend to be diffuse, ill-defined and hazy.

从放射学的观点来看,病毒性肺炎的浸润往往是弥漫性的界限不清的和模糊的。

Such patches consist of one or several small or large, smooth, well-defined areas devoid of papillae.

这种斑片包括一个或数个大小不一、光滑而边界清晰的区域,无明显突起。

definite ['definit] *a.* 明确的;肯定的

Whereas the red cells have a definite color, the leukocytes tend to be colorless.

红细胞有明确的颜色,而白细胞却近似无色。

There is thus a definite necessity for the rigid control of drinking-water.

因此,必须严格地控制饮水。

definitely ['definitli] *ad.* 明确,一定

The cathartic can definitely lead to the development of peritonitis during perforating diseases.

使用泻药在肠穿孔性疾病时肯定会导致腹膜炎的发生。

definition [defi'niʃən] *n.* 定义,定界,阐明;明确性

His definition helps distinguish tumor from other growth disturbances such as inflammation, repair, hyperplasia, and malformation.

他的定义有助于将肿瘤与其他诸如炎症、修复、增生和畸形等生长紊乱区分开来。

definitive [di'finitiv] *a.* 确定的,决定性的,最后的

Once the decision is made for operation, each consideration becomes important in preparing the individual for definitive treatment.

手术决定一经做出,在对病人所施手术的准备过程中每项考虑都至关重要。

The therapy should be definitive: prevent seizures, control blood pressure, and deliver.

应确定治疗方法:预防抽搐,控制血压,终止妊娠。

A definitive diagnosis of a congenital cytomegalovirus infection requires culturing cytomegalovirus from the urine of the infant.

先天性巨细胞病毒感染的确诊需要从小儿尿中培养出巨细胞病毒。

deflate [di'fleit] *v.* 放气;缩小

The globe of each eye had lost its fluid and deflated like a limp ballon to less than half size.

眼球失去了内含的液体,就像跑了气的软绵绵的气球一样体积小于原来的一半。

defoliant [diː'fəuliənt] *n.* 落叶剂

Litigation about Agent Orange, a defoliant and herbicide used by American forces in the Vietnam War, has provided the most extensive judicial discussion of toxic causation.

橙剂(一种美国部队在越南战争中使用的落叶剂和除草剂)立法向我们提供了最广泛的有毒物质因果关系的司法讨论。

A defoliant is any chemical sprayed or dusted on plants to cause its leaves to fall off.

落叶剂是喷洒在植物上使其叶子脱落的任何化学物。

deformability [diˌfɔːməˈbiləti] *n.* 变形能力

The ability of cell to change shape as they pass through a narrow space is called deformability, such as erythrocytes may change their shape during they pass through microvasculature.

细胞经过狭窄缝隙处时能改变自身形状的能力称为变形能力,如红细胞在通过微血管系统时可改变它们的自身形状。

deformation [ˌdiːfɔːˈmeiʃən] *n.* 畸形;变形(过程)

Elastic fibers contribute very little to resisting deformation and tearing of skin, although they appear to have a role in maintaining its elasticity.

虽然弹性纤维在维持皮肤弹性方面有作用,但对于恢复皮肤变形和防止皮肤撕裂方面则微不足道。

deformity [diˈfɔːmiti] *n.* 畸形

Rickets is a metabolic disorder of growing bone resulting in bony deformities.

佝偻病是生长期骨骼的代谢疾病,可形成骨骼畸形。

The final result is deformity of one or more valves, especially the mitral and aortic.

结局是一个或多个瓣膜变形,特别是二尖瓣和主动脉瓣。

First aid treatment is most essential in order to reduce pain and prevent deformity.

急救治疗在减少疼痛和预防畸形方面是必不可少的。

defy [diˈfai] *v.* 使不能,公然反对

Skin has defied successful transplantation because of its high immunogenicity.

由于皮肤有高度的致免疫性常使其移植手术不能成功。

degeneracy [diˈdʒenərəsi] *n.* 简并性,简并,退化

Based on the degeneracy properties in genetic codes, we propose a new idea on the similarity search.

根据遗传密码的简并特性,我们提出了一种相似性搜索的新思路。

degenerate [diˈdʒenəreit] *v.* 退化,变质,变性

Usually the cellular elements gradually degenerate and caseation necrosis occurs.

通常细胞的成分逐渐地变性并出现干酪样坏死。

degeneration [diˌdʒenəˈreiʃən] *n.* 退化,变性

A severe nutrition deficiency can bring on combined spinal cord degeneration and associated brain diseases.

严重的营养不良可同时引起脊髓的退行性病变及相关的脑病。

Degeneration may involve the deposition of calcium salts, fat and fibrous tissue in the affected organ or tissue.

受累的器官或组织中出现钙盐、脂肪及纤维组织的堆积,均属于变性范围。

No symptoms are caused by hyaline or cystic degeneration but the tumour may become so soft that diagnosis from an ovarian cyst may be difficult.

玻璃样变或囊性病变不引起症状,但肿瘤可能变得如此之软,以致和卵巢囊肿难以鉴别。

degenerative [diˈdʒenərətiv] *a.* 变性的,退化的

A very special problem in treatment of the elderly is the appropriate management of multiple-organ degenerative disease.

老年人治疗中的一个非常特殊的问题就是对多器官退行性疾病的适当处置。

Most joints transplanted freely developed severe degenerative change and poor function.

任意移植的关节大多都发生严重的退行性变化,而且功能很差。

degloving [diˈglʌviŋ] *a.* 脱套的(损伤)

The article explores the treatment of multi-finger degloving injury and its clinical features.
此文章探讨多指脱套伤的治疗及临床特点。

deglutition [ˌdiːgluːˈtiʃən] *n.* 吞咽

Deglutition syncope is less common, but may be seen in patients with underlying esophageal disease, especially esophageal spasm.
吞咽引起晕厥较少见,但可能见于有食管潜在疾病的病人,尤其是食管痉挛。

degradability [diˌgreidəˈbiliti] *n.* 可降解性

Collagen has great potential applications because of its unique construction of three-ply helix, predominant bio-compatibility and bio-degradability.
胶原具有广泛的应用前景,因为它有独特的 3 股螺旋结构、优越的生物相容性和生物降解性。

degradation [degrəˈdeiʃən] *n.* 降解(作用);退化

Hepatic enzymes activated by griseofulvin will cause degradation of warfarin.
被灰黄霉素激活的肝酶类可造成丙酮苄羟香豆素降解。
"Protected" in this sense means that bound C3b is protected from proteolytic degradation.
"保护"一词 在此指的是已结合的 C3b 可免受蛋白酶的降解。
Much of this change may result from a degradation of intracortical inhibition during senescence.
这种变化主要是由衰老时皮质内抑制的退化引起。

degrade [diˈgreid] *v.* 降解,退化

Most fungi can degrade organic materials and wastes.
大多数真菌能降解有机物和废物。
Human cerebral cortical function degrades gradually during old age.
人类大脑皮质的功能在老年期逐渐退化。

degranulation [digrænjuˈleiʃən] *n.* 去粒,脱粒

Leukocidin destroys human leukocytes by causing degranulation and membrane disruption.
杀白细胞素引起脱粒和细胞膜分裂,从而破坏人的白细胞。

dehiscence [diˈhisns] *n.* 裂开

Wound dehiscence is partial or total disruption of any or all layers of the operative wound.
手术伤口的任何一层或者全层,部分的或者全部的破裂,称作伤口裂开。
Wound dehiscence occurs in about 1% of abdominal surgical procedures.
大约有 1% 的腹部外科手术后发生伤口的裂开。

dehydrate [diːˈhaidreit] *v.* 使脱水,使失水

These patients may vomit profusely and become dehydrated and alkalotic.
这些病人可因大量呕吐以致失水和碱中毒。
The patient is now in a dehydrated condition.
病人现在处于脱水状态。

dehydration [ˌdiːhaiˈdreiʃən] *n.* 脱水(作用);失水

The rise in urea may partly reflect the degree of dehydration.
尿素的升高可以部分反映脱水的程度。
The terms hypertonic and hypotonic dehydration refer to the electrolyte concentration in water of outside the cell.
高渗与低渗脱水是指有关细胞外液中的电解质的浓度。

dehydroepiandrosterone [diːˈhaidrəuˌepiænˈdrɔstərəun] *n.* 脱氢表雄酮,脱氢异雄酮

Dehydroepiandrosterone is present in large amounts in the blood of young adults. Its concentration is lowered in many cases of depression.
脱氢表雄酮在年轻成年人的血液中是大量存在的,其浓度在抑郁症的许多病例中是下降的。

dehydrogenase [diˈhaidrədʒəneis] *n.* 脱氢酶

Oxidoreductase includes the enzymes formerly known either as dehydrogenases or as oxidases.
氧化还原酶包括过去称为脱氢酶或氧化酶等类的酶。
Lactate dehydrogenase is widely distributed in many tissues.
乳酸脱氢酶广泛分布于多种组织。

dehydrogenate [diː'haidrədʒəneit] *v.* 脱氢,去氢
Pyrrolizidine alkaloids are dehydrogenated to reactive pyrrole derivatives.
双吡咯烷类生物碱脱氢后形成活性吡咯衍生物。

deiodination [ˌdiːaiədi'neiʃən] *n.* 脱碘、去碘
The improved preparation was more efficient in deiodination and with less skin irritation and lower cost, thus it is worthy to be widely used.
改进后的制剂脱碘效果更好、对皮肤的刺激性更小、成本更低,因此值得广泛使用。
Deiodination is the foremost pathway of thyroid hormone metabolism.
脱碘是甲状腺激素代谢最为重要的途径。
The invention is a kind of high intensity compound deiodination sorbent.
本发明为一种高强度复合脱碘吸附剂。

delay [di'lei] *v.* 推迟,延误
In the presence of myelosuppression, treatment was reduced or delayed.
出现骨髓抑制时应减量或推迟治疗。
The delayed type of reaction to trichophytin is observed especially in acute kerion and dermatophytid reactions.
对毛癣菌反应的迟发型主要见于急性脓癣和癣菌疹反应。
n. 延迟,耽搁
Delays in obtaining organisms cultures and sensitivity tests resulted in delays in the institution of drugs that might have been appropriate based on the sensitivity patterns.
未及时进行病原菌的培养及药物敏感试验导致不能及时根据敏感试验结果选用合适的药物。
In order to protect the healthy eye from infection, it is covered without delay by a watch-glass dressing.
为了保护健康眼睛免遭感染,应及时戴上防护镜,用敷料覆盖。

delegate ['deligeit] *v.* 把…委托给
In such cases the task should be delegated to the most skilled or experienced operator.
对这类病例应指定由最有技术或有经验的施术者来操作。
Nurses have long performed tasks delegated to them by physicians.
护士长期以来都是执行医生所委托的任务。

deleterious [ˌdeli'tiəriəs] *a.* (对身心)有害的
Polluted air is deleterious to health.
污染的空气对健康有害。
However, pulmonary fat embolism per se usually is not physiologically deleterious unless it is massive.
然而,肺部脂肪栓塞本身通常在生理学上并非有害,除非它是大面积的。

deletion [di'liːʃən] *n.* (染色体的)缺失
Deletion means a loss of part of the DNA from a chromosome; it can lead to a disease or abnormality.
缺失是指染色体上部分 DNA 的丢失,可导致疾病或异常。
Chromosomal aberrations seen in solid tumours usually involve deletions in chromosomes.
实体性肿瘤的染色体畸变往往表现为染色体缺失。

deliberate [di'libərit] *a.* 蓄意的,故意的
The methods adopted for deliberate self-destruction vary from country to country and between the

sexes.
蓄意自毁者所采用的方法在不同的国家和不同的性别之间都有所不同。

deliberately [diˈlibəritli] *ad.* 有意地
One may deliberately retard the absorption of drugs by reducing the peripheral circulation.
可有意地通过减慢外周循环以延迟药物的吸收。

delicate [ˈdelikit] *a.* 微妙的,灵敏的,脆弱的
Communication between physician and the apprehensive and often confused patient is delicate and uncertain.
医生与忧心忡忡又往往迷惑不解的病人之间的沟通是很微妙又不确定的。
At this stage the eardrum must be opened to prevent the infection from spreading even deeper to the delicate structures within the internal ear.
在此阶段必须切开鼓膜,以防止感染更深地扩散到内耳的脆弱结构。

delineate [diˈlinieit] *v.* 描绘,叙述
The mass could not be delineated by abdominal examination.
腹部检查不能描绘出肿块的轮廓。
The pathophysiologic mechanisms that link advanced endometriosis and infertility have not been fully delineated.
晚期子宫内膜异位症和不孕症相联系的病理生理机制尚未完全阐明。

delinquency [diˈliŋkwənsi] *n.* 违法,少年犯罪
Delinquency is a term applied to various forms of misbehaviour amounting to legal offenced committed by children and young people.
犯罪行为一词用于各种形式的不正当行为,实际上指儿童和年轻人的违法行为。

delirious [diˈliriəs] *a.* 谵妄(性)的;妄想的
The delirious state may be acute or subacute,and is usually of fluctuating intensity.
谵妄状态可分为急性和亚急性(两种),但其强度经常变化。

delirium [diˈliriəm] *n.* 谵妄,发狂,妄想
Delirium rarely lasts longer than one week.
谵妄极少持续一周以上。
Delirium is less common in the middle-aged than in children and old people.
谵妄在中年人身上不如儿童和老年常见。

deliver [diˈlivə] *v.* 递送;释放;(使)分娩
Did you deliver my message to the doctor on duty?
你已将我的信交给了值班医生吗?
If the patient is to be delivered in her own home the doctor should go to see her as soon as labour begins.
如果患者在家分娩,一旦临产,医生就应前往诊视。
In the hospital most patients are delivered in the dorsal position,in which it is easier to maintain good aseptic technique.
在医院,多数病人取仰卧位分娩,这样较易保持良好的无菌技术。

delivery [diˈlivəri] *n.* 传送;分娩
Sixty per cent of premature deliveries occur for no known cause.
60%的早产原因不明。

deltoid [ˈdeltɔid] *n.* 三角肌
The posterior or anterior deltoid is the most powerful muscle during extension or flexion of the arm respectively.
后部三角肌和前部三角肌分别在臂的前屈和后伸过程中是最有力量的肌肉。

delusion [diˈljuːʒən] *n.* 妄想
Delusions and visual hallucinations also frequently occur with dementia.

妄想和幻觉也常出现于痴呆的病人。

A variety of delusions and hallucinations of a percecutory, depressive and somatic content are also present.

也可出现迫害、抑郁和有关躯体的种种妄想和幻觉。

delusional [di'ljuːʒənl] *a.* 妄想的

Organic delusional syndrome is characterized by clear consciousness.

器质性妄想综合征的特点是神志清醒。

demarcate ['diːmɑːkeit] *v.* 划分界线;区别

Smaller, more sharply demarcated ulcers are more likely to be benign.

较小的、分界比较明显的溃疡更可能是良性的。

The ulcer is shallow and sharply demarcated, with surrounding hyperemia.

溃疡表浅、边界清晰,周围有充血。

demarcation [diːmɑː'keiʃən] *n.* 分界,界线

There is a serious disagreement as to an exact demarcation of the properties of the six main classes.

关于六个主要类型在性质上的严格界线存在着严重分歧。

There is no clear line of demarcation between the jejunum and the ileum.

空肠与回肠之间无明显分界。

dematiaceous [diˌmæti'eisiəs] *a.* 着色的

Dematiaceous as a term is generally used to refer to a group of fungi that produce melanin in their cell walls.

"着色的"这个词一般用于描述一群能在其细胞壁产生黑色素的真菌。

demented [di'mentid] *a.* 发狂的

Many times patients with this condition appear depressed and demented.

患这种病的人常常显得忧郁和癫狂。

dementia [di'menʃiə] *n.* 痴呆

Individuals who have true dementia demonstrate consistently poor performance.

真性痴呆患者表现出一贯性的行为能力低下。

In dementia there is impairment of orientation, memory, comprehension and judgement.

痴呆症存在定向力、记忆力、理解力和判断力的损害。

Presenile dementia occurs in young or middle-aged people. The term is sometimes reserved for Alzheimer's disease and Pick's disease.

青年或中年可发生早老性痴呆,本词有时专用于阿尔茨海默氏病和皮克氏病。

demineralization [diːˌminərəlai'zeiʃən] *n.* 脱矿质(作用),去矿质(作用)

Congenital syphilis also produces extensive demineralization.

先天性梅毒也引起广泛性的脱矿质(作用)。

demographic [ˌdemə'græfik] *a.* 人口统计

Health information may include demographic information and personal characteristics, all of which may affect health status or health risks.

卫生信息可包括人口统计信息和个人特征,所有这些可能影响健康状况或健康风险。

Demographics is the study of the most recent statistical characteristics of a population.

人口统计学是对近期人口特征的统计学描述。

We could not know what the demographics is without more accurate figures.

由于缺乏更精确的数据,我们无法了解人口统计资料。

demonstrable ['demənstrəbl] *a.* 可表明的

Tetracycline has no demonstrable effects on the central nervous system.

四环素对中枢神经系统无明显作用。

Approximately 3 in 1000 live-born children die suddenly, without demonstrable cause during infancy.

大约3‰的活产儿在婴儿期无明显病因而突然死亡。

demonstrate [ˈdemənstreit] *v.* 论证,表明

An increase in size, number, and affinity of insulin receptors has been demonstrated in infants of the diabetic mothers.

糖尿病母亲的婴儿显示,胰岛素受体的大小、数目和亲和力增加。

demonstration [ˌdemənsˈtreiʃən] *n.* 论证;证实;示范;说明

The demonstration provides encouraging proof of specificity and effectiveness for this approach to cancer therapy.

此论证提供了这一探讨对癌症治疗的特异性和有效性的令人鼓舞的证明。

For demonstration of the fungus, two or three loose hairs are removed from the suspected areas with epilating forceps.

为了证明真菌感染,用拔毛镊从可疑部位拔2~3根松动的头发。

The students must learn from demonstrations and personal trials with expert advice.

学生必须通过示范学习和在专家指导下亲自试验来学习。

The diagnosis of bacteriuria is based on the demonstration of significant numbers of micro-organism in urine.

菌尿的诊断是基于在尿中发现足够数量的微生物。

demyelinating [diːˈmaiəlineitiŋ] *a.* 脱髓鞘的

The primary demyelinating disease may lead to multiple sclerosis.

原发性脱髓鞘性疾病可导致多发性硬化。

Chronic inflammatory demyelinating polyneuropathy is an acquired immune-mediated inflammatory disorder of the peripheral nervous system.

慢性脱髓鞘性多发性神经炎是一种周围神经系统获得性免疫介导的炎症性疾病。

demyelination [diːmaiəliˈneiʃən] *n.* 脱髓鞘(作用)

Multiple sclerosis is a spontaneous, acquired disease of the human central nervous system inflammatory demyelination.

多发性硬化是人类中枢神经系统自发的、获得性的、炎性的脱髓鞘疾病。

Immune-mediated, toxic, viral and genetic models of demyelination are now used to understand the manifold aspects of multiple sclerosis.

有关脱髓鞘病变免疫介导的、中毒的、病毒和遗传各种模式现在被用来帮助认识多发性硬化症多方面的特征。

denaturant [diːˈneitʃərənt] *n.* 变性剂,变性因素

The best known denaturant is heat.

最为熟知的变性因素是热。

denaturation [diːneitʃəˈreiʃən] *n.* 变性

If disruption goes as far as to cause loss of biological activity, the change is termed denaturation.

如果破坏达到引起生物学活性丧失的程度,这种改变称之为变性。

denature [diːˈneitʃə] *v.* 使变性

Strong acids and alkalis, as well as very concentrated salts and amines, also denature proteins.

强酸和强碱以及高浓度盐和胺也都可使蛋白质变性。

In this case, the enzymes and other proteins are denatured.

在这种情况下,酶和其他蛋白均发生变性。

dendrimers [ˈdendriməs] *n.* 树状聚合物

The progress in stabilizations and stabilization mechanisms of the metal nanoparticles by nonionic polymers, polyelectrolytes, amphiphilic polymers, double-hydrophilic polymers, and dendrimers is reviewed.

本文综述了非离子聚合物、聚电解质、两亲聚合物、双亲水聚合物及树状聚合物对金属纳

米粒子的稳定作用及其稳定机理的研究进展。

dendrite ['dendrait] *n.* 树突

Dendrites are treelike extensions at the beginning of a neuron that help increase the surface area of the cell body.

树突是树状扩展,起于一个神经元,有助于增加细胞体的表面积。

Dendrites play a critical role in integrating these synaptic inputs and in determining the extent to which action potentials are produced by the neuron.

树突在整合突触的传入冲动和决定神经元产生动作电位的程度上发挥关键作用。

dendritic [den'dritik] *a.* 树突状的

Dendritic cells capture microbial antigens from epithelia and tissues and transport the antigens to lymph nodes.

树突状细胞从上皮和组织内捕获微生物性抗原,然后将其运输到淋巴结。

Many studies have confirmed that the dendritic cell plays important roles in the occurrence and development of atherosclerosis.

许多研究已经证实树突状细胞在动脉粥样硬化的发生及发展过程中发挥重要的作用。

denervation [ˌdiːnəː'veiʃən] *n.* 去神经(法)

Denervation of the lung abolishes the cough reflex.

切除肺脏的神经可使咳嗽反射消失。

dengue ['deŋgi] *n.* 登革热

Dengue virus has four serotypes.

登革热病毒有四种血清型。

The Ministry of Health, with the assistance of WHO, is organizing a seminar for case management of dengue and dengue hemorrhagic fever for clinicians and nurses.

在世界卫生组织的协助下,卫生部正在为临床医师和护士组织一次登革热和登革出血热病例处理研讨会。

denitrification [diː,naitrifi'keiʃən] *n.* 反硝化作用

Biological nitrification and denitrification via nitrite for coke-plant wastewater was studied.

通过硝酸盐对焦化废水生物硝化和反硝化作用进行了研究。

Different carbon sources have different influence on denitrification.

不同的碳源对反硝化作用有不同的影响。

de novo [ˌdiː'nəuvəu] (拉)重新;更始

New protein-coding genes can originate either through modification of existing genes or de novo.

新的蛋白质编码基因可通过修改现有的基因或新创而产生。

dens [denz]【拉】*n.* 牙齿;齿状部分;齿突

So, as long as the slanting dens can be corrected and as long as the dens root can be made use of, doctors will reserve the natural tooth as much as they can.

所以,只要歪牙能够矫正,只要牙根能够利用,医生都会尽量保留天然牙齿。

dense [dens] *a.* 稠密的,浓厚的

People with the small dense forms of LDL (pattern B) respond to a low fat diet better than people with larger forms of LDL(pattern A).

具有小密集型低密度脂蛋白(B 型)的人们对低脂肪饮食的反应比那些具有较大型低密度脂蛋白(A 型)的人们好一些。

The chancre is characterized by a dense infiltration of round cells and plasma cells.

下疳的特征为稠密的圆细胞和浆细胞浸润。

densely ['densli] *ad.* 稠密地

The birth rate has begun declining in densely populated areas.

人口稠密地区的出生率已开始下降。

density ['densəti] *n.* 密度

The density of bones should be evaluated at the presence of renal diseases.
患肾脏疾病时，应对骨密度进行评估。

Prepare single-cell suspensions in the medium and adjust the final density to 1×10^7 viable cells/ml.
制备该培养基内的单细胞混悬液，并将其终密度调整到每毫升内有 1×10^7 个活细胞。

dental [ˈdentl] *a.* 牙的，齿的

The cavity is filled with dental pulp holding a number of blood vessels and nerves.
腔内充满了含有许多血管和神经的牙髓。

Dental caries is caused by the metabolism of the bacteria in plaque attached to the surface of the tooth.
龋齿由附着于牙齿表面牙斑上的细菌的代谢所致。

dentin(e) [ˈdentiːn] *n.* 牙质

Dentine is a substance harder than ordinary bone, and it forms the body of the tooth.
牙质是比普通骨头更硬的一种物质，它形成牙体。

The acid wears away the protein network of the enamel and dentine.
这种酸腐蚀作用破坏了牙釉质与牙本质的蛋白质网。

dentist [ˈdentist] *n.* 牙科医生

He is regarded as the best dentist in the hospital.
他被认为是那所医院里最好的牙科医师。

A dental technician constructs dentures, crowns, and orthodontic appliances in the laboratory for the dentist.
牙科技士在实验室内为牙科医生制备托牙、牙冠及正畸用具。

dentistry [ˈdentistri] *n.* 牙科学，牙科

A postgraduate course has been established at the Ohio State University College of Dentistry to study current concepts of occlusion.
俄亥俄州立大学牙科学院已开设了一门研究生课程来研究咬合面的现代概念。

denture [ˈdentʃə] *n.* 假牙，托牙（义齿）

In older people with dentures, it is often very hard for them to chew properly.
有假牙的老人常常难以正常咀嚼。

A complete denture replaces all the teeth in one jaw. A partial denture replaces some teeth because others still remain.
全口托牙是取代单颌的全副牙齿。部分托牙只取代缺失的牙齿，因为其他牙齿仍存留。

denudation [ˌdiːnjuːˈdeiʃən] *n.* 剥蚀

Alkylating agents are highly toxic to dividing mucosal cells, leading to oral mucosal ulceration and intestinal denudation.
烷化剂对正在分裂的黏膜细胞有高毒性，引起口腔黏膜溃疡和肠黏膜剥蚀脱落。

denude [diˈnjuːd] *v.* 剥去

Anal fissures represent denuded epithelium of the anal canal overlying the internal sphincter.
肛裂就是被覆在内括约肌表面之上的肛管上皮被剥脱了。

deny [diˈnai] *v.* 否认

Some patients deny pain but will complain of difficulty in breathing.
一些病人否认疼痛的感觉，但主诉呼吸困难。

deontology [ˌdiːɔnˈtɔlədʒi] *n.* 道义学

In medicine deontology includes consideration of the proper behaviour of a doctor towards his patients, whether a patient should be told if his condition is fatal or not.
在医学中，道义学包括医生如何恰当地对待病人的问题，例如当病人患绝症时医生是否可将病情告诉病人。

deoxygenate [diːˈɔksidʒineit] *v.* 脱氧，去氧

The veins carry deoxygenated blood from the capillaries back to the right side of the heart.
静脉把脱氧的血液从毛细血管带回到右心房。
Deoxygenated blood is blood that has circulated throughout tissues, is not devoid of oxygen, but contains diminished oxygen.
脱氧血是已循环经过全身组织的血液,不是不含氧,而是含氧量较低。

deoxyguanosine [diːˌɔksi ˈgwɑːnəˌsin] *n.* 脱氧鸟苷
We identified pathogenic mutations in deoxyguanosine kinase in 6 children with the hepatocerebral form of mtDNA depletion syndrome.
在6个患肝脑型 mtDNA 缺失综合征的儿童中,我们证实有脱氧鸟苷激酶的病理性突变。

deoxyribonucleic [diːˌɔksiˌraibəunjuːˈkliːik] *a.* 脱氧核糖的
Deoxyribonucleic acid is abbreviated DNA.
脱氧核糖核酸简写为 DNA。
Deoxyribonucleic acid is genetic material.
脱氧核糖核酸是遗传物质。

deoxyribose [diːˌɔksiˈraibəus] *n.* 脱氧核糖
Deoxyribose is one of the components of a nucleotide.
脱氧核糖是核苷酸的组成成分之一。
In the nucleotide, a nitrogenous base is joined to the deoxyribose.
在核苷酸中含氮的碱基与脱氧核糖相连。

dependence [diˈpendəns] *n.* 信赖性
Potent analgesics result in addiction and dependence.
强效镇痛药可导致成瘾和药物依赖。
In physical dependence withdrawal of the drug causes specific symptoms (withdraw symptoms), such as sweating, vomiting, or tremors, that are reversed by further doses.
躯体性赖药性的表现是:撤去药物可引起一些特殊的症状(戒断症状),诸如出汗、呕吐、震颤等,给药后又可消失。

dependent [diˈpendənt] *a.* 依靠的,依赖的
The body is dependent upon water for every essential function.
人体任何一种基本的功能都离不开水。
Capillary perfusion is dependent on numerous factors.
毛细血管的灌注取决于许多因素。
The well-being of each individual cell is dependent on the adequacy of its environment to furnish nutrition and carry away metabolites.
每个细胞的健康有赖于其周围环境供应充足的营养和运走代谢废物。

depersonalization [diːˌpəːsnəlaiˈzeiʃən] *n.* 人格解体
Depersonalization can occur in normal people under stress.
正常人处于强烈的(精神)压力下可以发生人格解体。

depict [diˈpikt] *v.* 描述;描画
Hospital regulations depict and enforce the duties of doctors and nurses.
医院章程描述和规定了医生和护士的职责。
In the exhibit, visually intriguing images and floor patterns graphically depict the burden of disease from tobacco.
在展览上,富于视觉冲击力的图片和地板设计生动地刻画了烟草造成的疾病负担。

deplete [diˈpliːt] *v.* 耗尽,使…枯竭
In pernicious anemia usually develops insidiously and progressively as the large hepatic stores of B_{12} are depleted.
恶性贫血时当肝脏中贮存的大量维生素 B_{12} 耗尽时,就会不知不觉地渐进性地出现贫血。
However, exposure to very large amounts of such reactive substances can deplete the glutathione.

然而,暴露于很大剂量的反应物质后会耗尽体内的谷胱甘肽。

depletion [diˈpliːʃən] *n.* 耗尽,枯竭,缺失

Chloride depletion tends to limit bicarbonate excretion.

氯化物耗竭可限制碳酸氢盐的排泄。

This effect apparently increased by mild starvation and protein depletion.

轻度饥饿和蛋白质耗尽时会明显的增强这种作用。

Clinical and laboratory findings of anemia of protein depletion mimic those in the hypometabolic states.

蛋白质缺失性贫血的临床症状和化验结果与代谢减退状态的情况相似。

depolarization [diːˌpəuləraiˈzeiʃən] *n.* 去极化

The first stage of the action potential, that is, the initial positive change in the membrane potential, is called depolarization.

动作电位的第一期,即膜内电位开始变正期,称为去极化。

deposit [diˈpɔzit] *v.* 沉积

Obstruction of the bile duct is associated with cholangitis, and eggs may be deposited in the liver.

胆管梗阻可并发胆管炎,而且虫卵会沉积于肝内。

n. 沉淀,沉着

Calcium deposit may be seen in an old tuberculous.

陈旧的结核病变中可见钙沉积。

deposition [ˌdepəˈziʃən] *n.* 沉积,沉积物

The deposition of calcium salts is irregular and may be sufficiently heavy.

钙盐的沉积多少不一,可达到相当大的量。

depot [ˈdepəu] *n.* 仓库

If excess carbohydrate is taken into the body it is deposited as fat in the fat depots.

如果机体摄取糖过多,就以脂肪形式存于脂库。

depress [diˈpres] *v.* 抑制,降低,使消沉

Large doses of corticosteroids have been shown to depress wound healing in animals.

在动物身上大剂量使用皮质激素已证明可抑制伤口愈合。

depressant [diˈpresənt] *a.* 抑制的,镇静的

This is the disadvantage of giving depressant drugs rapidly.

这就是快速给予抑制剂的缺点。

n. 抑制剂

Propranolol reduces cardiac output and is a cardiac depressant.

心得安减少心输出量,为心脏抑制剂。

depressed [diˈprest] *a.* 抑郁的;压低的;凹陷的

Depressed patients often respond slowly to questions.

患抑郁症的病人通常对(所问的)问题反应迟钝。

The plaque is generally flat, and may be centrally depressed or even clear.

斑块一般是扁平的,也可以是中心凹陷甚至是平滑光亮的。

depression [diˈpreʃən] *n.* 阻抑,压低; 凹陷; 抑郁(症)

The patient must be carefully observed for signs of delayed respiratory depression.

必须仔细观察病人是否有迟发性呼吸抑制的体征。

ST depressions were noted on the anterior wall leads of the ECG.

心电图前壁导联可见 ST 段压低。

Between the median and lateral folds are depressions called epiglottic valleculae.

正中襞和外侧襞之间各有一凹陷称会厌谷。

Childhood depression is not as rare as previously believed.

儿童期抑郁症不像以往所相信的那样稀少。

depressive [diˈpresiv] *a.* 抑郁的

New treatment strategies for depressive disorders are being developed and studied.

目前正在发展和研究对付抑郁性疾病的新的治疗策略。

deprivation [ˌdepriˈveiʃən] *n.* 丧失，缺乏

Protein deprivation may cause hypometabolism.

蛋白质缺乏可引起低代谢。

The neurons of the central nervous system cannot withstand deprivation of blood supply for more than a very few minutes.

中枢神经系统的神经细胞不能耐受超过数分钟时间的缺血。

deprive(of) [diˈpraiv] *v.* 剥夺，使丧失

This piece of tissue is deprived of its blood supply.

这块组织的血液供应中断了。

depurination [diːˌpjuəriˈneiʃən] *n.* 脱嘌呤

This cross-linking of DNA strands represents a much greater threat to cellular survival than do other effects, such as single-base alkylation and the resulting depurination and chain scission.

DNA 链交联对细胞存活的威胁远大于其他效应，如单碱基烷化及由此引起的脱嘌呤和断链作用。

deputy [ˈdepjuti] *n.* 代表

One associate administrator works as a deputy to the administrator.

一位助理院长代行院长职能。

a. 副的

Professor Lin is the deputy-director of this newly-built children' s hospital.

林教授是这所新建的儿童医院的副院长。

derange [diˈreindʒ] *v.* 搅乱，使紊乱，使…失去正常功能

Deranged metabolism of vitamin D seems to play a major role in the abnormal calcium metabolism of chronic renal failure.

维生素 D 的代谢紊乱似乎在导致慢性肾衰的钙代谢异常中起主要作用。

derangement [diˈrendʒmənt] *n.* 紊乱；（精神）错乱

Derangement of glucose metabolism after surgery is not specific to patients with diabetes mellitus.

外科手术后发生的糖代谢紊乱 并不是糖尿病患者所特有的。

MRI is an ideal method to diagnose internal derangement of temporomandibular joint.

MRI 是诊断颞下颌关节内紊乱症的理想方法。

deratization [diːˌrætiˈzeiʃən] *n.* 灭鼠

The deratization is done with effective, high attraction and slow action, baits.

用高吸引力和缓动的有效诱饵实施灭鼠。

The word deratization refers to extermination of rats, particularly aboard a merchant vessel.

"Deratization"一词是指消灭老鼠，特别是在商船上。

derivative [diˈrivətiv] *n.* 衍生物，衍化物

Coal derivatives, such as coal tar, produce skin cancer and cancer of the larynx and bronchus in coke oven workers.

煤的衍生物，如煤焦油，在焦炭炉工人中引起皮肤癌、喉癌和支气管癌。

Protein purified derivative is a more specific product and is the current recommended solution for tuberculin testing.

（结核菌）纯蛋白衍化物是一种更特异的产物，也是目前推荐做结核菌素试验的溶液。

derive [diˈraiv] *v.* 取得；衍化；导出

The vitamin A required by the human organism is derived from plants, fish, and other animals.

人体所需的维生素 A 来源于植物、鱼和其他动物。

Margarine is derived from vegetable oils.

人造黄油是用植物油做的。

dermagraft [ˈdəːməgraːft] *n.* 皮肤移植;植皮

Dermagraft patches are just 200 microns thick when taken from the growth incubator.

植皮补片从培育孵化器取出时的厚度仅200微米。

dermal [ˈdəːməl] *a.* 皮肤的;真皮的

The patient has been given a dermal sensitivity test. It's all right.

病人已做过皮肤敏感试验,一切正常。

The dermal vasculature consists principally of three important intercommunicating plexuses.

真皮血管系统主要由三个重要的互相联通的血管丛组成。

dermatitis [ˌdəːməˈtaitis] *n.* 皮炎

Inflammation of the skin is called dermatitis.

皮肤的炎症称作皮炎。

When dermatitis is induced by contact with an external agent, it is called contact dermatitis.

接触性皮炎就是与外界的物质接触后引起的皮炎。

dermatologist [ˌdəːməˈtɔlədʒist] *n.* 皮肤病学家,皮肤科医师

Dermatologist David Alkek sees too many cases like this woman's.

皮肤病学家戴维·阿尔开克见过如同这位妇女一样的病例真是太多了。

dermatology [ˌdəːməˈtɔlədʒi] *n.* 皮肤病学

Dermatology is the medical specialty concerned with the diagnosis and treatment of skin disorders.

皮肤病学是有关皮肤疾病的诊断和治疗的医学学科。

There is one great advantage in dermatology, namely, that of dealing with an organ that can be seen and felt.

皮肤病学的最大优点是需诊断的器官既能看到又能摸到。

dermatome [ˈdəːmətəum] *n.* 生皮节;植皮刀,皮区

The somite forms the myotome, sclerotome and perhaps dermatome.

体节形成生肌节、生骨节、或许还有生皮节。

Before the large flap transplantation, the dermatome of reception should be covered with 4-to-6-layer sterile bandage soaked by this product and the bandage should be replaced at least once a day within 1-3 days.

大型皮瓣移植:受皮区在移植前至少在1~3日内用本品浸润无菌纱布4~6层湿敷,每日更换一次。

dermatomyositis [ˌdəːmətəuˌmaiəˈsaitis] *n.* 皮肌炎

When symptoms of dermatomyositis improve spontaneously, periods of remission may occur.

当皮肌炎症状自发性改善时,缓解期可能出现。

Dermatomyositis is an idiopathic inflammatory myopathy with characteristic cutaneous findings.

皮肌炎是一种具有典型皮肤损害的特发性炎症性肌病。

dermatophyte [ˈdəːmətəfait] *n.* 皮肤癣菌,表皮寄生菌,皮肤真菌

This drug has strong bacteriostatic action on dermatophyte and mildew which can result in different kinds of skin affection.

此药对能引发各种皮肤感染的皮肤癣菌和霉菌具有强烈的抑菌作用。

The test could detect some common dermatophytes species of laboratory animal rapidly and specifically.

该试验可快速且特异性地检测出实验动物的一些常见皮肤真菌的种类。

dermatophytosis [ˌdəːmətəuˌfaiˈtəusis] *n.* 皮肤真菌病

By using PCR-RFLP, all of the 6 dermatophytoses were diagnosed to species level.

利用PCR-RFLP技术,在菌种水平上所有6个皮肤癣菌被诊断出来。

Superficial fungal infections caused by dermatophytes, dermatophytoses, are the most common skin infections.

由皮肤癣菌引起的浅部真菌感染(皮肤真菌病)是最常见的皮肤感染。

dermatosis [ˌdəːməˈtəusis] *n.* 皮肤病

Corticosterone for topical use, antiallergic drugs and antifungal drugs are still the main drugs used for dermatosis.

外用皮质激素、抗变态反应药和抗真菌药仍是皮肤病的主要用药。

Clinical practice proved that moist exposed therapy is not only effective for treating burn wounds, but also very efficacious for chronic refractory dermatosis.

临床实践证明,该疗法不仅用于烧伤创疡,同样也对慢性顽固性皮肤病有很好的疗效。

dermis [ˈdəːmis] *n.* 真皮

The inner layer of skin is known as dermis.

皮肤的内层称为真皮。

The dermis is beneath the epidermis.

真皮在表皮的下面。

dermoid [ˈdəːmɔid] *a.* 皮样的

A dermoid cyst may occur at any age, but is commonly found during reproductive life.

皮样囊肿可发生于任何年龄,但常见于生殖年龄。

dermoplasty [ˈdəːməˌplæsti] *n.* 植皮术

Nosebleeds are treated with septal dermoplasty.

进行鼻中隔植皮术治疗鼻出血。

Nasal dermoplasty is effective in controlling epistaxis in patients with hereditary hemorrhagic telangiectasia.

鼻植皮术在控制遗传性出血性毛细血管扩张症患者的鼻出血方面是有效的。

desaturation [diːˌsætʃəˈreiʃən] *n.* 减饱和作用,饱和不足

Approximately 80 percent of patients with chronic obstructive lung diseases have nocturnal oxygen desaturation during sleep.

大概有 80% 的慢阻肺患者,夜间睡眠时有氧饱和不足现象。

descend [diˈsend] *v.* 下降

The liver, spleen, and gallbladder should descend with respiration.

肝脏、脾脏和胆囊会随呼吸下移。

It then descends on the left side of the abdomen into the pelvis.

然后在腹腔左侧向下进入盆腔。

descending [diˈsendiŋ] *a.* 下降的;下行的

Movement of the food material is then downward on the left in the descending colon, and finally into the rectum.

接着,食物在左侧往下入降结肠,最后进入直肠。

describe [disˈkraib] *v.* 描写,叙述

The rare congenital form of anemia is best characterized and can be used to describe some aspects of this anemia in the acquired form.

罕见的先天性贫血最具特色,可用以描述获得性贫血的某些方面。

The migration of lymphocytes from primary to secondary lymphoid tissue has already been described.

淋巴细胞从初级到次级淋巴组织之间的迁移过程已被描述过了。

description [disˈkripʃən] *n.* 描述

A precise description of the local muscle weakness usually makes it possible to decide whether a peripheral nerve, cord, trunk or root is affected.

对局部肌无力的精确描述通常有可能确定该患者是周围神经、脊髓(神经索)、神经干或神经根受累。

This section contains brief descriptions of some common renal disorders.
这部分包括了一些常见肾脏疾病的简要介绍。

descriptive [di'skriptiv] *a.* 描述的，叙述的

"Hydronephrosis" is a descriptive term that denotes dilation of the collecting system.
肾盂积水是用来描述在集合管系统内产生扩张的名词。

desensitization [diːˌsensitai'zeiʃən] *n.* 脱敏(感)作用

If the allergy is confirmed, desensitization should precede penicillin therapy.
如果病人对青霉素过敏，那么在应用青霉素治疗之前先进行脱敏。

The mean number of small antral follicles noted in both ovaries was also unchanged after pituitary desensitization.
双侧卵巢小窦卵泡的平均数量在垂体降调节后也未改变。

deserve [di'zəːv] *v.* 值得，应受

The views of these young anthropologists deserve considering.
这些年轻的人类学家们的观点值得认真考虑。

desiccate ['desikeit] *v.* 使干燥

Anticholinergic agents have been avoided in the past because of their tendency to desiccate secretions.
抗胆碱能药物在过去避免应用，因它们可使分泌物减少。

desiccation [desi'keiʃən] *n.* 干燥；脱水

Desiccation of the microbial cell causes a cessation of metabolic activity.
微生物细胞的脱水可导致代谢活性停止。

design [di'zain] *v.* 设计；预定

All civilized societies establish and enforce measures designed to protect the health of their population.
一切文明社会都会建立和推广旨在保护人民健康的措施。

There are other masses of lymphoid tissue which are designed to filter not lymph, but tissue fluid.
另有一些淋巴组织构成的团块，其功能不是过滤淋巴，而是组织液。

The spleen is an organ which contains lymphoid tissue designed to filter flood.
脾脏是一个含有以过滤血液为目的的淋巴组织的器官。

Another example is a family of drugs designed to combat high blood pressure.
另一例子是研制出治疗高血压的系列药物。

designate ['dezigneit] *v.* 标明，指明，指定

Bouffé e Délirante is a term used to designate acute psychotic episodes originally thought to occur in psychopathic personalities.
突发性谵妄这一术语是用来指原先认为是见于精神病态人格的急性精神病发作。

These viruses were believed to be enteroviruses and were designated echovirus 28.
人们认为这些病毒是肠道病毒，并定名为埃可病毒28。

designation [ˌdezig'neiʃən] *n.* 名称，牌号

A designation may be the key by which a physician or other reader identifies the compound.
一个牌号有可能成为医生或其他读者识别该化合物的关键。

desirability [diˌzaiərə'biliti] *n.* 需要，要求

The correct approach to the problem of hospital treatment of the elderly must be based on a consideration of the desirability of rest.
正确探讨老年患者住院治疗问题，必须从休息的需要出发来考虑。

desirous [di'zaiərəs] *a.* 想望的，渴望的

In such a case the patient is often desirous to be operated upon.
在这种情况下，患者常常渴望接受手术。

desmoid ['desmɔid] *n.* 硬纤维瘤

A desmoid tumor is an aggressive soft tissue tumor that often invades and destroys surrounding healthy tissue and organs.

硬纤维瘤是一种具有侵袭性的软组织肿瘤，常常浸润并破坏周围的健康组织和器官。

The estimated incidence of desmoid tumor in the general population is 2 to 4 per million people per year, according to the Desmoid Tumor Research Foundation.

据硬纤维瘤研究基金会的数据，硬纤维瘤在人群中的发病率估计是每年 2 ~4/百万人。

desmoplasia [ˌdesməˈpleiziə] *n.* 促结缔组织增生

Desmoplasia refers to the formation of an abundant collagenous stroma stimulated by the parenchymal cells of the tumor.

促结缔组织增生是指肿瘤实质细胞引起的大量胶原性间质的形成。

Carcinoma, for example pancreatic carcinoma, usually elicits an intense non-neoplastic host reaction of desmoplasia.

癌，例如胰腺癌，常引起强烈的非肿瘤性的促结缔组织增生反应。

desmoplastic [ˌdezməˈplæstik] *a.* 促结缔组织增生的

Most demoplastic tumors are stony-hard.

多数促结缔组织增生性肿瘤质地坚硬。

Desmoplastic small round cell tumor is a rare malignant small cell neoplasm which tends to occur in adolescents and young adults.

结缔组织增生性小圆细胞肿瘤是一种十分罕见的恶性小细胞肿瘤，好发于青少年及年轻人。

despite [disˈpait] *prep.* 尽管，不管

Some patients with IDD escaped from chronic complications despite "poor control".

一部分 IDD 病人即使未控制血糖也不会发生慢性并发症。(IDD = insulin-dependent diabetes 胰岛素依赖性糖尿病)

Syphilis is still a major problem throughout the world despite the great strides made in its control.

尽管在控制梅毒方面取得了长足的进步，但梅毒仍旧是全世界一大问题。

despondency [disˈpɔndənsi] *n.* 忧郁，丧气

In lay terminology, it is a state of gloom, despondency or sadness which may or may not denote ill-health.

作为非专业性术语，该症是一种情绪低落、沮丧或悲哀的状态，可以是也可以不是健康不佳。

desquamate [ˈdeskwəmeit] *v.* 脱屑，脱皮

Scalded skin syndrome may have large bulli which desquamate following abrasion.

脱屑性皮肤综合征可有大疱，在擦伤后脱皮。

desquamation [deskwəˈmeiʃən] *n.* 脱屑，脱皮

The type of desquamation depends on the texture of the skin.

脱屑的方式取决于皮肤的质地。

Dyspigmentation may occur in these areas after desquamation.

脱屑后可在这些部位发生色素沉着异常。

desquamative [diˈskwæmətiv, ˈdeskwəmeitiv] *a.* 脱屑性的

Desquamative interstitial pneumonia is characterized by the accumulation of large amount of macrophages in the airspaces.

脱屑性间质性肺炎以肺泡腔内大量巨噬细胞聚集为特征。

In desquamative interstitial pneumonia, the alveolar septa are thickened by a sparse chronic inflammatory cell infiltration.

脱屑性间质性肺炎肺泡间隔增宽，伴少量慢性炎症细胞浸润。

destain [diːˈstein] *v.* 使脱色

This renders the cell difficult to stain or destain.

这就使细胞难以染色或者脱色。

destine [ˈdestin] *v.* 注定，预定

Scientists have extended the life span of human cells by working out how to overcome the mechanisms that destine them to age and die.

科学家们通过征服致使细胞注定衰老和死亡的机制来延长人类细胞的寿命。

destroy [disˈtrɔi] *v.* 破坏，消灭

The most important function of leukocytes is to destroy certain pathogens.

白细胞最重要的功能是消灭某些病原体。

Normally an organ called the spleen destroys the older red blood cells.

在正常情况下，衰老的红细胞是由一个叫做脾脏的器官破坏的。

destruction [disˈtrʌkʃən] *n.* 消灭，破坏

The basic principles are the same, that is, to prevent the spread and cause the destruction of pathogenic microorganisms.

其基本原理是一样的，都是防止致病微生物的传播和消灭致病微生物。

destructive [disˈtrʌktiv] *a.* 破坏(性)的，危害的

A chronically destructive process as the renal failure is, it may occur rapidly.

虽然肾衰竭是一个慢性破坏过程，它却可能迅速出现。

Chlorine is destructive to the mucous membranes of the respiratory passages.

氯对呼吸道黏膜有破坏作用。

detach [diˈtætʃ] *v.* 分开，分离

Generally the cells can be detached from suitable internal surfaces such as the serous membranes in useful numbers simply by washing the surfaces with physiological saline.

一般来说，单用生理盐水清洗表面就可使这些细胞由像浆膜那样适宜的内表面分离出可用的数量来。

When thin crusts become detached, the base may be dry, or red and moist; it will usually heal leaving a smooth, normal skin surface.

薄痂分离脱落时，其基底可以是干燥的或是红色的和潮湿的；此病通常能治愈，留下光滑的正常的皮肤表面。

detached [diˈtætʃt] *a.* 分离的

Once the tumor has invaded the serosa of its organ, it may become detached and mechanically disseminated.

肿瘤一旦侵入器官的浆膜，瘤细胞就可脱落并机械地播散。

detachment [diˈtætʃmənt] *n.* 分开，分离，脱离

Blindness from retinal detachment is a complication.

因视网膜剥离而导致失明则属于并发症。

Both sheath and needle are rotated together, completing the detachment of the tissue from its surroundings.

鞘管和针芯一起旋转，使组织与周围的联系分隔开来。

detail [ˈdiːteil] *n.* 细节，详情

Details of the theoretical background and practical technique are not included here but can be found in standard text books of cardiology.

详细的理论基础和实用技术此处不涉及，可查阅标准的心脏病教科书。

Katz has reviewed in detail the many component layers of the basement membrane zone.

Katz 详细观察了组成基底膜区的各层。

The hairs are examined first with a low-power objective and then with a high-power objective for detail.

头发先用低倍镜检查，然后再用高倍镜细看。

v. 详述，细说

This young scientist detailed the experiments leading up to his new discovery.
这位年轻的科学家详细讲述了将他引向新发现的实验。
The characteristics of magnetic resonance apparatus are fully detailed is our brochure.
磁共振装置的特性在我们的介绍手册中有详细的说明。
It is essential to obtain a clear and detailed description of the specific symptoms.
获取有关特有症状的清楚而又详细的描述是非常重要的。

detect [di'tekt] *v.* 察觉,发现;检出,查出
Physical examination rarely establishes the specific diagnosis but may be useful in detecting disease in other organ system.
体检很少能确立特定的诊断,但有助于发现某些器官的疾病。
Mature thymocytes in the medulla express CD44, which is not detected in cortical thymocytes.
髓质中成熟的胸腺细胞可表达 CD44 分子,这在皮质胸腺细胞中并未检出。

detectable [di'tektəbl] *a.* 可察觉的
18 months after mastectomy 66% controls were free of clinically detectable disease compared to 93% of patients given CMF.
切除乳腺 18 个月后,对照组中 66% 的患者没有临床上可检出的症状,而给了 CMF 组的患者则是 93% 没有可检出的症状。

detection [di'tekʃən] *n.* 探测,检测,发现
Another form of negative staining is used for detection of the capsules around cells.
另一种背景染色法用于检测包绕菌细胞的荚膜。
A clear advantage of home-testing is early detection.
家庭测验的一个明显优势就是早期发现。

detective [di'tektiv] *n.* 侦探
You need to understand that the physician is a medical detective.
你应当明白医生是医学上的侦探。

detector [di'tektə] *n.* 探测器
Smoke detectors are under used, being found in only 80 percent of homes.
烟雾探测器使用不足,只有 80% 的家庭使用。
A smoke detector detects the presence of smoke.
烟尘探测器可探测是否存在烟雾。
This detector can acquire multiple signals.
这个探测器能捕捉多种信号。

detergent [di'təːdʒənt] *n.* 去垢剂,清洁剂
Skin cleansers containing mild detergents may be used in place of soap.
含有温和去垢剂的洁肤剂可用来代替肥皂。
Eczema may be a manifestation of an allergy to certain foods, detergents, soaps and other chemicals.
湿疹可能是对某些食物、清洁剂、肥皂和其他一些化学物质产生变态反应的表现形式。

deteriorate [di'tiəriəreit] *v.* 恶化
Renal function begins to deteriorate.
肾功能开始恶化。
Deteriorating blood gases may indicate decreasing cardiovascular function rather than a progression of the pulmonary disease.
血气恶化可能表示心血管功能下降,而不是肺疾病的恶化。

deterioration [ˌditiəriə'reiʃən] *n.* 恶化,衰退
If deterioration is sudden, tension pneumothorax should be suspected.
如果病情恶化突然发生,则应考虑张力性气胸。
The patient showed marked deterioration in general intellectual functions.

病人显示出总的智力功能的明显衰退。

determinant [diˈtəːminənt] *n.* 决定因素 *a.* 决定性的

The actual size of the placenta and efficiency of placental function are among the most important determinants of fetal growth.

胎盘的实际大小及功能状况是影响胎儿生长的最重要的决定因素之一。

Although heredity is the principal determinant of sex in mammals, environmental factors must also be operative.

在哺乳动物中，虽然遗传对性别起决定作用，但是环境也起作用。

determination [diˌtəːmiˈneiʃən] *n.* 决定；测定

Flow determinations in the pulmonary circuits have not been possible using regular echocardiography.

应用常规超声心动图检查不可能测得肺循环血流的状况。

determine [diˈtəːmin] *v.* 决定；确定；测定

Every living organism has DNA, which determines the growth and function of the cells.

每一个活的生物都有 DNA，它决定着细胞的生长和功能。

Various epidemiologic studies have been carried out to determine the frequency and specific cause of sudden death in defined populations.

已进行多项流行病学调查以确定在特定的人群中突然死亡的发生率和原因。

Trauma and degenerative joint disease seem to be determining factors for the localization.

创伤和退行性病变的关节疾病似乎是病变定位的决定性因素。

deterrent [diˈterənt] *n.* 抑制因素

These are potential deterrents to wound healing.

这些都是伤口愈合的潜在性抑制因素。

Inadequate housing is a clear deterrent to home confinement.

住房不足显然是家庭分娩的禁忌。

detoxication [diːˌtɔksiˈkeiuʃən] *n.* 解毒

The results showed that the detoxication of citrate acid to Pb and tartaric acid to Cd was comparatively distinct.

结果表明柠檬酸对铅、酒石酸对镉均有较明显的解毒作用。

The injury causes, wounds care and detoxication methods for 41 cases of burns by ammonia of liquid state were analyzed and researched.

对 41 例液氨烧伤患者的致伤原因、创面处理及解毒方法进行了分析和研究。

detoxification [diːˌtɔksifiˈkeiʃən] *n.* 解毒（作用），解毒方法

Methadone is used in the detoxification from and treatment of narcotic addiction.

美沙酮用于麻醉药成瘾的解毒和治疗。

detoxify [diːˈtɔksifai] *v.* 解毒，去毒

The process of biotransformation usually inactivates or detoxifies (or both) the administered drugs.

生物转化过程通常使服用的药物失活或解毒（或二者兼而有之）。

The filtering unit detoxifies the blood so that it can be returned to the patient.

过滤设备可将血液解毒并使其返回至患者体内。

detrimental(to) [ˌdetriˈmentl] *a.* 有害的

Air pollution is detrimental to health.

空气污染有害于健康。

devastation [devəsˈteiʃən] *n.* 破坏

This could further result in the devastation of a shared food supply.

这将进一步导致已分享的食物的供应恶化。

develop [diˈveləp] *v.* 发展；发育；发生；培养；开发；产生，（开始）患（病）；研制；显影

As the infection developed, the dull ache in his joints became a sharp stabbing pain.
随着感染的发展,他关节的隐痛变成了强烈的刺痛。
The fetus is developing normally in the uterus.
胎儿在子宫里发育正常。
Wheals develop in a few seconds, but disappear slowly.
疹块可在几秒钟内发生,但消退缓慢。
They have provided good material for developing the reading skills.
他们提供了培养阅读技巧的好材料。
We must develop the natural resources of our country.
我们必须开发我们国家的自然资源。
An organism against which immunity has been developed will be coated with antibody if it enters the blood stream.
已经有免疫力对抗的细菌,一旦侵入血液,就会被抗体包围。
Persons subsiding on a marginal diet are prone to develop macrocytic anemia from folic acid deficiency.
进食很少的人易因叶酸缺乏而患巨红细胞性贫血。
A vaccine against the more common meningitis B will take far longer to develop, as the bacterium is more complicated.
一种抗更常见的乙型脑膜炎疫苗,由于这种细菌更复杂,研制起来须用更长时间。
He has developed the X-ray film taken for a lung cancer patient.
他已把给一位肺癌病人拍的 X 线片冲洗出来了。

development [di'veləpmənt] *n.* 发展;生长 ;发育;形成;产生;显影
Primary lymphoid organs are the major sites of lymphocyte development.
初级淋巴器官是淋巴细胞发育的主要场所。
The primary lesions may continue to full development or be modified by regression, trauma, or other extraneous factors.
原发损害可继续充分地发展,或因消退、损伤或其他外部因素而发生改变。
Gradually the blood pressure becomes stabilized at a higher level, as the result of development of arteriosclerosis.
由于已经产生了动脉硬化,所以血压会逐渐稳定在一个较高的水平上。
In conclusion, glucocorticoids have profound effects on mineral metabolism and bone cell function, which lead to the development of osteoporosis.
总之,糖皮质激素对矿物质代谢和骨细胞功能有着深远的影响,从而导致骨质疏松症的发生。

developmentally [diˌveləp'mentəli] *ad.* 发育地
The optic nerve is a fiber tract of the brain because developmentally the retina is a part of the brain.
视神经是脑的纤维束,因为在发育上视网膜是脑的一部分。

deviate ['diːvieit] *v.* 背离,偏离
Frontal sinuses are rarely symmetrical, because the septum between them frequently deviates from the median plane.
由于额窦间的中隔常不在正中,故很少对称。

deviation [ˌdiːvi'eiʃən] *n.* 偏差,误差
The more malignant the tumour, the more deviation from normal tissues.
肿瘤恶性度越高,与正常组织的差异就越大。
Alpha-fetoprotein concentration was considered to be elevated at 5 or more standard deviation above the mean.
甲胎蛋白浓度超过平均值 5 或 5 个以上的标准差即视为升高。

device [diˈvais] *n.* 器械,装置

Experienced physicians can gain much information using this device.

有经验的医生用这种仪器可了解很多的病情。

Though its employment requires knowledge and care, it is basically a simple device and easy to handle.

虽然使用它需要一定的知识和细心,但它基本上还是一种简单并容易操作的装置。

devise [diˈvaiz] *v.* 设计,发明

Imaging studies have been devised to minimize the likelihood of unsuccessful surgical explorations.

已设计了影像学检查的方法以便减少外科手术失败的可能性。

In order to improve sensitivity and specificity, tests have been devised using a treponemal antigen.

为了增加检测的灵敏度和特异性,人们设计了应用密螺旋体作抗原的试验。

devitalize [ˌdiːˈvaitəlaiz] *v.* 使衰弱;夺去生命

Small molecule amiloride modulates oncogenic RNA alternative splicing to devitalize human cancer cells.

小分子阿米洛利可调节致瘤性 RNA 的选择性剪接而杀死人的癌细胞。

It is essential to devitalize the teeth.

必须使牙失活。

devoid(of) [diˈvɔid] *a.* 缺乏的,没有的

Red blood cells are devoid of a nucleus.

红细胞没有核。

The drug is said to be efficacious for great pain and is devoid of any side effects.

据称该药对剧痛有效,而且没有任何副作用。

The patient's right arm is devoid of sensation of pain.

病人右臂失去痛觉。

devotion [diˈvəuʃən] *n.* 献身,忠诚

We highly respect him for his unselfish devotion to the development of medical science.

我们高度尊敬他对医学科学发展的无私奉献。

Dr. Li's utter devotion to the good of the people impressed us deeply.

李医生对人民利益的绝对忠诚给我们很深的印象。

dexamethasone [ˌdeksəˈmeθəsəun] *n.* 地塞米松

The dose of dexamethasone is seven times smaller than that of prednisone.

地塞米松的剂量是强的松的七分之一。

The patient cannot but administer dexamethasone in high dosage to reduce the swelling and save the sight.

此病人不得不用大剂量地塞米松来减轻水肿,并恢复视力。

dextran [ˈdekstrən] *n.* 葡聚糖

If neither whole blood nor plasma is immediately available, dextran may be used.

如果既没有立刻可用的全血又没有血浆,可使用葡聚糖。

Dextran expands the volume of plasma, although it is not a substitute for blood.

葡聚糖虽然不是血液的代用品,但可以扩充血浆的容积。

dextrin [ˈdekstrin] *n.* 糊精,葡聚糖

The sustained release formulations were prepared by using natural polymers like dextrin, guar gum and xanthan gum.

天然高分子物质如糊精、古尔胶和黄原胶被用于制备缓释制剂。

Starch converting enzymes are used in the production of malt dextrin, modified starches, or glucose and fructose syrups.

淀粉转化酶可以用于生产麦芽糊精、变性淀粉或葡萄糖和果糖糖浆。

dextrocardia [ˌdekstrəˈkɑːdiə] *n.* 右位心

Dextrocardia is a congenital defect in which the heart is situated on the right side of the body.

右位心是一种心脏位于身体右侧的先天性缺陷。

Medical diagnosis of congenital dextrocardia can be made by ECG or imaging.

心电图和影像学可以诊断先天性的右位心。

dextromethorphan [ˌdekstrəuˈmeθəfən] *n.* 美沙芬，右甲吗喃

Dextromethorphan is an antitussive agent.

右甲吗喃是一种镇咳药。

dextrose [ˈdekstrəus] *n.* 葡萄糖

An infusion of 1000 ml of 5% dextrose in water was started.

已开始输入 5% 葡萄糖 1000ml。

diabetes [daiəˈbiːtiːz] *n.* 糖尿病

There appears to be an inherited tendency to diabetes; the disorder may be triggered by various factors, including physical stress.

糖尿病似有遗传倾向，可由各种因素（如体力紧张）诱发。

The clinical picture of diabetes is due to diminished availability or effectiveness of insulin.

糖尿病的临床表现，是由于胰岛素的可利用性或有效性降低造成的。

diabetic [ˌdaiəˈbetik] *n.* 糖尿病患者

A diabetic must be careful of his diet.

糖尿病病人必须注意自己的饮食。

The first product is a skin graft that can heal foot ulcers in diabetics.

第一个产品是皮移植片，它能使糖尿病患者足部溃疡愈合。

a. 糖尿病的

Other causes of unconsciousness predisposing to aspiration lung abscess are convulsive seizures, anesthesia, diabetic coma, etc.

造成吸入性肺脓肿昏迷的其他原因有惊厥发作、麻醉、糖尿病性昏迷等。

diacylglycerol [daiæsilˈglisərɔl] *n.* 甘油二酯

A good yield of diacylglycerol-rich oil was obtained in a short reaction time under sonication and soft conditions.

在超声处理与温和的条件下，在较短反应时间内就得到了高产量的富含甘油二酯的油。

Diacylglycerol acyltransferase (DGAT) has been proposed as one of the drug targets for treating obesity and type 2 diabetes.

有人提出甘油二酯酰基转移酶可作为治疗肥胖和 2 型糖尿病的药物靶点之一。

The diacylglycerol(DAG) stays in the membrane, where it acts as an intracellular signaling molecule, activating protein kinase C, which further propagates the signal.

甘油二酯(DAG)呆在细胞膜内，在那里作为一种细胞内信号分子激活蛋白激酶 C，后者进一步转导信号。

diagnose [ˈdaiəgnəuz] *v.* 诊断

Those tumours arising in the skin are usually diagnosed and removed early.

发生于皮肤的那些肿瘤通常诊断和切除得早。

His illness was diagnosed as acute intestinal obstruction.

他的病被诊断为急性肠梗阻。

diagnosis [ˌdaiəgˈnəusis] *n.* 诊断

Investigations are used to confirm or deny a doubtful or difficult clinical diagnosis.

（用实验室）检查方法来确定或否定置疑的或困难的临床诊断。

Early diagnosis usually means high curability.

早期诊断常意味着很高的治愈率。

diagnostic [ˌdaiəgˈnɔstik] *a.* 诊断的

It is likely that, as diagnostic techniques improve, further causes of hypertension will be identified.

随着诊断技术的改进,很可能有更多的高血压病因得以查明。

A fluctuating level of consciousness is a major diagnostic criterion for delirium.

意识水平的波动是谵妄的一个主要诊断指标。

Bloody sputum in a chronic bronchitis patient is usually diagnostic of bronchiectasis.

慢性支气管炎病人的血痰,常作为诊断支气管扩张的依据。

diagram [ˈdaiəgræm] *n.* 图表

The diagram shows the forces acting on each block.

图中指出作用在每个物块上的力。

This is a very simplified and stylised diagram.

这是个非常简化和程序化的图表。

diakinesis [ˌdaiəkiˈniːsis] *n.* 丝球期,终变期

In diakinesis stage, the chromosomes reach maximal condensation.

在终变期,染色体达到最大程度的凝集。

Diakinesis is the last stage of the prophase in the first division of meiosis.

终变期是减数分裂第一次分裂前期的最后一个阶段。

dialysate [daiˈæliseit] *n.* 透析液;渗析液

Waste products in the bloodstream pass through the peritoneum into the dialysate.

血流中的代谢废物通过腹膜进入透析液。

A number of investigations showed that amino acid peritoneal dialysate in malnutrition CAPD (continuous ambulatory peritoneal dialysis) patients had benefit effects on improving nutrition status.

许多研究表明氨基酸腹膜透析液对改善营养不良的连续腹膜透析患者的营养状态有益。

dialysis [daiˈælisis] (*pl.* dialyses [daiˈælisiːz]) *n.* 透析,渗析

Severe renal failure is most easily managed by dialysis.

严重的肾衰用透析最易于控制。

Chronic dialysis and renal transplantation are routine in these patients.

这些病人按常规需进行长期的透析和肾移植手术。

dialyze [ˈdaiəlaiz] *v.* 渗析,透析

The dialyzing fluid contains none of the waste products of metabolism.

透析液中没有代谢废物。

This mixture was stored overnight at 5℃ and then dialyzed in the cold 0.05M sodium hydroxide.

将该混合物储存于5℃过夜,然后在冷的0.05M 氢氧化钠溶液中进行渗析。

dialyzer [ˈdaiəlaizə] *n.* 透析器

Haemodialysis is performed on patients whose kidneys have ceased to function; the process takes place in an artificial kidney, or dialyzer.

血液透析用于两侧肾脏已经丧失功能的病人,透析通过人工肾或透析机进行。

diameter [daiˈæmitə] *n.* 直径

The whole cell has a diameter of about one fiftieth of a millimetre.

完整细胞的直径约为1/50 毫米。

Snyder and Stellar reported an incidence rate of 20 per cent for rebleeding in ulcers greater than 2.5 cm in diameter.

Snyder 和 Stellar 报道,患有溃疡面直径大于2.5cm 时,其再出血的发病率为20% 。

diamond [ˈdaiəmənd] *n.* 菱形

The popliteal fossa is the diamond-shaped region at the posterior aspect of the knee.

腘窝为膝后方的一菱形区。

diapedesis [ˌdaiəpiˈdiːsis] (*pl.* diapedeses [ˌdaiəpiˈdiːsiːz]) *n.* 血细胞渗出

There is diapedesis of erythrocytes into the alveoli.

有红细胞渗出到肺泡内。

In the precence of infection large numbers of leucocytes reach the vaginal cavity, presumably by diapedesis through the vaginal wall.

感染时大量白细胞出现在阴道腔内,它可能是通过阴道壁渗出的。

diaphoresis [daiəfəˈriːsis] *n.* 出汗

Diaphoresis is the process of sweating, especially excessive sweating.

出汗是汗液分泌的过程,特别在大量汗液分泌时(更为明显)。

Myocardial infarction may be accompanied by diaphoresis, nausea and hypotension.

心肌梗死患者可伴有明显出汗、恶心和低血压。

diaphragm [ˈdaiəfræm] *n.* 膈,膈肌

The thorax is separated from the abdomen by the diaphragm.

胸腔与腹腔由膈肌分开。

diaphragmatic [ˌdaiəfrægˈmætik] *a.* 膈肌的

On admission Q waves were noted on the diaphragmatic wall leads.

入院时膈肌面壁导联有 Q 波。

diapophysis [ˌdaiəˈpɔfisis] *n.* 横突关节面

Under the guidance of CT, the needle punctures through the inner margin of diapophysis and gets in intervertebral disc.

在 CT 引导下,针经横突关节面内侧缘穿刺进入椎间盘内。

The total 27 cases of laminectomy and decompressive discectomy include internal fixation and diapophysis fusion for 23 cases.

进行全椎板切除及为减压的椎间盘切除的 27 例病人中有 23 例内固定加横突关节面融合的患者。

diarrh(o)ea [ˌdaiəˈriə] *n.* 腹泻

In this case, diarrhoea and vomiting are common and renal failure may develop.

在这种情况下,常有腹泻及呕吐,且可发展为肾功能衰竭。

Children are often liable to diarrhea, particularly if they are fed on artificial food.

儿童常易患腹泻,人工喂养的儿童尤其如此。

diaschisis [daiˈæskisis] *n.* 失联络现象

Diaschisis is a sudden loss of function in a portion of the brain connected to but at a distance of a damaged area.

失联络显像指远离损伤区域的大脑局部突发的功能丧失。

Crossed cerebellar diaschisis is a condition in which cerebellar hypometabolism is ascribed to functional disconnection of the contralateral hemisphere from the cerebral cortex.

交叉小脑失联络是由于小脑皮质与对侧大脑半球功能分离引起的小脑代谢减退。

diassociation [diəˌsəusiˈeiʃən] *n.* 分离,分裂

This increased optical density caused by a disassociation or melting of the DNA is called hyperchromicity.

这种由于 DNA 离解或融解引起的光密度增加,称之为增色效应。

The formation and disassociation of molecular clusters is off balance.

分子簇的形成与离解处于不平衡状态。

diastasis [daiˈæstəsis] *n.* 慢速充盈相,脱离

In physiology diastasis refers to the middle stage of diastole during a heartbeat cycle.

生理学上,慢速充盈相指心动周期时的舒张中期。

In pathology diastasis basically means separation of body parts that are joined together.

病理学上,脱离主要指身体相连部分的分离。

diastole [daiˈæstəli] *n.* 舒张(期)
During the period of diastole, the atrioventricular valves are open and the arterial valves are closed.
在(心)舒张期,房室瓣开放,动脉瓣关闭。

diastolic [daiəˈstɔlik] *a.* 舒张期的
No diastolic murmur was audible.
未听到舒张期杂音。
The normal diastolic blood pressure ranges between 65 and 85mmHg.
正常舒张压在 65 与 85mmHg 之间。

diastomyelia [dai,æstəmaiˈiːliə] *n.* 脊髓纵裂
Diastomyelia should be treated according to its type.
脊髓纵裂应按分型确定治疗方法。

diathesis [daiˈæθisis] *n.* 素质
Care should also be exercised in the immunization of children with a family history of an allergic diathesis.
对具有过敏素质家族史的儿童来说,在进行免疫时,需要格外的小心。
If anemia or bleeding diathesis is prominent, fresh frozen plasma or blood may be necessary.
如果贫血或出血素质明显,可能需用新鲜的冰冻血浆或血液。

diazepam [ˌdaiˈæzipæm] *n.* 安定,苯并二氮䓬
Diazepam, 8 to 40mg in divided doses, may make bed rest more tolerable.
分次给予剂量由 8 到 40 毫克的安定片能使病人更易卧床休息。
If emotional factors are important then a tranquillizer such as diazepam(valium) may be helpful.
如果情感因素起重要作用的话,服用镇静剂如苯并二氮䓬(安定)可能是有效的。

diencephalon [ˌdaienˈsefələn] *n.* 间脑
The diencephalon is a complex of structures within the brain; the major divisions of it are the thalamus and hypothalamus
间脑是脑内结构的复合体,主要分为丘脑和下丘脑。
The diencephalon relays sensory information between brain regions and controls many autonomic functions of the peripheral nervous system.
间脑负责大脑各区域之间的信息传递,并调控周围神经系统的许多自主功能。

diet [ˈdaiət] *n.* 饮食,节食
Antacids and diet often ameliorate symptoms but do not hasten healing.
制酸剂和饮食常可使症状缓解,但不能促使痊愈。
My mother and aunts are always trying new diets in order to reduce.
我母亲和姨母们为了减肥一直在试行新的饮食法。
The doctor put her on a diet.
医生让她吃规定的饮食。

dietary [ˈdaiətəri] *a.* 饮食的,食物的
The patient should stop smoking and adopt whatever dietary regime suits him best.
病人应戒烟,并采用最适合于他自己的食谱。
Thus, as long as the body is exposed to adequate sunlight, there is little or no dietary requirement for vitamin D.
因此只要机体能沐浴到充足的阳光,就很少需要或不需要食物供给维生素 D。

dietitian [daiəˈtiʃən] *n.* 营养学家
Nutritional management in patients with ARF requires close collaboration among physicians, nurses, and dietitians.
急性肾衰(ARF)病人的营养支持需要医生、护士和营养学家之间的密切合作。
The registered dietitian(RD), especially the clinical nutrition specialist, is the nutrition authority

on the health care team.
注册营养医师,特别是临床营养专家,是医疗小组的营养权威。

dietetics [ˌdaiəˈtetiks] *n.* 饮食学,营养学
Dietetics is the science concerned with the nutritional planning and preparation of foods.
营养学是关于营养计划的制订和食物烹调的科学。

differential [difəˈrenʃəl] *a.* (有)差别的,鉴别的
This aids in making the differential diagnosis.
此有助于鉴别诊断。
n. 差异,鉴别
The presence of an abdominal mass calls for a long list of differentials.
腹部肿块的出现需要与一系列疾病相鉴别。

differentiate [ˌdifəˈrenʃieit] *v.* 区分,鉴别;分化
Special laboratory tests should help to differentiate myeloencephalitis resulting from toxins or chemicals.
特殊化验应有助于鉴别由于毒素或化学物质引起的脑脊髓炎。
With time monocytes increase in number and differentiate into macrophages.
随着时间的推移,单核细胞逐渐增多并分化为巨噬细胞。
Gradually, the newly developing cells differentiate into the special cells that form the organs of the body.
新发育着的细胞渐渐分化成为形成身体器官的特殊细胞。

differentiation [ˌdifərenʃiˈeiʃən] *n.* 区别,鉴别;分化
Differentiation should also be made between affinity and intrinsic activity.
亲和力和内在活性间也应相区别。
The diagnosis of meningococcal meningitis requires differentiation from meningismus, other bacterial meningitides and viral meningoencephalitis.
脑膜炎双球菌脑膜炎在诊断时应与假性脑膜炎、其他细菌性脑膜炎和病毒性脑膜炎等相鉴别。
The affected cells grow differently and lack the differentiation characteristics of normal cells.
受影响的细胞生长方式发生变化,而不再具有正常细胞所特有的分化作用。

difficile [diːfiˈsiːl] *n.* 艰难(梭菌)
This paper described the cell killing activity of toxin A of clostridium difficile on four cell lines.
本文描述了艰难梭菌 A 毒素对 4 种培养细胞的细胞杀伤活性。

difficulty [ˈdifikəlti] *n.* 困难
During asthma, characteristically, there is great difficulty in breathing.
哮喘时,其特点是出现了呼吸的极度困难。

diffractometer [ˌdifrækˈtɔmitə] *n.* 衍射仪
XRD (X-ray diffraction) diffractometer is a very effective spectrum analyzer.
X 射线衍射仪是非常有效的光谱分析仪器。

diffuse¹ [diˈfjuːz] *v.* 扩散,散开
Products of the dead cells diffuse out and promote an acute inflammatory reaction.
死亡细胞的产物弥散出来,并引起急性炎性反应。
Isoniazid diffuses well throughout the body and reach therapeutic concentrations in serum.
异烟肼良好地分布全身,并在血清中达到治疗浓度。

diffuse² [diˈfjuːs] *a.* 扩散的,弥漫性的
The child's skull X-ray shows diffuse intracranial calcifications.
小儿头颅片显示颅内广泛钙化。
Ascitic leaks increase the incidence of wound infection, and may result in diffuse peritonitis.
腹水漏出可增大伤口感染率,因而可能导致弥漫性腹膜炎。

diffusible [di'fjuːzəbl] *a.* 可扩散的

Pyruvate is diffusible across the mitochondrial membrane by means of a carrier.

丙酮酸盐通过载体可穿过线粒体膜扩散。

These inductions are mediated by diffusible substances.

这些诱导是由某些可扩散的物质作为媒介促成的。

diffusion [di'fjuːʒən] *n.* 扩散

Diffusion of the drug into the interstitial component occurs rapidly.

药物迅速扩散到组织间隙。

There should occur a rapid diffusion of large numbers of bacilli by the air passages.

有大量的杆菌通过气道迅速播散。

digest [di'dʒest, dai'dʒest] *v.* 消化

All kinds of food begin to digest as soon as they enter the stomach.

各种食物一进胃内就开始消化。

The quantity of gastric juice secreted depends upon the amount and kind of food to be digested.

胃液分泌量的多少取决于被消化的食物的量和种类。

digestible [di'dʒestəbl] *a.* 可消化的,易消化的

A digestible lump of sugar as well as an indigestible coin would begin the tour of the alimentary canal in the oral cavity.

不管是可消化的糖块还是不可消化的硬币,其消化道之旅都必从口腔开始。

The digestible food and the indigestible coin are both pushed by the tongue into the pharynx.

可消化的食物和不可消化的硬币两者都是由舌头(向后)推入咽部的。

digestion [di'dʒestʃən, dai'dʒestʃən] *n.* 消化

Exercise is beneficial to the process of digestion.

运动有助于消化。

Digestion and absorption are the two chief functions of the digestive system.

消化和吸收是消化系统的两大重要功能。

digestive [di'dʒestiv, dai'dʒestiv] *a.* 消化的

The gastric glands, which cover most of the mucosa of the body, secrete large quantities of digestive juices.

覆盖胃体大部分的胃腺分泌大量消化液。

The alimentary canal is a muscular digestive tube extending through the body.

消化道是伸展贯穿于整个人体内的肌肉性的消化管道。

digit ['didʒit] *n.* 阿拉伯数字;手指;足趾

It is often tested at the bedside by asking the patient to recall several digits forward and backward.

通常在床边让病人顺着或倒着复述几个阿拉伯数字进行检查。

These arteriovenous anastomoses are best developed on the digits.

这些动静脉吻合支在手指或足趾的分布非常丰富。

The doctor on duty put a dressing on the mangled digit of the worker.

值班医生给这位工人血肉模糊的手指放上了敷料。

digital ['didʒitl] *a.* 指(趾)的;指纹样的;计数的,数字的

Digital rectal examination is a valuable diagnostic measure for the purpose of ruling out a large rectal cancer.

直肠指诊是用于排除大的直肠癌的一个有用的诊断方法。

Ten years ago I once saw a giant general-purpose transistorized digital computer in Beijing.

十年前我在北京曾经见过一台晶体管大型通用数字计算机。

Dr. Lin has bought a famous brand of digital camera.

林医生买了一个名牌数码照相机。

digitalis [ˌdidʒiˈteilis] *n.* 洋地黄

These vasodilators can successfully be used in conjunction with digitalis and diuretics.

这些血管扩张剂也能有效地与洋地黄和利尿剂联合使用。

With few exceptions, these patients should continue on digitalis therapy.

除少数例外,这些患者应该继续用洋地黄疗法。

digitalisation [ˌdidʒitəliˈseiʃən] *n.* 洋地黄化

Ventricular rate in atrial fibrillation is controlled by digitalisation.

房颤时的心室率可用洋地黄化控制。

Rapid digitalization is indicated when evidence of cardiac insufficiency is present.

当出现心功能不全症状时需急速给予洋地黄并达到洋地黄化。

digitoxin [didʒiˈtɔksin] *n.* 洋地黄毒甙

Digitoxin is a drug that increases heart muscle constraction and is used in heart failure.

洋地黄毒甙是可以增强心肌收缩的药物,常用来治疗心力衰竭。

Digitalis contains various substances, including digitoxin and digoxin, that stimulate heart muscle.

洋地黄含有洋地黄毒甙和地高辛等多种具有刺激心肌作用的成分。

dignity [ˈdignəti] *n.* 尊严,高尚,体面

Adequate pain control, maintenance of human dignity, and close contact with family are crucial.

最重要的是充分进行镇痛,保持人的尊严及与家人密切的联系。

digoxin [daiˈgɔksin, di-] *n.* 地高辛

Digoxin binds to plasma protein to the extent of 23 percent.

地高辛与血浆蛋白的结合率为23%。

dihydrofolic [ˌdaihaidrəuˈfəulik] *a.* 二氢叶酸的

In man and animals, ingested folic acid is reduced to dihydrofolic acid.

在人和动物体内摄入的叶酸被还原成二氢叶酸。

dihydromorphinone [daiˌhaidrəuˈmɔːfinəun] *n.* 二氢吗啡酮

Morphine and dihydromorphinone are equally efficacious.

吗啡和二氢吗啡酮的效能相等。

dihydropteridine [dai, haidrəuˈteridiːn] *n.* 二氢生物蝶呤

Here we report two cases of dihydropteridine reductase deficiency.

这里我们报道两个二氢生物蝶呤还原酶缺陷的病例。

The activity of dihydropteridine reductase is low.

二氢生物蝶呤还原酶的活性低。

dihydropyrimidine [dai, haidrəupəˈrimidiːn] *n.* 二氢嘧啶

Polymorphisms of the dihydropyrimidine dehydrogenase gene are associated with decreased enzyme activity and a significant risk of overwhelming drug toxicity.

二氢嘧啶脱氢酶基因的多态性与酶活性降低及强烈药物毒性的重大风险有关。

dihydroxycholecalciferol [ˈdaihai, drɔksi, kəulikælˈsifərɔl] *n.* 二羟胆钙化醇,二羟维生素 D

Calcium absorption is facilitated by 1,25-dihydroxycholecalciferol.

1,25-二羟维生素 D 可促进钙吸收。

Cholecalciferol is hydroxylated in the renal cortical cells to 1,25-dihydroxycholecalciferol.

胆骨化醇在肾皮质细胞内羟化为 1,25-二羟维生素 D.

dilatation [ˌdaileiˈteiʃən] *n.* 膨胀,扩张(术)

Alcohol produces dilatation of the skin vessels, flushing, and a sensation of warmth.

酒精引起皮肤血管扩张、面部潮红和温暖的感觉。

There was a moderate degree of right ventricular dilatation.

右心室轻度扩张。

The stomach is a dilatation of the alimentary canal between the esophagus and the duodenum.
胃是食管与十二指肠间的消化道扩张部分。

dilate [daiˈleit] *v.* 扩大,膨胀
If large quantities of blood enter, the heart chambers dilate greatly.
如果大量血液进入,心室腔大大扩张。
Her pupils are dilated, her mucous membranes dry.
她的瞳孔散大,黏膜干燥。

dila(ta)tion [daiˈleiʃən, ˌdailəˈteiʃən] *n.* 扩张,膨胀部分
Vascular dilation occurs directly after injury.
损伤后立即发生血管扩张。
The carotid sinus is a slight dilation of the proximal part of the internal carotid artery.
颈动脉窦为颈内动脉起始部的稍微膨大部分。
Acute toxic dilation of the colon with bleeding and perforation still has a high mortality.
伴有出血和穿孔的急性中毒性结肠扩张,死亡率仍很高。

dilator [daiˈleitə] *n.* 扩张剂
Epinephrine is a dilator of bronchial smooth muscle.
肾上腺素是一种支气管平滑肌的扩张药。

dilemma [diˈlemə] *n.* 困境,进退两难
The dilemma the doctor faced was whether he should tell the patient the truth.
医生面临的困境是要不要把事情的真相告诉病人。
Therapeutic abortion remains a dilemma for the medical profession.
治疗性流产对医务工作者来说仍是一个进退两难的事情。

diluent [ˈdiljuənt] *a.* 用以稀释的 *n.* 稀释剂
Blood counts are normally made by diluting a measured volume of blood with an appropriate diluent or lysing agent and counting in a chamber under the microscope.
血细胞计数,在正常情况下是把要测定的血量加入适当的稀释剂或细胞溶解剂后置于血细胞计数板的计数池内,在显微镜下计数。

dilute [daiˈljuːt] *v.* 稀释
The increase in interstitial fluid dilutes toxins.
间质内液体增加可稀释毒素。
Undue pressure that might cause tissue fluids to dilute the blood should be avoided while collecting the specimen.
采集血样时应尽量避免过度压挤造成组织液对血液的稀释。

dilution [daiˈljuːʃən] *n.* 稀释,稀释剂
The titer generally decreases by at least two dilutions within several months of adequate therapy for primary or secondary disease.
初期或二期梅毒患者经数月充分的治疗后,滴度一般至少降两个稀释度。

dim [dim] *a.* 暗淡的,模糊的
Reading in a dim light is bad for the eyes.
在暗淡的光线下阅读对眼睛有害。

dimension [diˈmenʃən] *n.* 维数,度数,尺寸
Two-dimensional echocardiography is particularly useful in assessing the dimensions of each cardiac chamber.
二维超声心动图在评估每个心腔大小时尤其有用。
Examination of other left ventricular dimensions after dilatation indicates that the greatest enlargement occurs at its mid-portion.
测量扩张后的左心室尺寸的数据表明其增大最明显的部位在中部。

dimensional [diˈmenʃənəl] *n.* 维度的

X-rays capture only a slice of the body's three-dimensional structure。
X 射线仅能获得身体某一部分的三维构造。
This subroutine sorts one or two dimensional arrays.
这个子程序可以对一维或者二维数组进行排序。

dimerize [ˈdaiməraiz] *v.* 形成二聚体
These receptors consist of a single subunit and dimerize on ligand binding.
这些受体含有单一亚单位,并在结合域形成二聚体。

dimethicone [ˌdaiməˈθikəun] *n.* 二甲基硅油
An overview of dimethicone for the treatment of head lice infestations is presented.
该文章对二甲基硅油治疗头虱传染进行了概述。
Dimethicone seems less irritant than existing treatments.
二甲基硅油似乎比现有的治疗方法刺激性要小。

dimethylbenzene [dai,meθilˈbenziːn] *n.* 二甲苯
This regulation prescribes the concentrations of benzene, toluene and dimethylbenzene in air for residential area by gas chromatograph method.
本条例规定用气相色谱法测定的居住区大气中苯、甲苯和二甲苯的浓度。
Gutted flap should be washed by current water, dehydrated by using graded ethanol, vitrified by dimethylbenzene and deposited in holly oil.
切取皮瓣流水冲洗,酒精梯度脱水,二甲苯透明,冬青油内保存。

diminish [diˈminiʃ] *v.* 减少,缩减
In case of acute pancreatic necrosis, both pancreatic and biliary secretions are diminished.
在急性胰腺坏死的病例,胰腺和胆汁的分泌都减少。
Diminished numbers of surface receptors lead to altered cellular responses.
表面受体数目减少可导致细胞反应改变。
They are arranged and numbered in order of diminishing size.
按由大渐小的次序排列并标上号码。

diminution [dimiˈnjuːʃən] *n.* 减少;缩减
There is generally diminution of self-control, foresight, creativity and spontaneity.
通常会出现自制力、预见力、创造力和自发性的降低。
Narrowing of airways is often associated with a diminution in maximal expiratory flow rate.
气道变窄后常使最大呼气流速降低。

dioxide [daiˈɔksaid] *n.* 二氧化物
Normal air around us consists of nitrogen, oxygen, carbon dioxide, and several other lesser-known gases.
我们周围的正常空气系由氮、氧、二氧化碳及几种不甚知名的其他气体组成。

dioxin [daiˈɔksin] *n.* 二噁英
Dioxin, being one of the most toxic chemical, can cause cancer, severe reproductive problem and immune system damage.
二噁英是毒性最强的化学物质之一,它可引起癌症、严重生殖障碍和免疫系统损伤。

dipeptide [daiˈpeptaid] *n.* 二肽
Two amino acids become joined by a peptide bond to form a dipeptide.
两个氨基酸分子通过肽键连接形成二肽。
The removal of a molecule of water from two amino acid molecules results in the formation of a dipeptide.
两个氨基酸分子通过失去一分子水缩合形成二肽。

diphasic [daiˈfeizik] *a.* 二相性的,双相的
The fever may follow a diphasic course.
发热可表现为双相热。

diphenhydramine [ˌdaifenˈhaidrəmiːn] *n.* 苯海拉明

Diphenhydramine is most effective in reversing the neuroleptic-induced dystonia.

苯海拉明对抗神经镇静剂引起的肌张力障碍是最有效的。

diphtheria [difˈθiəriə] *n.* 白喉

Patches on the tonsils and throat suggest diphtheria.

扁桃体和咽喉上的白色片状物使人想到是白喉。

The prompt administration of diphtheria antitoxin in adequate amounts is the first and most important step.

及时地给予适量的白喉抗毒素是首要的也是最重要的步骤。

diphtherotoxin [difˈθiərəˈtɔksin] *n.* 白喉毒素

No diphtherotoxin was detected in its soluble metabolites, indicating that cell wall defect might affect the production of diphtherotoxin.

在可溶性代谢物中检测不到白喉毒素，表明细胞壁缺陷可能影响白喉毒素的产生。

Diphtherotoxin in the stable L-form was detected with SDS-PAGE.

在稳定的 L 型细菌中用 SDS-PAGE 技术检测到白喉毒素。

diplegia [daiˈpliːdʒiə] *n.* 两侧瘫

The gait of 26 cerebral palsy children with spastic diplegia was analyzed.

对 26 例痉挛型脑瘫患儿进行了步态分析。

Cerebral diplegia is a form of cerebral palsy in which there is widespread damage of the brain cells that control the movements of the limbs.

大脑性两侧瘫指控制肢体运动的脑细胞遭受广泛损害所致的一种大脑性麻痹。

diplococcus [ˌdipləuˈkɔkəs] *n.* 双球菌

Gram-negative diplococcus was found in the samples from 11 (9.2%) Group B mothers.

革兰阴性双球菌可见于 11 例(9.2%)B 组产妇的涂片中。

A diplococcus is a round bacterium that typically occurs in pairs of two joined cells.

双球菌是一种圆形细菌，通常二个相连成对出现。

diploid [ˈdiplɔid] *n.* 二倍体

Diploid denotes that cells, nuclei, or organisms in which each chromosome except the Y sex chromosome is represented twice.

二倍体指除 Y 性染色体之外每条染色体都成双存在于细胞、细胞核或机体内。

a. 二倍的，二倍体的

An organism is said to be diploid if its chromosomes occurs in pairs.

如果某种生物的染色体均成对存在，那么这种生物就称作二倍体。

A mitotic cell division of a diploid cell produces two diploid cells.

一个二倍体的细胞经过一次有丝分裂产生两个二倍体细胞。

diplopia [diˈpləupiə] *n.* 复视

Diplopia is the most common visual symptom of disorders of ocular movements.

复视是由于眼球运动障碍引起的最常见的视觉症状。

Diplopia is usually due to a disturbance in the coordinated movements of the muscles that move the eyeball.

复视通常是由动眼肌的同步协调运动失调所致。

Whenever both eyes fail to record the same image on the brain, diplopia occurs.

当两只眼睛不能在脑中形成同一个映象时，就会发生复视。

diplotene [ˈdiplətiːn] *n.* 双线期

In diplotene the pairs of chromatids begin to separate from the tetrad.

双线期时，配对的染色单体开始从四分体中分离。

Prophase may be divided into successive stages termed leptotene, zygotene, pachytene, diplotene, and diakinesis.

前期可分为几个连续的阶段，分别称细线期、偶线期、粗线期、双线期和终变期。

dipolar [dai'pəulə] *a.* 双极的；偶极的

This type of ionized molecule with negative and positive charge is referred to as a dipolar ion or zwitterion.

这类带有负电荷和正电荷的离子称为偶极离子或两性离子。

dipyridamole [ˌdaipai'ridəməul] *n.* 双嘧啶氨醇，潘生丁

Dipyridamole dilates small resistance vessels.

潘生丁可以扩张小的阻力血管。

direction [di'rekʃən] *n.* 方向，指导；（复数）指示，医嘱；用法说明

His discovery gave this branch of science a new direction.

他的发现给这门科学指出了新的方向。

This doctorate candidate is writing a thesis under the direction of his supervisor.

这位博士生在他的导师指导下正在撰写论文。

For the bacterial type of pharyngitis, penicillin in certain forms can be given by mouth very effectively in accordance with a physician's directions.

对细菌型咽炎，有些类型的青霉素遵照医嘱口服很有效。

Before taking the medicine, you must read carefully the directions on the bottle.

服药之前，你必须仔细阅读药瓶上的用法说明。

directive [di'rektiv, dai'rektiv] *n.* 指令；方针 *a.* 指导的；管理的

DNA is considered to be a combination of chemical elements which initiates the directives or messages for all the activities of the cell including the transmission of hereditary characteristics.

DNA 被看作是由多种化学元素结合成的，它可对所有的细胞活动包括可传递遗传特征发出指令或信息。

director [di'rektə, dai'rektə] *n.* 处长，院长，所长，主任

The director of this hospital is a specialist in surgery.

这个医院的院长是一位外科学专家。

The director of this research institute has made a new invention recently.

这个研究所的所长最近又有一项新的发明。

Professor Wang is the director of the Center for Control and Prevention of Disease.

王教授是疾病控制和预防中心的主任。

disability [disə'biliti] *n.* 能力丧失，伤残

Chronic rheumatic heart disease causes disability.

慢性风湿性心脏病严重影响劳动力。

We don't believe that disease and disability need to be inevitable consequences of aging.

我们并不认为疾病和残疾是年事趋高的不可避免的结果。

The employment rates of people with disabilities are much lower than the employment rates of people without disabilities.

残疾人的就业率比非残疾人要低得多。

disable [dis'eibl] *v.* 使无能，使残废

The scientists transplanted healthy cortex tissue from fetal rats into the disabled animals.

科学家们将完好的胎鼠脑皮层组织移植到脑皮层受损伤的大鼠身上。

disaccharide [dai'sækəraid] *n.* 二糖，双糖

Monosaccharide and disaccharide contents in B_1, B_2, and B_3 were small.

B_1，B_2，B_3 中单糖和二糖的含量不多。

disadvantage [disəd'vɑːntidʒ] *n.* 不利（条件），损害；缺点

However, it has the disadvantage of causing increased pulmonary vascular resistance and increased right ventricular afterload.

然而,不利之处在于引起肺血管阻力升高,使右心室后负荷增高。

Despite the obvious disadvantage, this treatment has obtained wide acceptance.

尽管有明显的缺点,这个疗法还是得到广泛的使用。

disadvantageous [disˌædvɑːn'teidʒəs] *a.* 不利的

If an association is beneficial to one partner and at least not disadvantageous to the other, it is commensalism.

如果这种关系有利于一方,而对另一方至少无害,这就是共栖现象。

disagreement [disə'griːmənt] *n.* 不同意,不一致

Another area of disagreement is that of postoperative care.

另外的意见分歧是关于手术后护理的问题。

disalignment [ˌdisə'lainmənt] *n.* 不成直线,不成行列

A radiograph will show over lapping and disalignment of the skull bones (Spalding's sign).

放射线照片可以显示颅骨的重叠或排列不齐(的现象)(斯波耳丁氏征)。

disappearance [disə'piərəns] *n.* 消失

Therapy with this drug resulted in complete disappearance of symptoms.

用这个药治疗以后,症状完全消失。

disapprove ['disə'pruːv] *v.* 非难,不赞成

Self medication is often concealed by the patient, for fear this may be disapproved of by his doctor.

因为怕医生非难,病人常隐瞒自己用药。

disaster [di'zɑːstə] *n.* 灾难,严重事故

Environmental disasters can have an effect on agriculture, biodiversity, the economy and human health.

环境灾害对农业,生物多样性,经济和人类健康均可产生影响。

The Bhopal disaster also known as Bhopal Gas Tragedy was one of the world's worst industrial catastrophes.

博帕尔事件,也称为博帕尔毒气泄漏悲剧,是世界上最严重的工业灾难之一。

disc [disk] *n.* 盘 (disk)

Disc is a rounded flattened structure, such as an intervertebral disc or the optic disc.

盘是一个扁圆形结构,例如椎间盘、视神经盘。

The colour of the optic disc is usually similar in both eyes, but varies between individuals.

双侧眼底视盘的颜色通常近似,但在个体之间是有差异的。

The disc is subject to degeneration and tearing due to age and repetitive trauma.

随着年龄的增长和反复受到外伤,椎间盘很容易发生退行性病变和撕裂。

discard [dis'kɑːd] *v.* 丢弃,抛弃

We believe this classification should be completely discarded.

我们认为这种分类法应当全部放弃。

Things discarded from the diseased or the dead should be thoroughly disinfected.

患者或死者遗弃的物品应予以彻底消毒。

discern [di'səːn] *v.* 看出,分辨

Visual acuity means the degree of detail that the eye can discern in an image.

视敏度是指眼能分辨影像的细节的程度。

Clinical keenness and experience are often required to discern the real reason behind the patient's chief complaint.

要从病人的主诉中找出真正的原因常需临床的敏锐观察力和经验。

discharge [dis'tʃɑːdʒ] *v.* 排出,流出

The wound is still discharging pus.

伤口仍在流脓。

n. 流出物,排出物,释放

There may be a purulent discharge from the duct of the parotid gland.
腮腺导管可能有脓性排出物。
Nasal discharge may persist for several weeks as may a cough.
流鼻涕如同咳嗽一样可能持续几星期。
Infection in small children will cause both vaginitis and vulvitis, with evident discharge.
幼儿感染将引起阴道炎和外阴炎，且白带显著。
The patient will not be fit for work two or three weeks after discharge.
病人出院后两、三周内不宜工作。

discipline [ˈdisiplin] *n.* 学科
It is obvious, then, that the subject of this book, "human physiology", is but a small part of the vast discipline of physiology.
显然，本书的主题"人体生理学"只不过是广泛的生理学学科的一小部分。
Pediatrics and internal medicine are related disciplines.
儿科学和内科学是相关学科。

discitis [diskˈaitis] *n.* 椎间盘炎
Different treating methods bring about different results to discitis.
采用不同的方法治疗椎间盘炎其效果也会不同。
Three patients had bacterial discitis, and 2 had tuberculosis.
3 位病人患有细菌性椎间盘炎，2 位患有结核。

disclose [disˈkləuz] *v.* 揭开，揭露
It is a common misconception that the cause of death is invariably disclosed by adequate postmortem examination.
认为死亡的原因总是可由充分的尸检揭露出来是一种普遍的误解。
A number of reports failed to disclose any significant relationship between them.
若干报告未能揭示出它们之间任何有意义的关系。

disclosure [disˈkləuʒə] *n.* 公开
The Privacy Rule authorizes Privacy Boards to sometimes waive authorizations by individual patients for the disclosure of health information for research purposes.
隐私规则授权给隐私委员会，在为研究目的而公开卫生信息时有时可免除单个患者的授权。

discoidal [disˈkɔidəl] *a.* 盘状的，平圆形的；*n.* 圆盘
The discoidal particles represent a nascent form of HDLs that exist only transiently before being converted into the spherical form.
这种盘状颗粒代表高密度脂蛋白的初期形式，在变成球形结构以前仅仅短暂存在。

discoloration [disˌkʌləˈreiʃən] *n.* 变色，变色点
Hematomas produce elevation and discoloration of the wound edges, discomfort, and swelling.
血肿使伤口边缘隆起、变色，不适及肿胀。

discomfort [disˈkʌmfət] *n.* 不适
Epigastric discomfort or pain is a common symptom and is most frequently of intra-abdominal origin.
上腹部的不适或者疼痛是常见的症状，而且最常源于腹内。
Some 10 per cent of those taking griseofulvin will experience gastric discomfort.
服用灰黄霉素的人中约有 10% 的人感到胃部不适。

discontinuation [ˌdiskənˌtinjuˈeiʃən] *n.* 中断，停止
The reaction subsided following discontinuation of the drug.
用药停止后，反应即消退。

discontinue [ˌdiskənˈtinju] *v.* 中断，停止
If test results show abnormalities, the drug should be discontinued.
假如检查结果异常，应该停止给药。

Patients should be encouraged to discontinue smoking.
必须鼓励患者戒烟。

discontinuous [ˌdiskənˈtinjuəs] *a.* 间断的，不连续的
DNA synthesis is discontinuous.
DNA 合成是不连续的。

discord [ˈdiskɔːd] *n.* 不一致，不调和
Increased discord among married or separated parents had a similar effect.
已婚或分居父母之间的严重不和具有相似的结果。

discount [ˈdiskaunt] *v.* 不重视，打折扣
In any event, the seriousness of hepatitis must not be discounted because of the possibilities of complications in later life.
在任何情况下都不能忽视肝炎的严重性，因为以后还可能发生并发症。

discrepancy [disˈkrepənsi] *n.* 矛盾，不符，相差
There seems to be discrepancy in your figures.
你的数据好像有缺陷。
There is some discrepancy between the doctor' s diagnosis and the results of ultrasonic examination.
医生的诊断与超声波检查的结果有些不同。
Enormous discrepancies were observed in thse six cell types.
在这 6 个细胞类型中观察到了很大的差别。

discretion [disˈkreʃən] *n.* 谨慎
He has shown great discretion in the introduction of new material.
他对新资料的采用一向持谨慎态度。

discriminate [disˈkrimineit] *v.* 区别，辨别
Blood tests of liver function is used to evaluate functional status of liver and to discriminate among different types of liver disease.
血液检测肝功能用于评价肝功能状况和区别不同类型的肝病。
The immune system is a highly regulated and interdependent network of cells that must discriminate self from nonself and react to nonself with pleiotropic defensive responses.
免疫系统是一个具有高度受控的和相互依存的细胞网络系统，它必须从非己来识别自己，又必须与非己发生多效应的防御反应(的系统)。

discrimination [disˌkrimiˈneiʃən] *n.* 辨别，识别；歧视
The red blood cell peroxide hemolysis test does not offer increased sensitivity of disease discrimination.
红细胞过氧化物溶血试验不能增加鉴别此病的敏感性。

discriminator [diˈskrimineitə] *n.* 甄别器
The discriminator circuit owns the characters of very low-power and low operating voltage.
该甄别器电路具有微功耗、低工作电压的特点。
Microwave phase discriminator is used to translate the phase information to amplitude information which is easy to be processed.
微波鉴相器用于把相位信息转化成便于处理的幅度信息。

disease-free [diˈziːzˈfriː] *a.* 无病的
Results in this study showed that women given adjuvant chemotherapy had a longer disease-free interval than women given placebo.
研究的结果表明采用辅助性化疗的妇女比用安慰剂治疗的妇女的无病期长。
Adjuvant chemotherapy can prolong the disease-free period in women with breast cancer after radical mastectomy.
患乳腺癌的妇女，采用根治性乳腺切除术之后，用辅助性化疗可延长其无病期。

disequilibrium [ˈdisˌiːkwiˈlibriəm] *n.* 失去平衡

This permeability sets in motion the disequilibrium of Starling' s forces.

这种渗透性使得斯塔林氏压力失去了平衡。

There is considerable linkage disequilibrium across the entire HLA locus.

整个 HLA 基因座上存在相当多的连锁不平衡。

disfiguration [disfiːgjuˈreiʃən] *n.* 损形

Excision with skin graft of soar on the face can improve laxity and mobility of that portion, but it contributes little to remould the disfiguration.

面部瘢痕切除植皮只能改善功能(松弛和可动性),容貌损毁的改善远非理想。

There were various injury of tubulointerstitium and disfiguration of renal tubules in all cases.

所有病例均有不同程度的肾间质损害及肾小管功能的异常。

disfigure [disˈfigə] *v.* 使破相,毁损…的外形

Another potential use would be in surgery on faces badly disfigured by road accidents.

另一个有效的用途是用于因交通事故而严重毁损外形的面部手术上。

disfigurement [disˈfigəmənt] *n.* 损害

Cowpox is a far milder disease that carries little risk of death or disfigurement.

牛痘是一种不易造成死亡或损害的比较轻微的疾病。

disgust [disˈgʌst] *n.* 厌恶,憎恶

He/She looks at self in the mirror with disgust.

他/她用憎恶的心情观看镜中的自己。

disharmony [disˈhɑːməni] *n.* 不协调,不调和

To the patient disease means discomfort and disharmony with his environment.

对病人来说,疾病就是感觉不舒适以及与环境不协调。

disinfect [ˌdisinˈfekt] *v.* 消毒

Application of alcohol to the unbroken skin has a disinfecting effect.

酒精涂于完整的皮肤有消毒作用。

disinfectant [disinˈfektənt] *n.* 消毒剂

A germicide is essentially the same as a disinfectant.

灭菌剂与消毒剂基本上属同一类物质。

Chemical disinfectants have been employed widely in the prevention of spread of communicable disease.

化学消毒剂已经广泛用于预防传染病的蔓延。

disinfection [disinˈfekʃən] *n.* 消毒

The aim of disinfection is to destroy disease agents harmful in the human body.

消毒的目的是要消除人体的致病菌。

An example of disinfection by heat is the pasteurization of milk.

用巴氏灭菌法使牛奶消毒就是加热消毒的一例。

disintegrant [disˈintigrənt] *n.* 崩解剂

The present study deals with evaluation of crosslinked poly vinyl alcohol (PVA) as a potential disintegrant.

本研究评估交联聚乙烯醇作为潜在崩解剂的可能性。

The presence of moisture within pharmaceutical compacts containing a disintegrant influences drastically their mechanical properties.

潮湿度对于含有崩解剂药物的机械性能有较大影响。

disintegrate [disˈintigreit] *v.* 崩解,分解

In other tissues, necrotic cells absorb water and then disintegrate.

在另一些组织中,坏死细胞吸水,然后崩解。

disintegration [disˌintiˈgreiʃən] *n.* 分裂,分解,崩解,衰变

The disintegration of the vital functions of the cell has reached an irreversible stage.
该细胞的生命功能的丧失已达到不可逆转的阶段。
The final stage is a complete disintegration of the personality.
最终结局是整个人格的分裂。
These tissue disintegration products are derived from the local lesion.
这些组织分解产物来自局部损害。
Biological death occurs when changes in the organism lead to the disintegration of vital cells and tissues; death is then irreversible.
生物学死亡是指机体内的变化导致了生命细胞和组织产生了衰变,这种死亡是不可逆转的。

disintegrative [ˌdisinˈtigreitiv] *a.* 分裂的;分解的
The outcome of disintegrative psychosis is poor, most children becoming mentally retarded and incapable of speech.
分裂性精神病预后不良,大多数儿童成为精神发育迟缓以及不能言语。

disk [disk] *n.* 盘,板,圆片;软盘,磁盘
The computer disk was sent in a sealed container.
计算机软盘已装在密封的盒里寄出。
Have you recorded the data in disk?
你已把那些数据存储到磁盘上了吗?
In some patients, chest discomfort can be caused by cervical disk disease because of compression of nerve roots.
一些病人的胸部不适可能是由颈椎间盘疾病引起神经根受压所致。

dislocation [ˌdisləuˈkeiʃən] *n.* 脱位
Look for and splint all fractures and dislocations until the patient is brought to a hospital.
在护送病人去医院前,找出所有骨折和脱位处,并绑上夹板。
The patient has dislocation of the shoulder joint.
病人肩关节脱位。

dislodge [disˈlɔdʒ] *v.* 移去
Since the verrucae are usually firmly attached, they are not readily dislodged to produce embolic phenomena.
由于这些疣赘物常常牢固地附着在一起,故不易脱落而产生梗塞现象。

dismiss [disˈmis] *v.* 让…离开;解雇,开除;忽略
The patient was dismissed from the hospital when he was found free from leukemia.
这病人检查结果没有得白血病,他便获准出院。
The manager dismissed his secretary because of her incessant lateness.
由于他的秘书经常迟到,经理把她辞退了。
The potential complications of acute pharyngitis in young children may be much more serious than the disease itself; therefore, it should never be dismissed lightly.
幼儿患急性咽炎时便有患潜在并发症的可能性,它比咽炎本身更为严重,故绝对不可轻视。

dismutase [disˈmjuːteis] *n.* 歧化酶
Serum levels of ALT, AST and ALP were measured along with the examination of glutathione level, superoxide dismutase activity in liver tissue.
检测了 ALT、AST 和 ALP 中的血清浓度,同时还检测了肝组织中的谷胱甘肽浓度和超氧化物歧化酶活性。
The changes of superoxide dismutase were studied in both the model groups and treatment groups.
研究了模型组和治疗组超氧化物歧化酶的变化。

disomy [daiˈsəumi] *n.* 双躯干畸形;二体性

Disomy is the presence of two copies of a chromosome.

二体性是指含有一条染色体的两个拷贝。

In uniparental disomy, both copies of a chromosome come from the same parent.

单亲二体性中,一条染色体的两个拷贝都来自于一个亲本。

disorder [disˈɔːdə] *n.* 障碍,失调,紊乱,疾病

Periods of normal mood may not last more than a few months in the dysthymic disorder.

在精神抑郁症中,正常情绪时期不会持续几个月以上。

Study of the immune system has provided an understanding of the nature of many of the disorders of the immune response.

对免疫系统的研究有助于理解许多免疫反应疾病的性质。

Pericarditis may be the first manifestation of a connective tissue disorder.

心包炎可能是结缔组织出现病变的首要表现。

disorganisation [disˌɔːgənaiˈzeiʃən] *n.* 瓦解,结构破坏

Electron microscopy of cells which undergone necrosis shows severe disorganisation of structure.

电镜下,可看到已坏死细胞的结构严重崩解。

disorientation [dis, ɔːrienˈteiʃən] *n.* 定向障碍;迷失方向感

Disorientation is a common symptom of Alzheimer's Disease.

定向障碍是阿尔茨海默氏病的一个常见症状。

Topographical disorientation is a cognitive disorder marked by the inability to orient in the surroundings.

地形定向障碍是一种认知障碍,主要特征是对周围环境不能定向。

disparity [disˈpæriti] *n.* 差异

Shock has been defined as being characterized by a low arterial blood pressure, or a disparity in volume between blood and vascular bed.

休克一直被认为具有低动脉压特征,即以血容量与血管容量之间不匹配为特征。

dispensary [disˈpensəri] *n.* 药房

A dispensary is often part of an out-patient department in a hospital.

药房通常为医院门诊部的一部分。

Fetch two bottles of normal saline from the dispensary for transfusion.

去药房取两瓶生理盐水准备输液。

dispensation [ˌdispenˈseiʃən] *n.* 配方

Thus, during all that time, doctors were largely engaged in the unwitting dispensation of placebos on a massive scale.

因此,当时医生们主要从事大批量的配制不知成分的安慰剂(的工作)。

dispense (**with**) [disˈpens] *v.* 免除,豁免

Many of the liver's longer term functions, such as storage, may be dispensed with in the short term.

肝脏许多较长期的功能,如储存,在短期内可以被免除。

Treatment of such a condition cannot dispense with diuretics.

治疗这种病离不开利尿药。

dispermy [daiˈspəːmi] *n.* 双精受精

Informative cytogenetic markers in 21triploids were consistent with fertilization by dispermy.

21-三倍体的信息细胞遗传学标记与双精受精很一致。

disperse [disˈpəːs] *v.* 使散开,击溃

The larger melanosomes of dark skin are individually dispersed within the cytoplasm of keratinocytes.

深色皮肤中较大的黑素体呈单个分散在角质形成细胞的胞浆中。

The matter dispersed throughout some medium is called dispersion medium.
分散遍及某些介质中的物质称作分散介质。

displace [dis'pleis] *v.* 移置,取代,置换,移位

The more tightly bound drugs can displace the less firmly bound agents.
结合较牢固的药物可以置换结合不太牢固的药物。
Clofibrate displaces coumarin and phenytoin from binding sites.
安妥明能将香豆素和苯妥英从结合部位置换下来。

displacement [dis'pleismənt] *n.* 置换,移位

Angiography can demonstrate occlusion and displacement(e. g. tumor, hematoma).
血管造影能证实阻塞和移位(如肿瘤、血肿)。
Dislocation means the displacement of a bone from its normal position in a joint.
脱位是指关节处的骨头离开正常位置而移位。

display [di'splei] *v.* 展示;陈列;显露

Each NK cell has up to 11 receptors, which it can display in different combinations on the surface.
每一个自然杀伤细胞的受体可多达 11 个,它们与细胞表面进行了不同的结合来显示。
Collagen is uniform in width and each fiber displays characteristic cross striations with a periodicity of 68nm.
胶原的宽度一致,每一条纤维均呈现有 68nm 的周期性的特殊横纹。
A new way of generating antibodies is by phage display.
产生抗体的一种新方法是借助噬菌体展示技术来进行的。
The manner of display of the diseased areas is important.
暴露病变部位的方式很重要。

disposable [di'spəuzəbl] *a.* 一次性的

The syringes and needles they use for injection must be sterile and preferably disposable to minimize the risk of contamination.
他们用来注射的注射器和针头必须消毒,最好用一次性的注射器,以减少污染的危险性。
The disposable, needle-free injector expected to be on the market within two years will make life easier for thousands of diabetes sufferers.
这种一次性无针头注射器,预计在两年之内即可上市,届时将使数以千计的糖尿病患者的生活变得轻松一些。

disposal [dis'pəuzəl] *n.* 处理,处置;安排

The disposal of that rubbish by the factory pleased all neighbors.
工厂对那些垃圾进行了处理使得邻居们都感到满意。
In doing this, vital functions in relation to the maintenance of fluid and electrolyte balance and the disposal of waste material from the body are carried out.
在执行这项功能的过程中,还要行使与维持水和电解质平衡和由身体排除废物有关的重要功能。

dispose(of) [dis'pəuz] *v.* 处理,除去

It is estimated to dispose of about 30% of the glucose metabolized by the liver.
据估计通过肝脏代谢可以处理约 30% 的葡萄糖。
All discharges of the patient must be thoroughly disinfected before being disposed of.
病人所有的排泄物在处置前必须彻底消毒。

disposition [ˌdisprə'pɔːʃən] *n.* 安排;素质;性情

In children lassitude, anorexia, loss of weight, and change of disposition are present.
在儿童可出现如疲乏、厌食、体重减轻和性情改变(等症状)。

disproportionate [ˌdisprə'pɔːʃənit] *a.* 不相称的

Neurotic depression is characterized by disproportionate depression which has usually followed a distressing experience.

神经性抑郁症以不相称的抑郁为特征，通常发生于忧伤经历以后。

The disproportionate interventricular septal hypertrophy may cause subaortic obstruction with findings of progressive cardiac failure.

室间隔增厚过大可能导致主动脉下梗阻并伴有进行性心力衰竭的表现。

disprove [dis'pruːv] *v.* 反驳，证明…不成立

The diagnosis is confirmed or disproved by a laparotomy.

这个诊断可用剖腹术来证明或否定。

dispute [dis'pjuːt] *n.* 争论，争执，争议

The need for hospital admission for the severely ill elderly patient is not usually in dispute.

患有严重疾病的老年患者需住院治疗，对此通常没有争议。

This subject has been in considerable dispute.

这个主题有相当大的争论。

disregard [disri'gaːd] *v.* 忽视，不理；*n.* 忽视，不尊重

His behaviour was notably aberrant and a callous disregard for others.

他的行为明显异常，无情的漠视他人。

How to manage the behaviour of patients who disregard scheduled appointment times?

怎样管理忽视预约时间的病人的行为？

disrupt [dis'rʌpt] *v.* 干扰，妨碍

A stroke can disrupt the supply of oxygen to the brain.

脑卒中可导致大脑供氧中断。

Lack of sleep may disrupt natural hormonal balances, triggering overeating.

睡眠缺乏会打乱自身的激素平衡，促使饮食过量。

disruption [dis'rʌpʃən] *n.* 破裂，分裂

The wounds should be closed with special care to prevent disruption.

伤口应该特别小心地缝合以防止裂开。

Even the slight trauma of an injection can cause disruption of the muscle fibers and local necrosis.

即使轻微的注射损伤亦可引起肌纤维破裂和局灶性坏死。

disruptive [dis'rʌptiv] *a.* 分裂的，破坏（性）的

An impact against the head may produce primary disruptive damage of the brain.

对头部的碰撞可以产生脑部的初期破坏性损害。

disruptor [dis'rʌptə] *n.* 干扰物

Endocrine disruptors are chemicals that interfere with endocrine (or hormone system) in animals, including humans.

内分泌干扰物是一类能够影响动物（包括人类）内分泌或激素系统的化学物质。

This essay mainly discusses the effects of endocrine disruptors on aquatic animals.

该短文主要讨论了内分泌干扰物对于水生生物的作用。

dissection [di'sekʃən] *n.* 解剖，分割；撕裂，夹层

The more extensive dissections are required in the operation.

手术中需要更广泛的分离。

The renal vein required sharp dissection to free it from the tumour.

需要使用锐利的器械剥离肾静脉，使之摆脱肿瘤。

One of the severe vascular complications of hypertension is the dissection of the aorta.

高血压病所导致的严重血管并发症之一是主动脉夹层的形成。

disseminate [di'semineit] *v.* 播散

In severe cases, these changes can lead to disseminated intravascular coagulation.

在严重的情况下，这些变化可导致播散性血管内凝血。

dissemination [diˌsemiˈneiʃən] *n.* 播散，传播

Carcinoma of the colon is of slow growth and late dissemination.

结肠癌(的特点)是增生慢转移也慢。

Tuberculosis meningitis may be part of a general miliary dissemination of the infection.

结核性脑膜炎可能是感染全身的粟粒性扩散的一部分。

The enlarging necrotic patches may discharge into bronchi, with further dissemination throughout the lungs.

增大的坏死斑块可将坏死物排入支气管内，进一步播散至全肺。

dissipate [ˈdisipeit] *v.* 消散，消失

Excessive heat is dissipated by dilatation of the arterioles and evaporation of sweat which causes the skin to become pink, warm and moist.

过多的热量可通过小动脉扩张和汗液的蒸发而散发，并使皮肤红润、温热和潮湿。

If the stimuli are not dissipated, the retention of salt and water continues, and edema develops.

如果刺激因素未能消除，水钠潴留就会持续进展，发生水肿。

Together with increased cutaneous blood flow, increased sweat production can effectively dissipate excessive body heat.

皮肤血流量的增加和汗液分泌的增加起着有效的散热作用。

dissipation [ˌdisiˈpeiʃən] *n.* 消散，消退

With the dissipation of the fever, peripheral vasodilatation occurs and heat loss ensues.

随着发热的消退，周围血管舒张，并随之产生失热。

dissociation [diˌsəuʃiˈeiʃən] *n.* 分离；离解

A similar dissociation between the light reaction and the near response may be seen in patients with diabetes, encephalitis and midbrain neoplasma.

这种对于光反应和近反应类似的分离现象还可见于糖尿病、脑炎和中脑瘤等患者。

Oxygen reacts slowly at first, as shown by the flat part of the oxygen dissociation curve.

最初氧的结合反应缓慢，如氧解离曲线平坦部分所示。

The degree of dissociation of drugs play important roles in drugs transfering.

药物的解离度在药物的转运过程中起着重要作用。

dissolution [disəˈljuːʃən] *n.* 溶解，分解，液化

The rate of dissolution of a drug increases significantly as the size of drug particle decreases.

药物颗粒越小，溶解速率越快。

dissolvability [diˈzɔlvəˈbiliti] *n.* (可)溶性，溶解性

Due to its very strong dissolvability, it can dissolve organic matter, inorganic matter, resin, polymer, etc.

由于它具有极强的溶解性，能溶解有机物、无机物、树脂、聚合物等。

dissolve [diˈzɔlv] *v.* 使分解，使溶解

The chemical possesses a greater capability of being dissolved.

这种化学物质具有较大的易溶性。

The first step of cell division is prophase, during which the nucleus dissolves and the chromosomes begin migration to the midline of the cell.

细胞分裂的第一步是有丝分裂前期，这时细胞核解体，染色体开始迁移到细胞的中线。

distal(to) [ˈdistl] *a.* 远端的，远侧的

In these cases, a distal gastrectomy can be performed.

对于这些病例，可做一远端胃切除。

Blood flows into the aorta distal to the stenosis.

血液在狭窄部位的远侧注入主动脉。

distant [ˈdistənt] *a.* 远的，远部位的

Tumor recurrence in local, regional, or distant sites occurred in 30% of women given placebo.

用安慰剂的妇女，30%的人有局部、区域性或远部位肿瘤复发。

Distant gonorrhea complications only arise when the pathogen can rapidly become localized in the organs or tissue.

只有当病原菌能迅速局限在器官或组织中时才能引起远端淋病并发症。

distend [dis'tend] *v.* (使)扩张

The neck veins may be distended during expiration, yet they collapse quickly with inspiration.

在呼气时可见颈静脉扩张，在吸气时迅速塌陷。

In a late case the abdomen is distended and peristalsis may be visible.

在晚期病例，腹部鼓胀，可见肠蠕动。

distension [dis'tenʃən] *n.* 扩张，膨胀

(= distention)

There is progressive painful abdominal distention or repeated vomiting.

有进行性、疼痛性腹胀或反复呕吐。

Abdominal distension was noted in 11 children.

腹胀的小孩有 11 例。

Increased left atrial and pulmonary venous distension may lead to pulmonary vascular congestion.

左心房和肺静脉扩张的加重可导致肺部血管充血。

distil [dis'til] *v.* 蒸馏

Distilled water is purified water.

蒸馏水是纯净水。

As a result of the process, the final product is equivalent to distilled water.

由于这种处理的结果，最终的产品相当于蒸馏水。

distillate ['distileit] *n.* 蒸馏物

He concluded the distillation experiment by testing the purity of the distillate.

他以测定蒸馏物的纯度来结束他的蒸馏实验。

distillation [ˌdisti'leiʃən] *n.* 蒸馏

Distillation under reduced pressure was repeated until no more distillate came off below 40℃.

重复地进行减压蒸馏直到低于 40℃ 不再有蒸馏物蒸馏出为止。

Gasoline is produced by a series of refining processes beginning with the distillation of crude petroleum into fractions of different boiling ranges.

汽油是经过一系列的精炼过程而产生的，在开始时是将原油蒸馏后分成几个沸点范围完全不同的组分。

distinct [dis'tiŋkt] *a.* 与其他不同的，独特的

It is now recognised that cell death can take place in two distinct ways.

目前认为细胞死亡发生于两条不同的途径。

Decades of research suggests that tumours are distinct from one individual to another, with each tumour containing its own unique mutations.

数十年的研究提示肿瘤具有个体间的差别，每种肿瘤有其自身独特的一组突变。

distinctive [dis'tiŋktiv] *a.* 有特色的，区别的

These terms are distinctive enough to avoid confusion.

这些名称所具有的特殊性，足以防止混淆。

The bleeding from each kind of vessel, as a rule, shows distinctive character.

各种类型血管的出血通常具有不同的特征。

distinctly [dis'tiŋktli] *ad.* 清楚地

In asthma wheezing is distinctly audible.

哮喘时可清楚地听到喘鸣音。

distinguish [dis'tiŋgwiʃ] *v.* 区别，辨别

At least three types of epithelial cells can be distinguished in the thymic lobules.

在胸腺小叶中可辨别出至少三种类型的上皮细胞。

The various causes of chest pain can be distinguished by their likelihood to present in those different ways.

引起胸痛的各种原因可通过其不同的表现方式加以鉴别。

Before we discuss hereditary disease we need to distinguish them from other congenital diseases.

在讨论遗传性疾病之前，我们需要将它们与先天性疾病区别开来。

distinguished [dis'tiŋgwiʃt] *a.* 以…著名，杰出的

He is one of the most distinguished cardiac surgeons.

他是最著名的心脏外科医生之一。

Li Shi-zhen, a distinguished pharmacologist, was born in 1518.

杰出的药物学家李时珍诞生于 1518 年。

distort [dis'tɔːt] *v.* 使变形，扭曲

This murmur is caused by the flow of blood through the narrowed and distorted valve.

此杂音是由于血流通过狭窄变形的瓣膜时引起的。

EDTA is the preferred anticoagulant for blood counts, since morphology is less distorted and platelets are better preserved.

依地酸是适用于血细胞计数时用的抗凝剂，因为它不会使血细胞形态失真，而且会使血小板保存得较好。

distorted [dis'tɔːtid] *a.* 扭曲的；曲解的

The person's verbal response indicates the level of alertness, interest, and distorted thinking.

（通过对）患者的语言应答可推论出其敏捷性、兴趣和被扭曲的想法。

distortion [dis'tɔːʃən] *n.* 歪曲，失真，变形

In recalling the event, children may demonstrate several different types of memory distortions.

在回忆（创伤）事件时，儿童可显示数种不同的记忆扭曲。

In children disorders of adjustment reaction are associated with no significant distortion of development.

在儿童，这种调节反应紊乱不会伴有明显的发育障碍。

distractibility [ˌdistrækti'biliti] *n.* 注意力分散

In hyperkinetic syndrome of childhood the essential features are short-attention span and distractibility.

儿童多动症其基本特点是注意广度不足与注意力分散。

distraction [dis'trækʃən] *n.* 注意力分散，精神涣散

Immediate memory is highly vulnerable to distraction, requiring attention and vigilance to maintain the content.

瞬时记忆极易受到注意力分散的干扰，需要提高注意力和保持警醒以保留记忆的内容。

Environmental distractions can distort the messages sent between two people.

环境引起的精神涣散会使两人曲解相互传递的信息。

distress [dis'tres] *n.* 痛苦，窘迫

Treatment of ascites, other than to relieve distressing symptoms, is usually not indicated.

除了减轻痛苦症状外，腹水常常不需要治疗。

Physical examination revealed an anxious child in slight respiratory distress who complained of chest pain.

体检发现患儿表情焦虑不安，呈轻度呼吸窘迫状，并主诉胸痛。

distressful [dis'tresful] *a.* 使人痛苦的

The distressful news made the young mother's hair immediately stand on end.

这个悲痛的消息使年轻的母亲顿时毛发耸立。

distressing [dis'tresiŋ] *a.* 使人痛苦的，令人苦恼的

A single episode may last several days but is not always distressing.

一次发作可能持续数天,但并不总是痛苦的。

distribute [disˈtribju(ː)t] *v.* 分配,分布,分发

The oxygenated blood flows into the aorta to be distributed to all parts of the body.

氧合血流进主动脉,然后分布到全身各个部位。

The cells of the immune system are widely distributed throughout the body.

免疫系统的细胞广泛分布于全身。

distribution [ˌdistriˈbjuːʃən] *n.* 分配,分布

Lipid-soluble and lipid-insoluble drugs have different patterns of distribution.

脂溶性和非脂溶性药物有不同的分布模式。

Volume of distribution is defined as the amount of drug in the body in relation to the concentration of drug in the plasma.

分布容积表示体内的药量与血浆中药物浓度的关系。

All data were confirmed to be normal distribution by Shapiro-Wilk test.

所有数据都通过 Shapiro-Wilk 检验证实是正态分布的。

disturb [disˈtəːb] *v.* 扰乱,妨碍

Either too much or too little water will disturb brain function.

水分太多或太少都将使大脑的功能产生紊乱。

In shock this blood flow is disturbed.

休克时这种血液的流动发生障碍。

disturbance [disˈtəːbəns] *n.* 紊乱,障碍

These drugs commonly cause gastrointestinal disturbance as their major side effect.

这些药主要的副作用是常引起胃肠道功能紊乱。

Another problem reported in patients with single coronary artery is conduction disturbance.

独支冠状动脉患者的另一问题是传导障碍。

disulfide [daiˈsʌlfaid] *n.* 二硫化物

Since the chains may be covalently joined by the disulfide bonds of cystine, these bonds may have to be broken.

因为链与链之间可能由胱氨酸的二硫键共价连接,所以必须断裂这些键。

Immunoglobulins of all classes have a fundamental four-chain structure, consisting of two identical light and two identical heavy chains, which are held together by disulfide bonds.

所有类型免疫球蛋白有一基本的四链结构,由两条相同的轻链和两条相同的重链组成,其链间由二硫键连接在一起。

diuresis [ˌdaijuəˈriːsis] *n.* 利尿,多尿

Cardiac glycosides cause diuresis by increasing cardiac output and by increasing renal blood flow.

强心甙通过增加心输出量和肾血流量而引起利尿。

Sodium poor albumin infusions may be helpful in inducing diuresis.

低钠白蛋白输入可能有利于利尿。

diuretic [ˌdaijuəˈretik] *a.* 多尿的

In the diuretic phase, attention must be paid to adequate replacement of fluid and electrolytes.

在多尿期必须注意补充液体及电解质。

n. 利尿剂,利尿药

Various diuretics are extremely useful in the treatment of congestive heart failure.

各种利尿剂在充血性心力衰竭的治疗中极为有用。

diurnal [daiˈəːnəl] *a.* 白天的,一日间的

The present study examines the effect of diurnal rhythm on gene expression in the subcutaneous adipose tissue.

本研究检测了昼夜节律对皮下脂肪组织基因表达的影响。

diurnally [daiˈəːnəli] *ad.* 每日

Has the pain occurred diurnally?

疼痛是否每日发生?

divergence [daiˈvəːdʒəns] *n.* 分散,分歧

As for treatment there is divergence of views between them and me.

他们的治疗观点与我不同。

divergent [daiˈvəːdʒənt] *a.* 不同的

Divergent views are still expressed regarding the adequacy of this technique.

关于此项技术的切实可行性,目前仍有不同的看法。

diverse [daiˈvəːs] *a.* 多变化的,形形色色的

Symptoms of anxiety in children are often diverse and confusing.

儿童焦虑症状常常是多变和令人迷惑的。

At the conference the representatives put forward diverse proposals.

会上代表们提出了各种各样的建议。

M. pneumonia infection and lymphoid cells can result in diverse clinical manifestations.

肺炎支原体感染和淋巴样细胞可导致多种临床表现。

They are diverse in the region that binds to the antigen.

它们与抗原的结合区域是不同的。

diversion [daiˈvəːʃən] *n.* 转向,转移

His last argument was a diversion to make us forget the main point.

他最后的论点是在声东击西,想让我们忘掉要点。

The government is planning a South-to-North water diversion project.

政府正在计划一项南水北调工程。

diversity [daiˈvəːsiti] *n.* 多样性,差异

The great diversity of tumour types results in a wide spectrum of characteristics of tumour tissues and cells.

肿瘤类型的多样性导致肿瘤组织和细胞的特征差异很大。

There exists a diversity of opinion as to the clinical significance of this finding.

关于这一发现的临床意义存在有分歧意见。

Within the procaryotics, there is considerable diversity of cell shape and metabolic capability.

各种原核生物的细胞形态和代谢能力相差悬殊。

diverticulitis [daivə,tikjuˈlaitis] *n.* 憩室炎

Symptomatic duodenal diverticulitis is rare.

有症状的十二指肠憩室炎罕见。

Irregular and infrequent or difficult evacuation of the bowels can be a symptom of intestinal obstruction or diverticulitis.

不规则的、异常或困难排便可能是肠阻塞或憩室炎的症状。

diverticulosis [ˌdaivəːtikjuˈləusis] *n.* 憩室病(尤指肠憩室)

Fiber-rich choices for the elderly diet are important in preventing constipation and diverticulosis.

老人膳食中选择富含纤维的食物对预防便秘和肠憩室病是很重要的。

diverticulum [ˌdaivəˈtikjuləm] *n.* 憩室

If the surgeons didn't remove the diverticulum, it can cause pain and bleeding.

如果外科医师没有切除憩室,其可导致疼痛和出血。

The development of colonic diverticulum is thought to be the result of raised intraluminal colonic pressures.

结肠憩室的形成被认为是肠腔内压力升高所致。

divide [diˈvaid] *v.* 分裂

A cell can divide into two.

一个细胞可以分裂成两个。

division [di'viʒən] *n.* 分;分裂;部分

After a certain number of cell divisions, time on the biological clock runs out and the cells age and stop dividing.

细胞经过一定次数分裂后,其生物钟的时间耗尽,因而细胞衰老并停止分裂。

divorce [di'vɔːs] *v.* 离婚

Mr. Zhang divorced his wife three months ago.

张先生三个月前跟他的妻子离婚了。

He was recently divorced by his wife.

他的妻子最近和他离婚了。

Women who are divorced may also lose health insurance that they had through their husbands.

离婚妇女也同时失去通过她们的丈夫获得的健康保险。

n. 离婚

Their marriage ended in divorce in 2001.

他们的婚姻在 2001 年以离婚告终。

dizygotic [ˌdaizai'gɔtik] *a.* 两受精卵的;两合子的;双卵的

The rate of high blood pressure of the identical twins and the dizygotic twins was 7.5% and 7.0% respectively. The difference between the two had no statistical significance.

同卵双生儿与异卵双生儿血压偏高率分别为 7.5% 和 7.0%,两者差异无统计学意义。

dizziness ['dizinis] *n.* 头晕,头昏

Headaches, dizziness and mental disorders may be the result of cerebral artery sclerosis.

在大脑血管硬化后,可引发头痛、眩晕和精神变态(等症状)。

Patients use the term dizziness to decribe several unusual head sensations.

患者将各种异常的头部感觉都称之为头昏。

dizzy ['dizi] *a.* 头晕的

The patient still felt dizzy on getting out of bed.

病人起床后仍感到头晕。

DNA DNA(deoxyribonucleic acid) is the molecule that encodes genetic information.

DNA(脱氧核糖核酸)是编码(蕴藏)遗传信息的分子。

DNA is a double-stranded molecule held together by weak bonds between base pairs of nucleotides.

脱氧核糖核酸是双链分子,通过核苷酸中碱基对间氢键结合在一起。

DNA-adduct [DNA-ə'dʌkt] *n.* DNA-加合物

1,2,4-trihydroxybenzene has also been shown to cause DNA-adduct formation in murine bone marrow in vitro.

1,2,4-三羟基苯在体外试验时也表明可引起鼠骨髓内形成有 DNA 加合物。

doctor ['dɔktə] *n.* 医生,大夫

An old saying is "An apple a day keeps the doctor away".

古谚云:"日食一苹果,医生不找我"。

He is a famous doctor who has successfully perfomed many cases of very complicated heart surgery.

他是一位成功施行了许多例非常复杂心脏手术的著名医生。

Barium sulfate is to be used only under the direct supervision of a doctor.

硫酸钡只应在医生的直接指导下使用。

doctrine ['dɔktrin] *n.* 学说,教条

One year later, Wohler synthesized urea from ammonium cyanate and in so doing helped to discredit the doctrine of vitalism.

一年以后,Wohler 利用氰化铵合成了尿素,这样有助于推翻生机论的学说。

document [ˈdɔkjument] *v.* (用文件)证明,记载

A large literature documents the association of many types of cancers.

大量文献记载着许多型癌症之间的联系。

The diagnosis was documented by characteristic history, electrocardiogram, and enzyme changes.

诊断由典型病史、心电图和酶的变化所证实。

n. 文件,[计] 文档

In this kind of document, we use a specific bold type.

在这种文档中,我们使用一种特殊的粗体字。

Each document must be placed in its specific archive.

每个文件必须放在特定的文档。

documentation [ˌdɔkjumenˈteiʃən] *n.* 凭证,提供证据

Once the diagnosis of tuberculosis is suspected, the documentation consists of a positive tuberculin skin test.

一旦诊断疑为结核感染时,证实本病应包括阳性结核菌素皮肤试验。

Documentation of gestational age is fundamental to the management of the prolonged pregnancy.

孕龄资料是处理过期妊娠的关键。

dolor [ˈdɔlə] *n.* 痛

Dolor is one of the classical signs of inflammation in a tissue, the other three being calor (heat), rubor (redness), and tumor (swelling).

痛是组织发炎时的典型体征之一,其他 3 种体征是热、红和肿。

domain [dəuˈmein] *n.* (知识、活动的)领域;结构域

These persons have so internalized understanding of the domain that they have no need for rules, guidelines, or maxims.

这些人对该领域的理解已经非常深入,他们不再需要规则、指南或行为准则。

Research of CAPP software architecture is based on domain analysis.

CAPP 软件构建的研究是以结构域分析为基础的。

domed [dəumd] *a.* 半球形的,有穹顶的

The outer surface of the spleen is domed to fit underneath the diaphragm.

脾的外面呈穹顶状,与膈的下部形状相适应。

If at the mouths of hair follicles, follicular or lichenoid syphilids are apt to be conical; elsewhere on the skin, domed.

毛囊性或苔藓样丘疹如发生在毛囊口处,多为圆锥形,在他处皮肤上则呈圆顶状。

domestic [dəˈmestik] *a.* 本国的;家庭的

These pharmaceutic factories have produced enough antibiotics to satisfy domestic demands.

这些药厂已生产出足够的抗生素以满足国内的需要。

dominant [ˈdɔminənt] *a.* 优势的;显性的

Inheritance is either dominant or recessive.

遗传既可以是显性的,也可以是隐性的。

The gene transmitting tallness is called dominant and that transmitting shortness is recessive.

传递高的基因叫显性基因,而传递矮的基因叫隐性基因。

Conjunctivitis may be the first symptom, but sore throat is the dominant feature and may be slight or severe.

结膜炎可能为初期症状,但喉痛,无论轻重,则是主要特征。

dominate [ˈdɔmineit] *v.* 支配,控制

In other patients, encephalopathy, acute renal failure, or hepatic dysfunction may dominate the clinical picture.

在其他病人中,脑病、急性肾衰竭或肝功能失调可能支配着临床表现。

In some patients, pain in the extremities and joints may dominate the clinical picture.

在有些病人中肢体和关节痛可为最主要的临床表现。

donation [dəuˈneiʃən] *n.* 捐献,捐赠

Organ donation means that a person wishes his organs to be used after his death.

器官捐献是指一个人愿意在死后其器官能被利用。

donor [ˈdəunə] *n.* 供血者,供者,供体

The person from whom the blood is taken is called the donor.

献出血液的人叫作供血者。

Blood transfusion units now screen all donor blood for the presence of hepatitis B virus.

输血中心现在对所有的供血者进行乙型肝炎病毒的普查。

Approximately 30% of them were from living related donors and 70% from cadavers.

(供体中)30% 来自亲属活体供者,70% 来自尸体。

dopamine [ˈdəupəmiːn] *n.* 多巴胺,三羟酪胺(升压药)

Dopamine[5-10(μg/kg)/min] may be used to restore mean arterial blood pressure to≥60 mmHg or systolic pressure to ≥90mmHg.

多巴胺[5~10(微克/公斤)/分]可用来恢复平均动脉压为≥60 毫米汞柱或收缩压为≥90毫米汞柱。

A continuous infusion of dopamine or another ionotropic agent may also be needed for the management of shock.

对休克的处理,持续滴注多巴胺或其他电解质制剂是需要的。

dopaminergic [ˌdəupəmiˈnəːdʒik] *a.* 多巴胺能的

Several genes related to the function of dopaminergic neurons have been reported to be abnormal.

已有报道称几个与多巴胺能神经元功能相关的基因显示异常。

Parkinson's disease has been thought of as a dopaminergic disease.

帕金森氏病被认为是一种多巴胺能疾病。

Doppler [ˈdɔplə] *n.* 多普勒(超声成像)

Color Doppler is a technique that estimates the average velocity of blood flow within a vessel by color coding the information.

彩色多普勒这种技术可以将信息变成彩色编码来估计血管内血流的速度。

dormant [ˈdɔːmənt] *a.* 休眠的,暂停活动的

Occasionally a tumor, either benign or malignant, becomes inactive (dormant) for a period of time.

偶尔,良性或恶性肿瘤,在一个时期可处于非活动性(休眠)状态。

Anything from cosmic rays to radiation to diet may activate a dormant oncogen, but how remains unknown.

从宇宙射线到辐射,又到饮食中的某种因素能激活一种休眠的肿瘤基因,但它们是怎样激活基因的仍然不清楚。

dorsal [ˈdɔːsəl] *a.* 背的,背侧的

There are two groups of cavities: dorsal and ventral.

腔有两组:背侧腔和腹侧腔。

At all levels of the cord, the afferent fibers of the dorsal roots carry information from receptors.

在髓的所有水平切面,背根的传入纤维传递由感受器来的信息。

dorsally [ˈdɔːsəli] *ad.* 向背脊

The nerve fibers of this nucleus curve dorsally and caudally to cross the middle.

此核的神经纤维弯向背尾侧,且在中线交叉。

dorsiflexor [ˈdɔːsiˌfleksə] *n.* 足部背屈肌;背负肌

Mini-Taichiquan exercise can strengthen both dorsiflexors and plantar flexors, especially triceps surae, in the scope of ankle function.

简化太极拳运动可在踝关节功能范围内锻炼足部背屈和足底屈肌群,特别是小腿三头肌

的力量。

dosage [ˈdəusidʒ] *n.* 剂量

Excessive dosage of this drug can result in injury to the liver.

这种药使用过量会损害肝脏。

The dosage was reduced to a level which would work on the infected cells but not upset their normal metabolism.

药量已被减低到某一水平，既足以对付受感染的细胞，又不会干扰正常的新陈代谢。

dose [dəus] *n.* 量，(一次)剂量，一剂

Physicians chose the drugs and decided on doses and frequency of administration.

医生选药并确定给药的剂量和次数。

This product owns merits of being stable in quality, small in dose and high in efficacy.

本品具有质量稳定、服用量少、疗效显著等优点。

dot [dɔt] *n.* 小点，圆点

These dots are seen in 97 percent of all patients, and usually one to three days before the skin rash appears.

这些小点在97%的这类患者中均可见到，而且通常是在皮疹出现前一至三天内见到。

double-blind [ˈdʌbl-ˈblaind] *a.* 双盲的(统计学)

In this report, 38 prepubertal children completed a double-blind protocol.

在这个报告中，38 个青春期前的儿童完成了一项双盲科学实验计划。

In a double-blind trial neither the patient nor the clinician making the assessment of outcome knows which treatment has been given.

双盲试验中，病人和评价结果的临床医师都不知道所给予的治疗药物。

doublet [ˈdʌblit] *n.* 成对物，一对中的一个

Spontaneous deamination of 5-methylcytosine to thymidine in the CG doublet gives rise to C>T or G>A transitions.

CG 双体中的 5-甲基胞嘧啶自发去氨基变成胸腺嘧啶引起 C 到 T 或 G 到 A 的转换。

We can refer to these duplicated chromosomes as a doublet.

我们能够称这些复制的染色体为双体。

download [ˈdaunləud] *v.* 下载

The young doctor is downloading an important medical article from the Website of Yahoo.

这位青年医生正在从雅虎网站下载一篇重要的医学文章。

You can download many free softwares from Internet.

你可以从互联网上下载许多免费软件。

You must download on internet the driver files.

你必须在网上下载这个驱动文件。

downstream [ˈdaunstr iːm] *a.* 在下游的，在下阶段的

Our data collectively suggest that growth factors and their downstream tyrosine kinases can induce tyrosine phosphorylation of androgen receptor.

总之我们的资料表明，生长因子及其下游酪氨酸激酶能诱导雄激素受体的酪氨酸磷酸化。

doxorubicin [ˌdɔksəuˈruːbisin] *n.* 阿霉素

Tamoxifen reduced doxorubicin resistance in EAC/ADR cell in vitro.

他莫昔芬降低体外 EAC/ADR 细胞对阿霉素的耐药性。

doxycycline [ˌdɔksiˈsaikliːn] *n.* 多西环素，强力霉素

Prophylactic doxycycline has been reported to be effective in preventing traveler' s diarrhea in some areas.

根据报道预防药多西环素对某些地区的旅游者所患的腹泻也有预防作用。

draft [draːft] *n.* 饮剂

It may be advisable to accompany a helping of bacon or ham with a draft of orange juice.

进食咸肉或火腿时宜伴饮橘子水。

drain [drein] *v.* 排去(液体),引流,导液

The tears are drained away by small tubes and pass into the nose.

眼泪经小管排出,进入鼻腔。

If not promptly drained, the abscess may enlarge, killing more tissues in the process.

如未及时引流,脓肿可进一步增大,进而损毁更多的组织。

drainage ['dreinidʒ] *n.* 引流(法),导液(法)

The most important aspect of treatment is to establish surgical drainage.

治疗的最重要的方面是进行手术引流。

dramatically [drə'mætikəli] *ad.* 引人注目地

There are dramatically increasing trends in respiratory cancer among women in developed countries.

在发达国家里,妇女的呼吸道癌呈明显上升趋势。

The incidence of malaria dropped dramatically following the eradication programme.

采取根治方法之后,疟疾的发病率显著地下降了。

drape [dreip] *n.* 布单

Alcohol wash of the throat is followed by the placing of sterile surgical drapes over the area.

用酒精清洗喉部,然后在该区域范围铺上已消毒的手术布单。

draw [drɔː] *v.* 拉,拖;吸出;提取;划;皱,缩

The face of the newborn is pinched and drawn, resembling that of an old man or woman.

新生儿面孔现出难受和皱眉的表情,好像老头老太太。

No sharp line can be drawn between early and late congenital syphilis.

早发和晚发的先天性梅毒之间找不出明显的界线。

He draws a deep breath.

他深深地吸一口气。

The doctor draws out pus from the patient's pleural cavity by using a aspirator.

医生用吸引器从病人的胸膜腔抽出脓液。

The exhibition of medical apparatus and instruments drew over 20000 visitors.

这次医疗器械展览会吸引了 2 万多观众。

drawback ['drɔːbæk] *n.* 缺陷,缺点

A potential drawback of the candidate gene approach is that the wrong genes may be studied.

候选基因法的一个潜在缺陷是可能将错误的基因纳入研究。

Poor fuel economy is a common *drawback* among larger vehicles.

大型车辆的共同缺点是费油。

The only *drawback* of the plan is its expense.

该计划的唯一缺点是其花费。

dreadful ['dredful] *a.* 可怕的

Sulfa drugs can cure many dreadful diseases, including pneumonia, scarlet fever, and leprosy in a dramatic manner.

磺胺类药能奇迹般地治愈许多可怕的疾病如肺炎、猩红热和麻风病。

dress [dres] *v.* 穿衣;敷裹;换药

The patient dresses the finger himself daily, applying an antibiotic ointment or griseofulvin powder as recommended by Demis and Brown.

患者每天自己(换药和)包扎手指,如 Demis 和 Brown 所推荐的那样,敷用抗生素软膏或灰黄霉素粉。

In addition to relief of pain, treatment designed to prevent and care for shock should not wait until the burn can be properly dressed.

除了解除疼痛之外,防治休克和护理并不需要等到烧伤创面包扎之后才进行。

dressing ['dresiŋ] *n.* 敷料，敷裹

The finger should not come in contact with the sterile dressings.

手指不应该接触消毒敷料。

The dressing is held in place so as to keep the wound from being exposed.

把敷料固定，以免伤口暴露。

Dressings are inspected daily for evidence of bleeding.

每天检查敷料有无出血迹象。

drift [drift] *n.* 漂动，漂变

Random fluctuation in gene frequencies is referred to as genetic drift.

基因频率的随机波动称为遗传漂变。

drill [dril] *n.* 牙钻

Drill consists of a handpiece that takes variously shaped burs.

牙钻由可安装各种形状钻头的手执器构成。

Drills usually have a waterspray coolant.

牙钻通常附有喷水冷却的装置。

drilling ['driliŋ] *n.* 钻孔，钻井

If there is no response within 24 hours a broad-spectrum antibiotic should be used and surgery is indicated, involving evacuation of subperiosteal abscess and drilling of the bone.

如 24 小时内疗效不佳，应采用广谱抗生素和进行外科手术，包括除去骨膜下脓肿以及为骨头钻孔排脓。

Toxic gases are not only encountered in mining, oil drilling, and similar industries, but also, occasionally, in the home.

有毒气体不仅在采矿、石油钻井以及类似的工业中遇到，而且有时也可能在家庭中碰到。

drinking ['drɪŋkɪŋ] *n.* 饮水 饮用

Drinking water with high levels of arsenic can lead to neurological and cardiovascular complications.

饮水中含高浓度的砷可导致神经和心血管方面的并发症。

Many of these conditions are linked to unsafe drinking water, dirty living conditions and air pollution.

这当中的许多情况都和不安全的饮水、肮脏的居住环境和空气污染有关。

drip [drip] *v.* 滴下 n. 滴液，滴注

The patient was given glucose by intravenous drip.

用静脉滴注法给病人输葡萄糖。

dronabinol [drə'næbinɔl] *n.* 屈大麻酚（商标名：marinol）

Dronabinol is used to prevent the nausea and vomiting that may occur after treatment with cancer medicines.

屈大麻酚用于防止使用癌症药品治疗后可能出现的恶心和呕吐。

The dose of dronabinol will be different for different patients.

屈大麻酚的剂量随病人而有差异。

droplet ['drɔplit] *n.* 飞沫，小滴

Measles is a viral disease spread by droplet by infection.

麻疹是通过飞沫传染的病毒性疾病。

dropper ['drɔpə] *n.* 滴管

A convenient measuring dropper is supplied with every liquid.

每瓶口服液内配有一个方便的计量滴管。

You can try feeding the baby with your expressed milk from a cup or spoon or medicine dropper.

你可以试试用杯子或者勺子或者喂药器把吸出来的母乳喂给宝宝。

dropsy ['drɔpsi] *n.* 水肿，浮肿

In 1827, Richard observed that urea accumulated in the blood of patients with dropsy.
1827 年,Richard 已观察到在水肿病人的血液中有尿素蓄积。
Oedema is excessive accumulation of fluid in the body tissues; popularly known as dropsy.
水肿是由于人体组织内液体潴留过多,俗称浮肿。

drowning ['drauniŋ] *n.* 淹溺,淹死
Such emergencies include smoke asphyxiation, electric shock, or drowning.
这样的意外事故包括有烟窒息、触电或溺水。
Approximately 90% of drowning victims aspirate fluid into lungs.
溺死者中大约 90% 的人都将水吸入肺中。

drowsiness ['drauzinis] *n.* 倦睡;瞌睡
Delirium is common in the early stages, but tends later to give place to drowsiness and stupor which is followed by coma.
早期常有谵妄,但随后往往为倦睡或昏睡所替代,继之转为昏迷。
Minor adverse effects sometimes seen in nonintoxicated patients include dizziness and slight drowsiness.
有时在非中毒患者身上可能出现轻度的副作用,如瞌睡和轻度嗜睡。

drowsy ['draizi] *a.* 倦睡的,瞌睡的
The patient may appear alert one minute and confused and drowsy the next.
病人可表现为一会儿清醒,一会儿又糊涂和嗜睡。

drug [drʌg] *n.* 药,药物;麻醉剂;成瘾性毒品
Drugs are widely used for the prevention, diagnosis, and treatment of disease and for the relief of symptoms.
药物广泛用于疾病的预防、诊断和治疗以及解除症状。
The term medicine is sometimes preferred for therapeutic drugs in order to distinguish them from narcotics and other addictive drugs that are used illegally.
药品一词有时主要指治疗用药物,以区别于麻醉药和其他非法使用的成瘾药。
Drug abuse refers to the self-administration of a medicinal or pleasurable substance in a quantity or manner that impairs health or social functioning.
药物滥用是指自行服用一种药品或服用后令人愉快的物质,服用的剂量或方式不当以致有损健康或有碍履行社会职能。

drug-induced [ˌdrʌgin'djuːsd] *a.* 药物导致的
Penicillin is the most common cause of a drug-induced urticaria.
青霉素是引起药源性荨麻疹最常见的原因。

drug-resistant ['drʌgri'zistənt], drug-fast ['drngfɑːst] *a.* 抗药的,耐药的
At the end of 1-2 weeks the total count of fecal bacteria returns to normal or becomes higher than normal and the drug-susceptible microorganisms are replaced by drug-resistant ones.
在一、二周之后,其粪便中细菌的总量回升至正常值或高于正常值,同时其粪便中药敏微生物被抗药微生物所代替。

drunkenness ['drʌŋkənis] *n.* 醉酒
Pathological drunkenness is an acute psychotic episodes induced by relatively small amounts of alcohol.
病理性醉酒是由相当小剂量的酒精引起的一种急性心理症状。

dual ['dju(ː)əl] *a.* 双的,二重的
This molecule of RNA has a dual function.
这个 RNA 分子具有双重功能。

dubious ['djuːbjəs] *a.* 可疑的
There are fewer atypical or dubious protein banding patterns with isoelectric focusing techniques.
采用等电位聚焦法,非典型的或可疑的蛋白质呈带状图形的更少。

duct [dʌkt] *n.* 管,导管

The more complex glands require canals or ducts to carry the secretion to the surface.

较复杂的腺体需要管道即导管输送分泌物至表面。

Bile is drained from the liver cells by many small ducts that unite to form the main bile duct of the liver, the hepatic duct.

胆汁由肝细胞分泌经许多细小的管道流出,这些细小的管道再汇合成肝脏的主要胆管即肝管。

ductless [ˈdʌktlis] *a.* 无管的;无导管的

The glands that secrete such substances are called endocrine, or ductless glands.

分泌这种物质的腺体叫做内分泌腺,或无导管腺。

due [djuː] *a.* 预期的,约定的;应有的,适当的,由于(due to)

The next train to London is due here at 4 o'clock.

到伦敦的下一次列车预定四点到达。

Experiments on humans are due to start in three years and a treatment could be available by early next century.

人体实验预定在 3 年后开始,某种可应用的治疗方法可能于下世纪初产生。

After due consideration, he decided to receive the operation.

经过适当的考虑,他决定接受这次手术。

The accident was due to careless driving.

这起车祸起因于驾驶疏忽。

Indigestion is mostly due to irregular diet.

消化不良多由饮食不规律引起。

Diseases due to the bacteria, viruses, etc, are called infectious.

由细菌、病毒等引起的疾病叫做传染病。

dumb [dʌm] *a.* 哑的

She has been dumb from birth.

她自生下来就是哑巴。

dummy [ˈdʌmi] *n.* 虚拟物; *a.* 假的,虚拟的,模拟的

The dependent variable in this clinical trial is a dummy variable representing the missing data.

这一临床试验的因变量是代表缺失数据的虚拟变量。

They have carried out a double blind, double dummy, randomized, controlled trial of seratrodast on asthma treatment.

他们开展了塞曲司特治疗哮喘的双盲、双模拟、随机对照试验。

duodenal [djuəuˈdiːnəl] *a.* 十二指肠的

Patients with blood group O are more liable to duodenal ulceration than those in other groups.

O 型血的病人比其他血型的病人更易于患十二指肠溃疡。

Of these over two-thirds were found to have a gastric or, more often, a duodenal ulcer.

在这些病例中,三分之二以上是胃溃疡,更常见者为十二指肠溃疡。

duodenotomy [djuːəudiˈnɔtəmi] *n.* 十二指肠切开术

If a growth has to be removed from the inner wall of the duodenum, a duodenotomy is done.

如果必须从十二指肠内壁切除肿瘤,则要做十二指肠切开术。

Any time a surgeon incises the duodenum, he is performing a duodenotomy.

外科医生在切开十二指肠,可以说他正在做十二指肠切开术。

duodenum [ˌdjuəuˈdiːnəm] *n.* 十二指肠

The duodenum, the first ten inches of the small intestine, is shaped like a horse-shoe.

十二指肠是小肠开头 10 英寸的那一段,形状像马蹄铁。

The duodenum is the part of the small intestine that connects with the stomach.

十二指肠是小肠的一部分,它与胃相连。

duplicate [ˈdjuːplikit] *v.* 复制,复印

During cell division, the chromosomes duplicate themselves.

在细胞分裂过程中,染色体进行自我复制。

He duplicated a few copies of this article and handed her the original.

他将这篇文章复印了几份,并把原件交给了她。

a. 复制的;二重的

A duplicate copy of the file can be found on my desk.

我桌子上有一份这个文件的复本。

duplication [djuːpliˈkeiʃən] *n.* 成倍;重复

Intense competition for resources frequently results in wasteful duplication and ineffective use of the resources given.

人力和物力上激烈的竞争常常引起现有人力、物力方面的成倍浪费以及无效的使用。

dura [ˈdjuərə] *n.* 硬脑膜

His group placed epidural electrodes outside the dura through a small craniotomy.

他们以小型颅骨切开术在硬膜外放置硬膜外电极。

A blood clot is seen over the external surface of the dura. Thus, this is an epidural hematoma.

硬脑膜外表面可见一血块,此为硬膜外血肿。

dural [ˈdjuərəl] *a.* 硬脑膜的,硬脊膜的

Some cranial structures are sensitive to mechanical stimulation, such as the middle meningeal artery and dural sinuses.

某些颅脑结构对机械性刺激敏感,如脑膜中动脉和硬脑膜窦。

duration [djuəˈreiʃən] *n.* 持续时间;期间

The duration of therapy to be instituted depends on the nature of the disease to be treated.

治疗时间的长短取决于所治疗疾病的性质。

The acute rheumatic fever is of limited duration, but the carditis may lead to permanent valvular damage.

急性风湿热持续期有限,但心脏炎却会导致永久性瓣膜损害。

dust [dʌst] *n.* 灰尘,粉尘

Pneumoconiosis is an occupational lung disease and a restrictive lung disease caused by the inhalation of dust.

尘肺是由粉尘吸入引起的一种职业性肺病和限制性肺病。

An alveolar macrophage (or dust cell) is a type of macrophage found in the pulmonary alveolus.

肺巨噬细胞(或尘细胞)是见于肺泡的一种巨噬细胞。

dustibility [dʌstiˈbiliti] *n.* 可分散性,松散性

The finely divided products which have been treated according to the invention in practice have the advantages of improved dustibility.

根据源于实践的发明进行处理后的精细分化产物有着更好的可分散性。

dwarf [dwɔːf] *n.* 矮小,侏儒

Pituitary dwarfs have a deficiency of growth hormone due to a defect in the pituitary gland.

垂体性侏儒是由于垂体后叶的缺陷使生长激素分泌不足所致。

dwarfism [ˈdwɔːfizm] *n.* 侏儒症

In children absence of growth hormone results in failure to grow, producing dwarfism.

儿童期缺乏生长激素会引起生长迟滞,导致侏儒症。

Some valuable discoveries have resulted from gene splicing, one recent discovery was a hormone (human growth hormone) used to treat dwarfism.

通过基因拼接已经获得了一些很有价值的发现,一项最新的发现是一种用于治疗侏儒症的激素(人生长激素)。

dwindle [ˈdwindl] *v.* 减少,缩小

After menopause, when the supply of estrogen dwindles, women become more susceptible to cardiovascular disease.
绝经后，妇女雌激素水平降低，这时她们比较容易患心血管疾病。

dyad [ˈdaiæd] *n.* 双，对；二分体
At anaphase each tetrad separates into two dyads.
在后期每个四分体分开成为两个二分体。
A dyad consists of two sister chromatids.
一个二分体是由两条姐妹染色单体组成的。

dye [dai] *n.* 染色，染料
Bacteria have a high affinity for basic dyes.
细菌对碱性染料有高度的亲和力。

dynamic [daiˈnæmik] *a.* 动力学的，动态的
This transfer of substances, including water, to the tissue spaces is a dynamic process.
物质（包括水）转运至组织间隙是一种动力学过程。
The plasma membrane is seen as a dynamic everchanging structure.
质膜可看成是一种动态的，不断变化的结构。
Some agencies use 8 or 12 hours shifts, whereas others have gone to dynamic shifts with rotating hours.
一些机构的工作人员采用 8 或 12 小时轮班一次，而其他的则采取机动的轮流值班制度。

dysarthria [disˈɑːθriə] *n.* 构音障碍
Dysarthria refers to speech problems that are caused by the muscles involved with speaking or the nerves controlling them.
构音障碍指由控制发声的肌肉或支配这些肌肉的神经出现问题而导致的发声障碍。
Dysarthria may be the result of damages of the brain, nerve and muscles.
脑、神经和肌肉的损伤可以导致构音障碍。

dysbiosis [disˈbaiəsis] *n.* 微生态失调
Dysbiosis also called dysbacteriosis refers to a condition with microbial imbalances on or within the body.
微生态失调亦称菌群失调，是指机体体表或体内微生物失去平衡的一种状态。
Dysbiosis is most prominent in the digestive tract or on the skin, but can also occur on any exposed surface or mucous membrane.
微生态失调在消化道或皮肤表面最为突出，但也可发生于其他暴露的表面或黏膜。

dysbolism [ˈdisbəlizəm] *n.* 代谢障碍
We have made every effort to study dysbolism of laying broilers caused by feeding diets with high calcium and high sodium.
我们努力研究高钙高钠饮食所导致产卵肉用鸡的代谢障碍。
We study the status of insulin resistance, dysbolism of calcium ions and their relation in coronary heart diseases.
我们研究胰岛素抵抗状态、钙离子代谢障碍和它们与冠心病之间的关系。

dyscrasia [disˈkreizjə] *n.* 体液不调，恶液质
Adverse reactions to chloramphenicol include severe blood dyscrasias.
氯霉素的不良反应包括严重的血液病。

dysentery [ˈdisəntri] *n.* 痢疾
Infection with this parasite can cause amoebic dysentery.
感染这种寄生虫能引起阿米巴痢疾。
The patient has symptoms of toxic dysentery.
病人有中毒性痢疾症状。

dysequilibrium [ˌdisˌiːkwiˈlibriəm] *n.* 平衡失调

Dysequilibrium may be a presenting symptom of basal ganglia or frontal lobe lesions.

基底神经节区或额叶损伤都能引起平衡失调的症状。

dysfibrinogenemia [dis,faibrinədʒiˈniːmiə] *n.* 异常纤维蛋白原血症

Each dysfibrinogenemia is associated with slightly different effects on the thrombin time and on normal clotting.

每一种异常纤维蛋白原血症对于凝血酶时间和正常凝血的影响稍有不同。

Some dysfibrinogenemias cause abnormal bleeding or even thrombosis, while others have no effect on either bleeding or thrombosis.

有些异常纤维蛋白原血症引起异常出血甚至血栓形成，而另一些则对出血或血栓形成没有影响。

dysfunction [disˈfʌŋkʃən] *n.* 功能失调，功能异常

The therapy will reduce neurological dysfunction especially when given early.

这种治疗，特别是早期给药，将会减少神经系统功能异常。

Surface membrane dysfunction is frequently encountered following anoxia and certain poisons.

在缺氧和某些中毒之后，常见表面细胞膜功能失调。

dysgenesis [disˈdʒenisis] *n.* 发育不全

Gonadal dysgenesis is failure of the ovaries or testes to develop.

卵巢或睾丸发育障碍称为生殖腺发育不全。

dysgenics [disˈdʒeniks] *n.* 劣生学；种族退化学

The opposite of eugenics is dysgenics.

优生学的反面是劣生学。

Dysgenics refers to the deterioration in the health and well-being of a population by practices that allow the accumulation of deleterious alleles.

种族退化是指由于某个种群中的一些行为造成有害的等位基因积累从而使得该人群健康得以退化的现象。

dyskinesia [ˌdiskaiˈniːziə] *n.* （随意）运动障碍

Acquired forms of ciliary dyskinesia are seen in smokers and patients with bronchitis, viral infections, or other pulmonary diseases.

吸烟者和患支气管炎、病毒感染或其他肺病的病人都 可能出现获得性纤毛运动障碍。

Dyskinesia includes chorea, dystonia, and those involuntary movements occurring as side-effects to the use of L-dopa and the phenothiazines.

运动障碍包括有舞蹈症，张力障碍以及使用左旋多巴和吩噻嗪后出现的不随意运动的副作用。

dyskinesis [diskiˈniːsis] *n.* 反向运动；运动障碍

The drug has amazing effect on gastriointestinal dyskinesis.

这种药对胃肠动力障碍疾病有惊人的疗效。

Acute myocardial infarction frequently results in the production of regional dyskinesis.

急性心肌梗死常常导致心室壁局部反向运动。

dyskinetic [ˌdiskaiˈnetik] *a.* 运动障碍的

Patients with FD (functional dyspepsia) of dyskinetic type might have a significant decrease of preprandial and postprandial gallbladder emptying.

由运动障碍产生的功能性消化不良的患者会出现空腹及餐后胆囊排空明显地减少。

Intracardiac thrombi usually form on inflamed or damaged valves, on endocardium adjacent to a region of myocardial infarction (MI), in a dilated or dyskinetic cardiac chamber, or on prosthetic valves.

心脏内的栓塞通常发生在已有炎症或已被损伤的心瓣膜、心肌梗死区附近的心内膜、已发生运动障碍或已扩大的心腔内以及人工瓣膜等部位。

dyslipidemia [dislipiˈdemiə] *n.* 血脂异常；异常血脂症

The waist and triglyceride level are closely related with obesity and dyslipidemia, which are considered to be the main criteria in the diagnosis of central obesity.
腰围和甘油三酯水平,作为向心型肥胖的主要评判标准,与肥胖和脂代谢紊乱密切相关。
Gene therapy for dyslipidemia and diabetes is still in its infancy.
基因治疗血脂异常症和糖尿病仍处于初级阶段。

dysmenorrhea [ˌdismenəˈriːə] *n.* 痛经
Dysmenorrhea and signs and symptoms of premenstrual tension should be recorded as part of the menstrual history.
痛经及经前紧张综合征的症状和体征应在月经史中占一席之地。
The most common type is primary dysmenorrhea, which begins with the first period and has no apparent cause.
最常见的类型是原发性痛经,始于月经初潮,无明显原因。

dysmorphology [ˌdismɔːˈfɔlədʒi] *n.* 畸形学
Dysmorphology is the study of abnormalities of morphologic development.
畸形学是研究形态发育异常的学科。

dysostosis [ˌdisɔsˈtəusis] *n.* 骨发育障碍;骨发育不良
A dysostosis is a disorder of the development of bone, affecting ossification in particular.
骨发育不良是指骨发育失调,主要是影响骨化。
Clavicle-cranial dysostosis is a disorder involving the abnormal development of bones in the skull and collar area.
颅骨锁骨发育不良是指颅骨和锁骨区域骨的发育异常的疾病。

dyspareunia [ˌdispəˈruniə] *n.* 性交疼痛(症)
Dysmenorrhea and dyspareunia should be recorded at this point.
此时应记载痛经和性交痛(病史)。

dyspepsia [disˈpepsiə] *n.* 消化不良
When food is eaten too rapidly, dyspepsia may result.
进食太快时就会发生消化不良。
The term functional dyspepsia has also been used when clinical evaluation fails to reveal an explanation for indigestion.
当根据临床表现无法解释消化不良的原因时,也可用功能性消化不良这一术语来表示。

dyspeptic [disˈpeptik] *a.* 消化不良的
When confronted with dyspeptic symptoms of recent origin in a patient over 40 years the first necessity is to exclude gastric cancer.
40 岁以上的患者近期证实有消化不良的症状时,首先应排除的是胃癌。

dysphagia [disˈfeidʒiə] *n.* 吞咽困难
The thyroiditis is more common in women and occasionally causes dysphagia.
这种甲状腺炎在女性中很常见,偶尔引起吞咽困难。
Reddening and swelling of the mucosa and slight dysphagia symptoms may occur.
可能出现黏膜红肿和轻度吞咽困难的症状。

dysphonia [disˈfəuniə] *n.* 发声困难
We did not notice any open rhinolalia, dysphagia and dysphonia.
我们没有觉察到任何开放性鼻音、吞咽困难和发音困难。
If using your voice is difficult, then you know what dysphonia is.
当你很难发出声音,你就知道发声困难是什么意思了。

dysplasia [disˈpleiziə] *n.* 发育不良,发育异常
Mammary dysplasia may be associated with an increased incidence of cancer.
乳腺发育不良患者乳癌发病率可能增加。
Rickets or epiphyseal dysplasia may develop during rapid growth, as occurs in premature infants

and adolescents.
佝偻病或骨骼发育异常可能发生在快速生长期如在早产儿或青少年。

dyspnea [dis'pniːə] *n.* 呼吸困难，气短

Dyspnea is a common complaint of chronic heart failure. This symptom is first noted with exercise.
呼吸困难是慢性心力衰竭的常见主诉。此症状首先是在运动时注意到。
Accumulation of bubbles in the lungs may result in dyspnea, cough and chest pain.
气泡积聚在肺内可引起呼吸困难、咳嗽和胸痛。

dysraphism ['disrəfizəm] *n.* 闭合不全

MRI showed meningomyelocele associated with spinal dysraphism and tethered spinal cord syndrome.
MRI 显示脊髓脊膜膨出伴随神经管闭合不全及脊髓拴系综合征。
For example, vocal cord dysraphism, such as vocal nodules, would damage the health of vocal organs.
例如，声带闭合不全(如声带小结等)会损伤发声器官的健康。

dysrhaphism ['disrəfizəm] *n.* 脊柱裂；(神经管)闭合不全

"High spinal" (cervical and upper thoracic) dysrhaphism usually involves either a meningocele or a dermal sinus tract.
高位脊柱裂(颈段和上胸段)通常包括脑脊膜突出或皮肤窦道。
The clinical and radiologic findings in a child with sacral agenesis and extensive spinal dysrhaphism were reported.
已报道了一例骶骨发育不全和广泛脊柱裂患儿的临床和影像学检查结果。

dysrhythmia [dis'riθmiə] *n.* 节律障碍

Clinical manifestation of myocardial infarction include chest pain, hypotension, and cardiac dysrhythmias.
心肌梗死的临床表现包括胸痛、低血压和心律失常。
ECG is necessary to detect serious dysrhythmias that are frequent causes of morbidity and mortality with many drug overdoses.
很多药物过量时出现的严重心律失常是引起并发症和死亡的常见原因，所以需做心电图以便及时发现。

dyssomnia [dis'sɔmniə] *n.* 睡眠障碍

Let's talk about the effect of nursing intervention on patients with dyssomnia.
让我们谈谈护理干预对睡眠障碍病人的作用。
Dyssomnia was evaluated with a standard insomnia questionnaire.
用一种标准的失眠调查表评估睡眠障碍。

dysspermatogenesis [dis,spəːmətə(u)'dʒenisis] *n.* 生精障碍

The results showed that there were significant differences in serum FSH, LH, T, PRL levels between the severe dysspermatogenesis groups and the control groups.
结果显示在严重生精功能障碍的患者和对照组之间，其血清 FSH，LH，T，PRL 水平有很大差异

dysthymia [dis'θimiə] *n.* 精神抑郁症，胸腺功能障碍

Dysthymia is a depressed or irritable mood lasting at least a year.
精神抑郁症是一种持续至少一年的压抑和易激惹的情绪。

dysthymic [dis'θimik] *a.* 精神抑郁症的，胸腺功能障碍的

Symptoms of dysthymic disorder are less severe than major affective disorders.
精神抑郁症的症状比严重情感障碍要轻。
Dysthymic disorders is a chronic, mild condition.
精神抑郁症是一种慢性的轻微病症。

dystocia [dis'təuʃiə] *n.* 难产

The situation of shoulder dystocia brings fear to the heart of every doctor and midwife.

肩难产状态让每一位医生和助产士都深深感到担忧。

Post-term pregnancy has well-known risks associated with placental insufficiency and with dystocia.

众所周知，过期妊娠多伴随有胎盘功能不全和难产两种危险。

The results showed that the fetal dystocia accounted for 46.64%, obstetric-canal dystocia was 27.70% and parturition force dystocia occupied 25.68%.

结果表明胎儿性难产占46.62%，产道性难产占27.70%，产力异常性难产占25.68%。

dystonia [dis'təuniə] *n.* (肌)张力障碍

Local injection of botulinum toxin is effective in certain focal dystonias.

局部注射肉毒毒素对某些局部肌张力障碍有效。

The patient with acute dystonia may appear unable to get his tongue in his mouth.

急性肌张力障碍患者可能会难以将舌头缩回口腔内。

dystonic [dis'tɔnik] *a.* 张力障碍的

Dystonic cramps are where a muscle that is not needed for a movement is contracted.

肌张力异常性抽筋是指当进行某个动作时，不需要用到的肌肉却在收缩。

One of the disadvantages of the phenothiazines is their potential for dystonic effects.

吩噻嗪类药物的缺点之一在于其能产生潜在的张力障碍作用。

dystrophic [dis'trɔfic] *a.* 营养不良

The chemical reactions involved in dystrophic calcification are not understood.

营养不良性钙化涉及的化学反应还不清楚。

dystrophy ['distrəfi] *n.* 营养障碍，营养不良

Researchers can make bone marrow cells turn into muscle, causing mice with muscular dystrophy to produce correctly working muscle cells.

科学家们能使骨髓细胞转化为肌肉，使患有肌肉营养障碍的小白鼠产生可以正常工作的肌细胞。

The term dystrophy is applied to several unrelated conditions; for example, muscular dystrophy and dystrophia adiposogenitalis.

营养不良一词常用于一些相互间没有关联的病症，例如肌肉营养不良和肥胖性生殖营养不良。

dysuria [dis'juəriə] *n.* 排尿困难

The child began complaining of dysuria and urinary frequency.

患儿主诉排尿困难和尿频。

However, urinary symptoms, such as dysuria and urgency, were uncommon.

不过，泌尿系症状如排尿困难与尿急不多见。

E

earache [ˈiəreik] *n.* 耳痛

In a child who has a very high fever but who otherwise seems only moderately sick, acute earache is one of the first things to think about.

对一个体温非常高,但病情似乎只属于中等的患儿来说,急性耳痛是一个首先需要考虑的问题。

Apart from local causes, earache may be due to a lesion of the geniculate ganglion of the facial nerve or to herps zoster affecting the facial nerve.

耳的疼痛,除局部原因外,可能由面神经膝状神经节的损害或带状疱疹累及面神经所引起。

ear-drum [ˈiədrʌm] *n.* 鼓膜

What damage may high diving do to the ear-drum?

高位跳水会使鼓膜受到什么损害 ?

eccentric [ikˈsentrik] *n.* 离心的;怪僻的

People with schizoid personality disorder may be slightly eccentric or indicate avoidance of competitive situations.

有精神分裂样人格障碍的人可能稍微有点古怪或者表现出回避竞争性场合。

With volume overload when the ventricle is called on to deliver an elevated cardiac output for prolonged periods, it develops eccentric hypertrophy.

当(心室)容量负荷过高时,就需要心室长时间处于高心输出量状态之下,此时便会发生离心性心肌肥大。

ecchymosis [ekiˈməusis] (*pl.* ecchymoses[ˌekiˈməusiːz]) *n.* 瘀斑

Ecchymosis is a larger extravasation of blood into the skin.

瘀斑乃大量的血液外渗进入皮肤所致。

Skeletal metastasis usually leads to bone pain or periorbital ecchymosis and proptosis.

骨骼转移通常导致骨痛或眶周瘀斑和眼球突出。

echinocytosis [iˌkainəsaiˈtəusis] *n.* 棘状红细胞增多

The degree of echinocytosis was related to an increased blood viscosity at high shear rates.

棘状红细胞增多的程度与高剪切率时增加的血黏度有关。

echocardiogram [ˌekəuˈkɑːdiəgræm] *n.* 超声心动图

Echocardiogram revealed normal findings.

超声心动图所见正常。

A large left ventricle with poor function was confirmed by echocardiogram on the fifth hospital day.

入院第 5 天超声心动图证实左室大且功能不良。

echocardiographic [ˌekəuˌkɑːdiəuˈgrɑːfik] *a.* 超声心动图的

Radionucleide and echocardiographic studies can give additional information.

核素及超声心动图检查可提供更多的诊断依据。

echocardiography [ˌekəuˌkɑːdiˈɔgrəfi] *n.* 超声心动图(检查)

Echocardiography will demonstrate dilatation of the aortic root and the separation of the cusps.

超声心动图检查可见主动脉根部扩张,瓣叶分开。

Echocardiography is the most sensitive way of demonstrating pericardial fluid.

超声心动图检查是检测心包积液最敏感的方法。

echoencephalography [ˌekəuenˌsefə'lɔgrəfi] *n.* 脑回波检查法

An echoencephalography is a diagnostic procedure during which ultrasound is used to detect abnormalities in the brain.

脑回波检查法是一种应用超声检测脑内异常的诊断方法。

Two patients with apparently 'minor' head injury on echoencephalography subsequently developed an extradural hematoma.

两个在脑超声图检查显示明显轻微头部外伤的病人后来出现了硬膜外血肿。

echogenic [ˌekəu'dʒenik] *a.* 发生回波的

One of the cerebral hemispheres of the fetus is diffusely echogenic.

胎儿一侧大脑半球呈弥漫性回波。

A portion of the pancreas is shown as an echogenic structure between the stomach and the duodenum.

胰腺某一部分的回声结构显示在胃和十二指肠之间。

eclampsia [i'klæmpsiə] *n.* 惊厥,子痫

Approximately 10% of patients with eclampsia will show evidence of a consumptive coagulopathy.

约 10% 的子痫患者有消耗性凝血病。

Eclampsia includes seizures and coma that happen during pregnancy but are not due to preexisting or organic brain disorders.

子痫是指妊娠期发生的癫痫和昏迷,但并不是因为先前存在的或器质性的脑部病变。

eclipse [i'klips] *v.* 使失色

Besides,unhappiness is like a disease-it gradually eclipses interest in everything else.

此外,不愉快就像是一种疾病,它逐渐使人无论在哪方面都失去了兴趣。

eclipta [ik 'liptə] *n.* 鳢肠属;旱莲草粉末;墨旱莲

We establish a method called HPLC for determination of psoralen and isopsoralen in eclipta capsules .

我们确定了高效液相色谱(HPLC)法测定旱莲胶囊中补骨脂素和异补骨脂素含量。

We try to study effects of aqueous extract from eclipta prostrata on S180 solid tumor and immune system of mice.

我们尝试研究旱莲草水提物对小鼠的 S180 实体瘤的抗肿瘤作用及其免疫系统的影响。

ecologic [ˌekə'lɔdʒik] *a.* 生态(学)的

Such ecologic transformations can be responsible for exacerbations during antibiotic therapy.

在抗生素治疗期间,这种生态学的转变可导致病情恶化。

ecological [ˌekə'lɔdʒɪkəl] *a.* 生态的,生态学的

The ruin of large number of rainforest plants must destroy the ecological balance.

热带雨林植物的大量消失必然会导致生态平衡的破坏。

New progress has been made in the development of ecological environment.

生态环境建设取得了新的进展。

ecology [i'kɔlədʒi] *n.* 生态学

Ecology is a branch of biology that deals with the habits of living things,especially their relation to the environment.

生态学是生物学的一个分支,研究生物的习性,尤其是生物与环境的关系。

Ecology mainly concentrates on understanding the structure and function of ecosystem and their component parts.

生态学主要集中于了解生态系统的结构和功能及其组成成分。

e-commerce ['i-'kɔmərs] *n.* 电子商务

With the popularity of Internet and the development of IT,E-commerce is now in the ascendant.

随着互联网的普及以及信息技术的不断发展，电子商务的热潮方兴未艾。

The E-payment becomes the key part in the E-commerce.

电子支付成为电子商务中关键性的组成部分。

econazole [iˈkɔnəzəul] *n.* 益康唑

Econazole kills fungi and yeasts by interfering with their cell membranes.

益康唑通过干扰细胞膜而杀死真菌和酵母菌。

Econazole nitrate cream is a prescription drug used to treat some common types of fungal skin infections.

硝酸益康唑乳膏是用于治疗一些常见型皮肤真菌感染的处方用药。

economics [ˌiːkəˈnɔmiks] *n.* 经济学

Leaders of a hospital should have a knowledge of economics of management.

医院的领导应懂一些管理经济学方面的知识。

He is an associate professor of pharmaceutical economics and policy at the University of Southern California.

他是南加利福尼亚大学(讲授)药学经济学和政策的副教授。

ecosphere [ˈiːkəuˌsfiə] *n.* 生物圈

The former emphasizes the superiority of humans over other beings, while the latter calls for the equality among all the beings within the ecosphere.

前者强调人类对其他生物的统治，后者则呼吁生物圈里所有生物的平等。

The plan for construction of urban forestry ecosphere in Changsha City has been approved for implementation by the people's government of Changsha City.

《建造长沙市城市林业生物圈专项规划》已获长沙市人民政府批准实施。

ecosystem [ˌiːkəˈsistəm] *n.* 生态系统

The members of a living community exist together in a particular, balanced relationship or ecosystem.

生物群落的成员以一种特别的平衡的关系或称之为生态系统而生活在一起。

ecotoxicology [ˌiːkɔtɔksiˈkɔlədʒi] *n.* 生态毒理学

Ecotoxicology has been concentrating on understanding the effects of toxic chemicals on organisms.

生态毒理学集中于了解有毒化学物质对生物体的效应。

ectoderm [ˈektəudəːm] *n.* 外胚层

The ectoderm forms the skin.

外胚层形成皮肤。

Sense organs and some glands are also formed from the ectoderm.

感觉器官和一些腺体也来自外胚层。

ectohormone [ˌektəˈhɔːməun] *n.* 外激素

This paper surveyed the effect of ectohormone on the duration of instar of giant silkworm.

本文探讨了外源激素对天蚕蛾幼虫龄期的影响。

Ectohormone and feromone have not yet been applied to the prevention of the injurious insects on farmland.

外激素和信息素还没有应用于对农田害虫的防范。

ectopic [ekˈtɔpik] *a.* 异位的

Dietary phosphate restriction may reduce serum phosphate levels and prevent ectopic calcification.

限制饮食中的磷酸盐可降低血清中磷酸盐水平(以便)防止异位钙化。

The 24 hours of ECG monitoring shows that some people can have frequent ectopic beats even without any apparent heart disease.

24 小时心电图监测显示有些人虽然没有明显的心脏病，但仍可能经常出现异位搏动。

ectoplasm [ˈektəuplæzəm] *n.* (细胞)外质,外胞浆

Two-layer coupled oscillator system composed of endoplasm and ectoplasm plays important roles in such an information integration.

由内质和外质组成的双层耦合振荡器系统在这样的信息集成中发挥重要作用。

Ectoplasm may refer to the outer part of the cytoplasm in cell biology.

细胞外质在细胞生物学中是指细胞质的外层部分。

eczema [ˈekzimə] *n.* 湿疹

Eczema is an inflammatory itching disease of the skin.

湿疹是具有瘙痒感觉的一种皮炎。

Eczema may affect any and all parts of the skin surface.

湿疹可以发生在身体任何部位和所有皮肤表面。

eczematous [ekˈzemətəs] *a.* 湿疹的

Eczematous skin lesions are frequently present.

患者常有湿疹性皮肤损害。

edema [iːˈdiːmə] *n.* 水肿,浮肿 (=oedema)

With right ventricular failure the cyanosis deepens and peripheral edema becomes prominent.

有右心室衰竭时,发绀加重,外周水肿更明显。

Dyspnea rarely causes pulmonary edema by itself.

呼吸困难本身很少能引起肺水肿。

edematous [iˈdiːmətəs] *a.* 水肿的,浮肿的

The kidneys weighed 215g and 220g,and were described as being mildly congested and edematous.

两个肾分别重为 215g 和 220g,被认为是轻度充血和水肿。

In cases of haemolytic disease the placenta is large and edematous.

在溶血性疾病患者中,胎盘大而水肿。

edge [edʒ] *n.* 边缘,刃

Right ventricular hypertrophy follows and the increased thrust can be felt as a "lifting" impulse at the left sternal edge.

继之发生右心室肥大,增强的冲击力可在胸骨左缘触及抬举样搏动。

edible [ˈedibl] *a.* 可食的

This food is scarcely edible.

这种食物简直不能吃。

eduction [iːˈdʌkʃən] *n.* 排出

There is the effect that accelerates galactic eduction in lactation.

在哺乳期有促进乳汁排出的作用。

When a normal person increases in absorbing sylvite,uric potassium eduction also increases.

正常人摄入钾盐增加时,尿钾排出也增加。

effect [iˈfekt] *n.* 效果;影响 ;效应

This drug produced a quick effect.

该药迅速地产生了效果。

The medicine had no effect on him.

这种药对他无效。

A fixed effect model was used to combine the results of the two trials.

采用固定效应模型来合并这两项试验的结果。

v. 产生,实现

In these cases it is often difficult to effect a complete cure.

这样的病例常难于完全治愈。

The drug effected nothing.

此药无效。

effective [iˈfektiv] *a.* 有效的

The patient has finally received an effective treatment.

病人终于得到了有效治疗。

This drug is effective against indigestion.

此药对治疗消化不良有效。

effectively [iˈfektivli] *adv.* 事实上，实际上

Pediatric populations generate particular ethical concern because of a potential for lifelong discrimination that may effectively exclude them from educational opportunities.

儿童群体因为可能存在的终身歧视而产生特别的伦理学关注，事实上这可能会剥夺他们受教育机会。

A back injury effectively ended her career.

背部损伤实际上结束了她的职业生涯。

effector [iˈfektə] *n.* 效应物，效应基因；效应器

The agent causing the allosteric activation is termed an effector or modifier.

引起变构激活的因子称为效应物或变构剂。

efferent [ˈefərənt] *a.* 传出的

Nerves that carry impulses away from the brain or the spinal cord are known as efferent nerves.

将冲动由脑或脊髓传递出去的神经称为传出神经。

There are neurons in the sympathetic system which correspond to the efferent or motor neurons of the PNS (peripheral nerve system).

交感神经系统的神经元相当于周围神经系统的传出或运动神经元。

efficacious [ˌefiˈkeiʃəs] *a.* 有效力的

The drug is said to be efficacious for great pain and is devoid of any side-effect.

据称该药对剧痛有效，而且没有任何副作用。

A low sodium diet is efficacious in the treatment of cardiac edema and paroxysmal cardiac dyspnea.

在治疗心源性水肿和阵发性心源性呼吸困难时，采用低钠饮食是有效的。

efficacy [ˈefikəsi] *n.* 功效，效能

Efficacy is a measure of the inherent ability to exert an effect.

效能是衡量（药物）发挥效应所固有的能力。

The proper use of the drug never fails of its efficacy.

如使用适当，此药总是很有效力的。

The efficacy of aspirin in relieving headaches is well known.

阿司匹林有解除头痛的功效是人所共知的。

efficiency [iˈfiʃənsi] *n.* 效率

As more and more nephrons are destroyed, the kidney shrinks in size and its efficiency is gradually decreased.

由于愈来愈多的肾单位受到破坏，肾脏便缩小，其功能逐渐减退。

These new medical instruments in the hospital have raised efficiency many times.

医院的这些新医疗仪器把效率提高了许多倍。

efficient [iˈfiʃənt] *a.* 效率高的，有能力的

Efficient registered and practical nurses, technicians, and many others are members of the team.

小组中有正式注册的和有实际经验的能干护士、技术人员和其他成员。

She is an efficient obstetrician.

她是一位能力高超的产科医生。

efflux [ˈeflʌks] *n.* 释放

Under these conditions reperfusion of the area has produced a large potassium efflux.

在此情况下,缺血区再灌注释放出大量的钾。

effort [ˈefət] *n.* 努力,作用力

A patient with effort angina of 6 years' duration was admitted to the hospital.

一名有 6 年运动性心绞痛病史的病人被收入院。

effusion [iˈfjuːʒən] *n.* 渗漏液;渗出

This may be followed by an extensive effusion into the affected pleural sac.

此后在受累的胸腔内有大量的渗出液。

The one characteristic finding of pericardial effusion is percussion cannot outline the border of the heart.

心包渗出液的一个典型所见是叩诊不能描绘出心脏的边界。

In these cases, ascites and pleural effusions are unusual.

在这些病例中,腹水和胸膜渗液并不常见。

egg [eg] *n.* 卵

These hormones, however, can cause several eggs to be released, possibly leading to multiple births.

然而,这些激素能引起多个卵的排放,因而可能导致多胎。

eicosanoid [aiˈkəusəˌnɔid] *n.* 类二十烷酸,类花生酸

Eicosanoids are products of arachidonic acid metabolism including prostaglandins, leukotrienes and thromboxanes.

类二十烷酸是花生四烯酸的代谢产物,包括前列腺素、白三稀和血栓素。

ejaculatory [iˈdʒækjulətəri] *a.* 射精的

After spinal cord injury, most men experience fertility related problems including erectile and ejaculatory dysfunction, impaired spermatogenesis, abnormal sperm viability, motility, and morphology, genitourinary infection and endocrine abnormalities.

脊髓受损后的男性大多会发生以下问题:勃起和射精功能障碍、精子发生受损、异常精子活力、精子运动力和精子形态异常、泌尿生殖系统感染以及内分泌异常。

ejection [iːˈdʒekʃən] *n.* 排出;喷射

Grade Ⅱ systolic ejection murmur is present over the lower left precordium.

在心前区左下出现 Ⅱ级收缩期喷射性杂音。

elaborate [iˈlæbəreit] *v.* 精心制作;(从简单成分)合成;详尽描述

Enzymes may be elaborated by many parasites, of which some have the action of digestion.

许多寄生虫能制造酶,其中有些酶有消化作用。

10 of amino acids are designated "essential" since they cannot be elaborated within the body.

十种氨基酸被称为"必需氨基酸",因为它们不能在体内合成。

The existence of threshold doses for chemicals is important in evaluating their safety, as is elaborated in Chapter 7.

阈剂量的存在在化学物质安全性评价中是很重要的,如第七章所详细描述。

a. [iˈlæbərit]复杂的,精心做成的

The cell is usually an integral part of a more elaborate organ and organ system in a multicellular plant or animal.

在多细胞植物或动物中,细胞通常是组成比较复杂的器官和器官系统的组成部分。

elaboration [iˌlæbəˈreiʃən] *n.* 精心制作;从简单成分合成

The secretion of estrogen is dependent on the elaboration of gonadotropin.

雌激素分泌依赖于促性腺激素的生成。

High temperature is thought to be favourable for the elaboration of antibodies.

人们认为高温有利于抗体的产生。

elastic [iˈlæstik] *a.* 弹性的

Elastic tissue is found in the dermis of the skin, in arterial walls, and in the walls of the alveoli of

the lungs.
弹性组织见于皮肤表皮、动脉壁及肺泡壁。

Elastic cartilage is yellowish in colour and is found in the external ear.
弹性软骨微带黄色,见于外耳。

elasticity [ˌelæs'tisəti] *n.* 弹性,弹力;灵活性

Changes in the walls of arteries frequently lead to loss of elasticity.
动脉壁的变化常导致其失去弹性。

Our muscles can begin to lose strength and elasticity as early as age 20.
我们的肌肉可能早在 20 岁时就开始丧失收缩力和弹性。

elastin [i'læstin] *n.* 弹性蛋白

Elastin is fibrous.
弹性蛋白是纤维状的。

Elastin is one of important constituents of muscle.
弹性蛋白是肌肉的重要组成成分之一。

elbow ['elbəu] *n.* 肘

The human elbow is the region surrounding the elbow-joint — the ginglymus or hinge joint in the middle of the arm.
人类的肘是肘关节(手臂中间的屈戌关节)附近的区域。

elderly ['eldəli] *a.* 上了年纪的,老年的

Prolonged immobilization of elderly patients may have many harmful effects.
老年患者长期的卧床不动可能产生许多有害影响。

Bronchopneumonia is preceded by bronchial infection and is commonest in children and the elderly.
支气管肺炎发病之前有支气管感染,在儿童和老年人中最常见。

electric [i'lektrik] *a.* 电的

We can generate electric power by splitting atoms.
我们可以利用原子核裂变发电。

An electric current in metal is caused by the movement of electrons.
金属内电流是由电子运动引起的。

electricity [ilek'trisiti] *n.* 电,电流

ATP can be likened to electricity in that it can be made in many different ways, it can stored, and it can be used for many different purposes.
三磷酸腺苷可以比作电力,因为它可通过许多不同的途径产生,可贮存,也可用于许多不同的目的。

electrocardiogram [iˌlektrəu'kɑːdiəgræm] *n.* 心电图

A recording of the electrical activity of the heart on a moving paper strip is called electrocardiogram(ECG).
在移动的纸条上记录下来的心脏电活动曲线叫心电图。

The electrocardiogram is a very important tool for assessing the ability of the heart to transmit the cardiac impulse.
心电图是评价心脏传导冲动能力的一个很重要的工具。

electrocardiograph [i'lektrəu'kɑːdiəgrɑːf] *n.* 心电描记器,心电图仪

The original form of electrocardiograph was based on the principle of the string galvanometer.
心电描记器的最初形式是基于弦电流计的原理。

electrocardiographic [iˌlektrəuˌkɑːdiə'græfik] *a.* 心电描记器的

Careful electrocardiographic monitoring should be used during these differential processes.
鉴别过程中应进行仔细的心电图监测。

Electrocardiographic abnormalities during and after exercise may be especially valuable.

运动中和运动后的心电图异常可能特别有价值。

electroconvulsive [iˌlektrənkən'vʌlsiv] *a.* 电痉挛的

Electroconvulsive therapy (ECT) has been widely used since 1940.

电痉挛疗法自1940年后得以广泛地运用。

electrocution [iˌlektrəu'kjuːʃən] *n.* 触电死亡，电刑

Severe injury or death by electrocution is the result.

结果是由于电击而造成严重的伤害或死亡。

Nebraska was the only state still using electrocution as its sole means of execution.

内布拉斯加州是唯一一个仍然将电刑作为执行死刑唯一手段的州。

electrode [i'lektrəud] *n.* 电极

These electric currents can be picked up by electrodes and be recorded by electrocardiograph.

这些电流可用电极接收并由心电图仪记录下来。

A transducer-like probe (electrode) transmits electrical signals to a computer, which translates them into images on a video screen.

一枚似换能器的探针（电极）将电信号传送到电脑，电脑将其转译为图像出现在电视屏幕上。

electrodialysis [iˌlektrəudai'ælisis] *n.* 电渗析，电透析

Electrodialysis is also proving suitable for some sorts of liquid waste but not yet developed as a routine liquid waste treatment.

电渗析方法也被证实对某些种类的液体废物的处理是有效的，但尚未发展成一种常规应用的对液体废物进行处理的方法。

electroencephalogram [i'lektrəen'sefələgræm] *n.* 脑电图

An electroencephalogram (EEG) records electrical brain wave patterns that show brain activity.

脑电图可记录显示脑活动的电波模式。

The electroencephalogram (EEG) may be helpful in differentiating syncope from seizures.

脑电图（EEG）可能对晕厥与癫痫发作的鉴别有帮助。

electroencephalograph [iˌlektrɔen'sefələgrɑːf] *n.* 脑电描记器

The machine that records the electrical activity of the brain is known as an electroencephalograph.

记录脑电活动的仪器叫做脑电描记器。

electroencephalography [iˌlektrəuenˌsefə'lɔgrəfi] *n.* 脑电描记法

Berger in 1929 discovered a method of recording the electrical rhythms of the brain known as electroencephalography.

贝格尔于1929年发明了一种可以记录脑的电节律活动的方法，称作脑电描记法。

Electroencephalography is used to detect and locate structural disease, such as tumours in the brain.

脑电描记法用来探查和确定器质性疾病，如脑内肿瘤。

electrolysis [iˌlek'trɔlisis] *n.* 电解

Electrolysis is also used to plate one metal on another.

电解也用于将一种金属电镀在另一种金属上。

Water can be reduced to oxygen and hydrogen by electrolysis.

水通过电解可以分解为氧和氢。

electrolyte [i'lektrəulait] *n.* 电解质，电解（溶）液

Electrolyte is a substance that dissociates into ions in solution, and thus becomes capable of conducting electricity.

电解质是一物质，在溶液中离解为离子，因而变得能导电。

Laboratory studies for electrolytes were all within normal limits.

电解质检查全部在正常范围内。

electromagnetic [iˌlektrəumæg'netik] *a.* 电磁的

A diagram of the electromagnetic spectrum is shown in Figure 13-5.

图 13-5 显示电磁波谱的图表。

Spindel' s device uses an electromagnetic coil to vibrate the implanted magnet.

史平得尔的设计中使用了电磁线圈,用来振动已经植入的磁铁。

electromagnetism [iˌlektrəu'mægnətizəm] *n.* 电磁;电磁学

Everyone at MIT has to take two terms of physics, mechanics and electromagnetism.

麻省理工学院的所有学生都需要修两学期的物理、力学和电磁学。

In the new age, three basic requirements for electric sources are high reliability, high effect and low disturbance of electromagnetism.

新时代对电源的三大基本要求是:高可靠性、高效率、低电磁干扰。

electron [i'lektrən] *n.* 电子

A scanning electron microscope reveals the surfaces of objects at various magnifications.

扫描电子显微镜可显示不同放大倍数的物体的表面。

In some cases, examination of appropriately prepared specimens by electron microscopy (EM) is of diagnostic value.

对于某些病例,将样本适当处理后进行电镜检查可帮助诊断。

Most of the ATP generated in mitochondria is via the electron transport system.

线粒体中大多数三磷酸腺苷的产生是通过电子传递系统完成的。

electronegativity [iˌlektrəuˌnegə'tiviti] *n.* 阴电性,电负性

The ability to attract electrons from other atoms in a molecule is called electronegativity.

分子中一个原子从其它原子吸引电子的能力称为电负性。

Electronegativity is a measure of the ability of atoms to attract other atoms in the same molecule.

电负性是测定原子吸引同一分子中其他原子能力的一种方法。

electronic [ˌilek'trɔnik] *a.* 电子的

Informal processing of electronic waste may cause serious health and pollution problems.

对电子垃圾的随便处理可能会引起严重的健康和污染问题。

Electronic record systems can make health care more efficient and less expensive.

电子记录系统能使卫生保健的效率更高且花费更少。

electronically [ˌilek'trɔnikəli] *ad.* 用电子装置

By most automated technics, the Hb, RBC count, and MCV are electronically measured.

血红蛋白、红细胞计数及平均红细胞容积可通过自动化技术用电子装置测得。

electrophile [i'lektrəufail] *n.* 亲电子剂

Because electrophiles accept electrons, they are Lewis acids.

因为亲电子剂可以接受电子,所以它们是路易斯酸。

The alkene is working as an electron donor and bromine as an electrophile.

烯烃是作为电子供体,而溴则作为亲电体。

electrophilic [iˌlektrəu'filik] *a.* 亲电子的

The substrate of an electrophilic addition reaction must have a double bond or triple bond.

亲电加成反应的底物必须具有一个双键或三键。

Electrophilic reagents (electrophiles) are atoms, molecules, and ions that behave as electron acceptors.

亲电子剂是表现如同电子受体的一些原子、分子和离子。

electrophoresis [iˌlektrəufə'riːsis] *n.* 电泳

Serum protein electrophoresis can differentiate an acute from a chronic illness.

血清蛋白电泳可以鉴别疾病是急性或慢性。

electrophoretic [iˌlektrəufə'retik] *a.* 电泳的

When multiple sclerosis is suspected, fluid should be sent for determination of immunoglobulin

content and electrophoretic pattern.
当被怀疑为多发性硬化时,应取脑脊液测定其免疫球蛋白的含量并检测其电泳图形。

electrophysiological [iˌlektrəuˌfiziə'lɔdʒikəl] *a.* 电生理学的

This emphasizes the need to do complete electrophysiological studies in patients with the sick sinus syndrome.
这里应强调的是对病窦综合征病人需要进行全面的电生理研究。

Exacting electrophysiologic researches revealed that irritability of living tissue is a strictly electrical process.
严格的电生理学研究显示活组织的兴奋性是一精确的电的过程。

electrophysiology [iˌlektrəufizi'ɔlədʒi] *n.* 电生理学

Electrophysiology is the scientific approach to basic biologic problems.
电生理对基本生物学问题的科学性探讨。

electroshock [iˌlektrəuʃɔk] *n.* 电休克

Electroshock therapy is still used only as a last resort.
电休克疗法仍然只能作为最后采取的一种手段。

After five electroshock treatments her condition improved significantly.
经过五次电休克疗法治疗后,她的病情有明显改善。

In only a very small fraction of cases is electroshock prescribed.
只有很少一部分病例才用电休克疗法处理。

electrotherapy [iˌlektrɔ'θerəpi] *n.* 电疗法

Interrupted galvanism is a form of electrotherapy in which direct current, in impulses lasting for 30 to 100 milliseconds, is used to stimulate the activity of nerves or the muscles they supply.
断续流电疗法是一种电疗的方式,它采用直流电(其脉冲持续 30 ~ 100 毫秒)来刺激神经及其支配的肌肉。

electuary [i'lektjuəri] *n.* 煎膏剂,药糖剂

Solanum xanthocarpum is a spiny diffuse herb and used in medicine in various forms, such as decoction, electuary, etc.
茄属植物黄果茄是一种多刺伏卧草本植物,可以多种剂型入药,如汤剂、煎膏剂等。

Guanxingao is a kind of traditional Chinese rubber electuary medicine which is able to either cure or guard against coronary heart disease and angina pectoris.
冠心膏是一种传统中药橡胶煎膏剂,可以预防或治疗冠心病和心绞痛。

element ['elimənt] *n.* 元素

Hydrogen is the lightest element known.
氢是已知的最轻的元素。

Radium is a radioactive element.
镭是放射性元素。

elementary [ˌeli'mentəri] *a.* 基本的

There are four elementary tissues which make up the body as a whole.
构成整个身体的基本组织有四种。

elephantiasis [ˌelifən'taiəsis] *n.* 象皮病,象皮肿

Gross elephantiasis develops only in association with repeated infections in highly endemic areas.
显著的象皮肿只发生在该病高度流行的地区并经反复感染的患者身上。

eleutheroside [ˌelju: 'θerəusaid] *n.* 刺五加苷

Eleutheroside B is preferably prepared from leaves, flowers and fruits of acanthopanax.
最好是用刺五加叶、花、果实来制备刺五加苷 B。

Eleutheroside B has notably ecological, economic and social benefit.
刺五加苷 B 具有显著的生态效益、经济效益和社会效益。

elevate ['eliveit] *v.* 使升高,提高

The renal venous pressure was significantly elevated in this patient, simulating obstruction of the renal veins.
此病例的肾静脉压明显升高，类似肾静脉阻塞。
Elevating the inflamed part eases the pain and diminishes the inflamatory oedema.
抬高发炎的部位可以缓和疼痛并减轻炎症水肿。

elevated [ˈeliveitid] *a.* 升高的，提高的
Up to 22% of patients may exhibit elevated arterial blood pressure at initial presentation.
多达22%的病人在最初表现中可出现动脉血压增高。
Goiter is characterized by protruding eyeballs, quickened heart action, elevated temperature, nervousness, and insomnia.
甲状腺肿的特征是眼球突出、心跳加快、体温升高、精神紧张和失眠。

elevation [ˌeliˈveiʃən] *n.* 升高
There is no doubt that prolonged elevation of the blood pressure aggravates atheroma.
毫无疑问，长期血压升高能使粥样硬化加重。
In the more acute elevations of intracranial pressure, pulse rate may slow and blood pressure may climb.
在较急性的颅内压增高时，脉率可能减慢，血压可能增高。

elicit [iˈlisit] *v.* 引出，使发出
Careful daily examination of the joints, especially in the early morning, may elicit slight tenderness or limitation of motion.
每天仔细检查关节，特别是在清早，可显示出轻微压痛或活动受限。
The skeletal structure must be examined, particularly if a history of trauma is elicited.
骨骼结构必须检查，特别对有外伤史的病人更是如此。

eligibility [ˌelidʒəˈbiliti] *n.* 资格
Registry study designs often restrict eligibility for entry to individuals with certain characteristics (e. g. , age).
注册研究设计经常以某些特征(如年龄)限制个体的入选资格。

eligible [ˈelidʒibl] *a.* 合格的；有资格的
Some 26 subjects originally thought to be eligible showed too much improvement with therapy.
最初认为合格的大约有 26 名病人，随着治疗显示出明显的好转。

eliminate [iˈlimineit] *v.* 排除，清除，消灭
The primary function of immune system is to eliminate infections agents and to minimize the damage they cause.
免疫系统的主要功能是清除感染物和降低它所引起的损伤。
Cessation of cigarette smoking nearly always eliminates the cough of chronic bronchitis.
停止吸烟几乎总是能消除慢性支气管炎的咳嗽。
RNA synthesis is eliminated using actinomycin D.
采用放线菌素 D 可抑制 RNA 的合成。
You should try to eliminate some of the options which are unlikely.
你应努力排除那些不太可能的选择。
However, a part of the products of metabolism are eliminated also by other organs.
然而，一部分代谢物还由其他的器官排泄。

elimination [iˌlimiˈneiʃən] *n.* 除去，消除
The ideal treatment of cough is elimination of its underlying cause.
对咳嗽的理想治疗是去掉其潜在致病原因。
There was no relationship to food types; milk elimination caused no apparent effect.
(腹泻)与食物的类型无关；停用牛奶无明显效果。

elixirs [iˈliksəs] *n.* 酏剂

These elixirs often contain large quantities of sorbitol, which will increase the osmolar concentration.
这些酏剂常含有大量的山梨醇，这将增加容积渗透浓度。
Liquid medications, particularly elixirs and suspensions, are preferred for enteral administration.
液态药物，尤其是酏剂和悬液，常被优先用于肠内给药。

elliptocytosis [eˌliptəusaiˈtəusis] *n.* 椭圆形红细胞增多症
The vast majority of those with hereditary elliptocytosis require no treatment whatsoever.
绝大多数遗传性椭圆形红细胞增多症患者并不需要任何治疗。

elongate [ˈiːlɔŋgeit] *v.* 拉长
Some protozoa are oval or spherical, others are elongated.
有些原虫呈卵圆形或球形，有些为细长形。
The muscle fibers are composed of tens of thousands of thread-like myofibrils, which can contract, relax, and elongate.
肌纤维由成千上万的线样肌原纤维组成，后者能够收缩、松弛和延长。

elsholtzia [elˈʃɔltsiə] *n.* 香薷
We conducted the treatment and dialectical nursing for 50 patients with the elsholtzia drinking broth.
我们对50位患者进行了给予服用香薷饮汤剂的治疗和辨证护理。
The evaluation of bacteriostatic effects in vitro and dermal toxicity of elsholtzia essential oil was made.
对香薷精油的体外抑菌作用及皮肤毒性已进行了评价。

elucidate [iˈluːsideit] *v.* 阐明，说明(问题、困难)
The pathophysiologic changes common to all cases of diverticulosis of the colon have yet to be elucidated.
结肠憩室病所有病例中共同的病理生理变化，还有待充分阐明。

emaciation [imeisiˈeiʃən] *n.* 消瘦
Repeated attacks of asthma can lead to poor general health, emaciation.
哮喘反复发作可使病人全身健康状况不佳，消瘦。
If an animal is deprived of food, it loses weight quickly and finally dies of emaciation.
如果动物得不到食物供应，体重就很快减轻，最后死于消瘦。

embarrass [imˈbærəs] *v.* 阻碍
Pulmonary edema impairs gas exchange and may induce hypoxia, which embarrass cardiac function.
肺水肿减少气体交换，可能导致低氧血症，这将影响心脏功能。

embarrassed [imˈbærəst] *a.* 窘迫的
The patient's embarrassed manner as he entered increased the doctor's doubt.
病人进来时窘迫的神态增加了医生的怀疑。

embolectomy [ˌembɔˈlektəmi] *n.* 栓子切除术，栓子清除术
In some cases of pulmonary embolism, embolectomy may be life saving.
在一些肺动脉栓塞的病例中，采用栓子切除术能挽救生命。
Embolectomy is the emergency surgical removal of emboli which are blocking blood circulation.
栓子清除术是一种去除阻塞血液循环的栓子的紧急外科手术

embolic [emˈbɔlik] *a.* 栓塞的，栓子的
There is considerable evidence that tumor cells are often embolic in blood or lymphatic vessels without production of metastasis.
很多证据说明，肿瘤细胞栓子常在血管和淋巴管内而没有发生转移。

embolisation [ˌembəlaiˈseiʃənˌ-liˈz-] *n.* 栓塞治疗
Traditional treatment has normally involved open surgery to remove the faulty veins, but the new

embolisation process now offers an alternative that results in much less inside damage.
传统的治疗方法是去除紊乱血管的开放性手术，但是新方法采用栓塞技术可使手术损伤减小。

embolism [ˈembəlizm] *n.* 栓塞，栓子

Thrombosis of the veins of the lower limbs is the usual cause of serious pulmonary embolism.
下肢静脉血栓形成常引起严重的肺栓塞。

Pulmonary air embolism is a rare, life-threatening complication of permanent pacemaker implantation.
肺气体栓塞是置放永久性起搏器时罕见但危及生命的并发症。

embolization [ˌembəlaiˈzeiʃən] *n.* 栓塞，血栓形成

The mechanism of embolization of tumor cells is simple.
肿瘤细胞栓塞的机制简单。

Pulmonary embolization may result in further acute elevation of pulmonary arterial pressure.
肺血栓形成可导致肺动脉压的进一步急性上升。

embolize [ˈembəlaiz] *v.* 使栓塞，形成栓子

This thrombus on the wall of a ventricle may then break off and embolize to remote organs such as brain, kidney, or extremities, resulting in loss of function.
心室壁的血栓可能脱落，因而使较远部位的器官如大脑、肾脏或四肢产生栓塞，使这些器官丧失功能。

embolus [ˈembələs] (*pl.* emboli [ˈembəlai]) *n.* 栓子

Where such an embolus impacts, a combination of tissue necrosis and suppuration results.
在这种栓子阻塞部位，组织同时发生坏死和化脓。

Consequent pulmonary emboli are very common autopsy findings.
随后的肺栓塞在尸检中很常见。

embryo [ˈembriəu] *n.* 胚，胚胎

If the ovum released should be fertilized, the developing trophoblast around the embryo produces chorionic gonadotrophin.
如果被排出的卵子受了精，围绕胚胎发育的滋养层产生绒毛膜促性腺激素。

A clear fluid collects in the amniotic cavity surrounding the embryo.
透明的液体聚集在羊膜腔中胎儿的周围。

embryologic [ˌembriəˈlɔdʒik] *a.* 胚胎(学)的

Both lesions are the result of embryologic development defects.
这两种损害都是胚胎发育缺陷的结果。

embryonal [embriˈəunəl] *a.* 胚的，胚芽的

Some mechanisms of its embryonal toxicity are still unknown.
其胚胎毒性的一些机制还不知道。

Five-year relative survival for all embryonal cancers was 80%.
所有胚胎癌的 5 年相对生存率是 80%。

embryonic [ˌembriˈɔnik], embryonal [ˈembriənəl] *a.* 胚胎的；初期的

The pituitary has a double embryonic origin.
垂体有双重的胚胎起源。

The team of psychologists injected rats brain damaged from simulated heart attacks with embryonic mouse brain cells.
一组心理学家，给那些由模拟心脏病发作引起损伤的大鼠脑内注入小鼠的胚胎脑细胞。

embryotoxicity [ˈembriəuˌtɔkˈsisiti] *n.* 胚胎毒性

Some studies indicated that second hand smoking has effect on genotoxicity, reproductive toxicity and embryotoxicity.
一些研究表明二手烟具有遗传毒性、生殖毒性和胚胎毒性。

Currently no bioassays are available to assess the embryotoxicity of chemicals with terrestrial soil invertebrates.
目前还没有生物测定法用于评估化学品致陆地土壤无脊椎动物的胚胎毒性。

emerge [iˈməːdʒ] *v.* 出现
At all events the secretion emerging from the ducts is a viscid, mucous fluid.
在任何情况下从管道中排出的分泌物都是一种黏性液体。
Blood may be seen to emerge from one or the other ureter.
可以看到血从一侧或另一侧的输尿管流出。
The head of the child first emerged from the vagina.
婴儿头部首先在阴道口出现。

emergence [iˈməːdʒəns] *n.* 出现
Some of these threats are becoming more serious with the emergence of insecticide-resistant vectors.
随着抗杀虫剂病媒的出现,有些疾病的威胁越来越严重。
Public health experts are alarmed at the emergence of new strains of bacteria that cannot be destroyed by antibiotics.
公共卫生专家们因不能为抗生素消灭的新的菌株的出现而感到忧虑。

emergency [iˈməːdʒənsi] *n.* 紧急;急症
But for the emergency treatment, the patient might have lost both eyes.
若不是采取紧急治疗,病人的两眼很可能早已失明。
When a blood transfusion is required, it is usually a matter of emergency.
通常在紧急情况下才需要输血。
The purpose of this paper is to deal with the medical emergencies in renal disease.
本文的目的是探讨肾病急症。

emesis [ˈeməsis] *n.* 呕吐
Syrup of ipecac and copper sulfate cause emesis by local irritation of the stomach.
吐根糖浆和硫酸铜局部刺激胃而产生呕吐作用。
Severe headache is followed by coma, sometimes with emesis.
严重的头痛以后,常出现昏迷,有时伴有呕吐。

emetic [iˈmetik] *a.* 催吐的
Apomorphine is used as an emetic agent.
阿朴吗啡用作催吐药。
n. 催吐药
Apomorphine is a centrally-acting emetic.
阿朴吗啡是作用于神经中枢的一种催吐药。

emetine [ˈemətiːn] *n.* 依米丁,吐根碱
Emetine and dehydroemetine are cardiotoxic.
吐根碱及去氢吐根碱对心脏有毒性。

emigrate [ˈemigreit] *v.* 游出,渗出
Macrophages in inflamed tissues are derived mainly from emigrated, transformed blood monocytes.
炎症组织内的巨噬细胞主要由血液单核细胞游出后转变而来。

emigration [ˌemiˈgreiʃən] *n.* 游出,渗出
The emigration of leucocytes is an active process which occurs in two stages.
白细胞游出是一种主动的过程,有两个阶段。

eminently [ˈeminəntli] *ad.* 突出地
Modern burn treatment has been eminently successful in saving the lives of many people who only a few years ago would have died.

现代烧伤治疗方法已在拯救病人的生命方面获得了突出的成就,而这些病人,要是在几年前还是难免于死的。

emissary [ˈemisəri] *n.* 信使;使者 *a.* 密使的

Emissary veins connect the extracranial venous system with the intracranial venous sinuses.

导静脉连接颅外静脉系统和颅内静脉窦。

Morphologic changes in the dural sinuses and emissary veins of the posterior fossa relate closely to the development of the brain.

硬膜窦和后颅窝导静脉形态的改变与大脑的发育密切相关。

emission [iˈmiʃən] *n.* 散发,排放

Single photon emission computer tomography has developed rapidly since it was used in clinical practice at the end of 1970s.

单光子发射计算机断层显像自 20 世纪 70 年代末应用于临床以来发展迅速。

A number of environmental activists doubt that the Copenhagen summit will achieve binding emission reduction targets.

许多环保人士对哥本哈根峰会能否达成共同的减排目标表示质疑。

emit [iˈmit] *v.* 散发

The tank emitted an unpleasant odor.

水箱散发出一种难闻的气味。

All living cells of plants, animals and human beings emit biophotons which cannot be seen by the naked eye but can be measured by special equipment.

植物、动物和人的所有活细胞可发出不能肉眼看到、但可用特殊设备检测到的生物光子。

emodin [ˈemədin] *n.* 大黄素,泻素

All parameters increased significantly in the emodin treated group.

大黄素治疗组所有的指标都明显升高。

The crystal was determined as emodin by means of spectra.

经光谱法鉴定,所得结晶为大黄素。

Emodin in preparation was extracted by acid hydrolysis and organic solvent.

以酸水解和有机溶媒提取法来制备大黄素。

emotion [iˈməuʃən] *n.* 感情,情绪

Joy, grief, fear, hate, love, rage and excitement are emotions.

高兴、悲哀、恐惧、憎恨、喜爱、愤怒和兴奋都在情绪的范围。

emotional [iˈməuʃənəl] *a.* 情绪的,感情的

The heart rate is faster after meals, exercise and emotional excitement.

饭后、运动和情绪激动时,心率较快。

empathy [ˈempəθi] *n.* 移情作用;同感

These have significance for understanding the relationship between psychopathy, empathy, and antisocial behavior.

这些对理解精神病、移情与反社会行为之间的关系方面有重要意义。

emphasis [ˈemfəsis] *n.* 强调,重点

The prevention of infectious diseases is so important that it deserves special emphasis.

传染病的预防非常重要,值得特别重视。

This emphasis on clinical pharmacology is justified, since the effects of drugs are often characterized by significant interspecies variation.

强调临床药理学是理所当然的,因为物种各异而药物作用也各异。

emphasize [ˈemfəsaiz] *v.* 强调

They emphasized the importance of quality of life of the patients before the inevitable complications overtook them.

他们强调了在不可避免的并发症发生之前病人生活质量的重要性。

It is important to emphasize here that jaundice is not an essential symptom of hepatitis.
重要的是要在这里强调黄疸并非肝炎必具的症状。
Let it be emphasized that the lesion is silent in early stage of cancer of the stomach.
应该强调胃癌早期无任何症状。
It can never be too strongly emphasized that a serious attempt should be made to find underlying focus.
应该努力发现潜在的病灶,这一点怎样强调也不过分。

emphraxis [emˈfræksis] *n.* 阻塞,闭塞
The objective of our study is to discuss the clinical value and effectivity of self-made catheter system in treating sterilization caused by oviduct emphraxis.
本研究的目的是探讨应用自制导管系统治疗输卵管阻塞性不孕症的临床价值和疗效。
Different stenosis or emphraxis of below-popliteal arteries existed in all patients.
全部患者均存在腘动脉以下血管不同程度的狭窄或闭塞。

emphysema [ˌemfiˈsiːmə] *n.* 肺气肿
Both chronic bronchitis and emphysema result in airways narrowing.
慢性支气管炎和肺气肿都可以使气道狭窄。
When well developed, chronic bronchitis is usually accompanied by emphysema.
慢性支气管炎发展严重时通常伴有肺气肿。

emphysematous [ˌemfiˈsemətəs] *a.* 肺气肿的
Preoperative study of its right lung had shown that it was emphysematous and could not itself support life.
术前检查发现其右肺患有肺气肿,不能赖其维持生命。

empiric [emˈpirik] *a.* 经验主义的 *n.* 经验主义者
In the management of arthritic conditions, drugs are chosen on an empiric basis.
在治疗关节炎时,主要是根据经验选择药物。
In the management of these patients, empiric antibiotic therapy should be initiated.
在治疗这些患者时,开始应凭经验使用抗生素。

empty [ˈempti] *a.* 空的
This medicine must be taken on an empty stomach.
这种药必须空腹服用。
v. 倒空,排空
The veins empty themselves into the heart.
静脉血管将自己排空使血液流入心脏。

empyema [ˌempaiˈiːmə] *n.* 积脓;脓胸
Complications of bronchopneumonia include lung abscess, pleural effusion and empyema.
支气管肺炎的合并症有肺脓肿、胸腔积液及脓胸。
The rupture of the abscess into the pleural space with creation of empyema occurs only rarely.
脓肿破裂到胸膜间隙形成脓胸仅为罕见。

emulsification [iˌmʌlsifiˈkeiʃən] *n.* 乳化作用
In describing lipid digestion, you have to be clear about the concept of emulsification.
在叙述类脂消化时,必须弄清乳化作用的概念。

emulsify [iˈmʌlsifai] *v.* 使乳化
Fat does not dissolve in water, so in order to emulsify fat something special is needed.
脂肪不溶于水,所以,要乳化脂肪就需要某种特殊东西。
It was found that basic ionic water acted to emulsify cholesterol and triglycerides clearly.
已发现碱性离子水可明显乳化胆固醇和三油酸甘油酯。

emulsion [iˈmʌlʃən] *n.* 乳浊液;乳剂
The bile from the liver breaks up fat particles into very small particles to form an emulsion.

来自肝脏的胆汁可将脂肪颗粒分解为微粒，并形成乳剂。

enact [iˈnækt] *v.* 制定（法案）

The Patient Safety and Quality Improvement Act of 2005 (PSQIA) was enacted in response to a 1999 report by the Institute of Medicine.

2005 患者安全和质量改善法案（PSQIA）是针对医学研究所 1999 年的一项报告而制定的。

enamel [iˈnæməl] *n.* （牙）釉质

Acids are corrosive to the enamel and dentine of the teeth.

酸类对于牙釉质和骨质都有腐蚀作用。

The enamel protects the body of the tooth from the germs in the mouth.

（牙）釉质保护牙体使之不受口腔里的细菌的伤害。

enamine [ˈenəmiːn] *n.* 烯胺

Enamine catalysis has been used mostly in the context of carbonyl α-substitution reactions.

烯胺催化主要用于羰基 α-取代反应。

The mechanism involves the formation of a reactive enamine intermediate.

此机制涉及一种反应性烯胺中间体的形成。

enanthema [ˌenənˈθiːmə] *n.* 黏膜疹

An enanthema is a lesion of the mucous membranes.

黏膜疹是一种黏膜病变。

Could Parkinson's disease cause enanthema?

帕金森氏病能引起黏膜疹吗？

enantiomer [iˈnæntiəumə] *n.* 对映体

Chiral ligand-exchange chromatography (CLEC) is one of the basic chromatography methods for enantiomer separation.

手性配体交换色谱法是分离对映体的基本色谱法之一。

encapsulate [inˈkæpsjuleit] *v.* 用囊状物包裹

The lesions may become encapsulated by fibrous tissue.

病变已被纤维组织包裹。

The adult flute lives singly or in pairs encapsulated in the cystic spaces of the lung.

成虫单个或成双的在肺泡间形成囊肿。

Percussion may also differentiate the free fluid of ascites from the encapsulated fluid within an ovarian cyst.

采用叩诊的方法也能鉴别卵巢囊肿内包裹的液体和游离的腹水。

encapsulation [inˌkæpsjuˈleiʃən] *n.* 包膜（形成）

Some low-grade cancers may develop partial encapsulation by the same mechanism as in benign neoplasms.

某些低度的恶性肿瘤可以通过和良性肿瘤相同的机制形成部分包膜。

encelialgia [enˈseliəldʒiə] *n.* 内脏痛

Encelialgia refers to the pain located in any of the abdominal viscera.

内脏痛是指任何腹部脏器的疼痛。

Referred pain is a characteristic of encelialgia.

牵涉痛是内脏痛的一个特点。

encephalitis [enˌsefəˈlaitis] *n.* 脑炎

Type B encephalitis is characterized by headache, high fever, rigidity of the neck, etc.

乙型脑炎是以头痛、高烧、颈部强直等现象为特征的。

This patient is free from symptoms of encephalitis.

这个病人没有脑炎的症状。

encephalomalacia [enˌsefələuməˈleiʃiə] *n.* 脑软化症

Pulmonary hypoplasia and remote brainstem necrosis associated with multicystic encephalomalacia were found at autopsy.
尸检结果显示为肺发育不良和远程脑干坏死伴囊性脑软化。
The chicken was fed with low VE feedstuff to duplicate model of encephalomalacia.
用低维生素 E(VE)日粮饲喂雏鸡,复制脑软化症动物模型。

encephalomeningitis [enˌsefələuˌmeninˈdʒaitis] *n.* 脑膜 脑炎
Nonpurulent encephalomeningitis with larvae in the cerebrospinal fluid, choroid, and retina may also occur.
非化脓性脑膜脑炎病人在脑脊液、脉络膜及视网膜内可见幼虫。

encephalomyelitis [enˌsefələumaiəˈlaitis] *n.* 脑脊髓炎
Encephalomyelitis is sometimes part of an overwhelming virus infection.
脑脊髓炎有时是严重全身病毒感染的一部分。
Clinically apparent encephalomyelitis occurs in 1 of 1000 patients with measles.
临床上,患麻疹的病人中常常有 1/1000 典型的脑脊髓炎患者。

encephalomyeloradiculitis [enˌsefələuˌmaiələuræˌdikjuˈlaitis] *n.* 脑脊髓神经根炎
The clinical features of acute EBV myeloradiculitis, encephalomyeloradiculitis, and subacute meningomyeloradiculitis are distinctive.
急性 EBV 脊髓神经根炎、脑脊髓神经根炎和亚急性脊膜脊髓神经根炎的临床特征不同。
C57BR/cdJ mice developed encephalomyeloradiculitis following peripheral inoculation of the C strain of lactate dehydrogenase-elevating virus.
C57BR/cdJ 鼠外围接种 C 株乳酸脱氢酶活性病毒后出现脑脊髓神经根炎。

encephalon [enˈsefələn] (*pl.* encepla [enˈsefələ]) *n.* 脑
Since the scientific name for the brain is encephalon, infection of the brain is known as encephalitis.
由于大脑的科学名称是脑,当脑受到感染时通称为脑炎。

encephalopathy [enˌsefəˈlɔpəθi] *n.* 脑病
In other patients, encephalopathy, acute renal failure, or hepatic dysfunction may dominate the clinical picture.
在其他病人中,脑病、急性肾功能衰竭或肝功能失调可能为主要的临床表现。
Elevations in serum ammonia levels are common in cirrhosis and may account for some of the symptoms and findings associated with hepatic encephalopathy.
肝硬化病人的血氨水平升高,这可以解释肝性脑病的某些症状。

enchondroma [ˌenkɔnˈdrəumə] *n.* 内生软骨瘤
Enchondromas are the most common of the intraosseous cartilage tumors.
内生软骨瘤是最常见的骨内软骨肿瘤。
The term chondroma is sometimes used synonymously with enchondroma.
软骨瘤有时被用作内生软骨瘤的同义词。
The objective of our research is to evaluate the results of frozen allogenous bone grafting for the treatment of hand enchondroma.
本研究的目的是评价冷冻异体骨移植治疗手部内生软骨瘤的效果。

enclose [inˈkləuz] *v.* 围住,把…封入
Bacteria do store granules, but these are never enclosed by a membrane.
细菌的确能贮存颗粒,但这些颗粒无膜包绕。
The most striking and distinctive characteristic of eucaryotic cells is their possession of intracellular membrane enclosed organelles.
真核生物细胞最显著、最具有特征的性质是其具有细胞内膜性结构包绕的细胞器。

encode [inˈkəud] *v.* 编码,译成密码
DNA (deoxyribonucleic acid) is the molecule that encodes genetic information.

DNA(脱氧核糖核酸)是编码(蕴藏)遗传信息的分子。

The main tissue transplantation antigens are encoded by the polymorphic MHC locus.

主要组织移植抗原系由多态性的 MHC 位点编码。

Genes are specific sequences of bases that encode instructions on how to make proteins.

基因是含有指导蛋白质合成信息的特定碱基序列。

encompass [inˈkʌmpəs] *v.* 围绕,包括

Instead of being limited to family and close friends, it now may encompass the school and community.

这种情况现在可以包括学校和社区,而不仅限于家庭和好友。

The process of oocyte maturation encompasses several molecular and structural alterations in the cytoplasm.

卵母细胞成熟过程包括细胞质的某些分子和结构改变。

connective tissues encompass a wide variety of tissues in the body.

机体很多组织周围都有结缔组织环绕。

encounter [inˈkauntə] *v.* 遭遇,遇到

Adverse drug reactions are among the most frequent problems encountered clinically and represent a common cause for hospitalization.

药物的副作用是临床上常遇到的问题而且也是住院的常见原因。

Group A streptococci are encountered somewhat more frequently than other bacteria and are generally believed to be causally related with rheumatic fever.

A 组链球菌要比其他病菌稍微多见一些,一般认为它是引起风湿热的原因。

In toxicologic studies, the doses selected are usually larger than those are encountered by humans.

毒理学研究中选用的剂量往往比人们接触的剂量大。

encourage [inˈkʌridʒ] *v.* 鼓励,促进,支持

If the sick child of pharyngitis old enough, he should be encouraged to gargle, using saline solution.

如患咽炎的患儿够大,应鼓励他用盐水漱口。

These medicated wafers may encourage fungous infections of the mouth and the tongue.

这些糯米纸囊剂会促使口腔和舌头的真菌感染。

The past success of PTA has encouraged expanding indication.

PTA 以往的成功使其适应证范围扩大。

encrypt [enˈkript] *v.* 加密

They are best used to encrypt files on a hard disk.

它们最习惯于加密储存在硬盘上的文件。

Wireless hardware developers could use the software to encrypt their products.

无线硬件开发商可以用该软件为他们的产品加密。

endangiitis [ˌendændʒiˈaitis] *n.* 血管内膜炎

The fundamental pathological changes are the endangiitis and an infiltration usually containing a significant admixture of plasma cells.

基本病理改变表现为血管内膜炎和明显混合有浆细胞的细胞浸润。

Using the steady pressure and speed to infuse chemotherapeutic agents can significantly decrease the incidence of the vein endangiitis.

采用恒定的压力及速度进行静脉推注化疗药物能显著地降低静脉内膜炎的发生率。

endangium [enˈdændʒiəm] *n.* 血管内膜

Coronary artery endangium can be injured by interventional treatment.

介入治疗可能造成冠状动脉血管内膜损伤。

Insufficient apoptosis of vascular smooth muscle cells is the important mechanism of endangium

hyperplasia after balloon injury of the vessels.
血管平滑肌细胞凋亡不足是球囊损伤后血管内膜增生的重要机制。

endarterectomy [ˌendɑːtəˈrektəmi] *n.* 动脉内膜切除术

Endarterectomy is an effective way for the treatment of carotid artery stenosis.
动脉内膜剥脱术是治疗颈动脉硬化性狭窄的有效方法。

To prevent and treat ischemic stroke with carotid endarterectomy has become a routine surgical option, and its efficacy has been confirmed.
应用颈动脉内膜切除术预防和治疗缺血性卒中已成为一种常规的手术选择,其疗效已得到明确肯定。

endarteritis [ˌendɑːtəˈraitis] *n.* 动脉内膜炎

Endarteritis of the aorta may obstruct the mouths of the coronary arteries, supplying the heart.
主动脉内膜炎可堵塞营养心脏的冠状动脉口。

endeavour [inˈdevə] *n. v.* 努力,尽力

I have endeavoured in each succeeding edition to remedy this by submitting to the criticism of my learned friends those sections in which notable advances have occurred.
每次再版修订时,我都尽力补救这一缺陷,按照那些博学的友人的批评,去修改内容已有显著进展的章节。

It enables him to practise primary prevention, which endeavours to ensure that disorders do not develop.
这使他能够采取重要的预防措施,尽量保证疾病不会迁延。

endemic [enˈdemik] *a.* 地方流行的,(某地)特有的

Measles is a disease of cosmopolitan distribution, endemic in all but isolated populations.
麻疹分布于世界各地,除隔离的人群外,各地均可流行。

Strains endemic in hospital are often resistant to many antimicrobial drugs.
医院内特有的菌株常常对许多抗菌药物具有耐药性。

n. 地方流行病

They are working on a report of their investigation of the endemic.
他们正在写一份这种地方流行病的调查报告。

endergonic [ˌendəˈgɔnik] *a.* 吸收能量的,吸能的

During an endergonic reaction, energy input is required.
在吸能反应期间需要能量输入。

ending [ˈendiŋ] *n.* 结局;死亡;末梢

These receptors are nerve endings that discharge impulses according to the extent of stretch in the wall of the vessel in which they are imbedded.
这些感受器是嵌入血管壁的神经末梢,并依血管壁的扩张程度发出冲动。

endocardial [ˌendəuˈkɑːdiəl] *a.* 心内的;心内膜的

In patients with partial endocardial scar extension, the ablation was effective in eliminating some but not all arrhythmias.
在伴有部分心内膜瘢痕扩展的患者中,消融术能有效地消除一些(并非所有的)心律失常。

The tan to white areas of myocardial scarring seen from the endocardial surface represents a previous myocardial infarction.
心脏内膜表面的褐色到白色的心肌瘢痕区域显示了陈旧性的心肌梗死。

endocarditis [ˌendəukɑːˈdaitis] *n.* 心内膜炎

Endocarditis is most often due to rheumatic fever or results from bacterial infection (bacterial endocarditis).
心内膜炎主要因风湿热或细菌性感染 (细菌性心内膜炎)引起。

In acute bacterial endocarditis, the most common causative bacte rium is staphylo coccus aureus.

急性细菌性心内膜炎的最常见病原菌是金黄色葡萄球菌。
We knew that subacute bacterial endocarditis and tuberculous meningitis were always fatal.
我们知道亚急性细菌性心内膜炎和结核性脑膜炎都是致命的疾病。

endocardium [ˌendəu'kɑːdiəm] *n.* 心内膜
Endocarditis is defined as infection involving endocardium.
心内膜炎被定义为侵犯心内膜的感染。

endocervical [ˌendəu'səːvikəl] *a.* 子宫颈内的
Endocervical infections produce a discharge that is often purulent with a yellow-green color.
子宫颈内膜炎常出现分泌物，它通常呈现黄绿色。

endocrine ['endəukrain, 'endəukrin] *n.* 内分泌
There is no direct evidence linking the fetal endocrines to the initiation of human labor.
胎儿内分泌和分娩开始相联系的直接依据是没有的。
a. 内分泌的
Research has demonstrated a number of different types of cells with endocrine function.
研究证明许多不同类型的细胞都有内分泌功能。

endocrinology [ˌendəukri'nɔlədʒi] *n.* 内分泌学
Endocrinology is defined as the study of the ductless or endocrine glands and their internal secretions.
内分泌学的定义是：研究无管腺或称内分泌腺及它们的内分泌液的科学。
Endocrinology concerns the synthsis, secretion and action of hormones.
激素的合成、分泌和作用称为内分泌学。
A third area of medicine which has had major advances recently is the field of endocrinology.
最近已取得重大进展的医学的第三领域就是内分泌学领域。

endocytosis [ˌendəusai'təusis] *n.* 细胞摄粒作用，细胞吞饮作用
Taking things into cells is called endocytosis.
把物质摄入细胞称为细胞摄粒作用。
Endocytosis includes both phagocytosis and pinocytosis.
细胞吞饮作用包括吞噬作用和胞饮作用。
The hepatocyte contains several specialized receptor-mediated endocytosis systems that are of great physiologic importance.
肝细胞含有多种特殊的受体介导的细胞摄取作用的系统，该系统有很重要的生理功能。

endoderm ['endəudəːm] *n.* 内胚层
The endoderm forms organs inside the body.
内胚层形成体内器官。
The stomach and small intestine arise from the endoderm.
胃和小肠来自内胚层。

endodermal [ˌendəu'dəːməl] *a.* 内胚层的
Endodermal sinus tumor, also known as yolk sac tumor, is a member of the germ cell tumor group of cancers.
内胚窦瘤，又叫卵黄囊瘤，是生殖细胞肿瘤的一种。
The diagnosis of endodermal sinus tumor in pregnant women and in infants is complicated because of the extremely high levels of AFP in those two groups with normal condition.
诊断孕妇和婴儿的内胚窦瘤很复杂，因为这两种人群正常情况甲胎蛋白的水平就很高。

endoenzyme [ˌendəu'enzaim] *n.* 胞内酶
Endoenzyme was still active within pH 5.0 ~ 6.0 and 30 ~ 50℃.
胞内酶在 pH 5.0 ~ 6.0，30 ~ 50℃时仍然具有活性。
Would catalase be classified as an endoenzyme or an exoenzyme?
催化酶可归类为胞内酶还是胞外酶？

endogenous [en'dɔdʒənəs] *a.* 内源的,内生的

There is reason to believe that both endogenous and leukocytic pyrogen are the same.

有理由认为内源性致热质和白细胞致热质是同一类物质。

Tranylcypromine is effective in the symptomatic treatment of endogenous depression.

反苯环丙胺对内源性抑郁症有效。

endolymph ['endɔlimf] *n.* 内淋巴液

Endolymph fills the membranous labyrinth of the ear.

内淋巴液充满耳的膜迷路。

Endolymph has a high potassium concentration and is maintained by a pump mechanism.

内淋巴液的钾浓度很高,而且该高浓度是依靠离子泵的机制来维持的。

endolysin [en'dɔlisin] *n.* 细胞内溶素

Endolysin is an enzyme that degrades the bacterial peptidoglycan cell wall, resulting in lysis of the bacterial cell.

细胞内溶素是降解细菌的肽聚糖细胞壁从而导致细菌细胞裂解的一种酶。

Double-stranded DNA phages require two proteins for efficient host lysis: the endolysin and the holin.

双链 DNA 噬菌体引起高效的宿主细胞裂解需要两种蛋白质:细胞内溶素和穴蛋白。

endometrial [ˌendəu'miːtriəl] *a.* 子宫内膜的

Endometrial polyps may lead to abnormal uterine bleeding.

子宫内膜息肉可引起异常的子宫出血。

Embryo implantation depends on the quality of the ovum and endometrial receptivity.

胚胎着床取决卵子质量和子宫内膜容受性。

endometrioid [ˌendəu'miːtriɔid] *a.* 子宫内膜样的

About 85% endometrial carcinomas are endometrioid adenocarcinomas characterized by gland patterns resembling normal endometrial epithelium.

大约 85% 的子宫内膜癌是子宫内膜样腺癌,其特征是癌性腺体与正常子宫内膜上皮相似。

Endometrioid carcinoma may occur in ovaries; about 15% to 20% of cases coexist with endometriosis

子宫内膜样癌可发生于卵巢,约 15% 至 20% 病例同时合并子宫内膜异位症。

endometrioma [ˌendəuˌmiːtri'əumə] *n.* 子宫内膜瘤

Bilateral, large ovarian endometriomas frequently are not symptomatic unless rapture occurs.

两侧大的卵巢子宫内膜瘤常无症状,除非发生破裂。

endometriosis [ˌendəuˌmiːtri'əusis] *n.* 子宫内膜异位

Endometriosis has received widespread attention.

子宫内膜异位症曾受到广泛的注意。

The commonest site of endometriosis is the ovary, and in about 50% patients both ovaries are involved.

子宫内膜异位症的最常见部位为卵巢,大约半数病人两侧卵巢均受累。

After operations, 6 month follow-up visits were made for both 44 cases of ovarian endometriosis in the laparoscope group and 36 cases of such a disease in the laparotomy group.

术后,分别对腹腔镜组中卵巢子宫内膜异位症 44 例和开腹组中卵巢子宫内膜异位症 36 例进行了 6 个月的随访。

endometritis [ˌendəumə'traitis] *n.* 子宫内膜炎

Endometritis, sometimes restricted to the neck of the womb, is a reaction to bacterial attack upon the membrane, possibly following physical damage.

子宫内膜炎有时局限于子宫颈部,它是由于子宫内膜受损后被细菌感染后造成的。

Tuberculous endometritis is always secondary to tuberculous salpingitis and the prognosis for fer-

tility is very poor.
结核性子宫内膜炎常继发于结核性输卵管炎,易引起不孕。

endometrium [ˌendəu'miːtriəm] *n.* 子宫内膜

Cyclical changes in the histological structure of the endometrium are caused by the action of the ovarian hormones.
子宫内膜组织学结构的周期性改变是由于卵巢激素作用所致。

endomyocarditis [ˌendəuˌmaiəukɑː'daitis] *n.* 心肌(心)内膜炎

The principal causes of endomyocarditis are rheumatic fever and virus infections.
心肌内膜炎发生的主要病因是风湿热和病毒感染。

endonexin [ˌendəu'neksin] *n.* 内联蛋白

The protein was termed endonexin-2 as it shows 74% sequence identity with bovine endonexin.
这种蛋白过去称内联蛋白-2,因它的氨基酸序列 74% 与牛内联蛋白相同。
Based on this close relationship, the placental protein was named endonexin Ⅱ.
依据这种关系,该胎盘蛋白称为内联蛋白-2。

endonuclease [ˌendəu'njuːklieis] *n.* 核酸内切酶

Endonuclease is an enzyme that catalyze the hydrolysis of interior bonds of ribonucleotide or deoxyribonucleotide.
核酸内切酶是一种催化核(糖核)苷酸或脱氧核苷酸内键的水解酶。

endoperoxide [ˌendəupə'rɔksaid] *n.* 内过氧化物

Unlike the classical prostaglandins, the cyclic endoperoxides are potent inducers of platelet aggregation and release.
环内过氧化物与典型的前列腺素不同,前者是血小板的聚集和释放的强力的诱导剂。

endophyte ['endəufait] *n.* 内生菌,内生植物

Endophytes are organisms, often fungi and bacteria, that live between living plant cells.
内生菌是生活在活植物细胞间的生物,常常是真菌和细菌。
Endophytes or endophytic fungi are a kind of fungi that live inside plants.
内生真菌是生活在植物内部的一类真菌。

endoplasmic [ˌendəu'plæzmik] *a.* 内质的,内形成性的

The endoplasmic reticulum is a membranous network that extends throughout the cell.
内质网是广泛分布于细胞内的膜性网。
The bulk of the endoplasmic reticulum in most cells is encrusted with ribosomes.
绝大多数细胞的大部分内质网上镶嵌着核糖体。

endorphin [en'dɔːfin] *n.* (生化)内啡肽

The brain and the immune system can communicate directly through endorphins, hormones, and cytokines.
大脑和免疫系统之间可直接通过内啡肽、激素和细胞因子相互联系。
Endorphins are a series of peptides of 31 amino acids, isolated from the brain.
内啡肽是从脑(组织)分离出来的由 31 个氨基酸组成的一系列的肽。
These substances, all peptides, are termed endorphins for endogenous morphine.
这些内源性吗啡肽类统称为内啡肽。

endoscope ['endəskəup] *n.* 内[窥]镜

Fiber optics, visible light travelling through flexible glass cables, are being used in endoscopes.
纤维镜是用可见光经柔韧的玻璃丝做成的导线束来传导的,现已应用于内[窥]镜。
Using a longer endoscope it is possible to visualise a large portion of the small intestine.
利用一种更长的内[窥]镜有可能看到小肠的大部分。
Most endoscopes consist of a tube with a light at the end and an optical system for transmitting an image to the examiner's eye.
绝大多数内[窥]镜的基本结构都是由尾部带有光源的管子和把映象传送到检验者眼内

的光学系统组成。

endoscopy [enˈdɔskəpi] *n.* 内[窥]镜检查

Endoscopy will reveal secondary vesical changes.

内[窥]镜检查可见继发性膀胱改变。

Nonulcer dyspepsia refers to symptoms that suggest a diagnosis of peptic ulcer despite the documented absence of an ulcer by endoscopy.

非溃疡性消化不良是指有类似消化性溃疡的症状而内[窥]镜检查未发现溃疡。

endosome [ˈendəsəum] *n.* 核内体(含有脱氧核糖核酸)

Endosomes transport proteins between cellular compartments.

核内体可以在细胞腔隙之间转运蛋白质类物质。

endospore [ˈendəuspɔː] *n.* 芽孢,内孢子

Endospores are highly resistant resting forms that are produced within the cell.

芽孢是在细胞内部形成的具有高度抵抗力的休止形态。

On return of favourable conditions the endospore changes back to the vegetative form.

回到有利时机时,内孢子又可以恢复到生长状态。

endosteum [enˈdɔstiəm] *n.* 骨内膜

Other types of tissue found in bones include marrow, endosteum and periosteum, nerves, blood vessels and cartilage.

骨中可见其他类型的组织,包括骨髓、骨内膜和骨外膜、神经、血管和软骨等。

Periosteum and endosteum play roles in not only bone development and bone formation but also bone regeneration and bone reparation

骨外膜与骨内膜不仅在骨的发生和形成中,而且在骨再生和修复中都起作用。

endosymbiosis [ˌendəuˌsimbaiˈəusis] *n.* 内共生

Plant chloroplast may descend from cyanobacteria prokaryote according to endosymbiosis.

根据内生说植物叶绿体可能起源于蓝藻类的原核生物。

Chloroplast and mitochondria probably arose by endosymbiosis of photosynthetic cyanobacterium and an alpha proteobacteria, respectively.

叶绿体和线粒体可能分别起源于具有光合作用的蓝藻和 α-变形菌的内共生作用。

endothelial [ˌendəuˈθiːliəl] *a.* 内皮的

As a result of endothelial damage to capillaries, fluid is lost across capillaries and venules into interstitial space.

由于毛细血管内皮损伤,体液便通过毛细血管和小静脉进入间质空间而失去。

endothelium [ˌendəuˈθiːliəm] *n.* 内皮

Endothelium is derived from embryonic mesoderm.

内皮来源于胚胎的中胚层。

The host response is mediated by leukocytes, humoral factors and the vascular endothelium.

机体的反应由白细胞、体液因子和血管内皮介导。

Intact vascular endothelium maintains the fluidity of the blood.

完整的血管内皮维持着血液的流动性。

endotoxemia [ˌendəutɔkˈsiːmiə] *n.* 内毒素毒血症

Thus, in our model of pathogenesis, hypotension would develop in the phagocytic phase of endotoxemia.

因此在我们的发病机制的试验模式中,在内毒素毒血症的吞噬阶段可出现低血压。

endotoxic [ˌendəuˈtɔksik] *a.* 内毒素的

In these cases, endotoxic shock poses the greatest threat to the patient.

在这种情况下,内毒素性休克是对患者最大的威胁。

endotoxin [endəuˈtɔksin] *n.* 内毒素

Because this molecule is an integral part of the cell wall, it is often called endotoxin.

由于该分子是细胞壁的组成部分,故常称为内毒素。

Inflammation induced by endotoxin will be arbitrarily divided into three phases.

由内毒素诱发出来的炎症可以主观地分为三个时相。

endotracheal [ˌendəutrəˈki(ː)əl] *a.* 气管内的

High-volume, low-pressure endotracheal tubes prevent aspiration more effectively than other kinds of tubes.

高容量、低压的气管内导管较其他类型的导管能更有效地防止吸入。

Bronchial obstruction by endotracheal or tracheostomy tubes often occurs.

气管插管及气管切开后插管常会发生支气管阻塞。

endow [inˈdau] *v.* 捐赠,赋予

The rich businessman endowed the hospital with half his fortune.

这个富商把他的一半财产捐赠给了医院。

This scientist is a man highly endowed with original ideas.

这位科学家是一个具有非凡独创见解的人。

endpoint [ˈendˌpɔint] *n.* 端点,末端,终结点

The study endpoint was end-stage renal disease.

该研究的终点是终末肾病。

Our studies with these chemicals showed that cytotoxicity does not necessarily correlate with any of the genetic endpoints.

我们用这些化学药品进行的研究显示,细胞毒性不一定与某种遗传学终点相关。

end-stage [ˈend-steidʒ] *n.* 晚期

Lung transplantation offers selected patients with end-stage chronic obstructive pulmonary disease (COPD) an improved quality of life and possibly enhanced survival.

对患有晚期慢性阻塞性肺病的选择性病人,肺移植可改善其生活质量,并可能延长生存时间。

endurance [inˈdjuərəns] *n.* 忍耐,持久

Endurance is the ability to sustain a specified level of physical activity.

耐力就是持续地维持一种特定的躯体活动的能力。

Exercise cycle helps improve strength, range of motion, and endurance of your leg muscles.

自行车运动可以帮助改善腿部肌肉的力量、活动的范围以及耐力。

endure [inˈdjuə] *v.* 忍受;持续

In old age we understand better how to avoid troubles; in youth, how to endure them.

人到老年,我们更能懂得如何避免麻烦;年轻时则更能懂得如何忍受麻烦。

The serpiginous syphilitic ulcers may be palm-sized and endure for many years, with only minimal healing and with scarring.

蛇行性梅毒性溃疡可有手掌大小并持续多年,仅少部分愈合成瘢痕。

enema [ˈenimə] *n.* 灌肠法

Sigmoidoscopy and barium enema may cause endocarditis.

乙状结肠镜检查与钡灌肠可导致心内膜炎。

The enema will clean the bowels of all decomposing materials.

灌肠可以清除大肠内的一切腐败物质。

energy [ˈenədʒi] *n.* 能量,活力,能力

Two important energy sources circulate in the blood: free fatty acids and glucose.

有两种重要的能源物质随血液循环:即游离的脂肪酸和葡萄糖。

engage [inˈgeidʒ] *v.* 从事于;约定;入盆

It is shown in the examination that the head is engaged in the pelvis.

经检查显示:胎儿的头部已进入骨盆。

Macrophages can actively move about to engage in phagocytosis.

巨噬细胞能活跃地移动而参与吞噬作用。

engineering [ˌendʒiˈniəriŋ] *n.* 工程，工程学

Through the techniques of genetic engineering, he transfers genes from one organism to another.

运用基因工程技术，他可以将基因由一个机体转移到另一个机体。

The design of artificial liver is based on chemical engineering principles.

人工肝脏的设计是以化学工程的原理为基础的。

engorgement [inˈgɔːdʒmənt] *n.* 充血；肿胀

The purpose of this study was to test the effectiveness of milk removal as a method of reducing the discomfort of postpartum breast engorgement in non-breastfeeding women.

此项研究在于测试泌乳在非哺乳妇女作为减轻产后乳房肿胀不适的一种方法的效果。

Minimal engorgement was experienced by 46% of the subjects.

百分之四十六的受试者出现轻微的充血肿胀。

engulf [inˈgʌlf] *v.* 吞没，吞食

Macrophages can engulf a wider range of foreign material than polymorphs.

巨噬细胞较多形核白细胞吞噬异物的范围更加广泛。

In microautophagy, cytoplasmic components are engulfed by an invaginated vacuolar membrane.

在微自噬过程中，细胞质成分被一个内陷的泡膜所吞噬。

enhance [inˈhɑːns] *v.* 提高，增加

Several investigators have tried to enhance the accuracy of creatinine clearance rate by blocking tubular creatinine secretion with the H_2 receptor blocker.

数位研究者试图利用 H_2 受体拮抗剂阻断小管分泌肌酐以提高肌酐清除率的准确性。

Neostigmine enhances gastric contraction and secretion.

新斯的明可增加胃收缩和分泌。

Griseofulvin by mouth enhances the efficacy of the topical medications.

口服灰黄霉素可增强局部药物治疗的效能。

The growth of a tumor may be enhanced or retarded by hormones, drugs, chemicals, and infections.

肿瘤的生长可受激素、药物、化学制剂和各种感染的促进和抑制。

enhancement [inˈhɑːnsmənt] *n.* 增强作用，促进作用

Goals of therapy include support of vital signs, prevention of further absorption and enhancement of elimination of the toxins.

治疗的目的包括维持生命体征、防止毒物再吸收和促进毒物排泄。

enhancer [inˈhaːnsə] *n.* ［遗］增强子；强化剂；增加者

Enhancers are regulatory elements located either 5’ or 3’ of a gene or in its introns.

增强子是位于基因 5’或 3’末端或者其内含子区域的调节元件。

Mutation in enhancers can interfere with the normal expression of a gene.

增强子上的突变能干扰基因的正常表达。

enigma [iˈnigmə] *n.* 不可思议的人（或事情）

Always an enigma, cancers and inflammations of the pancreas are rendered more diagnosable.

常常令人费解，胰腺内的癌和炎症更易被诊断出来。

enkephalin [enˈkefəlin] *n.* 脑啡肽

The enkephalins function as neurotransmitters or neuromodulators at many location in the brain and spinal cord.

脑啡肽的功能是在脑和脊髓许多部位起着神经递质或神经调质的作用。

enlargement [inˈlɑːdʒmənt] *n.* 肥大，肿大

Proliferation of lymphocytes in lacrimal and salivary glands may cause bilateral painless enlargement.

泪腺和唾液腺淋巴细胞增生，可引起两侧腺体无痛性肿大。

Infection accounts for most instances of lymph node enlargement in children.

儿童淋巴结肿大,多数病例是由感染引起。

enormous [iˈnɔːməs] *a.* 巨大的,庞大的

Domestic violence is an enormous problem in the United States.

在美国,家庭暴力是一个很大的(社会)问题。

The economic effect as well as human impact of the new treatment could be enormous.

新疗法无论是对人类健康的效益或在经济上的效果都是巨大的。

Although the bacteria seem small,they are enormous in comparison with the viruses.

虽然细菌看起来很小,但和病毒一比较,却显得巨大了。

enormously [iˈnɔːməsli] *ad.* 巨大地,极大地

The ability of the endocrine system to cope with stress varies enormously in people.

人们的内分泌系统对付紧张的能力差异很大。

Sensitivity to alcohol varies enormously between individuals.

人类个体之间对于酒精的敏感性有极大的差异。

enrofloxacin [ˌenrəˈflɔksəsin] *n.* 恩诺沙星,恩氟沙星

Enrofloxacin is a kind of veterinary drug which is widely applied to prevention and treatment on animal infectious disease.

恩诺沙星作为动物专用抗菌药,已广泛用于动物感染性疾病的预防和治疗。

Among the 12 antibacterials, Ciprofloxacin, Enrofloxacin and Streptonivicin had better bacteriostasis effect on pathogenic bacterium in cow subclinical mastitis.

在12种抗菌药物中,环丙沙星,恩诺沙星和新生霉素对奶牛乳房炎病原菌具有较好的抑菌效果。

ensue [inˈsjuː] *v.* 随后发生

With the dissipation of the fever, peripheral vasodilation occurs and heat loss ensues.

随着发热的消退,周围血管舒张,并随后发生失热。

ensure [inˈʃuə] *v.* 保证,保护

This medicine will ensure you a good night's sleep.

这药将保证你晚上睡上一个好觉。

The mother should ensure that the head of the infant is not lower than the rest of the body during the rest period.

在婴儿休息时,母亲应注意使婴儿头部不低于身体的其他部位。

entail [inˈteil] *v.* 需要;使承受

This job entails a lot of hard work.

这工作需要大量的艰苦劳动。

Needle biopsy entails obtaining the tissue from the thyroid.

穿刺活检可从甲状腺获得(活的)组织。

This would enable improved identification of individuals and families at high risk for the development of malignancy, entailing intensive continued surveillance and probably earlier diagnosis.

这样可提高鉴别能力,以鉴定出有极大危险发生恶性肿瘤的个体和家族,使其接受持续不断的严密监护,且可能早期得到诊断。

enteral [ˈentərəl] *a.* 肠内的

Pristine enteral nutrition can help patients to recover who were operated on for esophageal disorders.

早期的肠内营养能够帮助食管手术病人术后康复。

Disturbance of enteral flora can lead to enteritis.

肠道的菌群紊乱能够导致肠炎。

enterectomy [ˌentəˈrektəmi] *n.* 肠切除术

Enterectomy is necessary if the necrosis happens in a part of intestine tube.

如果有部分肠管坏死必须行肠管切除术。

Earlier definitive diagnosis and enterectomy on time is the key point of the treatment for mesenteric venous thrombosis (MVT).

早期明确诊断和及时行肠切除是治疗肠系膜静脉血栓形成的关键。

enteric [en'terik] *a.* (小)肠的

Typhoid fever is the classical example of enteric fever caused by salmonellae.

伤寒是沙门氏菌属引起的肠热症的典型实例。

These diseases are clinically almost identical with enteric fever.

这些疾病在临床上和伤寒几乎相同。

enteric-coated [enˌterik'kəutid] *a.* 包有肠溶衣的

Fe in enteric-coated capsules is not well absorbed and has no place in therapy.

包有肠溶衣胶囊的铁不易被吸收,不宜用于治疗。

enteritis [ˌentə'raitis] *n.* 肠炎

Infective enteritis is caused by viruses or bacteria.

传染性肠炎是由病毒或细菌引起的。

Enteritis with diarrhea is observed in Reiter's disease.

莱特尔病中也出现肠炎性腹泻。

Enterobacteriaceae ['entərəuˌbæktəri'eisiiː] *n.* 肠杆菌科

Comparing the identification of staphylococcus, enterobacteriaceae, pseudomonas to traditional methods, the average rate of coincidence with bacterium genus is 97.9%.

葡萄球菌、肠杆菌科细菌、铜绿假单胞菌三种细菌的鉴定与传统方法相比,菌属鉴定平均符合率97.9%。

Enterobacteriaceae were sensitive to imipenem (100%).

肠杆菌科对亚胺培南敏感(100%)。

enteroclysis [ˌentə'rəukliːsis] *n.* 灌肠;肠造影法

The value of diagnosis of intestinal diseases by double-balloon enteroscopy and intestinal enteroclysis was evaluated in the paper.

该文评估了双气囊小肠镜和小肠造影检查对小肠疾病的诊断价值。

Some investigators advocate the use of CT enteroclysis, which provides a flexible method of viewing small bowel obstruction (SBO).

一些研究者主张使用CT肠造影术作为一种变通的方法来观察小肠梗阻。

enterocolitis [ˌentərəukə'laitis] *n.* 小肠结肠炎

The risk of radiation enterocolitis correlates with the radiation dose.

随着放射剂量的加大,发生放射性小肠结肠炎的危险也会增加。

enteroendocrine [ˌentərəu'endəukrain] *n.* 肠内分泌(细胞)

Glucagon-like peptide-2(GLP-2) is a polypeptide hormone produced and secreted from enteroendocrine L-cells, which can specifically promote the growth of intestinal mucosa.

胰高血糖素样肽-2(GLP-2)是由一种肠内分泌L细胞产生分泌出的多肽类激素,特别能促进肠黏膜生长。

The diet and gut microflora influence the distribution of enteroendocrine cells in the rat intestine.

在大鼠肠道中,其饮食和肠道微生物群落可影响肠内分泌细胞的分布。

enteroinvasive [ˌentərəuin'veisiv] *a.* 侵袭肠黏膜的,肠侵袭的

This paper reports the isolation and identification on a new strain of the enteroinvasive E. coli.

本文报告一新株侵袭性大肠杆菌的分离与鉴定。

The enteroinvasive E. coli causing an outbreak of food poisoning was first discovered and confirmed in China.

引起暴发性食物中毒的这种侵袭性大肠杆菌首次在中国发现并被证实。

enterokinase [ˌentərəu'kaineis] *n.* 肠激酶

Enteropeptidase (also called enterokinase) is an enzyme produced by cells of the duodenum and

involved in human digestion.
肠肽酶也称肠激酶,是十二指肠细胞产生的一种酶,参与人类消化过程。
Enterokinase converts trypsinogen into its active form trypsin, resulting in the subsequent activation of pancreatic digestive enzymes.
肠激酶可将胰蛋白酶原转变成其活性形式胰蛋白酶,继而引起胰腺消化酶的活化。

enteropathogenic ['entərəuˌpæθə'dʒenik] *a.* 肠致病的
Enteropathogenic and enterohaemorrhagic E. coli constitute a significant risk to human health worldwide.
肠致病性大肠杆菌和肠出血性大肠杆菌是全球人类健康重要的危险因子。
Mesophilic digestion is very effective in killing enteropathogenic bacteria.
中温消化对杀灭肠道致病菌非常有效。

enteropathy [entə'rɔpəθi] *n.* 肠病
In about 10% of cases, a more severe enteropathy resembling Crohn disease may develop.
约 10% 的病例可发生更严重的肠病,类似克罗恩病。

enteroscopy [ˌentə'rɔskəpi] *n.* 肠(窥)镜,肠镜检查
The diagnostic value and safety of pushing enteroscopy in intestinal diseases are discussed in the chapter.
该章讨论了推进式电子小肠镜对小肠疾病诊断价值和安全性。
They evaluated the safety, clinical efficacy and patient tolerance to the double-balloon enteroscopy in patients with small bowel diseases.
他们评估了双气囊电子小肠镜对小肠疾病患者安全性、临床效应和耐受性。

enterostomy [ˌentə'rɔstəmi] *n.* 肠造口术
Enterostomy is an operation in which the small intestine is brought through the abdominal wall and opened or is joined to the stomach or to another loop of small intestine.
肠造口术是将小肠经腹壁切口拉出并造口,或将其与胃或其他小肠肠袢相连接的一种手术。

enterotoxin [ˌentərəu'tɔksin] *n.* 肠毒素
Ingestion of the preformed enterotoxin causes rapid (2-6h) onset of vomiting and diarrhea.
食入已形成的肠毒素后会很快出现呕吐和腹泻(2 ~ 6 小时)。
Nearly all strains known to elaborate enterotoxins are coagulase-positive staphylococcus aureus.
几乎所有已知产生肠毒素的均为凝固酶阳性金黄色葡萄球菌。

enteroviral [ˌentərəu'vaiərəl] *a.* 肠病毒的
Immunity following enteroviral infection appears to be type-special and of long duration.
经肠病毒感染后产生的免疫反应似乎是一种特殊类型且持续时间较长。

enterovirus [ˌentərəu'vaiərəs] *n.* 肠道病毒
Enteroviruses are distributed worldwide and commonly cause asymptomatic infection.
肠道病毒在世界分布广泛而且常会引起无症状感染。

enterprise ['entəpraiz] *n.* 进取心;企业
He got the job because he showed the spirit of enterprise.
他显示了在事业上的进取心,所以获得这项工作。
Jian-min Pharmaceutical Factory is a famous enterprise in Wuhan.
健民制药厂是武汉的一家著名企业。

enthesiopathy [ˌenθisi'ɔpəθi] *n.* 末端病
Enthesiopathy of the FCU (Flexor Carpi Ulnaris) at the pisiform might exhibit abnormalities assessable for sonographic characterization.
豌豆骨附近的尺侧腕屈肌末端病可以通过超声影像学检查发现异常。

enthesis [en'θiːsis] *n.* 填补法;肌腱附着点;肌腱末端
Collectively, the fibrocartilages, bursa, fat pad and the enthesis itself constitute the enthesis or-

gan.
总之,肌腱末端器官是由纤维软骨、囊液、脂肪垫和肌腱附着点本身共同组成的。

enthesitis [enθiː'saitis] *n.* 肌腱附着点炎,肌腱末端病

However, a number of MRI studies have shown a link between enthesitis and synovitis in individual swollen joints in Psoriatic arthritis and spondyloarthropathies but not in RA.
然而,一些磁共振影像学研究已经显示:在银屑病性关节炎和脊柱关节病的肿胀关节中,肌腱附着点炎和滑膜炎之间存在着关联,而风湿性关节炎则未发现这种关联。

enthusiasm [in'θjuːziæzəm] *n.* 热情

His enthusiasm made everyone else interested.
他的热情使其他人都产生了兴趣。

After an initial early wave of enthusiasm, the problems of immunosuppression slowed application of the procedure.
在最初开始的热潮过去后,免疫抑制的问题减慢了这项技术的应用。

enthusiastic [inˌθjuːzi'æstik] *n.* 热情的

He doesn't know much about the subject, but he's very enthusiastic.
他对此项目虽然知道的不多,但却很热情。

entity ['entiti] *n.* 实体;存在;病种

Is there such an entity as shock?
究竟有没有休克这种实体?

The sick sinus syndrome is not a rare clinical entity.
病窦综合征并不是一种临床罕见疾病。

All these drug reactions may simulate entities not usually attributed to drugs.
所有这些药物反应都可模拟一般不由药物引起的疾病。

entropy ['entrəpi] *n.* 熵

The amount of disorder in a system is known as entropy.
在一个系统中的混乱度称为熵。

enucleate [i'njuːklieit] *v.* 去核

The enucleated cell eventually dies.
去核细胞最终会死亡。

enucleation [i'njuːkli'eiʃn] *n.* 剜出术

In ophthalmology enucleation is an operation in which the eyeball is removed but the other structures in the socket are left in place.
在眼科学中,眼球摘出术是指将眼球取出但仍保留眼眶内其他组织结构的手术。

enumerate [i'njuːməreit] *v.* 点,数;列举

The functions may be enumerated as follows.
那些功能可以列举如下。

enumeration [iˌnjuːmə'reiʃən] *n.* 计数;列举,查点,详表

Enumeration of the number of bacteria in the uria is therefore an extremely important diagnostic procedure.
因此,尿中细菌计数是一个极重要的诊断方法。

enuresis [ˌenjuə'riːsis] *n.* 遗尿

Enuresis can be caused by underlying disorders of the urinary tract but is usually functional in nature.
遗尿可因潜在的泌尿道内的疾病引起,但其本质却是功能性的。

Enuresis is a disorder most common in children, the main manifestation is a persistent involuntary voiding of urine by day or night.
遗尿症是一种常见于儿童的疾患,主要表现为白天或夜间不断的非自主性排尿。

envelope ['envələup] *n.* 包膜,细胞壁

The complex envelope provides the cell with its shape and the rigidity.
复杂的细胞壁给细胞提供了必要的形态和韧度。

environment [inˈvaiərənmənt] *n.* 环境

The group of science dealing with the environment and now especially with the effect of pollution is environmental science.
对环境的一系列研究，特别是现今对污染影响的研究，称为环境科学。

The well-being of each individual cell is dependent on the adequacy of its environment to furnish nutrition and carry away metabolites.
各个细胞的健康有赖于周围环境供应充足的营养物质和运走代谢的废物。

environmental [inˌvaiərənˈmentəl] *a.* 环境的

In tinea pedis, the nails may act as reservoir from which reinfection may occur under proper environmental conditions.
患足癣时，趾甲可作为真菌的贮存所，在适当的环境条件下可由此引发再感染。

Air, earth, water, and food are the major environmental media or vectors through which exposures to hazardous environmental agents may occur.
空气、土壤、水和食品是主要的环境传媒或传病介体，通过它们可发生与有害环境因子的接触。

Respiratory paralysis may be caused by too low a concentration of oxygen in the environmental air.
呼吸麻痹可因外界空气中氧的浓度过低引起。

enzymatic [enzaiˈmætik] *a.* 酶的；酶促的

Both enzymatic and chemical methods are used to break polypeptide chains into smaller polypeptide fragments.
酶学方法和化学方法都可用于将多肽链断裂为较小的多肽片段。

enzyme [ˈenzaim] *n.* 酶

Notably, enzymes generally exhibit marked specificity.
值得注意的是酶通常表现出明显的特异性。

eosinophil [ˌiːəuˈsinəfil] *n.* 嗜酸性细胞

The cerebrospinal fluid shows a raised protein concentration, and eosinophils are present.
脑脊液检查显示蛋白含量增高及有嗜酸性细胞存在。

Normal values for the differential leucocyte count are: segmented neutrophils 34 to 75%, band neutrophils 0 to 8%, lymphocytes 12 to 50%, monocytes 3 to 15%, eosinophils 0 to 5%, and basophils 0 to 3%.
白细胞分类计数的正常值为：中性分叶核粒细胞占34%～75%，中性杆状核粒细胞占0～8%，淋巴细胞占12%～50%，单核细胞占3%～15%，嗜酸粒细胞占0～5%，嗜碱粒细胞占0～3%。

eosinophilia [ˌiːəsinəˈfiliə] *n.* 嗜酸性粒细胞增多，嗜酸性

Drug-induced pulmonary eosinophilia was suspected and valproic acid was discontinued.
怀疑是药物引起的肺嗜酸粒细胞增多，故停用了丙戊酸。

In this article, the term eosinophilia is defined as an increase in peripheral blood eosinophilic leukocytes to more than 600 cells per microliter (μL) of blood.
在本文中，术语嗜酸粒细胞增多定义为外周血嗜酸性粒细胞增多大于600个/微升血。

eosinophilic [ˌiːəˌsinəˈfilik] *a.* 嗜酸性的

Eosinophilic infiltration of the endocardium with fibrosis has been reported in fatal trichinellosis.
有报告旋毛虫病死亡者心内膜有嗜酸性细胞浸润伴纤维化。

In the brain the temporal and occipital lobes are the favored sites of eosinophilic granulomas containing the flukes or ova.
有脑部易侵犯部位为颞叶及枕叶，形成含吸虫成虫或虫卵的嗜酸性肉芽肿。

ependymitis [ˌependiˈmaitis] *n.* (脑)室管膜炎

Granular ependymitis in syphilis often shows damage to the ependymal lining and proliferation of subependymal glia with hydrocephalus.
梅毒时颗粒性室管膜炎常表现为室管膜被衬上皮受损,室管膜下胶质细胞增生及脑积水。
Granular ependymitis is known to occur following tuberculosis and syphilis of the CNS.
已知颗粒性室管膜炎发生于中枢神经系统的结核和梅毒之后。

ependymoma [eˌpendiˈməumə] *n.* 室管膜瘤
Ependymomas typically occur near the fourth ventricle in the young adults.
在年轻人,室管膜瘤通常发生在第四脑室附近。
Ependymomas are slow-growing and usually benign growths on the lining of the spinal cord and parts of the brain.
室管膜瘤是在脊髓内面和部分脑内生长缓慢的良性肿瘤。

ephedra [iˈfedrə,ˈefə-] *n.* 麻黄,麻黄属
We want to know about the transplanting technique of ephedra sinica.
我们想要了解麻黄的移栽技术。
Artificial cultivation of ephedra sinica is a crucial aspect of its clinical medication.
麻黄人工栽培是其临床用药的一个至关重要的方面。

ephedrine [eˈfedrin;ˈefidriːn] *n.* 麻黄碱
Ephedrine can cause constriction of blood vessels and widening of the bronchial passages.
麻黄碱能使血管收缩和支气管舒张。
Currently,ephedrine is rarely used in the treatment of asthma.
现在,已很少(有人)用麻黄碱来治疗哮喘。

epiblast [ˈepiblæst] *n.* 外胚层;上胚层
The team reported that they found the new cells in the innermost cell layer,the epiblast,of one week old rodent embryos,rather than in very early stage embryo where ordinary ES cells are found.
这个研究小组报道称这些新细胞是在一周大的啮鼠动物的细胞层的最里层(外胚层)发现的,而不是在有胚胎干细胞的早期阶段胚胎里发现的。
The mature embryo is composed of radicle,coleorhiza,plumule,coleoptile,scutellum and epiblast. That is the typical structure of the mature embryo of grass family.
成熟胚有胚根、胚根鞘、胚芽、胚芽鞘、盾片及外胚叶等典型禾本科植物成熟胚的结构。

epicondyle [ˌepiˈkɔndail] *n.* 上髁
A trabecular microfracture of the lateral epicondyle,most likely caused by an impaction force,can be seen.
股骨外上髁可见骨小梁微骨折,这很可能是由压缩暴力所致。

epicondylitis [ˌepiˌkɔndiˈlaitis] *n.* 上髁炎
Epicondylitis is not associated with joint effusion because the process is extra-articular.
上髁炎因为是在关节外发生病变所以不伴有关节腔内积液。

epidemic [epiˈdemik] *n.* 流行,流行病
The disease is endemic but small epidemics may occur in schools and institutions.
本病呈地方性发病,但在大中学校中可发生小的流行。
Despite the new drug therapies being developed,the end of the AIDS epidemic is not in sight.
虽然目前正在开发不少新药疗法,但艾滋病的蔓延仍看不到尽头。
a. 流行的
Major epidemic diseases and other communicable diseases must be reported to the appropriate health authorities.
主要流行病和其他传染病必须报告给有关卫生当局。
Epidemic influenza (A) may occur every 2-3 year among persons in communities with declining immunity acquired during a previous outbreak.

流行性感冒(A 型)每 2 ~ 3 年可发生在前一次大流行的人群中获得免疫力下降的人身上。

epidemiological [ˌepiˌdiːmiəˈlɔdʒikəl] *a.* 流行病学的

WHO has described several broad yet distinct epidemiological patterns of HIV infections and AIDS cases.

世界卫生组织描述了 HIV 感染和艾滋病病例的若干种主要而又独特的流行病学类型。

epidemiology [ˌepiˌdiːmiˈɔlədʒi] *n.* 流行病学

Epidemiology is the science of studying the factors determining and influencing the frequency and distribution of disease.

流行病学是一门研究决定和影响疾病发生的频率和分布诸因素的科学。

Succeeding generations revealed in turn the broader medical and socio-economic epidemiology of the disease.

几代人陆续揭示了此病与医疗和社会、经济因素之间广泛的流行病学关系。

epidermis [ˌepiˈdəːmis] *n.* 表皮

The skin comprises two layers, the epidermis and the dermis.

皮肤包括表皮和真皮两层。

Three degrees are recognised: ①mild erythema, ②superficial destruction of the epidermis with blistering, ③deep destruction involving the whole epidermis.

(烧伤)可分为三度:①有轻微的红斑,②表皮层的表面受损,并带有水疱,③ 累及整个表皮深度的损坏。

epidermitis [ˌepidəːˈmaitis] *n.* 表皮炎

Exudative epidermitis is a generalized dermatitis that occurs in 5- to 60-day-old pigs.

渗出性皮炎是一种发生在 5 ~60 日龄幼猪中的常见皮炎。

Hospital infection is characterized by coagulase-negative staphylococci epidermitis, which takes up 30.77%.

医院感染以凝固酶阴性的表皮葡萄球菌为主,占 30.77%。

epidermophyton [ˌepiˌdəməˈfaitɔn] *n.* 表皮癣菌属

Emmons' critical review of dermatophyte taxonomy resulted in the three genera known today: Epidermophyton, Microsporum, and Trichophyton.

埃蒙斯对表皮癣菌分类法的重要评述形成大家今天所熟知的皮肤癣菌三个属:表皮癣菌属、小孢子菌属和毛癣菌属。

The minimum inhibitory concentration of Quxuanling varnish to epidermophyton floccosum was 1.80g/ml.

去癣灵涂剂对絮状表皮癣菌属的最低抑菌浓度是 1.80g/ml。

epididymitis [ˌepiˌdidiˈmaitis] *n.* 附睾炎

The cause of infectious epididymitis is divided into two groups according to the age of the patient.

依照患者年龄的不同其所患的附睾炎可以分为两种。

epidural [ˌepiˈdjuərəl] *a.* 硬膜外的

Complications from epidural anesthesia are the same as those for spinal anesthesia, with the exception of headache.

硬膜外麻醉的并发症,除头痛外,与脊髓麻醉相同。

Epidural administration of narcotics is an important advance in pain relief.

硬膜外腔给麻醉性镇痛药是镇痛的一个重要进展。

epigastric [epiˈgæstrik] *a.* 腹上部的

Gastric ulcer pain may be epigastric or occur anywhere in the anterior upper abdomen.

胃溃疡疼痛可发生在上腹部,也可在上腹前部的任何部位。

The abdominal pain of acute cholecystitis may begin gradually as mild vague epigastric distress.

急性胆囊炎的腹痛开始是轻微模糊的上腹不适。

epigastrium [ˌepiˈgæstriəm] *n.* 上腹部

On examination the main physical sign is tenderness in the epigastrium or right hypochondrium, but between attacks this may be absent.

在检查中主要的体征是在上腹部和右季肋部有压痛，但在发作间期可无此现象。

epigenetic [ˌepidʒiˈnetik] *a.* 渐生说的，后生说的，表观遗传的

Therefore, chemicals capable of producing such epigenetic effects may act in their target sites as nongenotoxic carcinogens.

因此，能产生这种渐生效应的化学物质可能在其靶部位起到非遗传性致癌物的作用。

Epigenetic changes have been found in tumors and some autoimmune diseases.

肿瘤和一些自身免疫性疾病都已经发现有表观遗传改变。

DNA methylation is an important epigenetic modification which regulates a number of biological processes.

DNA 甲基化是一种重要的表观遗传修饰，它调节许多生物学过程。

epigenetics [ˌepidʒiˈnetiks] *n.* 表观遗传，表观遗传学

Epigenetics is a type of gene regulation that can be passed from a cell to its daughters.

表观遗传是一种可以从细胞传递到其子细胞的基因调控方式。

Epigenetics studies how environmental factors can affect gene expression.

表观遗传学研究环境因素如何能影响基因表达。

epiglottis [epiˈglɔtis] *n.* 会厌

The epiglottis may be swollen to 8 to 10 times its normal size and appear bright red.

会厌可以肿大到正常大小的 8～10 倍，呈鲜红色。

Due to the action of the epiglottis there is little, if any, water in the lungs.

由于会厌的作用，肺里即使有水也很少。

epilepsy [ˈepilepsi] *n.* 癫痫

Focal (or symptomatic) epilepsy is a symptom of structural disease of the brain, and the nature of the fit depends upon the location of the disease in the brain.

病灶性（症状性）癫痫是脑结构疾病的症状，其发作特点因病灶在脑中的不同部位而不同。

When it is established that the patient is suffering from epilepsy, the next step in diagnosis is to try to establish its cause.

在确定病人患有癫痫时，诊断的下一步就是努力去确定其病因。

Both epilepsy type and age of patients provide important clues to etiology.

癫痫类型和病人年龄给病因的研究提供了重要的线索。

epileptic [ˌepiˈleptik] *a.* 癫痫的

An epileptic attack is the manifestation of a paroxysmal discharge of abnormal electrical rhythm in some part of the brain.

癫痫发作是脑的某部位异常电节律的阵发性放电现象。

Excessive amounts can cause blood sugar to plummet and trigger an epileptic seizure.

剂量太大会导致血糖骤然降低，诱发癫痫病。

Numerous factors—organic, psychological, sociological and pharmacological—may play a part in the causation of the psychoses observed in epileptics.

许多因素——器质性的、心理学的、社会学的和药物学的——可能在癫痫患者的精神因果关系中起一部分作用。

epileptiform [ˌepiˈleptifɔːm] *a.* 癫痫样的

EEG recordings showed recurrent and prolonged focal epileptiform paroxysms.

脑电图记录显示重复和持久的局部癫痫样发作。

The incidence of evoked epileptiform discharges is frequent.

诱发的癫痫样放电的发生率是频繁的。

epileptogenesis [ˌepiˌleptəuˈdʒenəsis] *n.* 癫痫产生,

Here we studied effects of GBP on epileptogenesis.

这里我们研究 GBP 在癫痫产生方面的作用。

Both clinical and experimental findings suggest that the initial insult triggers a self-promoted pathological process, currently named epileptogenesis.

临床和实验室结果均提示初期的损害诱发了自发的病理损害,通常称为癫痫发作。

epimerization [ˌepiməraiˈzeiʃən] *n.* 差向异构作用,差向异构化

The epimerization of several tetracycline derivatives was examined at several pH values.

在几个 pH 值下测定几种四环素衍生物的差向异构化。

The epimerization is a process that involves the conversion of glucose molecules.

差向异构化是一个涉及葡萄糖分子转换的过程。

epimestrol [ˌepiˈmestrəul] *n.* 表美雌醇

Epimestrol is an anterior pituitary activator.

表美雌醇是一种垂体前叶的激活剂。

epinephrine [ˌepiˈnefrin] *n.* 肾上腺素

Epinephrine produces vasoconstriction.

肾上腺素产生血管收缩作用。

Epinephrine stimulates the beta-adrenergic receptors in the bronchioles.

肾上腺素兴奋细支气管上的 β-肾上腺素能受体。

epiphysiodesis [iˌpifisiˈɔdisis] *n.* 骺骨干固定术

Other advantages to percutaneous epiphysiodesis include reduced operative time, shorter hospital stays, and faster return to activity.

经皮骺骨干固定术的其他优点包括手术时间减少、住院天数缩短、功能恢复更快。

epiphysis [iˈpifisis] (*pl.* epiphyses [iˈpifisiːz]) *n.* 松果体;(骨)骺

Each epiphysis has its own growth plate where growth occurs.

每个骨骺都有自己的生长平面,从那里开始骨骼的生长。

Slipped upper femoral epiphysis is a common adolescent hip disorder.

股骨上端骨骺滑移是青年人常发的髋部疾病之一。

episiotomy [iˌpiziˈɔtəmi] *n.* 会阴切开术

Episiotomy is necessary in some cases and a clean incision is always preferable to an irregular laceration.

有些病例需要做会阴切开术,有一个整齐的切口总是要比不规则撕裂好。

Anesthesia and hemostasis may not be required before episiotomy because the tissue is stretched.

因为局部组织已伸展开来,所以在外阴切开术前可不需要进行麻醉和止血。

episode [ˈepisəud] *n.* 插曲;发作

A single episode may last several days but is not always distressing.

一次发作可能持续数天,但并不总是痛苦的。

The child was found to have had four previous episodes of severe depression.

发现此患儿以往曾有 4 次严重抑郁发作。

The history of previous coronary episodes must be enquired into.

以前的冠状动脉疾病史,必须加以查询。

episodic [epiˈsɔdik] *a.* 发作性的

Depression is an episodic disorder.

抑郁症是一个具有发作性质的疾病。

episome [ˈepisəum] *n.* [遗]附加体;游离基因

An episome is an additional genetic element that can exist either as an autonomous entity or be inserted into the continuity of the chromosome of a host cell.

附加体是能以自主实体而存在,也能插入寄生细胞连续的染色体之中的一种附加遗传因素。

An episome is a DNA element that either can exist as an autonomously replicating sequence in the cytoplasm or can integrate into chromosomal DNA.

附加体是 DNA 元素,以细胞质中自主复制序列存在,也可整合进染色体 DNA 中。

epistasis [i'pistəsis] *n.* 上位

Epistasis means one gene interfers with or prevents the expression of another gene located at a different locus.

上位效应是指一个基因干扰或抑制位于另一位点基因的表型的现象。

epistaxis [ˌepi'stæksis] *n.* 鼻出血

While in the hospital, the child developed several episodes of epistaxis and began to bruise easily.

在住院期间,患儿发生过几次鼻出血并且易于出现皮肤瘀斑。

Mucous membrane bleeding, epistaxis, and other types of bleeding are found in plasmatic coagulation factor deficiencies.

黏膜出血、鼻出血和其他类型的出血在血浆凝血因子缺乏时可以出现。

epithelial [ˌepi'θiːliəl] *a.* 上皮的

There are two types of membrane, epithelial and fibrous.

膜有两种:上皮膜和纤维膜。

epithelioid [ˌepi'θiːliɔid] *a.* 上皮状的

The epithelioid cord extends from the apex of the bladder to the umbilicus.

上皮状索带从膀胱顶端伸延到脐。

epithelium [ˌepi'θiːliəm] *n.* 上皮细胞

Epithelium forms a protective covering for the body and all its organs.

上皮组织给人体及人体各器官形成一个保护性覆盖层。

A few substances are actively secreted from the blood into the tubules by the tubular epithelium.

少数物质被肾小管上皮细胞由血液主动分泌到肾小管内。

epitope ['epitəup] *n.* 表位,抗原决定簇

Epitope is an alternative term for antigenic determinant.

表位是抗原决定簇的另一名称。

Other uses of recombinant DNA technology are the cloning of defined epitopes into viral or bacterial hosts.

重组 DNA 技术的其他用途是将特定表位克隆至病毒或细菌宿主体内。

epluchage [eplu'tʃɑːdʒ] *n.* 清创术

A clinical observation was put on the treatment of serious cases of acute pancreatitis after epluchage and drainage by TCM combined with western medicine.

临床观察了采用中西医结合方法对重症急性胰腺炎进行清创引流术后的疗效。

Infection rates have no obvious difference when it is less than 8 hours after epluchage.

清创术后 8 小时以内,感染率无明显差别。

epoxide [i'pɔksaid] *n.* 环氧化物

Epoxide hydrolase functions in detoxication during drug metabolism.

环氧化物水解酶的功能是在药物代谢中起解毒作用。

A novel technology by using laser microstrip antenna on curved surface of teflon, polyimide and epoxide resins is introduced in this paper.

本文介绍的新技术是在聚四氟乙烯、聚酰亚胺和环氧树脂曲面基体上应用激光微带天线。

eptifibatide [ˌepti'fibətaid] *n.* 依替巴肽（抗血小板药）

Most doctors understand the pharmacokinetic and pharmacodynamic properties of eptifibatide in healthy subjects receiving the low-molecular-weight heparin.

大多数医师都了解在接受低分子量肝素的健康受试者中依替巴肽的药代动力学及药效学特性。

equalize [ˈiːkwəlaiz] *v.* 使相等

The effect, however, still is a tendency to equalize the concentrations of the various substances in a given area.

但是其效果仍然是使一特定的区域内各种物质的浓度趋向均等。

equation [iˈkweiʃən] *n.* 相等，平衡

Implicit in the preceding equation is that lymphatic flow can increase in the case of imbalance of forces and result in no accumulation of interstitial liquid.

已有的内在的平衡表现为在（产生淋巴液的各种）力量失衡的情况下淋巴回流增加，不会产生细胞间液体蓄积。

equilibrate [ˌiːkwiˈlaibreit] *v.*（使）平衡

My assumption that potassium would equilibrate was not supported by this analysis.

我认为钾会达到平衡的推测，没有得到这次分析结果的证实。

equilibrium [ˌiːkwiˈlibriəm] *n.* 平衡

Diffusion and movement of drugs continue until an equilibrium has been achieved on both sides of the membrane.

药物的扩散和运动一直持续到膜的两侧浓度达到平衡为止。

Enzymes do not alter the final equilibrium of a reaction but accelerate the attainment of that equilibrium.

酶并不改变反应的最终平衡，而是加速平衡的到达。

equip [iˈkwip] *v.* 装备，配备

Hospitals are equipped and staffed to provide modern health care.

医院配备了人员和器械，提供现代化的医疗服务。

All animal species are equipped to defend themselves against aggressors.

各种动物都具有防御侵害者的能力。

All the cells of the body are equipped with the necessary organelles for carrying on an independent existence.

机体的所有细胞都被赋予有它们所需要的用以维持独立生存的细胞器。

equivalent [iˈkwivələnt] *a.* 相等的，相当的

One thousand units of penicillin are equivalent to 0.6 mg.

1000 单位的青霉素等于 0.6mg。

All living cells contain nuclei or an equivalent nuclear substance.

所有的活细胞含有胞核或一个相应的核质。

eradicate [iˈrædikeit] *v.* 根除，消灭

The local growth of many cancers can be eradicated or controlled effectively.

很多恶性肿瘤的局部生长能被有效地根除或控制。

There are many treatment options to eradicate pathogenic microbes from drinking water.

有很多可供选择的处理方法用于清除饮水中的病原微生物。

eradication [irædiˈkeiʃən] *n.* 根除

Pasteur was the first scientist who contributed to the eradication of silkworms disease.

巴斯德是第一位为根除蚕病作出贡献的科学家。

erase [iˈreiz] *v.* [计算机] 擦除，删除

It will erase everything on your hard drive.

它将删除你硬盘上所有的东西。

If you make a mistake, use the delete button to erase backwards.

如果输入错误，可使用 Delete 按钮来向后删除。

erect [iˈrekt] *a.* 垂直的，竖起的

The patient is to sit erect, the arms hanging, loosely at the sides, head somewhat elevated.
患者要坐直,双臂放松垂直于两侧,头略抬起。

erectile [iˈrektail] *a.* 勃起的,有勃起能力的

The prevalence of erectile dysfunction is higher among the men with hypertension than among the normotensive men.
高血压男性中勃起障碍的发生率高于正常血压者。

Obesity and high cholesterol are also associated with erectile dysfunction.
肥胖和高胆固醇也与勃起功能障碍有关。

ergogenic [ˌəːgəuˈdʒenik] *a.* 生力的

According to Olympic rules, no drug may be taken that is ergogenic, namely, which enhances performance.
根据奥林匹克规则,那些生力的,即提高成绩的药物不能服用。

ergometric [əːgəuˈmetrik] *a.* 测力计的

The patients' steadystate working capacity is measured by bicycle ergometric examination.
病人的稳态心功能系用踏车测力计检查来测定的。

ergometrine [əːgəuˈmetrin] *n.* 麦角新碱

A prophylactic injection of ergometrine, preferably 0.5 mg intravenously, should be given.
应给予麦角新碱预防性注射,最好是0.5mg 静脉注射。

ergonomics [ˌəːgəuˈnɔmiks] *n.* 工效学

Ergonomics, a great subject, designed to serve the people.
工效学,一门服务于人的伟大学科。

Ergonomics is a new branch of science which studies the relations between human, machine and environment.
工效学是一门研究人-机-环境关系的新兴分支学科。

ergosterol [əːˈgɔstərɔl] *n.* 麦角甾固醇

Ergosterol is of plant origin and is the sterol found in fungi.
麦角固醇来源于植物,它是一种存在于真菌类中的固醇。

erode [iˈrəud] *v.* 侵蚀,腐蚀

Tissue necrosis compounds the development of sinus tracts and erodes major blood vessels.
组织坏死合并窦道形成并且侵蚀大血管。

Caseous hilar lymph nodes may erode into the bronchi.
干酪样肺门淋巴结可侵蚀支气管。

erosion [iˈrəuʒən] *n.* 侵蚀,腐蚀

Subtle bony changes of erosion or fracture are not seen on plain radiographs.
在 X 线平片中看不见极细微的骨侵蚀的骨折变化。

Such lesions are difficult to differentiate clinically from cervical erosions.
临床上,这种病变很难与子宫颈糜烂鉴别。

erosive [iˈrəusiv] *a.* 腐蚀的;冲蚀的;侵蚀性的;糜烂的

Bleeding from erosive gastritis was rarely life-threatening.
腐蚀性胃炎导致的出血罕有危及生命的。

Proton pump inhibitors (PPIs) can decrease the amount of acid produced in the stomach and help heal erosions in the lining of the esophagus known as erosive esophagitis.
质子泵抑制剂可以降低胃酸产生量,促进糜烂性食管炎糜烂面的愈合。

errhysis [ˈeraisis] *n.* 渗血

The ulcers caused by surface cancer necrosis may cause persistent errhysis.
表层癌坏死所致的溃疡可引起持续的渗血。

Extensive errhysis was a primary cause of hemorrhage in the liver transplantation. .
广泛渗血是肝移植出血一个主要原因。

erroneous [iˈrəunjəs] *a.* 错误的

The concept that enlargement of the thymus is an important cause of unexpected death is erroneous.

认为胸腺增大是意外死亡的重要原因的观念是错误的。

Another cause of erroneous diagnosis is the dominance of extracardiac problems which may obscure the cardiac lesion.

误诊的另一原因是心外的临床表现占优势，它可以掩盖心脏的损害。

erroneously [iˈrəunjəsli] *ad.* 错误地，不正确地

Disinfection and sterilization are terms which are often used erroneously and sometimes reversely.

消毒和灭菌的术语常被误用，有时甚至被颠倒了。

error [ˈerə] *n.* 错误，缺陷，误差

Sometimes it is unavoidable that a doctor makes an error in diagnosing a disease.

医生在诊断上的错误有时是难免的。

Acute gastritis is a common complaint, often due to some error in diet.

急性胃炎是一种常见病，往往由饮食不当引起。

Sampling error cannot be avoided or totally eliminated. It can be reduced by increasing sample size.

抽样误差不能避免或完全消除，误差可以通过增加样本而减少。

erupt [iˈrʌpt] *v.* 喷发；发出（疹）

When the rash is fully erupted, it tends to deepen in colour and then fade into a faint brown staining.

当皮疹完全发出时，颜色加深，然后隐退成淡褐色斑。

eruption [iˈrʌpʃən] *n.* 萌出，长出；发疹

Eruption of the temporary teeth is sometimes delayed and out of the normal order.

有时乳牙萌出推迟和排列不齐。

Measles must be differentiated from other disorders accompanied by an eruption.

麻疹应与伴有发疹的其他疾病相区别。

The eruption comes out first as a rule about the face and soon afterward on extremities and to a lesser extent on the trunk.

一般，皮疹最初是在脸部出现的，但不久就会出现在四肢，在躯干上也可出现，但为数不多。

erysipelas [eriˈsipiləs] *n.* 丹毒

Erysipelas is an infection of the skin and underlying tissues with the bacterium streptococcus pyogenes.

丹毒是由一种叫做丹毒链球菌引起的皮肤及皮下组织感染。

Erysipelas is an infection of the skin with involvement of cutaneous lymphatic vessels.

丹毒是一种侵及皮肤淋巴管的感染。

erysipeloid [ˌeriˈsipilɔid] *n.* 类丹毒

Erysipeloid is an acute bacterial infection of traumatized skin and other organs.

类丹毒是一种由外伤引起的皮肤的或其他器官的一种急性细菌感染。

Erysipeloid form is the typical clinical form of cutaneous leishmaniasis.

类丹毒是皮肤利什曼病的典型临床形式。

erythema [eriˈθiːmə] *n.* 红斑，红皮病

Erythema nodosum does occur in pulmonary tuberculosis.

结节性红斑可以出现于肺结核。

They manifest themselves by induration, erythema, and pain.

它们本身表现为硬结、皮肤变红和疼痛。

erythematous [eriˈθemətəs] *a.* 红斑的

Pharynx was not erythematous and had no exudate.
咽部无红斑及渗出物。

erythroblast [iˈriθrəublæst] *n.* 成红细胞,有核红细胞

Erythroblasts are normally present in the bloodforming tissue of the bone marrow, but they may appear in the circulation in a variety of diseases.
在正常情况下,成红细胞存在于骨髓造血组织中。但在某些疾病时也可以出现于循环中。

erythrocyte [iˈriθrəusait] *n.* 红细胞

Erythrocytes carry oxygen from the lungs to the tissues.
红细胞把氧从肺带到组织。
Today we recognize that the erythrocyte is far from inert.
今天我们认识到,红细胞决不是不活泼的。

erythrocytosis [iˌriθrəusaiˈtəusis] *n.* 红细胞增多

Relative erythrocytosis does not represent a true increase in total red blood cell mass.
相对性红细胞增多症并不是红细胞总数真正增多。

erythroderma [iˌriθrəuˈdəːmə] *n.* 红皮病

Erythroderma affects men three times as often as women.
红皮病的发病率男性约为女性的三倍。
Generalized erythroderma in a septic patient suggests toxic shock syndrome.
败血症病人出现全身红皮病提示毒性休克综合征。

erythrogenesis [iˌriθrəuˈdʒenisis], erythropoiesis [iˌriθrəupɔiˈiːsis] *n.* 红细胞生成

Erythrogenesis normally occurs in the blood-forming tissue of the bone marrow.
在正常情况下,红细胞的生成部位在骨髓的造血组织中。

erythrogenic [iˌriθrəuˈdʒenik] *n.* 红细胞发生的,红疹的

The rash is due to an erythrogenic toxin causing a vascular irritation.
疹子是由红疹毒素刺激血管引起的。

erythroid [ˈeriθrɔid] *a.* 红色的,红细胞系的

The major issue is that the marrow erythroid mass fails to expand appropriately in response to the anemia.
其主要问题为骨髓红细胞系在贫血时不能相应增长。

erythroleukemia [iˌriθrəuljuːˈkiːmiə] *n.* 红白血病

HMBA can inhibit erythroleukemia cell proliferation and induce differentiation.
HMBA 能抑制红白血病细胞增殖并能诱导分化。
In order to study whether erythroleukemia was really a subtype of acute leukemia, the clinical laboratory characteristics and development of disease in 21 cases of erythroleukemia were analyzed.
为了研究红白血病是否为急性白血病的一个真正亚型,我们分析了 21 例红白血病患者的临床实验特征与疾病的进展。

erythromycin [iˌriθrəuˈmaisin] *n.* 红霉素

Erythromycin is largely excreted in the bile, while the urinary excretion is negligible.
红霉素主要经胆汁排泄,而在尿中排泄很少。

erythropenia [iˌriθrəuˈpiːniə] *n.* 红细胞减少

Erythropenia is a reduction in the number of red blood cells (erythrocytes) in the blood. This usually, but not invariably, occurs in anaemia.
红细胞减少是血液中红细胞数量下降。常见于贫血,但也有例外。

erythrophagia [iˌriθrəuˈfeidʒiə] *n.* 噬红细胞现象

Erythrophagia refers to the destruction of red blood cells by cells such as macrophages.
噬红细胞现象是指诸如巨噬细胞的细胞对红细胞的破坏。
A sarcomatous variant of malignant histiocytosis is reported to have less cohesive and pleomorphic

neoplastic cells with erythrophagia.
有报道称，肉瘤样变型的恶性组织细胞增多症中肿瘤细胞黏附性差，多形并存在噬红细胞现象。

erythropoiesis [iˌriθrəupɔiˈiːsis] *n.* 红细胞生成
A number of clues should lead the clinican to suspect that chloramphenicol is interfering with erythropoiesis.
一系列的线索应促使临床医生推测氯霉素能干扰红细胞生成。
Man uses about 25mg/day of Fe for normal erythropoiesis.
为了维持正常的红细胞生成男子每日利用铁约25mg。
Sideroblastic anemias are particularly characterized by evidence of ineffective erythropoiesis.
铁粒幼细胞性贫血所具有的特点就是红细胞的无效生成。

erythropoietic [iˌriθrəupɔiˈetik] *a.* 红细胞生成的
A decrease in erythropoietic activity may be a partial factor in the anemia.
红细胞生成活动减少可能是此种贫血的部分原因。

erythropoietin [iˌriθrəuˈpɔiitin] *n.* 红细胞生成素
Erythropoietin is a glycoprotein that acts through specific receptors on RBC precursors.
红细胞生成素是一种作用于红细胞前体上的特定受体的糖蛋白。
Erythropoietin increases the rate of red cell production (erythropoiesis) and is the mechanism by which the rate of erythropoiesis is controlled.
红细胞生成素能加快并控制红细胞的生成速度。

erythropsia [eriˈθrɔpsiə] *n.* 红视症
Erythropsia is a rare symptom sometimes experienced after removal of a cataract and also in snow blindness.
红视症是一种少见的症状，有时出现在白内障手术之后，也可以出现在雪盲时。

eschar [ˈeskɑː] *n.* 焦痂
Acids, on the other hand, cause coagulation necrosis and eschar formation, which limits further penetration.
另一方面，酸性物质可以引起凝固性坏死和有焦痂形成，它阻挡了酸的进一步渗入。

Escherichia [ˌeʃəˈrikiə] *n.* 埃[舍里]希氏杆菌属
At 13 months of age the child had an episode of prolonged diarrhea due to a rare strain of enteropathogenic Escherichia coli.
病儿于13个月时，因肠道致病性大肠埃[舍里]希氏杆菌的一种罕见菌株所致，曾发生过迁延性腹泻。

esophageal [iˌsɔfəˈdʒiːəl] *a.* 食管的
A history of gastrointestinal bleeding in a patient with liver disease may suggest esophageal varices.
肝病患者如有胃肠出血史可能提示食管静脉曲张。
Esophageal cancer appears to be induced by quite disparate agents among geographic hot spots.
食管癌在各高发地区中引起发病的因素千差万别。
Esophageal pain may be accompanied by dysphagia and regurgitation.
食管病变引起的疼痛可伴有吞咽困难和反胃。

esophagitis [iːˌsɔfəˈdʒaitis] *n.* 食管炎
Esophagitis is inflammation of the esophagus. It may be acute or chronic.
食管炎是指食管的炎症，可以是慢性的或是急性的。
The most common cause of esophagitis is gastroesophageal reflux.
食管炎最常见的病因是胃食管反流。

esophagram [iˈsɔfəgræm] *n.* 食管钡餐
Esophagram can be used to find early carcinoma of esophagus and esophageal varix.

食管钡餐可以发现早期食管癌及食管静脉曲张等病变。

esophagus [iˈsɔfəgəs] *n.* 食管，食道

The esophagus is the muscular tube extending from the pharynx to the stomach.

食管是从咽延伸到胃的一条肌性管状器官。

The heart is an organ which lies in front of the esophagus.

心脏是位于食管前面的一个器官。

essence [ˈesəns] *n.* 精髓，本质

We all see all there is to see, but the trained eye observes, and that is the essence of inspection in physical examination.

人人都能看见凡可看到的一切，可是只有经过训练的眼睛才能觉察一切，而这一点正是体检中望诊的本质。

essential [iˈsenʃəl] *a.* 基本的，必需的，原发的，特发的

The disease in all its essential characteristics corresponds to acute pancreatitis.

该病在所有主要特征方面和急性胰腺炎是一致的。

Cholesterol is essential for the synthesis of adrenal, ovarian, and testicular steroid hormones.

胆固醇为合成肾上腺、卵巢和睾丸三种甾体激素的必需原料。

The proportion of patients with so-called essential hypertension will thus become smaller.

所谓特发性高血压的比例，因此将变得较小。

essentially [iˈsenʃəli] *ad.* 实质上，基本上

The albuminoids are characterized by being essentially insoluble in most common reagents.

类白蛋白的特性是基本不溶于最常用的试剂中。

establish [isˈtæbliʃ] *v.* 制订，建立

In 1960 an international conference was held in Denver to establish a standard numbering-system for human chromosomes.

1960 年在丹佛举行了国际会议以制订 一个标准的人类染色体记录系统。

Isolation of a virus does not necessarily establish its etiological role in the myocardial disease.

分离出某种病毒也不能肯定地确定该心肌病就是由这种病毒引起的。

The diagnosis is easily established by direct microscopic examination.

通过直接显微镜检查是容易确诊的。

established [isˈtæbliʃt] *a.* 确认的

It is advisable to be cautious before substituting them for established and safe ones.

用新药取代已知的和安全的药物时以小心为宜。

ester [ˈestə] *n.* 酯

Dietory lipid is mostly triacylglycerol, along with some cholesterol and its esters, and phospholipids.

饮食中的脂类大部分是三酰甘油，还有一些胆固醇、胆固醇酯和磷脂。

esterase [ˈestəreis] *n.* 酯酶

Blood contains an esterase which is capable of hydrolyzing the vitamin A ester.

血液含有一种能水解维生素 A 酯的酯酶。

esterification [eˌsterifiˈkeiʃən] *n.* 酯化（作用）

The rate of hydrolysis is for the most part significantly lower than the esterification rate.

多数情况下，水解速度明显低于酯化速度。

The esterification mechanism of unsaturated carboxylic acid was analyzed in this paper.

这篇文章分析了不饱和羧酸酯化反应的机制。

esterolytic [ˌestərəˈlitik] *a.* 酯水解的

Here we report esterolytic enzymes in mouse liver.

这里我们报道在老鼠肝脏中酯水解的酶。

We detected esterolytic enzymes in human subcutaneous adipocytes.

我们在人类皮下脂肪细胞中发现了酯水解的酶。

estimate ['estimeit] *v.* 估计,估价

We estimated that the hospital would admit 800 in-patients.

我们估计这所医院能容纳 800 个住院病人。

It is estimated that 38 million serologic tests for syphilis are performed yearly in the United States.

在美国一年内完成的梅毒血清试验,估计有 3800 万例。

The earthquake was estimated to be 7.8 on the Richter Scale.

这次地震估计为里氏 7.8 级。

Breast cancer, the most common cause of cancer death in women, resulted in an estimated 46 000 deaths in 1994.

乳腺癌是妇女最常见的肿瘤死亡原因,1994 年的死亡数字估计为 46 000 人。

estimation [ˌesti'meiʃən] *n.* 估计,测定

Incidentally these reactions are a basis for the estimation of ascorbic acid in biological fluids.

碰巧这些反应是测定生物体液中抗坏血酸水平的基础。

estradiol [ˌestrə'daiɔl] *n.* 雌二醇

The relevant hormone determining results show: prolactin, estradiol and progesterone content in serum have regularly changed during reproductive and non reproductive phase.

相关激素测定的结果表明:血清中泌乳素、雌二醇和孕酮含量在生殖期和非生殖期呈现规律性变化。

These neurons regulate the secretion of gonadotrophin hormones, which in turn control the secretion of estradiol from the ovaries.

这些神经元调节促性腺激素的分泌,而促性腺激素又来调控来自卵巢的雌二醇的分泌。

estrogen ['estrədʒən, 'iːstrədʒən] *n.* 雌激素

At puberty the tubes, uterus and vagina enlarge in response to increased estrogen stimulation.

在青春期,对雌激素刺激增多的反应是输卵管、子宫和阴道的扩大。

The cortex is capable of producing androgens and estrogens.

皮质能够产生雄性和雌性激素。

estrone ['estrəun] *n.* 雌酮;雌素酮

In premenopausal women, more than 95% of serum estradiol and most of serum estrone is derived from ovarian sėcretion.

在绝经前的妇女,血清中超过 95% 的雌激素及绝大多数的雌酮是由卵巢分泌而来。

The estrogen in vertebrates is produced in the ovary, which includes B-estradiol, estrone, and estriol.

脊椎动物的雌激素产生于卵巢中,主要包括 B 雌二醇,雌素酮与雌激素三醇。

etanercept [i'tænəːsept] *n.* 依那西普(可溶性 TNF 受体-IgG1Fc 融合蛋白)

Etanercept provided significant improvement in symptom severity.

依那西普显著改善了病情的严重程度。

ethacrynic [ˌeθə'krinik] *a.* 利尿的

Furosemide and ethacrynic acid are extremely potent diuretics and are effective when given orally or paraenterally.

呋喃苯胺酸和利尿酸是口服或注射都有效的强力的利尿剂。

ethambutol [e'θæmbjutɔl] *n.* 乙胺丁醇

Researchers compared the efficiency of using the moxifloxacin and ethambutol antibiotics in 170 TB patients in Rio de Janeiro, Brazil.

研究人员比较了巴西里约热内卢的 170 位结核病患者服用莫西沙星和乙胺丁醇的效果。

The most common anti-TB medicines are isoniazid, rifampicin, pyrazinamide and ethambutol.

最常用的抗结核药品是异烟肼、利福平、吡嗪酰胺和乙胺丁醇。

ethanol [ˈeθənɔːl] *n.* 乙醇，酒精

Many yeasts convert sugar to ethanol and carbon dioxide.

许多酵母菌能将糖转变为乙醇和二氧化碳。

ether [ˈiːθə] *n.* 醚，乙醚

Ether also has laxative action when administered by mouth.

口服乙醚还有松弛作用。

Ether irritates the respiratory tract and affects the circulation.

醚能刺激呼吸道并影响循环系统。

Ethernet [ˈiːθə，net] *n.* 以太网

Ethernet and Local Talk networks use a linear bus topology.

以太网和 Local Talk 网络使用的是总线型拓扑。

There are challenges for deploying Gigabit Ethernet.

应用千兆位以太网仍有挑战。

ethical [ˈeθikəl] *a.* 伦理的，道德的

As a matter of practical necessity，nurses cannot avoid ethical decision making.

由于实际需要，护士不可避免地要作出符合职业道德的决定。

ethics [ˈeθiks] *n.* 伦理学，道德标准

Some chapters in this book will also deal with problems such as falls，incontinence，ethics，and long-term care.

本书的某些章节还将讨论像跌倒、失禁、伦理、长期护理等问题。

A nurse may also disagree with a physician about questions of ethics.

关于道德标准问题护士也可能与医生看法不一致。

ethnicity [eθˈnisiti] *n.* 种族，族群

Population admixture is simply a manifestation of confounding by ethnicity，which can occur if both baseline disease risk and genotype frequency vary across ethnicity.

人群混合只是种族混杂的一种表现形式，当疾病的基线风险和基因型频率出现种族差异时，即可呈现。

ethyl [ˈeθil，ˈiːθail] *n.* 乙基，乙烷基

With ethyl chloride，spray a small spot on the dorsolateral aspect just proximal to the nail to be anesthetized.

在指背面靠指甲处用氯乙烷喷雾来麻醉。

ethylaldehyde [ˈeθiˈl ældihaid] *n.* 乙醛

Use immunohistochemical staining and ethylaldehyde acid-induced biomonoamine fluorescence to determine the distribution of sympathetic nerve terminals in human cervical capsule tissues.

用免疫组化染色法和乙醛酸诱发生物单胺荧光法来测定人颈椎关节囊交感神经纤维的分布情况。

What is the molecular formula for ethylaldehyde?

乙醛的化学分子式是什么？

ethylbenzene [ˌeθilˈbenziːn] *n.* 乙基苯

Preliminary results on toluene，xylene and ethylbenzene were already published in 1985.

对于甲苯、二甲苯和乙基苯的初步研究结果已于 1985 年发表。

ethylene [ˈeθiliːn] *n.* 乙烯

Ethylene oxide and beta-propiolactone are germicidal gases or vapors capable of killing bacterial spores.

氧乙烯和乙丙内酯是具有杀死菌孢能力的气体或蒸气。

ethylenediamine [ˌeθiliːn，daiəˈmiːn] *n.* 乙二胺

Reaction of 4 with ethylenediamine and tris(2-aminoethyl)amine resulted in the formation of bis- and tris-ebselen derivatives，respectively.

化合物 4 与乙二胺和三(2-氨乙基)胺反应分别形成 2、3-依布硒衍生物。

PEI and ethylenediamine as modifiers were bonded on AC surface for specific selective extraction of quercetin from Oldenlandia diffusa.

聚醚酰亚胺和乙二胺以修饰剂的形式结合在活性炭表面可特异性用于白花蛇舌草中槲皮素的萃取。

etiologic(al) [ˌiːtiəˈlɔdʒik(əl)] *a.* 病因学的,病原学的

This symptom has been credited with specific etiologic significance.

这种症状被认为具有特殊的病原学意义。

Etiologic factors responsible for cancer of the stomach are far from being clear.

胃癌的致病因素还远未了解清楚。

Disturbances of immune mechanisms are believed to play an important etiologic role.

免疫功能紊乱被认为起着重要的病因学作用。

etiologically [ˌiːtiəˈlɔdʒikəli] *ad.* 在病因学上

Etiologically, cancer is a group of diseases rather than a single disease entity.

从病因上看,癌是一类疾病,而不是一种单一的疾病。

etiology [iːtiˈɔlədʒi] *n.* 病因学,病因

Regardless of the etiology, hypertension may be divided into benign and malignant types.

如果不考虑病因学,高血压可分为良性和恶性两型。

The etiology of such weight loss may be medical or psychiatric.

此种体重减轻的病因可能是内科的或心理的。

It is possible that numerous etiologies may lead to the expression of depressive symptoms.

可能的是,多种病因可导致抑郁症状的出现。

etiopathogenesis [ˌiːtiəuˌpæθəˈdʒenisis] *n.* 发病机制

We are presently going through a revaluation of the knowledge acquired in the last decades regarding the etiopathogenesis of type 1 diabetes mellitus.

我们目前正在对过去几十年中获得的关于 1 型糖尿病发病机制的认识重新进行评估。

Gastric cancer is one of the few malignant neoplasms for which an infectious agent has been recognized as playing a dominant role in its etiopathogenesis.

感染性因子被认为在少数恶性肿瘤的发病机制中起主要作用,胃癌是其中之一。

eubacteria [juːbækˈtiəriə] *n.* 真细菌

Dietary FOS did not influence caecal microflora counts but it selectively increased Bifidobacteria and eubacteria.

饮食添加剂低聚果糖不影响盲肠菌群的总数,但选择性地使双歧杆菌和真细菌明显增多。

A pair of universal primer for eubacteria targeting conserved region in 16S rRNA gene were designed.

针对 16S rRNA 基因的保守区,设计了一对真细菌的通用引物。

eucaryotic [ˌjuːkæriˈɔtik] *a.* 真核生物的

The algae, fungi and protozoa, as well as plant and animal cells, are termed eucaryotic cells.

藻类、真菌和原虫类以及动植物的细胞均被称为真核生物细胞。

euchromatin [juːˈkrəumətin] *n.* 常染色质

Euchromatin forms the main body of the chromosome.

常染色质构成了染色体的主体。

Euchromatin has a relatively high density of genes.

常染色质区基因具有相对高的密度。

eucommia [juːˈkɔmiə] *n.* 杜仲;杜仲属

Eucommia as well as its utilization is very important.

杜仲及对其利用很重要。

Molecular cloning of a HMG-CoA reductase gene from eucommia ulmoides oliver is a problem we have to face.

杜仲的 HMG 辅酶 A 还原酶基因的分子克隆是我们要面对的一个问题。

eugenic [juːˈdʒenik] *a.* 优生的

Eugenic policies became quite popular in Europe and North America during the early decades of the twentieth century.

在 20 世纪早期,优生政策在欧洲和北美已很流行。

eugenics [juːˈdʒeniks] *n.* 优生学

Eugenics is aimed at improving the genotype.

优生学的目的在于改善基因型。

Eugenics is the study of improving a species by artificial selection; usually refers to the selective breeding of humans.

优生学是研究用人工选择手段提高物种质量的一门学科,通常指人类的选择性婚配。

Eugenics is mainly concerned with the detection and, where possible, the elimination of genetic disease in man.

优生学主要是检查人类遗传病,并在可能的情况下,消除它们。

eukaryote [juˈkæriəut] *n.* 真核生物

Structurally speaking, cells are either prokaryotes or eukaryotes.

从结构上讲,细胞要么是原核生物细胞,要么是真核生物细胞。

Eukaryotes have a special network of minute filaments and tubules.

真核生物有由细丝和小管构成的特殊网络(结构)。

euphoria [juːˈfɔːriə] *n.* 精神愉快,欣快

Codeine produces very little euphoria.

可待因的欣快作用甚小。

euphoric [juːˈfɔrik] *a.* 欣快症的

As hypoxemia develops, the patient becomes restless and then euphoric.

随着缺氧症的发展,病人显得烦躁,进而又出现欣快症。

euploid [ˈjuːplɔid] *n.* 整倍体;*a.* 整倍体的

An exact multiple of the haploid chromosome number is called euploid.

单倍染色体数目的整数倍被称为整倍体。

For example, if the haploid number is 7, the euploid number would be 7, 14, 21, 28, etc, and there would be equal numbers of each different chromosome.

例如,如果单倍体(染色体)数目是 7,整倍体将是 7、14、21、28 等,并且每条不同染色体的数目相同。

euthanasia [ˌjuːθəˈneizjə] *n.* 安乐死;安然去世

The question of euthanasia raises serious moral issues.

安乐死的问题引起一些重要的道德问题。

Euthanasia and physician-assisted suicide are still legally prohibited acts in the United States.

在美国,安乐死和医生帮助的自杀仍然在法律上被禁止。

eutrophication [juːˌtrɔfiˈkeiʃən] *n.* 富营养化

Eutrophication is the primary problem of the water quality in lake and reservoir.

富营养化是湖泊和水库水质的主要问题。

It is of significance to study the eutrophication of water and protect water environment.

研究水体富营养化和保护水环境有重要意义。

evacuate [iˈvækjueit] *v.* 排空,排除

From the rectum the food material is evacuated from the body through the anus.

食物从直肠经肛门被排出体外。

Hematomas in this area must be evacuated early, before ventilation is compromised.

这一部位的血肿应在危及通气之前及早清除。

evacuation [iˌvækjuˈeiʃən] *n.* 排空，排除

The first cause is delay in evacuation of an abscess.

第一个原因是脓肿排空延缓。

Treatment in most cases involves evacuation of the clot under sterile conditions.

在大多数情况下，处理包括在无菌条件下进行血凝块清除。

evade [iˈveid] *v.* 逃避，回避

Viruses have evolved various strategies to evade recognition by antibody.

病毒具有多种逃避抗体识别的策略。

evaluate [iˈvæljueit] *v.* 估价，评价

There have been only limited clinical methods of evaluating estrogen production.

评价雌激素产生的临床方法是很有限的。

These patients were evaluated with coronary angiography before renal transplantation.

这些病人在肾移植前用血管造影作了检查。

Twenty patients with various forms of renal disease were evaluated.

研究了患有各型肾病的 20 例病人。

evaluation [iˌvæljuˈeiʃən] *n.* 估价，评价

A longer period of evaluation on more patients will be required.

需要对更多的病人进行较长时间的评价。

evaporate [iˈvæpəreit] *v.* 蒸发

Solvents have a much lower vapor pressure but still evaporate promptly when applied as a thin film.

溶剂的蒸气压低得多，但用来作为薄膜时仍能快速蒸发。

evaporation [iˌvæpəˈreiʃən] *n.* 蒸发

The evaporation of sweat from the surface of the body also helps to cool the body.

体表汗液蒸发也帮助身体变凉。

From the evaporation of water people know that liquid can turn into gases under certain conditions.

根据水的蒸发现象，人们知道液体在一定条件下能够转变成气体。

eventually [iˈventjuəli] *ad.* 终于，最后

Extra tissue fluid and some of the cell waste enter the lymphatic capillaries and are eventually returned to the blood stream.

多余的组织液和某些细胞代谢产物进入毛细淋巴管，最终回流至血液循环。

For example, proliferating B cells eventually mature into antibody-producing plasma cells.

例如，增殖的 B 细胞最终成为成熟的产生抗体的浆细胞。

evidence [ˈevidəns] *n.* 证据，迹象

Epidemiological evidence also suggests that there is an increased risk of bladder, kidney, and liver cancer following the ingestion of arsenic.

流行病学的证据也提示在摄入砷后，膀胱癌、肾癌和肝癌发生的危险度有所增加。

At surgery a gallbladder with stones or evidence of disease should be removed.

手术中如发现胆囊有结石或患病的证据，应当切除。

There is recent statistical evidence that in women the hormones taken as oral contraceptives may predispose to this type of thrombosis.

最近有统计资料证明，妇女口服激素避孕药，可诱发这种类型的血栓。

Unipolar depression is a form of recurrent depressive illness without evidence of manic features.

单相抑郁症为一种没有躁狂特点迹象的复发性抑郁症的类型。

evident [ˈevidənt] *a.* 明显的

People require less sleep as they grow older, and this becomes increasingly evident after age 55.

人们随着年龄增大需要睡眠的时间减少，而这在 55 岁后越来越明显。

In patients in whom no myocardial cause is evident a gastrointestinal evaluation may be helpful.
对于没有明显心肌疾病的病人，胃肠道检查是有帮助的。

evoke [iˈvəuk] *v.* 引起

Many different types of injury may evoke inflammation.
许多不同类型的损伤均可引起炎症。

evolution [ivəˈluʃən] *n.* 进化，发展

The theory of evolution by Darwin explains the origin of mankind.
达尔文的进化论解释了人类的起源。

Great changes have been made in medicine with the evolution of immunology.
随着免疫学的发展，医学出现了许多重大变化。

evolutionary [ˌiːvəˈluːʃənəri] *a.* 进化的

Transitional forms might represent repeated episodes of the evolutionary process.
过渡期形态可能是进化过程的重现。

Asexual reproduction has certain distinct evalutionary advantages.
无性繁殖具有某些明显的进化优势。

evolve [iˈvɔlv] *v.* 发展，演化

Each of the processes may have evolved for defence against injury.
每一过程可有抗损害的防御作用。

Application of increasingly advanced new technology has allowed the field of embryo evaluation to evolve rapidly and dramatically over the past five years.
过去五年中，越来越多高新技术的应用已经使胚胎评估领域得到了快速而显著地发展。

In this section, we discuss some of the ways that genes and genomes have evolved over time to produce the vast diversity of modern-day life forms on our planet.
本节中我们讨论基因和基因组随时间进化而使我们的星球产生当今多样化生命形式的一些方式。

exacerbate [ekˈsæsəbeit] *v.* 使（疾病或症状）加重，恶化

Clothing which applies pressure to the skin appears to exacerbate the urticarial wheals.
使皮肤受压的衣服可能使荨麻疹疹块加重。

School failure can exacerbate the already low self-esteem of depressed children.
在学校成绩不佳，可使抑郁儿童本已很低的自尊心进一步降低。

exacerbation [ekˌsæsəˈbeiʃən] *n.* 加重，恶化

Mucopurulent exacerbation in association with infections are not frequent.
感染使咳黏液脓痰加重的情况较少。

The exacerbation of the condition was brought on by a severe attack of cold.
一场重感冒引起病情的恶化。

exaggerate [igˈzædʒəreit] *v.* 夸张，言过其实

Urgency is an exaggerated desire to urinate.
尿急是过分的急于排尿。

We cannot exaggerate the importance of the careful physical examination.
认真进行体检的重要性无论怎样强调也不过分。

In one case electronmicrographic studies showed a picture suggestive of an exaggerated immune response, rather than a deficient one.
在一个患者身上，电子显微镜图像显示免疫应答增强，而不是免疫缺陷。

In second febrile period the symptoms of cough and fever are exaggerated and there is the concomitant appearance of physical findings suggestive of viral pneumonia.
在第二期，即热病期，咳嗽和发烧的症状加剧，同时有提示病毒性肺炎的物理学检查所见。

exaggeration [igˌzædʒəˈreiʃən] *n.* 夸张，夸大的事例

The statement that this doctor can cure all kinds of diseases was definitely an exaggeration.

说是这位医生能治愈所有疾病，这肯定是夸大其词。

Progeria is an exaggeration of the normal aging process affecting all individuals.

早衰是侵袭所有个体的过分的正常衰老过程。

exanthem [ek'sænθəm] *n.* 皮疹

3 cases of West Nile virus infection appeared punctate exanthem.

有三例西尼罗河病毒感染者出现斑点状皮疹。

The incidence of exanthem in the control group was significantly higher than that in the experimental group.

对照组的皮疹发生率显著高于实验组。

exasperate [ig'zæspəreit] *vt.* 使恶化

His condition is exasperated owing to leaving hospital too soon.

他因过早出院而病情恶化。

Their clinical conditions have been exasperated due to the lack of timely treatment over a prolonged period.

由于长期得不到及时治疗，他们的病情恶化了。

exceed [ik'siːd] *v.* 超过，胜过

As the number of candidates exceeds the number of places, medical schools in the U. S. have introduced selection procedures.

由于申报入学的人数超过了学校能够接受的人数，美国的医学院采用了择优录取的办法。

The mammary gland grows when the rate of proliferation exceeds the rate of cell death.

当增殖速率超过细胞死亡速率时，乳腺会增大。

exception [ik'sepʃən] *n.* 例外

Blood loss of less than 500ml is rarely associated with systemic signs; exceptions include bleeding in the elderly or in the anemic patient.

失血量不到 500ml 很少引起全身症状，但当老年人或白血病人发生失血时则属例外。

The STS is invariably strongly reactive, but an exception occurs when very high titers of antibody are present.

梅毒血清试验总是阳性，但在抗体滴度非常高时可出现例外。

The diagnosis of gonorrhea is based without exception on the detection of the pathogen.

淋病的诊断无一例外地基于病原体的检出。

exceptional [ik'sepʃənəl] *a.* 例外的，异常的，特殊的

An ovarian biopsy is necessary to make such a diagnosis in the exceptional case.

卵巢活组织检查用于异常病例的诊断是必要的。

exceptionally [ik'sepʃənəli] *ad.* 特别地，格外地

The incidence of iron deficiency anemia in children in the underdeveloped countries is exceptionally high.

儿童缺铁性贫血的发病率在不发达国家内特别高。

excess [ik'ses] *a.* 过量的，额外的

These tumors sometimes are associated with syndromes of excess hormone production.

这些肿瘤有时与过多的激素分泌的综合征有联系。

The excess glucose will be transformed into glycogen in the liver and the muscles.

过剩的葡萄糖将在肝脏和肌肉中转变成糖原。

excessive [ik'sesiv] *a.* 过多的，过分的

Brain cells require an adequate, but not excessive, amount of sugar to metabolize normally.

大脑细胞需要适量的而不是过量的糖，以进行正常的新陈代谢。

Statistical evidence certainly supports the idea that excessive smoking is an important factor for lung cancer.

统计数据明确地证实了过度抽烟是引起肺癌的重要因素这一想法。

During intestinal obstruction, on auscultation excessive bowel sounds may be heard.
肠梗阻时,听诊可听到肠鸣音亢进。

excise [ekˈsaiz] *v.* 切除,割去

An infection that is unlikely to respond to nonsurgical treatment usually must be excised or drained.
对非外科治疗效果不好的感染通常必须进行切除或引流术。

The sensor significantly improves the precision with which surgeons can excise brain tumours, and enables them to operate through smaller flaps in the skull.
这种传感器可以显著地提高外科医生切除脑肿瘤的准确性,并且使他们在颅骨内通过更小的皮瓣进行手术。

excision [ekˈsiʒən] *n.* 切除(术)

One of the fine arts of surgery is to know when to intervene with excision.
外科治疗的技巧之一就是了解何时进行切除。

Excision of part of the common bile duct is much less common.
总胆管的部分切除术是很少做的。

excisional [ekˈsiʒənəl] *a.* 切除的

An additional benefit of excisional biopsy would be determining the antibiotic sensitivity of the infecting atypical mycobacterium.
切除淋巴结作活组织检查的另一优点是可确定致病的非典型分枝杆菌对抗生素的敏感性。

Surgical diagnosis may be made by excisional biopsy in peripheral lesions.
周围性病变可通过活检而取得外科诊断。

excitability [ikˌsaitəˈbiliti] *n.* 兴奋性

One of the most essential symptoms of life is excitability, i. e. , the ability to respond to irritation.
生命的最基本特征之一是兴奋,也就是对刺激具有反应的能力。

excitation [ˌeksaiˈteiʃən] *n.* 兴奋

During excitation a polarized membrane becomes momentarily depolarized and an action is set up.
兴奋时,已经极化的细胞膜又暂时的去极化,产生了动作电位。

excite [ikˈsait] *v.* 引起,激发

These factors increase the tension within the stomach and thus excite pain.
这些因素增加了胃的张力,于是激起痛感。

excitement [ikˈsaitmənt] *n.* 兴奋,激动

When the news was reported there was a lot of excitement.
当消息传来时,立即引起了极大的兴奋。

Under the stress of excitement, the child's condition could go unrecognized until too late.
在极度兴奋状态下,孩子的情况可能一直到很晚才被察觉。

exclude [iksˈkluːd] *v.* 排除

When confronted with dyspeptic symptoms of recent origin in a patient over 40 years the first necessity is to exclude gastric cancer.
每当40岁以上的病人具有近期消化不良的症状时,首先必须排除胃癌。

exclusion [iksˈkluːʒən] *n.* 排斥,排除

The diagnosis is made on an exclusion basis in that no other etiological factor is found.
在基本上排除其他病因时,才能下这个诊断。

The diagnosis is established by exclusion of other organic causes.
这个诊断,由于排除了其他器质性的病因而确定了。

exclusive [iksˈkluːsiv] *a.* 唯一的,独有的

Infants who enjoy prolonged and exclusive breast feeding have been found to have good iron sta-

tus.
能享受长期、全部母乳喂养的婴儿已被发现具有良好的铁质状态。

exclusively [iks'klu:sivli] *ad.* 专门;仅仅;全部

This operating room is exclusively for heart surgery.
这间手术室是专为心脏手术用的。

Sudden deaths from congenital heart disease are encountered almost exclusively in infancy and early childhood.
先天性心脏病引起的突然死亡几乎仅仅在婴儿和幼儿时期见到。

Some illnesses are confined exclusively or principally to a single anatomic compartment.
有些疾病完全或主要被限制在某单一的解剖部位。

excreta [eks'kri:tə] *n.* 排泄物

Excreta and body fluids of these patients should be disposed of in an area used only for this purpose.
这些病人的排泄物和体液必须在指定的专用地点进行处理。

Those countries that have not yet implemented programmes for improvement of drinking-water supply and sanitation towards the global goal of safe water and adequate excreta disposal for all will have done so.
尽管有些国家尚未履行改善饮水供应和饮水卫生的计划,以便达到全球安全用水和无害处理排泄物的目标,他们也要这样做。

excrete [eks'kri:t] *v.* 排泄,分泌

Since xanthine and hypoxanthine are more soluble than uric acid, they are easily excreted.
由于黄嘌呤和次黄嘌呤比尿酸更易溶于水,因此它们易被机体排泄。

Cholesterol is excreted at amounts between 300 and 1500 mg per day.
胆固醇每天的排泄量为 300 ~ 1500mg。

excretion [eks'kri:ʃən] *n.* 排泄,分泌

Stone formation occurs also as a result of increased calcium excretion.
结石形成也可作为钙排泄增加的结果。

The daily excretion of uric acid amounts to about 0.6gm.
尿酸的每天排出量可达约 0.6 克。

excretory [eks'kri:təri] *a.* 排泄的

The work of the excretory organs prevents the products of metabolism from accumulating in the organism.
排泄器官的作用能使代谢物不淤积在机体内。

Each gland has an excretory tube that extends to the surface and opens at a pore.
每一腺体都有一根分泌管伸展到皮肤表面,并开口于一小孔。

excruciating [ik'skru:ʃieitiŋ] *a.* 极度的,剧烈的(痛)

The patient complains of excruciating pain.
病人主诉难以忍受的疼痛。

I've had an excruciating migraine all day.
我一整天均有剧烈的偏头痛。

exemplify [ig'zemplifai] *v.* 举例说明,作为…例子

This case exemplifies the serious effects of angina pectoris.
这一病例典型地说明了心绞痛的严重后果。

The description of these closely related compounds have exemplified some special feature of toxicology that deserves emphasis.
对这些紧密相关化合物的阐述,已举例说明了其某些需要强调的毒理学特性。

The cerebral cortex can exert a profound influence, exemplified by amenorrhoea due to emotional disturbance.

大脑皮质能产生很大的影响，由于情绪不稳定引起闭经为一例证。

exergonic [ˌeksəˈgɔnik] *a.* 能量释放的，放能的

Exergonic reactions are enormously important in living cells.

在生活的细胞中，放能反应是极其重要的。

During an exergonic reaction, energy is released.

在放能反应期间，能量被释放出来。

exert [igˈzəːt] *v.* 施加，产生，发挥

Drugs that interact with receptor sites may exert their effects in extremely small doses.

与受体部位相互作用的药物在极小剂量时就能发挥效用。

exertion [igˈzəːʃən] *n.* 努力，费力

Often hypertension occurs temporarily as a result of excitement or exertion.

过于激动或劳累常可造成暂时性的高血压。

Large meals and cold weather reduce the amount of exertion necessary to precipitate pain.

饱食及寒冷天气可以降低诱发疼痛所需的负荷量。

exertional [igˈzəːʃənəl] *a.* 劳累性的

Left atrial pressure may be elevated only with exertion in mild heart failure, resulting in exertional dyspnea.

轻度心力衰竭患者如过度用力，可使左心房压力升高并导致劳累性呼吸困难。

exfetation [ˌexfiˈteiʃən] *n.* 宫外孕

If treatment is not proper, it can cause exfetation which is seriously minatory to women's health.

假如治疗不恰当，可引起宫外孕，严重威胁女性身体健康。

It can result in oviduct obstruction and lead to complications including sterility, exfetation, habitual abortion or even pelvic infection.

可造成输卵管闭塞，导致日后不育、宫外孕、习惯性流产、甚至盆腔炎等并发症。

exfoliation [eksˌfəuliˈeiʃən] *n.* 剥落，剥落物，表皮脱落，鳞片样脱皮

The skin manifestations include generalized erythematous rash with exfoliation.

皮肤的临床表现包括全身性的红斑疹和表皮脱落。

Regular exfoliation and massaging can help tone and firm skin.

定期磨砂和按摩有助于紧致肌肤。

exfoliative [eksˈfəulieitiv] *a.* 脱落(上皮)的

Biopsy and exfoliative cytology can give histological confirmation.

活检和脱落上皮细胞的细胞学检查可以从组织学上加以肯定。

exhalation [ˌekshəˈleiʃən] *n.* 呼出，呼气；蒸发；发散物(如气体、气味等)

The normal adult breathing rate is about 17 to 19 inhalations and exhalations per minute.

正常成年人的呼吸频率为每分钟约 17 到 19 次。

exhale [eksˈheil] *v.* 呼出；发散出；蒸发，发散

Moreover, exhaled air is always saturated with watery vapours.

此外，呼出的空气中总是饱和着水蒸气。

exhaust [igˈzɔːst] *n.* (排出的)废气

Exhaust emission of vehicle engines is one of the primary air pollution sources.

机动车引擎的废气排放是大气主要污染源之一。

Air pollution is quite serious in China today due to high total pollution exhaust emission level.

目前中国的大气污染十分严重，主要由于废气排放总量处于较高水平。

exhausted [igˈzɔːstid] *a.* 精疲力竭的

The patient felt very exhausted with the functional exercise.

功能训练以后，病人感到非常疲乏。

exhaustion [igˈzɔːstʃən] *n.* 衰竭，虚脱；耗尽

The extreme nervous exhaustion influenza causes is very suggestive.

流感引起的极度神经衰弱具有重要的参考价值。

Heat exhaustion is most common in new arrivals in a hot climate and is treated by giving drinks or intravenous injections of salted water.

热衰竭最常见于那些新到热带的人，可给予饮水或静脉注射盐水进行治疗。

exhaustive [ig'zɔːstiv] *a.* 彻底的，详尽的

There is a group of patients with chronic, nonspecific low back pain in whom no anatomic or pathologic lesion can be found despite exhaustive investigation.

有一类慢性的、非特异性的背部下方疼痛的病人，即使进行彻底地检查也未发现解剖学或病理学上的病变。

exhort [ig'zɔːt] *v.* 规劝；激励

If the shoulders do not descend after the birth of the head the mother should be exhorted to bear down.

当胎头娩出后，如果胎肩不下降的话，应当嘱咐妈妈向下用力。

exicipient [ik'sipiənt] *n.* 赋形剂

The agent may be admixed with a pharmaceutically acceptable carrier, diluent or exicipient.

这种制剂可与药用载体、稀释剂或赋形剂相混合。

Such exicipients have been admixed to and tested as nasal adjuvant for diphtheria and tetanus toxoid.

这些赋形剂经与鼻用佐剂混合，并对其用于白喉和破伤风类毒素进行了测试。

existence [ig'zistəns] *n.* 存在，生存

The existence of this form of conjunctivitis is of short duration without danger to the eye.

这种类型的结膜炎病程短，对眼睛无危害性。

The prerequisite to the diagnosis of myocarditis is the awareness of its existence and alertness to its manifestations.

诊断心肌炎的前提是想到这一疾病并对其临床表现有所警觉。

exocrine ['eksəkrain] *n.*, *a.* 外分泌（的）；外分泌腺（的）

Endocrine is thus to be distinguished from exocrine.

因此内分泌（腺）可与外分泌（腺）相区别。

exocytosis [ˌeksəusai'təusis] *n.* 出胞作用，胞吐（作用）

The exocyst plays a crucial role in the targeting of secretory vesicles to the plasma membrane during exocytosis.

在出胞作用过程中，胞吐囊在靶向运送分泌囊泡至质膜中发挥关键作用。

Many neurotransmitters transmit their information by the exocytosis means of synapse.

很多神经递质是通过突触的胞吐形式来传递所载信息。

exoenzyme [ˌeksəu'enzaim] *n.* 胞外酶

Either the endoenzyme or the exoenzyme has an excellent effect on degradation of caprolactam.

无论是胞内酶还是胞外酶对己内酰胺都有很好的降解效果。

Exoenzymes are enzymes produced within the cell and then released to the outside of the cell to begin the process of extracellular digestion.

胞外酶是在细胞内产生并释放到细胞外进行胞外消化的酶类。

exogenous [ek'sɔdʒinəs] *a.* 外源的，外生的

Poisoning is injury by an exogenous chemical agent.

中毒是由一种外源性化学剂引起的（体内）损伤。

In normal persons, pain serves to protect the body from exogenous injury and internal disease.

对正常人而言，疼痛是用来保护人体使其免受外源性损伤及内部疾患的。

Obese individuals are resistant to both endogenous and exogenous insulin.

肥胖病人对内源性和外源性胰岛素均不敏感。

exon ['eksɔn] *n.* 外显子

The protein-coding parts of the gene are called exons.

基因中编码蛋白质的部分序列被称为外显子。

Exons are expressed.

外显子能表达。

exonuclease [ˌeksəu'njuːklieis] *n.* 核酸外切酶

Exonuclease is the enzyme that catalyse the hydrolysis of terminal bonds of ribonucleotide or deoxyribonucleotide chains, releasing mononucleotide.

核酸外切酶是可以催化核(糖核)苷酸或去氧核苷酸链末端键水解的酶,可释放出单核苷酸。

exophthalmos [ˌeksɔf'θælmɔs] *n.* 眼球突出,突眼

Exophthalmos is usually bilateral but may be asymmetrical.

突眼通常是双侧性的但也可以是不对称的。

The eye is diplaced forwards(exophthalmos) and in more severe cases there is optic nerve compression.

眼球会凸向前方(突眼),严重时会导致视神经受压。

exorphins [ig'zɔːfiːns] *n.* 外啡肽

Gluten exorphins are a group of opioid peptides which are formed during digestion of the gluten protein.

谷蛋白外啡肽是一组在谷蛋白消化过程中产生的阿片样肽。

The invention solves the problem that the traditional exorphins preparing method has high preparing cost and is easy to produce harmful substances in the preparing process.

本发明解决了现有的外啡肽制备方法成本高、制备过程中容易产生有害物质的问题。

exostosis [ˌeksɔs'təusis] *n.* 外生骨疣(*pl.* exostoses[ˌeksɔs'təusiːz])

To avoid the complications, a less radical drilling of exostoses is proposed.

为了避免并发症,提出了一项不怎么激进的钻孔法来治疗外生骨疣。

exotoxin [ˌeksəu'tɔksin] *n.* 外毒素

Exotoxin genes were abundant in both bloodstream (11-23 genes) and wound (8-19 genes) isolates.

外毒素基因在血流(11-23 基因)和创伤组织(8-19 基因)中都很丰富。

Helicobacter pylori blocks the proliferation of human $CD4^+$ T cells, facilitated by vacuolating exotoxin and γ-glutamyl transpeptidase.

空泡外毒素和 γ 谷氨酰转肽酶可促进幽门螺杆菌抑制人类 $CD4^+$ T 细胞增殖。

expand [iks'pænd] *v.* 扩大,扩充

Microsurgery is basically a technique for expanding the visual horizon of the surgeon.

显微外科是扩大外科医生视野的基本技术。

These operations have expanded their understanding of the brain and nerve damage.

这些手术使他们对于脑和神经损伤有了进一步的了解。

expansion [iks'pænʃən] *n.* 扩大,扩充

To the clinical surgeon there is a vast expansion of what he can offer his patients in whatever surgical specialty he resides.

对临床外科医生来说,不论他从事外科哪一专业,都能为病人提供广泛的服务。

expectancy [iks'pektənsi] *n.* 期待,期望;预期

With advances in modern medicine, the average person in quite a number of countries can now look forward to a life expectancy of 71 years.

随着现代医学的进展,许多国家里的普通人现在可期望活到 71 岁。

From the point of view of health, however, action may be taken to reduce age-specific mortality in order to improve life expectancy.

然而从卫生观点看,可以采取措施降低年龄死亡专率以提高预期寿命。

The proportion of abortions in those affected does not exceed normal expectancy.
那些患者的流产率不超过正常预期范围。

expectant [iks'pektənt] *a.* 期待的;预期的
Although the only cure for preeclampsia is delivery, there are times when expectant therapy is justified.
尽管终止妊娠是治愈子痫前期唯一的方法,但有时需要采用期待疗法。

expectedness [iks'pektidnis] *n.* 预期程度
For marketed products regulated by FDA, AEs are categorized for reporting purposes according to the seriousness and expectedness of the event.
对 FDA 监管的上市产品,为便于报告,不良事件应根据该事件的严重性和预期程度进行分类。

expectorant [eks'pektərənt] *n.* 祛痰剂
Licorice has been used for centuries as an expectorant to loosen phlegm.
甘草用作祛痰剂来化痰已有几个世纪了。
a. 化痰的
Humid moist air prevents the drying of mucus and it further assists the expectorant process.
湿润的空气防止黏液干燥,并进一步促进化痰过程。

expectorate [ek'spektəreit] *v.* 咳出(痰等);吐(唾液、血等)
Some patients raise a very ill-smelling sputum; some expectorate only in the morning and "clear their tubes for the day".
有些病人咳出带有臭味的痰,有些只在早晨咳出痰而一天不再咳痰了。

expectoration [ekˌspektə'reiʃən] *n.* 吐痰,咳出物
The patient has suffered from a cough and expectoration without obvious cause for more than a few weeks.
这位病人无明显原因咳嗽和咳痰达数周以上。

expedite ['ekspidait] *v.* 加急;迅速执行
The registry is in compliance with regulations regarding expedited and periodic adverse drug reaction reporting.
注册登记遵照加急和定期不良药物反应报告的规则。

expenditure [iks'penditʃə] *n.* 消费,费用
Staying in bed keeps energy expenditure at a minimum.
卧床可使能量的消耗保持在最低限度。

expense [ik'spens] *n.* 费用,耗费;代价,损失,牺牲
They live on or in and at the expense of host, develop inside the body of host, vertibrate as well as invertibrate.
它们寄生于宿主的体内或体表并损耗宿主,既在无脊椎动物又在脊椎动物宿主体内生长。

expensive [iks'pensiv] *a.* 贵的
This drug is effective and not expensive, either.
这种药有效,而且也不贵。
This medicine is rather more expensive than that.
这种药比那种贵得多。

experimental [eksˌperi'mentl] *a.* 实验的,试验的
Many experimental animals inherit the tendency to develop tumors.
许多实验动物由于遗传而具有发生肿瘤的倾向。
No polyvalent vaccine is available, but experimental vaccines have been effective against a single type of rhinovirus.
现在还没有抗多种病毒的疫苗,但是,对单一类型的鼻病毒,试验疫苗还是有抵抗效能的。

experimentally [ikˌsperi'mentli] *ad.* 用实验,在试验上

It can be shown experimentally that cells use oxygen and give off carbon dioxide.
可用实验来显示细胞利用氧气和排除二氧化碳。

experimentation [eksˌperimenˈteiʃən] *n.* 实验(法)
There is no evidence from animal experimentation that a mechanical injury is capable of causing cancer to develop in a normal animal.
尚无动物实验证据表明机械性损伤能在正常动物体内引起癌症。

expert [ˈekspəːt] *n.* 专家
Dr. Li is an expert in X-ray.
李医生是一位 X 线专家。
a. 熟练的
Mr. Wang is an expert technician.
王先生是一位熟练的技术员。

expertise [ˌekspəːˈtiːz] *n.* 专门知识(或技能)
This technique calls for more sophisticated apparatus and a great degree of expertise on the part of the operator.
这种技术要求较灵敏的仪器设备和操作者的高度熟练技能。

expiration [ˌekspiˈreiʃən] *n.* 呼气,呼出;满期,截止
There is tachypnea with a relatively prolonged expiration.
出现呼吸急促,同时呼气时间相对延长。
The expiration of used air from the lungs leaves space for the fresh air to go in.
浊气从肺中呼出腾出空间给新鲜空气进入。
The cooperation will bring many benefits to both sides at the expiration of the agreement.
这次合作在协议满期时将给双方带来许多好处。
The expiration date for this medicine is Sept. 15 2004.
这药的失效期是 2004 年 9 月 15 日。

expiratory [ˌiksˈpaiərətəri] *a.* 呼气的
The remaining 400 ml are lost through the expiratory air.
残余的 400ml 通过呼气消失。
The chief manifestation of asthma is severe paroxysmal dyspnea of the expiratory type.
哮喘病的主要表现为严重呼出型阵发性呼吸困难。

expire [ikˈspaiə] *v.* 呼出,呼气;满期,终止
Finally, there is an increase in CO_2 expired after a meal has been consumed.
最终,在用餐后呼出的二氧化碳有所增加。
Those expired drugs have no effect.
那些过期的药物已经失效。

explain [ikˈsplein] *v.* 解释,说明
The doctor, not wishing to make her nervous, did not fully explain the seriousness of her condition.
医生不愿使她精神紧张,并没有充分地给她说明病情的严重性。

explicable [ikˈsplikəbl] *a.* 可解释的,可说明的
Specific arithmetical retardation is not explicable in terms of general mental retardation or of inadequate schooling.
特异性计算迟钝不能以一般精神发育迟滞或缺乏教育来解释。

explicit [iksˈplisit] *a.* 清楚的,明显的
After evaluation, an explicit treatment plan should be developed for patient.
在准确评估病情之后需要对病人制订一个清楚的治疗方案。

exploit [iksˈplɔit] *v.* 开发,剥削
In general, it is still the largest and scarcest animals that are most heavily exploited.

一般说来,受到最严重掠杀的,仍然是那些最大的和最珍稀的动物。

Abundant resources of medicinal herbs in the mountainous areas are to be further exploited.

山区丰富的中草药资源有待进一步开发。

exploration [ˌeksplɔːˈreiʃən] *n.* 探索,探查

Since a pelvic tumour may be malignant, surgical exploration or laparoscopy is essential.

由于盆腔肿瘤可能为恶性,手术探查或腹腔镜检查就非常必要。

exploratory [eksˈplɔːrətəri] *a.* 探查(性)的

The doctors thought it necessary to perform an exploratory thoracotomy.

医生们认为有必要做剖胸探查。

explore [iksˈplɔː] *v.* 探索,钻研

Exploring the situation on the basis of blood examination is simply searching in the wrong place.

根据血液检查来探索其情况,简直是找错了位置。

explosion [iksˈpləuʒən] *n.* 爆炸;暴发;激增

An explosion of new ideas and doctrines has flooded the medical literature.

大量的新观念和学说涌现于医学文献中。

explosive [iksˈpləusiv] *a.* 爆炸(性)的,突发的

Although the clinical onset of aplastic anemia is usually insidious, occasionally it is explosive.

虽然再生障碍性贫血的临床发作通常是不知不觉的,但偶然也会是暴发性的。

The cough is described as explosive and occurring in clusters and it persists as a major clinical symptom.

咳嗽呈爆破音,成串出现,并作为一个主要临床症状而持续存在。

exponentially [ˌekspəuˈnenʃəli] *adv.* 以指数方式

A virus typically will spread exponentially at first.

病毒开始通常以指数方式扩散。

The number of microorganisms in a culture will grow exponentially until an essential nutrient is exhausted.

培养基中的微生物将以指数方式生长直到一种必须营养素耗尽。

expose [ikˈspəuz] *v.* 暴露,使受(危险、风险等)

Don't expose the medicine to direct sunshine.

不要让此药受到日光的直接照晒。

Medical X-rays are exposing the public to increasingly higher levels of radiation.

医用 X 线使大众受到愈来愈高剂量辐射的风险。

It is sad that children are now heavily exposed to junk food and lacking adequate exercise.

可悲的是,如今孩子们过多地食用垃圾食品,而且缺乏足够的体育锻炼。

exposure [iksˈpəuʒə] *n.* 暴露,照射(X 线)

Exposure to light sets off a complex response inside the bodies of animals and humans.

动物和人接触光线会引起体内复杂的反应。

It is important to isolate the patient in order to protect him from exposure to bacterial infection.

隔离病人使他不致接触细菌感染,这样做是重要的。

express [ikˈspres] *v.* 表示,表达,压出

Decreased erythropoietin production is expressed as a peripheral reticulocytopenia and a subnormal marrow response.

促红细胞生成素的生成减少表现为外周网织红细胞减少和骨髓反应异常。

A small proportion of α、β、T cells express neither CD4 nor CD8.

少量的 α、β、T 细胞既不表达 CD4 也不表达 CD8。

Especially when the gland is not enlarged, one also expresses material for microscopic investigation.

特别是腺体未肿大时,也应挤出材料用于显微镜检查。

expressivity [ˌekspreˈsiviti] *n.* 表现度,表现性

An infant's or young child's first infection with many of the respiratory viruses may give rise to great expressivity in clinical disease.

婴儿或幼童首次被一些呼吸道病毒感染时可能发生极为严重的症状。

expulsion [iksˈpʌlʃən] *n.* 驱逐,逼出

Expulsion may be helped by a reversed wave of peristalsis in the oesophagus.

食道的逆向蠕动波有助于胃内容物的迫出。

There are cases in which the fetus dies in utero before labour starts and this is usually followed by expulsion of the fetus from the uterus within a few days.

有些病例在分娩开始前胎儿已死在宫内,通常胎儿在几天内从子宫排出。

exquisite [ˈekskwizit] *a.* 精致的;极度的;敏锐的

A typical regulator loop therefore has both positive and negative component, providing exquisite control over hormone levels and action.

因而典型的调控环路由正负两部分组成,精确地控制激素的水平及作用。

exquisitely [ˈekskwizitli] *ad.* 非常

Some medically important bacteria are exquisitely sensitive to killing by the mere presence of oxygen.

一些医学上很重要的致病细菌极易被纯氧的环境杀死。

exsauguinate [eksˈsæŋgwineit] *v.* 放血;使充血

If the twins are uniovular bleeding from the cord might exsauguinate the second twin through the anastomosis in the placenta.

如果是单卵双胎,脐带的出血可能通过胎盘的血管的吻合使其第二个胎儿失血。

extensive [iksˈtensiv] *a.* 广大的,广泛的,广博的

This may be followed by an extensive effusion into the affected pleural sac.

此后在受累的胸腔内有大量的渗出液。

Coronary bypass operations require extensive resources.

冠状动脉旁路手术需要大量人力、物力。

Human serum has come into extensive use.

人类血清已被广泛地使用。

Nurses have been given extensive training to prepare them to provide expert nursing care.

为了培养护士们熟练的护理技术,她们都已接受了广泛的训练。

extensively [iksˈtensivli] *ad.* 广大地,广泛地

Digoxin is excreted extensively unchanged by the kidney.

地高辛大量以原型从肾脏排泄。

Phenyl butazone (98%) and diazepam (96%) bind to plasma proteins extensively.

保泰松(98%)和安定(96%)都表现出极高的血浆蛋白结合率。

extensor [ikˈstensə; ek-] *n.* 伸直肌,伸肌群

The extensor mechanism of the fingers, hand, wrist, and forearm is extremely intricate.

手指、手、腕、前臂的伸肌群机制是非常复杂的。

extent [iksˈtent] *n.* 广度,宽度,长度,范围,程度

The extent of the osmotic pressure depends upon the number of nondiffusable particles in solution on each side of the membrane.

渗透压的大小取决于半透膜两侧溶液中不能弥散的颗粒数。

There are marked variations in the extent of the disease and in its effect on the person.

疾病的程度以及它对人的影响有显著的差别。

Pathogenic organisms are only pathogenic by virtue of their ability to evade host defence mechanisms to some extent.

病原微生物是指那些在一定程度上具有入侵宿主防御机制的病原体。

After a diagnosis is established, the extent of metastatic tumor should be determined.
诊断明确后，需确定肿瘤转移范围。

external [eksˈtəːnəl] *a.* 外部的

In addition the skin performs an essential sensory function, receiving many impulses from the external environment.
此外，皮肤还具有重要的感觉功能，接受来自外界的多种刺激。

The external portions of the intrapilary hyphae segment into chains of ectothrix spores.
毛发内菌丝的外段分裂成发外孢子链。

extirpate [ˈekstəːpeit] *v.* 摘除

Lymph nodes may be invaded by cancer and should be completely extirpated.
淋巴结可被癌症侵袭，这时必须全部摘除。

extra-abdominal [ˌekstrəæbˈdɔminl] *a.* 腹外的

The presence of these alimentary symptoms helps to exclude extra-abdominal and abdominal wall causes.
这些消化道症状的存在，有助于排除腹外和腹壁的原因。

extra-articular [ˌekstrəɑːˈtikjulə] *a.* 关节外的

The extra-articular manifestations are very important in determining both the morbidity and mortality of the disease.
关节以外的表现非常重要，可以决定本病的致残率与死亡率。

extracardiac [ekstrəˈkɑːdiæk] *a.* 心外的

Another cause of erroneous diagnosis is the dominance of extracardiac problems which may obscure the cardiac lesion.
误诊的另一原因是心外的临床表现占优势，它可以掩盖心脏所受的损害。

extracardial [ˌekstrəˈkɑːdiəl] *a.* 心外的

Extracardial heart failure may also be due to mechanical disorders.
心外心力衰竭也可能是机械性障碍所致。

extracellular [ˌekstrəˈseljulə] *a.* 细胞外的

Extracellular fluid is the fluid surrounding cells.
细胞外液是指在细胞周围的体液。

In addition there is the increase in blood volume and extracellular fluid.
此外，还有血容量和细胞外液的增加。

extracorporeal [ekstrəkɔːˈpɔːriəl] *a.* 体外的

It would theoretically be possible to create a small extracorporeal circulation.
从理论上说创造一个小体外循环是可能的。

extracranial [ˌekstrəˈkreinjəl] *a.* 颅外的

The author will describe the methods used to define diseases of the extracranial carotid arteries.
作者将阐述用以确诊颅外颈动脉疾病的方法。

extract[1] [iksˈtrækt] *v.* 取出，拔出；提出

In the remaining 4 cases the stone was extracted easily without serious complication.
其余 4 例结石取出均顺利，且无严重的合并症。

The vaccines consist of substances extracted from infectious agents.
该疫苗系由传染因子中提出的物质制成的。

extract[2] [ˈekstrækt] *n.* 浸膏；提出物

Extract is made by evaporating a solution of the drug in water, alcohol, or ether.
浸膏是经过蒸发药物的水溶液、酒精溶液或醚溶液制成的。

The patient told the nurse that he had taken the liquid extract of sennae.
病人告诉护士，他已服用了番泻叶流浸膏。

extraction [ikˈstrækʃən, ekˈstrækʃən] *n.* 摘出术；拔出，取出；浸出，提取出

In many cases stones in the biliary or urinary tract, usually requiring operative extraction can be passed out spontaneously after taking herbal medicine.
许多病例中，通常需手术取出的胆道或尿道结石，服用中草药后可自动排出。
For some products, the use of microorganisms has replaced chemical synthesis or extraction from animal or plant sources.
就某些产品而言，微生物的运用已取代了化学合成或从动物和植物原料的提取。
A 22-month-old infant of Italian extraction was referred because of anemia and splenomegaly.
一个 1 岁 10 个月的意大利血统幼儿，因贫血和脾脏肿大而被转来就诊。

extradural [ˌekstrəˈdjuərəl] *a.* 硬膜外的
Epidural anesthesia is accomplished by injecting a local anesthetic into the extradural space.
将局麻药注入硬膜外腔即产生硬膜外麻醉。

extrahepatic [ˌekstrəhiˈpætik] *a.* 肝外的
The laboratory studies and the liver biopsy in this patient are most compatible with extrahepatic biliary atresia.
此病人实验室的和肝活体组织的检查结果与肝外胆道闭锁最为相符。

extraneous [eksˈtreinjəs] *a.* 外部的，无关的
All extraneous diversions such as flowers, radios, televisions and food are prohibited from being put in ICU (intensive care unit).
所有无关紧要的消遣品，如花、收音机、电视机、食品等不许放入重症监护室。

extraordinarily [iksˈtrɔːdinərili] *ad.* 异常地，特别地
At present, extraordinarily complicated research projects can be undertaken by the academic surgeons at relatively little cost.
目前，从事学术研究的外科医生们能以相对小的代价来从事异常复杂的研究项目。

extraordinary [ˌekstrəˈɔːdinəri] *a.* 非常的，特别的
He is a most extraordinary scientist in medical genetics.
他在医学遗传学方面是一位极不平凡的科学家。
The extraordinary changes in cardiovascular and renal function that occur during pregnancy have fascinated clinical investigators.
妊娠期间，心血管和肾脏功能的异常改变令临床研究者感到意外。
In nodular syphilid, extraordinary and characteristic circular or serpiginous patterns are produced.
结节性梅毒症可形成非常特殊的和有特征性的环状或蛇行状的图形。

extrapancreatic [ˌekstrəˌpænkriˈætik] *a.* 胰腺外的
The presence of insulin immunoreactivity in extrapancreatic tissues and fluids suggests multiple sites of insulin production.
胰腺外组织及液体中胰岛素的免疫反应性提示胰岛素产生的多个不同部位。
The extrapancreatic nerve is composed mostly of unmyelinated nerve fibers with a smaller component of myelinated nerve fibers.
胰腺外神经主要由无髓鞘神经纤维及少数的有髓神经纤维构成。

extrapolate [eksˈtræpəleit] *v.* 推断，外推
The results of such laboratory studies can be extrapolated to the field, however, this assumption is seldom tested.
这些实验研究的结果，可以外推到现场，然而这种设想很少有人测试过。
Keya (1949) demonstrated that many of the positive effects of dietary restriction could be extrapolated to humans.
Keya (1949) 已证明膳食限制在多方面的正面效应可能外推到人类。

extrapolation [eksˌtræpəˈleiʃən] *n.* 外推法
This will allow us to move independently into the low-dose extrapolations.

这将允许我们独立地转入对低剂量的外推(研究)。

extrapyramidal [ˌekstrəpiˈræmidəl] *a.* 锥体束外的

Thioridazine is less likely to produce extrapyramidal side effects.

甲硫达嗪很少引起对于锥体外系统的副作用。

extrasystole [ˌekstrəˈsistəli] *n.* 期外收缩,过早收缩

Extrasystole may be produced by any heart disease, by nicotine from smoking, or by coffeine from excessive tea or coffee consumption.

期外收缩可以由各种心脏病或吸烟的尼古丁引起,或大量饮茶或咖啡引起。

Atrial extrasystoles usually cause no symptoms but give the sensation of a missed beat or an abnormally strong beat.

房性早搏通常不引起任何症状,但病人会感觉到心脏停搏一次或一次异常强烈的心跳。

extrauterine [ˌekstrəˈjuːtərain] *a.* 子宫外的

The large majority (95%) of extrauterine pregnancies (also called an ectopic pregnancy) occur in the fallopian tube and, however, they can occur in other locations, such as in the ovary, cervix, or abdominal cavity.

大部分(95%)的宫外孕(又称作异位妊娠)都发生在输卵管,然而也可以发生在卵巢、宫颈或腹腔。

extravasation [eksˌtrævəˈseiʃən] *n.* 外渗;外渗物(如血液)

Colchicine can cause severe extravasation if it infiltrates into subcutaneous tissues.

如果秋水仙碱浸润皮下组织,可引起严重的渗出。

The spleen has the function of keeping the blood circulating in the vessels and preventing extravasation.

脾具有使血液行于脉中而不溢出脉外的功能。

extreme [iksˈtriːm] *n.* 极端,极度;(*pl.*)极端不同的性质

Store this drug at room temperature, do not expose to extremes of temperature.

将此药贮存在室温之中,勿使接触高温或低温。

Acute bronchitis occurs most commonly at the extremes of life, i. e. in the young infant and in the elderly person.

急性支气管炎最常发生于生命的极期,即幼婴和老年人。

Clinical and physiologic observations have shown the extremes of presentations of the patient with chronic obstructive lung disease and respiratory failure.

临床和生理学观察表明,慢性阻塞性肺病和呼吸衰竭的病人有完全不同的表现。

extremity [iksˈtremiti] *n.* 末端;肢

The extremities are normal in appearance with good range of motion.

四肢外观正常,活动范围正常。

Venous blood flows from the extremities to the heart.

静脉血从四肢流向心脏。

There is no reaction to pain in her right extremities.

她的右肢并无疼痛反应。

extremophile [ikˈstriːməfail] *n.* 极端微生物

The research on the adaptation mechanism of extremophiles will promote the understanding of deep sea biosphere.

关于极端微生物适应机制的研究将促进我们对深海生物圈的了解。

Halophilic microorganisms are found as normal inhabitants of highly saline environments and thus are considered to be extremophiles.

嗜盐微生物被发现是高盐环境中的正常栖息者,因而被认为是极端微生物。

extrinsic [eksˈtrinsik] *a.* 外在的

The muscles of the larynx are divided into extrinsic and intrinsic groups.

喉肌分为喉外肌群和喉内肌群。

extrude [eks'truːd] *v.* 挤出，伸出

If the baby has been extruded through a complete rupture, it is first removed.

如婴儿已通过完全破裂口排出，则先将其移走。

At ovulation the follicle ruptures and extrudes its oocyte surrounded by its zona pellucida and corona radiata cells.

排卵时，卵泡破裂并排出其卵母细胞及其周围的透明带和放射冠细胞。

extubation [ˌekstju'beiʃən] *n.* 除管法

Recovery from anesthesia begins with the discontinuation of anesthetic drugs and extubation of the trachea.

随着麻醉剂的终止和气管拔管，病人就开始从麻醉中恢复。

exudate ['eksjudeit] *n.* 渗出物，渗出液

Macrophages are activated by factors present in the inflammatory exudate.

巨噬细胞被炎性渗出物内的因子激活。

Cultures of any exudates are made from samples collected prior to therapy.

任何渗出液的培养均应使用治疗前收集的标本去做。

exudation [ˌeksjuː'deiʃən] *n.* 渗出

Exudation is an important local defence mechanism.

渗出是一种重要的局部防御机制。

exudative [ig'zjuːdətiv] *a.* 渗出的

The lesions spread rapidly and are exudative.

病变迅速蔓延，而且是渗出性的。

exude [ig'zjuːd] *v.* 渗出

Sweat exudes through the pores.

汗从（汗腺的）毛孔中渗出。

The cervix is red and swollen, the mucous membrane protrudes from the cervical canal, and greenish-yellow pus exudes.

宫颈红肿，黏膜自宫颈管突出，有黄绿色脓液流出。

ex vivo [eks'viːveu] [拉] 在生物体外，体外

The ex vivo expansion of human hematopoietic stem cells (HSCs) is a rapidly developing area with a broad range of biomedical applications .

体外扩增造血干细胞是一个快速发展的领域，具有广泛的生物医学应用前景。

In this research the feasibility and curative effects of gelatin coated national Pt-Ir alloy stent mediated local drug delivery were studied in vivo and ex vivo.

本研究对明胶蛋白涂层的国产铂-铱合金支架介导的局部给药可行性及疗效进行了体内及体外两方面的实验研究。

eyelid ['ailid] *n.* 眼睑

The eyelids defend the eyeballs from dust and many other foreign bodies.

眼睑保护眼球，以防灰尘及其他异物。

F

facet [ˈfæsit] *n.* 小平面;某一方面

An effort has been made to elucidate some facets of progesterone production.

已做出一番努力来阐明黄体酮产生的某些原因。

facial [ˈfeiʃəl] *a.* 面的

The patient was noted to have early morning facial edema.

病人在清晨有面部浮肿。

facilitate [fəˈsiliteit] *v.* 使容易;促进

The use of this instrument will facilitate the diagnosis.

这种仪器的应用将促进诊断。

Some substances can diffuse through the cell membrane only by a special mechanism called facilitated diffusion.

某些物质只能依靠一种称为易化弥散的特殊机制,通过细胞膜进行弥散。

facility [fəˈsiliti] *n.* (*pl.*)设备,工具;机构

The practice of medicine without adequate laboratory facilities denies the patient some important advantages.

行医没有充足的化验设备,会使病人丧失一些重要的(对诊断等的)有利条件。

Facilities for treating shock should be ready.

应该准备好抢救休克的各种器械。

Patients are usually grouped in health care facilities according to problems, needs, and age.

病人在医疗卫生机构里通常按照病种、需要和年龄进行分类安排。

factor [ˈfæktə] *n.* 因素

In addition to methadone dosage, other factors must be considered.

除去美沙酮的剂量外,还必须考虑其他因素。

The primary factor causing food security problem is environmental pollution.

造成食品安全问题的主要因素是环境污染。

facultative [ˈfækəltətiv] *adj.* 兼性的;特许的

It was found that bacteria in aerobic granules were diverse and some of them were facultative aerobes.

研究发现含氧颗粒中的细菌是多样化的,其中有些是兼性需氧菌。

A new strain of acid-tolerant facultative anaerobic cellulose-degrading bacteria was isolated.

新的耐酸兼性厌氧且降解纤维素的菌株被分离出来了。

fade [feid] *v.* 消退,消失

This patient's excitement has faded.

此病人的激动情绪已消退了。

The rashes all over the face and body of the sick child have gradually faded.

病孩面部和全身的疹子已逐渐消退。

faeces [ˈfiːsiːz] *n.* 粪便;排泄物;糟粕(=feces)

Once this symptom happens, blood appears in the vomit and faeces.

一旦出现此种症状,呕吐物和粪便中就会带血。

In cats, it resides in the wall of the small intestine and passes out of the host in its faeces.

在猫科动物,它一般停留在小肠壁,并通过粪便排出宿主体外。

fail [feil] *v.* 衰竭;缺乏

Thrombi may form rapidly as the circulation is failing immediately before death.

当临死前循环衰竭时,血栓可以迅速形成。

v. (to)失败; 未做成

Failing to maintain an erection can also be a sign of some underlying conditions or diseases.

不能维持勃起可能是一些潜在疾病的征兆。

The advice "getting enough sleep to get rid of stress" is not new but is something that most people fail to follow.

"用足够的睡眠来摆脱压力"这条建议并不新鲜,但大多数人都做不到。

failover [feil'əuvər] *n.* [计算机]故障转移

Constant system availability is assured by available failover capabilities.

故障转移能力确保了持续的系统可用性。

For failover cluster installations, this base drive must be a clustered drive.

对于故障转移群集安装,此基准驱动器必须是群集驱动器。

failure ['feiljə] *n.* 失败;缺乏;衰竭

Greater than 10^5 organisms per gram of tissue correspond to a greater than 50% graft failure.

当每克组织的细菌数超过 10^5 时,移植失败率就相应地超过 50% 。

The resulting failure of protein synthesis has been corrected in experimental situations.

所产生的蛋白合成缺乏已经在实验情况中得到纠正。

Congestive heart failure is classed according to functional capacity.

充血性心力衰竭根据心功能状况进行分级。

faint [feint] *a.* 虚弱的,微弱的

Certain drugs produce extremely slow or faint breathing or cessation of breathing.

某些药物引起极慢或微弱的呼吸,甚至使呼吸停止。

The macular eruption is seldom noticed in blacks and is so faint that it is frequently not recognized in others.

斑疹在黑人身上很少被注意到,它很不清楚即使在其他人身上也难识别。

n. 晕厥

This patient went off in a faint yesterday afternoon.

昨天下午这个病人曾昏了过去。

fainting ['feintiŋ] *n.* 晕厥

Fainting while in the supine position should always suggest a seizure.

在仰卧位时发生晕厥现象常提示有癫痫发作。

Fainting commonly occurs in otherwise healthy people and may be caused by an emotional shock, by standing for prolong periods, or by injury and profuse bleeding.

晕厥常见于在其他方面较健康的人,它可由于情绪打击、长时间站立、或由于外伤和大出血引起。

faintness ['feintnis] *n.* 昏厥

If the hemorrhage is extensive, there may be faintness.

如果大出血,可能出现昏厥。

fall [fɔːl] *n.* 跌倒

Falls can be a problem for all ages.

跌倒是各种年龄的人都可能遇到的问题。

fallacy ['fæləsi] *n.* 谬误;幻觉

The experiment proved the fallacy of this reasoning.

实验证明了这一推论的错误。

fallopia [fə'lɔpiə] *n.* 何首乌属

Polygonum multiflorum belongs to fallopia.

何首乌归于何首乌属。

The content of emodin in fallopia was also determined by the same method.

同法测定了何首乌中大黄素的含量。

fallopian [fə'ləupiən] *a.* 输卵的

The normal fallopian tube is rarely palpable even under ideal conditions of examination.

即使在理想的检查条件下，正常输卵管也难于触及。

Hysterosalpingogram is the most common way for the fallopian tube patency test, which uses x-ray to trace the passage of fluid through the tube.

子宫输卵管造影是现在最常用的输卵管通畅试验方法，它是利用X-射线跟踪流体通过输卵管情况来判断的。

fallout ['fɔːlaut] *n.* 微粒回降

The exhaust gases and soot from automobiles are rich in carcinogenic agents. The same is true of radiation fallout.

汽车排出的废气和烟雾含有大量的致癌物质。放射线微粒回降物亦然。

famciclovir [ˌfæm'siːklɔviə] *n.* 法昔洛韦（商标名：famvir）

Famciclovir is used to treat the symptoms of herpes zoster (also known as shingles), a herpes virus infection of the skin.

法昔洛韦用于治疗皮肤疱疹病毒感染的带状疱疹症状。

familial [fə'miljəl] *a.* 家族的，家庭的

Hypertrophic cardiomyopathy is sometimes familial.

肥厚型心肌病有时可为家族性的。

familiar [fə'miljə] *a.* 熟悉的；通晓的；亲近的

Almost everyone is familiar with the word "contagious".

几乎每个人都熟悉"接触传染"这个词。

Digital camera is now familiar to many people.

数码相机现在已为许多人所熟悉。

Non-liquefaction of semen is one of the familiar reasons resulting in male infertility.

精液不液化是引起男性不育的常见原因之一。

familiarity [fəˌmili'æriti] *n.* 熟悉，通晓

Familiarity with this condition leads to correct diagnosis.

熟悉这种病状将有利于正确的诊断。

Familiarity with the pathogenesis and diagnosis of this disorder is essential to good management.

掌握此病病因和诊断，对正确处理是必要的。

familiarize [fə'miljəraiz] *v.* 使熟悉，使通晓

A nurse must be familiarized with the conditions and procedures in patient care.

护士必须熟悉病人护理的条件与程序。

family ['fæmili] *n.* 家，家族

Stress proteins are classified into four families based upon their sequence homology and molecular mass.

应激蛋白常可根据其序列的同源性和分子量的大小而将其分为四个家族。

fantastic [fæn'tæstik] *a.* 极大的；奇异的

The era of transplantation has produced the most fantastic change in the history of biology and medicine.

器官移植时代，使生物学史和医学史上产生了极大的变化。

fantasy ['fæntəsi] *n.* 想象力，幻想

By some estimates, approximately half of our waking thoughts consist of daydreams and fantasies.

根据估算，我们醒着时思考的问题中差不多一半都包含着白日梦与幻想。

farsightedness ['fɑː'saitidnis] *n.* 远视

The implantable lenses can be designed to correct optical problems, such as farsightedness or nearsightedness.
植入的透镜可设计用来矫正视力问题,如远视和近视。

fascial [ˈfeiʃəl] *a.* 筋膜的

If an ascitic leak develops, the wound should be explored and the fascial defect closed.
如果发生腹水漏,应探查伤口,缝闭筋膜缺损。

fasciitis [fəˈsaitis] *n.* 筋膜炎

Nodular fasciitis is a rapidly growing mass, with high cellularity and mitotic activity that can be misdiagnosed as a soft tissue sarcoma.
结节性筋膜炎是一种生长迅速的肿块,细胞丰富,核分裂活性高,常误诊为软组织肉瘤。

Pseudosarcomas of soft tissue are fibroblastic/myofibroblastic and matrix-forming proliferations, including nodular fasciitis, proliferative fasciitis and myositis, and so on.
软组织假肉瘤是指纤维母细胞/肌纤维母细胞的并产生基质的增生性病变,包括结节性筋膜炎、增生性筋膜炎和增生性肌炎等等。

fasciotomy [fæʃiˈɔtəmi] *n.* 筋膜切开术

The purpose of this study is to determine whether an adductor fasciotomy will alleviate the pain and improve the function in patients with a chronic "groin pull".
这个实验的目的在于判定内收肌群筋膜切开术能否减轻慢性腹股沟牵拉患者的疼痛和改善其功能。

fashion [ˈfæʃən] *n.* 方式

I initially postulated that after 40 minutes of ischemia, potassium would have equilibrated between the intracellular and the extracellular fluid in the fashion described above.
我原推测,在缺血 40 分钟之后,钾会按照上述方式,在细胞内液和细胞外液之间达到平衡。

fastidious [fæsˈtidiəs] *adj.* 难养的,苛刻的

Fastidious bacteria resistance in Guangzhou district was investigated.
对广州地区难养菌的耐药性进行了调查。

A fastidious organism is any organism that has a complex nutritional requirement.
难以培养的微生物指的是对营养成分有复杂要求的微生物。

fasting [ˈfɑːstiŋ] *n.* 禁食,节制饮食

During the first 24h of fasting, circulating glucose, fatty acids, and triglycerides and liver and muscle glycogen are used as fuel sources.
禁食的头 24 小时内,循环中的葡萄糖、脂肪酸、甘油三酯以及肝脏和肌肉中的糖原可用作能量来源。

The specimen for a blood glucose test is usually drawn in the morning before breakfast and is called a fasting blood glucose.
进行血糖测试的标本通常在清晨早餐前抽取,称为空腹血糖。

fat [fæt] *n.* 脂肪

People who exercise while dieting lose more body fat.
一边节食一边锻炼的人会失去身体上更多的脂肪。

fatal [ˈfeitəl] *a.* 致命的,致死的

The loss of fluid and protein and secondary electrolyte changes lead to shock, which may prove fatal unless promptly treated.
液体和蛋白质流失以及继发性电解质变化会导致休克,除非迅速治疗,否则这种休克就是致命的。

Chronic nephritis can lead to sometimes fatal condition known as uremia, which means an accumulation of urinary constituents in the blood.
慢性肾炎有时能导致称为尿毒症的致命情况,即血液中有尿液成分的积聚。

fatality [fə'tæliti] *n.* 死亡(事故),致命性

Failure to recognize this important concept will result in fatality.

认识不到这一重要概念会引起致命后果。

The cause of death is the disease, injury, or combination of abnormalities responsible for the fatality.

死亡原因是可引起致命的疾病、损伤或各种异常现象。

Fatalities as a direct result of an acute attack of asthma are rare.

哮喘的急性发作可直接致死的病例是罕见的。

father ['fɑːðə] *v.* 确定…的生父

Investigation fathered the baby on him.

调查结果证明,他就是那个婴儿的生父。

fatigability [ˌfætigə'biliti] *n.* 易疲(劳)性

The subjective manifestation of active pulmonary tuberculosis are general malaise, easy fatigability, prostration, mild fever, night sweats, loss of appetite, persistent cough, etc.

活动期肺结核的主观症状是全身不适、易疲劳、虚脱、轻度发烧、盗汗、食欲不振、持续性咳嗽等。

fatigue [fə'tiːg] *n.* 疲劳

The number of men and women experiencing fatigue for six months or longer was about equal.

经受6个月或更长时间疲劳症的男性女性人数基本相等。

v. 使疲劳

The patient is easily fatigued with the slightest physical activities.

病人稍微从事体力活动就容易感到疲劳。

fatty ['fæti] *a.* 脂肪的,油脂的

The doctor advised him specifically not to eat fatty food.

医生特别劝他不要吃多脂肪的食物。

The bulk of the content of the cyst is usually made up of fatty material.

这种囊肿的内含物通常大部分由脂肪物质构成。

faulty ['fɔːlti] *a.* 有错误的,有缺点的

Abnormal sounds are called murmurs and are due to faulty action of the valves.

不正常的心音叫做杂音,是由于瓣膜功能有缺陷造成的。

Excess water within the body indicates that the number and distribution of electrolytes are faulty.

体内过量的水显示电解质含量和分布有毛病。

favism ['fɑːvizəm] *n.* 蚕豆病

Favism is an X chromosome-linked recessive hereditary metabolic disorder which has a prevalence of between 3% and 35% amongst the Asian population.

蚕豆病是一种X染色体连锁的隐形遗传代谢病,其在亚洲人群的患病率为3%到35%之间。

favor ['feivə] *v.* 支持,赞成,有利于

Debate over which test is preferred continues, but the trend of evidence favors the use of MRI.

有关何种检查更适合的争论仍在继续,但有关资料倾向于支持使用MRI方法来检查。

Although these nodules may arise anywhere on the skin, the most favored site is the trunk or scalp.

虽然这些结节可以发生于皮肤的任何部位,但最好发的部位是躯干或头皮。

favorable ['feivərəbl] *a.* 良好的,有利的,赞成的

In this case, when no cause can be determined, the prognosis is usually favorable.

在这种情况下,如果找不到任何原因,常表明预后良好。

The spores serve to produce new organisms when material containing them again is placed in surroundings favourable to bacterial growths.

当含有芽孢的物质又处于有利于细菌生长的环境中时，这种芽孢便会产生新的有机体。

favorably [ˈfeivərəbli] *ad.* 有利地

Acidic compounds are excreted more favorably if the urine is alkaline.

尿液为碱性时，更有利于酸性药物的排泄。

It is too soon to tell if actual survival will be favourably affected as well, or if important long-term side effects will emerge.

要认定对实际存活有好处，或断言会出现严重的持久的副作用，都还为时过早。

favorite [ˈfeivərit] *n.* 特别喜爱的人（或物）

The new book "Medical Psychology" is a great favorite with students.

《医学心理学》是学生们非常喜爱的一本新书。

a. 特别喜爱的

What is your favorite color?

你最喜爱的颜色是什么？

In late syphilis the mucous membranes are attacked, the tongue being a favorite site.

晚期梅毒常累及黏膜，舌为其好发部位。

feasibility [ˌfiːzəˈbiliti] *n.* 可行性

This two-and-one-half-day conference focused on the feasibility and practical implications of the routine use of dietary restriction in safety assessment.

这两天半的会议重点讨论了膳食限制在安全评估中常规应用的可行性和实际影响。

feasible [ˈfiːzəbl] *a.* 可实行的，可行的

Perhaps none of these suggestions will prove to be feasible.

或许这些建议没有一个将被证明是可行的。

In emergencies, or when the oral route is not feasible because of vomiting, the parenteral preparation may be used.

紧急时或因呕吐而不能经口给药时，不妨使用非经口药物。

feat [fiːt] *n.* 功绩，业绩

Man's first landing on the moon was a feat of great daring.

人类首次登上月球是具有伟大勇敢精神的业绩。

feathery [ˈfeðəri] *a.* 羽毛状的

Feathery degeneration of hepatocytes is a kind of parenchymal changes of cholestasis.

肝细胞的羽毛状变性是一种胆汁淤积时肝实质的病变。

Feathery degeneration of hepatocytes is due to retention of bile acids.

肝细胞的羽毛状变性是由于胆酸淤积导致的。

feature [ˈfiːtʃə] *n.* 特征，特色；（期刊的）特辑

The professor is describing the anatomic and physiologic features of muscular contraction.

教授正在讲述肌肉收缩的解剖学和生理学的特征。

Constipation is a universal feature of complete obstruction.

完全性肠梗阻时便秘是普遍出现的症状。

Examining the patient, the physician noticed some changes in his feature.

医生在检查患者时，发现其病象有些变化。

Prof. Smith is one of the editors of this feature.

史密斯教授是本特辑的编者之一。

v. 以…为特色

The prosthesis features less friction, greater movement and faster rate of recovery.

这种假体修复术的特点是摩擦较少，活动度较大，恢复速度较快。

The newly-designed apparatus is chiefly featured by its high sensitivity.

这种新设计的仪器的主要特点是其高度的灵敏性。

febrile [ˈfiːbrail] *a.* 热性的，发热的

No apparent cause can be found for such febrile reaction which usually persists for only a few days.

这种发热的反应一般仅持续数日，不能找到明显的原因。

Febrile patients whose response was slow experienced a high immediate mortality.

对治疗反应慢的发热患者，即刻死亡率高。

fecal [ˈfiːkəl] *a.* 粪便的

Constipation due to inactivity and unawareness of rectal distension leads to fecal impaction.

由于不活动和感觉不到便意引起的便秘导致粪便阻塞。

These patients were asked to complete a questionnaire about urinary and fecal incontinence, associated symptoms, and other health issues.

这些病人被要求填写一份关于大小便失禁、相关症状以及其他健康问题的问卷。

feces [ˈfiːsiːz] (*pl.*) *n.* 粪便

Examination of the feces often gives the clue to the cause of diarrhoea.

粪便检查常常为查明造成腹泻的原因提供线索。

However, some lead is eliminated in bile, feces and sweat.

然而，有些铅是由胆汁、粪便和汗水中排泄出来的。

feeble [ˈfiːbl] *a.* 虚弱的

The pulse is feeble or apparently absent.

此时脉搏已很微弱或明显地消失。

feedback [ˈfiːdbæk] *n.* 反馈

This genetic activity is controlled mainly by internal feedback mechanisms within the cell.

这种基因活性主要受细胞内部反馈机制的控制。

The level of cortisol is thought to control directly the secretion of ACTH (adrenocorticotropic hormone) through a negative feedback.

通常认为氢化可的松的浓度可通过负反馈机制直接调控促肾上腺皮质激素的分泌。

feeding [ˈfiːdiŋ] *n.* 喂养，饲养

Feeding is an important problem in bringing up healthy children.

喂养法是哺育健康儿童的一个重要课题。

felon [ˈfelən] *n.* 化脓性指头炎

An acute felon associated with or without paronychia is an unusual and more aggressive manifestation of this drug-dependent nail dystrophy.

伴或不伴甲沟炎的急性脓性指头炎是一种罕见的但更具侵袭性药物依赖性甲营养不良的表现。

We report a case of felon infected by methicillin-resistant S. aureus.

我们报道了一起甲氧西林耐药的金黄色酿脓葡萄球菌感染的脓性指头炎的病例。

female [ˈfiːmeil] *a.* 女性的，妇女的

This ward area is for the female patients.

这个病区是为妇女病人设的。

There are quite a number of female doctors in the department of genecology and obstetrics.

妇产科里很有一些女医生。

femoral [ˈfemərəl] *a.* 股骨的，股的

Femoral hernias occur more commonly in females because of the wider female pelvis.

股疝较常发生于女性，因女性的骨盆较宽。

The external iliac arteries continue into the thigh, where the name of these tubes is changed to femoral.

髂外动脉延伸入大腿，此处这些脉管改称为股动脉。

femur [ˈfiːmə] *n.* 股骨

The report also highlights the high death of elderly patients with fractured femurs.

报告也着重指出患有股骨骨折的老年患者的死亡率是很高的。

fenestrated [fiˈnestreitid] *adj.* 开窗的，穿孔的

Glomerular filter consists of fenestrated endothelium, basement membrane, and foot processes of epithelial cells.

肾小球滤过膜由有孔的内皮、基底膜和上皮细胞的足突构成。

The cytoplasm of endothelial cells of blood vessels is not intact, but fenestrated.

血管内皮细胞的胞质不是完整的，而是有窗孔的。

fenugreek [ˈfenjugriːk] *n.* 胡芦巴；胡芦巴的种子

Fenugreek seed comprises seed coat, endosperm and embryo.

胡芦巴的种子包括种皮、胚乳和胚芽。

We put fenugreek leaves in warm water for 10 minutes and then ground it into powders.

将胡芦巴子叶浸于暖水约 10 分钟，然后磨成粉状。

feosol [ˈfiːəsɔl] *n.* 硫酸亚铁(ferrous sulfate 制剂的商品名)

Feosol provides the iron needed by the body to produce red blood cells.

硫酸亚铁提供身体所需的铁以生产红细胞。

ferment [fəˈment] *v.* (使)发酵

Lactic acid bacteria are capable of fermenting lactose, converting it into lactic acid.

乳酸菌能酵解乳糖，使它转化成乳酸。

fermentation [ˌfəːmenˈteiʃən] *n.* 发酵

Note that alcoholic fermentation is also a form of glycolysis.

注意，乙醇发酵也是酵解的一种形式。

Chloromycetin is produced by either chemical synthesis or fermentation.

氯霉素或者用化学合成法生产，或者用发酵法生产。

ferritin [ˈferitin] *n.* 铁蛋白

Serum ferritin is the best method for detecting storage depletion in outpatients and for screening hospital patients.

血清铁蛋白的检测适用于门诊病人和住院病人的普查，它是能够检测铁贮存缺乏的最好方法。

Example of metalloproteins are ferritin, containing iron, and ceruloplasmin, containing copper.

金属蛋白的例子有：铁蛋白(含有铁)和血浆铜蓝蛋白(含有铜)。

ferrokinetic [ˌferəukaiˈnetik] *a.* 铁动力学的

Ferrokinetic studies provide evidence of ineffective erythropoiesis, inferring that abnormal erythroid maturation results in increased intramedullary death of RBCs.

铁动力学检查提供红细胞无效生成的证据，表明红细胞不能正常成熟，以致在髓内的死亡增多。

ferrous [ˈferəs] *a.* 亚铁的

Similar preparations used to treat anaemia include ferrous fumarate and ferrous succinate.

治疗贫血的类似制剂还有延胡索酸亚铁和琥珀酸亚铁。

Fe can be provided by ferrous sulfate or ferrous gluconate, best given orally between meals since food or antacids may reduce absorption.

硫酸亚铁和葡萄糖酸亚铁可提供铁，最好在两餐之间口服，因食物和抗酸药可降低其吸收。

fertility [fəːˈtiliti] *n.* 生育力

Fertility is the capacity to conceive or induce conception.

生育力是受孕或导致受孕的能力。

Aroma-Scan has already proposed a handheld fertility monitor.

Aroma-Scan 已提出生产一种手提的生育力检测器。

fertilization [ˌfəːtilaiˈzeiʃən] *n.* 受精

Normally, the ovum migrates from one of the fallopian tubes to the uterine cavity about 72 hours after fertilization.

正常情况下，卵子在受精后 72 小时左右从一侧输卵管游走到达宫腔。

New and advanced technologies to help a woman become pregnant include in vitro fertilization, intracytoplasmic sperm injection, and other similar procedures.

帮助妇女怀孕的新而先进的技术包括体外受精，卵胞浆内单精子注射，和其他类似的方法。

fertilize [ˈfəːtilaiz] *v.* 使受精

To fertilize an ovum refers to the entering of a sperm into the ovum.

使卵受精是指精子进入一卵细胞内。

The fertilized ovum derives half of its developmental characteristics from the mother and half from the fertilizing sperm of the father.

受精卵从其父母亲那各获得一半的发育特性。

fetal [ˈfiːtl] *a.* 胎儿的

The fetal heart tones resemble the ticktock of a watch heard through a pillow.

胎儿心音类似从枕头下面听到的钟表滴答声。

Thymus manufactures lymphocytes and is essential to fetal growth.

胸腺制造淋巴细胞，对胎儿成长必不可少。

fetid [ˈfetid] *a.* 恶臭的

Fetid breath may be due to the expelled air, gases thrown off from the digestive tract, or to a diseased mouth.

口臭可由呼吸道、消化道排出的气体或口腔的疾病引起。

The patients with intestinal bacterial infection usually have fetid diarrhea.

肠道细菌感染的患者常有腹泻并伴大便恶臭。

α-fetoprotein [ˌfiːtəuˈprəutiːn] *n.* 甲胎蛋白

α-fetoprotein is normally present at high concentration in fetal and maternal serum.

甲胎蛋白（AFP）在正常胎儿和母亲的血清中含有很高的浓度。

fetotoxicity [ˈfiːtəˌtɔkˈsisiti] *n.* 胎儿毒性

The present study evaluated the effects of this chemical on fetotoxicity.

本文评估了这种化学物质的胎儿毒性效应。

Five compounds known to induce fetotoxicity were administered during organogenesis.

在器官发生期给药，已知有五种化合物对胎儿有毒。

fetotoxin [ˈfiːtə ˈtɔksin] *n.* 胚胎毒物

Fetotoxin is a chemical that can cause health effects in a developing fetus or embryo.

胚胎毒物是一类会对发育中的胚胎或胎儿产生不良健康效应的化学物质。

In contrast, a fetotoxin may cause adverse effects at any time in pregnancy.

相反，一种胚胎毒物可以在怀孕中的任何时期引起不良健康作用。

fetus [ˈfiːtəs] *n.* 胎儿

The fetus is a chimera carrying human leukocyte antigen (HLA) alleles from both parents.

胎儿是携带父母双方人类白细胞抗原（HLA）等位基因的嵌合体。

The formation of blood cells is an important function of the spleen in the fetus.

胎儿脾脏的重要功能是产生各种血细胞。

fever [ˈfiːvə] *n.* 发热（烧）

Fever is one of the commonest manifestations of disease, its feature is a rise in body temperature produced by a disturbance in the mechanisms regulating it.

发热是疾病最普通的体征之一，其特征是体温调节机制紊乱而使体温升高。

Symptomatic therapy of viral pneumonia includes bed rest, acetylsalicylic acid for fever, and the use of humidity for younger children and infants.

病毒性肺炎的对症治疗包括卧床休息，乙酰水杨酸解热，以及对幼童和婴儿使用湿敷解热。

fiber [ˈfaibə] *n.* 纤维

Fiber is receiving increasing attention as a dietary factor in disease prevention and treatment.

纤维作为一种食物要素在疾病的预防与治疗中越来越为人所关注。

Collagen fibers are loosely arranged in the upper(papillary) portion of the dermis.

胶原纤维疏松地排列在真皮上部（乳头层）。

fiberoptic [faibəˈrɔptik] *a.* 纤维镜的；纤维光学的

Modern methods of fiberoptic gastroscopy and cytologic examination are increasing diagnostic accuracy to over 90%.

现代的检查方法，如纤维胃镜检查和细胞学检查将诊断准确率提高到 90% 以上。

fibril [ˈfaibril] *n.* 原纤维，纤丝

The specific polypeptide chains are secreted by the cell and assembled into collagen fibrils.

这种特殊的多肽链被细胞分泌出来并聚集成胶原纤维。

Our objective is to investigate the relationship between disk area and retinal nerve fibril layer thickness in patients with large cup.

我们的目的是要研究大视杯人群视盘面积和视网膜神经纤维厚度的关系。

fibrillar [ˈfaibrilə] *a.* 原纤维的

The principal constituent of the dermis is the fibrillar structural protein, collagen.

真皮的主要成分是原纤维结构蛋白——胶原。

fibrillation [ˌfaibriˈleiʃən] *n.* 纤维性颤动

Ventricular rate in atrial fibrillation is controlled by digitalisation.

房颤时的心室率可用洋地黄化控制。

fibrin [ˈfaibrin] *n.* 纤维蛋白

The clotting mechanism is the conversion of plasma fibrinogen into the insoluble fibrin.

凝血机制是血浆纤维蛋白原转变成不溶解的纤维蛋白。

fibrinogen [faiˈbrinədʒən] *n.* 纤维蛋白原

These substances are required to bring about the change of fibrinogen to fibrin.

为把纤维蛋白原变成纤维蛋白，这些物质是必需的。

The liver gives rise to serum albumin and serum globulin as well as fibrinogen and heparin.

肝脏产生血清白蛋白、血清球蛋白，还有纤维蛋白原和肝素。

fibrinoid [ˈfaibrinɔid] *a.* 纤维素样的

Fibrinoid degeneration actually is a kind of necrosis.

纤维素样变性实际上是一种坏死。

Fibrinoid necrosis is usually seen in immune reactions involving blood vessels.

纤维素样坏死常见于免疫反应时，并累及血管。

fibrinolysin [ˌfaibriˈnɔlisin] *n.* 纤维蛋白溶酶

We know that thrombi are constantly forming and being broken down by fibrinolysins.

我们知道血栓在不断形成并不断被纤维蛋白溶酶分解。

fibrinolysis [ˌfaibriˈnɔlisis] *n.* 纤维蛋白溶解，纤溶，纤维素分解

Drugs causing fibrinolysis have been utilized therapeutically.

纤维蛋白溶解药物已经被用于临床治疗。

A case of primary systemic fibrinolysis(PSF) has been successfully treated with cyclosporin A.

使用环孢素 A 成功治疗原发性全身性纤维蛋白溶解症 1 例。

The clinical signification of dysregulation of coagulation and fibrinolysis system in Dengue hemorrhagic fever and Dengue shock syndrome has been determined.

登革热出血热和登革热休克综合征患者凝血和纤溶系统的失调的临床意义已被确定。

fibrinolytic [ˌfaibrinəuˈlitik] *a.* 溶解纤维蛋白的

Nosebleeds are treated with anti-fibrinolytic agents.
鼻出血可用抗纤维蛋白溶解剂治疗。
The patient did not have any known contraindications to fibrinolytic therapy.
该例患者对溶解纤维蛋白治疗无任何已知的禁忌证。

fibrinous [ˈfaibrinəs] *a.* 纤维素性的
A fibrinous exudate is characteristic of inflammation in the lining of body cavities, such as the meninges, pericardium and pleura.
纤维素性渗出是体腔被衬上皮(如脑膜、心包膜和胸膜)炎症的特征。
Conversion of the fibrinous exudate to scar tissue within the pericardial sac leads to obliteration of the pericardial space.
在心包腔内纤维素性渗出物转变为瘢痕组织可导致心包腔闭锁。

fibroadenoma [ˌfaibrəu,ædəˈnəumə] *n.* 纤维腺瘤
Fibroadenomas are the most common benign tumor of the female breast, and they are frequently multiple and bilateral.
纤维腺瘤是女性乳腺最常见的良性肿瘤,常常双侧多发。
The breast-specific biphasic tumors——fibroadenoma and phyllodes tumor arise from intralobular stroma.
纤维腺瘤和叶状肿瘤是乳腺特异性的双向分化的肿瘤,起源于乳腺小叶内的间质。

fibrocartilage [ˈfaibrəuˈkɑːtilidʒ] *n.* 纤维软骨
The triangular fibrocartilage complex(TFCC) with its ulnar foveal attachment is the primary stabilizer of the distal radioulnar joint(DRUJ).
三角纤维软骨复合体及其尺侧的中间凹注视附属物是桡尺远端关节主要的稳定装置。

fibroid [ˈfaibrɔid] *n.* 纤维瘤
In most cases fibroids are multiple.
大多数病例中纤维瘤是多发性的。

fibroma [faiˈbrəumə] (*pl.* fibromas 或 fibromata[faiˈbrəumətə]) *n.* 纤维瘤
Fibromas are another benign tumor of the heart, also presenting mainly in childhood.
另一种心脏的肿瘤是纤维瘤,它主要发生于儿童时期。

fibromyalgia [ˌfaibrəumaiˈældʒiə] *n.* 纤维肌痛
Because patients with fibromyalgia complain of chronic fatigue, and because most patients with chronic fatigue syndrome have, on examination, multiple tender points, both designations are believed to describe the same entity.
患有纤维肌痛的病人主诉有慢性疲劳,而患有慢性疲劳综合征的病人检查身体常有多处压痛点,因此有人认为这两种病情描述的是同一种疾病。

fibromyoma [ˌfaibrəumaiˈəumə] (*pl.* fibromyomata[ˌfaibrəumaiˈəumətə]) *n.* 纤维肌瘤
Fibromyomata are the commonest new growths of the uterus and one of the most common tumours of the human body.
子宫纤维肌瘤是子宫最常见的新生物,也是人体最常见的肿瘤之一。

fibronectin [ˌfaibrəuˈnektin] *n.* 纤维结合素
Moreover, the anchoring fibronectin molecules of old fibroblasts are larger and have less ability to bind native collagens than do those of young fibroblasts.
然而衰老的成纤维细胞的锚状纤维结合素的分子较大,它与天然胶原的结合力也比年轻的成纤维细胞要差。

fibronection [ˈfaibrəuˈnekʃən] *n.* 纤维连接蛋白
Fibronection and IL-2(interleukin-2) are useful in clinical diagnosis and prognosis of nasopharyngeal carcinoma.
纤维蛋白连接素和白细胞介素 2 有助于鼻咽癌的临床诊断和预后。

fibrosa [faiˈbrəusə] *n.* 纤维膜

Fibrosa is the outermost connective tissue covering of any organ, vessel, or other structure.
纤维膜是被覆于某种器官、血管或其他结构最外面的结缔组织。

Osteitis fibrosa is a complication of hyperparathyroidism in which the bones turn soft and become deformed.
纤维性骨炎是甲状旁腺功能亢进的一种并发症,表现为骨骼变软和变形。

fibrosarcoma [ˌfaibrəusɑːˈkəumə] *n.* 纤维肉瘤

Infantile fibrosarcoma is rare and represents less than 1% of all cancers in children.
婴儿纤维肉瘤罕见,在儿童所有癌症中发病率不足 1% 。

fibrose [ˈfaibrəus] *v.* 纤维化

The scarred appendix is a fibrosed appendix, not chronic appendicitis.
这种瘢痕性阑尾是纤维化了的阑尾,而不是慢性阑尾炎。

fibrosis [faiˈbrəusis] *n.* 纤维增生,纤维化,纤维变性

Renal carcinoma may stimulate fibrosis such as that seen in periureteral fibrosis.
肾癌可刺激纤维增生,如见于输尿管周围的纤维增生一样。

The primary complex heals with fibrosis and frequently, calcifies without therapy.
原发综合征愈合并纤维化,常常不经治疗即可钙化。

fibrous [ˈfaibrəs] *a.* 纤维性的

Fibrous membranes are composed of connective tissue only.
纤维膜仅由结缔组织构成。

fibula [ˈfibjulə] *n.* 腓骨

During yesterday's match against Stoke City, Aaron Ramsey sustained fractures to the tibia and fibula in his right leg. In the evening he underwent an operation.
在昨天同斯托克城的比赛中,阿伦拉姆齐右腿胫骨和腓骨骨折,晚上他进行了手术。

It is the fibula in the ankle that has to be checked, that is what I have been told.
据我所知,他需要进一步检查的是踝关节附近的腓骨。

fibular [ˈfibjulə] *a.* 腓骨的

Fibular osteotomy remains a challenging aspect of mandibular microsurgical reconstruction, dependent largely on surgeon's experience, intraoperative judgment, and technical speed.
腓骨截骨术仍然是下颌骨显微外科重建术中的一个具有挑战性的方面,它主要依赖于外科医生的经验,术中判断和操作速度。

ficolin [ˈfiːkəulin] *n.* 纤维胶原素,纤维胶凝蛋白

Ficolins are carbohydrate-binding proteins that initiate the lectin pathway of complement activation.
纤维胶原素是糖结合蛋白,它能启动补体激活的凝集素途径。

Ficolin is a collagenous lectin which plays a crucial role in innate immunity.
纤维胶原素是一种在天然免疫中起关键作用的胶原凝聚素。

fidelity [fiˈdeliti] *n.* 精确,逼真

The tRNA molecule is essential to the two steps that determine the fidelity of protein synthesis.
在决定蛋白质合成的精确性的两个步骤中,tRNA 是必不可少的。

figure [ˈfigə] *n.* 图形,图表(Fig.);数字

Fig. 1 illustrates deeply stained cytoplasm and prominent nuclei.
图 1 显示着色很深的细胞浆和明显的细胞核。

Results of some of these tests are illustrated in Figure 5.
测验的某些结果如图 5 所示。

Thus, compared with a natural incidence of infertility which is appoximately 15%, this figure is exceedingly high.
于是,与不育的自然发生率约 15% 相比较,这个数字就是很高了。

filament [ˈfiləment] *n.* 丝,丝状体

This filament,lying between the cell membrane and the cell wall,is actually a bundle of flagella.

轴丝位于细胞膜和细胞壁之间,实际上它是细胞两极发出的鞭毛束。

filarial [fiˈlɛəriəl] *a.* 丝虫的

This was an ideal method to be used in filarial infection surveillance.

这是用于丝虫感染监测的一种理想方法。

Infection occurs when filarial parasites are transmitted to humans through mosquitoes.

当丝虫通过蚊子传播给人时会出现感染。

filariasis [ˌfiləˈraiəsis] *n.* 丝虫病

Filariasis in the tropics,polyarteritis nodosa and plumonary embolism should also be considered.

还应考虑热带地区的丝虫病、多发性结节性动脉炎和肺栓塞。

file [fail] *n.* 档案,卷宗,文件

Did you see my file,Alice?

你见到我的文件了吗? 爱丽斯?

He read all the files on this case.

他阅读了有关这个案件的全部卷宗。

v. 把...归档[(+away)]

She filed all these documents carefully.

她把所有这些文件仔细归档。

File away all these documents carefully,please.

请将这些文件仔细归档。

filial [ˈfiljəl] *a.* 子女的;后代的,子代的

In genetics the first filial generation is represented by F1.

在遗传学中用 F1 表示子一代。

filler [ˈfilə] *n.* 填充剂,填充物

When inorganic filler content was increased,a remarkable increase in the static modulus and dynamic modulus were observed.

无机填充剂的含量增加时,静态模量和动态模量都会显著增加。

Participants from the Injectable Filler Safety(IFS)Study were reinterviewed to obtain data on the course of adverse reactions and the therapy.

为了获得不良反应和治疗过程中的数据,对"注射填料安全研究"课题的参与者进行了回访。

filling [ˈfiliŋ] *n.* 填充,充盈

The department of stomatology of our hospital has bought many new types of filling instruments.

我们医院的口腔科购置了许多新型的填充器械。

In many forms of edema,the effective arterial blood volume,an parameter of the filling of the arterial tree,is reduced.

在多种类型的水肿中,有效的动脉血容量作为一种动脉树充盈度的参数是降低的。

Even in the absence of structural heart disease,the extremely high heart rates may impair cardiac filling and output.

即使在没有器质性心脏病的情况下,极快的心率也能降低心脏充盈(度)和搏出(量)。

filopodium [filəˈpeudiəm] *n.* (*pl.* filopodia)丝状假足,伪足

In conclusion,continuous exposure to tetracaine at small concentrations delayed neurite growth,reduced the number of filopodia,and decreased actin content.

因此,低浓度丁卡因的持续接触可延迟轴突的生长,减少伪足的数量,和降低肌动蛋白的含量。

filter [ˈfiltə] *n.* 滤器,滤纸

In addition,mycoplasmas are very small cells that can pass through many filters that retain other

bacteria.
此外，支原体的细胞很小，能通过其他细菌所不能通过的许多滤器。
v. 滤过
Some of the rays are filtered out in passing through the atmosphere.
有些光线在穿过大气层时被滤掉。
The lymph nodes function as a sort of filtering structures in the human body.
人体淋巴结起着过滤装置的作用。

filtrable [ˈfiltrəbl] *a.* 可滤过的
The causal agent is a filtrable virus, distinct from that of measles.
这种病原体是与麻疹的病原体不同的滤过性病毒。

filtration [filˈtreiʃən] *n.* 过滤
The spleen is involved in blood filtration.
脾具有过滤血液的功能。
Other factors can influence the efficiency of filtration.
其他一些因素均可影响过滤的效果。

fimbria [ˈfimbriə] (*pl.* fimbriae) *n.* 菌毛，纤毛
Fimbriae are straight filaments, thinner and shorter than flagella, extending out from the surface of the cell.
菌毛为笔直的丝状物，比鞭毛要细而短些；它由细胞的表面向外伸出。

fimbrioplasty [ˈfimbriəu,plæsti] *n.* 输卵管伞端成形术
Fimbrioplasty is one of several reconstructive procedures designed to correct infertility.
输卵管伞端成形术是治疗不孕中几个重建手术方式之一。
The fimbrioplasty is preferred to salpingostomy, since salpingostomy does not play the same role as the fimbriated extremity of fallopian tube does.
比起输卵管造口术，输卵管伞端成形术更适用，因输卵管造口术不能解决输卵管伞端起的重要作用。

finalize [ˈfainəlaiz] *v.* 予以最终形式，使定案
The diagnosis of leukemia should never be finalized and told to parents until the bone marrow is examined.
在未作骨髓检查前，白血病的诊断决不应该是最后的诊断，也不应该告诉患儿的双亲。

finasteride [fiˈnæstəraid] *n.* 非那司提
Finasteride, which comes as a tablet, is used to treat benign prostatic hypertrophy (BPH).
非那司提为片剂形式，用于治疗良性前列腺肥大。

finding [faindiŋ] *n.* (*pl.*) 调查（或研究）的结果
The findings of the commission are satisfactory.
该委员会的调查结果是令人满意的。

fine [fain] *a.* 精致的，细微的
Auscultation reveals fine inspiratory rales throughout.
听诊时全肺出现吸气期小水泡音。
It is well known that exposure to particulate matter, especially to fine and ultra-fine particles, enhances the risk of cardio-respiratory diseases.
众所周知暴露于微粒物质，特别是细颗粒和超细颗粒，可增加心肺疾病的风险。
The neurofibril is a fine, cytoplasmic thread that extends from the cell body into the process of a neuron.
神经原纤维是一种胞浆细丝，它从神经元的胞体延伸至突起。

fingernail [ˈfiŋgəneil] *n.* 指甲
We must keep our fingernail clean.
我们必须保持我们的手指甲干净。

If our fingernails are long, dirt can get under them.
如果我们的手指甲长,脏东西能进入到它下面。

fingerprinting [ˌfiŋgəˈprintiŋ] *n.* 指纹法
Fingerprinting means the identification of multiple specific alleles on a person's DNA to produce a unique identifier for that person.
指纹法是通过对一个人 DNA 中特定等位基因的鉴定而产生一种独特的确定个体身份的方法。

finite [ˈfainait] *a.* 有限的,限定的
In severe ischemia ischemic cells swell from a finite volume.
严重缺血时,缺血细胞的肿胀来自有限的液体。

firm[1] [fəːm] *a.* 坚固的,结实的,稳固的;坚决的
Papules may be of soft or firm consistency.
丘疹的质地可软可硬。

firm[2] [fəːm] *n.* 商号,企业
I am equally obliged to Messrs Churchill Livingstone for the forbearance and helpfulness that I have for twenty-five years experienced from this great publishing firm.
我同样对 Churchill Livingstone 公司表示感谢,25 年来的经验使我感受到了这个大出版企业对我的耐心和帮助。

firmicutes [fəːˈmikjuːtiːz] *n.* (*pl.*)硬壁菌门
Firmicutes play an important role in beer, wine, and cider spoilage.
硬壁菌门在啤酒、白酒和苹果汁的变质中起重要作用。
Firmicutes are gram-positive bacteria with a low mole% G+C content and they constitute one of the main phyla within the bacteria.
硬壁菌是革兰阳性菌,G+C 百分摩尔含量低,在细菌中是主要菌门之一。

firmness [ˈfəːmnis] *n.* 坚固,结实
It may be necessary to palpate the lesion for firmness and fluctuation.
用扪诊的方法检查受损害部位的硬度和弹性可能是必要的。

first-pass [ˈfəːst-pɑːs] *n.* 首过
"First-pass effect" may be defined as the loss of drug as it passes through the liver for the first time.
首过效应系指药物首次通过肝脏时的损失。

fish-flesh [fiʃ-fleʃ] *a.* 鱼肉样的
On cut section, sarcoma is usually homogeneous and fish-flesh.
在切面上,肉瘤通常是均质的,呈鱼肉状。
Typically fibrosarcomas are unencapsulated, infiltrative, soft, fish-flesh masses with hemorrhage and necrosis.
典型的纤维肉瘤是无包膜、浸润性生长、质软和鱼肉状,常伴有坏死和出血。

fission [ˈfiʃən] *n.* 分裂;裂殖(法);(原子)核裂变
Bacteria reproduce by fission or simple splitting into parts.
细菌是用分裂或分成几个部分的方法来繁殖的。

fissure [ˈfiʃə] *n.* 裂伤
Fissures of the perianal skin may be associated with pruritus ani.
肛周皮肤的裂伤与肛门瘙痒有关。

fist [fist] *n.* 拳头
The heart is about the size of the closed fist.
心脏约为捏紧的拳头那样大小。

fistula [ˈfistjulə] (*pl.* fistulas 或 fistulae [ˈfistjuliə]) *n.* 瘘,瘘管
When the abscess is opened or when it ruptures, a fistula is formed.

当脓肿被切开或破裂时，就形成了一个瘘。

Fistulas located near the bladder neck may be troublesome.

存在于膀胱颈附近部位的瘘管是麻烦的。

fistulize [ˈfistjulaiz] *v.* 造瘘，造口

For almost a century the fistulizing procedures were the most popular in glaucoma.

过去将近一个世纪，造口术是青光眼手术中最普通的一种。

fistulous [ˈfistjuləs] *a.* 瘘管的

The double pylorus consists of fistulous communication between the gastric antrum and the duodenum.

双幽门是由胃窦与十二指肠之间形成瘘管所致。

Dural arteriovenous fistulous malformations are classified into three types based upon their anatomical similarities.

硬脑膜动静脉瘘样血管畸形依据解剖结构相似性可分为三种类型。

fit [fit] *n.* 突发，阵发，发作

When death occurs as the result of a fit it is usually the accidental result of the loss of consciousness.

当病人由于(癫痫)发作而死亡时，通常为意识丧失的偶然结果。

While risk of fits remains the patient must on no account be left unattended.

当依旧有发作的危险时，病人决不可无人照顾。

fitness [ˈfitnis] *n.* 适合度，适应性

Most deleterious dominant mutations have a fitness value between 0 and 1.

大多数有害显性突变的适合度在 0 ~ 1 之间。

fix [fiks] *v.* 固定，确定

The date for the heart surgery of this child is not completely fixed yet.

这个小孩心脏手术的日期尚未完全确定。

One end of a muscle is attached to a roughened area on bone or cartilage, while the other is fixed in a similar manner to an adjacent bone.

肌肉的一端附着在骨或软骨上的粗糙面，而另一端则以类似的方式附着在相邻的骨上。

Other viruses may gain access to cells indirectly via antibody and C3b fixed to the virus.

其他病毒可借助固定在病毒上的抗体和 C3b 分子间接进入细胞。

fixation [fikˈseiʃən] *n.* 固定，定位

We interpret these structural changes as a result of poor fixation.

我们把这些结构变化解释为固定不良的结果。

Her fixation point was on the left.

她的注视点在左边。

More important, the technique would provide enough stability to do away with external fixation devices, which often cause infections.

更为重要的是，该技术将提供足够的稳定性而取消常常引起感染的外部固定器械。

fixative [ˈfiksətiv] *n.* 固定液

The lethally injured cells placed immediately in fixative are dead but not necrotic.

致死性损伤的细胞立即放入固定液，这些细胞是死亡的，但不是坏死的。

10% neutral formalin is the most common used fixative.

10% 中性福尔马林是最常用的固定剂。

fixed [fikst] *a.* 固定的；不变的；不易挥发的

Fixed drug eruptions recur in the same location as circular areas of erythema.

固定性药疹常在同一部位复发，表现为圆形红斑。

In meningovascular neurosyphilis, the eyes may show fixed pupils.

脑膜血管性神经梅毒时，眼可出现瞳孔固定。

flabbiness [ˈflæbinis] *n.* 松弛

The infant may develop anorexia, flabbiness of subcutaneous tissues, and loss of muscle tone.

婴儿可能出现食欲缺乏、皮下组织松弛和肌肉张力缺失。

flaccid [ˈflæksid] *a.* 弛缓的

Flaccid paralysis is the most obvious clinical expression of the neuronal changes.

弛缓性麻痹系神经元变性在临床上最显著的表现。

flaccidity [flækˈsiditi] *n.* 软弱，没气力；松弛

Periods of hypertonicity may alternate with bouts of flaccidity.

周期性的张力过高可能与弛缓相交替。

This condition is affecting your spleen, causing your muscle atrophy and flaccidity.

这种情况会影响你的脾脏，造成肌肉萎缩和松弛。

flag [flæg] *n.* 旗帜；标记

Each type of NK cell can be inhibited by one or more HLA flags.

每种类型的天然杀伤细胞均能为 1 个或多个人体白细胞抗原标记所抑制。

flagellate [ˈflædʒəleit] *n.* 鞭毛虫

Flagellates are organisms with one or more whip-like organelles called flagella.

鞭毛虫是那些具有一根或多根称为鞭毛的鞭状细胞器结构的生物。

The word *flagellate* describes a particular construction of eukaryotic organism and its means of motion.

鞭毛虫这个词表达了真核生物的一种特殊结构及其运动方式。

flagellum [fləˈdʒeləm] （*pl.* flagella[fləˈdʒelə] ）*n.* 鞭毛，鞭节

Flagella are fine, whiplike organelles.

鞭毛是细小的鞭样的细胞器。

Flagella are involved in cellular swimming.

鞭毛参与细胞的游动。

flank [flæŋk] *n.* 胁；胁腹；侧面

In occipitoposterior position, the fetal heart sounds may be heard either in the flank or near the midline.

在枕后位时，胎心音可在母体胁腹或近中线处听到。

flap [flæp] *n.* 瓣，片

Surgery such as free skin flap transfer is now being performed routinely.

诸如游离皮瓣移植这类手术，现在已成为常规手术。

flask [flɑːsk] *n.* 烧瓶

Next, Pasteur removed the spinal cord of a rhabdovirus infected rabbit and dried it in a flask at room temperature.

接着，巴斯德把受棒状病毒感染兔的脊髓移出，在室温下的烧瓶中干燥。

As the cells fill up with mucus they have the appearance of a goblet or flask and are known as the goblet cells.

当这些细胞充满黏液时，它们有高脚杯或长颈瓶的外观，因而被称为杯状细胞。

flat [flæt] *a.* 平的，扁平的

The outer cells of the epidermis are flat and horny.

表皮的外层细胞呈扁平而角化。

Flat feet need treatment(exercises) only if they cause pain.

扁平足只有在出现疼痛时才有必要治疗。

Wheals are evanescent, edematous, flat elevations of various sizes.

风团是易消散的、水肿性的、大小 不等的平顶隆起。

flatten [ˈflætn] *v.* （使）变平

Expanding the ring flattens the cornea to correct a short sighted eye.

环舒张使角膜扁平以校正近视。

Note should be made of the general appearance of the abdomen, whether distended or flattened.

应注意腹部的一般外形，是膨胀还是平坦。

flatuence [ˈflætjuləns] *n.* 肠胃胀气

Excessive crying may cause aerophagia, which results in flatulence and abdominal distention.

过度哭闹会引起吞气症，导致气胀和腹胀。

One symptom of chronic gastritis is flatulence.

慢性胃炎的症状之一就是气胀。

flatulent [ˈflætjulənt] *a.* 胃肠胀气的

Fructooligosaccharide has light flatulent phenomenon at 30 times adult dosage.

给予 30 倍成人剂量的低聚果糖有轻微的胃肠胀气现象。

Flatulent dyspepsia is one of the commonest ailments of man.

胀气性消化不良是人类最常见的疾病之一。

flavin [ˈfleivin] *n.* 黄素

The flavin coenzymes take part in a large number of oxidation-reduction reactions.

黄素辅酶参与大量的氧化还原反应。

flavivirus [ˌfleivi ˈvaiərəs] *n.* 黄热病毒属（登革热）

Many flaviviruses are transmitted via arthropod vectors to humans.

很多黄热病毒通过节肢动物媒介而传播给人类。

West Nile Virus (WNV) is a member of the flavivirus genus.

西尼罗河病毒是黄热病毒属的一种。

flavo(u)r [ˈfleivə] *v.* 给…调味，加味于…

The dosage of flavored children's aspirin is now limited to 1.25 grain per tablet.

小儿服用的有香味的阿司匹林的剂量现在被限制为每片 1.25 格令。（注：1 格令 = 0.065 克）

n. 香料、香味、风味

Glutamic acid and its ions and salts, called glutamates, are flavor-enhancing compounds which provide an umami (savory) taste to food.

谷氨酸及其离子和盐（称谷氨酸盐）是增味剂，可以给食物添加鲜味。

When you have a cold, any food and drink sometimes has very little flavour to you.

患感冒时，任何食物和饮料有时对你都毫无滋味。

flavo(u)ring [ˈfleivəriŋ] *n.* 调味品，调味香料

Some flavorings have little food value.

有些调味品没有什么营养价值。

flaw [flɔː] *n.* 缺点；瑕疵；裂缝

Researchers reported that the tests can detect flaws in the skin cells of patient with Alzheimer's.

研究人员报道这套试验可探测到阿尔茨海默病患者皮肤细胞中的缺陷。

flexibility [ˌfleksəˈbiliti] *n.* 屈曲性；柔韧性；灵活性

As strength and flexibility improve, the patient gradually returns to normal activities.

随着力量和灵活性的不断提高，病人逐渐地恢复正常活动。

flexible [ˈfleksəbl] *a.* 易弯的，能屈的

Both erythrocytes and leucocytes are flexible.

红细胞和白细胞都具有伸缩性。

flexion [ˈflekʃən] *n.* 弯曲，弯曲部分

The degree of flexion of the head can often be made out by abdominal palpation.

胎头的俯屈程度常可通过腹部触诊得知。

In the patients operated on, all tight structures were released to obtain full flexion.

手术治疗的病人，术中凡紧张的结构均予松解，以获得充分的屈曲。

flexor [ˈfleksə] *n.* 屈肌

Management of flexor tendon injuries is one of the most demanding tasks in hand surgery.

对屈肌肌腱损伤的处理是手外科中要求最高的任务之一。

The aim of this study is to investigate the influence of hip proprioceptors on the organisation of the flexor reflex elicited by nociceptive stimulation in individuals with spinal cord injury.

这项研究的目的是要探究脊髓损伤的患者由伤害性刺激引起的屈肌反射对臀部本体感受器的影响。

float [fləut] *v.* 悬浮,飘浮

Prions are free-floating proteins.

朊病毒是一种自由悬浮的蛋白质。

Platelets are disc-shapped cells floating in blood.

血小板是飘浮在血液中的碟状细胞。

flocculant [ˈflɔkjulənt] *n.* 絮凝剂

The effectiveness of chitosan as a coagulant flocculant in surface water treatment has been studied.

对壳聚糖在地表水处理中作为絮凝剂的有效性已进行了研究。

Differential scanning calorimetry study and flocculant assay revealed high temperature stability of exopolysaccharide(EPS) up to 97℃.

差示扫描量热法研究和絮凝剂测量显示表多糖的高温稳定性可达 97℃。

flora [ˈflɔːrə] *n.* 菌丛

The intestinal flora of infants fed on human milk endows special benefits.

人乳喂养的婴儿的肠道菌丛具有特殊益处。

Solutions of some chemical compounds are used to reduce the microbial flora of the oral cavity.

有些化合物的溶液可以用来减少口腔中存在的菌丛。

floxuridine [flɔkˈsjuːridin] *n.* 氟尿嘧啶脱氧核苷

Floxuridine, belonging to the group of medicines known as antimetabolites, is used to treat some kinds of cancer.

氟尿嘧啶脱氧核苷属抗代谢物药类,用于治疗一些癌症。

Floxuridine interferes with the growth of cancer cells, which are eventually destroyed.

氟尿嘧啶脱氧核苷干扰癌细胞的生长并最终将其消灭。

The doctor should talk to the patient about the good floxuridine will do as well as the risks of using it.

医生应当告诉病人有关氟尿嘧啶脱氧核苷的治疗作用和使用此药的风险。

flucloxacillin [ˌfluːklɔksəˈsilin] *n.* 氟氯青霉素

The organism may not be penicillin sensitive, so flucloxacillin is the drug of choice.

本菌对青霉素不敏感,因而可选用氟氯青霉素治疗。

fluctuant [ˈflʌktjuənt] *a.* 波动的

Clinically an abscess first manifests itself as a hard, red, painful swelling which later softens and becomes fluctuant.

临床(可见)脓肿最初呈硬、红肿块,以后变软,并有波动性(变化)。

fluctuate [ˈflʌktjueit] *v.* 波动

The disease tends to fluctuate in severity.

该病的严重程度往往有波动。

Normal temperature fluctuates not only with the time of the day but also with the part of the body.

正常体温不仅在一天的时间内有波动,而且在身体各个部位也有变化。

fluctuation [ˌflʌktjuˈeiʃən] *n.* 波动

Fluctuation is a late sign of pyogenic abscess of breast.

波动是乳腺化脓性脓肿的晚期体征。

The symptoms last for several weeks or longer, during which time they may show marked fluctuations in intensity.

症状持续数周或更长，在此期间病情的严重程度可有明显的波动。

Therefore, data on the expected incidence of the different types of tumors in the control animals and on its fluctuations are available.

因此，关于对照动物的不同肿瘤的预期发生率及其波动范围的数据都是可利用的。

flucytosine [flu'saitəsiːn] *n.* 氟胞嘧啶

Flucytosine has been shown to be effective in the treatment of various systemic fungal infections.

氟胞嘧啶已被证实对各种全身性霉菌感染的治疗有效。

fluid [fluid] *n.* 液体，液

There are other masses of lymphoid tissue which are designed to filter not lymph, but tissue fluid.

另外还有一些淋巴组织构成的团块，其功能不是过滤淋巴液，而是组织液。

fluke [fluːk] *n.* 吸虫

The fluke matures in two to three weeks and begins to lay eggs.

2～3周时吸虫成熟并开始排卵。

fluorescence [fluə'resəns] *n.* 荧光

We studied on the theory and method in detecting colorectal cancer with laser-induced fluorescence.

我们研究了用激光诱导荧光检测大肠癌的理论与方法。

Ethanol solution can emit visible fluorescence when induced by UV light.

乙醇溶液在紫外光照射下可以发射荧光。

fluorescent [ˌfluə'resnt] *a.* 荧光的

Indirect fluorescent antibody test and hemagglutination test are of practical importance.

间接荧光抗体试验和血细胞凝集试验具有实际重要性。

fluoride ['fluəraid] *n.* 氟化物

The water supply of this city contains adequate amounts of fluoride.

这个城市供应的自来水含有适量的氟化物。

Fluoride may cause health problems if present in public or private water supplies in amounts greater than the drinking water standard set by EPA.

如果公共或私人供水中氟化物的量高于美国环保署规定的饮用水标准，则可能引起健康问题。

Skeletal fluorosis is a bone disease caused by excessive intake of fluoride.

氟骨症是由摄入过量氟所引起的一种骨疾病。

fluorimetry [ˌfluːə'rimitri] *n.* 荧光测定法

Fluorimetry is a type of electromagnetic spectroscopy which analyzes fluorescence from a sample.

荧光测定法是一种分析样品荧光的电磁光谱方法。

This paper deals with advanced aspects of fluorimetry as applied to clinical chemistry.

本文论述了荧光测定法应用于临床化学分析的先进方面。

fluorochrome ['fluərəkrɔm] *n.* 荧色物，[试剂] 荧光染料

A fluorochrome commonly conjugated with antibodies for use in indirect immunofluorescence.

荧光染料通常连接到抗体上用于间接免疫荧光法。

The fluorochrome of the sex-linkaged cocoon fluorescent color variety "Yingguang" is studied by the UV spectral photometry and paper chromatography.

用紫外光谱分析和纸层析法，对性连锁的蚕茧荧光染料品种"荧光"的荧光素进行了研究。

fluoroscopy [fluə'rɔskəpi] *n.* X 线透视检查，荧光镜检查

Fluoroscopy is a type of medical imaging that shows a continuous x-ray image on a monitor, much like an x-ray movie.

X 线透视检查是一种能在监视器上显示连续性 X 线图像的医学成像术，很像 X 线电影。

Angiography is the use of fluoroscopy to view the cardiovascular system.

血管造影是利用 X 线透视检查来查看心血管系统。

fluorosis [fluə'rəusis] *n.* 氟中毒

Dental fluorosis is characterized by mottled enamel, which is opaque and may be stained.

牙齿氟中毒的特点是：出现斑釉色，即釉质无光泽并被着色。

Changes in fatty acid composition of phospholipid in SH-SY5Y Cells are caused by fluorosis.

氟中毒引起 SH-SY5Y 神经细胞磷脂的脂肪酸组成改变。

The chronic fluorosis appeared after 16-30 days.

慢性氟中毒在 16 ~ 30 天后出现。

fluorouracil [ˌfluərə'juərəsil]（缩 5-Fu）*n.* 氟尿嘧啶（抗肿瘤药）

Fluorouracil is also applied as a cream to treat certain skin conditions, including skin cancer.

氟尿嘧啶也可以霜剂的形式治疗某些皮肤病，包括皮肤癌。

A few toxicants, e. g. ,5-fluorouracil, thallium, and lead, are known to be absorbable from the intestine by active transport system.

已知少数毒物，如 5-氟尿嘧啶、铊和铅，可以通过主动转运系统经肠道吸收。

flush [flʌʃ] *n.* 红润，潮红

Hectic flush occurs in such wasting diseases as pulmonary tuberculosis.

痨病患者的面色潮红见于消耗性疾病，如肺结核。

Episodic flushing, especially of the face, lasting some 10 to 30 minutes, is a consistent sign of carcinoid syndrome.

特别是面部的持续 10 ~ 30 分钟的阵发性潮红，是类癌综合征始终如一的体征。

Bronchial asthma is characterized by respiratory distress, flushing and cyanosis.

支气管哮喘表现为呼吸困难、面红和发绀。

flutamide ['flutəmaid] *n.* 氟他胺，氟硝丁酰胺

Flutamide, taken by mouth in tablet form, is used to treat prostate cancer.

氟他胺为片剂，口服用于治疗前列腺癌。

flutter ['flʌtə] *n.* 扑动

Atrial flutter and fibrillation may be transient.

心房扑动和纤颤可能是暂时的。

focal ['fəukəl] *a.* 病灶的，灶（性）的

Some cells show what appears to be areas of focal degeneration.

有的细胞显示有灶性退行性变化。

Atheromatous narrowing of the arteries which supply the brain predisposes to focal loss of neurons.

分布在脑内的动脉的粥样硬化性狭窄易引起局部的神经细胞丧失。

focus(on) ['fəukəs]（*pl.* focuses 或 foci['fəusai]）*n.* 焦距，焦点，（病）灶

A near-sighted eye has a shorter focus than a normal eye.

近视眼的焦距比正常眼睛要短。

Focus is on the problem of environmental pollution.

焦点（或重点）放在环境污染的问题上。

The combination of a focus with regional lymph node involvement is called the primary complex.

病灶伴有局部淋巴结侵犯称为“原发性综合病变”。

The foci of ectopic endometrium are actually continuous with the normal endometrium.

异位子宫内膜病灶和正常的子宫内膜实际上是连接的。

v. 聚焦，集中

The medical specialists focus their attention on the problem of environmental pollution.

医学专家们把他们的注意力集中在环境污染的问题上。

foe [fəu] *n.* 敌人,危害物

Dirt is a dangerous foe to health.

污物对健康极为有害。

foetal [ˈfiːtl] *a.* 胎儿的

Foetal haemoglobin is low in sickle cell anemia.

镰状细胞性贫血的胎儿血红蛋白是低的。

The influence of foetal gender has been found.

已经发现对胎儿性别的影响。

fog [fɔg] *n.* 雾

The wind soon dispelled the fog.

风很快把雾吹散了。

He disappeared in the dense fog.

他消失在浓雾里。

folate [ˈfəuleit] *n.* 叶酸

Chronic malaria depletes folates store especially during pregnancy.

慢性疟疾使叶酸的储量减少,特别在妊娠期。

Parenteral administration of folate will overcome these deficiencies.

肠道外给予叶酸治疗可纠正这些缺乏症。

folic acid [ˈfəulikˈæsid] *n.* 叶酸

Folic acid is one of the water soluble vitamins.

叶酸是水溶性维生素之一。

follicle [ˈfɔlikl] *n.* 小囊,卵泡

The whole structure of the follicle takes on a yellow colour and is therefore known as the corpus luteum.

整个卵泡结构呈现黄色,故称为黄体。

A boil is an abscess of a hair follicle or a sebaceous gland, caused by the staphylococcus aureus.

疖是金黄色葡萄球菌引起的毛囊(即皮脂腺)脓肿。

follicular [fɔˈlikjulə] *a.* 滤泡性的,卵泡的

The hallmark of all follicular adenomas is the presence of an intact, well-formed capsule encircling the tumor.

滤泡性腺瘤的特征是具有完整而良好的包膜围绕肿瘤。

Follicular cyst is one of the common non-neoplastic cysts closely related with gynecologic endocrine dysfunction

卵泡囊肿是妇科一种常见的非肿瘤性囊肿,与内分泌功能紊乱密切相关。

folliculitis [fəˌlikjuˈlaitis] *n.* 毛囊炎

The infective rate in those suffering from rosacea, folliculitis, acne vulgaris or seborrheic dermatitis was higher than the normal ones.

面部皮肤有酒糟鼻、毛囊炎、痤疮或脂溢性皮炎的患者感染率高于面部皮肤健康者。

They studied on the neutrophilic folliculitis and the spectrum of pyoderma gangrenosum in inflammatory bowel disease.

他们研究了炎症性肠病中的中性粒细胞性毛囊炎和坏疽性脓皮病谱。

follow [ˈfɔləu] *v.* 接着,跟随;遵循

Disease often follows starvation because the body is weakened.

饥饿后常常生病,因为此时身体变虚弱了。

Constrictive pericarditis never follows acute rheumatic fever.

急性风湿热决不会引起缩窄性心包炎。

A patient must follow the doctor's advice.

病人必须遵从医嘱。

The doctor followed the patient for 2 months and found a quick postoperative recovery.

医生对病人进行了两个月的随访，发现手术后的恢复很快。

The main points of Freud's theory are as follows.

弗洛伊德学说的主要论点如下。

following [ˈfɔləuiŋ] *a.* 接着的；下列的；下述的

The atmospheric oxidation of methyl-tert-butyl ether can be summarized in the following formulas.

甲基-叔-丁基酯的大气氧化作用可以归纳为如下公式。

The epidermis may be divided into the following zones: basal layer, malpighian or prickle layer, granular layer, and horny layer, or stratum corneam.

表皮可分为下列各层：基底层、马尔匹基层或棘层、颗粒层和角化层或角质层。

A typical low-pitched rumbling diastolic murmur commences immediately following the opening snap.

典型低调的隆隆样舒张期杂音在开瓣音之后立即出现。

The following are terms of immunology. Please translate them into Chinese.

下面是免疫学名词，请将它们翻译成中文。

The professor asked the interns the following questions about genetic heritance.

教授问了实习医生一些有关基因遗传的下列问题。

follow-up [ˈfɔləuˌʌp] *n.* 随访

The patients must be cooperative and amenable to careful follow-up.

患者必须合作并密切配合随诊。

Despite intensive treatment and close follow-up, the patient had frequent severe asthma attacks.

尽管进行了深入细致的治疗和密切的随访，病人仍常出现严重哮喘发作。

fontanel(le) [ˌfɔntəˈnel] *n.* 囟，囟门

The degree of flexion or extension of the head can be found by palpation of the fontanelles.

头的屈曲或仰伸程度可通过触诊囟门发现。

food [fuːd] *n.* 食物，食品

They must find food to eat.

他们必须要找到食物充饥。

This is the kind of food everyone likes.

这是一种每个人都喜欢的食物。

foodstuff [ˈfuːdstʌf] *n.* 食物

Biochemistry involves a study of the major foodstuffs and their utilization by the body.

生物化学包含对主要食物及身体利用这些食物的研究。

Under these circumstances, the total energy obtained from foodstuff breakdown is greatly reduced.

在这些情况下，由食物分解所获取的总能量明显降低。

foramen [fəˈreimən] (*pl.* foramina [fəˈræminə]) *n.* 孔

Each transverse process of vertebra is pierced by a foramen.

每个脊椎横突都是穿孔的。

The nerves of the brain come out through foramina in the skull wall.

脑的神经通过颅壁的孔延伸出来。

forceps [ˈfɔːseps] *n.* 钳，产钳

If forceps delivery is attempted the head should be pressed down as far as possible by abdominal pressure from an assistant.

如试图用产钳助产，应让助手在腹部加压将胎头尽可能压低。

forearm [ˈfɔːrɑːm] *n.* 前臂

The forearm has been in cast for 3 days already.
前臂石膏固定已有三天了。

foregoing [fɔːˈgəuiŋ] *a.* 前述的，前面的

The foregoing have all been included in the proposals.
前面所提到的（事项）已经全部包括在本提案之中。

foreign [ˈfɔrin] *a.* 异质的，外来的

A foreign body known to have been swallowed may become lodged in the recesses of the hypopharynx.
已知的异物被吞下可停留在下咽部的隐窝中。

Respiratory obstruction may be caused by such foreign objects as chunks of food or trinkets.
呼吸道堵塞可能由食物团块或小玩物等异物引起。

The recognition of foreign antigen is the hallmark of the specific adaptive immune response.
外来抗原的识别是特异的适应性免疫应答的特点。

foreignness [ˈfɔrinis] *n.* 外国（人）的特性，外来性，异物性

Americans are willing to accept new things and foreignness.
美国人喜欢接受新事物和外来的东西

Five important factors in the effective functioning of antigens are foreignness, degradability, molecular weight, structural stability, and complexity.
异物性、可降解性、分子量、结构稳定性和复杂性是影响抗原有效功能的五大因素。

forelimb [ˈfɔːlim] *n.* 前肢

The doctor said the problem lied in its forelimb and it would not die.
医生说问题在于它的前肢上，不过它不会死的。

We also found that retinoic acid was unnecessary for hindlimb budding, but was needed for forelimb budding.
同时我们也发现视黄酸只对前肢的发育有决定作用，后肢则没有。

forelock [ˈfɔːlɔk] *n.* 额毛，额发

A case with congenital sensorineural hearing loss, characteristic blue irises, white forelock and congenital leucoderma is described as Waardenburg syndrome (WS).
报告 1 例 Waardenburg 综合征，具有先天性感觉神经性耳聋、特征性的蓝色虹膜、前额白发以及先天性白斑。

forerunner [ˈfɔːrʌnə] *n.* 先驱，前兆

Whether this stage of chloramphenicol toxicity is a forerunner of aplastic anemia is unknown.
氯霉素的此期毒性是否就是再障贫血的前期，尚不清楚。

forever [fəˈrevə(r)] *ad.* 不断地，永恒地

Why are you forever asking the same questions?
为什么你老是提相同的问题？

We will carry on Dr. Bethune's spirit of selflessness forever.
我们将永远继承白求恩医生无私的精神。

form [fɔːm] *n.* 表格 *v.* 形成

In this paper, we introduce a system being able to read statistical forms.
在本文中，我们介绍一个能阅读统计表格的系统。

They wanted to know what gives such cells the ability to form tumours.
他们想知道究竟是什么使这些细胞能够形成肿瘤。

formaldehyde [fɔːˈmældihaid] *n.* 甲醛

Formaldehyde is an organic compound, known to be a human carcinogen.
甲醛是一种有机化合物，被认为是一种人类的致癌物。

After Vladimir Lenin died in 1924, his brain was preserved in a formaldehyde solution.
弗拉基米尔·列宁于 1924 年去世，他的大脑被保存在甲醛溶液里。

formality [fɔːˈmæliti] *n.* 形式

She was already assured of the job and the interview was only a formality.

她已被告知获得该项工作，而面谈只不过是一种形式。

format [ˈfɔːmæt] *n.* （出版物的）版式，形式，格式

Particularly welcome is the self-teaching format of the book.

本书便于自学的编排方式特别受欢迎。

Therefore, the fastest way to store and retrieve this data is in binary format.

因此，存储并检索此数据的最快方式是运用二进制格式。

formidable [ˈfɔːmidəbl] *a.* 可怕的，难以克服的

Childbirth and the immediate postpartum period impose a formidable stress on the maternal coagulation system.

分娩和产褥初期对母体的凝血系统可能产生可怕的影响。

formula [ˈfɔːmjulə] *n.* 分子式，公式；处方，婴儿食物配方

The formula for water is H_2O.

水的分子式是 H_2O。

The most widely used formula for relating height and weight is the body mass index(BMI), which is weight/(height)^2.

有关身高和体重的最常用公式是体重指数（BMI），即体重/身高的平方。

These are drugs of official formula.

这些都属法定处方药品。

This child was put on soy formula because of a strong family history of allergy.

这小儿有明显的家族过敏史，所以用豆制品配制的食物喂养。

formulate [ˈfɔːmjuleit] *v.* 使公式化，系统地阐述

The generally accepted criteria of diagnosis are those formulated by Smith.

一般公认的诊断标准是由史密斯所阐述的。

fornix [ˈfɔːniks] *n.* 穹隆

The fornix is a major efferent tract of the hippocampus, a structure critical for normal memory function.

穹隆是一个主要的海马传出束，是正常记忆功能的重要结构。

The role of structural degradation of the fornix in memory dysfunction in mild cognitive impairment has remained unclear.

穹隆的结构退化在轻度认知受损时记忆功能异常中的作用尚不明确。

fortnight [ˈfɔːtnait] *n.* 两周

Isolate patients who are sputum-positive for first fortnight of treatment.

对痰阳性患者首先隔离治疗两周。

During acute glomerulonephritis the pyrexia subsides in two to three days and in the great majority recovery is complete in a fortnight or so.

急性肾小球肾炎时，发烧经 2 ~ 3 天消退，而且大部分患者在二周左右即可完全康复。

fossa [ˈfɔsə]（*pl.* fossae[ˈfɔsiː]）*n.* 窝，凹

Skull fractures in the anterior cranial fossae deserve special comment.

颅前窝的颅骨骨折需要进行特别评论。

foul [faul] *a.* 难闻的，恶臭的

During infectious hepatitis the breath is extremely foul-smelling, as is the odor of the stools.

当患有传染性肝炎时，其呼气有难闻的气味，犹如粪便的恶臭。

foundation [faunˈdeiʃən] *n.* 基础，基金，基金会

This project was supported by National Natural Science Foundation of China (Grant No. 30325614)

此项目得到（中国）国家自然科学基金的资助。（资助编号:30325614）

founder [ˈfaundə] *n.* 奠基者，创立者，创始人，起始

As chairperson and founder of the music therapy department at Berklee College of Music, would you explain what music therapy is?

作为波克丽音乐学院音乐治疗系的主任和音乐疗法的创始人，您可以解释一下什么是音乐疗法么？

Most founder mutations are recessive: only a person with two copies of the affected gene, one from each parent, will suffer from the disease.

大部分起始突变都是隐性的：只有来源父母双方的两份基因都受到影响时才会发病。

fowl [faul] *n.* 禽，家禽

Avian influenza is a disease of bird including domestic fowl characterized by respiratory, gastrointestinal and encephalitic symptoms.

禽流感是一种包括家禽在内的鸟类的一种疾患，其特征有呼吸系统、胃肠道和脑炎性症状。

fraction [ˈfrækʃən] *n.* 部分；分数

A minor fraction of deaths in infancy is caused by mechanical asphyxia.

婴儿期的死亡只有很少部分是由机械性窒息引起。

fracture [ˈfræktʃə] *n.* 骨折

A careful search for fractures should be performed in all patients with a significant history of head trauma.

对于所有有明显头部外伤史的病人，都应该仔细检查是否有骨折。

v. 断裂，折断

Fractured ribs over the liver should suggest liver injury.

肝区肋骨有断裂时应考虑肝损伤。

fragile [ˈfrædʒail] *a.* 脆的，易碎的

Fragile X syndrome is caused by dynamic mutation.

脆性 X 染色体综合征是由动态突变引起的。

Chromosome fragile sites are gaps or breaks in chromosomes.

染色体脆性位点是染色体上的小沟或裂隙。

fragility [frəˈdʒiliti] *n.* 脆性，脆弱

The basic abnormility of the red cell can be demonstrated by osmotic fragility studies.

红细胞的基本异常可以从渗透压脆性试验中得到证实。

Scurvy is a disease characterized by muscular pain, weakness, hemorrhages, fragility of bones and loosening and decay of the teeth.

坏血病的特征是肌肉疼痛、虚弱、出血、骨质脆弱、牙齿松动变质。

fragment [ˈfrægmənt] *n.* 断片，碎片

Such cloned DNA fragments could provide the basis for simple and rapid tests for the presence of that type of organism in a clinical specimen.

这种克隆的 DNA 片段，为简便快速地检测临床标本中微生物的型别奠定了基础。

The bicuspids and molars serve to grind and crush the food into very fine fragments.

前磨牙和磨牙可用以将食物磨压成很细的碎片。

fragmentation [ˌfrægmənˈteiʃən] *n.* 分裂，破碎，断裂

In circumstances of chronic intravascular hemolysis, RBC fragmentation may produce Fe lack by chronic hemoglobinuria and hemosiderinuria.

在慢性血管内溶血的情况下，红细胞的碎裂可因慢性血红蛋白尿和含铁血黄素尿而造成缺铁。

frail [freil] *a.* 脆弱的，虚弱的

Although the worst effects of air pollution were on those who were frail, elderly or sick, healthy individuals were affected too.

尽管空气污染最坏的作用体现在那些身体虚弱、年老或生病的人身上,但健康人亦受其影响。

frameshift [ˈfreimʃift] *n.* 移码突变

Such mutations are called "frameshifts".

这种突变称为移码突变。

framework [ˈfreimwəːk] *n.* 结构;构架组织;支架

Scleral framework is the larger and coarser part of the angle of the iris which is adjacent to the sclera.

巩膜构架组织是虹膜角的较大和较粗的部分,它靠近巩膜。

The capsule of the spleen, as well as its framework, is more elastic than that of the lymph nodes.

脾的被膜和基本结构较淋巴结(的被膜和构架)更富弹性。

frank [fræŋk] *a.* 症状明显的

If bleeding, frank or occult, has occured anemia is added to this.

如果已有出血,不论是明显出血还是潜血,其外观皆表现为贫血。

At autopsy, the patient's own emphysematous right lung contained frank abscesses with an almost pure growth of Pseudomonas.

尸检发现,患有肺气肿的右肺有明显的脓肿,并有一块几乎纯粹的假单胞菌的增生物。

frankincense [ˈfræŋkinsens] *n.* 乳香

The phoenix was said to build its own funeral pyre out of myrrh, frankincense and other spices.

凤凰据说是燃烧没药、乳香和其他香料来建立其葬火。

Frankincense is a sweet smelling gum resin.

乳香是一种芳香气味的树胶脂。

free [friː] *a.* 游离的

At a given total plasma concentration only a portion of the total amount of drug is free in the plasma water.

在一定总血浆浓度中,药物总量中只有一部分在血浆中是游离的。

Free frucrose is taken in fruit and honey.

游离果糖可从水果和蜂蜜中摄入。

fremitus [ˈfremitəs] *n.* 震颤

The vibrations produced over the chest wall by vocal sound are called vocal fremitus.

由语音产生的胸壁震动称作语音震颤。

freon [ˈfriːɔn] *n.* 氟利昂

Freon is a widely used coolant in refrigerators and air conditioners.

氟利昂是冰箱和空调中广泛使用的制冷剂。

Freon was used in a wide variety of applications, until growing evidence suggested that it was contributing to damage in the ozone layer which protects the Earth.

人们曾广泛地使用氟利昂,直至越来越多的证据表明该物质导致地球保护层—臭氧层的破坏。

frequency [ˈfriːkwənsi] *n.* 频繁,次数,频率

The frequency of AA genotype was higher in the control subjects(97%) as compared to all in the patient group.

对照组受试者的 AA 基因型频率(97%)显著高于所有病例组成员。

The important aspect of gastric ulcers is the frequency of malignancy.

胃溃疡的重要特征是常呈恶性。

frequent [ˈfriːkwənt] *a.* 常见的,经常的

Otitis media is also a frequent complication of measles, influenza, scarlet fever and other infections.

中耳炎是麻疹、流行性感冒、猩红热和其他感染的常见并发症。

Exposure to hazards in the workplace and the environment is a frequent occurrence.
在工作场所内和环境中接触有害物质是经常发生的。
In aplastic anemia hemorrhages into ocular fundi are frequent.
再生障碍贫血时常有眼底出血。

frequently [ˈfriːkwəntli] *ad.* 常见地,经常地
The cornea is referred to frequently as the"window"of the eye.
角膜常常被称为眼睛的窗户。
The cases of lead encephalopathy were noted more frequently in summer than in winter.
铅毒性脑病的病例在夏天要比冬天多见。

freshener [ˈfreʃnə] *n.* 清新剂
Electronic nose could quantify the effectiveness of air fresheners for aerosol manufacturers.
电子鼻可帮助气雾剂制造商们用来量化空气清新剂的效果。

friability [ˌfraiəˈbiliti] *n.* 易碎性,脆性
A cervical chancre differs from a carcinoma in the lesser degree of friability and lesser tendency to bleed on examination.
宫颈下疳与癌的区别在于前者脆性程度较轻,检查时出血倾向较小。
The physical parameters(crushing strength and friability) of all formulated batches were within acceptable limits.
所有批次制剂的物理参数(抗压强度和脆碎度)均在可接受的范围内。
Both types of pellets were evaluated for particle size,flow,friability,dissolution and content uniformity.
评估了两种类型的丹药的颗粒大小、流动性、脆碎度、溶出度和均匀度。

friction [ˈfrikʃən] *n.* 摩擦
The heart changes its shape and size during each beat and friction damage is prevented by the arrangement of pericardium and its serous fluid.
每一次心跳时,心脏都改变其形状和大小,而有了心包和心包液则可防止摩擦损伤。
Excoriations are caused by scratching with the fingernails by other mechanical trauma,and even from constant friction.
表皮剥脱是由手指搔抓或由其他机械性外伤,甚至由经常不断的摩擦而引起的。

frightening [ˈfraitniŋ] *a.* 令人吃惊的
Even relatively small amounts of blood is a frightening symptom.
即使有少量的出血也是一个严重的症状。

frontal [ˈfrʌntəl] *a.* 额的
Errors of refraction and muscle imbalance may lead to frontal headache in persons involved in close work or prolonged study.
屈光不正和肌平衡失调可导致视近工作或长时间学习者额部头痛。

frontalis [frʌnˈteilis;ˈfrʌntəlis] *a.* 额的
Frequently no ocular cause can be found and the frontal headache must be ascribed to overuse of the frontalis muscle or to anxiety.
前额疼痛常不能从眼睛上找到原因,必须用额肌使用过度或经常忧虑来解释。

frostbite [ˈfrɔstbait] *n.* 冻疮,霜害
Frostbite or sunburn may also initiate such inflammatory responses as heat and pain.
冻疮或晒斑也可引起发热和疼痛等炎症反应。

fructan [ˈfrʌktən] *n.* 果聚糖
The body weights of animals did not change significantly indicating that the administration of garlic fructans is well-tolerated.
动物的体重并没有显著变化,表明动物对大蒜果聚糖有良好的耐受性。
This behavior suggests a relationship between 1-FFT enzymatic activity and the concentration of

fructans.

这种反应表明了 1-果糖基转移酶的活性和果聚糖浓度之间的关系。

fructose [ˈfrʌktəus] *n.* 果糖,左旋糖

Fructose is largely derived from dietary sucrose.

果糖主要来自饮食中的蔗糖。

fruitful [ˈfruːtful] *a.* 富有成效的,丰富的

A particularly fruitful approach has been chromosome walking.

染色体步移一直是一种特别有效的方法。

A recent dialog between wildlife management biologists and toxicologists promised fruitful results in modeling effects of chemicals on populations.

最近,一场野生生物管理学家与毒理学家的对话有望就化学物质对种群的模式作用获得丰富的成果。

frustrate [ˈfrʌstreit] *v.* 阻挠,使感到灰心

Malnutrition remains one of the most frustrating and troublesome complications of ARF.

营养不良仍然是急性肾衰(ARF)最难以纠正和最麻烦的并发症之一。

frustration [frʌsˈtreiʃən] *n.* 挫折

One is bound to suffer frustrations and setbacks.

每个人都会遇到这样或那样的坎坷与挫折。

fuel [fjuəl] *n.* 燃料

Consumers need to spend more on food and fuel now.

如今,消费者需要在食品和燃料上花费更多。

The fuel might be wood, charcoal or any other burnable material.

燃料可以是木材、木炭或者其他任何可燃的物质。

fugax [ˈfjuːgæks] *a.* 一时的,暂时的

Amaurosis fugax is characterized by unilateral transient diminution or loss of vision that develops over seconds, remains for 1-5 minutes at most, and resolves in 10-20 minutes.

一过性黑矇以单眼短暂性视力下降或丧失为特征,可在数秒钟发生,最多持续 1 ~5 分钟,10 ~20 分钟消退。

Proctalgia fugax is a severe, episodic rectal and sacrococcygeal pain.

痉挛性肛部痛是一种严重的偶然发生的直肠和骶尾部疼痛。

fulfill [fulˈfil] *v.* 实现,完成

It has not fulfilled all the early expectations.

这并没有实现所有先前的设想。

fullerene [ˈfuləriːn] *n.* 碳簇

Since the discovery of fullerenes in 1985 and carbon nanotube in 1991, they have attracted increasing attention because of their particular structure, and their unique physical, chemical and electric properties.

自 1985 年发现碳簇和 1991 年发现碳纳米管以来,这两个纳米材料就因它们独特的结构、特有的物理、化学、电学性质而备受人们关注。

full-term [ˈfulˈtəːm] *a.* 足月的

She gave a full-term birth to a boy last night.

她昨夜产下一个足月男孩。

Breast milk is the natural food for full-term infants during the first months of life.

母乳对足月的婴儿在头几个月是天然的食物。

fulminant [ˈfʌlminənt] *a.* 暴发性的

Rarely, a more fulminant form occurs with high fevers, severe abdominal pain, and profuse diarrhea, mostly seen in children.

暴发性阿米巴肠炎罕见,多发生于儿童,表现为高热、剧烈腹痛和严重腹泻。

fulminating ['fʌlmineitiŋ] *a.* 暴发性的

A fulminating attack of rheumatic fever of a child may hit the myocardium heavily.

儿童暴发性的风湿热发作可使心肌受到严重损伤。

The onset of acute meningitis may be fulminating, acute, or less commonly, insidious.

急性脑炎的发病可呈暴发性、急性或在少数情况下呈隐袭性。

function ['fʌŋkʃən] *v.* (器官等)活动;起作用

Dopamine functions as a neurotransmitter in the central nervous system, but not in the periphery.

多巴胺作为一种神经递质对中枢神经系统起作用,而不是作用于外周(神经)。

The darker cells may function in a manner similar to that of cells of the dermal duct.

深染细胞的作用方式与真皮导管细胞相似。

n. 功能

I realized this when learning about the structure and function of the stomach.

我也是学习了胃部的结构和功能后才意识到这点的。

A tissue is a group of similar cells which have an identical general function.

组织是一组具有相同的一般功能的类似细胞。

functional ['fʌŋkʃənəl] *a.* 功能的;起作用的

Congestive heart failure is classed according to functional capacity.

充血性心力衰竭根据心功能状况进行分级。

A functional disease is one in which the function of a part of the body is impaired.

功能性疾病就是人体某一部分的功能受到损伤。

Collateral vessels are silent blood vessels that become functional in hypoxic emergencies.

侧支血管为静息血管,仅在缺氧的紧急情况下才发挥作用。

functionality [ˌfʌŋkʃə'næliti] *n.* 功能,具有功能性

By the age of 20 the thymus, the only organ which produces T-cells, is down to 1% functionality.

到 20 岁时,体内生产 T 细胞的惟一器官胸腺仅具有 1% 的功能作用。

functionally ['fʌŋkʃənəli] *ad.* 功能上

The close linkage of functionally related gene is surely of value to the organism.

功能上有关联的基因的紧密连锁,对机体无疑是重要的。

fundamental [ˌfʌndə'mentəl] *a.* 基本的,基础的

A Gene is the fundamental physical and functional unit of heredity.

基因是遗传的基本结构单位和功能单位。

fundoplication ['fʌndəupli'keiʃən] *n.* 胃底折叠术

Fundoplication is a surgical procedure to treat gastroesophageal reflux disease (GERD) and hiatus hernia.

胃底折叠术是治疗胃食管反流疾病和食管裂孔疝的一种外科手术。

In the Nissen fundoplication, the fundus wraps all the way 360 degrees around the esophagus.

在 Nissen 胃底折叠术中,胃底折叠区围绕食管一周,即 360 度折叠。

fundus ['fʌndəs] (*pl.* fundi ['fʌndai]) *n.* 底,基底

The stomach is divided into a fundus, a body and a pyloric portion.

胃分为胃底、胃体和幽门部。

If twins are present the uterus also appears wide but the height of the fundus will be higher than normal.

如为双胎,子宫也较宽,但宫底比正常要高。

funduscopic ['fʌndəskəupik] *a.* 眼底镜的

The funduscopic examination is an integral part of the neurologic examination, and papilledema is always sought.

眼底镜检查是神经系统检查的一个组成部分,往往要检查有无乳头水肿。

funduscopy [ˌfʌn'dʌskəpi] *n.* 眼底镜检查

Funduscopy and visual fields by confrontation were unremarkable.
眼底镜检查和对诊法查视野无异常。

fungal [ˈfʌŋgəl] *a.* 真菌的,霉菌的
Endocarditis due to fungal infection is invariably fatal.
由真菌感染引起的心内膜炎其结果总是致命的。
When clinically appropriate, tuberculosis and fungal cultures should be requested.
在临床需要时,应要求对患者进行结核菌或霉菌的培养。

fungicide [ˈfʌndʒisaid] *n.* 杀真菌剂
A fungicide kills fungi, a virucide inactivates viruses.
杀真菌剂杀死真菌,杀病毒剂使病毒失去活力。

funguria [fʌŋˈgjuəriə] *n.* 霉菌尿
Those pathogens associated with funguria include Candida albicans.
与霉菌尿相关的致病菌包括白假丝酵母菌。

fungus [ˈfʌŋgəs] (*pl.* fungi [ˈfʌŋgai]) *n.* 真菌
The fungi are immotile, nonphotosynthetic protists.
真菌是无活动力、无光合作用的原生生物。
The true fungi are another large group of simple plants.
真菌是简单植物中的另一大类。

funnel [ˈfʌnəl] *n.* 漏斗
In funnel chest the body of the sternum, usually only the lower end, is curved backwards.
在漏斗胸(患者),其胸骨体下端常向后背方向弯曲。

furazolidone [ˌfjuərəˈzɔlidəun] *n.* 呋喃唑酮(抗菌药)
Other antibiotics, including chloramphenicol and furazolidone, and slightly less effective than tetracycline.
其他抗生素包括氯霉素及呋喃唑酮等的疗效要比四环素稍微差一些。

furnace [ˈfəːnis] *n.* 炉,灶
In 1993 there were 184 hazardous waste incinerators in the United States. About 164 plants burn hazardous wastes as fuel in cement kilns, boilers, and industrial furnaces.
1993 年,在美国约有 184 座有害废物焚化炉。约 164 个工厂在水泥窑、锅炉及工业加热炉中用有害废料作燃料。

furnish [ˈfəːniʃ] *v.* 供应,提供,装备
The physician should assume the responsibility to furnish or arrange for physical, emotional, and spiritual support.
医生应该承担起为病人提供或安排身体的、情感的和精神上支持的责任。
Investigations have furnished ideas as to how foods are broken down and how they are built in living cells.
研究显示了食物如何在活细胞内被分解和合成。
The well-being of each individual cell is dependent on the adequacy of its environment to furnish nutrition and carry away metabolites.
各个细胞的健康有赖于周围环境供应充足的营养和运走代谢产物。

furosemide [fjuəˈrəusəmaid] *n.* 速尿,速尿灵
Furosemide is chemically related to the thiazide diuretics.
速尿灵的化学结构与噻嗪类利尿剂类似。

furthermore [fəːðəˈmɔː] *ad.* 而且,此外
Furthermore, it guides the next step system design and development in the collaborated environment to reduce the project risk.
而且,它将指导在协作环境中的下一步系统设计和开发工作,从而减少项目风险。
Furthermore, no study has investigated the relationship between platelet reactivity and inflamma-

tion in unstable angina patients.

此外,还没有研究涉及不稳定心绞痛病人血小板反应性和炎症的关系。

furuncle ['fjuərʌŋkl] *n.* 疖

A more extensive and invasive follicular infection with some involvement of subcutaneous tissue is termed a furuncle.

当毛囊感染扩展并侵及皮下组织时称为疖。

fuse [fjuːz] *v.* 熔合,熔化

Lysosomes can be observed fusing with membrane vesicles that have budded in from the surface membrane.

可观察到溶酶体可以与由表面膜(结构)内陷形成的膜性小泡相溶合。

fusiform ['fjuːzifɔːm] *a.* 梭形的;纺锭状的;两端渐细的

In general,the endothelial cells in different arterial segments were fusiform. Their long axes were consistent with the direction of the blood flow.

在不同动脉段内皮细胞一般呈梭形(核区较隆起),其长轴与血流的方向一致。

It is further helpful to classify aneurysms into saccular and fusiform.

更有帮助的是把动脉瘤分成囊形和梭形两类

fusion ['fjuːʒən] *n.* 融合,融合物

Bacteria fusion promises to be a major advance in research involving microbial genetics.

细菌融合有望成为微生物遗传学研究中的一大进展。

This linguistic fusion is now a familiar dialect spoken by young people in cities across Britain.

现在,这种语言融合已成为英国各个城市年轻人都常使用的方言。

futility [fju'tiləti] *n.* 无益,无效

Periods of depression are marked by worry,pessimism,low output of energy and a sense of futility.

抑郁期明显的特征表现为焦虑、悲观、缺乏活力和徒劳无益的感觉。

G

gadolinium [ˈɡædəliniəm] *n.* 钆

Like most rare earths, gadolinium forms trivalent ions which have fluorescent properties.

像多数稀土元素一样,钆形成三价离子,具有发荧光的特性。

Paramagnetic ions, such as gadolinium, move differently within a magnetic field. This trait makes gadolinium useful for magnetic resonance imaging(MRI).

顺磁离子如钆在磁场内以不同的方式移动,这种特性使钆可用于磁共振成像。

gait [ɡeit] *n.* 步态,步法

This produced a gait disturbance and a loss of memory.

这会产生步态紊乱和记忆力丧失。

Under the supervision of a therapist, the patient progresses from needing gait aids and constant supervision to the maximum level of independent gait compatible with safety.

在治疗师的指导下,病人从需要(别人)帮助来行走和不断指导逐渐有进步以至最大限度地独立安全地行走。

galactorrhea [ɡəˌlæktəuˈriːə] *n.* 溢乳

The syndrome of amenorrhea in association with galactorrhea has been known since ancient times.

早在古代就已经知道在闭经时伴随有溢乳为特征的综合征。

Amenorrhea-galactorrhea syndrome is a rare endocrine disorder, primarily characterized by the abnormal production of breast milk, anovulation, and amenorrhea.

闭经溢乳综合征是少见的内分泌紊乱性疾病,以乳汁产生异常,无排卵及闭经为主要特征。

galactose [ɡəˈlæktəus] *n.* 半乳糖

Glucose and galactose enter the cell interior by a sodium-dependent active transport process.

葡萄糖和半乳糖可以通过钠依赖性的主动转运机制进入细胞内。

galactosemia [ɡəˌlæktəˈsimiə] *n.* [遗] 半乳糖血(症)

Galactosemia results from the inability to metabolize galactose.

半乳糖血症发病原因是无法代谢半乳糖。

Infants with galactosemia should not be breastfed, but should receive a non - lactose-containing formula.

患半乳糖血症的婴儿不能母乳喂养,需要进食含非乳糖的配方奶。

gallbladder [ˈɡɔːlblædə] *n.* 胆囊

Cholecystitis is inflammation of the gallbladder.

胆囊炎是胆囊的炎症。

Gallbladder attacks can cause excessive vomiting.

胆囊疾病的发作能造成剧烈呕吐。

gallium [ˈɡæliəm] *n.* 镓(化学元素)

Gallium 67(67Ga) imaging is of value in determining the extent of a variety of neoplasms when appropriate treatment decisions are to be made.

镓 67 成像技术有助于明确各种肿瘤的发展程度,方便医生来制订合适的治疗方案。

Today, almost all gallium is used for microelectronics.

现在几乎所有的镓被用于微电子。

Several gallium salts are used, or are in development, as both pharmaceuticals and radiopharmaceuticals in medicine.
在医学上几种镓盐被用作或正被开发为药物和放射性药物。

gallop [ˈgæləp] *n.* 奔马律(心脏的一种异常节律)
In the presence of right ventricular failure there are often an early diastolic gallop.
右心室衰竭时常有舒张早期奔马律。
The decreased distensibility of the thick left ventricle commonly produces a presystolic gallop.
厚的左心室扩张性下降,常产生收缩期前奔马律(第四心音)。

gallstone [ˈgɔːlstəun] *n.* 胆石
Usually the presence of a gallstone call for the excision of the gallbladder.
胆结石的出现通常要求切除胆囊。
Recurrent episodes of cholecystitis are usually associated with gallstones.
反复发作的急性胆囊炎,一般均合并胆石症。

galvanometer [ˌgælvəˈnɔmitə] *n.* 电流计
In its original form the instrument was based on the principle of the string galvanometer, which was invented in 1903 by a Dutch physiologist.
该仪器原始的形式是以线圈电流计原理为基础,由荷兰生理学家于 1903 年发明的。

gamete [ˈgæmiːt] *n.* 配子
During the formation of gametes the chromosome number is reduced by one-half.
配子形成中,染色体的数目减半。
Gametes are referred to as sexually reproductive cells: the sperm and egg.
配子是指有性生殖细胞即精子和卵子。

gametogenesis [gəmiːtəuˈdʒenisis] *n.* 配子形成,配子发生
Gametogenesis is the formation of the ova or sperm.
配子形成是指精子或卵子的形成。

gamma [ˈgæmə] *n.* 伽马
Gamma rays and neutrons can produce harmful effects in living organisms.
r 射线和中子都能损害生物组织。
Gamma knife is operated by a team of professional personnel who must have received specialized training.
伽马刀要由一些经过专门训练的专业人员操作。

gammopathy [ˈgæməˌpəθi] *n.* 丙种球蛋白病
A monoclonal gammopathy of undetermined significance (MGUS) occurs in up to 2 percent of persons 50 years of age or older.
意义未明的单克隆丙种球蛋白病(MGUS)在 50 岁或以上年龄的人群中发生多达 2%。

ganciclovir [gænˈsaikləvir] *n.* 丙氧鸟苷,更昔洛韦
He was treated empirically with gancyclovir, and multiple blood and CSF cultures were negative.
他在接受经验性的丙氧鸟苷治疗,多次血培养和脑脊液培养均是阴性。
Ganciclovir is used to treat the symptoms of cytomegalovirus (CMV) infection of the eyes in people whose immune system is not working fully.
丙氧鸟苷用于治疗那些免疫系统异常、眼部感染巨细胞病毒的人的症状。

ganglion [ˈgæŋgliən] (*pl.* **ganglia** [ˈgæŋgliə]) *n.* 神经节,腱鞘囊肿
Pain nerve endings are free nerve endings whose cell stations lie in the posterior root ganglia.
痛觉神经末梢是游离的神经末梢,其细胞位于脊背根神经节。
Other rare complications include premature cataracts, pseudotumor cerebri, and calcifications of the basal ganglia.
其他少见的并发症包括早产儿白内障、脑假瘤、基底神经节钙化。
We now have different means to treat ganglion cysts, typically by surgical excision.

我们现在有不同的方式去处理腱鞘囊肿，通常是外科切除。

ganglionectomy [ˌgæŋgliə'nektəmi] *n.* 神经节切除术

Ganglionectomy is a procedure in which your healthcare provider removes a cyst from your hand, wrist, foot, or other part of your body.

神经节切除术是一种切除手、腕、足或身体其他部分囊肿的手术。

Dorsal root ganglionectomy may be performed open or percutaneously for the relief of cancer and non-cancer related chronic pain.

背根神经节切除术可以开放式手术或经皮手术，来缓解癌症或非癌症相关的慢性疼痛。

ganglioneuroblastoma ['gæŋgliəˌnjuərəublæs'təumə] *n.* 成神经节细胞瘤

Ganglioneuroblastoma is a variant of neuroblastoma.

成神经节细胞瘤是神经母细胞瘤的变种。

ganglioneuroma [ˌgæŋgliənju'rəumə] *n.* 神经节瘤

Ganglioneuroma is a tumor of the sympathetic nerve fibers arising from neural crest cells.

神经节瘤是一种交感神经纤维肿瘤，起源于神经嵴细胞。

ganglioside ['gæŋgliəsaid] *n.* 神经节苷脂

Anti-ganglioside antibodies that react to self-gangliosides are found in autoimmune neuropathies.

在自身免疫性神经病中，对自身神经节苷脂的反应会产生抗神经节苷脂抗体。

Gangliosides are the group of glycosphingolipids.

神经节苷脂类是一组鞘糖脂类。

gangliosidosis [ˌgæŋgliəsai'dəusis] *n.* 神经节苷脂沉积症

GM1 gangliosidosis is an inherited disorder that progressively destroys nerve cells (neurons) in the brain and spinal cord.

GM1 神经节苷脂沉积症是一种遗传性疾病，缓慢破坏脑和脊髓内的神经细胞(神经元)。

The GM2 gangliosidoses are a group of related genetic disorders.

GM2 神经节苷脂沉积症是一组相关的遗传性疾病。

gangrene ['gæŋgriːn] *n.* 坏疽

Necrosis with putrefaction is called gangrene.

伴有腐败的坏死称为坏疽。

Gangrene can result from a number of disorders involving the arteries, among them diabetes.

许多累及动脉的疾病会产生坏疽，糖尿病是其中之一。

gangrenous ['gæŋgrinəs] *a.* 坏疽性的

As noted above, an infarct of the intestine rapidly becomes gangrenous.

如上所述，肠的梗死迅速产生坏疽性变化。

He agreed to have an operation to amputate his left foot which had become gangrenous.

他同意做手术，截除坏疽的左脚。

gantry ['gæntri] *n.* 支架

This paper investigated the effect of gantry angle on sprial CT coronal imaging of paranasal sinus.

这篇文章探讨螺旋 CT 副鼻窦冠状扫描时机架摆动角度对冠状成像质量的影响。

We rotate the gantry within the angle to modulate the fields.

我们在一定角度内旋转机架以调整视野。

garbage ['gɑːbidʒ] *n.* 垃圾，废料

It has been estimated that about 15% of the total environmental mercury contamination comes from garbage incineration.

据估算在环境的汞污染中约有 15% 来自垃圾焚烧产生的灰烬。

gardenoside ['gɑːdnəusaid] *n.* 栀子苷，栀子甙；栀子

Our aim is to optimize the extraction process of gardenoside in gardenia.

我们的目的是优化栀子中栀子苷的提取工艺。

Crystallization is a simple and rapid method to isolate gardenoside.

重结晶是一种简单、快速分离栀子苷的办法。

gargle [ˈɡɑːɡl] *v.* 嗽口

The patient must gargle with the solution every morning.

病人每天早晨必须用这溶液嗽口。

n. 含嗽液

Gargle is a solution used for rinsing or medicating the mouth and throat.

含漱液是用于漱洗或治疗口腔和咽喉的溶液。

gas [ɡæs] *n.* 气体，毒气

Plants also release the gas into the atmosphere.

植物也会向大气中释放这种气体。

Any substance is made of atom, whether it is solid, liquid or gas.

任何物质，不论是固体、液体还是气体，都是由原子组成的。

gaseous [ˈɡeisjəs] *a.* 气(体)的，气态的

There are three states of matter: solid, liquid and gaseous.

物质的存在有三种状态：固态、液态和气态。

gasoline [ˈɡæsəliːn] *n.* 汽油

Once gasoline is produced at a refinery, it is distributed through a series of transport and storage pathways.

一旦汽油在一家汽油精炼厂中生产出来，它将通过一系列的运输和储存途径进行分配。

Hydrocarbons such as gasoline are found in all households and in many workplaces.

在无数的家庭和众多的工地都可以找到碳氢化合物如汽油。

gastrectomy [ɡæsˈtrektəmi] *n.* 胃切除术

When a stomach ulcer has perforated, a partial gastrectomy may be indicated.

当胃溃疡穿孔时，需进行部分胃切除术。

Total gastrectomy is the treatment of choice for Zollinger-Ellison syndrome unresponsive to medical management.

Zollinger-Ellison 综合征病人在用药治疗无效时可选择全胃切除术。

gastric [ˈɡæstrik] *a.* 胃的

Pepsin is an enzyme found in the gastric juice.

胃蛋白酶是胃液中所见的一种酶。

The highest incidence of gastric ulcer is in adolescence and early adult life.

胃溃疡最高发病率是在青春期或成年初期。

gastrin [ˈɡæstrin] *n.* 胃泌素

In duodenal ulcers there is evidence of an increase in gastrin production which increase acid production from the gastric parietal cells.

有证据表明十二指肠溃疡可能是胃泌素分泌增多所致，它可使胃壁细胞分泌过多的盐酸。

gastrinoma [ˌɡæstriˈnəumə] *n.* 促胃液素瘤；胃泌素瘤

Diagnosis earlier in case of gastrinoma was the key point for prognosis.

胃泌素瘤的早期诊断是预后的关键点。

Twelve cases of gastrinoma found in the recent 30 years in our hospital were analyzed.

对本院最近 30 年收治的 12 例胃泌素瘤病例进行了分析。

gastritis [ɡæsˈtraitis] *n.* 胃炎

Soft food is easy of digestion and suitable for the gastritis patient.

松软的食物容易消化，适于胃炎患者食用。

In the opinion of most doctors, the treatment of chronic gastritis is to remove the cause.

根据大多数医生的意见，治疗慢性胃炎是祛除病因。

gastrocnemius [ˌɡæstrəuˈkniːmiəs] *n.* 腓肠肌

Dancing Dobermann disease is a type of myopathy that primarily affects the gastrocnemius muscle in Dobermanns.

杜宾舞蹈病是一种主要影响杜宾犬的腓肠肌的肌肉病变。

No significant loss in the function of the leg and ankle was observed after transposition of the gastrocnemius muscle.

腓肠肌移位后对小腿及踝关节功能无明显影响。

gastroenteritis [ˌgæstrəuˌ entə'raitis] *n.* 胃肠炎

More commonly the stomach and the small intestine are both involved, so that the illness is known as gastroenteritis.

较常见的是胃和小肠二者都发炎,所以此病称为胃肠炎。

Estimates of the responsibility of these viral agents in producing gastroenteritis have ranged between 40% and 90%.

这些病毒引起急性胃肠炎估计范围在 40% ~90% 之间。

gastrointestinal [ˌgæstrəuin'testinəl] *a.* 胃肠道的

Alteration of function of the gastrointestinal tract seems tobe directly influenced by the emotional state of the individual.

胃肠道功能的改变似乎受个人情绪状态的直接影响。

Occasionally, endocarditis may follow instrumentation in the gastrointestinal tract.

偶尔心内膜炎可发生于胃肠道器械检查术后。

gastrojejunostomy [ˌgæstrɔˌdʒiːdʒu'nɔstəmi] *n.* 胃空肠吻合术

Gastrojejunostomy is done in preference to gastroduodenostomy if the latter operation is technically difficult or in special operations to avoid a backflow of bile into the stomach.

如果进行胃十二指肠手术在技术上有困难,或者要避免手术后胆汁反流到胃内,则以施行胃空肠吻合术为好。

gastroparesis [ˌgæstrəupə 'riːsis] *n.* 胃轻瘫

The symptoms of gastroparesis showed gastric fullness, but no obvious pain in the abdomen.

胃瘫表现为胃潴留,而无明显腹痛。

The causes and treatment of gastroparesis after transabdominal proximal subtotal gastrectomy (TPSG) was discussed in the study.

该研究讨论了经腹近端胃大部切除术后胃瘫的病因及治疗方法。

gastroschisis [gæs'trɔskisis] *n.* 腹裂

The clinical materials of 5 newborns with gastroschisis were analyzed retrospectively.

本文回顾性分析了 5 例新生儿腹裂的临床资料。

The authors consider that staged silo repair is a simple and safe approach to neonatal gastroschisis.

作者认为应用硅塑囊分期修复术治疗新生儿腹裂是一种简单、安全有效的方法。

gastroscope ['gæstrəskəup] *n.* 胃(窥)镜

As gastroscope can usually be introduced into the duodenum it is also known as gastroduodenoscope.

因胃镜亦可用来检查十二指肠部位,故也可将其称作胃十二指肠镜。

gastroscopy [gæs'trɔskəpi] *n.* 胃镜检查

The flexible gastroscopy can detect many early cases of gastric carcinoma.

可弯曲性胃镜检查能发现许多胃癌早期病例。

gastrostomy [gæs'trɔstəmi] *n.* 胃造口术

A gastrostomy is the kindest way to give fluids and food.

胃造口术是供给液体和食物最好的方法。

Percutaneous gastrostomy (PEG) is useful for long-term enteral feeding.

经皮胃造口术(PEG)常适用于长期进行肠道饲养。

gastrulation [ˌgæstru'leiʃən] *n.* 原肠胚形成

The quantity of yolk affects the movement of cell populations during gastrulation.
原肠胚形成期间，卵黄量可影响细胞群的移动。

gate [geit] *v.* 给装大门；门控

MSCT with retrospectively ECG-gating permits the detection of significant coronary arteries stenosis with high accuracy if image quality is satisfactory.
回顾性心电门控多层螺旋 CT 在显像质量较好的情况下，对检查明显的冠状动脉狭窄具有较高的准确性。

gauze [gɔːz] *n.* 纱布

The gauze should be immersed in antiseptic solution for a few minutes.
应该把纱布在消毒液中浸泡几分钟。

gavage [gəˈvɑːʒ] *n.* [法]管饲法

The experiment animals were treated with erigeron breviscapus (50mg/kg) dissolved in 0.9% NaCl by gavage for 7 days.
实验动物用灯盏花素（每公斤体重 50 毫克）溶于 0.9% 的食盐水中管饲 7 天的方式进行处理。

gaze [geiz] *v.* 凝视，注视

He neglected the subject though gazing at it.
尽管他凝视着这项内容，但还是忽视了。

I happened to gaze out the ward window and a severely burned patient caught my eyes.
我无意往病房窗外一看，一名严重烧伤病人映入我眼帘。

n. 凝视；注视

Eye tracking is the process of measuring either the point of gaze ("where we are looking") or the motion of an eye relative to the head.
眼球追踪是测量我们凝视的点（我们看着的地方）或者相对于头部来说眼睛移动的过程。

gecko [ˈgekəu] *n.* 蛤蚧；壁虎

We must establish the quality standard for gecko capsule.
我们必须建立蛤蚧胶囊的质量标准。

Analysis of the chemical constituents of gecko is useful for the research.
蛤蚧成分分析对这项科研很有用。

gel [dʒel] *n.* 凝胶

The single cell gel electrophoresis is a new technique to evaluate the genetic damage in exposed populations.
单细胞凝胶电泳是评价暴露人群遗传学损伤的一种新技术。

Voltaren Gel is used to relieve the pain of osteoarthritis in the knees, ankles, feet, elbows, wrists, and hands.
扶他林凝胶用于缓解膝、踝、脚、肘、腕和手等部位骨关节炎引起的疼痛。

gelatin [ˈdʒelətin] *n.* 明胶

Gelatin has been used in medicine as a source of protein in the treatment of malnutrition.
明胶在医学上作为一种蛋白质的来源常可用来治疗营养不良。

gelatinization [dʒəˌlætinaiˈzeiʃən] *n.* 凝胶化，糊化，胶凝作用

Gelatinization influences gastric emptying, but does not influence absorption.
胶凝作用影响胃排空但不影响吸收。

Amylose plays an important role during the initial stages of corn starch gelatinization.
直链淀粉在玉米淀粉凝胶化的初始阶段起重要作用。

gelatinous [dʒiˈlætinəs] *a.* 胶状的

Grossly the tumour has a gelatinous appearance and texture.
用肉眼看，肿瘤呈胶状外观和质地。

gemstone [ˈdʒemstəun] *n.* 宝石

Gemstone spectral CT is one of the most advanced CT scanners currently, its spectrum images have higher clinical value in determining tissue homologies.

宝石能谱 CT 是目前最先进的 CT 之一，其能谱成像对判断组织同源性有较高的临床价值。

gene [dʒiːn] *n.* 基因，遗传因子

Gene is a segment of a DNA molecule that contains all the information required for synthesis of a product.

基因是 DNA 分子的一个片段，它含有合成一个产物需要的所有信息。

Operator gene serves as a starting point for reading the genetic code and controls the activity of the structural gene by interacting with repressor.

操纵基因是作为阅读遗传密码的起始点，并通过和阻遏物的相互作用来控制结构基因的活动。

The production of each enzyme is thought to be under the control of a particular gene.

各种酶被认为是在特定的基因控制下产生的。

The discovery that genes can cause cancer opens a whole new understanding of the way cancer develops.

基因能引起癌症这一发现开创了对癌症产生方式的全新理解。

general [ˈdʒenərəl] *a.* 全身性的；全面的；普遍的

To trace the general circulation, let us begin with the venous blood which is returned to the right atrium by the superior and inferior venae cavae.

追踪全身循环，让我们从通过上、下腔静脉回到右心房的静脉血开始。

AIDS is a matter of general interest to the public.

艾滋病是大众普遍关心的事。

generalizability [ˌdʒenərəˌlaizəˈbiliti] *n.* 普遍性

The representativeness of the actual population to the target population is referred to as generalizability.

实际人群对目标人群的代表性被称为普遍性。

generalizable [ˈdʒenərəlaizəbl] *a.* 可归纳的，可推广的

It is critical in quantitative analysis to get statistically reliable and generalizable results.

定量分析中关键的一点是要得到统计学上可依赖和可概括性的结果。

These methods are generalizable to other medical imaging techniques.

这些方法可推广用于其他医学影像技术。

generalization [dʒenərəlaiˈzeiʃən] *n.* 概括；判断

This theory, like so many ideas in science, has been a slowly developing generalization.

这个理论像许多科学思想一样，是经缓慢发展而概括出来的。

An exception to this generalization is the coronary arteries, which sometimes undergo arteriosclerosis rather early in life, especially in men.

这种概括的一个例外是冠状动脉；有时它在一生中很早就发生硬化，尤其是男性。

generalize [ˈdʒenərəlaiz] *v.* 弥漫，扩散；全身化

Pain that suddenly becomes generalized and stays that way suggests peritonitis.

疼痛突然变为弥漫性并持续不止，提示为腹膜炎。

The patient rapidly developed generalized edema with ascites.

病人迅速发展为全身性水肿并有腹水。

Appendicitis usually starts as a generalized pain across the abdomen.

阑尾炎开始时通常是全腹疼痛。

generate [ˈdʒenəreit] *v.* 发（电）；产生；引起

The machine generates electricity.

这台机器发电。

Their electricity comes from a new generating station.
他们的电力来自一座新的发电站。
The presence of an invading virus generates specific antibodies.
病毒侵入体内可以产生特异性抗体。

generator [ˈdʒenəreitə] *n.* 发电机;发生器
Generator is the important component of the X-ray tube, and also the important part of the CT tube.
发生器是 X 线球管的重要部件,也是 CT 球管的重要构成部分。
Transistor high frequency generator has the characteristics of fast heating speed, high efficiency and low power consumption.
晶体管式高频发生器具有加热速度快,效率高,耗电少的特点。
99mTc can be obtained from 99Mo in a nuclide generator.
通过核素发生器可以由 99 钼获取 99m 锝。

genesis [ˈdʒenisis] (*pl.* **geneses** [ˈdʒenisiːz]) *n.* 发生
These all play a role in the genesis of the acute inflammatory reaction.
所有这些都能在急性炎症发生中起作用。

genetic [dʒiˈnetik] *a.* 遗传(学)的
Identical twins are persons who possess the same exact genetic makeup of blood group and other genes.
单卵性双胞胎是指其血型和其他基因中的遗传结构完全相同的(两个)人。
There are also many genetic abnormalities of haemoglobin.
血红蛋白也有许多遗传异常。
Data on genetic factors in arteriosclerosis are very limited.
关于动脉硬化的遗传学因素的数据极少。

genetically [dʒiˈnetikəli] *ad.* 遗传学地;遗传地
In human color blindness is genetically regulated by a recessive gene.
人类色盲在遗传上是由隐性基因控制的。
There is no medical evidence to date that genetically modified foods are not safe to eat.
到目前为止没有医学证据表明食用基因改造的食物是不安全的。

geneticist [dʒiˈnetisist] *n.* 遗传学家
Mendel was a famous geneticist.
孟德尔是一位著名的遗传学家。

genetics [dʒiˈnetiks] *n.* 遗传学
Genetics has its own special language.
遗传学有其自身独特的语言。
Genetics is a branch of biology.
遗传学是生物学的一个分支。
Genetics includes the study of how human characteristics are inherited from one's parents.
遗传学包括对人类性状如何从亲代传递给子代的研究。

genital [ˈdʒenitl] *a.* 生殖的;生殖器的
In postmenopausal women, carcinomas of the genital tract figure prominently in differential diagnosis of abnormal uterine bleeding.
在绝经后妇女异常的子宫出血鉴别诊断中应着重考虑生殖道癌肿。
It is quite difficult to diagnose genital tuberculosis. The most important test is endometrial curettage, testing the menstrual blood taken from the uterus.
生殖器结核的诊断困难,最重要的检查是子宫内膜诊刮,检查源于子宫内的经血。

genitalia [ˌdʒeniˈteiliə] *n.* 生殖器
Adult flukes have been found in other organs, including the genitalia and muscle.

成年吸虫也见于其他器官，包括会阴部和肌肉。

genitourinary [ˌdʒenitəuˈjuərinəri] *n.* 泌尿生殖器的

Cryptorchidism is a common congenital abnormality of pediatric genitourinary system.

隐症是一种常见的小儿泌尿生殖系统先天畸形。

To our knowledge, this is the first case of kidney rupture as the consequence of genitourinary tuberculosis.

根据我们所知，这是第一个因泌尿生殖器结核诱发的肾脏自发性破裂的病例。

genome [ˈdʒiːnəum] *n.* 基因组

The nucleic acid comprising the entire genetic information of an organism is called genome.

包含有一个机体全部遗传信息的核酸称为基因组。

The human genome project is an international effort, started in the mid 1980s.

人类基因组工程是一项国际间共同努力的工作，它开始于 20 世纪 80 年代中期。

The current goal of the Human Genome Project is to obtain the sequence of all 3 billion bp of human DNA.

人类基因组工程当前的目标是获得人类 DNA 分子中 30 亿碱基对的排列顺序。

The genome can be rapidly scanned to find the mutations.

基因组可以快速地进行扫描以便找到基因突变的位点。

genomics [dʒiˈnɔmiks] 基因组学

Genomics is the study of genes and their function.

基因组学是研究基因及其功能的学科。

genotoxic [ˌdʒenəuˈtɔksik] *a.* 遗传毒性的

Our recent studies have shown that two environmental metal pollutants, lead and mercury, induce genotoxic DNA damage.

我们当前的研究已显示出有两种环境污染物，如铅和汞，可以诱发有遗传毒性的对 DNA 的损伤。

genotoxicity [ˌdʒenəutɔkˈsisiti] *n.* 基因毒性

We investigated the lipid peroxidation, liver cell injury and genotoxicity using the human hepatocellular carcinoma cell line.

我们用人肝细胞癌株来研究脂质过氧化、肝细胞损伤和基因毒性。

genotype [ˈdʒenətaip] *n.* 基因型，遗传型

The entire genetic constitution of an individual is termed its genotype.

一个个体的全部基因组成称为其基因型。

The human male has the genotype XY.

人类男性的基因型为 XY。

gentamicin [ˌdʒentəˈmaisin] *n.* 庆大霉素

Gentamicin(gentamycin) is used in serious infections by gram-negative organisms.

庆大霉素用于革兰氏阴性菌的严重感染。

Gentamicin should be added to broaden coverage for polymicrobial peritonitis.

加用庆大霉素后可以拓宽抗菌谱以便控制由多种细菌引起的腹膜炎。

gentian [ˈdʒenʃiən] *n.* 龙胆紫

The heat fixed smear is covered with a solution of gentian or crystal violet.

用龙胆紫或结晶紫溶液覆盖于加热固定的标本片上。

If the skin is scratched, put some gentian violet potion on it.

如果皮肤抓伤了，擦点龙胆紫药水。

In recent years, gentiana spot blight disease is the main disease of Chinese herbal medicine gentian.

龙胆草斑枯病是近几年中药材龙胆草的最主要病害。

genuine [ˈdʒenjuin] *a.* 真正的，名副其实的；纯血统的

Some medical research work requires mice of genuine breed.
某些医学研究工作需要纯种小鼠。
Dr. Bethune is the genuine friend of Chinese people.
白求恩大夫是中国人民的真正朋友。

genus ['dʒiːnəs] (*pl.* **genera** ['dʒenərə]) *n.* 种属,类
Thus, this manual serves as a guide or key for the rapid naming of a genus or species.
因此,该手册可作为细菌种属快速命名的指南或依据。
Paleontology has taught us that species or genera have disappeared from this planet.
古生物学曾告诉我们,一些物种或种属已经从本行星上消失。
Schistosomiasis is a tropical disease caused by blood flukes of the genus Schistosoma.
血吸虫病是一种热带病,由血吸虫属的血液吸虫引起。

geographic [dʒiə'græfik] *a.* 地理的
The importance of the various viruses in the causation of pneumonia varies from year to year in each geographic area.
不同的病毒在引起肺炎方面的重要性在每个地理区域每年都不同。

geometric [dʒiəu'metrik] *a.* 几何学的
The range of normal ferritin in most laboratories is 30 to 300ng/ml and the geometric mean is 88 in men and 49 in women.
血清铁蛋白的正常范围,在大多数实验室为 30 ~ 300ng/ml,几何均数男性为 88,女性为 49。

geophagia [dʒiə'feidʒiə] *n.* 食土癖
There was no history of geophagia.
无食土癖病史。

geriatric [dʒeri'ætrik] *a.* 老年病学的,老年的
These schemes have been adopted by the majority of geriatric departments.
这些方案已被大多数老年病学部门所采纳。

geriatrics [ˌdʒeri'ætriks] *n.* 老年病学
Geriatrics is a branch of medicine that deals with the problems and diseases of old age and aging people.
老年病学是医学的分支,它研究老年人和衰老者的各种问题和疾病。

germ [dʒəːm] *n.* 细菌,病原菌;胚,胚芽
The wound must be kept clean so that germs do not infect it.
伤口必须保持干净,以免细菌感染。
The mutation has occurred in a germ cell and is transmitted to the descendents of the affected individual.
生殖细胞已发生突变,且传递给患者后代。

germicide [dʒəːmi'said] *n.* 杀菌剂
A germicide is essentially the same as a disinfectant.
杀菌剂本质上与消毒剂相同。

germinal ['dʒəːminəl] *a.* 发生的,胚种的
The individual with the hereditary form already carries one mutation(germinal) that may lead to cancer but must get one more mutation(somatic) in order to develop the cancer.
具有遗传型的个体,早已有一个致癌的(生殖细胞的) 突变,但还必须再获得一个(体细胞的) 突变,才能发癌。

germinoma [dʒəːmi'nəumə] *n.* 生殖细胞瘤
Germinomas are gonadal neoplasms that rarely occur extragonadally in the midline structures of the human body.
生殖细胞瘤是性腺肿瘤,很少发生于性腺外的人体中线部位。

OCT4 expresses variably in primary intracranial germinomas and may be a probable prognostic marker for intracranial germinoma.

OCT4 在原发性颅内生殖细胞瘤中表达不一致,可能成为颅内生殖细胞瘤的预后标记物。

germline [ˈdʒəːmlain] *n.* 种系,生殖细胞系,胚性

A germline mutation is any detectable and heritable variation in the lineage of germ cells.

种系突变是生殖细胞系中任何可检测的和可遗传的变异。

The new germline stem cells displayed all the markers indicative of fully mature sperm.

新的生殖系干细胞显示完全成熟精子的所有标记。

Defensive mechanisms based upon germline-encoded receptors constitute a system of innate immunity.

基于胚系基因编码的受体所建立的防御机制构成了天然免疫系统。

gerontology [dʒerənˈtɔlədʒi] *n.* 老年学,老年医学

Gerontology is a scientific study of the phenomena of aging and of the problems of the aged.

老年学是对老年人的问题和衰老现象的科学研究。

gestation [dʒesˈteiʃən] *n.* 妊娠,怀孕

Tubal gestation appears to have become more common in the last fifteen years, now occurring once in about 130 pregnancies.

近 15 年来输卵管妊娠更为常见,目前,约 130 次妊娠中发生 1 次输卵管妊娠。

gestational [dʒesˈteiʃənəl] *a.* 妊娠的

Ultrasound is useful in distinguishing ectopic from early intrauterine pregnancy, in which gestational ring can be detected.

超声检查有助于鉴别异位妊娠与早期宫内妊娠,妊娠时能检出妊娠环。

Gestational hypertension is usually defined as having a blood pressure higher than 140/90 after 20 weeks of gestation without the presence of protein in the urine.

妊娠期高血压通常定义为妊娠 20 周后血压高于 140/90,而且尿里不含蛋白。

giardiasis [ˌdʒiːɑːˈdaiəsis] *n.* 贾第鞭毛虫病

Giardiasis is an infection of the small bowel by a single-celled organism called Giardia lamblia.

贾第虫病是一种称为贾第鞭毛虫的单细胞生物所引起的小肠感染。

Giardiasis can be found among 20-30% of people in developing countries.

在发展中国家,贾第鞭毛虫病可见于 20% ~30% 的人群。

gigantism [ˈdʒaigæntizəm] *n.* 巨大,巨大发育

Fetal gigantism has long been associated with maternal diabetes.

长期以来人们就认识到巨大胎儿与母亲糖尿病有关。

gingivitis [ˌdʒindʒiˈvaitis] *n.* 牙龈炎

Gingivitis, inflammation of the gum tissue, is a term used to describe non-destructive periodontal disease.

牙龈炎,即牙龈组织的炎症,这一术语用于描述非破坏性的牙周组织疾病。

The symptoms of gingivitis are non-specific and manifest in the gum tissue as the classic signs of inflammation, such as swollen gums, and purple gums.

牙龈炎的症状是非特异性的,其牙龈组织表现出典型的炎症症状,例如牙龈肿胀和发紫。

ginseng [ˈdʒinseŋ] *n.* 高丽参,人参

American ginseng grows naturally in forests in many eastern states.

在美国许多东部地区的森林中生长着天然西洋参。

ginsenoside [ˈdʒinsinəusaid] *n.* 人参皂苷

Please establish as soon as possible the determination method of ginsenoside content in Lizhongtang formula granule.

请尽快建立一个理中汤配方颗粒中人参皂苷含量的测定方法。

The study on the microbiological transformation of ginsenoside is a great challenge for us.

人参皂苷微生物转化的研究对我们来说是个难题。

girdle [ˈgəːdl] *n.* 带；托带；引力带

This tissue is found mainly around the shoulder girdle.

这种组织主要见于肩胛带周围。

The appendicular skeleton consists of the shoulder girdle and bones of upper extremities and the pelvic girdle and bones of lower extremities.

四肢骨骼由肩胛带和上肢骨及骨盆带和下肢骨构成。

gland [glænd] *n.* 腺体

The glands of the body manufacture substances which are distributed to all parts of the body.

身体的腺体制造各种物质，这些物质被送到身体的各个部位。

glandular [ˈglændjulə] *a.* 腺的

The pituitary consists of two lobes—the larger anterior lobe, of glandular structure, and the smaller posterior lobe.

垂体由两叶组成，即较大的具有腺体结构的前叶和较小的后叶。

glaucoma [glɔːˈkəumə] *n.* 青光眼

Each type of glaucoma requires a special operation.

每种类型的青光眼都有自己特殊的手术。

In all types of glaucoma the eventual problem is to reduce the intraocular pressure.

所有类型的青光眼其（治疗的）基本问题是降低眼内压。

Open-angle glaucoma rarely causes ocular pain or corneal edema.

开角型青光眼很少出现眼痛和角膜水肿。

glenohumeral [ˌgliːnəuˈhjuːmərəl] *a.* 盂肱的

Arthrography of the glenohumeral joint and MRI scan are of great value in the diagnosis of traumatic rotator cuff ruptures.

盂肱关节造影和磁共振成像对外伤性肩袖破裂的诊断有重要价值。

The surgery with post-surgical rehabilitation or non surgical therapy is the common treatment strategies for glenohumeral instability.

对盂肱关节不稳定性的常见治疗方案包括手术治疗（术后康复治疗）及非手术性治疗。

glibenclamide [glaiˈbenkləmaid] *n.* 优降糖

Glibenclamide is used to treat diabetes.

优降糖用于治疗糖尿病。

glidant [ˈglaidənt] *n.* 助流剂

Glidant is a substance that is added to a powder to improve its flowability.

助流剂是一种加在粉末中以改善其流动性的物质。

The formulation includes active ingredient lactase, excipient diluent agent, corrective, binder, glidant and lubricant and so on.

配方组成包括活性成分乳糖酶、辅料稀释剂、矫味剂、黏合剂、助流剂和润滑剂等。

gliocyte [ˈglaiəusait] *n.* 胶质细胞

Gliocytes are small phagocytic neuroglial cells.

胶质细胞是一种小的具有吞噬功能的神经胶质细胞。

Gliocytes are directly related to the formation and storage of glycogen.

胶质细胞与糖原的合成和储存有直接的关系。

glioma [glaiˈəumə] *n.* 神经胶质瘤

The purpose of this study is to explore the infiltrative and metastatic mechanism of brain glioma.

本研究的目的在于探讨脑胶质瘤的浸润，转移机制。

global [ˈgləubəl] *a.* 全球的，全世界的

The rapid spread of SARS (severe acute respiratory syndrome) in early 2003 was a global challenge to us.

2003 年年初严重急性呼吸系统综合征的迅速蔓延对我们是一次全球性的挑战。

globalization [ˌgləubəlaiˈzeiʃən] *n.* 全球化

The world is moving further toward multi-polarization and economic globalization.

世界多极化和经济全球化趋势进一步发展。

The present globalization of the drug issue has posed a grave menace to human well-being and development.

当今世界,全球化的毒品问题已对人类的健康和发展构成重大威胁。

With the development of economy and globalization, there are a great deal of crises such as greenhouse effect, air pollution and acid rain.

随着经济的发展和全球化,出现温室效应、空气污染和酸雨,给人类带来空前危机。

globulin [ˈglɔbjulin] *n.* 球蛋白

Globulins, as a class, are defined as proteins which are insoluble in water, soluble in weak salt solutions.

球蛋白类是指不溶于水、溶于弱盐液的蛋白质。

Immune γ globulin(500-750mg in adults) protects contacts of infectious hepatitis.

免疫 γ 球蛋白(成人为 500 ~ 750mg)对接触传染性肝炎者有保护作用。

glomerular [gləuˈmerjulə] *a.* 肾小球的

The glomerular membrane offers a complete barrier to the passage of blood cells.

肾小球膜是防止血细胞通过的一个完善的屏障。

Osmotic diuretics are given by intravenous infusion and are excreted by glomerular filtration.

渗透性利尿剂通过静脉滴注给药,并由肾小管滤过排泄。

glomerulonephritis [gləuˌmerjuləuneˈfraitis] *n.* 肾小球性肾炎

These manifestations may be due to renal emboli or glomerulonephritis.

这些现象可能由肾栓塞或肾小球肾炎引起。

glomerulopathy [gləuˌmerjuˈlɔpəθi] *n.* 肾小球病

Glomerulopathy is a term used to describe a noninflammatory disorder affecting the glomeruli of the nephron.

肾小球病这一术语用于描述累及肾单位中肾小球的非炎症性疾病。

It is clear that immune mechanisms involve most forms of primary glomerulopathy and many of the secondary glomerular disorders.

很显然,免疫机制参与了大多数原发性肾小球病和许多继发性肾小球疾病的发生。

glomerulosclerosis [gləuˌmerjuləuskliəˈrəusis] *n.* 肾小球硬化

Glomerulosclerosis refers to a hardening of the glomerulus in the kidney and scarring of the kidneys' tiny blood vessels.

肾小球硬化是指肾小球变硬,以及肾内微小血管的瘢痕形成。

ECM deposition and hyalinization lead to glomerulosclerosis in response to chronic injury.

作为对慢性损伤的反应,ECM 的沉积和玻璃样变导致肾小球硬化。

glomerulus [gləuˈmerjuləs] (*pl.* **glomeruli** [gləuˈmerjulai]) *n.* 小球;肾小球

At the beginning of each nephron, an afferent arteriole terminates in a small knot of capillaries, the glomerulus.

在每个肾单位的开端,一根传入小动脉终止于一小团毛细血管,即肾小球。

glucagon [ˈgluːkəgɔn] *n.* 胰高血糖素

Glucagon is a hormone secreted by the islets in the pancreas.

胰高血糖素是胰腺中胰岛分泌的一种激素。

glucocorticoid [ˌgluːkəuˈkɔːtikɔid] *n.* 糖(肾上腺)皮质激素,糖皮质类固醇

Conversely, adrenal hemorrhage during bacterial sepsis may cause glucocorticoid production to cease.

相反,细菌性脓毒病感染时,肾上腺出血可导致糖皮质激素生成停止。

Glucocorticoids should be avoided in the majority of patients with infectious mononucleosis.
患传染性单核细胞增多症应避免使用糖皮质类固醇。

gluconate ['gluːkəneit] *n.* 葡萄糖酸盐
Calcium gluconate often gives relief from pain.
葡萄糖酸钙常常可以缓解疼痛。

gluconeogenesis [ˌgluːkəuˌniːəu'dʒenisis] *n.* 葡糖异生作用
The hepatic cellular gluconeogenesis and the carbon flow rate in pyruvate recycling significantly increased in B group compared to C group.
B 组与 C 组相比较,B 组肝细胞葡糖异生和丙酮酸循环的碳流量均明显增强。
Seventy-two hours after major burns, there was increased gluconeogenesis.
大面积烧伤 72 小时后,肝脏糖原异生增加。

glucose ['gluːkəus] *n.* 葡萄糖
Glucose is used by the muscles to release energy.
肌肉利用葡萄糖以释放能量。
Since carbohydrate is not metabolized, the blood glucose level rises.
由于碳水化合物没有被代谢而引起血糖升高。

glucuronic acid [gluːkjuə'rɔnik'æsid] *n.* 葡萄糖醛酸
Phenytoin in the liver is first hydroxylated and then conjugated with glucuronic acid.
苯妥英钠在肝脏首先被羟化,然后再与葡萄糖醛酸相结合。

glutamate ['gluːtəmeit] *n.* 谷氨酸;谷氨酸盐
Glutamate is an excitatory neurotransmitter.
谷氨酸是一种兴奋性的神经递质。
The term glutamate is often used interchangeably with glutamic acid.
谷氨酸盐一词常可与谷氨酸一词混用。

glutaminase [gluː'tæmineis] *n.* 谷氨酰胺酶
The biosynthetic enzyme genes identified included heme oxygenase, glutaminase and glutamic acid decarboxylase.
被鉴定的生物合成酶基因包括血红素加氧酶、谷氨酰胺酶和谷氨酸脱羧酶。
Glutaminase is considered as the main glutamate(Glu)-producing enzyme.
谷氨酰胺酶被认为是主要的产生谷氨酸的酶。

glutamine ['gluːtəmiːn] *n.* 谷氨酰胺
Glutamine is a glucogenic amino acid.
谷氨酰胺是一种成糖氨基酸。
Glutamine is an important carrier of urinary ammonia and is broken down in the kidney by glutaminase.
谷氨酰胺是一种尿氨的重要的载体,它在肾脏内被谷酰胺酶分解。

glutaraldehyde [ˌgluːtə'rældəhaid] *n.* 戊二醛
Glutaraldehyde is an organic compound with the formula $CH_2(CH_2CHO)_2$.
戊二醛是一种有机化合物,其分子式是 $CH_2(CH_2CHO)_2$。
Glutaraldehyde is used to disinfect the medical and dental facilities.
戊二醛是用来消毒医疗和牙科设备。

glutaric acidemia [gluː'tærik ,æsi'diːmiə] *n.* 戊二酸血症
Glutaric Acidemia type I is an inherited neurometabolic childhood disease.
I 型戊二酸血症是一种遗传性的神经代谢性儿童疾病。
Glutaric acidemia type I is caused by inherited deficiency of glutaryl-CoA dehydrogenase.
I 型戊二酸血症是由于遗传性的戊二酰辅酶 A 脱氢酶缺乏所致。

glutaric aciduria [gluː'tærik ,æsi'djuəriə] *n.* 戊二酸尿症
Glutaric aciduria type Ⅰ is a rare organic aciduria.

Ⅰ型戊二酸尿症是一种少见的有机酸尿症。

Glutaric aciduria type I is caused by inherited deficiency of glutaryl-CoA dehydrogenase.

Ⅰ型戊二酸尿症是由于遗传性的戊二酰辅酶 A 脱氢酶缺乏所致。

glutathione [ˌgluːtə'θaiəun] *n.* 谷胱甘肽

Glutathione is the major naturally-occurring antioxidant present in our cells.

谷胱甘肽是人体细胞内自然生成的主要抗氧化剂。

The only organ that can effectively absorb glutathione is the lungs.

能够有效吸收谷胱甘肽的唯一器官是肺。

glutathione-S-transferase [ˌgluːtə'θaiəun-es-'trænsfəˌreis] *n.* 谷胱甘肽-S-硫转移酶

The present study investigated the distribution of glutathione-S-transferase M1 (GSTM1) gene polymorphism in health Yao and Han nationalities of Guangdong province.

本文探讨了广东地区瑶族和汉族健康人群中谷胱甘肽硫转移酶 M1 (GSTM1) 基因多态性的分布。

Glutathione-S-transferase can constitute up to 10% of cytosolic protein in some mammalian organs.

在某些哺乳动物器官,谷胱甘肽-S-硫转移酶可构成多达 10% 的细胞蛋白质。

gluteal ['gluːtiəl] *a.* 臀肌的;臀的

The gluteal region in infants is small and is composed primarily of fat.

婴儿的臀部较小,主要由脂肪组成。

Contracture of middle gluteal muscle was the mechanism of GMC (gluteal muscle contracture) with obliquity of pelvis.

臀中肌挛缩是伴骨盆倾斜的臀肌挛缩症的发病机制。

glycan ['glaikæn] *n.* 多糖,聚糖

Glycomics is an emerging field of life science, which focuses on glycan structures and function.

糖组学是生命科学的新兴研究领域,主要研究多糖的结构与功能。

The α-mannosidase is a key enzyme of N-glycan synthesis and metabolism, which functions on removing the mannose residue of glycan.

α-甘露糖苷酶是一种参与 N-聚糖合成与代谢的关键酶,它的功能是除去 N-多糖中的甘露糖残留。

glycation [glai'keiʃən] *n.* 糖化,加糖作用

The accumulation of advanced glycation end products is a key mediator of renal tubular hypertrophy in diabetic nephropathy.

晚期糖基化最终产物的蓄积是糖尿病肾病肾小管肥大的重要中介物质。

Hyperglycemia contributes to greater platelet reactivity by promoting glycation of platelet proteins.

高血糖症通过促进血小板蛋白的糖化作用而增强血小板的活性。

glycerin ['glisərin] *n.* 甘油,丙三醇

The vesicles contain a clear tenacious fluid of the consistency of glycerin.

水疱含有清亮的黏稠的甘油一样的液体。

glycerite ['glisərait] *n.* 甘油剂

Glycerite is a medicinal preparation made by mixing or dissolving a substance in glycerin.

甘油剂是将物质混合或溶解于甘油中制成的药物制剂。

We first proposed using the concentration-adjustable glycerite as an ultrasonic transmitting medium.

我们首先推荐使用浓度可调的甘油剂作为超声传输的介质。

glycerol ['glisərɔl] *n.* 甘油

Fatty acids and glycerol may combine and form different kinds of fats, each having its own qualities.

脂肪酸和甘油可结合形成不同的脂肪,并各有各的特性。

glycine [ˈɡlaisiːn] *n.* 甘氨酸

The simplest amino acid is glycine.

最简单的氨基酸是甘氨酸。

Glycine and alanine can react to form two different dipeptides, glycylalanine and alanylglycine.

甘氨酸与丙氨酸能反应形成两种不同的二肽,即甘氨酰丙氨酸与丙氨酰甘氨酸。

glycogen [ˈɡlikəudʒen, ˈɡlaikəudʒen] *n.* 糖原

Glycogen occurs in almost all tissues but brain is an exception.

除脑外,几乎所有组织都含有糖原。

The liver is also concerned with converting sugars into glycogen and forming urea.

肝还参与把糖变为糖原和形成尿素的活动。

glycogenesis [ɡlaikəuˈdʒenisis] *n.* 糖原合成

The formation of glycogen from food is glycogenesis.

从食物中形成糖原称为糖原生成。

Glycogenolysis and glycogenesis are completely different.

糖原分解与糖原合成完全不同。

glycogenolysis [ɡlaikəudʒeˈnɔlisis] *n.* 糖原分解

Glycogenolysis in liver supports blood glucose concentration.

肝脏中的糖原分解维持血糖浓度。

glycogenosis [ˌɡlaikəudʒiˈnəusis] (*pl.* **glycogenoses** [ˌɡlaikəudʒiˈnəusiːz]) *n.* 糖原沉积病

The inherited defects of glycogen metabolism are collectively known as the glycogenoses.

糖原代谢的遗传缺陷总称为糖原沉积病。

glycolipid [ˌɡlaikəuˈlipid] *n.* 糖脂

The blood group substances A, B and H are present as glycolipid on the surface of erythrocytes, as well as on the surface of many epithelial cells and most endothelial cells.

血型物质 A、B 和 H 是存在于红细胞膜表面的糖脂,也存在于许多上皮细胞和大多数内皮细胞膜的表面。

glycolysis [ɡlaiˈkɔlisis] *n.* 糖酵解

Glycolysis can be both aerobic and anaerobic.

糖酵解可以是有氧或无氧代谢。

The splitting of glucose, known as glycolysis, occurs in all cells except for a few bacteria.

葡萄糖分解称为糖酵解,可发生于除少数细菌外的所有细胞。

glycome [ˈɡlaikəum] *n.* 糖组

The glycome is the entire complement of sugars, whether free or present in more complex molecules, of an organism.

糖组指存在于一个生物体内的整套聚糖,不管是游离还是结合于复合分子中。

The glycome exceeds the complexity of the proteome as a result of the even greater diversity of the glycome's constituent carbohydrates.

糖组比蛋白组更复杂,因为糖组的组分碳水化合物更复杂多样。

glycoprotein [ˌɡlaikəuˈprəutiːn] *n.* 糖蛋白

Glycoprotein or enzyme changes can help differentiate between bacteria and viral illnesses.

糖蛋白变化或酶变化有助于区分细菌性疾病和病毒性疾病。

The zona pellucida is a glycoprotein membrane surrounding the plasma of an oocyte.

透明带是围绕在卵母细胞胞浆外的糖蛋白膜。

glycosaminoglycan [ˌɡlaikəusəˌmiːnəuˈɡlaikæn] *n.* 氨基多糖,氨基葡聚糖

The compounds such as the chondroitin sulfates, dermatan sulfates, heparan sulfates, and heparin, keratan sulfates, and hyaluronic acid all are glycosaminoglycan.

硫酸软骨素、硫酸肤质、硫酸乙酰肝素、肝素、硫酸角质以及透明质酸等化合物都属于氨基

多糖类。

glycoside [ˈɡlaikəsaid] *n.* (葡萄)糖苷

Cardiac glycosides increase cardiac output by having a positive inotropic effect.

强心甙借助其正性肌力作用而增加心输出量。

glycosuria [ˌɡlaikəuˈsjuəriə] *n.* 糖尿

The presence of glucose in the urine in abnormally large amounts is termed glycosuria.

尿中含有异常大量的葡萄糖时称作糖尿。

Diabetes mellitus is a chronic familial disease characterized by hyperglycemia and glycosuria.

糖尿病是一种以高血糖和糖尿为特征的慢性家族性疾病。

glycosylation [ˌɡlaikəusiˈleiʃən] *n.* 糖基化

Glycosylation is an effective method of improving functional property of protein.

糖基化是改善蛋白质功能特性的一种有效方法。

N-glycosylation of proteins is an important post-translation modifying process in organism.

蛋白质 N-糖基化是机体中一种重要的翻译后修饰过程。

glycyrrhizin [glisiˈraizin] *n.* 甘草酸,甘草甜素

Glycyrrhizin is the main pharmacologically active component in licorice.

甘草酸是甘草的主要药理活性成分。

The aim of this research was to explore the direct cardiac activity of glycyrrhizin and glycyrrhetinic acid.

该研究的目的是探讨甘草酸和甘草次酸对心脏的直接作用。

gnawing [ˈnɔːiŋ] *n.* 持续性痛 *a.* 痛苦的

The pain is more or less constant, of moderate intensity, and frequently is described as a persistent pulling, gnawing, or aching discomfort.

疼痛大致是持续性的,呈中等强度,并常被描述为持续性牵拉痛或酸痛不适。

At night gnawing pain pierces my bones. My veins have no rest.

夜间持续性痛刺透我骨,我的脉络都不得安息。

gnotobiology [ˌnəutəubaiˈɔlədʒi] *n.* 悉生生物学,无菌生物学

Gnotobiology is the study of animals in the absence of microorganisms.

悉生生物学是研究无菌动物的学科。

Gnotobiology is one of important fields in modern bioscience.

悉生生物学是现代生命科学中的重要领域之一。

gnotobiote [ˌnəutəuˈbaiəut] *n.* 悉生动物

A germ-free animal infected with one or more microorganisms in order to study the microorganism in a controlled situation is termed gnotobiote.

让无菌动物感染上一种或多种微生物,以便在控制的条件下研究这些微生物,这种动物称作悉生动物。

Gnotobiote is widely used for the research on relationship between microbes and host.

悉生动物广泛用于研究微生物与宿主的相互关系。

gnotobiotics [ˌnəutəubaiˈɔtiks] *n.* 悉生生物工程学

The science gnotobiotics involves with maintaining a microbiologically controlled environment.

悉生生物工程学是有关维护以微生物来控制的环境的学科。

goiter [ˈɡɔitə] *n.* 甲状腺肿

Goiter is an enlargement of the thyroid gland, causing a swelling in the front of the neck.

甲状腺肿是甲状腺的增大,引起前颈肿胀。

goitrogen [ˈɡɔitrədʒən] *n.* 致甲状腺肿物质

Goitrogens are substances that suppress the function of the thyroid gland by interfering with iodine uptake, which can, as a result, cause an enlargement of the thyroid.

致甲状腺肿物质是一类通过干扰碘摄入来抑制甲状腺功能,最终导致甲状腺肿大的物质。

It's true that there are certain foods that contain goitrogens, which are compounds that make it more difficult for the thyroid gland to create its hormones.

确实有些食物中含有致甲状腺肿物质，这些物质会使甲状腺激素的生成变得十分困难。

gonad [ˈɡɔnæd] *n.* 性腺，生殖腺

For example, luteinizing hormone(LH) receptors are almost exclusively on the gonads.

例如，黄体生成素受体几乎全部在性腺上。

The outside layer(cortex) of the adrenal gland arises from mesodermal tissue closely related to the gonads.

肾上腺外层(皮质)来自与生殖腺紧密相关的中胚层。

gonadal [ˈɡɔnædəl] *a.* 性腺的

There is no evidence that gonadal or parathyroid hormones participate in the metabolic responses to infection.

没有证据表明性激素或甲状旁腺激素参与了对感染的代谢反应。

Gonadal agenesis refers to incomplete development of gonad.

性腺发育不全意味着性腺发育的不完全。

gonadectomy [ˌɡɔnəˈdektəmi] *n.* 性腺切除术

Gonadectomy is recommended to avoid the risk of malignancy which is of the order of 5%.

推荐性腺切除术以避免出现几率约为5%的恶性肿瘤。

gonadotrophic [ˌɡɔnədəuˈtrɔfik] *a.* 促性腺的

Dysfunctional uterine bleeding is caused by temporary alteration in the output or balance of either the gonadotrophic or the ovarian hormones.

功能失调性子宫出血，是由于促性腺激素或卵巢激素在释放或平衡方面暂时性变化而引起的。

gonadotropin [ˌɡɔnədəuˈtrəupin] *n.* 促性腺激素(=gonadotrophin)

The hypothalamus controls the output of gonadotropins from the pituitary gland.

下丘脑控制着来自垂体的促性腺激素的释放。

The main gonadotrophins are follicle-stimulating hormone and luteinizing hormone.

主要的促性腺激素是促卵泡激素和促黄体生成激素。

gonococcus [ˌɡɔnəuˈkɔkəs] (*pl.* **gonococci** [ˌɡɔnəuˈkɔksai]) *n.* 淋球菌

Species of Gram-negative cocci such as gonococci and meningococci are very sensitive to desiccation.

有些革兰氏阴性球菌，如淋球菌和脑膜炎球菌，对于干燥特别敏感。

gonorrhoea [ˌɡɔnəˈriːə] *n.* 淋病

Gonorrhoea may cause distant focal lesions and can infect the eyes of an infant during birth.

淋病可以引起远处局灶性病损，分娩时可使婴儿眼睛受到感染。

Prophylaxis may be given after exposure, such as after contact with a person with gonorrhoea.

预防治疗也可在接触后，如在接触淋病病人后给药。

gout [ɡaut] *n.* 痛风

Gout is a disease causing painful swellings in joints, especially toes, knees and fingers.

痛风是可以引起关节，特别是足趾、膝盖和手指关节肿痛的一种疾病。

Allopurinol is used to lower uric acid levels in primary gout.

别嘌呤醇可降低原发性痛风(患者)的尿酸水平。

gouty [ˈɡauti] *a.* 患痛风的，痛风性的

Secondary pyogenic infection of gouty joints is uncommon.

痛风关节的继发性化脓感染不常见。

The prevalence of gouty arthritis is 0.1% to 0.4%.

痛风性关节炎的患病率为0.1%到0.4%。

governance [ˈɡʌvənəns] *n.* 管理

The plan for patient registry governance and oversight should clearly address such issues as overall direction and operations, scientific content, ethics, safety, data access, publications, and change management.
患者登记研究的管理和监督计划应明晰解决诸如总体方向和操作、科学内涵、伦理、安全性、数据访问、公布和变更处置等问题。

gradation [grəˈdeiʃən] *n.* 分等,等级
Congenital infection with cytomegalovirus can result in all gradations of severity of involvement.
巨细胞病毒先天感染其累及的严重程度可以有各种等级。

gradient [ˈgreidiənt] *n.* 梯度,倾斜度
Facilitated diffusion also occurs solely in the direction of the concentration gradient.
促进弥散也只能沿着浓度梯度的方向进行。

gradient-echo [ˈgreidiəntˈekəu] *n.* 梯度回波
Gradient-echo cine technique is usually used for cardiac MR imaging.
梯度回波电影技术通常用于心脏的磁共振成像。

grading [ˈgreidiŋ] *n.* 分级
The tumor grading is according to the differentiation of the tumor cells.
肿瘤的分级是依据肿瘤细胞的分化程度。
Sometimes, the tumor grading is associated with the patients' prognosis.
有时,肿瘤的分级与病人的预后相关。

graft [grɑːft] *n.* 移植,移植物
It became necessary to make skin grafts to cover up the burn surface.
需要做植皮,以覆盖烧伤面。
These transplants were performed with high graft and patient survival rates.
所进行的这些移植术的移植物存活率和病人存活率均较高。

gram-negative [græmˈnegətiv] *a.* 革兰阴性的
These structures are found on both Gram-positive and Gram-negative bacilli.
这种结构在革兰阳性或阴性杆菌中都有。
Occasionally, gram-negative organisms are responsible for exacerbations of bronchitis.
偶尔,革兰阴性菌也是导致支气管炎恶化的原因。

gram-positive [græmˈpɔzətiv] *a.* 革兰阳性的
As seen by rRNA homologies, most of the mycoplasmas are related to the Gram-positive organisms.
由 rRNA 的同源性可见,大多数支原体与革兰阳性菌有联系。
In such cases the Gram stains may still show clumps of gram-positive cocci.
在这类病例中,革兰氏染色仍可发现革兰氏阳性球菌凝块。

grant [grɑːnt] *n.* 拨款,资助
This study was supported by grants from National Tenth Five-year Projects Plan(No. 2001BA701A20)
本研究获得国家十五规划计划的资助。(资助编号:2001BA701A20)

granula [ˈgrænjulə] *n.* 颗粒剂
Anxin granula has the effect of resisting cardiocyte apoptosis and can be used to prevent and treat HF.
安心颗粒有抑制心肌细胞凋亡的作用,可用于心力衰竭的防治。
KuShen Granula has an effect of anti-inflammation and restraining immunity
苦参颗粒有抗炎及抑制免疫的作用。

granular [ˈgrænjulə] *a.* 粒状的,颗粒状的
Mid-stream urine specimen obtained from acute glomerulonephritis patient may reveal bacterial infection and granular casts.
急性肾小球性肾炎患者的中段尿标本可以见到细菌感染和颗粒管型。

When platelets aggregate they secret certain granular constituents in a process analogous to secretion reactions in other cells.
当血小板聚集时,它们有与其他细胞分泌反应相类似的过程,分泌一定的颗粒成分。

granule ['grænjuːl] *n.* 颗粒
Bacteria do store granules, but these are never enclosed by a membrane.
细菌确能贮存颗粒,但这些颗粒无膜包绕。
Recent data from a number of laboratories indicate that the intrinsic death pathway plays an important role in executing apoptosis of granule neurons.
来自一些实验室的最新资料显示,内源性死亡通路在颗粒神经元凋亡执行中起重要作用。

granulocyte ['grænjuləusait] *n.* 粒细胞,粒性白细胞
Granulocytes and mononuclear phagocytes migrate simultaneously from blood to the site of inflammation.
粒细胞和单核吞噬细胞同时从血液中涌入炎症部位。

granulocytic [ˌgrænjuləu'sitik] *a.* 粒细胞的,粒性白细胞的
A subset of idiopathic cases progresses to frank leukemia(usually acute granulocytic leukemia).
有些特发性病例发展成症状明显的白血病(通常为急性粒细胞性白血病)。

granulocytopenia [ˌgrænjuləuˌsaitəu'piːniə] *n.* 粒细胞减少,粒细胞缺乏症
Both the thrombocytopenia and the granulocytopenia are usually self-limited and resolve over 3 to 6 weeks.
血小板减少与粒细胞减少两者通常有自限性,持续约 3 ~6 周。

granuloma [ˌgrænju'ləumə] *n.* 肉芽肿,肉芽瘤
Such a chronic inflammatory mass is traditionally called a granuloma.
这种慢性炎性肿块传统上称为肉芽肿。
The basic pathologic lesion in chronic schistosomiasis is the egg granuloma.
慢性血吸虫病的基本病理病变是虫卵肉芽肿。

granulomatosis ['grænjuˌləumə'təusis] *n.* 肉芽肿病
End-stage renal disease occurs in up to 20% of patients with these diagnoses, which include Wegener' s granulomatosis and microscopic polyangiitis.
在诊断为这种疾病的患者中,有 20% 的患者发生终末期肾病,其中包括韦格纳氏肉芽肿病和微型多血管炎。
CT manifestations of Wegener granulomatosis of lung was presented in the symposium.
研讨会上展示了韦格肉芽肿的 CT 表现。

granulomatous [ˌgrænju'lɔmətəs] *a.* 肉芽肿的,肉芽瘤的
Reinfection with M. tuberculosis is thus followed by an immediate brisk granulomatous response.
结核杆菌再感染就会引起迅速的肉芽肿性反应。

granulopoiesis [ˌgrænjuləpɔi'iːsis] *n.* 粒细胞生成
Attempts to stimulate granulopoiesis with corticosterosis or other therapy are usually ineffectual.
试用皮质类固醇激素刺激粒细胞生成,或采用其他疗法,一般均不奏效。

granulysin [ˌgrænju'laisin] *n.* 颗粒溶解素,粒溶素,粒溶蛋白
Granulysin is a cytotoxic protein present in the cytotoxic granules of cytotoxic CD8 T cells and NK cells.
颗粒溶解素是一种细胞毒蛋白,存在于细胞毒 CD8 T 细胞和 NK 细胞的细胞毒颗粒中。
T-cell release of granulysin contributes to host defense in leprosy.
在麻风病中,T 细胞释放的颗粒溶解素有利于宿主防御功能。

granzyme ['grænzaim] *n.* 颗粒酶
Granzymes are serine proteases present in cytotoxic CD8 T cells and NK cells and are involved in inducing apoptosis in the target cell.
颗粒酶是存在于细胞毒性 CD8 T 细胞和 NK 细胞中的丝氨酸蛋白酶,参与诱导靶细胞

凋亡。

Cells were perforated, granzyme B will be able to enter and destroy infected cells.

细胞穿孔后,颗粒酶 B 就能够进入并破坏受感染的细胞。

grapeseed ['greipsi:d] *n.* 葡萄籽

The study on the protective effects and mechanisms of grapeseed Procyanidins on cerebral injury in mice is ongoing.

正在进行葡萄籽原花青素对小鼠脑损伤的保护作用及机制的研究。

It is not easy to extract and refine the grapeseed oil

提取和精制葡萄籽油不是那么容易的。

graph [græf, grɑ:f] *n.* 曲线图,图表

The graph shows the effect of age on blood pressure.

此曲线图表示年龄对血压的影响。

grasp [grɑ:sp] *v.*, *n.* 抓住,紧握;理解,领会

The loose nail is now grasped with a hemostat and lifted out.

用止血钳将松脱的指甲夹紧再将其拔出。

grassroots ['grɑ:sru:ts] *n.* 基层

A network of medical care at the grassroots level has been initially established in the rural areas of China.

目前,中国农村基层医疗卫生网已经初步形成。

gravely ['greivli] *ad.* 严重地,重大地

Patients who are gravely ill should have the advantage of both drugs in combination.

严重的病人可从两种药物的联合使用中得到好处。

gravitate ['græviteit] *v.* (使)下沉,(使)受重力作用

If the patient is in bed, ankle oedema may be minimal but fluid gravitates to the sacral region.

若病人卧床,其踝部水肿可能极轻,但液体则沉积于骶部。

gravity ['græviti] *n.* 重力;严重性

There is little relation between the severity of chest discomfort and the gravity of its cause.

胸部不适的程度与其原发病灶的严重程度关系不大。

The normal kidney regulates the specific gravity of the urine according as the body needs.

正常人的肾脏可以按照人体的需要来调节其尿的比重。

gray [grei] *a.* 灰色的

Hyphae and spores are green against a gray background.

菌丝和孢子在灰黑色背景上呈绿色。

v. 变成灰色

Lerner has likened the pathogenesis of graying of the hair to that of vitiligo.

Lerner 把毛发变灰的发病机制比作白癜风的发病机制。

n. (神经)灰质

In the brain gray matter forms the cerebral cortex and the outer layer of the cerebellum; in the spinal cord the gray matter lies centrally and is surrounded by white matter.

在脑部灰质形成大脑皮质和小脑外皮层;在脊髓内灰质居于中央,四周被白质包围。

grief [gri:f] *n.* 悲痛,悲伤

Grief means keen mental suffering or distress over affliction of loss, deep sorrow, painful regret.

悲伤意味着强烈的精神痛苦,或丧失(亲人)的折磨,深切的伤心,痛苦的懊悔。

grip [grip] *n.* 流行性感冒,流感

The more neglected the prevention, the higher the attack rate of grip.

越是忽略了预防,流感发病率越高。

griseofulvin [ˌgrisiəu'fʌlvin] *n.* 灰黄霉素

Griseofulvin is well absorbed from the gut and is given in a daily dose of 250mg(child) or 500mg (adult).

灰黄霉素经肠道可很好吸收,儿童每日的剂量为250mg,成人为500mg。

Mild and temporary side-effects such as headache, skin rashes, and digestive upsets may occur when griseofulvin is administered by mouth.

口服灰黄霉素可有轻微的和暂时的副作用,如头痛、皮疹和胃肠道不适。

groin [grɔin] *n.* 腹股沟

Sometimes, a person with CLL (Chronic Lymphocytic Leukemia) may notice enlarged lymph nodes in the neck, armpit or groin and then go to see a doctor.

有时,患有慢性淋巴细胞性白血病的人会注意到自己颈部、腋下或腹股沟等部位的肿大的淋巴结,然后去医院看病。

The other half got stents——tiny wire mesh tubes threaded into the neck artery from an incision in the arm or groin.

另一半患者则接受支架术:将微小金属丝网管从手臂或者腹股沟的切口进入动脉到达颈动脉。

groove [gruːv] *n.* 沟

RESULTS: The angle between the transverse foramen and the vertebral artery groove in atlas was (67.875±5.394)°on the left side and (69.844±4.546)°on the right side.

结果:寰椎横突孔与椎动脉沟的成角左侧为(67.875±5.394)°,右侧为(69.844±4.546)°。

The medial and lateral subcutaneous fat of the nasolabial groove was 1.3 mm and 4.5mm in thickness respectively.

测得鼻唇沟内侧脂肪厚度为1.3mm,外侧为4.5mm。

gross [grəus] *a.* 肉眼(不用显微镜)能看到的,大的,显著的

At first only gross changes and later microscopic findings were demonstrated.

开始仅显示出大的肉眼看到的变化,后来则显示出镜下的变化。

In such instances, gross autopsy findings usually consist only of pulmonary edema and visceral congestion.

在这样的情况下,尸检肉眼观通常仅能发现肺水肿和内脏充血。

Staining techniques are revealing less gross abnormalities and variations in chromosomes.

染色技术显示较不明显的染色体异常和变异。

grossly [ˈgrəusli] *ad.* 显著地,严重地

The wound was grossly contaminated.

伤口已经严重污染。

This is a grossly inaccurate and inadequate method.

这个方法非常不准确,而且不适用。

ground [graund] *n.* 基础

Ground substance is the matrix of connective tissue, in which various cells and fibres are embedded.

基质是结缔组织的细胞间质,其中包埋有各种细胞和纤维。

v. 把…基于(on)

I'm sure that his arguments are grounded on facts.

我敢肯定他的论点是以事实为基础的。

groundwater [ˈgraundˌwɔːtə] *n.* 地下水

Groundwater is being pumped out much faster than it is being replenished.

地下水被抽取的速度远快于其补充的速度。

Arsenic is an element that can be released into groundwater by soil and rocks.

砷是一种元素,它可以通过土壤和岩石渗入地下水。

growth [grəuθ] *n.* 生长,发育

Growth hormone differs from other pituitary hormones (such as thyrotropin, luteinizing hormone

and adrenocorticotropic hormone) which have specific target organ.
生长激素有别于其他的垂体激素(如促甲状腺素、黄体生成素及促肾上腺皮质激素),这些激素都有特异的靶器官。

guanine [ˈgwɑːniːn] *n.* 鸟嘌呤

The interaction between Mg^{2+} and Ca^{2+} with guanine is stronger than that between Na^+ and K^+ with guanine.
鸟嘌呤中 Mg^{2+} 与 Ca^{2+} 的相互作用比 Na^+ 与 K^+ 之间的相互作用强。

Guanine is the most likely acceptor of the phosphate group.
鸟嘌呤是磷酸基团最可能的受体。

The guanine nucleotide exchange factors(GEFs) are proteins that can remove the bound GDP from G proteins, this allows GTP to bind and activate the G protein.
鸟嘌呤核苷酸交换因子(GEFs)是能够从 G 蛋白中移除结合的 GDP,从而允许 GTP 结合和激活 G 蛋白的蛋白质。

guarantee [gærən'tiː] *v.*, *n.* 保证

This food is guaranteed additive-free.
这种食品保证不含添加剂。

Thus, vaccination does not guarantee immunization.
因此,接种疫苗并不能保证会产生免疫。

To guarantee the cure of gonorrhea, similar follow-up tests are necessary.
为了确保治愈淋病,类似的追踪试验是必要的。

The manufacture's guarantee says that they will replace any defective parts for nothing.
厂方的保单上说明他们将免费更换一切不合格的零部件。

guidance [ˈgaidəns] *n.* 指引,指导

If ultrasonic guidance is utilized to direct the biopsy needle into the suspected lesion, the last step is not required.
如果利用超声波的引导将活检的针头插入可疑的病变部位的话,最后的一步也就不需要了。

guideline [ˈgaidlain] *n.* 方针,指导方针,准则

Guidelines have been developed to assist physicians in screening youth at risk.
已经建立了指导方针来帮助医生对高危青年(群体)的普查。

At the outset it must be noted that treatment guidelines are in the process of change, particularly in relation to concurrent HIV infection.
在开始时必须指出,治疗的准则正在变化的过程中,特别是关于同时伴有 HIV 感染的患者。

guinea-pig [ˈginipig] *n.* 豚鼠,荷兰猪

We kept many guinea-pigs for experiments.
我们养了许多豚鼠供试验用。

gum [gʌm] *n.* 牙龈,齿龈

The first eight deciduous teeth to make their appearance through the gums are the incisors.
最先从齿龈中长出的八个乳齿是切齿。

Symptoms of scurvy are bleeding gums, loose teeth, and poor healing of wounds.
坏血病的症状是齿龈出血、牙齿松动和伤口愈合不良。

gumma [ˈgʌmə] *n.* 树胶样肿,梅毒瘤

Gummas are nodular lesions probably related to the development of delayed hypersensitivity to the bacteria.
树胶样肿是结节状病变,可能与细菌引起的迟发型超敏反应有关。

They wanted to evaluate the imaging manifestations of cerebral gumma.
他们曾想评估大脑梅毒瘤的影像学表现。

gut [gʌt] *n.* 肠

Along the entire extent of the digestive tract, special substances are secreted into the gut, especially when food is present.

沿着整个消化道,一些特殊的物质分泌进入肠道,特别是在有食物的时候。

In the early stages of shock the small vessels in organs such as the gut are severely constricted.

在休克早期,脏器中如肠中的小血管剧烈收缩。

gutta [ˈgʌtə] (*pl.* **guttae** [ˈgʌtiː]) *n.* [拉] 滴,滴剂

Gutta is the form in which medicines are applied to the eyes and ears.

在医药中滴剂是用于眼睛和耳道的一种剂型。

gynaecomastia [ˌgainikəuˈmæstiə] *n.* 男子女性型乳房(=gynecomastia)

Gynecomastia is the most common breast pathology.

男子女性化乳房是一种最常见的乳房病理学变化。

This is a case of 19 years male who presented with micropenis, marked gynaecomastia and weight gain.

这是一个 19 岁的男性病例,表现为小阴茎、显著的男子女性化乳房和体重增加。

gynecologic [ˌgainikəˈlɔdʒik] *a.* 妇科(学)的

The patient' s age is a most important factor in the evaluation of gynecologic signs and symptoms.

患者的年龄对评价妇科症状和体征是一个非常重要的因素。

gynecology [ˌgainiˈkɔlədʒi] *n.* 妇科学

Gynecology is the branch of medicine which treats diseases of the genital tract in women.

妇产科学是论述妇女生殖道疾病的一门医学学科。

HBV infection was prevalent in the digestive department, while the incidence of latent syphilis was high in the department of gynecology.

乙型肝炎为消化科的高发疾病,而潜伏梅毒为妇科的高发疾病。

gynecomastia [ˌgainikəuˈmæstiə] *n.* 男性乳房发育

Gynecomastia is the abnormal development of mammary glands in males resulting in breast enlargement.

男性乳房发育是男性乳腺的异常发育,导致乳房增大。

In the male with hepatic failure, impaired estrogen metabolism and consequent hyperestrogenemia may lead to hypogonadism and gynecomastia.

在肝功能衰竭的男性患者中,雌激素代谢障碍和随后的高雌激素血症导致性腺功能减退和男性乳房发育。

gyration [dʒaiˈreiʃən] *n.* 旋转,回旋

In this case, a charged particle has a simple cyclotron gyration.

在这种情况下,带电粒子有一个简单的回旋回转。

This paper advances a non-contact detection technology of discontinuous gyration surface's radial jumping error.

这篇论文提出一种能够实现非连续回转面径向跳动误差检测的非接触检测方法。

H

habitat [ˈhæbitæt] *n.* 栖息地

Water makes an excellent habitat for a cold-blooded animal.

水是冷血动物理想的栖息地。

habitually [həˈbitjuəli] *ad.* 习惯性地，习以为常地

She habitually spent the hours from 9 p. m. to midnight in reading popular science.

她习惯性地把晚上九点至午夜的时间用于阅读科普读物。

haem [hiːm] *n.* 血红素

Haem is an iron-containing pigment.

血红素是一种含铁的色素。

In haemoglobin the prosthetic group is haem.

血红蛋白的辅基是血红素。

haemorrhoid [ˈhemərɔid] *n.* 痔

The main causes of haemorrhoid include: chronic constipation and straining, prolonged sitting, advanced age.

痔的主要原因包括：慢性便秘和用力排便、久坐、高龄。

What should haemorrhoid notice in dietary respect?

痔疮在饮食方面应该注意什么？

haemostasis [ˌhiːməuˈsteisis, ˌhem-] *n.* 止血法

Haemostasis is a process by which bleeding is stopped and blood is kept within a damaged blood vessel。

止血法是让出血停止的过程，并使血液留在受损的血管中。

Haemostasis is maintained in the body via three mechanisms: vascular spasm, platelet plug formation and blood coagulation.

在人体内止血通过三个机制完成：血管收缩、血小板血栓形成和血液凝固。

half-life [ˈhɑːflaif] *n.* 半衰期

The continuous enterohepatic cycling will increase the half-life of this agent in the body.

持续的肝肠循环会延长该药物在体内的半衰期。

The half-life of a drug or its elimination half-life is the time required to reduce its concentration in the blood by one half.

药物的半衰期或者说它的清除半衰期，是指药物在血液中的浓度降低一半所需要的时间。

hallmark [ˈhɔːlmɑːk] *n.* 标志；特点

A high serum iron is the early hallmark of chloramphenicol toxicity.

血清铁升高是氯霉素的毒性的早期指标。

hallucination [həˌluːsiˈneiʃən] *n.* 幻觉

An hallucination is a sensory experience for which there is no adequate external stimulus.

幻觉是在没有充分的外部刺激时产生的感觉。

Hallucinations occur when the brain is experiencing the inner reality while awake.

幻觉是人在醒着时大脑在历经内在现实时出现的。

hallucinogen [həˈluːsinədʒən] *n.* 致幻(觉)剂

Reserpine, methyldopa, and some hallucinogens may cause a depressive syndrome.

利血平、甲基多巴和某些致幻剂可造成抑郁综合征。

LSD and mescaline are both strong hallucinogens.
麦角酸二乙基酰胺和墨斯卡灵都是强有力的致幻剂。

hallucinosis [həˌluːsiˈnəusis] *n.* 幻觉症

The typical age of onset of alcohol hallucinosis is about 40.
酒精幻觉症的典型初发年龄约为 40 岁。

Hallucinosis is attributable principally to misuse of alcohol or other centrally acting drugs.
幻觉症主要归因于滥用酒精或其他作用于(神经)中枢的药物。

hallux [ˈhæləks] *n.* 大踇趾

20 cases of severed hallux were successfully replanted in our department.
我们科室成功地对 20 例离断踇趾进行了再植手术。

Chronic and extensive inflammation of the paratenon leads to stenosed tenosynovitis, producing the functional hallux rigidity.
肌腱旁组织的慢性和广泛的感染会引起狭窄性腱鞘炎,引起功能性的踇趾强直。

halo [ˈheiləu] *n.* 晕,空晕

Usually there is a clear halo around the intra-nuclear viral inclusion.
通常在核内病毒包涵体周围有一个清晰的空晕。

In chromophobe renal carcinoma, the neoplastic cells have pale eosinophilic cytoplasm with a perinuclear halo.
在嫌色性肾细胞癌中,肿瘤细胞具有淡染的嗜酸性胞质及核周空晕。

halogen [ˈhælədʒən] *n.* 卤素

The halogens are bromine, chlorine, fluorine, and iodine.
卤素是指溴、氯、氟和碘等元素。

haloperidol [ˌhæləuˈperidɔl] *n.* 氟哌啶醇

Haloperidol is a preferred agent for the treatment of delirium.
氟哌啶醇是治疗谵妄的首选药物。

Haloperidol is a butyrophenone neuroleptic agent.
氟哌啶醇是丁酰苯类安定药。

halophile [ˈhæləfail] *n.* 嗜盐菌

Many researchers study on the characteristics and application of extreme halophiles.
许多研究人员研究极端嗜盐菌的特性及其应用。

Halophile and salt-tolerant yeast have wide perspective and practicability on the treatment of wastewater with high salinity.
嗜盐菌和耐盐酵母菌在处理高含盐废水方面有广阔的应用前景。

halt [hɔːlt] *v.* (使)停止

It would be useful to halt virus replication.
阻止病毒复制将会有用。

hamartoma [ˌhæmɑːˈtəumə] *n.* 错构瘤

It is believed that tumors formerly classified as chondroma, osteochondroma or lipochondromas probably would be classified as hamartomas by present criteria.
现认为以前分类为软骨瘤、骨软骨瘤或脂肪软骨瘤的肿瘤,按目前标准来分类可分到错构瘤中。

hamper [ˈhæmpə] *v.* 妨碍,阻止

The emergence of drug-resistant strains has hampered the effect of chloroquine.
抗药菌株的出现已经影响到氯喹的疗效。

hamstring [ˈhæmstriŋ] *n.* 腘绳肌腱,腘旁腱

An attempt to produce passive extension of the knee with the hip fully flexed evokes spasm of the hamstrings and causes pain.
在髋部完全屈曲时,试图让膝部被动伸展,则可引起腘旁腱的痉挛而造成疼痛。

handbook [ˈhændbuk] *n.* 手册

This "Handbook of Legal Medicine" is the first excellent text in its field.

这本《法医学手册》是该领域里第一本优秀的教科书。

handicap [ˈhændikæp] *n.* 障碍,缺陷,残疾

Poor health is a serious handicap to a medical worker.

健康不良对于一个医务工作者来说,是一个严重的障碍。

A handicap may be the result of an accident or a disease, or it may be congenital.

残疾可由事故或疾病引起,也可能是先天性的。

Deafness can be a serious handicap.

失去听力是一种严重的残疾。

Handicap refers to a disadvantage resulting from an impairment or a disability that limits or prevents the fulfillment of a normal role.

残疾是指由损伤或残疾所造成的缺陷因而不能或限制了完成正常的任务。

handle [ˈhændl] *v.* 触,操纵,处理

Tularemia may also be transmitted to man by handling infected rabbits.

土拉菌病也可通过接触感染的兔子而传给人。

Severe burns are among the most difficult of all medical problems to handle.

严重烧伤是所有医学难题中最难处理的问题之一。

hantavirus [ˌhæntəˈvaiərəs] *n.* 汉坦病毒

The mice that transmit the hantavirus often take refuge in farmers' fields, barns and even homes.

传播汉坦病毒的小鼠往往栖身于农田、谷仓、甚至家中。

The virus which causes hemorrhagic fever is hantavirus.

引起出血热的病毒是汉坦病毒。

haploid [ˈhæplɔid] *a.* 单倍的 *n.* 单倍体(指一个个体或细胞只具有单套的同源染色体)

A meiotic cell division of a diploid cell results in two haploid cells.

一个二倍体的细胞经过一次减数分裂产生两个单倍体细胞。

A haploid human cell has 23 chromosomes.

一个单倍体人类细胞有 23 条染色体。

haploinsufficiency [ˌhæpləinsəˈfiʃənsi] *n.* 单倍不足,单一等位基因不足性

Haploinsufficiency means the inability of a single copy of the genetic material to carry out the functions normally performed by two copies.

单一等位基因不足性指单拷贝的遗传物质不足以维持通常由两个拷贝来完成的功能。

TS is associated with an astounding array of potential abnormalities, most of them thought to be caused by haploinsufficiency of genes that are normally expressed by both X chromosomes.

特纳综合征与一组惊人的潜在异常有关,大部分的这些异常被认为是由于两个 x 染色体正常表达的基因单倍不足所引起。

haplotype [ˈhæplətaip] *n.* 单倍型,单形体

A haplotype is defined as a series of alleles found at a linked locus on a chromosome.

单倍型定义为在一条染色体的基因座连锁上发现的一系列等位基因。

It is known that studies using haplotype information generally outperform those using single-marker analysis.

已知使用单体型信息研究通常优于使用单个标记分析。

hapten [ˈhæptən] *n.* 半抗原

A molecule that must combine with an endogenous protein to elicit an allergic reaction is called a hapten.

必须与内源蛋白质结合才能引发过敏反应的分子被称为半抗原。

Haptens are small molecules that become immunogenic only when covalently coupled to immunogenic protein carriers.

半抗原都是小分子，只有共价结合到免疫源性蛋白载体之后才能成为免疫源性（物质）。

haptoglobin [ˌhæptəuˈgləubin] *n.* [生化]结合珠蛋白

His serum haptoglobin disappeared or reduced.

他血清中的结合珠蛋白消失了或减少了。

In cattle, the most sensitive acute phase protein was haptoglobin (HP).

结合珠蛋白（HP）是奶牛最为敏感的急性期蛋白。

harbour [ˈhɑːbə] *v.* 聚藏

An incubating carrier is a person harbouring the causative organism.

一个潜伏期的带菌者是一个隐藏着致病微生物的人。

The patient himself may harbour the hemolytic streptococcus germ.

病人本人可能带有溶血性链球菌。

hardness [ˈhɑːdnis] *n.* 硬度，硬性

Water hardness is primarily the amount of calcium and magnesium in the water.

水的硬度主要是水中钙镁的量。

Moderate water hardness seems to work the best for breeding and coloration.

硬度适中的水似乎对育种和染色最有利。

hardware [ˈhɑːdwɛə] *n.* 硬件

I know nothing about computer hardware.

我对计算机硬件一窍不通。

a computer system is composed of software and hardware in the light of its working mode.

从计算机的工作模式看，计算机系统是由软件和硬件组成的。

harmonization [ˌhɑːmənaiˈzeiʃən] *n.* 协调；和谐

International Conference on Harmonization (ICH) guideline E1 outlines the size of the human database needed for licensing a medicine for non-life-threatening conditions.

国际协调会指南 E1 概述了人类数据库的大小，用于非危及生命情况的药物注册批准。

harmony [ˈhɑːməni] *n.* 和谐，协调

The parts of your body work together in harmony.

人体各部分工作协调一致。

harness [ˈhɑːnis] *v.* 利用；驾驭

Nuclear medicine, a diagnostic tool, is efficient, precise and sophisticated and we' re dedicated to harnessing its power.

核医学是一种高效、精准、尖端的诊断工具，我们致力于利用它的这种威力。

emerging evidence supports the potential for harnessing the cytotoxic power of eosinophils and redirecting it to kill solid tumors.

新出现的证据支持这种可能性，即利用嗜酸性粒细胞的毒性去杀死实体瘤。

hatch [hætʃ] *v.* 孵化

When sufficient spring rain falls to form a lake, once every two to five years, these eggs hatch.

当足够的春雨汇成湖泊时，每隔二至五年这些卵便孵化一次。

hazard [ˈhæzəd] *n.* 危险，危害；公害

When this procedure is used, the above described hazards are virtually eliminated.

使用这个方法时，上述的危险基本上得到消除。

Polluted environs are a positive health hazard.

污染了的环境，对于健康构成绝对的危害。

Though often beneficial, mindless use of antibiotics is not without hazard.

使用抗生素虽然常常有利，但如盲目使用，就不免有害。

hazardous [ˈhæzədəs] *a.* 危险的

Smoking has been firmly proved to be hazardous to health.

已有很有力的证据证明吸烟对健康危害极大。

In the case, the removal of an enzyme inducer could be hazardous.
在这种情况下,撤去酶诱导剂可能是很危险的。

haze [heiz] *n.* 霾 *v.* 使雾气笼罩

The haze poses serious health hazards, especially to those with a history of respiratory illness.
霾可造成严重的健康危害,特别是对那些有呼吸系统疾病史的人。

Some health problems linked to the haze are caused mainly by fine dust particles irritating the nose, throat, lungs, eyes and skin.
与霾有关的健康问题主要是由于细粉尘颗粒刺激鼻、咽喉、肺、眼和皮肤引起。

The mountain villages were hazed by mist in the morning.
清晨的山村笼罩在雾气之中。

hazy [ˈheizi] *a.* 模糊的

From the radiologic point of view, the infiltrates in viral pneumonia tend to be diffuse, ill-defined and hazy.
从放射学的观点来看,病毒性肺炎的浸润往往是弥漫性的,界限不清和模糊。

headache [ˈhedeik] *n.* 头痛

Headache is one of the most common ailments of man, it is a symptom rather than a disorder in itself.
头痛是人们最常见的疾病,它是一种症状而其本身并非一种病变。

I have a terrible headache.
我头痛得很厉害。

She has a history of headaches of five years' duration, but none as bad as the present one.
她有 5 年的头痛病史,但没有一次像现在痛得这样厉害。

heading [ˈhediŋ] *n.* 名称,标题

A remarkable series of defense mechanisms against injury can be considered under several different headings.
一系列奇异的对付损伤的防御机制可被纳入不同的标题下讨论。

heal [hiːl] *v.* 治愈,愈合,痊愈

"Inactive rheumatic heart disease" represents the stage of healed structural lesions.
"非活动性的风湿性心脏病"表示组织损伤处于愈合时期。

Many psychiatrists have observed the healing effect of physical work.
许多精神病医生观察到体力活动的医疗作用。

Once the myocardial infarct has healed, the patient may live for 15 to 20 years in good health.
一旦心肌梗死痊愈,病人可以健康存活 15 ~ 20 年。

healing [ˈhiːliŋ] *n.* 愈合

Antacids and diet often ameliorate symptoms but do not hasten healing.
制酸剂和饮食常可使症状缓解,但不能促使痊愈。

health [helθ] *n.* 健康;卫生;体质

Health is better than wealth.
健康胜于财富。

Promote physical culture and build up people's health.
发展体育运动增强人民体质。

Everyone should pay attention to public health.
每个人都应注意公共卫生。

healthful [ˈhelθfəl] *a.* 卫生的,有益于健康的

A healthful environment is essential to our personal health.
合乎卫生的环境对我们的个人健康是必不可少的。

healthy [ˈhelθiː] *a.* 健康的,健壮的

Nowadays most children are quite healthy.

现在绝大多数儿童都很健康。

People should protect their health by eating healthier foods, stopping smoking and exercising more.

人们应吃更有利健康的食物、戒烟和多锻炼来保护自己的健康。

hearing [ˈhiəriŋ] *n.* 听,听力,听觉

Hearing aids are very helpful for the person with hearing loss.

助听器对于听力丧失的人来说非常有用。

Wearing earphones at high volume and going to noisy bars were two of the reasons cited for the hearing problem.

使用大音量耳机和去喧闹的酒吧被认为是导致听力下降问题的两大原因。

heartburn [ˈhɑːtbəːn] *n.* 烧心感,胃灼热

Gastroesophageal reflux disease is usually manifestated by dysphagia and heartburn.

胃食管反流性疾病常表现为吞咽困难和烧心感。

Dyspepsia consists of various symptoms in the upper abdomen, such as discomfort, early satiation, bloating, heartburn, belching, nausea, vomiting, or pain.

消化不良包含上腹部的多种症状,如不适、早期饱胀感、腹胀、胃灼热、嗳气、恶心、呕吐和疼痛。

heat [hiːt] *n.* 热,热度

All the energy in the system becomes dissipated as heat.

系统中的所有能量都转化为热能消散了。

Hypothermia happens when the body cannot produce as much heat as it loses.

当身体无法产生足够热量来补充其损失的时候,体温就会下降。

heated [ˈhiːtid] *a.* 激烈的,热烈的

Cigarette smoking is the etiologic agent that has aroused the greatest interest and the most heated debates.

抽烟是引起最大兴趣和最激烈讨论的致病因素。

heatstroke [ˈhiːtstrəuk] *n.* 中暑

Heatstroke is potentially fatal unless treated immediately.

中暑如不给予及时的治疗,也能致死。

hebephrenia [ˌhebiˈfriːniə] *n.* 青春期痴呆

Hebephrenia typically starts in adolescense or young adulthood.

青春期痴呆典型的发病始于青春期或成年初期。

heel [hiːl] *n.* 脚跟

Training in the collection of capillary blood from finger or infant's heel, is first given.

首先要训练的是采集手指或婴儿脚跟毛细血管的血液。

hegar [ˈhegər] *n.* 黑加(征);黑格氏(征)

Hegar's sign is a non-sensitive indication of pregnancy in women—its absence does not exclude pregnancy.

黑加征指示妊娠并不敏感,但没有黑加征并不能排除妊娠。

height [hait] *n.* 高度,顶点

The normal child increases in both height and weight, but the increase of the two is not always parallel.

正常儿童的身高和体重两者同时增加,但其增加量未必是平行的。

The reaction generally occurs 6 to 8 hours after injection, but may not reach its height for several days.

通常这种反应在注射后 6 ~ 8 小时发生,但不会在几天内达到顶点。

helical [ˈhelikəl] *a.* 螺旋形的

Flagella are long, hollow, helical filaments, usually several times the length of the cell.

鞭毛是长而空心的螺旋形的丝状物,其长度通常为细胞长度的数倍。

helicopter [ˈhelikɔptə] *n.* 直升飞机

Helicopters also fly considerably slower than the twin-engine airplanes commonly used in medical evacuation.

直升飞机比在医疗疏散人群时使用的双引擎飞机的飞行速度要慢。

helix [ˈhiːliks] (*pl.* **helices** [ˈhelisiːz]) *n.* 螺旋,螺旋构型

DNA is a double helix.

DNA 是一种双螺旋结构。

The α-helix can form its spiral in either a left-handed sense or right-handed sense.

α-螺旋可形成左手或右手螺旋。

helminth [ˈhelminθ] *n.* 肠虫,蠕虫

Helminths, or worms, are composed of many cells and are visible to the naked eyes.

肠虫或蠕虫是由许多细胞组成的,肉眼即可看到。

helper [ˈhelpə] *n.* 帮助者,辅助者

T cells that cooperate with B cells to enhance the production of antibodies are called helper T cells.

和 B 细胞合作以增强抗体产生的 T 细胞被称为辅助性 T 细胞。

hemachromatosis [ˌhiːməˌkrəuməˈtəusis] *n.* 血色病,血色素沉着

Cardiac magnetic resonance (MR) of this patient revealed deposition of iron in the myocardium and established the diagnosis of hemachromatosis-related cardiomyopathy.

该患者的心脏磁共振(MR)显示心肌铁沉积,从而确诊血色病相关性心肌病。

Previously, hepatic iron overload resembling that in hereditary hemachromatosis has been found in beta 2-microglobulin knockout (beta 2m-/-) mice.

以前在 beta-2 微球蛋白基因敲除(beta 2m-/-)小鼠中已经发现,肝脏铁负荷超载类似于遗传性血色病的表现。

hemagglutination [ˌhiməgluːtiˈneiʃən] *n.* 血细胞凝集试验

Indirect fluorescent antibody test and hemagglutination test are of practical importance.

间接荧光抗体试验和血细胞凝集试验具有实用的重要性。

hemagglutinin [ˌhiːməˈgluːtinin] *n.* 血凝素,血凝集素

The hemagglutinin causes the agglutinations of erythrocytes of several species.

血凝素可导致几个种属的红细胞凝集。

hemangioblastoma [hiːˌmændʒiəublæsˈtəumə] *n.* 脑血管母细胞瘤

10 cases of cerebral haemangioblastoma proved by surgery were analyzed retrospectively.

回顾性分析了 10 例经手术证实为脑血管母细胞瘤的病案。

hemangioendothelioma [hiˌmændʒiəuˈendəuˌθiːliˈəumə] *n.* 血管内皮细胞瘤

Epithelioid hemangioendothelioma is a rare pulmonary neoplasm with less than 40 cases described worldwide.

上皮样血管内皮细胞瘤是罕见的肺部肿瘤,全世界报道不足 40 例。

Epitheloid hemangioendothelioma of the liver is a rare mesenchymal tumor, the recommended treatment of which is either liver resection or hepatic transplantation, if no metastasis is found.

肝脏上皮样血管内皮细胞瘤是罕见的间质性肿瘤,在没有发现转移的情况下推荐的治疗方法是肝切除或者肝移植。

hemangioma [hiːˌmændʒiˈəumə] *n.* 血管瘤

Hemangiomas are less common than lipomas in the small intestine.

小肠内血管瘤比脂瘤较为少见。

hemangiopericytoma [hiˈmændʒiəuˌperisaiˈtəumə] *n.* 血管外皮细胞瘤

Hemangiopericytomas are rare soft-tissue tumors originating from extravascular cells (pericytes).

血管外皮细胞瘤是一种少见的软组织肿瘤,起源于血管外皮细胞。

hematemesis [ˌhiməˈtemisis] *n.* 呕血

The most striking symptoms of esophageal varicose vein are melena and hematemesis.

食道静脉曲张最突出的症状是黑粪和呕血。

Hematemesis is the vomiting of blood, usually from the upper gastrointestinal tract.

呕血是指血由口呕出，通常源自上消化道。

hematinic [ˌheməˈtinik] *n.* 补血药

Hematinics are used, often in combination with vitamins and folic acid, to prevent and treat anemia due to iron deficiency.

补血药在用于预防和治疗缺铁性贫血时，常与维生素类和叶酸联合使用。

In treatment of iron-reutilization anemia hematinics have no value.

在治疗铁再利用性贫血时补血药没有任何治疗价值。

hematochezia [ˌhiːmətəuˈkiːziə] *n.* 便血

The most common cause of hematochezia is bleeding from hemorroids precipitated by straining or passage of hard stools.

便血的最常见原因是用力排便或排硬粪便引起的痔疮出血。

There was no associated vomiting, melena, hematochezia, or constipation.

不伴有呕吐、黑便、便血或便秘。

hematocrit [hiˈmætəkrit, ˈhemətəkrit] *n.* 红细胞压积，血细胞比容

If there is shock with an elevated hematocrit, then the plasma volume loss of peritonitis is suggested.

如果休克伴有红细胞压积升高，则提示腹膜炎伴有血浆容量损失。

Ordinarily, anemia refers to a decrease in the total number of circulating erythrocytes, or a decrease in the concentration of hemoglobin in blood, or a decrease in the hematocrit compared to a normal group.

一般说来，贫血是指循环红细胞总数减少，或血液中血红蛋白浓度降低，或和正常组相比血比容下降。

hematogenous [ˌhiːməˈtɔdʒinəs] *a.* 血源性的

Hematogenous pneumonia is seen in those with soft tissue infections.

血源性肺炎见于软组织感染者。

The liver is involved either by direct extension of the tumor or through hematogenous spread.

肝脏受累可由肿瘤直接扩散或通过血源传播所致。

hematologic [ˌhimətəˈlɔdʒik] *a.* 血液的

Bone marrow aspiration and biopsy should be done early in suspected hematologic diseases.

疑有血液病时应早抽取骨髓作活检。

hematology [ˌhiməˈtɔlədʒi] *n.* 血液学

Hematology is the science dealing with the morphology of blood and blood-forming tissues, and with their physiology and pathology.

血液学是研究有关血液的形态和造血组织以及血液的生理学、病理学的科学。

hematoma [ˌhiːməˈtəumə] *n.* 血肿

Wound hematoma is a collection of blood and clots in the wound.

血液和凝血块积聚在伤口内称伤口血肿。

A hematoma is a localized collection of blood outside the blood vessels, usually in liquid form within the tissue.

血肿是指血液在血管外局部积聚，通常是以液体状态存在于组织中。

hematopoiesis [ˌhimətəupɔiˈiːsis] *n.* 造血，造血作用，生血作用，血细胞生成

Hematopoiesis is the generation of all the cellular elements of blood, and in humans occurs in the bone marrow.

造血作用就是产生血中的所有细胞成分，在人类是出现在骨髓。

Hematopoiesis of the other blood elements occurs in the fetal spleen.
其他血液成分的生成发生在胎儿脾脏。

hematopoietic [ˌhiːmətəupɔiˈetik] *a.* 生血的，造血的

Occupational and environmental exposure to cadmium is also associated with development of cancer of the prostate, kidney, liver, hematopoietic system and stomach.
镉的职业性接触与环境接触也与前列腺、肾、肝、造血系统和胃的癌的发生有关联。

hematopoietin [ˌhimətəupɔiˈiːtin] *n.* 促红细胞生成素

The hematopoietin family is a large family of structurally related cytokines that includes growth factors and many interleukins with roles in both adaptive and innate immunity.
促红细胞生成素家族是一个结构上相关的细胞因子大家族，这些细胞因子包括生长因子和很多白介素，它们在适应性免疫和固有免疫起作用。

hematotoxic [ˌhiːmətəˈtɔksik] *a.* 血液毒性的

Workers exposed to benzene solvent showed a range of hematotoxic effects including anemia, leucopenia, and thrombocytopenia.
接触苯溶液的工人表现出一定范围的血液毒性效应，包括：贫血、白细胞减少和血小板减少。

hematotoxicity [ˈhemətəˌtɔkˈsisiti] *n.* 血液毒性

The hematotoxicity of benzene exposure has been well known for a century.
一个世纪以来，由苯暴露所导致的血液毒性已为大家所熟知。

Use of anthracyclines is often limited in older patients due to cardiac toxicity and hematotoxicity.
蒽环类药物的心脏毒性和血液毒性限制了其在老年病人中的应用。

hematotoxicology [ˈhemətəˌtɔksiˈkɔlədʒi] *n.* 血液毒理学

Animal hematotoxicology: a practical guide for toxicologists and biomedical researchers.
动物血液毒理学：毒理学家和生物医学研究者的实用指南。

The prolonged effects of extracted microcystins on hematotoxicology were investigated.
研究了微囊藻毒素提取物在血液毒理学方面的长期效应。

hematuria [ˌhiːməˈtjuriə] *n.* 血尿

He has been suffering from proteinuria, hematuria and hepatic injury for three years.
他患蛋白尿、血尿和肝脏损害已有 3 年了。

Hematuria may be found at the initial presentation in patients with idiopathic nephrotic syndrome.
血尿可见于特发性肾病综合征患者的最初表现中。

heme [hiːm] *n.* 血红素，亚铁血红素

Deficient or defective heme or globin synthesis produces a hypochromic-microcytic RBC population.
血红素或球蛋白合成不足或有缺陷可产生低色素小细胞性红细胞群。

Free erythrocyte protoporphyrin is measurably increased in circumstances of altered heme synthesis.
在血红素合成有改变的情况下，游离红细胞原卟啉可增加到能测出的水平。

hemianesthesia [ˌhemiˌænisˈθiːziə] *n.* 偏身感觉障碍；半身麻木

We reported a patient with stroke due to the ischemia in the vascular territory of the right middle cerebral artery who had left spatial neglect and left hemianesthesia.
我们报道了一例右侧大脑中动脉分布区缺血性卒中的患者，表现左侧空间忽略和左侧偏身感觉障碍。

heat stimulation to the left vestibule can reduce the impairments of right-brain-damaged patients with left unilateral neglect, including left hemianesthesia.
左侧前庭热刺激可减轻对左单侧忽略的右脑受损病人的损害，包括左侧偏身感觉障碍。

hemianopia [ˌhemiəˈnəupiə] *n.* 偏盲

Homonymous hemianopia is a visual field defect involving either the two right or the two left halves of the visual fields of both eyes.
同侧偏盲是一种视野缺失，累及双眼右侧半或左侧半视野。
Brain damage disrupts these complicated processes, resulting in severe visual impairments including hemianopia.
脑损伤破坏了这些复杂的通路过程，导致严重的视力受损，包括偏盲。

hemiarthroplasty [ˌhiːməˈtemisis, ˌhem-] *n.* 半关节成形术
On the following day, the patient was operated on with epidural anesthesia for the right hemiarthroplasty.
次日患者在硬膜外麻醉下接受了右侧半关节成形术。
It is possible that some fractures previously treated with hemiarthroplasty may be cured successfully with locking plates.
一些以前需要行半关节置换的骨折可能通过锁定钢板成功治愈。

hemidecortication [ˌhemidiːˌkɔːtiˈkeiʃən] *n.* 偏侧大脑皮层切除术
Large neocortical lesions, such as hemidecortication, are detrimental to motor and cognitive skills.
较大的新皮层损伤，如偏侧大脑皮层切除术，对运动和认知技能有伤害。
Patients who have undergone left hemidecortication for infantile hemiplegia have mild linguistic defects.
进行了左侧偏侧大脑皮层切除术的婴儿偏瘫病人有轻微的语言障碍。

hemimelia [ˌhemiˈmiliə] *n.* 半肢畸形
The infant, born at 29 weeks of gestation, has tetralogy of Fallot and tibial hemimelia.
这个婴儿在孕 29 周出生，患有法洛四联征和胫侧半肢畸形。
Fibular hemimelia is a congenital disorder characterized by partial or total absence of the fibula.
腓侧半肢畸形是一种先天性疾病，以腓骨的部分或者全部缺失为特点。

hemipelvectomy [ˌhemipelˈvektəmi] *n.* 偏侧骨盆切除术；半骨盆切除术
A hemipelvectomy is a high level pelvic amputation.
半骨盆切除术是高位的骨盆切除。
Hemipelvectomy was performed for 7 sarcomas and 6 carcinomas.
对 7 位肉瘤患者和 6 位癌患者施行了半骨盆切除术。

hemiplegia [ˌhemiˈpliːdʒiə] *n.* 偏瘫
Findings of EEG and cranial CT in 21 children with hemiplegia type of viral encephalitis were analyzed.
对 21 例偏瘫型病毒性脑炎患儿的脑电图和头颅计算机断层扫描进行了分析。
In this paper, we study the correlative technology of applying robot to the rehabilitation training of the patients with hemiplegia for their upper-limb multiple-motion.
本文对机器人用于偏瘫患者上肢复合运动康复训练中的相关技术进行探讨研究。

hemirachischisis [ˌhemirəˈkiskəsis] *n.* 隐性脊柱裂
The patients with primary enuresis complicating with hemirachischisis were treated with routine manipulations as well as the massage and manual method on acupoints.
并发隐性脊柱裂的原发性遗尿病人可通过常规的推拿和在穴位上按摩以及用手工方法治疗。
Hemirachischisis is a one-sided, incomplete fusion of the lumbar vertebrae, detectable by radiography.
隐性脊柱裂是一侧腰椎的不完全融合，可用放射摄影术检测出来。

hemisphere [ˈhemisfiə] *n.* 半球
The outer nerve tissue of the cerebral hemisphere is gray matter and is called the cerebral cortex.
大脑半球的外部神经组织是灰质，叫做大脑皮质。
Inside the hemispheres are two spaces extending in a somewhat irregular fashion.

半球内有两个间隙,伸展样式不太规则。

hemispheric [ˌhemiˈsferik] *a.* 半球的

Neglect syndrome is less common following left hemispheric damage.

大脑左半球损伤后出现忽视症状并不常见。

This exercise is thought to help increase inter-hemispheric communication.

这项运动被认为可以加强两脑半球间的交流。

hemizygous [ˌhemiˈzaigəs] *a.* [遗]半合子的

Both single genes and chromosome segments may be hemizygous.

单独的基因和染色体片段都有可能是半合子。

Bilateral sensorineural hearing loss, which is never congenital in onset, occurs in 90% of hemizygous males with X-linked AS.

双侧感觉神经性听力失聪虽从不先天性发病,但 90% 的伴有 X 染色体连锁的 AS 的杂合子男性却患此病。

hemobilia [ˌhiːməuˈbiljə] *n.* 胆道出血

Hemobilia is manifested by upper gastrointestinal bleeding.

胆道出血表现为上消化道出血。

The patients with massive hemobilia are often diagnosed by angiography and treated by interventional embolization.

胆道大出血的患者常以血管造影进行诊断并行介入栓塞治疗。

hemocatheresis [ˌhiːməkəˈθerisis] *n.* 红细胞破坏

This process is carried out in the red pulp and is referred to as ' hemocatheresis'.

在红髓中发生的这个过程称"红细胞破坏"。

hemoccult [ˈhiːməkʌlt] *n.* 隐血

The remainder of the examination was unremarkable and stool hemoccult testing was negative.

其他检查无特殊表现,大便隐血试验为阴性。

hemochromatosis [ˈhiːməˌkrəuməˈtəusis] *n.* 血色沉着病

This patient suffers from hemochromatosis, a treatable condition which displays similar symptoms of liver cirrhosis.

这个病人得的是一种可治愈的血色素沉着症,其症状和肝硬化相似。

Hemochromatosis is a liver disease caused by iron overload.

血色沉着病是由于铁过量造成的肝脏疾病。

hemodiafiltration [ˌhiːməuˌdaiəfilˈtreiʃən] *n.* 血液透析滤过

An increased prevalence of spontaneous bleeding manifestation has been observed since the beginning of maintenance hemodiafiltration.

自从开展维持性血液透析滤过以来,自发性出血的情况增多了。

hemodialysis [ˌhiːmədaiˈælisis] *n.* 血液透析,血液渗析

Hemodialysis is performed on patients whose kidneys have ceased to function, the process takes place in an artificial kidney, or dialyser.

血液透析用于两侧肾已丧失功能的病人,透析通过用人工肾或透析机来进行。

Hemodialysis can prolong survival and provide partial rehabilitation.

血液透析能延长存活期并且使部分病人康复。

hemodynamic [ˌhiːmədaiˈnæmik] *a.* 血流动力学的

The hemodynamic mechanism is a very simple one.

血流动力学机制很简单。

This arrhythmia may produce a rapid ventricular rate, resulting in hemodynamic deterioration.

这种心律失常可以产生快速性心室率,结果引起血流动力学的恶化。

hemodynamically [ˌhiːməudaiˈnæmikəli] *ad.* 在血流动力学上

The lesion which is present is not hemodynamically significant.

所出现的损伤在血流动力学上是不重要的。

hemodynamics [ˌhimoudaiˈnæmiks] *n.* (用作单或复)血液动力学

No study has yet demonstrated an objective improvement in hemodynamics, lung mechanics, or gas exchange following phlebotomy.

现在还没有研究资料表明静脉切开后可以客观地改善血液动力学、肺机械功能或气体交换。

hemoglobin [ˌhiːməuˈgləubin] *n.* 血红蛋白

The normal amount of hemoglobin varies from about 14 to 16 grams per 100 cc. of blood.

血红蛋白常数在每 100 立方厘米血液中约为 14 ~ 16 克不等。

Anoxia can occur as a result of lack of available hemoglobin.

缺氧的发生可由于缺少血红蛋白的有效供应。

hemoglobinopathy [ˌhiːməuˌgləubiˈnɔpəθi] *n.* 血红蛋白病

Variant hemoglobins (hemoglobinopathy) can be used to trace past human migrations and to study genetic relationships among populations.

变异的血红蛋白(血红蛋白病)能用于追溯过去的人类迁移和研究人群间的遗传关系。

Hemoglobinopathies such as thalassemias and sickle cell anemia, important genetic diseases of people, have not been seen in other animals.

有些人类的重大遗传性血红蛋白病(例如地中海贫血和镰状细胞性贫血)没有在其他动物中发现。

hemoglobinuria [ˌhiːməuˌgləubiˈnjuəriə] *n.* 血红蛋白尿

In circumstances of chronic intravascular hemolysis, RBC fragmentation may produce Fe lack by chronic hemoglobinuria and hemosiderinuria.

在慢性血管内溶血的情况下,红细胞的碎裂可因慢性血红蛋白尿和含铁血黄素尿而造成缺铁。

March hemoglobinuria is observed in distance rumers and is most likely related to damage to red cells as they pass through vessels in the soles of the feet.

行军性血红蛋白尿多见于长跑运动员,主要与红细胞通过足底部的血管时受损有关。

hemolysis [hiːˈmɔlisis] *n.* 溶血,血细胞溶解

Anemia is due to hemolysis, hemorrhage, and azotemia and may be severe.

贫血可由溶血、出血和氮质血症引起,可以很严重。

When RBC values fall at a rate>10% without hemorrhage, hemolysis is established as a causative factor.

当红细胞的下降大于 10% 而又没有出血时,可确定溶血是一致病因素。

hemolytic [ˌhiːməˈlitik] *a.* 溶血的

A hemolytic anemia is due to red-cell destruction.

溶血性贫血是由红细胞的破坏引起的。

The fetus probably dies from cardiac failure caused by the severe hemolytic anemia rather than from placental insufficiency.

胎儿可能死于严重溶血性贫血引起的心衰,而不大可能死于胎盘功能不全。

hemolyticuremic [hiˌmɔlitikjuˈremik] *a.* 溶血性尿毒的

Children with severe colitis due to S. dysenteriae I are prone to develop the hemolyticuremic syndrome.

儿童患志贺痢疾杆菌 I 引起的严重结肠炎易发展为溶血性尿毒综合征。

hemoperfusion [ˌhiːməupəˈfjuːʒən] *n.* 血液灌流

Hemoperfusion has been used in poisoning, hepatic failure, and in treatment of uremia and its complications.

血液灌流已用于中毒,肝功能衰竭和尿毒症及其并发症的治疗。

hemopericardium [ˈhiːməˌperiˈkɑːdiəm] *n.* 血心包;心包积血

Hemodynamic deterioration cues that an emergency operation is needed to relieve hemopericardium.
血流动力学恶化提示需行急诊手术解除心包积血。
Hemopericardium is one of the complications after cardiosurgery.
心包积血是心脏外科手术的并发症之一。

hemoperitoneum [ˌhiːməuˌperitəu'niːəm] *n.* 腹腔积血
Massive hemoperitoneum and contractive spleen on CT might be indicated rupture of solid organ.
CT 示腹腔大量积血与脾脏缩小提示可能有实质性器官破裂。
The objective is to explore the status and role of non-operative management of blunt abdominal trauma with hemoperitoneum.
(该文)旨在探讨对伴有内出血的钝性腹部损伤进行非手术治疗的现状和作用。

hemophilia [ˌhiːmə'filiə] *n.* 血友病
Hemophilia is an example of a genetically heterogeneous syndrome.
血友病是一种遗传异质性综合征的一个范例。
In many countries hundreds of thousands of people suffer from such common blood diseases as aplastic anemia, hemophilia and platelet deficiency.
在许多国家,有成千上万的人患有再生障碍性贫血、血友病、血小板减少等常见的血液病。

hemophiliac [ˌhiːmə'filiæk] *n.* 血友病患者
Hematuria is relatively common in hemophiliacs.
血尿在血友病患者中较为常见。
Not surprisingly, there are now fewer cases of AIDS among hemophiliacs and people given blood transfusion.
并不奇怪的是现在在血友病患者和被输血的人中间艾滋病病例比较少。

hemopoiesis [ˌhiːməupɔi'iːsis] *n.* 造血作用
It facilitated the growth of stem cells of marrow hemopoiesis, largely increased the amount of monocells and promoted its particle differentiation.
它可促进骨髓造血干细胞生长,大量增加单细胞数量,并促进其粒子分化。
In all cases of the observed group there were remission of clinical symptom, significant weight gain, serum albumin increase and recovery of marrow hemopoiesis.
观察组所有病例都有临床症状的缓解、明显的体重增加、血清白蛋白增加和骨髓造血作用的恢复。

hemoptysis [hiː'mɔptisis] *n.* 咯血
The cough was nonproductive with no hemoptysis.
咳嗽无痰,亦无咯血。
Haemoptysis is the expectoration of blood or of blood-stained sputum from the larynx, bronchi, trachea, or lungs。
咯血是指咳出来自喉部、支气管、气管或肺组织的血液或血痰。
There are many conditions involving haemoptysis that include bronchitis, pneumonia (most common), and lung neoplasm.
许多情况可以引起咯血,其中包括支气管炎、肺炎(最常见),及肺部肿瘤。

hemorrhage ['heməridʒ] *n.* 出血
This causes widespread petechial hemorrhages in the skin and various tissues.
这就引起皮肤和各种组织广泛的点状出血。
Vasopressin may stop hemorrhage from varices.
垂体加压素可阻止静脉曲张出血。

hemorrhagic [ˌhemə'redʒik] *a.* 出血的
In later deaths small hemorrhagic infarcts are seen in the white matter of the cord.
晚期死亡病例,在脊髓白质内可见小的出血性梗死。

The necrotic wall of the intestine is congested, edematous and hemorrhagic.
坏死的肠壁上有充血、水肿及出血(的现象)。

hemorrhoid [ˈheməɾɔid] *n.* 痔

They interpret this as(being) due to hemorrhoids rather than a possible carcinoma of the colon.
他们认为是痔疮所致,而不认为有结肠癌的可能。

hemorrhoidal [ˌheməˈrɔidl] *a.* 痔的

Enlargement of the hemorrhoidal veins may produce symptomatic hemorrhoids.
痔静脉的扩张可引起有症状的痔。

hemorrhoidectomy [ˌhemərɔiˈdektəmi] *n.* 痔切除术

The results of hemorrhoidectomy are excellent.
痔切除术的效果极好。

hemosiderin [ˌhiːməuˈsidərin] *n.* 含铁血黄素,血铁黄素

Iron deficiency may also be secondary to increased urinary loss of hemosiderin.
铁的缺乏也可能是继发于尿液中含铁血黄素丢失量的增加。

Hemosiderin deposition in the liver is a common feature of hemochromatosis and is the cause of liver failure in the disease.
肝中含铁血黄素沉积是血色素沉着症的一个共同特征,是导致疾病中肝功能衰竭的原因。

hemosiderinuria [ˌhiːməuˌsidəriˈnjuəriə] *n.* 含铁血黄素尿症

In circumstances of chronic intravascular hemolysis, RBC fragmentation may produce Fe lack by chronic hemoglobinuria and hemosiderinuria.
在慢性血管内溶血的情况下,红细胞的碎裂可因慢性血红蛋白尿和含铁血黄素尿而造成缺铁。

hemostasis [hiˈmɔstəsis] *n.* 止血(法),瘀血

Wound hematoma is almost always caused by imperfect hemostasis.
伤口血肿差不多都是由止血不完善所致。

When the injury is extensive, the blood clotting mechanism is activated to assist in hemostasis.
当损伤面扩大时,血液凝固机制增强(被激活),从而有助于止血。

There are some methods of hemostasis for you to grasp.
你要掌握某些止血方法。

hemostatic [hiːməˈstætik] *a.* 止血的

The entire hemostatic mechanism can be devided into three components: extravascular effects, vascular effects, and intravascular effects.
整个止血机制分为三个组成部分:血管外作用,血管性作用和血管内作用。

The most important screening tests of the primary hemostatic system are a bleeding time and a platelet count.
用于检查基本止血系统功能最重要的指标是出血时间和血小板计数。

Hemostatics are used to control bleeding due to various causes and may be used in treating bleeding disorders, such as haemophilia.
止血剂用于控制各种原因引起的出血,也可用来治疗出血性疾病,如血友病。

hemothorax [ˌhiːməuˈθɔːræks] *n.* 血胸

Hemorrhagic pleuritis or hemothorax may result from trauma.
出血性胸膜炎或血胸可由外伤引起。

Blood in the pleural cavity is called hemothorax which is usually due to injury.
血液存在于胸膜腔内时叫作血胸,它常由损伤引起。

hepadnaviridae [hepˌædnəˈviridiː] *n.* 嗜肝 DNA 病毒科

HBV belongs to hepadnaviridae with a partially double stranded and circular DNA genome.
HBV 属于嗜肝 DNA 病毒科,具有部分双链环状的 DNA 基因组。

The hepatitis B virus(HBV) and other members of the hepadnaviridae replicate by reverse tran-

scription of RNA.
乙肝病毒以及其他嗜肝 DNA 病毒通过 RNA 的逆转录过程而复制。

heparan [ˈhepəræn] *n.* 乙酰肝素

Platelet factor 4 binding to the heparan sulfate would prevent the antithrombin III interaction with glycosaminoglycan and thus would prevent enhancement of the rate of thrombin inactivation.
血小板因子 4 和硫酸乙酰肝素结合时可阻止抗凝血酶Ⅲ和葡糖胺聚糖之间的相互作用，从而防止了凝血酶失活的速度加快。

heparin [ˈhepərin] *n.* 肝素

Commercial heparin is a sulfated mucopolysaccharide.
通常的商品肝素是一种硫酸化黏多糖。

Small amount of heparin, a powerful anticoagulant, are normally present in the blood.
肝素是一种很强的抗凝剂，正常血液中就有少量存在。

hepatic [hiˈpætik] *a.* 肝的

Hepatic coma may be precipitated by protein in the gut.
肠内蛋白沉积也可能诱发肝昏迷。

Don't inform the patient of the fact that he has hepatic carcinoma.
不要告诉病人他患肝癌的事实。

hepaticojejunostomy [hiˌpætikəuˌdʒidʒuːˈnɔstəmi] *n.* 肝管空肠吻合术

Hypoalbuminemia is the most important risk factor for outcome after hepaticojejunostomy.
低白蛋白血症是肝内胆管空肠吻合术术后结局的最重要危险因素。

Main surgical treatments of bile duct reoperation include lobar resection with Roux-en-Y hepaticojejunostomy and T-tube drainage.
胆管再次手术的主要外科治疗包括肝叶切除连同 Roux-en-Y 胆管空肠吻合术和 T 管引流。

hepatitis [ˌhepəˈtaitis] *n.* 肝炎

Chronic hepatitis may be defined as inflammation of the liver continuing without improvement for at least six months.
慢性肝炎可下定义为病程至少持续 6 个月而症状无改善的肝脏炎症。

Ameobic hepatitis is common on a world basis and usually presents as a hepatic abscess.
阿米巴肝炎是世界范围内的常见病，一般表现为肝脓肿。

hepatization [ˌhepətaiˈzeiʃən] *n.* 肝样变

The four stages of lobar pneumonia consist of congestion, red hepatization, gray hepatization and resolution.
大叶性肺炎的四期分为：充血期、红色肝样变期、灰色肝样变期和溶解消散期。

Hepatization in the lobar pneumonia refers to a uniformed consolidation with a liver-like consistency of the involved lobe.
大叶性肺炎的肝样变是指病变肺叶均匀一致的实变，质地像肝脏。

hepatoblastoma [hepətəublæsˈtəumə] *n.* 肝胚细胞瘤

Hepatoblastoma is the most common malignant liver tumour in infants and young children.
肝胚细胞瘤是婴幼儿中一种最常见的恶性肝肿瘤。

Adult and paediatric patients with hepatoblastoma appear to have worse outcomes.
患肝胚细胞瘤的成人和儿童患者似乎后果更糟。

hepatocellular [ˌhepətəuˈseljulə] *a.* 肝细胞的

To date, fatal hepatocellular damage has been reported in three patients.
至今，有致命的肝细胞损伤的患者已有 3 例报道。

Clonorchiasis has no causal relationship with hepatocellular cancer.
华支睾吸虫病与肝细胞癌无病因上的联系。

hepatocyte [ˈhepətəsait] *n.* 肝细胞

They studied on the relationship between hepatitis B virus and hepatocyte apoptosis.

他们研究了乙肝病毒与肝细胞凋亡之间的关系。

Excessive vitamin A and zinc intake could affect the cell cycle of hepatocyte.

过量摄入维生素 A 和锌可能影响肝细胞的细胞周期。

hepatoma [ˌhepəˈtəumə] *n.* 肝肿瘤，肝细胞瘤

Carcinoma arising within the liver may be hepatoma, cholangioma, or mixed origin.

发生于肝脏内的癌瘤可以是肝肿瘤、胆管瘤或混合型。

hepatomegaly [ˌhepətəˈmegəli] *n.* 肝大

There is usually a marked degree of hepatomegaly.

通常有明显的肝肿大。

hepatosis [ˌhepəˈtəusis] *n.* 肝功能障碍

We report herein a case of vitiligo in a cow, apparently associated with hepatosis.

我们在此报告一头患白癜风的牛，显然与肝病相关。

This experiment has certain significance in revealing the mechanism of hepatosis induced by CCl_4 poisoning.

本实验对于阐明四氯化碳中毒性肝病发病机制有一定的意义。

hepatosplenomegaly [ˌhepətəuˌspliːnəuˈmegəli] *n.* 肝脾（肿）大

In such case, abdomen was soft with no hepatosplenomegaly.

在这种情况下，腹软，肝脾不肿大。

The most prominent clinical finding of myelosclerosis is hepatosplenomegaly.

骨髓硬化症的最突出的临床表现是肝脾肿大。

hepatotoxicant [ˈhepətəˈtɔksikənt] *n.* 肝毒物

Tumor necrosis factor receptor knockout (TNFR KO) mice were used to examine the role of tumor necrosis factor-α (TNFα) signaling during acute hepatotoxicant exposure.

采用肿瘤坏死因子受体敲除（TNFR KO）小鼠研究在急性肝毒物暴露下肿瘤坏死因子 α（TNFα）信号传导的作用。

This expression profile analysis could be one of the useful tools for evaluating a potential hepatotoxicant in the drug development process.

这个表达谱分析可以成为一个有用的工具，用作评估药物开发过程中的潜在肝毒物。

hepatotoxicity [ˌhepətəutɔkˈsisiti] *n.* 肝毒性，肝中毒，肝脏毒性，肝细胞毒性

Hepatotoxicity is one of the most common adverse reactions during anti-tuberculosis treatment.

肝毒性是抗结核药物治疗中最常见的毒副作用之一

Legalon is the antidote of choice in patients with acute hepatotoxicity from amatoxin poisoning.

利肝隆是毒伞毒素中毒所致急性肝中毒病人的常用解毒药。

heptamer [ˈheptəmə] *n.* 七聚物

Another exciting agent, and the one probably closest to human testing, would alter the heptamer itself.

可能最接近人体试验的另一种激动剂，可改变七聚体本身。

herald [ˈherəld] *n.* 先驱，预示

Such symptoms are usually considered as a herald of measles.

这种症状常常被看成是麻疹的先兆。

v. 宣布；预示…的来临

Significant hepatomegaly and splenomegaly herald the presence of portal hypertension.

显著的肝肿大及脾肿大预示门脉高压的发生。

Lengthening of the menstrual cycle may herald the approach of secondary amenorrhea.

月经周期的延长，也许预示继发性无月经的到来。

herb [həːb] *n.* 草，草药

The cost of medicinal herbs is far less than that of chemical drugs.

草药的价格比化学药物低得多。

This herb lowers the blood pressure, in similar manner to that western drug.

这草药降低血压,作用和那西药相似。

The amount of the useful parts of the herb is not constant throughout the year.

草本植物所含有用部分的量不是全年都一样的。

herbal [ˈhəːbəl] *a.* 草本植物的

Despite the existence of herbal medicines for many centuries, only a relatively small number of plant species—about 5000—have been studied.

虽说草药已有数百年的历史,但只有比较少数的植物种类(大约 5000 种)受到研究。

The muscle relaxant helps reduce muscle tension during abdominal operations under acupuncture or herbal anaesthesia.

在针刺或草药麻醉下的腹部手术时肌肉松弛药有助于缓解肌肉张力。

herbalism [ˈhəːbəlizəm] *n.* 本草学

Herbalism is a traditional medicine or folk medicine practice based on the use of plants and plant extracts.

本草学是在植物和植物提取物使用基础上形成的传统医药或民间医药实践。

Herbalism has been practised all over the world for thousands of years.

草药医术在世界各地实际应用已达数千年之久。

herbicide [ˈhəːbiˌsaid] *n.* 除草剂

Paraquat is an effective and widely used herbicide.

百草枯是一种高效且应用广泛的除草剂。

He attributed this to a dilution effect of the herbicide.

他把这归因于除草剂的稀释效果。

hereditary [hiˈreditəri] *a.* 遗传的

Thalassemia major is a hereditary chronic hemolytic anemia due to a biochemical defect in the synthesis of hemoglobin.

重型海洋性贫血是由于血红蛋白合成的生化缺陷而引起的遗传性慢性溶血性贫血。

Patients with hereditary diseases can be treated through gene therapy.

患遗传性疾病的病人能通过基因疗法进行治疗。

hemophilia is a hereditary bleeding disorder caused by deficiency of a coagulation factor.

血友病是一种遗传性出血性疾病,因缺乏某种凝血因子而引起。

heredity [hiˈrediti] *n.* 遗传,遗传特征

A Gene is the fundamental physical and functional unit of heredity.

基因是遗传的基本结构单位和功能单位。

Menstruation normally begins between the ages of 11 and 14, but this will be affected by heredity and the nutritional state of the patient.

正常人月经在 11 ~ 14 岁开始,但可受遗传及营养状态的影响。

Heredity, obesity, metabolic disease all play a role in coronary artery disease.

遗传、肥胖、代谢疾病都对冠状动脉病有致病作用。

herein [hiərˈin] *ad.* 此中,于此

We herein present this experience as a study of the long term efficacy of kidney transplantation in this population.

本文这里提供的经验是对这类患者肾移植长期效果的一项研究。

heritable [ˈheritəbl] *a.* 可遗传的

Duodenal ulcers are more prevalent in persons with blood group O than in those with other blood groups, suggesting some heritable basis.

O 型血的人比其他血型的人更易患十二指肠溃疡,提示了某种遗传因素。

hermaphrodite [həːˈmæfrədait] *n.* [动、植] 雌雄同体;阴阳人;两性体

It is also a hermaphrodite, fertilising itself to produce clones.
它还是一种雌雄同体动物,通过自体受精来得以繁殖。
Or was she, perhaps, a hermaphrodite, with both male and female chromosomes?
或者,她也许是同时拥有男女双性染色体的双性人?

hermaphroditism [həːˈmæfrəˌdaitizəm] *n.* 两性畸形
Among human beings, hermaphroditism is an extremely rare anomaly in which gonads for both sexes are present.
在人类,两性畸形(雌雄同体性)是极其罕见的异常现象。
In some patients, both ovarian and testicular tissues are present, a condition known as hermaphroditism.
某些患者同时存在卵巢和睾丸组织,这种情况称为两性畸形。

hernia [ˈhəːniə] *n.* 疝,突出
The definitive treatment of hernia is early operative repair.
疝的根本治疗是早期手术修复。
This is the way to differentiate a direct from an indirect hernia.
这是鉴别直疝和斜疝的方法。

herniation [ˌhəːniˈeiʃən] *n.* 突出,疝形成
Herniation of intervertebral disk may impinge on nerve roots.
椎间盘突出可侵犯神经根。

heroin [ˈherəuin] *n.* 海洛因
These drugs include almost all the sleeping pills, the principal offenders being the barbiturates, heroin, morphine, and other narcotics.
这类药物几乎包括所有的安眠药,主要有巴比妥类、海洛因、吗啡及其他麻醉药。

herpes [ˈhəːpiːz] *n.* 疱疹
This child has a herpes simplex infection involving the central nervous system.
这小孩患单纯疱疹感染并累及中枢神经系统。
They plan soon to examine the herpes viruses which cause many different kinds of infections.
他们打算不久以后观察引起多种感染的疱疹病毒。

herpes-zoster [ˈhəːpiːz-ˈzɔstə] *n.* 带状疱疹
Herpes-zoster in children is often painless, but older people are more likely to get zoster as they age, and the disease tends to be more severe.
儿童带状疱疹通常无疼痛,但老年人随着年龄的增长更容易出现带状疱疹,病情也更严重。
Herpes-zoster occurs only in people who have been previously infected with varicella zoster virus (VZV).
带状疱疹只发生在以前感染过水痘-带状疱疹病毒的人群。

hesitation [ˌheziˈteiʃən] *n.* 犹豫
There is much more hesitation from clinicians to adjust doses based on genetic testing than on indirect clinical measures of renal and liver function.
与按照肾和肝功能的间接临床测试来调整药物剂量相比,临床医生更加犹豫依据基因检测结果来调整剂量。

hesperetin [heˈsperitin] *n.* 橙皮素
Hesperetin had no inhibition to recombinant PI3-K.
橙皮素对重组人 PI3-K 没有抑制作用。
a slight reduction of hepatic cholesterol by hesperetin was also observed in the control group.
我们也观察到对照组给予橙皮素后肝脏胆固醇有轻度降低。

hesperidin [heˈsperidin] *n.* 橙皮苷
Orange juice contains hesperidin, a naringin-like substance.

橙汁中包含着橙皮苷,一种类似于柑橘苷的物质。

a new successive process to extract pectin and hesperidin from orange peel has been introduced.

引入了从柑橘皮中提取果胶和橙皮苷的新的连续加工方法。

heterochromatin [ˌhetərəu'krəumətin] *n.* 异染色质

Heterochromatin is chromatin that is either devoid genes or has inactive genes.

异染色质是不含基因或只有失活基因的染色质。

heterocrania [ˌhetərə'kreiniə] *n.* 偏头痛

This is called heterocrania, an illness by no means mild, even though it intermits or appears to be slight.

这被称作偏头痛,尽管这种疾病只是间歇发作或者症状较轻,但它绝不是轻微的疾病。

Heterocrania lasted from 6 to 24 hours and consisted of onesided throbbing head pain, gastric upset, and sensitivity to light, sound, and smells.

偏头痛可持续 6 到 24 个小时,伴有单侧头部跳痛、胃内不适,同时对光、声、气味敏感。

heterocrine ['hetərəkriːn] *a.* 多种分泌的

Many glands have both exocrine and endocrine secretions, as for instance the pancreas, and may therefore be called heterocrine glands.

许多腺体既有外分泌又有内分泌,例如胰腺,因此可被称为多种分泌腺。

heterodimeric [ˌhetərəu'daimərik] *a.* 异二聚体的,杂二聚体的

The integrin family consists of heterodimeric moleculer with α and β chains.

整合素家族由 α 和 β 链组成异二聚体分子。

heterogeneity [ˌhetərəudʒi'niːiti] *n.* 异质性,不均一性

The majority of inherited human diseases exhibit genetic heterogeneity.

大多数遗传病存在遗传异质性。

We did not detect significant heterogeneity between the studies, and thus we conducted analyses using the fixed effect models.

我们没有检测到各研究间显著的异质性,因此我们使用固定效应模型进行分析。

heterogeneous [ˌhetərə'dʒiːniəs] *a.* 异质的,多相的

Finally, a number of heterogeneous entities are called granulomas.

最后,一些异质性疾病被称为肉芽肿。

The pathophysiological causes of intrauterine growth retardation are heterogenous.

宫内生长迟缓的病理生理原因是多源的。

Many neoplastic lesions in the MRI showed similar heterogeneous intensity signal, so bringing difficulty for diagnosis and differential diagnosis.

许多肿瘤性病变在 MRI 上表现为相似的混杂信号,因此对诊断和鉴别诊断带来困难。

heteromorphism [ˌhetərəu'mɔːfizəm] *n.* 异形;[遗]异态性

Q banding is particularly useful for detecting occasional variants in chromosome morphology or staining, called heteromorphisms.

Q 带在染色体形态学或染色,即异态性方面,对检测偶见的变异型特别有用。

The Objective is to investigate the relationship between chromosome heteromorphism and early reproduction inability.

目的是探讨染色体异态性与早期生殖障碍的关系。

heterophil ['hetərəfil] *a.* 嗜异性的,嗜染性的

Heterophil antibodies may be absent, and atypical lymphocytes may not be present at the onset of the neurologic event.

在神经系统症状出现时可以缺少异嗜性抗体,也可以不出现异型淋巴细胞。

heteroplasmy [ˌhetərəu'plæzmi] *n.* 异质性

Heteroplasmy is a common phenomenon in mitochondrial DNA somatic mutations of human tumors.

异质性是人类肿瘤线粒体 DNA 体细胞突变的普遍现象。

Nuclear transfer could result in heteroplasmy in cloned embryos and offspring, affecting the phenotypes of the individuals and even causing mitochondrial diseases.

核移植可能导致克隆胚胎及后代的异质性,从而影响个体的表型甚至导致线粒体疾病。

heteroploid [ˈhetərəplɔid] *n.* 异倍体,非整倍体 *a.* 异倍体的,非整倍体的

A chromosome complement with any chromosome number other than 46 is said to be heteroploid.

(人)染色体组的染色体数目不是 46 的话,就被称为异倍体。

Chromosome numbers which deviate from the normal number of chromosomes for a species are said to be heteroploid.

染色体数目偏离了该物种的正常染色体数,被叫做异倍体。

heterosexual [ˌhetərəˈsekʃuəl] *a.* 异性的,异性恋的

Another key factor involved in heterosexual transmission of human immunodeficiency virus(HIV) is the likelihood of exposure to an infected partner.

异性之间人类免疫缺陷病毒传播的另一个关键因素,可能是接触到一个已感染的性伙伴。

For example, the incidence of AIDS is higher among homosexual than among heterosexual men.

例如,同性恋中患艾滋病的发病率要比异性恋的男性高。

heterotroph [ˈhetərəutrɔf] *n.* 异养生物

Heterotrophs derive their energy by taking in foods.

异养生物通过进食获得能量。

All the millions of animal and fungal species are heterotrophs.

所有数以万计的动物和真菌均为异养生物。

heterozygosity [ˌhetərəuzaiˈɡɔsiti] *n.* 杂合性

Loss of heterozygosity(LOH) in a cell is the loss of normal function of one allele of a gene in which the other allele was already inactivated.

细胞中杂合性缺失是指一个基因的一个等位基因丢失正常功能,而该基因的另一个等位基因已经失活。

heterozygous [ˌhetərəuˈzaiɡəs] *a.* 杂合的

If both alleles at a locus are different, he or she is heterozygous.

如果在一个位点的两个等位基因不同,那么他或她是杂合的。

The genotype Aa is heterozygous.

基因型 Aa 是杂合的。

hexane [hekˈsein] *n.*【化】己烷

Hexane is a hydrocarbon with the chemical formula C_6H_{14}.

己烷是一种碳水化合物,化学分子式为 C_6H_{14}。

Pure hexane is a colorless liquid with a slightly disagreeable odor.

纯己烷是一种无色液体,有点难闻的气味。

hexose [ˈheksəus] *n.* 己糖

It is suggested that SPS(sucrose phosphate synthase) could be activated by hexose and feedback-inhibited by sucrose.

有人提出,蔗糖磷酸合成酶可被己糖激活而被蔗糖反馈抑制。

Vitamin C, a hexose lactone, plays an extensive role in plant and most animals.

维生素 C,是一种己糖内酯化合物,在植物和大多数动物体内具有广泛作用。

hiatal [haiˈeitəl] *a.* 裂孔的;非等粒的;空隙的

Common disorders include gastritis, peptic ulcer, hiatal hernia, and cancer.

胃部常见的疾病有胃炎、消化性溃疡、食管裂孔疝和胃癌等。

The occurrence of peptic ulcer in some patients with hiatal hernia may necessitate consideration of both diagnoses.

在一些裂孔病患者会发生消化性溃疡时,这时应考虑两种疾患的诊断。

hiatus [haiˈeitəs] *n.* 裂孔

Bleeding from hiatus hernia and gastric carcinoma is usually insidious(but not always).

裂孔疝和胃癌的出血常常是隐性的(但不总是如此)。

hiccup [ˈhikʌp] *n.* 打嗝;*v.* 打嗝

A young baby may frequently get a bout of hiccups during or soon after a feed.

小婴儿进食过程中或刚刚进食后经常会打嗝。

The neonatal form of non ketotic hyperglycinemia presents in the first days of life with encephalopathy, seizures, myoclonus and characteristic "hiccups".

新生儿期的非酮性高甘氨酸血症发生在出生后头几天,表现为脑病、癫痫、肌阵挛和特征性的打嗝。

hierarchy [ˈhaiərɑːki] *n.* 等级体系,(染色体)级系

Events similar to the early stage may be controlled through a hierarchy of genes.

其过程类似于早期阶段可以通过基因系统来控制。

highlight [ˈhailait] *v.* 集中注意力于,使突出,强调

The purpose of this article is to highlight the potentially deleterious effect of atropine on the ischemic myocardium.

本文的目的主要是讨论阿托品对缺血心肌潜在的有害作用。

The fact that the present study only involved a small number of test subjects highlights the need for a more extensive study and research.

目前的研究只涉及少数的受测试人员这一事实强调需要更广泛的调查研究。

Our results highlight the significant influence of the time of exposure to cadmium on the morphological changes and alert about the risk of cadmium's ability to accumulate in testes.

我们的结果突出显示镉暴露时间的长短对形态学改变的显著影响,并对镉在睾丸中蓄积的危险性提出了警示。

hilar [ˈhailə] *n.* 肺门的,门的

The hilar lymph nodes are usually enlarged in the secondary pulmonary tuberculosis.

继发性肺结核时肺门淋巴结常肿大。

The hilar vasculature must be carefully examined in the patient with renal cell carcinoma.

肾细胞癌患者肾门部的血管一定要仔细检查。

hinder [ˈhində] *v.* 阻止,妨碍

The binding of bilirubin is hindered by many pharmacologic agents.

许多药物可阻碍胆红素的结合。

The slow onset of tuberculosis frequently hinders its early diagnosis.

结核病的发作迟缓常妨碍其早期诊断。

hindlimb [ˈhaindlim] *n.* 下肢,后肢

Alcohol was administered before the injection of sodium chloride into the soles of mice hindlimb feet.

在注射氯化钠到小鼠后肢足底之前,先给予酒精。

Estimate the associations between occupational stress and prevalence of musculoskeletal disorders in hindlimb.

评估职业压力与下肢肌肉骨骼疾病患病率之间的联系。

hint [hint] *v.* 暗示,提示

No one has hinted that our water quality wasn't the best in the region.

一直没有人向我们暗示过在该地区我们的水质存在问题。

If you give me a hint, I am sure that I can guess the answer.

如果你给我一点暗示,我确信我定能猜得出来。

hip [hip] *n.* 髋(部)

The patient should have an X-ray of the hip bone.

病人髋骨应照 X 线片。

hippocampal [ˌhipəuˈkæmpəl] *a.* 海马的(**hippocampus** [ˌhipəuˈkæmpəs] *n.* 海马)

Recent experimental evidence shows that elevated cortisol concentration damage hippocampal neurones.

近来的实验证据显示出皮质醇浓度升高时可损伤海马神经元。

Hippocampal damage may induce mental dysfunction, such as cognitive deficits.

海马损伤可诱发精神障碍如识别的缺陷。

hippocampus[ˌhipəuˈkæmpəs] *n.* 海马

This investigation aimed to isolate neural stem cells from neonatal hippocampus and induce them to differentiate into cholinergic neurons.

本研究的目的是要将神经干细胞从新生海马中分离出来,并诱导其分化成为胆碱能神经元。

hirsutism [ˈhəːsjuːtizəm] *n.* 多毛(症)(尤指妇女多毛症)

Removal of the tumor results in the return of menstruation although the signs of masculinization such as hirsutism may be slow to disappear.

肿瘤的切除虽然可使患者的月经恢复,但是其男性化的体征如多毛症等可能消失得较慢。

histamine [ˈhistəmiːn] *n.* 组(织)胺

Histamine is present in considerable amounts in the cells of the human skin.

组胺在人体皮肤细胞中存在有相当的量。

histidine [ˈhistidiːn] *n.* 组氨酸

In addition to glycine, acceptor amino acids for xenobiotic conjugation include arginine and histidine.

除苷氨酸外,供外源化合物结合的受体氨基酸还有精氨酸和组氨酸。

histiocyte [ˈhistiəˌsait] *n.* 组织细胞(=histocyte)

The lymph node shows reactive follicular hyperplasia with irregular clusters of epithelioid histiocytes.

淋巴结出现反应性滤泡增生并伴有不规则的上皮样组织细胞团。

histocompatibility [ˌhistəukəmˌpætəˈbiləti] *n.* 组织相容性,组织适合性

Histocompatibility means identify in all transplantation antigen in immunology.

组织相容性是指所有被移植的抗原都具有免疫学上的一致性。

histogenesis [ˌhistəuˈdʒenisis] *n.* 组织发生

The two most popular theories of histogenesis are the transport theory and the coelomic metaplasia theory.

两个最流行的组织发生学说是转移学说和体腔化生学说。

histological [ˌhistəˈlɔdʒikəl] *a.* 组织学的

Biopsy and exfoliative cytology can give histological confirmation.

活检和脱落上皮的细胞学检查可以从组织学上(对该病)予以肯定。

histologically [ˌhistəˈlɔdʒikəli] *ad.* 组织学上地,组织结构上地

Histologically, the outlines of the dead cells are usually visible.

组织学检查,死亡细胞的轮廓往往可见。

histology [hisˈtɔlədʒi] *n.* 组织学

The diagnosis may be made separately by macroscopic appearance, by histology, and by cytology.

可以根据肉眼外观、组织学方法和细胞学方法分别作出诊断。

histone [ˈhistəun] *n.* 组蛋白

Histones are the most abundant proteins in the nucleus.

组蛋白是细胞核中最丰富的蛋白质。

Histones are the structureal proteins of chromatin.

组蛋白是染色质的结构蛋白质。

histopathological [ˌhistəˌpæθəˈlɔdʒikəl] *a.* 组织病理学的

Histopathological grading of ependymoma has been controversial with respect to its reproducibility and clinical significance.

室管膜瘤的组织病理学分级在其再现性和临床意义方面是有争议的。

The detection of small quantities of invasive or metastatic cells by normal histopathological staining with haematoxylin and eosin is not always sensitive.

用苏木素和伊红进行的常规组织病理学染色对少量侵袭性或转移性细胞的检测并不一定都敏感。

histopathology [ˌhistəupəˈθɔlədʒi] *n.* 组织病理学,病理组织学

Published reports on the histopathology found in patients with the sick sinus syndrome are relatively few.

已公布的关于病窦综合征病人组织病理学发现的报告较少。

Histopathology was routinely performed on the skin and subcutaneous tissue, the brain, pituitary gland, and any other organs or tissues with pathological lesions.

对于皮肤和皮下组织、脑、脑垂体及具有病理损伤的其他任何器官或组织,都要常规作病理组织学检查。

histoplasma [ˌhistəˈplæzmə] *n.* 组织胞浆菌属

PAS stain highlights Histoplasma capsulatum infection in the liver.

PAS 染色显示肝内荚膜组织胞浆菌感染。

The objective is to detect the Histoplasma capsulatum(HC) which causes a capsulatum disease.

目的是检测引起荚膜组织胞浆菌病的病原菌荚膜组织胞浆菌(HC)。

histoplasmin [ˌhistəˈplæzmin] *n.* 组织胞浆菌素

196 patients of pulmonary tuberculosis and 53 patients of non-tuberculosis pulmonary disease were tested with histoplasmin.

对 196 例肺结核和 53 例非结核的肺病病人进行了组织胞浆菌素的皮肤试验。

33.67% TB patients reacted to histoplasmin with skin test.

结核患者组织胞浆菌素皮试阳性率为 33.67%,

histoplasmosis [ˌhistəuplæzˈməusis] *n.* 组织胞浆菌病

Histoplasmosis is a fungal infection that primarily affects the lungs but may also affect other organs.

组织胞浆菌病是一种真菌感染,主要影响肺部,但也可能影响其他器官。

Disseminated histoplasmosis infection may be diagnosed using an antigen test, and can be fatal if left untreated.

弥散性组织胞浆菌感染可使用抗原试验进行诊断,如果不进行治疗可能是致命的。

hives [haivz] *n.* 荨麻疹

Hives manifests as pruritic, palpable, erythematous skin lesions.

荨麻疹表现为瘙痒性的可触及的红色皮损。

Normally, peanuts, shell fish, eggs, and possibly milk cause severe and almost immediate hives or angioedema.

通常,花生、甲壳类动物、蛋类、或许牛奶均能引起严重的、几乎是立即出现的荨麻疹或血管性水肿。

hoarse [hɔːs] *a.* 沙哑的,嘶哑的

He has a sore throat and a hoarse voice.

他喉咙疼痛,嗓音嘶哑。

He was not hoarse, however, because the vocal chords were not involved.

然而,他的声音并没有嘶哑,因为声带并没有受炎症牵连。

hoarseness [ˈhɔːsnis] *n.* (声音)嘶哑

A foreign body in the larynx causes hoarseness.

喉部异物可引起声音嘶哑。

The child may have a little hoarseness.

患儿可能有些(声音)嘶哑。

hollow [ˈhɔləu] *v.* 内陷,(使)变空

When older people lose their teeth, their cheeks hollow in, and they do not look so well.

老年人牙齿脱落时,面颊塌陷,看起来不那么好看。

Peristaltic movement is set off by distension of the hollow intestine.

中空肠道的扩张引起(肠壁)蠕动。

holocarboxylase [ˌhɔləukaːˈbɔksileis] *n.* 羧化全酶

This binding is catalyzed by holocarboxylase synthetase.

这个结合被羧化全酶催化。

Holocarboxylase synthetase deficiency is multiple carboxylase deficiency.

羧化全酶合成酶缺乏是多种羧化酶缺乏。

holoendemic [ˌhɔləuenˈdemik] *a.* 全地方病的,全地区流行的

In hyperendemic and in holoendemic areas malaria takes a toll of older infants and young children.

在高流行地区及大面积流行地区的儿童及少年常因患疟疾而死亡。

holoenzyme [ˌhɔləuˈenzaim] *n.* 全酶

1,8-dihydroxyanthraquinone is an effective inhibitor of CK2 holoenzyme.

1,8-二羟基蒽醌是肌酸激酶2(creatine kinase)全酶的有效抑制剂。

Baicalein was shown to strongly inhibit the holoenzyme activity of CK2.

黄芩甙能显著抑制CK2全酶的活性。

holter [ˈhault] *n.* 霍尔特,即Norman J. Holter美国理学博士

The ECG abnormalities may be recorded by continuous ECG monitoring or ambulatory Holter monitoring and are reversed by nitroglycerin.

心电图的异常情况可用持续心电图监测或动态心电图监护仪来记录,服用三硝酸甘油酯可得到扭转。

[注] Holter于1961年发明ambulatory electrocardiograph动态心电图监测,一般称作ambulatory Holter monitor(或monitoring),日常中文称为长程心电图,英文可简称为Holter。

homeobox [ˈhəumiəuˈbɔks] *n.* 同源(异型)盒

Thyroid transcription factor 1 (TTF-1) is a homeobox domain transcription factor of the NKX2 family.

甲状腺转录因子1是含一同源盒域的转录因子,属于NKX2家族。

homeopathy [ˌhəumiˈɔpəθi] *n.* 顺势疗法,同种疗法

Homeopathy is a system of medicine which involves treating the individual with highly diluted substances, given mainly in tablet form, with the aim of triggering the body's natural system of healing.

顺势疗法是一种医疗体系,指用高度稀释的物质来治疗病人,主要以片剂形式给予,其目的是激发机体的天然康复系统。

Homeopathy is an absurd pseudoscience, which survives today as a "complementary" or "alternative" medicine, despite there being no reliable scientific evidence that it works.

顺势疗法是一种荒唐的伪科学,尽管没有可信赖的科学证据显示其有效,它仍然作为一种替代疗法而存在至今。

homeostasis [ˌhəumiəˈsteisis] *n.* 体内平衡,自身稳定

Each organ system of the body plays its specific role in homeostasis.

身体每个器官系统在体内平衡中起着各自的特殊作用。

Homeostasis is a dynamic form of equilibrium in the body's internal environment.

稳态是机体内环境动态平衡的一种形式。

homeotic [ˌhəumiˈɔtik] *a.* 同源(异型)的

The methylation of histone H3-K27 was proved to be linked to several silencing phenomena including homeotic-gene silencing, X inactivation and genomic imprinting.

组蛋白 H3 第 27 位赖氨酸的甲基化与同源盒基因沉默、X 染色体失活、基因印迹等基因沉默现象有关。

A natural homeotic mutant of Xanthoceras sorbifolia was discovered in seedling nursery of Beijing Forestry University.

在北京林业大学苗圃内发现了一个文冠果的同源异型自然变异株。

homicide [ˈhɔmisaid] *n.* 杀人;杀人者

Death by homicide frequently resembles sudden death from natural causes.

他杀造成的死亡常常类似由自然原因引起的突然死亡。

Firearm homicides and suicides now exceed deaths from motor vehicle accidents.

现在用枪杀人及自杀所致的死亡超过了车祸所致的死亡。

homing [ˈhəumiŋ] *n.* 回家,归巢

Homing is the process by which lymphocytes leave the circulation and enter a lymph node.

归巢是淋巴细胞由循环系统进入淋巴结内的过程。

homocysteine [ˌhɔməusisˈtiːin] *n.* 高半胱氨酸,同型半胱氨酸

Cobalamin is essential in the conversion of homocysteine to methionine.

维生素 B_{12}在同型半胱氨酸转化为甲硫氨酸的过程中是必不可少的。

Folic acid can lower blood levels of homocysteine, a substance that increases the risk of heart disease.

叶酸能降低血液中高半胱氨酸的水平,这种物质能增加患心脏病的危险性。

homocysteinemia [ˌhəuməuˌsistiˈniːmiə] *n.* 同型半胱氨酸血症

The MTHFR polymorphism is linked to homocysteinemia, which in turn affects thrombosis risk.

MTHFR 多态性与同型半胱氨酸血症相关,后者进而影响血栓形成的风险。

homocystinuria [ˌhəuməusistiˈnjuːriə] *n.* 高胱氨酸尿

Homocystinuria is a rare autosomal-recessive disorder.

高胱氨酸尿症为一种少见的常染色体隐性遗传性疾病。

Homocystinuria is a genetic disease with multiple systemic complications.

高胱氨酸尿症是伴有多种全身并发症的遗传性疾病。

homogenate [hɔˈmɔdʒineit] *n.* 匀浆,均浆

Good thermal contact between homogenate and the surface of the disc is required.

在匀浆和碟片的表面之间需要有良好的热接触。

In liver homogenates, we measured the activities of superoxide dismutase and catalase.

我们检测了在肝脏匀浆中的超氧化物歧化酶和过氧化氢酶的活性。

homogeneity [ˌhɔməudʒeˈniːiti] *n.* 同质;同种;同次性

MRI has strict demands on strength, stablity and homogeneity of magnetic filed.

MRI 对磁场的强度、稳定性和均匀性有严格的要求。

Culture of seed cells is a basic element of tissue engineering, cells mainly come from self-cell, variant of the same homogeneity, cells of heterogeneity, and so on.

种子细胞的培养是组织工程的基本要素,细胞主要来源于自体、同种异体、异种细胞等。

homogeneous [ˌhəuməuˈdʒiːniəs] *a.* 均匀的,同种的,同质的

Study results were pooled when the data were sufficiently homogeneous.

当数据足以同质时,研究结果进行了合并。

A material that is homogeneous is uniform in composition or character.

同质的物质其构成或特性是一致的。

homogenous [hɔˈmɔdʒinəs] *a.* 同源的,同质的,均一的

The cell is not a homogenous mass, it is divided into smaller structures, called organelles.

细胞不是一种同种物质的聚合体,它还可以分为更小的结构,称作细胞器。

On first examination the cytoplasm appears to be a uniformly homogenous substance.

起初观察时,细胞质看来是相同的均一物质。

homograft [ˈhəuməgrɑːft] *n.* 同种移植物

Homograft is the tissue or organ transplanted from a donor of the same species but different genetic makeup.

从种族相同但基因构成不同的供体获得移植的组织或器官称为同种移植物。

Homograft valve is increasingly used for aortic valve replacement in young patient as a first choice.

同种移植瓣膜被越来越多地用于年轻患者主动脉瓣置换的第一选择。

homologous [hɔˈmɔləgəs] *a.* 相应的,类似的,同源的

In human cell containing 46 chromosomes each cell contains 23 pairs of homologous chromosomes.

人类体细胞含有 46 条染色体,每个细胞含有 23 对同源染色体。

In most organisms the chromosomes occur in pairs, each member of which is homologous.

大多数生物的染色体是成对的,每一对的两条染色体(也)是同源的。

homologue [ˈhɔməlɔg] *n.* 同族体,相当或相同的事物

Computer scanning and analysis show that the nucleotide sequence of DNA fragment is unique, being no significant homologue with that of other Plasmodium genes published.

计算机检索和分析表明,该 DNA 片段与其他已测序列的疟原虫基因无明显同源性,是一个新克隆的间日疟原虫 DNA 片段。

They planned to study the effects of benzene and its homologue on the menstruation and reproductive function of female workers.

他们计划研究苯及其同系物对妇女接触者月经及生殖功能的影响。

homology [hɔˈmɔlədʒi] *n.* 同种性,同源性

The five viruses of hepatitis are distinct and show no homology of structure, virus family, or replicative cycle.

5 种肝炎病毒是不同的,并且显示不同的结构、病毒属或复制周期。

Homology is any similarity between characters that is due to their shared ancestry.

同源性是指由于拥有共同的祖先而在特征上具有某种相似性。

Protein homology is biological homology between proteins, meaning that the proteins are derived from a common "ancestor".

蛋白同源性是蛋白之间的生物同源性,意味着这些蛋白来源于共同的"祖先"。

homoplasmy [ˈhəuməuˌplæzmi] *n.* 同型异源性

Pathogenic tRNA mutations can reach homoplasmy and show very different penetrance among patients.

致病性的 tRNA 突变能够引起同型异源性,并在病人中显示出非常不同的外显率。

Homoplasmy is the presence of a mutation affecting all of the mitochondrial DNA (mtDNA) copies in a mammalian cell or chloroplast DNA in a plant cell.

同型异源性是指一种突变的发生会影响哺乳动物细胞中所有的线粒体 DNA 拷贝或植物细胞叶绿体 DNA。

homosexual [ˌhəuməuˈsekʃuəl] *a.* 同性恋的

AIDS was first recognized as a distinct disease entity among homosexual men in the United States in 1981.

艾滋病于 1981 年首次在美国被公认为男性同性恋者中一种独特的病种。

Most homosexual men with gonococcal infection have rectal symptoms.

大多数有淋球菌感染的同性恋的男性多有直肠的症状。

Kaposi's sarcoma occurs with greater frequency in homosexuals with AIDS.

Kaposi 肉瘤多发于患艾滋病的同性恋者。

homosexuality [ˌhəuməuˌseksju'æliti] *n.* 同性恋

Early effeminate behaviour in boys can be a precursor or predictor of adult homosexuality.

男孩早期出现女性行为可成为成年时同性恋的一种先兆或预报。

The increased incidence of these conditions is related to the numbers of sexual partners and sexual practices and not to homosexuality itself.

在这种情况下发病的增高与性伴侣和性活动的数量有关,而与同性恋本身无关。

homozygous [ˌhɔmə'zaigəus] *a.* 纯合的,纯合子的

If both alleles at a locus are identical,the individual is homozygous at that locus.

如果在一个位点的两个等位基因相同,那么此个体在该位点是纯合的。

A recessive gene appears to affect the phenotype only if it is present in a homozygous condition.

隐性基因只有在纯合的状态时才能影响表型。

honeysuckle ['hʌniˌsʌkl] *n.* [植]金银花;忍冬

Honeysuckle has a twining habit.

金银花有盘绕的习性。

I think honeysuckle was the saddest odor of all.

我认为金银花是所有的花香味中最难闻的一种。

hookworm ['hukwəːm] *n.* 钩虫

The larval hookworms enter the body by burrowing through the skin,usually that of the sole of the foot.

钩蚴通常经脚底皮肤钻入人体。

hopper ['hɔpə] *n.* 加料斗

Bulk feed hopper with conveyor is the best alterative when a vibratory hopper cannot be used.

当振动加料斗不能使用时,带有输送器的散装饲料加料斗是最好的选择。

The hopper is easy to mount and remove,ensuring a hygienic environment for packaging of medication.

加料斗易于安装和移动,确保了药物包装的卫生环境。

horizon [hə'raizən] *n.* 地平线;眼界,见识

The course in medical history opened up new horizons for the students.

医学史课程使学生们开了眼界。

Microsurgery is basically a technique for expanding the visual horizon of the surgeon.

显微外科主要是扩大外科医生视野的一种技术。

horizontal [ˌhɔri'zɔntəl] *a.* 地平线的,水平的

The horizontal axis in the graph represents age in years.

曲线图中的水平轴代表年龄。

hormesis [hɔː'miːsis] *n.* 低剂量辐射兴奋效应

The term hormesis has been most widely used in the toxicology field.

低剂量辐射兴奋效应这一术语已经极广泛地应用于毒物学领域。

Hormesis refers to a biphasic dose response to an environmental agent characterized by a low dose stimulation or beneficial effect and a high dose inhibitory or toxic effect.

低剂量辐射兴奋效应指针对环境中试剂的一种两相剂量反应,即低剂量兴奋(有益作用)和高剂量抑制(毒性作用)。

hormonal [hɔː'məunəl] *a.* 激素的,内分泌的

The myometrium is under both neural and hormonal control.

子宫肌层是在神经及激素支配之下。

As a result,a hormonal release is triggered,which alters the perception of pain.

以上过程触发了激素的释放,致使改变疼痛的知觉。

hormone ['hɔːməun] *n.* 激素

Hormones are necessary for good health, as they cause necessary reactions of many kinds in the body.

激素是良好健康必不可少的,因为它们可引起身体中各种必要的反应。

Technically, vitamin D could be considered a hormone rather than a vitamin.

从专业上讲,维生素 D 可被看作是激素,而不是维生素。

There is no evidence that gonadal or parathyroid hormones participate in the metabolic responses to infection.

没有证据表明性激素或甲状旁腺激素参与了对感染的代谢反应。

hospital [ˈhɔspitəl] *n.* 医院

Less than a century ago, many people refused to go to a hospital for care.

还不到一百年以前,许多人不愿去医院治病。

Today's hospitals provide good and complete medical services and as much comfort for the patient as possible.

今天的医院为病人提供良好的医疗服务,而且尽可能让病人舒适。

hospitalization [ˌhɔspitəlaiˈzeiʃən] *n.* 入院,住院(期)

However, some situations require hospitalization.

但有些情况需要入院治疗。

During hospitalization the patient developed acute chest pain with ECG signs as above.

住院过程中病人出现急性胸痛,心电图征象如上述。

A percutaneous renal biopsy was performed on the 9th day of hospitalization.

住院第 9 天做了经皮肾活检。

hospitalize [ˈhɔspitəlaiz] *v.* (送病人)住院

Since the patient's blood pressure is extremely high, he must be hospitalized at once.

由于这病人的血压特别高,他必须立即住院。

host [həust] *n.* 主人;寄主,宿主

The embryos of the worm may gain access to the human host in polluted drinking water.

蠕虫胚胎可随污染了的饮水侵入人类宿主体内。

hostile (to) [ˈhɔstail] *a.* 敌对的,不友善的

Sunshine is hostile to disease germs.

阳光对于病菌有抑制或杀灭的作用。

hostility [hɔsˈtiliti] *n.* 敌意

Hostility is the urge to harm another person in the expression of anger.

敌意是以愤怒的形式来伤害他人的强烈欲望。

household [ˈhaushəuld] *n.* 家庭,户;家务

The medical team conducted a survey of schistosomiasis household by household.

医疗队挨家挨户地对血吸虫病进行了调查。

a. 家庭的

The refrigerant in a household refrigerator also undergoes a cyclic process.

家用冰箱的致冷剂也经历循环过程。

housekeeping [ˈhauskiːpiŋ] *n.* 家政;家务管理;家用开支

Housekeeping proteins are present in every cell and have fundamental roles in the maintenance of cell structure and function.

持家蛋白在所有细胞中均有表达,它们为维持细胞结构和功能起着基本作用。

Housekeeping genes are genes that are always expressed because the proteins they produce are essential for the cells to function.

持家基因是那些持续表达的基因,因为它们产生的蛋白质是细胞必须的。

Houttuynia [hauˈtuiniə] *n.* 鱼腥草

The summary deals with the recent study of the chemical compositions, pharmacological action

and clinical application of Houttuynia.
摘要概述了近期对鱼腥草的化学成分、药理和临床应用的研究进展。
Three different methods like boiling, alcohol reflux extracting and ultrasonic extracting are respectively adopted to extract the total flavones of Houttuynia.
分别采用水煮法、乙醇回流提取法及超声波提取法提取鱼腥草的总黄酮。

Houttuynin [hau'tuinin] *n.* 鱼腥草素
Houttuynin was extracted from houttuynia cordata thunb with the method of solvent extraction process.
利用溶剂提取法从鱼腥草中提取鱼腥草素。
We should improve the synthetic method of houttuynin so as to adapt it to the industrial production.
我们应改进鱼腥草素的合成方法,以适应工业化生产。

huge [hjuːdʒ] *a.* 极大的,巨大的
We know that such crops as corn require huge amounts of nitrogen fertilizers.
我们知道像玉米这类农作物需要大量氮肥。
He won a huge success in his research work.
他的研究工作已获得了巨大成功。

humanitarianism [hjuˌmæni'tɛəriənizm] *n.* 人道主义
The duty of our medical workers is to heal the wounded, rescue the dying, and practise revolutionary humanitarianism.
我们医务工作者的职责是救死扶伤实行革命的人道主义。

humanity [hjuː'mæniti] *n.* 人类,人性,(*pl.*)人文学科
Advances in medicine benefit all humanity.
医学的进步造福全人类。
It is an act of humanity to heal the wounded.
救死扶伤是一种人道主义的行为。
The candidate for medical school in USA must complete at least 3 years of higher education in college, with special emphasis on social sciences and the humanities.
在美国报考医学院的学生必须在大学修满三年的高等教育,并把重点放在社会科学和人文学科上。

humeral ['hjuːmərəl] *a.* 肱骨的,肩的
The fixation patterns of humeral head prosthesis shaft include cemented one and cementless one.
肱骨头假体柄的固定方式有骨水泥和非骨水泥两种。
Cubitus varus is the most difficult problem in the treatment of humeral supracondylar fracture in children.
发生肘内翻畸形是治疗儿童的肱骨髁上骨折中最难解决的问题。

humerus ['hjuːmərəs] *n.* 肱骨
Nonoperative management is appropriate for the majority of proximal humerus fractures.
非手术治疗适用于大部分肱骨近端骨折。
Bone marrow edema was found in 48 parts: 43 at hips, 3 at tibial plateaus, and 2 at the head of humerus.
有 48 个部位发生骨髓水肿,其中 43 个位于髋关节,3 个在胫骨平台和 2 个在肱骨头。

humic ['hjuːmik] *a.* 腐殖的
Humic substances are known to coat membrane filters.
腐殖质是已知能够覆盖滤膜的物质。
Ultimate analysis provides a useful inventory of the distribution of the major elements in humic substances.
元素分析提供腐殖物质中主要元素分布的有用资料。

humidity [hjuːˈmiditi] *n.* 湿度，湿气

Surgical asepsis also includes maintaining proper temperature and humidity and may include sterilization of the air.

手术无菌也包括维持正常温度和湿度，甚至包括对空气的灭菌处理。

Heat stroke typically occurs in individuals exercising at humidities that are higher than normal.

中暑一般是人在周围温度高于正常环境而且处于活动的状态时发生的。

Humidity therapy may be delivered in a variety of ways.

湿疗可用多种方法进行。

humoral [ˈhjuːmərəl] *a.* 体液的

Chronic rejection is a late cause of renal deterioration mediated by humoral factors.

慢性排斥反应是体液因素介导的晚期引起肾脏恶化的原因。

humorally [ˈhjuːmərəli] *ad.* 体液状地；湿性地

Chemical substances called hormones are liberated into the blood from particular glands, and carried humorally to exert special effects on distant structures.

被称作激素的化学物质由特殊的腺体释放并进入血中，呈液态状运输，对远处的部位发挥特殊作用。

hurt [həːt] *v.* 损害

Radiation can hurt us directly and indirectly.

辐射可以直接或间接地损害我们。

hyaline [ˈhaiəliːn] *a.* 透明的，玻璃样的

It gives the impression of hyaline degeneration.

它给人以玻璃样变性的印象。

The walls of arterioles usually become thickened and hyaline in arterial hypertension.

在动脉高压时，小动脉壁常常增厚而且呈玻璃样变。

It is not unusual to find the bronchiolar and alveolar walls bordered by a homogeneous acidophilic hyaline membrane.

常可见在细支气管和肺泡壁形成同质嗜酸性透明膜边。

hybrid [ˈhaibrid] *a.* 杂种的

In this way, genetic characteristics can be "recombined" to bring about entirely new hybrid forms of life.

按照这种方式，基因特征可以"重新组合"再产生新一代的杂种个体。

hybridization [ˌhaibridaiˈzeiʃən] *n.* 杂交，杂化

Hepatitis D virus(HDV) RNA can be readily detected by molecular hybridization in the serum of infected individuals.

用分子杂交技术在感染个体血清中能很容易地检出 HDV RNA(丁型肝炎病毒核糖核酸)。

hybridoma [ˌhaibriˈdəumə] *n.* 杂交瘤

By this procedure, Milstein and Kohler developed a hybridoma that made a specific antibody.

米尔斯坦和科勒用此方法培养出一个杂种瘤，后来成为一种特效抗体。

In a word, hybridoma technology-a potent new biotechnology with widespread practical applications to agriculture, medicine and industry.

总之，杂交瘤技术是一种强有力的新的生物技术，它能广泛地应用于农业、医学和工业。

hydatidiform [ˌhaidəˈtidifɔːm] *a.* 囊状的，棘球囊状的

This group of lesions includes hydatidiform mole, invasive mole(chorioadenoma destruens), and choriocarcinoma.

这一组病变包括葡萄胎、侵蚀性葡萄胎(破坏性绒毛膜腺瘤)及绒毛膜癌。

hydramnios [haiˈdræmniəs] *n.* 羊水过多

Hydramnios may occur with twins, adding to the size and confusing the diagnosis.

羊水过多也可发生于双胞胎,它可使子宫更大并可造成误诊。

hydrate [ˈhaidreit] *n.* 水合物

Nitric acid forms hydrates with water.

硝酸与水形成水合物。

v. 水合

Thromboxane A_2 is hydrated in the blood to thromboxane B_2.

血小板凝集素 A_2 在血中水合为血小板凝集素 B_2。

hydration [haiˈdreiʃən] *n.* 水合(作用);输液

In the emergency room,he received intravenous hydration.

在急诊室他接受了静脉输液。

Hydration is very important for the conformation and utility of nucleic acids.

水合作用对核酸的构造和效用都是非常重要的。

Hydration sometimes helps to reduce the concentration of toxic substances in the tissues.

水化作用有时可帮助减少组织中有毒物质的浓度。

hydrocarbon [ˌhaidrəuˈkɑːbən] *n.* 烃,碳氢化合物

Gasoline is a complex mixture of volatile hydrocarbons containing as many as 1000 chemical substances.

汽油是一种复杂的有挥发性的羟类混合物,含有多达上千种化学物质。

The female sex hormones resemble very much the carcinogenic hydrocarbons in structure.

雌性激素与致癌性碳氢化合物在结构上颇为近似。

hydrocephalus [ˌhaidrəuˈsefələs] *n.* 脑积水

Hydrocephalus due to ventricular block is called obstructive hydrocephalus.

由脑室受阻引起的脑水肿称为阻塞性脑水肿。

Brain tumor should always be considered in the differential diagnosis of hydrocephalus.

在脑积水鉴别诊断时,应常考虑到脑瘤。

hydrochloric [ˌhaidrəˈklɔrik] *a.* 氯化氢的

The gastric juice itself has two main components:hydrochloric acid and enzymes.

胃液本身有两种主要成分:盐酸和一些酶。

Chlorine was prepared in 1774 by heating hydrochloric acid with manganese dioxide.

在 1774 年把盐酸和二氧化锰混合加热制得了氯气。

hydrocortisone [ˌhaidrəuˈkɔːtisəun] *n.* 氢化可的松

Hydrocortisone is given early and in large doses intravenously.

及时静脉注射给予大剂量的氢化可的松。

Hydrocortisone,the principal glucocorticoid secreted by the adrenal gland,is used for its anti-inflammatory action.

氢化可的松是由肾上腺分泌的一种主要的糖皮质激素,因其抗炎作用而被(广泛)使用。

hydrogel [ˈhaidrədʒel] *n.* 水凝胶

The crosslinking ratio is one of the most important factors that affect the swelling of hydrogels.

交联率是影响水凝胶膨胀的最重要因素之一。

Hydrogels used in drug delivery are usually formed outside of the body.

药物传递用的水凝胶通常在体外形成。

hydrolysis [haiˈdrɔlisis] *n.* 水解(作用)

A drug such as penicillin G or erythromycin may be destroyed by acid hydrolysis.

药物如青霉素 G 或红霉素可由酸水解而被破坏。

Active transport requires the expenditure of energy,no doubt involving the hydrolysis of ATP (ATP,adenosine triphosphate).

主动转运需要耗能,无疑涉及三磷酸腺苷的水解。

hydrolyze [ˈhaidrəlaiz] *v.* (使)水解

Fats are hydrolyzed by lipase, converting them to glycerol and fatty acids.
脂肪被脂酶水解转变为甘油和脂肪酸。
Procaine, a local anesthetic, is also hydrolyzed by pseudocholinesterase.
普鲁卡因是一种局部麻醉药，它也是由假胆碱酯酶水解的。

hydronephrosis [ˌhaidrəuniˈfrəusis] *n.* 肾盂积水
Obstruction of the ureter causes hydroureter and subsequently hydronephrosis.
输尿管梗阻会引起输尿管积水，继而出现肾盂积水。
The location and cause of obstructing processes in patients with hydronephrosis can be much better defined by CT scan than by ultrasound.
对于肾盂积水的患者，采用 CT 检查要比超声波检查更能明确梗阻的部位和原因。

hydrophilic [ˌhaidrəuˈfilik] *a.* 吸水的，亲水的
Glycosides possess both lipophilic residues and hydrophilic residues.
配糖体具有亲酯性和亲水性残基。
The blood-brain barrier prevents the access of hydrophilic chemicals to the brain except for those that can be actively transported.
血-脑屏障能阻止亲水性的化学物质进入脑，除非这些化学物质能被主动运输到脑。

hydrophobia [ˌhaidrəuˈfəubiə] *n.* 恐水病，狂犬病
Early-stage symptoms of rabies are malaise, headache and fever, progressing to acute pain, violent movements, uncontrolled excitement, depression, and hydrophobia.
狂犬病的早期症状是不适、头痛和发热，发展到急性疼痛、剧烈运动、不受控制的兴奋、抑郁和恐水症。
Rabies and hydrophobia are not the same; patients can develop hydrophobia for a variety of reasons, most likely due to a psychiatric disorder.
狂犬病和恐水症并不相同，病人可由于多种原因而发生恐水症，最可能是由于一种精神疾病。

hydrophobic [ˌhaidrəuˈfəubik] *a.* 疏水的，恐水的
The lipids contain hydrophilic and hydrophobic regions with a single molecule.
脂质在单一分子内含亲水和疏水区域。

hydropic [haiˈdrɔpik] *a.* 水肿的，浮肿的
Cloudy swelling is closely related to hydropic or vacuolar degeneration, described below.
混浊肿胀与下述的水肿或空泡变性有密切关系。
Death of a hydropic fetus usually occurs in haemolytic disease.
水肿胎儿的死亡通常发生在患溶血性疾病时。

hydrops [ˈhaidrɔps] *n.* 积水；水肿
Hydrops fetalis is an excess accumulation of fluid in the fetus.
胎儿水肿是液体在胎儿体内的过度积聚。
Hydrops develops when too much fluid leaves the bloodstream and goes into the tissues.
当过多的液体离开血流进入组织就会发展成积水。

hydroscopicity [ˌhaidrəskəˈpisiti] *n.* 吸水性
Bismuth nitrate pentahydrate belongs to five-color triclinic system crystal, owns hydroscopicity and sour flavor.
五水硝酸铋为五色三斜晶系结晶，有吸湿性并具有酸味。
The hydroscopicity of wood is closely related to the condition of internal wood surface, chemical composition and microstructure of wood.
木材的吸水性与木材内表面、化学成分和微观结构密切相关。

hydrosphere [ˈhaidrəsfiə] *n.* 水圈；水界
These dissolved materials thus pass from the lithosphere to the hydrosphere.
这些可溶性物质就从岩石圈转移到水圈。

All the water of the earth's surface is included in the hydrosphere.
地球表面的水都属于水圈的范畴。

hydrothorax [ˌhaidrəuˈθɔːræks] *n.* 胸膜积水，水胸
Hydrothorax is a chronic collection of serous fluid in the pleural cavity.
水胸是胸腔内慢性积聚浆液。

hydrotropy [haiˈdrɔtrəpi] *n.* 水溶助长性
The actual mechanism of hydrotropy is still not clear.
水溶助长性的具体机制尚不清楚。
The present investigation illustrates the application of mixed hydrotropy.
本研究阐明了混合水溶助长性的应用。

hydroxide [haiˈdrɔksaid] *n.* 氢氧化物
The hairs are placed on a slide and covered with a drop of a 10 to 20 per cent solution of potassium hydroxide.
先将头发放在载玻片上，然后滴一滴 10% ~20% 的氢氧化钾溶液。

hydroxybenzene [ˈhaiˌdrɔksibenziːn] *n.* 苯酚
The domestic demand of hydroxybenzene is about 10 tons per year.
国内苯酚的需求量大约是每年 10 吨。
The menthol and hydroxybenzene in complex boric acid powder were determined by GC.
用气相色谱法测定复方硼酸散中薄荷醇和苯酚的含量。

hydroxyeicosatetraenoic-acid [haiˌdrɔksiaiˌkəusətetrəiːˈnəuik-ˈæsid] *n.* 羟基二十碳四烯酸
It is known that hydroxyeicosatetraenoic-acid (HETE) is chemotactic for leukocytes.
已知羟基二十碳四烯酸对白细胞有趋化作用。

hydroxylase [haiˈdrɔksileis] *n.* 羟化酶
The most common enzyme defect is of 21-hydroxylase.
21-羟化酶的缺乏是最常见的酶缺乏病。
It is now possible to test for 21-hydroxylase deficiency by identifying mutations in affected genes.
现在可以通过鉴定受累基因的突变来检测 21-羟化酶缺乏症。

hydroxypiperaquine [ˌhaidrɔksipiˈperəkwin] *n.* 羟基哌喹
In this experiment, teratogenic effect of Hydroxypiperaquine Phosphate has been studied in mice.
该实验研究了磷酸羟基哌喹对小鼠的致畸效应。
This report presents the effects of three antimalaria agents-chloroquine, piperaquine and hydroxypiperaquine.
该报告展示了氯喹、哌喹和羟基哌喹三种抗疟药的效果。

hydroxypropylstarch [haiˌdrɔksiˈprəupilstɑːtʃ] *n.* 羟丙基淀粉
A new hydroxypropylstarch polymer has been used together with poly ethyleneglycol to obtain two liquid phases in aqueous solution.
一种新的羟丙基淀粉聚合物与聚乙二醇联合使用可得到水溶液中的两种液相。
The partition behaviour of cutinase on poly ethyleneglycol (PEG)-hydroxypropylstarch aqueous two-phase systems was characterized.
角质酶的特点是可在聚乙二醇-羟丙基淀粉水两相系统中产生分割作用。

hydroxyzine [haiˈdrɔksiziːn] *n.* 羟嗪（安定药，解痉药，抗组胺药）
Hydroxyzine is the most effective drug for controlling the pruritus of urticaria.
羟嗪是控制荨麻疹瘙痒症最有效的药物。

hygiene [ˈhaidʒiːn] *n.* 卫生，卫生学
Poor hygiene is one of the factors which bring about TB (tuberculosis).
卫生条件差是引起结核病的因素之一。
We should pay attention to public and private hygienes and reduce the incidence of disease.
我们应当讲究公共卫生和个人卫生以减少疾病的发生。

It is also the duty of medical workers to popularize knowledge of hygiene.
普及卫生知识也是医务人员的职责。

hygienic [haiˈdʒiːnik] *a.* 卫生的

Such health hazards tend to be forgotten in the affluent, hygienic, temperate, well fed west.
此类卫生公害常被生活富裕、讲究卫生、有节制的、营养充足的西方(人)所遗忘。

hygroscopicity [ˌhaigrəskɔˈpisiti] *n.* 吸湿性,吸水性

Hygroscopicity is an important physical property of drug materials.
吸水性是药物材料的一项重要物理性质。

This barrier property depends on the water vapor diffusion coefficient and the material hydroscopicity properties.
这个防护性能取决于水蒸气扩散系数和材料吸水性能。

hymenoptera [ˌhaiməˈnɔptərə] *n.* 膜翅目(昆虫)

However, food additives, inhalant allergens, and hymenoptera antigens are some of the possible etiological factors.
然而,食物添加剂、吸入性变应原及膜翅目昆虫抗原也是一些可能的病原学因素。

hyoscine [ˈhaiəsiːn] *n.* 莨菪

Proprietary drugs often contain certain potent substances such as hyoscine or vitamin B_{12}.
专卖药品常含有某种强效的物质,如莨菪或维生素 B_{12}。

hyperacidity [ˈhaipəːrəˈsiditi] *n.* 酸过多,胃酸过多

Hyperacidity of the gastric juice is one of the causes of the initial necrosis of the mucous membrane.
胃液中的胃酸过高是黏膜初次坏死的原因之一。

hyperactivity [ˌhaipərækˈtiviti] *n.* 功能亢进,极度活跃

This reaction appears to reflect cellular hyperactivity rather than regression.
这个反应看来反映的是细胞功能亢进而不是退化。

Researchers have been looking for the cause of attention deficit hyperactivity disorder.
研究者正在寻找注意力缺陷多动障碍(ADHD)的原因。

Inattention, hyperactivity and impulsivity are core symptoms of ADHD.
注意力不集中、多动和冲动是注意力缺陷多动障碍(ADHD)的核心症状。

hyperacute [ˌhaipərəˈkjuːt] *a.* 超急性的

Hyperacute rejection is due to preformed cytotoxic antibodies against donor lymphocytes or renal cells.
超急性的排斥反应是由于预先形成的抗供者淋巴细胞或肾细胞的细胞毒抗体所致。

hyperalgesia [ˌhaipərælˈdʒiːziə] *n.* 痛觉过敏

Opioid-induced hyperalgesia is a clinical phenomenon, characterized by increasing in pain in patients who are receiving increasing doses of opioids.
阿片样物质引起的痛觉过敏这种临床现象的主要特征是当病人服用的阿片样物质剂量加大,疼痛的程度就加深。

Mechanical hyperalgesia is a clinically-relevant form of pain sensitization.
机械性痛觉过敏是一种痛觉临床相关形式。

hyperammonemia [ˌhaipə(ː)ˌræməuˈniːmiə] *n.* 血氨过多,高氨血症

MCAD deficiency patients may present acutely with hyperammonemia, hypoglycemia, encephalopathy, and hepatomegaly.
MCAD 缺乏症病人可以急性表现为高氨血症、低血糖、脑病和肝大。

The exercise protocols have the potential of aggravating hyperammonemia.
这个运动方案有加重血氨过多的可能。

hyperbaric [haipəˈbɛərik] *a.* 高压的

Air pressure at the hyperbaric chamber is raised rapidly from 2 atm. to 3 atm.

高压氧舱内的气压迅速从两个大气压升高到三个大气压。

hyperbilirubinemia [ˌhaipə(ː)biliˌruːbiˈniːmiə] *n.* 血胆红素过多,高胆红素血症

Hyperbilirubinemia may result from decreased bilirubin clearance or bilirubin overproduction.

血胆红素过多症可由胆红素清除率减少或产生量过多引起。

Gilbert's syndrome is the only common form of congenital non-hemolytic hyperbilirubinemia.

Gilbert 综合征是最常见的可以引起先天性非溶血性高胆红素血症的疾病。

hypercalcemia [ˌhaipə(ː)kælˈsiːmiə] *n.* 血钙过多,高钙血症

Prednisolone is given to treat hypercalcemia.

给予强的松龙治疗高钙血症。

Malignancy is the cause of two thirds of the cases of hypercalcemia seen in hospitalized patients.

在住院病人患有高钙血症的病例中约有 2/3 是由恶性肿瘤引起的。

hypercalciuria [ˌhaipəkælsiˈjuəriə] *n.* 高尿钙症

Finally, the high serum calcium leads directly to hypercalciuria which predisposes the patient to formation of renal stones.

最后,高血清钙直接导致高尿钙症,使患者易形成肾结石。

hypercapnia [ˌhaipə(ː)ˈkæpniə] *n.* (血内)碳酸过多,高碳酸血症

For persistent hypoxemia or hypercapnia, intubation may be required.

对于持续低氧血症或高碳酸血症,需要进行气管插管。

It is possible to seperate the time course of adaptation to hypercapnia into acute and chronic phases.

可以根据患者对高碳酸血症适应的时间的先后分为急性期和慢性期。

hypercholesterolemia [ˌhaipəkəˌlestərəuˈliːmjə] *n.* 血胆脂醇过多

Too much cholesterol in the blood is called high blood cholesterol or hypercholesterolemia.

血液中的胆固醇含量过高称为高胆固醇血症。

Hypercholesterolemia is associated with increased relative weight in girls.

高胆固醇与女孩体重的相对增加有关。

hyperdense [ˈhaipədens] *n.* 高密度

In the suprasellar region, there was a round hyperdense lesion on non-contrast enhanced CT which subsequently exhibited intense enhancement.

平扫 CT 可见鞍上区一圆形高密度病变,增强检查明显强化。

hyperecho [ˌhaipəˈekəu] *n.* 高回声

The ultrasonographs of spleen metastatic carcinomas were of four types: echoless, hypoecho, hyperecho and bull's eye sign.

脾脏转移癌的超声图像呈现四种类型:无回声、低回声、高回声及牛眼征。

hyperemesis [ˌhaipə(ː)ˈremisis] *n.* 剧吐

Hyperemesis is diagnosed when the vomiting is intractable and leads to dehydration and at least a 5% to 10% loss of body weight.

难治性呕吐引起脱水及体重至少下降 5% 到 10% 可诊断为剧吐。

Some psychosocial factors are related to psychosomatic symptoms of women with hyperemesis gravidarum, which provides a theoretical basis for psychological intervention during pregnancy.

妊娠剧烈呕吐患者的身心症状水平与心理社会因素有一定的关系,这为妊娠期的心理行为干预提供了理论依据。

hyperemia [ˌhaipəˈriːmiə] *n.* 充血

Histamine causes active hyperemia and increased vascular permeability lasting 10-15 minutes.

组胺引起主动性充血和血管通透性增高持续 10 ~ 15 分钟。

hyperemic [ˌhaipəˈiːmik] *a.* 充血的

The dead muscle is tan-yellow with a surrounding hyperemic border.

坏死心肌呈黄褐色且周边有充血的边界。

The microabscesses have yellow centers and prominent hyperemic borders.
微小脓肿中心是黄色，外周明显充血。

hyperflexion [ˌhaipəˈflekʃən] *n.* 屈曲过度

Hyperflexion of the fetus or contortionist attitude of its limbs give supporting evidence of fetal death.
胎儿过度的屈曲或肢体扭曲可以支持胎儿死亡的诊断。

hypergammaglobulinemia [ˌhaipəgəˌmægləuˌbjuliˈniːmiə] *n.* 高丙球蛋白血症

Most hypergammaglobulinemias are caused by an excess of immunoglobulin M(IgM).
大多数高丙球蛋白血症是由于免疫球蛋白 M(IgM)过多引起。

We have characterized some key parameters of hypergammaglobulinemia provoked by systemic and persistent viral infection.
我们已经描述了全身持续性病毒感染所致高丙球蛋白血症的一些关键参数。

hyperglycemia [ˌhaipəglaiˈsiːmiə] *n.* 高血糖

Local stasis in the renal veins can be caused by an osmotic diuresis due to hyperglycemia.
高血糖症渗透性利尿可引起肾静脉处局部淤滞。

Diabetes mellitus is a clinical syndrome involving a variety of metabolic disorders characterized by hyperglycemia.
糖尿病是一种有多种代谢异常且具有高血糖特征的临床综合征。

hyperglycinemia [ˌhaipəˌglaisiˈniːmiə] *n.* 高甘氨酸血症

Non ketotic hyperglycinemia is a rare inborn error of glycine metabolism.
非酮性高甘氨酸血症是一种少见的先天性甘氨酸代谢异常。

Nonketotic hyperglycinemia is a clinical syndrome consisting of severe hyperglycemia, hyperosmolarity, and intracellular dehydration without ketoacidosis.
非酮症高甘氨酸血症是一种临床综合征，包括严重的高血糖、高渗透压、细胞内脱水，但没有酮症酸中毒。

hyperimmune [ˌhaipə(ː)riˈmjuːn] *n.* 超免疫的，高价免疫的

For maximum protection hyperimmune serum and vaccine are required.
最好的预防措施需用高价免疫血清和疫苗。

hyperimmunization [ˌhaipəˌimjuːnaiˈzeiʃən] *n.* 超免疫，超免疫法

Repeated immunization to achieve a heightened state of immunity is called hyperimmunization.
重复免疫获得的一种免疫增强状态称为超免疫。

The rabbit hyperimmunization model has previously been used to evaluate candidate hypoallergenic protein ingredients.
家兔免疫增强模型以前曾用来评价候选的低过敏源性蛋白成分。

hyperinflation [ˌhaipəinˈfleiʃən] *n.* 过度充气

Since there is no significant tissue destruction and elastic loss, senile emphysema is better to be named senile hyperinflation.
因为没有明显的组织破坏和弹性丧失，老年性肺气肿最好称为老年性过度充气。

Compensatory emphysema is better to be designated as compensatory hyperinflation because of no destruction of the septal walls.
因为没有肺泡间隔的破坏，代偿性肺气肿最好命名为代偿性过度充气。

hyperinsulinemia [ˌhaipə(ː)ˌrinsjuliˈniːmiə] *n.* 高胰岛素血症

This hyperinsulinemia is associated with a decrease concentration of insulin receptors in target cells of insulin action.
高胰岛素血症与受胰岛素作用的靶细胞上的胰岛素受体的浓度下降有关。

hyperintensity [ˌhaipəinˈtensiti] *n.* 高信号

The cerebrospinal fluid shows hyperintensity on T2WI images.
脑脊液在 T2 加权图像上显示为高信号。

Signal of hepatic cysts varied from low intensity to slightly hyperintensity.
肝囊肿表现多样，从低信号到稍高信号不等。

hyperkalemia [ˌhaipə(ː)kəˈliːmiə] *n.* 血钾过多，高钾血症

The most important clinical effects of hyperkalemia are cardiac conduction changes and arrhythmias.
高钾血症最重要的临床影响是心脏传导改变和心律不齐。

Metabolic acidosis can further exacerbate the hyperkalemia.
代谢性酸中毒可使高钾血症患者的病情进一步恶化。

hyperkinetic [ˌhaipəkaiˈnetik] *a.* 运动过度的，运动功能亢进的

The hyperkinetic syndrome of childhood is associated with marked conduct disturbance but not developmental delay.
童年运动过度综合征伴有明显的行为障碍而不是发育延缓。

hyperlipemia [ˌhaipə(ː)liˈpiːmiə] *n.* 血脂过多，高脂血（症）（= hyperlipidemia, hyperlipoidemia）

Patients with uremic hyperlipemia demonstrate elevations of the very low density lipoproteins (VLDL).
尿毒症性高脂血症患者表现出极低密度脂蛋白浓度升高。

hyperlipidemia [ˌhaipə(ː)ˌlipiˈdiːmiə] *n.* 高脂血症，血脂过多

Hyperlipidemias may be primary and familial or secondary to other identifiable disorders or to the use of drugs.
高脂血症可以是原发的、家族性的、继发于其他疾病或由于用药所引起的。

The first-line management of any primary hyperlipidemia should always be dietary modification.
对任何原发性高脂血症患者的最先的治疗措施常为饮食调整。

hyperlipidemic [ˌhaipəˌlipiˈdiːmik] *a.* 高血脂的

Specific hyperlipidemic syndromes should be treated.
明显的高血脂症应予治疗。

hypermagnesemia [ˌhaipə(ː)mægniˈsiːmiə] *n.* 高镁血，血镁过多

Hypermagnesemia causes respiratory suppression and cardiac arrhythmias.
高镁血症可引起呼吸抑制和心律失常。

hypermedia [ˌhaipəˈmiːdiə] *n.* 超媒体

Hypermedia is the multimedia display of hypertext.
超媒体是超文本的多媒体表现。

Hypertext and hypermedia have as a major property a non-linear information link.
超文本和超媒体有一个主要特征，即非线性的信息连接。

hypermenorrhea [ˌhaipəˌmenəˈriːə] *n.* 月经过多

Hypermenorrhea is most often due to anatomic abnormalities of the uterus, such as uterine myomas.
月经过多常由于子宫结构异常如子宫肌瘤引起。

Abnormal uterine bleeding may occur in the form of hypermenorrhea.
不正常子宫出血可能以月经过多形式出现。

hyperopia [ˌhaipəˈrəupiə] *n.* 远视

One defect that is often responsible for eyestrain in children is hyperopia.
常常造成儿童眼疲劳的一种缺陷是远视。

Hyperopia can be corrected by convex, convergent lenses.
远视可通过凸透镜得到矫正。

hyperostosis [ˌhaipərɔsˈtəusis] *n.* 骨质增生，骨肥厚

The method is characterized by resecting hyperostosis of the mandibular angle, the bulky masseter and the buccal fat pad through intraoral or combined extra-intraoral approach.

这个方法的特点是通过口内或结合口外途径切除下颌角肥厚部位，过大的咬肌以及颊脂垫。

hyperoxaluria [ˌhaipəːˌrɔksəˈljuəriə] *n.* 尿草酸盐过多，高草酸盐尿

Acquired hyperoxaluria is due to increased absorption of oxalate.

获得性高草酸盐尿是由于草酸盐的吸收增加引起的。

Primary hyperoxaluria refers to two peroxisomal enzyme deficiencies.

原发性高草酸尿涉及二种过氧化物酶的缺陷。

hyperoxide [ˌhaipə(ː)ˈrɔksaid] *n.* 超氧化物

Hyperoxide-SHP was first discovered in 1818 by the French chemist Louis Jacques.

超氧化物-SHP 由一位法国化学家路易·雅克于 1818 年首次发现。

Hyperoxide is a compound having a relatively large percentage of oxygen.

超氧化物是一类含氧百分比相当高的化合物。

hyperparathyroidism [haipəːˌpærəˈθairɔidizəm] *n.* 甲状旁腺功能亢进

Primary hyperparathyroidism is generally associated with adenomas of one or more parathyroid glands that secrete an excess of parathormone.

原发性甲状旁腺功能亢进通常与一个或一个以上的甲状旁腺腺瘤分泌过多的甲状旁腺素有关。

Secondary hyperparathyroidism is usually associated with hyperplasia of the parathyroid glands.

继发性甲状旁腺功能亢进通常与甲状旁腺的增生有关。

hyperplasia [haipəˈpleiziə] *n.* 增殖，肥大

The primary medial hyperplasia is one of the arterial diseases.

原发性的内膜增殖是一种动脉疾病。

A number of reports have documented the relationship of endometrial hyperplasia to endometrial carcinoma.

不少报告证实了宫内膜增生与子宫内膜癌的关系。

hyperplastic [ˌhaipə(ː)ˈplæstik] *a.* 增生的

Hyperplastic polyps are rarely greater than 5mm.

增生性息肉很少有直径大于 5 毫米的。

hyperpnea [ˌhaipəːˈpniːə] *n.* 呼吸过度，呼吸深快

Arterial pressure tends to rise with hyperpnea.

当通气过度时动脉血压会有上升的趋势。

hyperprolactinemia [ˌhaipəprəuˌlæktiˈniːmiə] *n.* 高泌乳素血症

Aripiprazole is often recommended as the drug of choice in patients who develop antipsychotic-induced hyperprolactinemia.

阿立哌唑常被推荐作为抗精神病药引起的高泌乳素血症的首选药。

Disorder of the dopamine system has been linked with Parkinson ' s disease, Tourette ' s syndrome, schizophrenia, hyperprolactinemia and addiction.

帕金森氏病、妥瑞氏综合征、精神分裂症、高泌乳素血症以及药物成瘾等疾病都与多巴胺系统紊乱有关。

hyperpyrexia [ˌhaipə(ː)paiˈreksiə] *n.* 高热

The hallmark of the clinical picture of leukemia is progressive pallor, hyperpyrexia, and bleeding manifestations.

白血病临床表现的特点是进行性苍白、高热和出血。

hyperreactivity [ˌhaipəˌriækˈtiviti] *n.* 高反应性

Bronchial hyperreactivity has long been recognized as a hallmark of chronic asthma.

支气管高反应性一直被认为是慢性哮喘的一个标志。

Airway sensory hyperreactivity is linked to capsaicin sensitivity.

气道感觉高反应性与辣椒素敏感性有关。

hyperreflexia [ˌhaipəriˈfleksiə] *n.* 反射亢进

Autonomic hyperreflexia is a reaction of the autonomic nervous system to overstimulation.

自主性反射亢进是自主神经系统对过度刺激的一种反应。

The most common cause of autonomic hyperreflexia is spinal cord injury.

自主性反射亢进最常见的原因是脊髓损伤。

hypersecrete [ˌhaipəsiːˈkriːt] *v.* 分泌过多

Children with peptic ulcers, like adults on the average, hypersecrete gastric acid.

患消化性溃疡的儿童也像一般的成年人那样,可以分泌过多的胃酸。

hypersecretion [ˈhaipəsiˈkriːʃən] *n.* 分泌亢进,分泌物过多;痰多

No cause is usually found though duodenal ulcer is associated with gastric hypersecretion.

虽然十二指肠溃疡伴有胃酸分泌亢进,但通常找不到发病原因。

Bronchopulmonary drainage should be maintained in patients with hypersecretion.

痰多的病人应持续作支气管肺引流。

hypersensitivity [ˌhaipəˌsensiˈtiviti] *n.* 过敏(性)

These effects are classed as hypersensitivity reactions.

这些作用归类为过敏反应。

Quinidine may produce cinchonism and cutaneous hypersensitivity reactions.

奎尼丁可产生金鸡纳反应和皮肤过敏反应。

hypersomnia [ˌhaipəˈsɔmniə] *n.* 睡眠过度,嗜睡

Many patients with hypersomnia usually have excessive daytime sleepiness.

嗜睡症患者经常白天睡意过多。

The authors recommend that hypersomnia should be treated as a potential risk factor for suicidal behavior.

作者建议嗜睡应被看成自杀行为的潜在危险因素。

hypersplenism [ˌhaipə(ː)ˈsplenizəm] *n.* 脾功能亢进

Hypersplenism contributes to anemia, thrombocytopenia, and leukopenia.

脾功能亢进可引起贫血、血小板减少以及白细胞减少。

Leukopenia occurs occasionally, but anemia can hardly ever be attributed to hypersplenism.

脾功能亢进时偶尔可出现血中白细胞减少,但却极少引起贫血。

hyperstimulation [ˌhaipəˌstimjuˈleiʃən] *n.* 刺激过度;超排卵;卵巢过度刺激综合征

The impact of ovarian hyperstimulation syndrome on thyroid function in women without thyroid disorders was investigated.

研究了卵巢过度刺激综合征在无甲状腺疾病妇女中对甲状腺功能影响。

About 10% of women going through IVF treatment will experience ovarian hyperstimulation syndrome.

大约 10% 妇女在体外受精治疗中会出现卵巢过度刺激综合征。

hypersusceptibility [ˈhaipəsəˌseptəˈbiliti] *n.* 过敏

Hypersusceptibility test will be considered before CT contrast examination.

在 CT 造影检查前可考虑进行过敏试验。

hypertension [ˌhaipəˈtenʃən] *n.* 高血压;压力过高

The rare development of pulmonary hypertension is due to recurrent small emboli.

经常发生的小栓子可引起罕见的肺动脉高压。

Cirrhosis accounts for 80% of the portal hypertension seen in Britain.

在英国 80% 的门脉高压的原因为肝硬化。

hypertensive [ˌhaipəˈtensiv] *a.* 高血压的

The early hypertrophic changes are usually observed only in young hypertensive subjects.

早期的肥厚性变化通常仅见于年轻高血压患者。

n. 高血压患者

In all these sites, the change is usually more severe in hypertensives.
所有这些部位的病变,在高血压患者往往更加严重。

hypertext [ˌhaipəˈtekst] *n.* 超文本

In essence, hypertext is a large distributed document.
本质上,超文本是一种大型分布式文档。

Hypertext system is mainly determined through non-linear links of information.
超文本系统主要通过信息的非线性链接决定。

hyperthermia [ˌhaipəˈθəːmiə] *n.* 高温,高热

Malignant hyperthermia marked by rapid rise in body temperature, signs of increased muscle metabolism, and usually, rigidity.
恶性高热的特点是体温的迅速上升,肌肉代谢升高征并通常伴有强直。

Hyperthermia, an elevation of core temperature without elevation of the hypothalamic set point, is due to inadequate heat dissipation.
高温是体内中心温度升高而下丘脑体温调定点并未上移,这种状态是由于散热不够引起的。

hyperthymia [ˌhaipəˈθaimiə] *n.* 情感增盛

Hyperthymia and dysthymia constitute the cyclothymic personality type which is associated with manic-depressive disease.
情绪高涨和情绪低落两者构成了与狂躁抑郁症有关的具有周期性情绪波动的人格类型。

hyperthyroidism [ˌhaipəˈθairɔidizəm] *n.* 甲状腺功能亢进

Hyperthyroidism is predominantly a disease of adult women, with peak incidence between 30 and 50 years of age.
甲状腺功能亢进主要见于成年妇女,其发病高峰在 30 到 50 岁之间。

High output heart failure is often produced by a variety of systemic diseases, including hyperthyroidism.
高排出量心力衰竭常由各种全身性疾病引起,其中包括甲状腺功能亢进。

hypertonic [ˌhaipəˈtɔnik] *a.* 高渗的,张力过强的

If hypertonic saline is injected intravenously, the cerebrospinal fluid pressure falls profoundly for a period of 2-4 hours.
如果静脉内注入高渗盐水,脑脊液压可显著下降达 2 ~4 小时。

Hypertonic solution means a solution having a greater tonicity than the blood.
高张性溶液是指高于血液张力的溶液。

hypertonicity [ˌhaipəːtəuˈnisiti] *n.* 高渗性;高张性;过度紧张

Physical examination reveals hypertonicity and muscular rigidity.
体格检查发现张力过高和肌肉僵硬。

Botulinum A toxin has been widely applied to the treatment of muscular hypertonicity.
肉毒杆菌毒素已被广泛应用于治疗肌肉张力过高。

hypertriglyceridemia [ˌhaipətraiˌglisəraiˈdiːmiə] *n.* 高甘油三酯血症

Hypertriglyceridemia is associated with an increased risk of cardiovascular events and acute pancreatitis.
高甘油三酯血症与心血管事件和急性胰腺炎的风险增高有关。

Hypertriglyceridemia(hTG), a condition in which triglyceride levels are elevated, is a common disorder in the United States.
高甘油三酯血症这种甘油三酯水平升高的疾病在美国是一种常见病。

hypertrophic [ˌhaipəˈtrɔfik] *a.* 肥厚的,肥大的

These hypertrophic changes give way to fibrous replacement of muscle.
这些病变不再是肥厚,而是肌组织为纤维组织所取代。

hypertrophy [haiˈpəːtrəufi] *n.* 肥大

There was a mild degree of left ventricular hypertrophy.
左心室轻度肥厚。
Right ventricular hypertrophy develops in response to elevated pulmonary arterial pressures.
右心室的肥大随着肺动脉压的升高而发生。

hyperuricemia [ˌhaipəjuəriˈsiːmiə] *n.* 血尿酸过多，高尿酸血症
Hyperuricemia is usually mild in ARF and does not require specific intervention.
急性肾衰（ARF）患者通常患有轻度的血尿酸升高，它并不需要特殊的治疗。
Hyperuricemia is commoner without clinical gout than with it.
高尿酸血症不合并痛风者较合并痛风者更为多见。

hypervariable [haipə(ː)ˈvɛəriəbl] *a.* 超变的，高变的
Hypervariable regions form the antigen-binding sites.
超变区形成了抗原结合位点。

hyperventilate [ˌhaipə(ː)ˈventileit] *v.* 通气过度，过度呼吸
The patient was fearful, hyperventilating and scratching her trunk and extremities.
患者呈现恐惧及通气过度的状态，并不时搔抓其躯干和四肢。

hyperventilation [ˌhaipə(ː)ˌventiˈleiʃən] *n.* 过度通气，过度呼吸
Hyperventilation is a relatively common cause of syncope and is usually in young women during periods of stress.
过度通气相对来说是一种晕厥的常见原因，常易发生于高度紧张的年轻女性。
Careful intubation allows controlled hyperventilation to lower intracranial pressure quickly.
通过仔细进行气管插管来控制过度通气能很快降低颅内压。

hypervitaminosis [haipəˌvaitəmiˈnəusis] *n.* 维生素过多症
Hypervitaminosis A (excess ingestion of vitamin A) produces toxic effects.
维生素 A 过多（症）可产生毒性作用。

hypesthesia [ˌhaipisˈθiːzjə] *n.* 感觉减退，感觉迟钝
Involvement of major nerve trunks is less common, but diffuse hypesthesia is common in advanced disease.
大的神经干受损很少见，但是晚期疾病常常出现弥散性的感觉迟钝。

hypha [ˈhaifə] *n.* 菌丝（*pl.* hyphae [ˈhaifiː]）
A hypha is a long, branching filamentous structure of a fungus.
菌丝是真菌的一种长长的、分枝丝状结构。
In most fungi, hyphae are the main mode of vegetative growth, and are collectively called a mycelium.
在多数真菌中，菌丝是真菌中植物性生长的主要方式，统称为菌丝体。

hypnagogic [ˌhipnəˈgɔdʒik] *a.* 使瞌睡的，催眠的，入睡前发生的
The syndrome of sleep disorders includes hypnagogic hallucinations and frightening.
睡眠障碍的症状包括入睡前幻觉和恐惧。

hypnosis [hipˈnəusis] *n.* 催眠，催眠状态
Hypnosis is a condition of artificially produced sleep or of a trance resembling sleep.
催眠是指人工产生的睡眠或似睡非睡的恍惚状态。
Since aspirin does not cause hypnosis or euphoria, its sites of action have been postulated to be subcortical.
因阿司匹林不产生催眠或欣快感，所以推测它的作用部位在皮质下。

hypnotic [hipˈnɔtik] *a.* 催眠的，催眠性的
Salicylamide and acetophenetidin, when combined and injected, elicited marked hypnotic activity.
水杨酸胺和非那西汀混合后进行注射可产生催眠作用。
n. 催眠药

Sedatives and hypnotics may be divided into barbiturates and nonbarbiturates.
镇静药和催眠药可分成巴比妥类和非巴比妥类。

Hypnotics can't be prescribed casually without analysis of sleep complaints.
没有对失眠症状进行分析,不能随意开安眠药。

hypoalbuminemia [ˌhaipəuælˌbjumiˈniːmiə] *n.* 白蛋白减少

The primary abnormality in nephrotic sydrome is proteinuria with hypoalbuminemia, and edema usually being present.
肾病综合征的主要异常表现是蛋白尿、低蛋白血症,且常出现水肿。

hypocalcemia [ˌhaipəukælˈsiːmiə] *n.* 血钙过少;低钙血(症)

In the neonatal period birth injury, associated with cerebral anoxia, hypoglycaemia, or hypocalcemia, may lead to convulsions.
在新生儿时期伴有脑缺氧、低血糖或低血钙的产伤可引起抽搐。

hypocapnia [ˌhaipəuˈkæpniə] *n.* 低碳酸血症

Do hyperoxaemia and hypocapnia add to the risk of brain injury after intrapartum asphyxia?
高氧血症和低碳酸血症会增加产时窒息后的大脑损伤风险吗?

Central sleep apnea(CSA) was associated with atrial fibrillation, hypocapnia, and diuretic use.
中枢性睡眠呼吸暂停与房颤、低碳酸血症和利尿剂的使用有关。

hypochloremia [ˌhaipəukləːˈriːmiə] *n.* 低氯血症

They have been shown to be effective in patients with hypoalbuminemia, hyponatremia, hypochloremia, hypokalemia, and reductions in GFR.
已发现它们对于有低白蛋白血症、低钠血症、低氯血症、低钾血症以及 GFR 降低的患者有效。

hypochloremic [ˌhaipəukləːˈriːmik] *a.* 低氯血症的

Diuresis can lead to hypochloremic alkalosis.
利尿可导致低氯性碱中毒。

hypochondrium [ˌhaipəˈkɔndriəm] *n.* 季肋部;疑难症

On examination the main physical sign is tenderness in the epigastrium or right hypochondrium, but between attacks this may be absent.
检查中主要的体征是在上腹部或右季肋部有压痛,但发作间期并无此现象。

Hypochondria refer to excessive worry about having a serious illness.
疑病症是指过度担心自己罹患严重疾病的一种神经症。

Many patients with hypochondria present many symptoms, such as gastro-intestinal problems, palpitations, or muscle fatigue.
疑病症患者常有胃肠道不适、心悸和肌肉疲劳等症状。

hypochromia [ˌhaipəuˈkrəumiə] *n.* 血红蛋白过少;着色不足

Hypochromia is a characteristic feature of disorders of hemoglobin synthesis, most commonly iron deficiency.
血红蛋白过少是由于血红蛋白的合成障碍引起,但通常发生于铁缺乏时。

It's difficult to recognize hypochromia until the hemoglobin concentration decreases to less than the 8 to 9g/dl range.
在血红蛋白浓度低于 8 ~9g/dl 之前,血红蛋白过少很难被发现。

hypochromic [ˌhaipəuˈkrəumik] *a.* 低色素的,血红蛋白过少的

Deficient or dedefective heme or globin synthesis produces a hypochromic-microcytic RBC population.
血红素或球蛋白合成不足或有缺陷就会产生低色素小红细胞性的红细胞群。

hypocotyl [ˌhaipəuˈkɔtil] *n.* 子叶下轴,[植] 下胚轴

It doesn't fall into the sea or the mud from the mother tree until its hypocotyl matures.
直至胚轴成熟后它才离开母树落入海水或淤泥中。

As the development of the hypocotyl continues, the characteristic crook in the upper portion becomes apparent.

随着下胚轴继续发育,上部特有的弯曲显得更为明显。

hypodense [ˈhaipəudens] *n.* 低密度

Both hepatic carcinoma and hemangiomas show hypodense in plain CT scan.

CT 平扫时,肝癌和肝血管瘤都表现为低密度。

In the delayed phase, the wall, septations and edematous zone of the abscess are all isodense, only the necrotic areas are not enhanced and was hypodense.

延迟期脓肿壁、分隔及水肿带均呈等密度,仅坏死区无强化呈低密度。

hypodermic [haipəˈdəːmik] *a.* 皮下的,皮下组织的

The nurse will use surgical aseptic technique when administering a hypodermic injection to a patient.

在对病人进行皮下注射时,护士就用得上外科无菌操作。

A shot that can be given superficially is administered with a hypodermic needle.

给予浅表性注射时,可用皮下针头。

hypoecho [ˌhaipəuˈekəu] *n.* 低回声

The ultrasonographs of spleen infarct were cuneiform or irregular and they were even or uneven hypoecho.

脾梗死超声图像呈现楔形或不规则形,并且呈均匀或不均匀低回声。

Primary liver cancer is usually manifested as hypoecho and uneven distribution of light spot.

原发性肝癌通常表现为低回声和光点的不均匀分布。

hypofibrinogenamia [ˌhaipəufaiˌbrinəudʒiˈniːmiə] *n.* 血纤维蛋白原过少

In these cases there is no urgent call for interference, unless the complication of hypofibrinogenamia occurs.

对这些病例不要急于干预,除非出现了低纤维蛋白原血症的并发症。

hypogammaglobulinemia [ˌhaipəuˌgæməˌglɔbjuːliˈniːmiə] *n.* 血丙种球蛋白过少,低丙种球蛋白血症

Hypogammaglobulinemia is characterised by a markedly reduced or absent IgA and IgM content in the serum and jejunal secretions.

血清和空肠液中 IgA 和 IgM 的含量显著减少或缺乏时可称之为低丙种球蛋白血症。

Infants with transient hypogammaglobulinemia have normal amounts of circulating mature B lymphocytes.

患暂时性低丙种球蛋白血症婴儿的循环血中含有正常数量的成熟 B 淋巴细胞。

hypogastrium [ˌhaipəuˈgæstriəm] *n.* 腹下区

The pain of posterior urethral calculi may expand to the hypogastrium and below.

后尿道结石所致的疼痛可扩展到腹下区及以下的部位。

The pain is dull and poorly localized to the epigastrium, periumbilical regions, or hypogastrium, depending on the embryonic origin of the organ involved.

依据患病器官胚胎起源部位,疼痛为钝性且难以准确定位在上腹部、脐周区或腹下区。

hypoglycemia [ˌhaipəuglaiˈsiːmiə] *n.* 血糖过少

The baby had transient hypoglycemia in the newborn nursery but otherwise did well.

在新生儿室婴儿有短暂的低血糖症,其它尚好。

hypoglycemic [ˌhaipəuglaiˈsiːmik] *a.* 低血糖的

Hypoglycemic coma can be induced by the over administration of insulin or oral hypoglycemic agents.

低血糖性昏迷可由过量服用胰岛素或口服降糖药引起。

n. 降血糖药

The two recently introduced sulfonylurea oral hypoglycemics are glyburide and glipzide.

最近问世的两种磺酰脲类口服降血糖药为优降糖和吡磺环己脲。

hypogonadism [ˌhaipəuˈɡəunədizəm] *n.* 性腺功能减退(症),性腺发育不足

Hypogonadism is a prominent feature of zinc deficiency.

性腺功能减退是锌缺乏的一个显著特征。

Hypogonadism occurs in approximately one third of symptomatic men with hemochromatosis but is much less frequent in women.

性腺功能减退见于约 1/3 的有症状的男性血色病患者,而较少见于女性患者。

hypogonadotrophic [ˌhaipəˌɡəunædəuˈtrəufik] *a.* 促性腺分泌不足的

Hyperprolactinemia causes hypogonadotrophic hypogonadism.

高泌乳素血症引起促性腺分泌不足的性腺功能减退。

The causal association of childhood obesity and hypogonadotrophic hypogonadism needs to be studied to unravel the cause.

需要研究儿童肥胖症与性腺素分泌不足性性腺功能减退之间的因果关系以揭示其原因。

hypointensity [ˌhaipəuinˈtensiti] *n.* 低信号

Primary hepatic carcinoma always demonstrates hypointensity on T1WI images.

原发性肝癌在 T1 加权图像上通常表现为低信号。

On sagittal and axial T2WI,5 cases were of high signal or heterogeneous high signal,5 cases were of heterogeneous hypointensity or hypointensity.

在 T2WI 矢状面和轴面 5 例表现为高信号或混杂高信号,5 例表现为混杂低信号或低信号。

hypokalemia [ˌhaipəukeiˈliːmiə] *n.* 血钾过少,低钾血症

Hypokalemia is the single most useful clue to the diagnosis of primary aldosteronism.

低钾血症是诊断原发性醛固酮增多症的唯一最有用的线索。

Severe symptomatic hypokalemia requires larger doses(20-40mmol/h),with cardiac monitoring and frequent plasma K levels.

严重的有症状的低钾血症需大剂量补钾(20～40 毫摩尔/小时),同时要监测心电图和血钾水平。

hypokalemic [ˌhaipəukeiˈliːmik] *a.* 血钾过少的,低钾血的

Prolonged use of strong laxatives leads to severe hypokalemic alkalosis.

长期使用强烈的泻药可导致严重的低血钾性碱中毒。

hypolipidemic [ˌhaipəulipiˈdemik] *a.* 低血脂的,降血脂的

The pharmaceutical industry has provided us with a number of hypolipidemic agents.

制药工业为我们提供了一系列降血脂药物。

Another agent with reported hypolipidemic effects is neomycin.

另一个据报道具有降血脂作用的药物是新霉素。

hypomania [ˌhaipəuˈmeiniə] *n.* 轻度躁狂(症)

Mania and hypomania involve dysfunctional beliefs about the self,others,and the world,as well as about affective regulation.

躁狂和轻躁狂涉及对自身、他人、世界以及对情感调节的异常信念。

Hypomania-prone individuals tend to describe more recent events.

有轻躁狂倾向的个体倾向描述较近期发生的事件。

hypomenorrhea [ˌhaipəuˌmenəˈriə] *n.* 月经过少

Hypomenorrhea may occur premenopausally or during oral contraceptive usage.

月经过少可发生于绝经前或使用口服避孕药期间。

hypometabolism [ˌhaipəumeˈtæbəlizəm] *n.* 代谢低下

Protein deprivation may cause hypometabolism.

蛋白质缺乏可导致代谢低下。

hypomethylation [haipəuˌmeθiˈleiʃən] *n.* 低甲基化

Hypomethylation of retrotransposons can cause altered gene expression in humans.
逆转录转座子低甲基化可引起人类基因表达的改变。
Hypomethylation is also observed at a number of single-copy genes.
低甲基化也见于一些单拷贝基因。

hyponatremia [ˌhaipəunəˈtriːmiə] *n.* 低钠血症
When hyponatremia is present in the presence of edema, rigid water restriction is also advised.
如果有水肿的同时又有低钠血症,则应严格控制水的摄入。

hypophosphatasia [ˈhaipəuˌfɔsfəˈteizjə] *n.* 低磷酸酯酶症
Hypophosphatasia is a rare and sometimes fatal metabolic bone disease.
低磷酸酯酶症是一种罕见的,有时甚至可致命的代谢性骨病。
Hypophosphatasia is an inherited disorder that affects the development of bones and teeth.
低磷酸酯酶症是一种遗传性疾病,影响骨骼和牙齿的发育。

hypophosphatemia [ˌhaipəuˌfɔsfəˈtiːmiə] *n.* 低磷酸盐血症,血磷酸盐过少
Hypophosphatemia is a low level of phosphorus in the blood.
低磷酸盐血症是指血中磷的水平较低。
Fanconi's syndrome has renal tubular injury with severe hypophosphatemia.
Fanconi 综合征有肾小管损伤,同时伴有严重的低磷酸盐血症。

hypophysectomy [haiˌpɔfiˈsektəmi] *n.* 垂体切除术
Hypophysectomy is the treatment of choice for pituitary-dependent Cushing's Syndrome.
对垂体依赖性库欣综合征应选用垂体切除术。

hypophysis [haiˈpɔfisis] *n.* 垂体
Mammary gland is the target organ of endocrine; its physiological function is regulated and controlled by the hypothalamic-hypophysis-ovarian axis.
乳腺是内分泌腺的靶器官,其生理功能受到下丘脑垂体卵巢轴的调控。
The ACTH test can evaluate the function of adrenocortical and the regulation of hypophysis adrenal axis.
促肾上腺皮质激素(ACTH)试验能评估肾上腺皮质的功能和脑下垂体肾上腺轴的调节功能。

hypopituitarism [ˌhaipəupiˈtjuːitərizm] *n.* 垂体功能减退
An exogenous, psychotic episode in the patient was induced by multi-hormonal reduction due to hypopituitarism and disappeared after hormonal replacement therapy.
病人外源性精神症状发作由垂体功能减退导致多种激素减少引起,并且经激素替代治疗之后消失。
Hypopituitarism is associated with increased cardiovascular mortality.
垂体功能减退与心血管死亡率增加有关联。

hypoplasia [haipəuˈpleiziə] *n.* 发育不全,再生不良
The mechanisms of normochromic-normocytic anemias involved are hypoproliferation, hypoplasia and myelophthisis.
正色正常红细胞性贫血的机制为增殖不足,再生不良及全骨髓萎缩。

hypoplastic [ˌhaipəuˈplæstik] *a.* 发育不全的,细胞减少的
The receptor cells are present but are hypoplastic, and do not project above the surrounding supporting cells.
可出现受体细胞,但数量减少,它并不能覆盖周围的支持细胞。
Normochromic-normocytic anemias with defective production pose a hypoproliferative or hypoplastic mechanism.
生成不足所致的正色正常红细胞性贫血的产生机制是增生不足或发育不全。

hypoproliferation [haipəuprəulifəˈreiʃən] *n.* 增殖不足
In hypoproliferation normal humoral stimulus(erythropoietin) is lacking.

增殖不足的机制是缺乏正常的体液刺激因素(促红细胞生成素)。

hyposensitization [ˌhaipəuˌsensitaiˈzeiʃən] *n.* 脱敏(作用)

Inhalation of salmeterol fluticasone combined with specific hyposensitization is an effective method to prevent and treat bronchial asthma.

吸入沙美特罗替卡松同时结合特异性脱敏可有效防治支气管哮喘。

All the patients were treated by specific hyposensitization therapy.

所有患者均采用特异性脱敏治疗。

hypospermia [ˌhaipəuˈspəːmiə] *n.* 精子减少症

Hypospermia, a medical term meaning low ejaculating volume, should not be confused with oligospermia, which means low sperm count.

精子减少症是指射精量减少的临床术语,不应与精子计数减少的少精子症混淆。

Maxocum was designed by our specialists not only to increase low sperm count but also to cure sperm issues like azoospermia, hypospermia and oligospermia.

由我们专家研制的 Maxocum 不仅能提高精子数量,还能治愈无精症、精子减少症以及少精子症。

hypotension [haipəuˈtenʃən] *n.* 低血压;压力过低

Myocardial infarction may also occur during hypotension(including surgery).

心肌梗死也可发生于低血压时(包括外科手术时)。

Another disadvantage of regional anesthesia is hypotension due to sympathetic blockade.

区域麻醉的另外一个缺点是交感阻滞引起的低血压。

hypotensive [ˌhaipəuˈtensiv] *a.* 低血压的

The drug may increase hypotension in patient already hypotensive.

该药对已患低血压的病人可能加重低血压。

Histamine augments the hypotensive effects of acetylcholine.

组织胺增强乙酰胆碱的降血压作用。

hypothalamic [ˌhaipəuˌθəˈlæmik] *a.* 下丘脑的

Lesions in the hypothalamic-posterior pituitary system produce diabetes insipidus.

下丘脑垂体后叶系统的病变可产生尿崩症。

Lesion in or near the hypothalamic posterior pituitery system may produce diabetes insipidus.

下丘脑垂体后叶系统内部或邻近的病变可产生尿崩症。

hypothalamus [ˌhaipəuˈθæləməs] *n.* 下丘脑

The hypothalamus plays a key role in controlling both water intake and water loss.

下丘脑在控制水分摄入和排泄中起着关键作用。

It is well established that the thermoregulatory center resides in the anterior hypothalamus.

人们已确认温度调节中枢位于下丘脑前部。

hypothermia [haipəuˈθəːmiə] *n.* 低温,降温

One advance was hypothermia, the artificial lowering of the body temperature.

一个进展是降温法(低温麻醉),即用人工方法降低体温。

But hypothermia could not be used safely in long and intricate surgery.

但是,低温法不能安全地使用于时间长的复杂手术。

hypothesis [haiˈpɔθisis] (*pl.* hypotheses [haiˈpɔθisiːz]) *n.* 假设;前提

Most of the research regarding this hypothesis has been done in experimental animal.

关于这一假设的大部分实验是在实验动物身上做的。

The specific etiology of this abnormality remains unknown although certain hypotheses have been proposed.

虽然提出了一些假说,此种畸形的特定病因学仍不清楚。

hypothesize [haiˈpɔθisaiz] *v.* 假设,假定

Low birth weight has been associated with occupation, and a link with exercise was hypothesized

by Briend in 1980.
低出生体重婴儿与母亲的职业有关，而与运动相关的假设已在 1980 年由 Briend 提出。

hypothetical [ˌhaipəu'θetikəl] *a.* 假设的

Often an expert is asked to answer a special type of question, the "hypothetical question".
专家经常会被要求回答一种特殊类型的问题，即："假设的问题"。

hypothyroidism [ˌhaipəu'θairɔidizəm] *n.* 甲状腺功能减退

Hypo-or hyperthyroidism was confirmed in our animals by measuring plasma T4 levels at the beginning of the study (Table 1).
甲状腺功能减退或甲状腺功能亢进在实验开始时通过测量动物的血浆 T4 水平得到证实（见表 1）。

Disturbances in the secretion of thyroxine are classed under two headings: ①hypothyroidism, or lack of secretion, and ②hyperthyroidism, or excess of secretion.
甲状腺分泌失调分为两种情况：①甲状腺功能减退，即分泌缺乏；②甲状腺功能亢进，即分泌过多。

hypotonic [haipəu'tɔnik] *a.* 低张的，低渗的

Hypotonic solutions produce a flow of water into cells.
（细胞外的）低渗溶液可以使水向细胞内流动。

Hypotonic duodenography can be used to distinguish infiltrative from inflammatory lesions of the duodenum.
低张性十二指肠造影术可用来鉴别十二指肠浸润性和炎性的损伤。

After a precipitous delivery, the uterus may be hypotonic and hemorrhage from the placental implantation site.
急产后，子宫张力低，此时可能从胎盘植入部位出血。

hypovitaminosis [haipəuˌvaitəmi'nəusis] *n.* 维生素缺乏症

Hypovitaminosis A (vitamin A deficiency) leads to night blindness.
维生素 A 缺乏症导致夜盲症。

hypovolemia [ˌhaipəuvə'liːmiə] *n.* 血容量减少，低血容量

Abnormally decreased volume of circulating fluid in the body is termed hypovolemia.
体内循环液体（如血浆）容量异常的减少称之为低血容量。

Noncardiac causes of hypotension should be considered: hypovolemia, acute arrhythmia, or sepsis.
非心源性低血压应考虑是低血容量、急性心律失常或败血症。

hypoxemia [ˌhaipɔk'siːmiə] *n.* 血氧过少，低氧血症

Pulmonary embolism may be associated with hemoptysis, tachycardia and hypoxemia.
肺栓塞可表现为咯血、心动过速和低氧血症。

Ventilation with O_2 may promptly reverse hypoxemia and acidosis.
给氧可迅速纠正低氧血症和酸中毒。

hypoxia [hai'pɔksiə] *n.* 缺氧，低氧症

The clinical expression of anemia results from tissue hypoxia.
贫血的临床表现是组织缺氧所致。

Arterial blood gases should be monitored and respiratory assistance provided if hypoxia occurs.
如果发生缺氧应检测动脉血氧并提供辅助呼吸。

hypoxic [hai'pɔksik] *a.* 缺氧的

Consciousness may be retained until the patient becomes severely hypoxic.
意识可以保持清醒直到病人严重缺氧。

hysterectomy [ˌhistə'rektəmi] *n.* 子宫切除术

Subtotal hysterectomy may not stop bleeding if the rupture involves the cervix.
如果破裂累及宫颈，做子宫次全切除术不能完全止血。

hysteria [hisˈtiəriə] *n.* 癔症，歇斯底里

Many clinicians still prefer to retain "hysteria" as a diagnostic category.

许多医生仍然喜欢将"歇斯底里"作为一种诊断项目。

The term hysteria is also used to describe a state of tension or excitement in which there is a temporary loss of control over the emotions.

"歇斯底里"一词也用于描述紧张或激动状态，其中存在有感情的暂时失控。

hysterical [hisˈterikəl] *a.* 癔症的，歇斯底里的

Hysterical symptoms (neurosis) may develop under stress.

在紧张状态下可发生癔症的症状（神经症）。

Hysterical tremor is a difficult diagnosis, but a key feature is that the tremor dramatically diminishes or disappears when the patient's attention is distracted.

癔症性震颤很难诊断，但它的一个主要特征是当病人的注意力被分散时震颤明显减轻或消失。

hysterosalpingography [ˌhistərəˌsælpiŋˈgɔgrəfi] *n.* 子宫输卵管造影术

Hysterosalpingography is a radiologic procedure to investigate the shape of the uterine cavity and the shape and patency of the fallopian tubes.

子宫输卵管造影术是一种放射学操作，用于检查子宫腔的形状与输卵管的形状和通畅性。

The effects of three non-ionic contrast media were similar in hysterosalpingography.

三种非离子型造影剂在子宫输卵管造影中的效果相似。

hysteroscopic [ˌhistərəsˈkɔpik] *a.* 宫腔镜检的

We reported two cases of interstitial pregnancy successfully treated with a combined hysteroscopic and laparoscopic approach.

我们报道了两例运用宫腹腔镜联合术成功治疗间质部妊娠的例子。

One hundred and sixty-nine patients were examined with a combined laparoscopic and hysteroscopic technique to detect tubal, peritubal, peritoneal, or intrauterine causes of infertility.

一百六十九个病人运用宫腹腔镜联合术来检测输卵管、输卵管周围、腹膜或宫内等所引起的不孕不育的原因。

hysteroscopy [histəˈrɔskəpi] *n.* 宫腔镜检查

Hysteroscopy is a diagnostic procedure that makes possible the examination of the inside of the uterus without making an abdominal incision.

宫腔镜检查是一种诊断程序，使不用开腹就可检查子宫内部成为可能。

Hysteroscopy is used to diagnose and treat abnormal vaginal bleeding.

宫腔镜检常被用于诊断和治疗异常阴道出血。

hysterotomy [ˌhistəˈrɔtəmi] *n.* 子宫切开术

When the uterus extends above the umbilicus, the physician may empty the uterus by abdominal hysterotomy.

当子宫增大达到脐以上时，医生就可以行腹部子宫切开术以排空子宫内容。

I

iatrogenic [aiˌætrəuˈdʒenik] *a.* 医源性

Iatrogenic is now applied to any adverse condition in a patient occurring as the result of treatment by a physician.

“医源性”现在用来表示经医生处理而使病人出现的任何有害状况。

The application of some hi-tech such as CT or MRI may generate more iatrogenic diseases.

一些高新技术如 CT、磁共振等的应用可能引起更多的医源性疾病。

None of these 16 patients suffered from iatrogenic injury to the bile duct after surgical tretment. .

16 位患者经手术治疗后无一例发生医源性胆管损伤。

ibuprofen [ˌaibjuˈprəufən] *n.* 异丁苯乙酸,布洛芬

Ibuprofen toxicity is mild, including nausea, vomiting, abdominal pain.

异丁苯乙酸的中毒症状较轻,包括恶心、呕吐和腹痛。

The hypothalamic set point is reset downward by the inhibition of local prostaglandin synthesis by aspirin and ibuprofen.

通过阿司匹林和布洛芬抑制局部前列腺素合成使下丘脑体温调定点下调。

ichthammol [ikˈθæmɔl] *n.* 鱼石脂

Ichthammol is an ammoniated coal tar product, used in ointment form for certain skin diseases.

鱼石脂是一种含有氨煤焦油的产品,多以软膏剂的形式用于某些皮肤病。

ichthyosis [ˌikθiˈəusis] (*pl.* ichthyoses [ˌikθiˈəusiz]) *n.* (鱼)鳞癣,干皮病

The ichthyoses are several hereditary diseases of diverse genetic and biochemical manifestations.

干皮病是一种有多种遗传和生物化学表现的遗传病。

icterus [ˈiktərəs] *n.* 黄疸

Icterus refers to the yellow pigmentation of the skin or scleras by bilirubin.

黄疸是指皮肤或巩膜被胆红素黄染。

In biliary obstructive disease, icterus may be severe and still not cause pruritus.

在胆管阻塞性疾病中,黄疸可以很严重而不引起瘙痒。

ideally [aiˈdiəli] *ad.* 理想地

Ideally, the physician should be able to prescribe a dose that will produce a maximum antithrombotic effect with a minimum risk of hemorrhage.

理想的是,医生应当开出既能发挥最大的抗血栓作用,又能使发生出血的危险最小的药物剂量。

identical [aiˈdentikəl] *a.* 同一的,相同的

The clottable and antigenic fibrinogens were nearly identical.

凝血性和抗原性纤维蛋白原几乎相同。

The treatment for this disease is identical with that for gastric ulcer.

此病的疗法与胃溃疡的疗法相同。

identifiable [aiˈdentifaiəbl] *a.* 可看作是相同的;可辨认的;明显的

Some toxins have identifiable enzyme activity.

某些毒素具有明显的酶的活性。

identification [aiˌdentifiˈkeiʃən] *n.* 识别,鉴定

True identification requires microscopic examination.

可靠的鉴别需要显微镜检查。

In most cases of meningococcal meningitis, the diagnosis is readily established by the specific identification of the organism.

大多数脑膜炎双球菌脑膜炎病例,通过对细菌做特殊的鉴定易于确诊。

For the purpose of identification, the name and age of the patient are noted on his bed card.

为了辨认,病人的姓名和年龄都记录在病床卡片上。

identify [ai'dentifai] *v.* 识别,鉴定,验明;明确

The liver has been identified as the major site of conversion of progesterone to carbohydrates.

肝脏作为孕酮转化为碳水化合物的主要部位,已被确认。

Thus far, no meningococci resistant to penicillin or chloramphenicol have been identified.

至今还没有发现过对青霉素或氯霉素有抗药性的脑膜炎双球菌。

The causative organism should be identified by this technique.

应当用这种技术鉴定病原体。

The shape of a cell or cells often helps in identifying an organism or a part of a living thing.

细胞的形状往往有助于辨明是什么生物体或生物体的哪一部分。

identity [ai'dentiti] *n.* 同一(性),一致(性);鉴定

The cytologic identity of cancer cells in the lung argues forcefully for a primary lung cancer.

在肺内癌细胞的细胞学鉴定有力地证明是原发性肺癌。

Therefore, the identity of a particular product can be determined surely only from the original label of the package in which it was sold or by chemical analysis.

因此,对于某一产品的特性,只有根据出售时包装上原有的标签说明,或进行化学分析,才能确定。

idiopathic [ˌidiə'pæθik] *a.* 自发的,特发的

These patients are said to have primary, essential or idiopathic hypertension.

这些患者被认为患原发性、特发性或自发性高血压病。

The leading cause of death in children with idiopathic nephrotic syndrome is infection.

特发性肾病综合征患儿死亡的首要原因是感染。

idiosyncratic [ˌidiəusiŋ'krætik] *a.* 特异反应性的

The acute psychotic episodes are regarded as individual idiosyncratic reactions to alcohol.

这些急性精神病性发作被认为是个人对酒精的特异性反应。

idiotope ['idiətəup] *n.* 独特位,独特型决定位

Idiotope is a single antigenic determinant on an antibody V region.

独特位就是抗体可变区中的单个抗原决定簇。

ignorant ['ignərənt] *a.* 无知的,愚昧的;不知道的

The patient was ignorant of the time when the first attack occurred.

病人并不知道第一次发病的时间。

No one can be a good physician who has no idea of surgical operations, and a surgeon is nothing if ignorant of medicine.

缺乏外科手术概念,不能成为好的内科医师;而不懂内科学的人则根本称不上外科医师。

ignore [ig'nɔː(r)] *v.* 不顾,忽视

Ignoring the need to investigate even a mild anemia is a serious error.

忽略对哪怕是轻微的贫血的探究也是一个严重错误。

ileitis [ˌili'aitis] *n.* 回肠炎

Backwash ileitis is most commonly a radiologic term referring to the dilated terminal ileum seen on barium contrast studies.

反流性回肠炎是一个常用的放射学术语,常指在钡剂造影时见到的已经扩张了的回肠末端。

ileocecal [iliəu'siːkəl] *a.* 回盲肠的

Ileum, in its turn, opens into the large intestine, or colon, at the ileocecal valve.

回肠又在回盲瓣处开口于大肠,即结肠。

ileocolic [ˌiliəuˈkɔlik] ,ileocolonic [ˌiliəukəˈlɔnik] *a.* 回肠结肠的

The contents of the ileum, the lowermost segment of the small intestine, are forced by peristaltic action through the ileocolic valve and into the ascending colon.

小肠最低部分(回肠)的内容物,由于肠蠕动作用而通过回肠结肠瓣,被推入到升结肠。

Unlike idiopathic ileocolic intussusception, most postoperative intussusceptions are ileoileal or jejunojejunal.

不像特发性回肠-结肠型套叠那样,多数术后肠套叠为回肠-回肠型或空肠-空肠型。

ileocolitis [ˌiliəukɔˈlaitis] *n.* 回肠结肠炎

Ileocolitis refers to Crohn disease involving both the ileum and large bowel.

回肠结肠炎是指疾病累及了回肠和大肠两者的克罗恩病。

ileostomy [ˌiliˈɔstəmi] *n.* 回肠造口术

Total colectomy with ileostomy is the elective operation performed in most centers.

在大多数医疗中心以全结肠切除和回肠造口术作为选择性手术。

ileum [ˈiliəm] *n.* 回肠

Jejunum is about seven and a half feet long and continues into the ileum.

空肠长约7.5英尺,继续延伸至回肠。

ileus [ˈiliəs] *n.* 肠梗阻

Intestinal obstruction early in the postoperative period may be the result of paralytic ileus or mechanical obstruction.

手术后早期肠梗阻可能是肠麻痹或机械性阻塞的结果。

The clinical features of hypokalemia are muscle weakness, ileus, polyuria and ECG changes.

低钾血症的临床特征为肌无力、肠梗阻、多尿和心电图变化。

iliac [ˈiliæk] *a.* 髂的,髂骨的

In the pages that follow, we will describe the methods used to define disease of the external iliac arteries.

在下文中,我们将叙述用以诊断髂外动脉疾病的方法。

In iliac abscess, particularly when psoas muscle is involved, severe pain may be referred to the hip, thigh, or knee.

髂部脓肿,特别是当腰大肌受累时,严重的疼痛可牵涉到髋部,大腿或膝部。

ill-defined [ˈildiˈfaind] *a.* 不明了的,界限不清的

The factors that are released after renal mass ablation remain ill-defined.

肾脏肿块切除后释放的因子,其情况仍然不是很明确。

From the radiologic point of view, the infiltrates in viral pneumonia tend to be diffuse, ill-defined and hazy.

从放射学的观点来看,病毒性肺炎的浸润往往是弥漫性的、界限不清和模糊的。

illegal [iˈliːgəl] *a.* 非法的,违法的

Driving faster than the speed limit is illegal.

超速驾驶是违法的。

Injection drug users are a hidden population, engaging in an illegal activity of which society disapproves.

静脉药成瘾者是躲藏在暗处的一群人,他们专门从事社会所不允许的非法活动。

illegible [iˈledʒəbəl] *a.* 无法辨读的,不清楚的

The teacher told the student that his paper was illegible.

老师对这个学生说他的论文无法辨读。

illicit [iˈlisit] *a.* 违法的,不正当的

Most current illicit drug users are multiple drug users.

目前大部分非法吸毒者使用着多种毒品。

HIV transmission occurs when infected needles are shared by people using illicit drugs.
当使用违禁药品的人共用了已污染的针头就会染上 HIV。

illness [ˈilnis] *n.* 疾病

Illness accompanying recurrent infections with a given virus are usually less severe and are more likely to involve the upper respiratory tract.
伴有某种病毒反复感染的疾病通常不严重，而且多可能累及上呼吸道。

Radiation illness is a condition resulting from exposure of the whole body to a dose of over 1 Gy of ionizing radiation.
放射病是全身暴露于超过 1 戈瑞剂量的电离辐射而发生的一种状态。

Psychosomatic illness is a disorder in which the physical symptoms are caused by psychological factors.
心身疾病是由心理因素引起身体(物理)症状的一种疾患。

illuminate [iˈljuːmineit] *v.* 照亮，照明，启发

Endoscopes are flexible, tubelike instruments used to illuminate medical problems in the dark, interior areas of the human body.
内镜是一种能弯曲的管状仪器，它可用来照亮人体内部暗处的病灶。

illumination [iˌljuːmiˈneiʃən] *n.* 照明；照亮

Examination should be conducted in a well-lighted room, and daylight is the ideal illumination.
体检应在明亮的房间里进行，而日光是最理想的。

illusion [iˈljuːʒən] *n.* 错觉，幻觉

An illusion is a misinterpretation of sensory experience.
错觉是对感官体验的错误理解。

illustrate [ˈiləstreit] *v.* 举例说明，图解

The article is illustrated by charts and diagrams.
文章附有图表说明。

Fig. 1 illustrates endometriosis occurring in the vagina.
图 1 说明在阴道出现的子宫内膜异位。

illustrative [ˈiləstreitiv] *a.* 用作说明的

The example below may be illustrative.
下面的例子可能说明问题。

The chart is illustrative of the life cycle of the round worm.
图表说明蛔虫的生活史。

image [ˈimidʒ] *n.* 影像，图像

Rays of object pass through the lens and vitreous body to form an image on the retina.
物体的光线通过晶体和玻璃体，有视网膜上形成一个图像。

Mirror image is an image with right and left relations reversed.
镜中的影像是一个左右关系完全相反的影像。

imagination [iˌmædʒiˈneiʃən] *n.* 想象；想象力

I must confess, however, that my imagination runs a bit short than I try to conceive an artificial liver.
然而我必须承认，当我力图设想一个人工肝脏时，我的想象力就有点不足了。

imagine [iˈmædʒin] *v.* 想象

The patient imagines the beam hitting the tumor cells and causing them to shrink.
病人在想象该光束正在袭击肿瘤细胞并使其缩小。

imaging [ˈimidʒiŋ] *n.* 影像，图像

Imaging is crucial to the identification of lesions of the nervous system in disease.
对于神经系统疾病的病变的鉴别，影像起决定性作用。

In the last two decades, imaging of the kidney has undergone significant changes.

在过去的二十年中，肾脏的造影技术已经有了显著的变化。

Before ordering any diagnostic imaging examination, the requesting physician must have a clear idea of the question he or she seeks to answer.

在申请任何影像学检查来协助诊断之前，医生必须对需要解决的问题本身有清楚的认识。

imbalance [im'bæləns] *n.* 不平衡，失调

Endocrine imbalances resulting from thyroid dysfunction and menopause may cause pruritus.

由甲状腺功能不良和绝经产生的内分泌失衡可引起瘙痒。

Imbalance between production and clearance may result either from excess release of bilirubin into the bloodstream or from some diseases that impair the hepatic uptake, metabolism of bilirubin.

胆红素生成和排泄之间的不平衡可以是由于过多的胆红素释放入血液中，也可以是由于某些疾病影响肝脏对胆红素的摄取和代谢。

imbed [im'bed] *v.* 将…嵌入，包埋，植入

The teeth are imbedded in special sockets of the upper and lower jaws.

牙齿被嵌在上下颚的特殊牙槽内。

After reaching the uterus, the little ball of cells becomes imbedded in the now greatly thickened uterine lining.

小卵子细胞到达子宫后，就会在现已大为增厚的子宫内膜中定居。

imidazole [ˌimi'dæzəul] *n.* 咪唑，异吡唑

Antifungal agents such as the imidazoles also have been used in the treatment of mycosis.

抗霉菌药物如咪唑类也已用于治疗霉菌病。

The imidazoles are active in vitro against many fungi.

咪唑类在体外试验中对许多霉菌有对抗作用。

imipramine [i'miprəmiːn] *n.* 丙咪嗪

Children were treated with imipramine up to a maximum of 5mg/kg/day.

儿童用药的最大剂量是每天每公斤体重 5 毫克的丙咪嗪。

imitate ['imiteit] *v.* 模仿，模拟

All these can be done without having to imitate a single living metabolic function.

这些都不必在模拟任一有生命的代谢功能条件下来完成。

immature [ˌimə'tjuə] *a.* 发育未全的，未成熟的

The metastatic tumor was composed of immature tumor cells.

转移瘤系由未成熟的肿瘤细胞组成。

If hemorrhage was massive and acute, occasional normoblasts and immature WBCs may be seen in the circulation.

如果出血量大而且是急性的，偶尔可在循环中见到幼红细胞和未成熟的白细胞。

immediate [i'miːdjət] *a.* 立即的，直接的，紧靠的

Severe trauma often brings on shock and requires immediate treatment.

严重创伤常引起休克，需要立即治疗。

A rapid response following the injection of antigen is termed immediate allergic reaction.

注射抗原后很快发生反应称之为速发性变态反应。

The immediate treatment of domestic violence is focused on treating physical injuries, and on providing emotional support.

对家庭暴力的紧急处理应着重于治疗身体的伤害和提供精神支持。

immense [i'mens] *a.* 广大的，巨大的

An ocean is an immense body of water.

海洋是一个特别巨大的水体。

immerse [i'məːs] *v.* 使沉浸于

We are immersed in a festival atmosphere.

我们沉浸在节日的气氛中。

Usually a thin piece of an organ is taken and <u>immersed</u> in a drop of the liquid part of blood(plasma). Under proper conditions the culture will show all signs of life.

通常,取一薄片器官浸泡在血液的液态部分(血浆)中。在适当的条件下,培养物会显示生命的所有特征。

immersion [iˈməːʃən] *n.* 浸入

Infection occurs during <u>immersion</u> in fresh water containing schistosome cercariae.

感染发生于人体进入带有血吸虫尾蚴的淡水中时。

immigrant [ˈimigrənt] *n.* 移民,侨民

Geographical survey should be included in the taking of the history when confronted with a sick visitor or <u>immigrant</u> to this country.

当检查来自外地或外国的病人时,应将该患者来自的地域概况列入其病史采集的内容。

T. Schoenleinii is rarely seen in the United States and usually only in <u>immigrants</u>, whereas it is predominant in the Middle East.

许兰毛癣菌在美国已少见,通常仅见于移民,但它在中东则是占优势的。

imminent [ˈiminənt] *a.* 急迫的,危急的

When the head no longer recedes between contractions, this indicates that it has passed through the pelvic floor and that delivery is <u>imminent</u>.

当胎头在宫缩间隔期不再回缩时,表明胎头已通过盆底并即将娩出。

immobile [iˈməubail] *a.* 不能活动的

Fungi are <u>immobile</u> but lack other plant like traits.

真菌不能活动,但又缺乏其他植物似的特征。

immobility [ˌiməuˈbiliti] *n.* 不动,固定

The main causes of <u>immobility</u> are weakness, stiffness, pain, imbalance, and psychological problems.

不能动的主要原因有身体虚弱、强直、疼痛、不平衡和心理问题。

Deep venous thrombosis and pulmonary embolism due to <u>immobility</u> remain significant causes of death in hospitalized patients.

由于长期卧床不动引起的深静脉血栓形成和肺栓塞是住院病人死亡的重要原因。

immobilization [iˌməubilaiˈzeiʃən] *n.* 不动,固定

Prolonged <u>immobilization</u> of elderly patients may have many harmful effects.

老年患者长期的卧床不动可能产生许多有害影响。

immortal [iˈmɔːtəl] *a.* 不朽的,永生的,不死的,不灭的

The resulting hybridoma cell is <u>immortal</u> and synthesizes homogeneous, specific antibodies.

产生的杂交瘤细胞是永生化的,并可合成均一性、特异性抗体。

immune [iˈmjuːn] *a.* 免疫的,有免疫力的

Equally important to this subject are the various cells that constitute the <u>immune</u> system.

构成免疫系统的各种细胞在此学科中也同样重要。

The lymphocytes participating in the <u>immune</u> response have antigen-specific receptors on their surface membrane.

参与免疫反应的淋巴细胞在它们的表面膜上有抗原特异受体。

immunity [iˈmjuːniti] *n.* 免疫(力)

Recurrent hepatitis is extremely rare and <u>immunity</u> probably lifelong.

肝炎复发十分少见,免疫可能是终身的。

Natural <u>immunity</u> is that with which an individual is born.

先天免疫是一个人生来就有的免疫。

immunization [ˌimjunaiˈzeiʃən] *n.* 免疫法

Primary tuberculosis is seldom seen because of a high level of <u>immunization</u>.

因为高水平的免疫措施,原发性结核病已很少见。

Active immunization has been found to be effective in preventing or modifying the severity of infection.

人们已发现自动免疫能有效地预防感染或减轻感染的严重程度。

immunize [ˈimjunaiz] *v.* 使免疫

One attack of scarlet fever will immunize the patient against it for life.

猩红热发病一次即可使病人对它终身免疫。

The babies immunized with vaccine before birth produce more antibodies than the other babies.

出生前用疫苗免疫过的婴儿比一般婴儿能产生更多的抗体。

immunoabsorbent [ˌimjunəuæbˈsɔːbənt] *n.* 免疫吸附

The presence of Ab to a particular Ag in the serum of a patient can be determined using enzyme-linked immunoabsorbent assays(ELISA).

患者血清中针对某一特定抗原的抗体的存在可用酶联免疫吸附法进行测定。

immunoadsorption [ˌimjunəuædˈsɔːpʃən] *n.* 免疫吸附

Immunoadsorption is of particular value because the adsorbed material can be recovered from the complex by careful treatments.

免疫吸附有特殊的意义,因为经过细致的处理后已经被吸附的物质又能从复合物中复原。

immunoassay [ˌimjunəuˈæsei] *n.* 免疫测定

This can be done by a number of methods including enzyme immunoassay.

这可用多种方法包括酶免疫测定来检查。

Enzyme-linked immunoassays are sensitive and specific,and will become generally available.

酶联免疫试验是灵敏的,且具有特异性,将被广泛使用。

immunobiology [ˌimjunəubaiˈɔlədʒi] *n.* 免疫生物学

Immunobiology is the study of the biological basis for host defense against infection.

免疫生物学研究的是宿主防御感染的生物学基础。

The results give new insight into the immunobiology of IL-10 and suggest that the IL-10 may become a therapeutic agent.

这些结果使我们对 IL-10 的免疫生物学有了新的认识,并提出 IL-10 可以成为一种治疗药物。

immunoblotting [ˈimjunəuˌblɔtiŋ] *n.* 免疫印迹

Immunoblotting is used to assay for the presence of molecules in a mixture.

免疫印迹可用于测定某种混合物中分子的存在。

The results of immunoblotting and double immunofluorescence showed that partial induced cells expressed CK and S-100 simultaneously.

免疫印迹法和双重免疫荧光标记的结果显示部分诱导细胞同时表达 CK 与 S-100。

immunocompetence [ˌimjunəuˈkɔmpitəns] *n.* 免疫活性,免疫全能

Its mechanism is probably related to the enhancement of immunocompetence, anti-inflammation and improvement of local microcirculation.

推测其机制可能与提高机体免疫活性、抗菌消炎和改善局部微循环有关。

Immunocompetence is a common conception in biomedical and animal sciences,and refers to the ability of organisms against diseases.

免疫全能是生物医学和动物科学的一个常见的概念,意指机体对疾病的抵抗能力。

immunocompetent [ˌimjunəuˈkɔmpitənt] *a.* 免疫全能的,免疫活性的

Being immunocompetent refers to being in a normal state of body immunity.

免疫全能指机体免疫功能处于正常状态。

Immunocompetent state is the ability of the body to produce a normal immune response following exposure to an antigen.

免疫全能状态是指机体接触抗原后产生正常的免疫应答的能力。

immunocomplex [iˌmjuːnəuˈkɔmpleks] *n.* 免疫复合物

The deposition of immunocomplexes in tissues such as blood vessel walls may directly cause inflammation and tissue damage.

免疫复合物在血管壁等组织的沉积可直接导致炎症和组织损伤。

immunocompromised [ˌimjunəuˈkɔmprəmaizd] *a.* 免疫受损的，免疫力低下［削弱］的，免疫功能不全的

Immunocompromised state of a body may lead to many opportunistic infections.

机体在免疫低下的情况下可受到许多机会感染。

CMV is usually seen in immunocompromised hosts and can be widespread in many organs.

巨细胞病毒通常在免疫缺陷宿主中可见，并能在多个器官中扩散。

immunocytochemistry [ˌimjunəu, saitəuˈkemistri] *n.* 免疫细胞化学

NF-κB was analyzed using immunocytochemistry.

用免疫细胞化学方法分析了 NF-κB。

The current protocols for blocking background staining in immunohistochemistry are reported.

阻断免疫细胞化学中背景着色的实验指南已有报道。

immunodeficiency [iˌmjuːnəudiˈfiʃənsi] *n.* 免疫缺陷

AIDS is caused by infection with the human immunodeficiency virus (HIV).

艾滋病是由人类免疫缺陷病毒(HIV)感染引起。

The primary diagnostic features of the immunodeficiency include hypogammaglobulinemia and impaired functional antibody.

这种免疫缺陷的基本诊断特征包括丙种球蛋白减少和抗体功能受损。

immunodominant [ˌimjunəuˈdɔminənt] *adj.* 免疫优性的，免疫显性的。

Immunodominant epitopes are those epitopes in an antigen that are preferentially recognized by T cells.

免疫显性表位就是指抗原中那些优先被 T 细胞识别的表位。

immunoediting [ˌimjunəuˈeditiŋ] *n.* 免疫编辑

In this review, we discuss the roles of the IFNs, not only in cancer immunosurveillance but also in the broader process of cancer immunoediting.

在这篇综述中，我们不仅讨论了 IFNs 在肿瘤免疫监视中的作用，而且讨论了 IFNs 在更为广泛的肿瘤免疫编辑过程中的作用。

immunoelectron [ˌimjunəuiˈlektrɔn] *n.* 免疫电子

Specific antibodies can be used to reveal ultramicroscopic structures in cells by the technique of immunoelectron microscopy.

借助免疫电子显微镜，特异性抗体可以用来揭示细胞内超微结构。

The prospects of colloidal gold immunoelectron microscopy technique were discussed in this paper.

本文讨论了胶体金免疫电镜技术的前景。

immunoelectrophoresis [ˌimjuːnəuilektrəufəˈriːsis] *n.* 免疫电泳

In immunoelectrophoresis, Ags are placed in a well cut in a gel and electrophoresed.

在免疫电泳中，抗原被放入凝胶内的孔中并电泳。

immunoenhancement [ˌimjunəuinˈhaːnsmənt] *n.* 免疫增强(法)

The immunoenhancement induced by 25mg/kg LBP3a is more effective than that induced by a 12.5 and 50mg/kg.

25mg/kg LBP3a 诱导的免疫增强作用比 12.5 和 50mg/kg 诱导的更有效。

Increased heterophil count during hibernation provided the only support for winter immunoenhancement.

冬眠期间异嗜白细胞计数的增加为冬季免疫增强提供了唯一的支撑。

immunoevasin [ˌimjunəuiˈveisin] *n.* 免疫逃逸素

Immunoevasins are proteins expressed by some viruses that enable the virus to evade immune recognition by preventing the appearance of peptide:MHC I complexes on the infected cell.
免疫逃逸素是某些病毒表达的蛋白质，通过阻止肽-MHC I 复合物出现在被感染细胞而能够使病毒逃逸免疫识别。

immunofluorescence [ˌimjunəuˌfluəˈresəns] *n.* 免疫荧光（法）
The immunofluorescence tests can be used to identify particular cells in suspension.
免疫荧光技术可用于鉴定特定的悬浮细胞。
The proportion of circulating T cells in the mononuclear cell fraction can be determined by immunofluorescence with CD2 or CD3 monoclonal antibodies.
循环的 T 细胞在单核细胞组分中所占的比例可用单克隆抗体 CD2 或 CD3 的免疫荧光法进行测定。

immunofluorescent [ˌimjunəufluəˈresnt] *a.* 免疫荧光的
Granular immunofluorescent deposits of IgG are seen along the glomerular basement membrane.
在肾小球的基底膜上可以看到有颗粒状的具有免疫荧光的 IgG 沉积。

immunogen [iˈmjuːnədʒin] *n.* 免疫原
An immunogen is a substance that is able to provoke an adaptive immune response.
免疫原是一种能刺激产生适应性免疫应答的物质。
All immunogens are antigens, but not all antigens are immunogens.
所有免疫原都是抗原，但并非所有抗原都是免疫原。
An immunogen is any molecule that can elicit an adaptive immune response on injection into a person or animal.
任何一种分子当其注射到人或者动物体内能激发适应性免疫反应时即被称为免疫原。

immunogenetics [iˌmjuːnəudʒiˈnetiks] *n.* 免疫遗传学
The study of their involement in the mechanisms of the normal and autoimmune response is termed immunogenetics.
对于涉及那些与正常的和自身免疫应答机制有关的研究的科学称为免疫遗传学。

immunogenic [ˌimjunəuˈdʒenik] *a.* 免疫源的，致免疫的
Parasites express many antigens which are usually immunogenic.
寄生虫表达的许多抗原通常是免疫源。
Most tumor associated antigens are either absent or weakly immunogenic through being expressed at low levels.
许多肿瘤相关抗原或者是缺失的或者是通过低水平的表达而为弱免疫源性。

immunogenicity [ˌimjunəudʒeˈnisiti] *n.* 免疫源性
Skin has defied successful transplantation because of its high immunogenicity.
皮肤由于具有高度免疫源性常使其移植不能成功。
This significantly decreases but does not eliminate the immunogenicity of the antibody.
这可显著减小但并不能消除抗体的免疫源性。

immunoglobulin [ˌimjunəuˈglɔbjulin] *n.* 免疫球蛋白
The blood count may show nonspecific eosinophilia; immunoglobulin M may be elevated.
血象可能显示非特异性嗜酸粒细胞增多，免疫球蛋白 M 也可能增高。
These neoplastic cells produce only one type of immunoglobulin molecule.
这些肿瘤细胞仅产生一种类型的免疫球蛋白分子。

immunohistochemistry [ˌimjunəu,histəuˈkemistri] *n.* 免疫组织化学法
Immunohistochemistry is widely used in the routine diagnosis of surgical pathology.
免疫组织化学法广泛应用于外科病理学的常规诊断中。
Immunohistochemistry is helpful for determining the origin of a tumor.
免疫组织化学法有助于确定肿瘤的来源。

immunolabel [ˌimju:neuˈleibl] *n.*, *v.* 免疫标记

In sham-operated rats, nNOS immunolabelling was strongly localized in Leydig cells (Fig. 2a).

在假手术大鼠，nNOS 免疫标记强烈定位于睾丸间质细胞（见图 2a）。

immunology [imju'nɔlədʒi] *n.* 免疫学

Edward Jenner's vaccination laid the basis for modern immunology.

爱德华·詹纳尔的种痘法为现代免疫学奠定了基础。

Modern immunology would not be what it is today without the contribution of transplantation research.

如果没有移植研究所做的贡献，现代免疫学将不是今天这个情况。

immunomodulator [ˌimjunəu'mɔdjuleitə] *n.* 免疫调节剂

The immunomodulator, FTY720, has been shown to be beneficial in experimental models of organ transplantation and autoimmunity.

免疫调节剂 FTY720 已经在器官移植和自体免疫实验模型中显示出了它的益处。

An immunomodulator is a substance which has an effect on the immune system. There are two types of effects - immunostimulation and immunosuppression.

免疫调节剂是对免疫系统有影响的物质，它有两类效应——免疫刺激和免疫抑制。

immunopathology [imjunəpə'θɔlədʒi] *n.* 免疫病理（学）

Emphasis is placed on diagnosis, pathogenesis, immunopathology and other areas.

重点放在诊断、发病机制、免疫病理及其他领域中。

immunophilin [ˌimjunəu'filin] *n.* 抑免蛋白，免疫亲和素，亲免蛋白，亲免素

Immunophilins are proteins in T cells that are bound by the immunosuppressive drugs cyclosporine A, tacrolimus, and rapamycin.

抑免蛋白是 T 细胞中能被免疫抑制药物环孢素 A、他克莫司和雷帕霉素结合的蛋白。

Two distinct signal transmission pathways in T lymphocytes are inhibited by complexes formed between an immunophilin and either FK506 or rapamycin.

T 淋巴细胞中两个截然不同的信号传导途径被抑免蛋白与 FK506 或与雷帕霉素结合形成的复合物所抑制。

immunoprecipitation [ˌimjunəupriˌsipi'teiʃən] *n.* 免疫沉淀反应

The tyrosine phosphorylation of leptin receptor was revealed by immunoprecipitation.

用免疫沉淀法显示了瘦素受体的酪氨酸磷酸化。

immunoprophylaxis [ˌimjunəuˌprɔfi'læksis] *n.* 免疫预防（法）

Immunoprophylaxis is the use of vaccine, toxoids, and immune serum to protect susceptible people against specific diseases.

免疫预防是用疫苗、类毒素及免疫血清来保护易感人群抵抗某些特殊疾病。

immunoproteasome [ˌimjunəu'prəutiːsəum] *n.* 免疫蛋白酶体

The immunoproteasome is a form of proteasome found in cells exposed to interferons and contains three different subunits compared with the normal proteasome.

免疫蛋白酶体是暴露于干扰素的细胞中的一种蛋白酶，与普通的蛋白酶比较含有三个不同的亚基。

immunoradiometric [ˌimjunəuˌreidiə'metrik] *a.* 免疫放射分析法的

Immunoradiometric assay is a method for measuring certain plasma proteins by using radiolabeled antibodies.

免疫放射分析法是一种通过使用放射性标记抗体来测定某些血浆蛋白的方法。

Immunoradiometric assay has been used in a variety of situations to measure and characterize peptides of the hypothalamic pituitary adrenal axis.

免疫放射分析技术已被用于测定不同条件下肽的浓度，并描述其在下丘脑-垂体-肾上腺轴中的特性。

immunoreactive [ˌimjunəuri'æktiv] *a.* 免疫反应的

The Dutch screening programme consists of two biochemical measurements of immunoreactive trypsinogen .
荷兰人的筛选计划中包含了 2 个有免疫反应的胰蛋白酶原的生化方法。
Immunoreactive trypsinogen is a biomarker for cystic fibrosis.
有免疫反应的胰蛋白酶原是囊性纤维症的生物标记。

immunoregulation [ˌimjunəuˌregjuˈleiʃən] *n.* 免疫调节,免疫控制作用
The immunoregulation effect of the astragalus was various.
黄芪的免疫调节作用是多方面的。
Selective immunoregulation may be a new approach to the treatment of immune diseases.
选择性免疫调控可能是治疗免疫性疾病的一种新方法。

immunoselection [ˌimjunəuˌsiˈlekʃən] *n.* 免疫选择
Tumor cells avoid immunosurveillance through immunoselection.
肿瘤细胞通过免疫选择逃避机体的免疫监视。

immunostimulation [ˌimjunəuˌstimjuˈleiʃən] *n.* 免疫刺激
Stimulation of an immune response is known as immunostimulation.
激发免疫反应的刺激被称为免疫刺激。
The results suggested the role of CpG motifs in immunostimulation and gene therapy.
结果表明了 CpG 基序在免疫刺激和基因治疗中的作用。

immunosuppressant [ˌimjuːnəusəˈpresənt] *a.* 抑制免疫的
Antineoplastic agents may be teratogenic, carcinogenic, and immunosuppressant.
抗肿瘤药可能致畸、致癌和抑制免疫。
n. 免疫抑制剂
Azathioprine is an effective immunosuppressant in the early phases of immune responses.
在免疫反应早期,硫唑嘌呤是一种有效的免疫抑制剂。

immunosuppression [iˌmjuːnəsəˈpreʃən] *n.* 免疫抑制
The discovery of the universal method for specific immunosuppression is very important for transplantation.
特异免疫抑制通用方法的发现对于移植术是非常重要的。
Generalized and prolonged immunosuppression increases susceptibility to infection.
全身性和持续性的免疫抑制可增加机体对感染的敏感性。

immunosuppressive [ˌimjuːnəusəˈpresiv] *a.* 抑制免疫的
Immunosuppressive agents are used in autoimmune diseases.
免疫抑制剂可用于治疗自身免疫性疾病。
n. 免疫抑制剂
Immunosuppressive is a drug used to counteract the response of the immune system to reject a transplanted organ.
免疫抑制剂可用来对抗(中和)免疫系统排斥被移植器官的反应。

immunotherapy [ˌimjuːnəuˈθerəpi] *n.* 免疫疗法
Scientists are devoting more attention to immunotherapy today.
今日科学家们对免疫疗法正在投入更多关注。
Not until such tests are available will it be possible to perform immunotherapy as a safe clinical procedure.
直到这种试验行之有效时,把免疫疗法作为安全的临床方法应用才是可能的。

immunotolerance [ˌimjunəuˈtɔlərəns] *n.* 免疫耐受性
Induction of immunotolerance can also be achieved in adult animals.
免疫耐受性也可以在成年动物身上诱发成功。

immunotoxicology [ˌimjunəutɔksiˈkɔlədʒi] *n.* 免疫毒理学
Immunotoxicology is the study of immune dysfunction resulting from exposure of an organism to a

xenobiotic.

免疫毒理学是研究生物体暴露于有害异物所致的免疫异常。

Therefore, developmental immunotoxicology assessment should address the possibility that environmentally induced changes in immune response balance may occur.

因此,发育免疫毒理学评估应该注意环境因素导致免疫应答平衡发生改变的可能性。

immunotoxin [ˌimjunəu'tɔksin] *n.* 免疫毒素

Immunotoxin is a novel class of targeted agents in recent years.

免疫毒素是近年来新兴的一种特异性靶向治疗药物。

The development situation and application prospect of immunotoxin therapy in oral diseases are reviewed in this paper.

本文综述了免疫毒素在口腔相关疾病治疗中的研究进展和应用前景。

Immunotoxins are antibodies that are chemically coupled to toxic proteins usually derived from plants or microbes.

免疫毒素是与毒性蛋白化学偶联的抗体,这些毒性蛋白通常源自植物或微生物。

impact ['impækt] *n.* 冲击(力),碰撞

Small blood vessels are easily damaged by a blunt impact.

小血管容易由于钝的冲击力而受到损伤。

impacted [im'pæktid] *a.* 嵌入的,嵌塞的;(牙)阻生的

The impacted material is called an embolus.

阻塞的物质称为栓子。

If there be an impacted stone in the cystic duct, it may be distended to a paper thinness.

如果胆囊管有胆石阻塞,胆囊壁可能膨胀得像一张纸那样薄。

Impacted fractures are those in which the broken ends of the bone are driven into each other.

嵌入骨折是骨骼的断端互相挤压穿插在一起。

impaction [im'pækʃən] *n.* 嵌塞,栓塞

By embolism is meant the transference of abnormal material by the bloodstream and its impaction in a vessel.

栓塞是指异常的物质被血流转运并阻塞血管的过程。

impair [im'pεə] *v.* 削弱;损伤

Deficiency of these substances presumably impairs nucleic acid synthesis.

这些物质的缺乏可能削弱核酸的合成。

Many drugs used in the treatment of cancer impair DNA replication.

许多用于治疗癌症的药物损伤 DNA 的复制。

impairment [im'pεəmənt] *n.* 削弱,损伤

Impairment of blood flow by pressure on the calves appears to be an important predisposing factor.

由于小腿压迫所致的血流障碍似乎是一个重要的诱发因素。

Significant impairment of more than one organ system profoundly influences operative risk.

一个以上器官系统的重大损害会对手术的危险性产生深远的影响。

Impairment is defined as any loss or abnormality of psychological, physiological, or anatomical structure or function.

损伤的定义是心理、生理或解剖的结构或功能的丧失或异常。

impart [im'pɑːt] *v.* 把…分给,给予

Certain drugs may impart a beechnut or orange color to the urine.

某些药物可使尿液呈山毛榉坚果色或橘黄色。

The disease is imparted to human beings by the bite of rat flea.

本病通过鼠蚤的叮咬传染给人。

impede [im'piːd] *v.* 阻碍,妨碍

The platelet mass can grow to sufficient size to impede blood flow without being dislodged.
血小板团块可增大到足以阻碍血液流动而又不能被挪动。
One of his coronary arterials was 37 percent blocked, seriously impeding the blood flow to his heart.
他有一根冠状动脉的37%已被堵塞,从而严重地阻碍着血流进入心脏。

impend [im'pend] *v.* 逼近,即将发生
No early impressions of impending disaster showed up till the close of the operation.
直到手术结束,没有出现过灾难即将来临的早期征象。

imperative [im'perətiv] *a.* 绝对必要的,强制的
Early identification and diagnosis for this disease are imperative.
此病的早期识别和诊断是很必要的。
Rest should be imperative if the temperature rises above 38℃.
如果体温高于38℃,就应强制休息。

imperceptible [impə'septəbl] *a.* 感觉不到的,难以察觉的
There is an imperceptible transition from acute inflammatory reaction to the melting away of the angry signs.
从炎症的急性反应到肿痛发炎症状的消失有一个难以察觉的转变过程。
The bone scan may show lesions that are imperceptible by the usual skeleton survey.
骨扫描可显示通常骨骼检查方法难以识别的损害。

imperfect [im'pəːfikt] *a.* 不完美的,有缺陷的
Some people are born with imperfect blood clotting mechanism.
有些人从出生起凝血机制就不完善。

imperforate [im'pəːfəreit] *a.* 无孔的,闭锁的;无齿孔的
This time also is the best time to find and treat the imperforate hymen.
这时也是发现并治疗处女膜闭锁的最好时机!
Imperforate anus is perhaps not the best description of the anorectal malformations under discussion.
肛门闭锁一词对于讨论肛门直肠畸形并不太确切。

impetigo [ˌimpi'taigəu] *n.* 脓疱病
The skin rash is compatible with impetigo which responds quickly to intramuscular penicillin.
皮肤的皮疹与脓疱疮一样,对青霉素肌肉注射反应迅速。

impinge [im'pindʒ] *v.* 冲击,撞击
When the waves impinge on the tympanic membrane, it vibrates with the waves.
当声波冲击到鼓膜时,鼓膜随声波振动。
Until tumors are large enough to impinge on preexisting nerves, pain does not result.
只是在肿瘤长大到足以压迫原有组织的神经时,才会产生疼痛。

implant [im'plɑːnt] *v.* 嵌入,植入,移植
The development of contact lenses and permanently implanted artificial lenses has opened a new world of sight.
隐形眼镜和永久性植入的人工晶体的产生为他们开创了一个视力新世界。
n. 植入物
The reasons for the tidal wave move to intraocular lens implants are clear.
人工晶体植入潮的(出现)原因是显而易见的。

implantable [im'plɑːntəbl] *a.* 可移植的
The implantable lenses can be designed to correct previous problems, such as nearsightedness.
植入的人工晶体可以设计用来矫正以前的视力问题,如近视。

implantation [implɑːn'teiʃən] *n.* 植入,移植
Many new patients will require an artificial pacemaker implantation annually.

每年许多新病人需要植入人工起搏器。

Patients with liver cancer can now benefit from the implantation of a device that dispenses 5-fluorouracil directly to the organ.

肝癌患者现在能受益于一种植入体内的装置，该装置可将 5-氟尿嘧啶直接送到器官(肝脏)。

implement [ˈimplimənt] *v.* 贯彻，履行

Although medicinal iron is cheap, its use may be culturally unacceptable or difficult to implement.

尽管药用铁剂价格便宜，但其使用可能因文化背景原因不能接受或难于实施。

implicate [ˈimplikeit] *v.* 使…牵连，与…有关

Vitamin A has also been implicated in protein synthesis.

维生素 A 还参与蛋白质的合成。

Lifestyle factors had long been implicated in the incidence of heart disease.

长期以来人们意识到心脏病的发病率与生活方式因素有关。

implication [ˌimpliˈkeiʃən] *n.* 暗示，含义

The present results have important implications for the treatment of the sensory, motor, and cognitive declines that accompany old age.

本研究结果对治疗伴随老年而来的感觉、运动和认知的衰退具有重要意义。

Words, especially medical terms, inevitably carry different implications for different people.

说话中的词语，特别是医学术语，不可避免地对不同的人具有不同的含义。

The patient needs considerable reassurance about symptoms and their implications.

应该尽可能使病人对症状及其后果消除疑虑。

implicit [imˈplisit] *a.* 隐含的

There is an implicit requirement from the perspective of promoting public health: any individual who believes a serious risk may be associated with exposure to a medical product should be encouraged to report this AE directly to FDA.

从促进公众健康的角度出发，一个隐含的要求是：任何个人若认为某个严重风险与暴露于一种医疗产品有关，应被鼓励向 FDA 直接报告这一不良事件。

imply [imˈplai] *v.* 含有…的意见，暗示

Obesity implies more than twenty percent excess above ideal body weight.

肥胖这一术语的含义是超过理想体重的百分之二十。

Negative results of the serological tests do not necessarily imply that this organism is not responsible for the disease.

血清学试验阴性结果未必就能说明这种微生物与疾病无关。

impose(on) [imˈpəuz] *v.* 强加

We must not impose our views on others.

我们不能把自己的观点强加于人。

An abnormal load is imposed on the heart in this situation.

此时，异常的负担加在心脏上。

impotence [ˈimpətəns] *n.* 阳痿

Impotence and loss of micturition control are serious complications of this operation.

阳痿和排尿失禁是该手术两个严重的并发症。

Impotence is rarely of endocrine origin. More frequently it accompanies a neurologic or emotional disorder.

阳痿很少是内分泌起因，而常常是由神经性或情绪上的紊乱所致。

impotent [ˈimpətənt] *a.* 阳痿的

An impotent man may be very fertile, because his testes produce many spermatozoa.

一个阳痿患者很可能能生育，因为他的睾丸仍能产生许多精子。

impractical [im'præktikəl] *a.* 不切实际的

This technique is impractical except for research purposes.

这技术除了为研究目的外是不实际的。

impression [im'preʃən] *n.* 印象;(牙)印模

His healing art made a lasting impression on me.

他的医术给我留下了持久的印象。

A soft impression material is placed over the teeth or jaw and sets within several minites. After removal from the mouth a plaster model is made.

将一种软的印模材料覆盖于牙齿或颌骨上数分钟后,再从口腔中取下,即制成石膏模型。

imprinting [im'printiŋ] *n.* 印记,印迹

Imprinting reflects a functional change in a gene.

印迹反映了基因内的功能性变化。

Imprinting affects only a minority of genes.

印迹只影响少部分基因。

More striking evidence for genetic imprinting comes from studies on early mouse embryos.

遗传印记更有力的证据来自于对小鼠早期胚胎的研究。

improper [im'prɔpə] *a.* 不适当的

Acute inflammation of the stomach may be brought on by improper eating habits.

不良的饮食习惯可引起急性胃炎。

impulse ['impʌls] *n.* 冲动;搏动

Acetylcholine is known to transmit nerve impulses.

已知乙酰胆碱可传导神经冲动。

The heart revealed the apical impulse to be in the fifth left intercostal space just outside the mid-clavicular line.

心脏检查显示心尖搏动在锁骨中线外左侧第五肋间。

impulsiveness [im'pʌlsivnis] *n.* 冲动,冲击

Impulsiveness, marked mood fluctuations and aggressiveness are also common symptoms.

冲动性、显著的情绪波动和攻击性行为也是常见的症状。

impulsivity [impʌl'siviti] *n.* 冲动,冲动性,易冲动

The researchers found that different kinds of impulsivity correlated with working memory.

研究人员发现,不同的冲动与工作记忆有关。

Inherited traits, such as impulsivity, can make a person more or less willing to have sex at an earlier age.

遗传特质,例如冲动性,会或多或少影响一个人是否会在较小的年龄时就发生性行为。

impurity [im'pjuəriti] *n.* 不纯,杂质

The fine hairs of the nostrils form a sieve, by means of which the air is cleared of its coarser impurities.

鼻孔的纤毛形成一个筛子,空气里所含较粗糙的杂质通过它时被清除掉。

Some impurities are carried away through the skin by the sweat.

汗水通过皮肤运走某些废物。

imputation [ˌimpjuː'teiʃən] *n.* 插补,归责

The development history of the laws for the tort act in medical field is somewhat the evolution history of imputation principle.

在医学领域,侵权行为法的发展历史,在一定意义上是归责原则的演进史。

inability [ˌinə'biliti] *n.* 无能,不能

Inability to catabolize other amino acids has been documented in a few cases.

已经在几个病例中记录了不能分解其他氨基酸的情况。

Acute renal failure implies the sudden inability of the kidney to perform any of its functions.

急性肾衰竭的含义是肾功能突然衰竭。

inactivate [in'æktiveit] *v.* 灭活，使不活动

Conventional inactivated vaccines and live attenuated vaccines have received most attention.

传统的灭活疫苗和减弱的活疫苗已受到普遍注意。

Prostaglandins are inactivated rapidly in the pulmonary, hepatic, and renal vascular beds.

前列腺素在肺、肝和肾的血管床迅速失活。

inactivation [inˌækti'veiʃən] *n.* 灭活，失活

Lung is involved in activation as well as inactivation of numerous physiologic and pharmacologic substances.

肺与许多生理和药理物质的激活和失活有关。

inactive [in'æktiv] *a.* 不活跃的，非活动性的

Exacerbations are liable to occur even when the rheumatic heart disease has become chronic and almost inactive.

即使风湿性心脏病变成慢性或几乎已停止了活动，病情仍可能恶化。

An inactive histologic appearance is no guarantee against recurrence.

不活动性的组织学表现，不足以成为不复发的保证。

inactivity [ˌinæk'tiviti] *n.* 不活动，静止

Constipation due to inactivity and unawareness of rectal distension leads to faecal impaction.

由于不活动和感觉不到便意引起的便秘导致粪便阻塞。

inadequacy [in'ædikwəsi] *n.* 不充足，不适当

General practice cannot escape its share of blame for these inadequacies.

对于这些不足之处，综合医疗（指非专科医疗）不能推卸它的责任。

inadequate [in'ædikwit] *a.* 不充足的

This food is inadequate in protein, vitamins and minerals.

此食物的蛋白质、维生素和矿物质含量均不足。

The inadequate supply of donor organ/tissues has led to consideration of animals as donors.

供者器官/组织来源不足导致人们考虑以动物作为供者。

inadvertent [ˌinəd'vəːtənt] *a.* 非故意的

When the registry sites report AEs directly to FDA, this process can risk inadvertent duplication of information for adverse drug events recorded both by the registry and the company.

当登记点直接向 FDA 报告不良事件时，这个处理方式可能面临着登记处和公司无意中重复记录药物不良事件的风险。

inanimate [in'ænimit] *a.* 无生命的

The term generally applies to preparations, usually liquids, intended for use on inanimate objects.

这个术语一般用于制剂，通常为液体，旨在用于无生命的物体。

inapparent [inə'pærənt] *a.* 隐性的，不显性的；不明显的

Active immunity can be acquired naturally by an attack of the infective disease, or by an inapparent infection, or it may be acquired artificially by innoculation with vaccines.

主动免疫可通过传染性疾病或不明显的感染而自然地获得，或者通过疫苗的接种而人工获得。

inappropriate [ˌinə'prəupriət] *a.* 不适当的

Spinal anesthesia is inappropriate for thyroidectomy.

脊髓麻醉不适用于甲状腺切除术。

inattention [ˌinə'tenʃən] *n.* 不注意，疏忽，粗心

The errors that people naturally make are often errors of inattention.

人们常犯的错误往往是因为粗心造成。

Inattention is a core symptom of ADHD.

注意力不集中是注意力缺陷多动障碍（ADHD）的一个核心症状。

inborn [ˈinbɔːn] *a.* 先天的，生来的

Inherited immunity is also called inborn immunity.

遗传免疫也称先天免疫。

inbred [inˈbred] *a.* 近交的，近亲繁殖的

An advantage of dietary control is that this enhances the reproducibility that was the basis for using inbred strains(or their hybrids) in the first place.

膳食限制的一个优点是可增强繁殖力，这就是首先使用近交株（或其杂种）的基础。

incapable [inˈkeipəbl] *a.* 不能的

The center by itself is incapable of mediating the act of vomiting.

此中枢本身不能产生呕吐的动作。

Patients are easily confused, disoriented, and incapable of recalling new information.

病人易出现意识模糊，定向力障碍以及不能回忆起新发生的事。

incapacitate [inkəˈpæsiteit] *v.* （使）无能力，（使）残疾

Traditional treatment is very slow, with many patients incapacitated for months.

传统治疗方法缓慢，使很多病人长达数月不能行动。

incapacitation [ˌinkəpæsiˈteiʃən] *n.* 无能力

The incapacitation of the microbe thus effected may or may not jeopardize its survival as a species.

使微生物丧失能力的这种作用，可能危及也可能不危及其作为物种的生存。

incentive [inˈsentiv] *n.* 刺激；动机

Factors that motivate participation include the importance, or scientific credibility of the patient registry, as well as the risks and burdens of participation and any incentives for participation.

激励参与的因素包括患者登记的重要性或科学可信性，以及参与的风险和负担和任何参与的动机。

a. 激励的

China Medicine Corporation adopts new incentive compensation plans.

中国医药公司采用新的激励补偿计划。

inception [inˈsepʃən] *n.* 开始

The patient is usually able to describe the onset of pain as being gradual or sudden at the inception.

患者通常能够描述疼痛发作的开始是逐渐的还是突然的。

incessant [inˈsesnt] *a.* 不断的，连续的

The incessant noise from the factory disturbed our attempts to fall asleep.

工厂一刻不停地传来噪音扰得我们无法入睡。

incessantly [inˈsesntli] *ad.* 不停地

This patient poured out his fears and feelings incessantly.

病人不停地倾诉他的恐惧和感受。

incidence [ˈinsidəns] *n.* 发生率，发病率

Small hematomas may resorb, but they increase the incidence of wound infection.

小的血肿可被再次吸收，但却增加了伤口的感染率。

This age group showed an incidence of 3.1 cases of peptic ulcer per 1000.

在这个年龄组中消化性溃疡的发病率为 3.1‰。

incident [ˈinsidənt] *n.* 事件，事故

He says the incident had soured the atmosphere of meeting.

他表示这一事件破坏了会谈的氛围。

The Yucheng rice oil poisoning incident in central Taiwan was one of the two known major human PCB intoxication episodes.

在台湾中部城市玉成发生的米糠油中毒事件是两个已知人类 PCB 中毒事件之一。

incident(**to**) [ˈinsidənt] *a.* 伴随而来的

Many people have been x-rayed incident to mass screening surveys for pulmonary disease.

许多人进行了配合群众性肺病普查的 X 线透视。

incidental [ˌinsiˈdentəl] *a.* 附带发生的，易发生的

Those undergoing cholecystectomy for trauma or cholecystectomy incidental to other procedures were excluded.

那些因外伤或其他手术而附带做胆囊切除术的病例不包括在内。

incineration [insinəˈreiʃən] *n.* 焚化，焚烧，火葬

Incineration is used for the destruction of carcasses.

火葬用于消除尸体。

Emissions from hazardous waste incineration include polychlorinated dioxins and furans, two of the most potentially toxic chemicals that are extremely persistent in the environment.

有害废物灰烬发散物含有聚氯二英和氧杂茂，这是两种最有潜在毒性的化学物质，在一段很长时期内存在于环境中。

incipient [inˈsipiənt] *a.* 初发的，初期的

The typical incipient chancre is a small red papule or a crusted superficial erosion.

下疳开始时的典型症状是一个红色小丘疹或带痂的表浅糜烂。

incise [inˈsaiz] *v.* 切，切开

An incised wound is one produced by pressure and friction against the tissue by an object having a sharp edge.

切伤是具有锐利边缘物体对组织的压力和摩擦而引起的一种创伤。

incision [inˈsiʒən] *n.* 切口，切开

The fetus is removed by means of an incision into uterus, usually by way of abdominal wall.

常通过腹壁，用切开子宫的方法将胎儿取出。

The length of the incision made should be sufficient to allow both hands in.

切口的长度要足以能容纳双手。

incisional [inˈsiʒənəl] *a.* 切口的，切开的

Incisional and ventral hernias comprise about 20%.

切口疝和腹壁疝约占 20%。

incite [inˈsait] *v.* 刺激，引起，诱发

Biologic agents such as bacteria are often the inciting agents.

细菌这类生物因子常是诱发因子。

inclination [ˌinkliˈneiʃən] *n.* 倾斜，斜度；倾向，爱好

Few gynaecologists have the time or inclination to conduct a detailed general medical examination.

很少的妇产科医生有时间或有意向对病人进行仔细的全身体检。

inclusion [inˈkluːʒən] *n.* 包含，包括；内含物

Inclusion conjunctivitis often is associated with venereal infection.

包涵体结膜炎常与性病的传染有关。

Adenovirus intranuclear inclusions are found in epithelial cells and histocytes.

在上皮细胞及组织细胞内可见腺病毒核内包涵体。

incompatible(**with**) [ˌinkɔmˈpætəbl] *a.* 不相容的，不能共存的

Total absence of one chromosome from all body cells is almost invariably incompatible with survival.

全部体细胞的一条染色体完全缺失几乎必然会导致死亡。

incompetence [inˈkɔmpitəns] *n.* 无能力；关闭不全

Sometimes rheumatic scarring distorts the valve and shortens chordae, producing incompetence.

风湿性瘢痕有时使瓣膜变形和腱索缩短，造成关闭不全。

Early diastolic murmurs result from semilunar valve incompetence and begin at the valve closure sound.

早期舒张期杂音是半月瓣关闭不全所致，在瓣膜关闭声开始时出现。

incompetent [inˈkɔmpitənt] *a.* 不合格的，功能不全的

If the ileocecal valve is incompetent, the small bowel will appear distended.

如果回盲瓣功能不全，小肠就会扩张。

incomplete [ˌinkɔmˈpliːt] *a.* 不完全的，不完善的

Evidence supporting the use of anti-oxidants such as vitamins E and C is still incomplete.

支持使用抗氧化剂（如维生素 E 和 C）的证据仍然不充分。

Finally there is an incomplete coat of peritoneum that covers only the upper portion of the bladder.

最后是仅仅覆盖在膀胱上部的一个不完全的腹膜层。

All methods of classifying disease help to organize the ways in which we try to cope with the incomplete understanding we have.

把所有的划分疾病的方法综合起来，能帮助我们找出处理划分疾病时所持有的不完全认识的途径。

inconceivable [ˌinkɔnˈsivəbl] *a.* 不可想象的，不可思议的

This, in our present state of knowledge, is not inconceivable.

就我们现有的知识而言，这不是不可思议的。

inconclusive [ˌinkənˈkluːsiv] *a.* 无确定结果的，非决定性的

Attempts to detect early chemical evidence of protein malnutrition have been inconclusive.

想测定早期蛋白质营养不良的化学变化的尝试未得到什么结果。

In some patients, the above studies may be inconclusive.

在某些患者，以上的研究也许是非决定性的。

inconsistency [ˌinkənˈsistənsi] *n.* 不协调，不一致

Inconsistencies were found among experienced technologists in up to 33% and among inexperienced technologists in up to 93%.

在有经验的技术员中不一致性达到近 33%，而在缺乏经验的技术员中不一致性达到近 93%。

inconsistent [ˌinkənˈsistənt] *a.* 不协调的，不一致的

This therapy has given inconsistent results.

本疗法产生不一致的效果。

incontinence [inˈkɔntinəns] *n.* 失禁，无节制，不能自制

With further deterioration, incontinence usually develops and adds to the degradation.

随着进一步恶化，常常发生（大小便）失禁，从而增加衰退进程。

Failure of voluntary control of the anal sphincters with involuntary passage of feces is called fecal incontinence.

不能有意控制肛门括约肌而不随意排出粪便称为大便失禁。

inconvenient [ˌinkənˈviːnjənt] *a.* 不便的，有困难的

Twenty-four hour collections are inconvenient and difficult for most patients.

对于大多数病人而言，收集 24 小时标本既不方便又很困难。

incorporate [inˈkɔːpəreit] *v.* 结合，合并

Assessing of treatments will become incorporated into clinicians' patient rounds.

对治疗的评估，将同临床医护人员对病人的查房结合在一起进行。

incorrectly [ˌinkəˈrektli] *ad.* 错误地，不正确地

The term anemia has been used incorrectly as a diagnosis.

贫血这一术语一直错误地被作为一种诊断来使用。

increased [inˈkriːst] *a.* 增加的

This is due in part to increased life expectancy.
这部分原因是人的预期寿命增加了。

He put up his prices to offset the increased cost of materials.
他提高了售价以补偿材料成本的增加。

increasingly [inˈkriːsiŋli] *ad.* 日益,愈来愈…

Patients are increasingly afraid,with reason,that treatment may be worse than the disease.
病人们有理由越来越害怕治疗会比疾病本身更糟糕。

This specialist has become increasingly important in helping to maintain inhalation equipment and its proper functioning.
这类专家在维护吸入装置及其正常功能方面显得愈来愈重要了。

increment [ˈinkrimənt] *n.* 增加

A relatively large increment in serum creatinine concentration reflects a relatively small decrement in GFR in patients with pre-existing chronic renal insufficiency.
对已有慢性肾功能不全的病人而言,血清肌酐浓度的增长反映出 GFR 的降低较小。

incretin [inˈkriːtin] *n.* 肠促胰岛素

At present,several incretin mimetics and DPP-Ⅳ inhibitors are undergoing late-stage clinical trials for the treatment of type 2 diabetes.
目前,正在进行用几种肠促胰岛素类似物和 DPP-Ⅳ抑制剂来治疗 2 型糖尿病的后期临床试验。

Glucagon-like peptide-1 is one of the most important members of incretin,which has an unusual therapeutic potential in type 2 diabetes mellitus and obesity.
胰高血糖素样肽 1 是重要的肠促胰岛素成员之一,对 2 型糖尿病及肥胖症有显著疗效。

incretion [inˈkriːʃən] *n.* 内分泌; 内分泌物

Diabetic mellitus is a common incretion disease,caused by absolutely or relatively absence of insulin that maintains the blood glucose level.
糖尿病是一种常见的内分泌疾病,是由于体内绝对或相对缺乏维持葡萄糖水平的胰岛素而引起的。

Many nutritionists see Vitamin B group as decompression agents which can adjust incretion,balance emotions and relax the nerve system.
许多营养学家将 B 族维生素视为减压剂,它可以调节内分泌,平衡情绪,松弛神经。

incubate [ˈinkjubeit] *v.* 培养、孵化;潜伏

Cover the tube with foil to prevent light inactivation of mitomycin C and incubate in a waterbath shaker at 37℃ for 45 min.
用金属薄箔将试管封盖以防止光线灭活丝裂霉素 C,并在 37℃ 水浴振荡器内培养 45 分钟。

An asymptomatic neonate with reactive serologic tests for syphilis may have incubating disease.
一个无症状的新生儿有阳性梅毒血清反应,可能有潜伏性梅毒。

incubation [ˌinkjuˈbeiʃən] *n.* 潜伏;孵化

The incubation period usually is 8 to 14 days but varies from five days to five weeks.
潜伏期通常为 8 ~ 14 天,但也可变动于 5 天至 5 周之间。

The development of the embryo in the egg of oviparous animals is incubation.
胚胎在卵生动物的卵中发育即为孵化。

incubator [ˈinkjubeitə] *n.* 孵化器;恒温器

Healthy tissue cells are injected into this scalfold,which is then put into an incubator that replicates conditions in the womb.
健康组织细胞被投入这种支架中,然后被放进一个模拟子宫条件的孵化器内。

The temperature within the incubator is regulated so that the infant's temperature is maintained between 35.5 to 36.6℃.

调节保温箱内的温度使婴儿体温维持在35.5～36.6℃之间。

incurable [inˈkjuərəbl] *a.* 不能治愈的

Though this disease is incurable, its progress can be slowed.

此病虽然不能治愈，但能延缓其发展。

Up to now, AIDS is an incurable disease.

直到目前，艾滋病是一种不能治愈的疾病。

indefinite [inˈdefinit] *a.* 不确定的，无限期的

Some information appears to be stored accurately for an indefinite time, whereas other items fade or become distorted.

有些信息似乎可被准确地记忆很长时间，而其他内容则逐渐被淡忘或被歪曲。

indefinitely [inˈdefinitli] *ad.* 无限期地；不明确地，模糊地

Some viruses may persist indefinitely by the integration of their DNA with that of the host cell.

某些病毒，靠自己的DNA与宿主细胞的DNA整合而能永久的存在。

Abnormal ECG rhythms commonly associated with epilepsy may persist indefinitely even for years after the patient has ceased to have attacks.

癫痫常伴发的异常脑电波节律可长期地存在，甚至在患者停止发作后仍持续数年之久。

indel [ˈindel] *n.* 插入缺失

Two major types of sequence variation have been associated with variation in human phenotype: single nucleotide polymorphisms (SNPs) and insertions/deletions (indels).

与人类表型变异相关的有两类主要序列变异：单核苷酸多态性和插入/缺失。

In comparison to base pair substitutions, indels are much less frequent in the genome and are of particularly low frequency in coding regions of genes.

与碱基对的置换相比较，插入/缺失在基因组出现的频率更低，在基因编码区尤然。

independence [ˌindiˈpendəns] *n.* 独立(性)，自主(性)

Return to independence with mobility first requires the achievement of sitting balance, which is necessary to perform a transfer from bed to standing or bed to chair.

病人恢复独立行动首先需要坐稳，才能够从卧床转为站立或从卧床转为坐轮椅。

index [ˈindeks] *n.* 指标；指数

Arterial blood pressure is the best index to the degree of shock.

动脉血压是了解休克程度的最好指标。

The lower the therapeutic index, the greater the possibility of causing toxicity.

治疗指数越低，引起中毒的可能性越大。

indicate [ˈindikeit] *v.* 指示；表明；需要

If the disease is recognized early, operation is indicated.

此病如果发现得早，则适于手术治疗。

The patient was badly wounded in the abdomen and a laparotomy was indicated at once.

该病人腹部受了重伤，需要立即做剖腹术。

indication [ˌindiˈkeiʃən] *n.* 指示；指征，适应证

The ratio of the right to left ventricular pressure may be a valuable indication of the size of the defect.

右心室与左心室压力的比值可能是缺损大小的一个有价值的指标。

Indications for this procedure will be listed below.

适用本方法的指征列举如下。

The appearance of headache and blushing are indications of the efficacy of these medications.

头痛及面部潮红是这类药物显效的表现。

Thus failure to gain weight adequately should be regarded as an indication to carry out some other placental function tests.

因此，未能适当增加体重应认为是进行其他胎盘功能试验的一项适应证。

indicative(of) [in'dikətiv] *a.* 指示的，预示的

The presence of epigastric or right upper quadrant pain is indicative of severe preeclampsia.

上腹部或右上腹部的疼痛的出现表明为重度子痫前期。

Somatic hallucinations or conversion are indicative of other mental disorders.

躯体幻觉或转换表示有其他精神疾病。

indicator ['indikeitə] *n.* 指示器，指示物

A rise in serum creatinine or blood urea nitrogen is an indicator of severe disease.

血清肌酐和血液尿素氮的升高指示疾病严重。

Recent memory is a relatively sensitive indicator of organic impairment.

近记忆是器质性损伤的一个较敏感的指标。

Myoglobin has been found to be an extremely sensitive indicator of myocardial necrosis.

人们发现肌红蛋白是心肌坏死的一种极为灵敏的指示物。

indigestion [ˌindi'dʒestʃən] *n.* 消化不良，不消化

Large amounts of alcohol may produce indigestion.

大量酒精可造成消化不良。

Indigestion is a popular, rather than a scientific or medical term.

不消化是一个通俗的称谓，而不是科学或医学的术语。

indirect [ˌindi'rektˌ-dai-] *a.* 间接的；不直截了当的

Longevity is an indirect indicator of population health.

人口寿命是间接反映人口健康状况的一项指标。

In fact, any organism that adapts to organisms around it will act as an indirect coevolutionary agent to some degree.

实际上，任何生物，只要能与其周边生物相适应，就可以在某种程度上起到间接协同进化的作用。

How serious are the risks of indirect exposure to tobacco smoking!

吸二手烟的危害可真大呀！

indiscretion [ˌindis'kreʃən] *n.* 不慎重

The attacks of peptic ulceration may persist for days or weeks and are often related to dietary indiscretion or periods of intence worry or strain.

消化性溃疡的发作可持续数日或数周，常与饮食不慎、长期过度忧虑或紧张有关。

Acute gastritis is caused usually by dietary indiscretions, excessive intake of alcohol, irritating drugs, food poisoning and infectious diseases.

急性胃炎通常是由饮食不当、饮酒过量、刺激性药物、食物中毒和传染性疾病引起的。

indiscriminate [ˌindis'krimineit] *a.* 不加区别的，不选择的

In any circumstance, the indiscriminate use of anti-microbial drugs is to be avoided.

在任何情况下都应避免不加区别地使用抗菌类药物。

indispensable(to) [ˌindis'pensəbl] *a.* 不可缺少的，必需的

The special senses are our guardians. As such they are indispensable to us.

特种感觉（五官觉）是我们的保卫者，因而是我们须臾不可离的。

Laboratory examinations are often indispensable in correct diagnosis.

化验检查对正确诊断往往是必不可少的。

indistinguishable [indis'tiŋgwiʃəbl] *a.* 难区分的

On inspection alone, cystic tumours may be indistinguishable from ascites.

仅望诊不能将囊肿与腹水加以区别。

individual [indi'vidjuəl, indi'vidʒuəl] *a.* 个人的，个体的，个别的

This living thing is highly organized, in that different parts of the individual cell carry on special life functions.

这种生物的机体组织是很健全的，因为每个细胞的不同部分完成专门的生命功能。

n. 个人,个体

The same disease may show variations under different conditions and in different individuals.

同一疾病在不同情况下和在不同的个人身上其表现不尽相同。

In the healthy individual there is little danger of the intake of sodium being inadequate.

健康个体摄入钠不足的危害性很小。

Individuals suffering from frequent severe fits are least likely to be completely cured.

发作频繁而严重的患者最难以完全治愈。

individuality [indiˌvidjuˈæliti] *n.* 个性,个人的特征;个体

The concept of personal individuality would not be what it is today without the contribution of transplantation research.

没有移植研究的贡献,对人的个体(特殊性)的概念将不是今天这个样子。

individualization [ˌindiˌvidjuəlaiˈzeiʃən] *n.* 个体化

These data will demonstrate whether dosage individualization can improve outcomes and decrease short- and long-term adverse effects.

这些资料将证明个体化给药能否改善药物效果并减少短期和长期的不良反应。

individualize [indiˈvidjuəlaiz] *v.* 使适应个别需要,使个体化

ICU(intensive care unit) nursing is individualized nursing care and is much more than sitting at a desk in front of a monitor.

监护室护理是个别护理,远不只是坐在监测仪前。

Therapy must be individualized to the patient's observed response to the drug.

必须根据所观察到病人对这药的反应进行适应个别需要的治疗。

indolent [ˈindələnt] *n.* 惰性的

Mucosa associated lymphoid tissue lymphoma is a kind of indolent lymphoma.

粘膜相关淋巴组织淋巴瘤是一种惰性淋巴瘤。

Indolent Lymphomas are slow growing, low-grade cancers and less responsive to treatments like chemotherapy, radiation, and immunotherapy in the early stage.

惰性淋巴瘤是生长缓慢的低级别癌,早期对化疗、放疗和免疫治疗不敏感。

indomethacin [ˌindəuˈmeθəsin] *n.* 消炎痛

Antiinflammatory agents(eg. indomethacin) can precipitate bronchoconstriction in some asthmatic persons.

有些哮喘病人使用了抗炎药(如消炎痛)会诱发支气管收缩。

indoor [ˈindɔː] *a.* 室内的

We believed that the dynamic indoor environment would enter our lives in the future.

我们坚信动态室内环境理念必将最终步入我们的生活。

Therefore, people attach more importance to indoor air pollution.

因此,室内空气污染受到人们的日益重视。

induce [inˈdjuːs] *v.* 引起,导致;诱导

Sodium poor albumin infusions may be helpful in inducing diuresis.

低钠白蛋白输入可能有助于利尿。

General anesthesia can be induced by giving drugs intravenously, by inhalation, or by a combination of both methods.

经静脉、吸入或两种方式联合给药都能诱导全身麻醉。

Interferons induce a state of antiviral resistance in uninfected tissue cells.

干扰素可诱发未感染组织细胞的抗病毒性。

Phenytoin is also effective in digitalis induced arrhythmias.

苯妥英对洋地黄引起的心律失常也有效。

inducement [inˈdjuːsmənt] *n.* 诱导,引诱,诱因,动机

Analgesia follows after a period of inducement and stimulation, thereby ensuring safe operations on the head, chest, abdomen or limbs.

经过一段时间的诱导和刺激之后便产生了无痛感，从而保证头、胸、腹或四肢等部位的手术可以安全进行。

inducer [in'djuːsə] *n.* 诱导剂

Phenobarbital and some other classical inducers are known to decrease the storage of DDT in man.

已知苯巴比妥和另一些经典的诱导剂可减少 DDT 在人体内的贮存量。

inducible [in'djuːsəbl] *a.* 可诱导的

Inducible transgenesis provides a valuable technique for the analysis of gene function in vivo.

诱导性转基因技术为在体分析基因功能提供了一种有用的方法。

Inducible NOS (also known as NOS-2) is a nitric oxide synthase which is inducible in a wide range of cells and tissues.

诱导型 NOS(也称 NOS-2) 是一种可在很多种细胞和组织中诱导表达的一氧化氮合酶。

induction [in'dʌkʃən] *n.* 诱导，引产

Many biochemical reactions in the body are the consequence of enzyme induction.

体内许多生化反应都是酶诱导的结果。

Treatment by induction of ovulation may be required if the patient complains of infertility.

如果病人陈诉不孕，则可能需要诱发排卵。

The goal of expectant management is to delay delivery until fetal viability is assured and the cervix is favorable for the induction of labour.

期待疗法的目的是延缓分娩直至胎儿有成活可能及宫颈条件适合引产。

induration [ˌindjuə'reiʃən] *n.* 硬结

Erythema extending >2cm beyond the margin of the wound, localized tenderness and induration are all findings suggestive of a wound infection.

伤口边缘大于 2 厘米的红肿、局部压痛和硬结均表明伤口感染。

industrial [in'dʌstriəl] *a.* 工业的，产业的

As new industrial processes and products evolve, occupational asthma may become more common.

随着工业进程和产品发展，职业性哮喘越来越普遍。

Chronic bronchitis is a common disorder particularly among smokers and those who live in large industrial cities where the air is polluted.

慢性支气管炎是一种常见病，特别是在吸烟者和生活在空气受到污染的大工业城市者多见。

industry ['indʌstri] *n.* 工业

Toxic gases are not only encountered in mining, oil drilling, and similar industries, but also, occasionally, in the home.

有毒气体不仅在采矿、石油钻井以及类似的工业中遇到，而且也可在家庭中遇到。

Pricing decisions made within the private-sector pharmaceutical industry can have a major impact on vaccine use.

由私人药厂决定的价格会对疫苗的使用产生较大的影响。

indwelling ['indweliŋ] *a.* 留置的

Fungal urine cultures in those patients with indwelling urinary catheters may require different interpretations.

对那些已留置导尿管的病人，其尿霉菌的培养可能需要做不同的解释。

ineffective [ˌini'fektiv] *a.* 无效的，无能的

In pernicious anemia serum bilirubin may be elevated because of ineffective erythropoiesis.

恶性贫血时由于红细胞生成不起作用故血清胆红素可以升高。

inefficacy [in'efikəsi] *n.* 无效

The objective of our study is to find out the cause of inefficacy of platelets transfusion in these patients.

我们此项研究的目的是要找出对这些病人输注血小板无效的原因。

However, this can also be due to the inefficacy of the drug and at this time we may wish to change the treatment to prevent disease progression.

然而,这也可以是因药物无效所致,那么此时我们希望改变治疗方案从而防止疾病的进展。

inefficiency [iniˈfiʃənsi] *n.* 无能,效率低

Health reform is caused by the widespread perception of inefficiency within the health services.

医疗改革的根由是人们普遍认识到已经存在的效率低下的医疗服务的问题。

inert [iˈnəːt] *a.* 惰性的,无作用的

The membranes are not inert but actively regulate the transport of crystalloids.

细胞膜不是惰性的,而是主动调节类晶体的运送。

Estriol is biologically relatively inert.

在生物学上,雌三醇是比较不活泼的。

inevitable [inˈevitəbl] *a.* 不可避免的

Infection is almost inevitable in the absence of thorough sterilization.

消毒不彻底,感染就几乎无法避免。

Drugs may produce symptoms in a variety of ways. Inevitable side effects may accompany the use of a drug like a shadow.

药物可以产生各种各样的症状,不可避免的副作用像影子一般地伴随着药物的使用而出现。

inevitably [inˈevitəbli] *ad.* 不可避免地;必然地

Such individuals are prone to manic-depressive psychosis but it does not occur inevitably.

这种人易患躁狂抑郁性精神病,但不是必然发病。

inexhaustible [ˌinigˈzɔːstəbl] *a.* 用不完的,无穷无尽的

The masses of the people have inexhaustible creative power and an eager desire to change all backward conditions.

人民群众有无穷无尽的创造力,有改变落后面貌的迫切愿望。

inexpensive [ˌiniksˈpensiv] *a.* 花费不多的,价格公道的

Noninvasive methods eventually may be expected to remedy this situation by allowing painless and relatively inexpensive interrogation of blood vessels to detect preclinical disease.

非侵害性方法,是通过无痛的、相对经济的血管检查法,探测临床前期疾病,从而可望矫正这一状况。

infancy [ˈinfənsi] *n.* 婴儿期(两岁以内),幼年期;初期

Nearly one third of cases of blindness dates from infancy.

将近 1/3 的盲症是从婴儿期开始的。

The use of computers and automatic equipment in medicine is still in its infancy.

电子计算机和自动装置在医学中的应用,还只是在它的幼年时代。

infantile [ˈinfəntail] *a.* 婴儿的,幼稚的

The application, with friction, of warm oil to every portion of the body is invaluable in acute infantile cases.

在身体各部外敷温油膏,并进行揉擦,对急性本病的幼儿是极有价值的。

infantilism [inˈfæntilizəm] *n.* 幼稚型;呆小病

There will also be absence of breast development in cases of pituitary infantilism.

垂体性侏儒症患者的乳房也可能有不发育的现象。

infarct [inˈfɑːkt] *n.* 梗死,梗塞

Infarct is an area of necrosis in a tissue due to ischemia resulting from obstruction of circulation to the area, mostly by a thrombus or embolus.

梗死是组织中一坏死区,大多是由于通到该区的血液循环被一血栓或栓子阻塞发生缺血而引起。

In women, septic pulmonary infarcts with abscess formation and cavitation should always suggest puerperal sepsis or infected abortion.

在妇女,脓毒性肺梗死有脓肿形成和空洞,应总是联想到产后脓毒血症或感染性流产。

infarction [inˈfɑːkʃən] *n.* 梗死,梗塞(形成)

Myocardial infarction may also occur during hypotension (including surgery).

心肌梗死也可发生于低血压时(包括外科手术时)。

Pulmonary infarction also causes collapse of lung tissue.

肺部的梗死形成也能引起肺组织萎陷。

infect [inˈfekt] *v.* 感染,传染

If a person is not infected with mycobacterium tuberculosis, the tuberculin skin test may be negative.

如果一个人没有感染上结核分枝杆菌,其结核菌素皮试可以是阴性的。

This is an important factor in the softening seen in infected organs at autopsy.

这是在尸检中所见的受感染器官软化的重要因素。

infection [inˈfekʃən] *n.* 感染,传染

Antibody appears at the onset of the illness and a rising titre indicates recent infection.

疾病开始时即有抗体生成,抗体滴定度的升高表明近期有感染。

Patients with diabetes mellitus are prone to development of cutaneous infection, bacteriuria, tuberculosis and moniliasis.

糖尿病病人易发生皮肤感染、菌尿、结核和念珠菌病。

infectious [inˈfekʃəs] *a.* 传染性的

Immune γ-globulin (500-750 mg in adults) protects contacts of infectious hepatitis.

免疫 γ-球蛋白(成人为 500 ~ 750 mg)对接触传染性肝炎者有保护作用。

Viruses are the smallest known infectious agents.

病毒是人们所知道的最小的传染因子。

infective [inˈfektiv] *a.* 传染性的,感染性的

The infective agents transmit infection and confer specific immunity.

致病因子传播感染并形成特殊的免疫性。

infectivity [ˌinfekˈtiviti] *n.* 传染性,传染力

This review will discuss the mechanisms of HIV infectivity.

这篇综述将讨论 HIV 传染性的机制。

He will focus on HIV infectivity.

他将专注于 HIV 的传染性。

Infectivity is the ability to produce infection; specifically, a tendency to spread rapidly from host to host.

传染性就是引起感染的能力,特别是从一个宿主向另一个宿主快速传播的趋势。

infectomics [infekˈtɔmiks] *n.* 感染组学

In this review, we focus on the events that are considered important in infectomics.

在这篇综述中,我们集中于感染组学中被认为重要的事件。

The interactions between microbial pathogens and their hosts may be globally and integratively understood by using infectomics.

使用感染组学可整体和全面地理解微生物病原体与宿主之间的相互作用。

infer [inˈfəː] *v.* 推论,推断

By this means the correct diagnosis can be inferred.

通过这种方法可以做出正确的诊断。

inference [ˈinfərəns] *n.* 推论,推断

The doctor selects the items which appear to him to be significant and from these he makes inferences.

医生选择那些在他看来比较重要的项目并从中做出推断。

His observations,his selections and his inferences are influenced by many factors.

他的观察、选择和推论受许多因素的影响。

inferior [inˈfiəriə] *a.* 下方的,下部的

The rectum is inferior to the small intestine.

直肠位于小肠的下方。

The local consumption coagulopathy is manifested anatomically as inferior vena caval thrombosis.

局部消耗性血凝病在解剖上表现为下腔静脉血栓形成。

infertility [ˌinfəˈtiliti] *n.* 不生育,不育症

Approximately 30% of patients undergoing laparoscopy for infertility have endometriosis.

因不孕症做腹腔镜检查的病例中,约 30% 为子宫内膜异位症。

After an almost 10-year episode of secondary infertility the patient had an operation for a right tubal pregnancy last year.

经过 10 年继发性不孕以后,患者去年因右侧输卵管妊娠接受了手术。

infestation [infesˈteiʃən] *n.* (昆虫)感染,体表感染

The infections and infestations are both exotic.

感染和体表感染都是外来的。

The microscope is required for the discovery of eggs or larval forms of most worm infestations.

大多数蠕虫感染的虫卵或幼虫都要用显微镜才能发现。

infiltrate[1] [inˈfiltreit] *v.* 浸润

Usually,malignant tumors invade,infiltrate,and destroy the adjacent normal tissues.

通常恶性肿瘤侵入、浸润和破坏邻近的正常组织。

It is a deep infiltrating ulcer which slowly eats away the bones and soft tissues.

它是一种深陷的、浸润性溃疡,逐渐地腐蚀掉骨和软组织。

infiltrate[2] [ˈinfiltreit] *n.* 渗入物,浸润物

Leukemic infiltrates of the retina and optic disc occasionally occur.

视网膜和视神经盘受白血病浸润偶可发生。

Chest X-ray revealed bilateral infiltrates in the upper lobes.

胸片显示双肺上叶浸润。

infiltration [ˌinfilˈtreiʃən] *n.* 浸润

The extent of such infiltration is of very practical importance in terms of therapy.

这种浸润范围在肿瘤的治疗上具有很重要的实际意义。

Cellular infiltration is the migration and accumulation of cells within the tissue.

细胞浸润是细胞(如炎性细胞)迁移和聚集在组织内。

infiltrative [inˈfiltrətiv] *adj.* 浸润性的;渗透性的

He has been diagnosed with infiltrative pulmonary tuberculosis.

他已被诊断为浸润性肺结核。

The tumor nodule shows infiltrative changes along the left border,with the invasive acinar growth pattern of this carcinoma shown on the nodule (hematoxylin and eosin).

显示肿瘤结节沿其左侧边缘有浸润性变化,在结节上(苏木精伊红染色)呈侵袭性腺泡生长方式。

infirm [inˈfəːm] *a.* 体弱的,虚弱的

The elderly infirm tend to suffer a decline in their functional capabilities and their self-sufficiency.

老年体弱者容易形成身体功能衰退和自我充实感下降。

inflame [in'fleim] *v.* (使)发炎

An inflamed tissue is characterized by redness, swelling, pain, heat and loss of function.

发炎的组织以红、肿、痛、热和功能丧失为特征。

An abscess may form when an inflamed appendix ruptures.

阑尾发炎破裂可形成脓肿。

inflammation [ˌinflə'meiʃən] *n.* 炎症

Inflammation of veins (phlebitis) also promotes thrombosis.

静脉的炎症(静脉炎)也可促进血栓形成。

The gall bladder is removed 2-3 months later after the inflammation has settled.

在炎症被控制后 2 ~ 3 月施行胆囊切除。

inflammatory [in'flæmətəri] *a.* 炎性的

There is no inflammatory reaction.

没有炎症反应。

Fever can be a prominent symptom of all infectious and inflammatory diseases.

发热可能是所有感染性和炎性疾病的突出症状。

inflatable [in'fleitəbl] *a.* 可膨胀的;可充气的

An inflatable vest can make emergency CPR—cardiopulmonary resuscitation —more effective.

一种充气式背心可使心肺复苏(CPR)的急救更为有效。

inflate [in'fleit] *v.* 使膨胀,使充气

In the procedure, a tiny ballon is inflated at the blockage site, expanding it without the need for surgery.

操作时,给插至阻塞部位的微小气囊充气,使该部位扩张而无需手术。

Conventional ventilation techniques during CPR require the lungs to be inflated 10 to 12 times per minute.

在心肺复苏(CPR)中,常规的通气方法须使肺部每分钟充气 10 ~ 12 次。

inflation [in'fleiʃən] *n.* 充气,膨胀,吹张,吹张法

Because lung tissue has a natural tendency to collapse at low volumes, additional pressure must be applied to achieve a given volume on the inflation limb.

由于肺组织在低容量时有自然塌陷的趋势,所以必须加压后才能使充气的膨胀支达到预定的容量。

influence ['influəns] n. *v.* 影响

The substances which influence osmotic pressure are those of molecular size too great to pass through the membrane.

影响渗透压的是那些分子太大不能透过膜的物质。

The publication of information allows citizens to determine what chemicals directly influence the quality of life where they work and live.

这些资料公布之后才能使公众了解在他们工作和生活的环境中有哪些化学物质直接影响他们的生活质量。

influenza [influ'enzə] *n.* 流行性感冒

Influenza is an acute respiratory illness caused by infection with influenza viruses.

流行性感冒是由流感病毒感染所引起的一种急性呼吸道传染病。

The major problem posed by influenza consists of its complications, the most common of which is pneumonia.

流行性感冒引起的主要问题在于其并发症,其中最常见的是肺炎。

influx ['inflʌks] *n.* 流入,注入

The influx of Ca^{2+} following acetylcholine is not mediated via cyclic AMP.

乙酰胆碱所引起的钙内流并不是经由 cAMP 介导的。

informality [infɔːˈmæliti] *n.* 简便，非正式

The very features of this big hospital are accessibility, informality, familiarity, continuity of care.

这个大医院的主要特征是就医方便、不拘形式、亲切随和、持续照顾等。

information [ˌinfəˈmeiʃən] *n.* 通知；情报；资料；信息

True microorganisms always contain DNA as the repository of their genetic information.

真正的微生物总是含有 DNA 作为它们的遗传信息的贮藏所。

Candidates for the certifying examination received an information booklet several weeks before the examination.

在考试前几星期，参加资格考试的人员收到了一本有关资料的小册子。

information superhighway [infəˈmeiʃən suːpəˈhaiwei] *n.* 信息高速公路

The information superhighway goes all around the world.

信息高速公路贯通全球。

The sheer size of the Internet makes it a candidate for the backbone of the information superhighway.

因特网规模的快速增长使得其可以作为信息高速公路骨干网的候选对象。

informative [inˈfɔːmətiv] *a.* 提供资料的；有益的

Hopefully, guest scientists and staff here will find these sessions informative and useful.

希望被邀请来的科学家们以及这里的同仁，都会感到这次会议是内容丰富和有裨益的。

infraclavicular [ˌinfrəkləˈvikjulə] *a.* 锁骨下的

Only the infraclavicular branches are approachable through the axilla.

只有锁骨下分支通过腋窝。

infrared [ˈinfrəˈred] *a.* 红外(线)的

This was caused by the action of infrared rays on a body.

这是由红外线作用于机体引起的。

n. 红外线

The spectral region in the red or near infrared will be emphasized.

着重研究的光谱区域是红或近红外波段。

infrastructure [ˌinfrəˈstrʌktʃə] *n.* 基础结构，内部结构

This study was designed to examine the impact of organizational infrastructure on the use of aspirin and beta-blockers during and after AMI (acute myocardial infarction).

本研究的目的是为了检测急性心肌梗死发生当时和以后组织内部结构对使用阿司匹林和β-受体阻断剂的影响。

infrequent [inˈfriːkwənt] *a.* 偶尔有的，不常见的

Plasma cells are infrequent in the blood.

浆细胞在血液中罕见。

The corymbose syphilid is another infrequent variant, usually occurring late in the secondary stage.

伞房花形梅毒疹是另一种不常见的变异体，通常在二期(梅毒)后期出现。

infrequently [inˈfriːkwəntli] *ad.* 不经常地，偶尔

When the dosage is adapted to the patient, marked side effects are seen only infrequently.

当剂量对患者适合时，只在少数情况下才出现明显的副作用。

infusion [inˈfjuːʒən] *n.* 输入，输注

Anesthesia usually begins by starting an intravenous infusion and applying a blood pressure cuff.

通常，麻醉工作始于给予静脉输液和系上血压表袖带时。

In pneumococcal meningitis, 20 to 40 million u of penicillin G may be given daily by constant infusion drip.

对于肺炎双球菌性脑膜炎可每天恒速滴注青霉素 G 2000 万 ~4000 万单位。

ingest [inˈdʒest] *v.* 食入，咽下

The availability of the ingested calcium depends on its absorption from the upper small intestine.
摄入钙的有效性取决于小肠上段对钙的吸收程度。
Another example is the necrosis of macrophages which have ingested silica particles.
另一个例子是吞噬硅粒的巨噬细胞坏死。

ingestion [inˈdʒestʃən] *n.* 摄入,食入,摄食
Infectious hepatitis virus is transmitted by ingestion of contaminated food and occasionally by blood transfusion or injection.
传染性肝炎病毒是通过摄入污染了的食物传染的,偶尔也通过输血或注射传染。
Bacillus dysenteriae produce a toxin in food which causes diarrhea 8 ~ 14 h after ingestion of contaminated meat.
痢疾杆菌在食物中产生毒素,可在食入污染肉类后 8 ~ 14 小时引起腹泻。

ingredient [ˌinˈgriːdjənt] *n.* 组成部分,成分
By these routes of administration the active ingredient is absorbed into the venous circulation.
通过这些途径,有效成分被吸收入静脉循环。
Insulin is a key ingredient in the metabolic process.
胰岛素是新陈代谢过程中一种主要的组成部分。

inguinal [ˈiŋgwinəl] *a.* 腹股沟的
In normal adults, inguinal lymph nodes may be easily palpable, ranging from 0.5-2cm in size.
正常人的腹股沟淋巴结容易被摸到,约为 0.5 ~ 2 厘米大小。

inhabit [inˈhæbit] *v.* 居住于
More than five billion people inhabit the earth.
五十多亿人口居住在地球上。
Certain viruses inhabit tissue for the life of the host, causing little harm as long as the host's immune system is intact.
某些病毒存在于组织中长达宿主的一生,只要宿主的免疫系统保持完整就不大会产生危害。

inhabitant [inˈhæbitənt] *n.* 居民;栖居的动物;寄居菌
The infecting bacteria, such as Escherichia coli and nonhemolytic streptococci, are normal inhabitants.
传染的细菌如大肠杆菌和非溶血性链球菌等为肠道内正常存在的细菌。
Most spore forming bacteria are inhabitants of soil.
绝大多数形成芽孢的细菌是土壤寄居菌。

inhalant [inˈheilənt] *n.* 吸入剂
Penicillin is also used as an aerosol inhalant.
青霉素还用作气雾吸入剂。

inhalation [ˌinhəˈleiʃən] *n.* 吸入(法);吸入剂
Miners are susceptible to lung damage caused by the constant inhalation of stonedust.
矿工们由于经常吸入石尘而易使肺部受到损伤。
A trained inhalation therapist should be a member of the ICU (intensive care unit) team.
监护室成员应包括一位训练有素的气雾治疗师。

inhale [inˈheil] *v.* 吸入
This patient inhaled the medicine half an hour ago.
这个病人半小时前吸入此药。
Post primary infection may be exogenous, i. e. caused by organisms in inhaled dust, etc.
原发后感染可为外源性的,由吸入含菌的灰尘等引起。

inhaler [inˈheilə] *n.* 吸入器;滤气器;吸入者
The patient should be allowed to select the best inhaler device for himself or herself.
应允许病人选择最适合他们的吸入器。

inherent [inˈhiərənt] *a.* 固有的

Metabolism is an inherent function of every cell of the body.

新陈代谢是身体每个细胞固有的功能。

Drugs do not create functions but merely stimulate or inhibit functions already inherent in the cells.

药物不能赋予细胞新的功能,而仅仅兴奋或抑制细胞固有的功能。

inherently [inˈhiərəntli] *ad.* 固有地,内在地

These two causes are inherently related to one another.

这两种病因相互之间有着固有的联系。

inherit [inˈherit] *v.* 遗传

Scientists have been reporting that a tendency to become an alcoholic can be inherited.

科学家们报道说,成为酗酒者的倾向是可以遗传的。

The inherited defects of glycogen metabolism are collectively known as the glycogenoses.

糖原代谢的遗传缺陷总称为糖原沉积病。

inheritable [inˈheritəbl] *a.* 可遗传的

Cancer of the eye occurring in childhood, adenomas of the thyroid and parathyroids are considered inheritable neoplasms.

儿童期发生的眼癌、甲状腺和甲状旁腺瘤都被认为是可遗传的赘生物。

inheritance [inˈheritəns] *n.* 遗传,遗产

The phenomenon of polygenic inheritance is an extension of Mendelian theory.

多基因遗传现象是孟德尔定律的延伸。

In autosomal dominant inheritance, disease severity may be uniform or variable.

常染色体显性遗传病的严重程度可能相同或不同。

inhibit [inˈhibit] *v.* 抑制

Sometimes the metabolites are able to inhibit the further metabolism of the parent drug.

有时代谢产物能抑制母体药物的进一步代谢。

A soft catheter should be passed, as a full bladder has an inhibiting effect on the uterine contractions.

应采用柔软的导管进行导尿,因为膀胱在充盈后可能妨碍子宫的收缩。

inhibition [inhiˈbiːʃən] *n.* 抑制

Enzyme inhibition is obviously the other face, the converse of the preceding.

酶的抑制显然是另一回事,与前述正相反。

inhibitor [inˈhibitə] *n.* 抑制剂,抑制物

Monoamine oxidase inhibitors include iproniazid, isocarboxacid, phenelzine, and tranylcypromine.

单胺氧化酶抑制剂包括异丙肼、马普兰、苯乙肼和苯环丙胺。

There may be a phosphatesensitive bacterial growth inhibitor in amniotic fluid.

在羊水内可能存在有一种对磷酸盐敏感的细菌生长抑制物。

inhibitory [inˈhibitəri] *a.* 抑制的

The inhibitory transmitter depresses the neuron rather than exciting it.

抑制性递质抑制神经元而不是兴奋它。

inimicable [iˈnimikəbl], inimical [iˈnimikəl] *a.* 有害的;不利的

The action of the salivary amylase is soon suspended due to the high acidity which is inimicable to the action of the salivary amylase.

由于强酸度不利于唾液淀粉酶起作用,唾液淀粉酶的作用很快暂停。

initial [iˈniʃəl] *a.* 最初的,开始的

These enzymes are responsible for the initial stages in the metabolism of many drugs.

这些酶对许多药物代谢的最初阶段起重大作用。

A 27-year-old woman with chondrosarcoma of the ethmoid sinus extending to the anterior fossa had initial symptoms of blurred vision on the left and slight proptosis.

一位患有筛窦软骨肉瘤并侵犯颅前窝的 27 岁女性出现左眼视力模糊及轻微突眼的始发症状。

The fever was not down after the initial injection, nor was it after the second one.

第一次注射后热度并未下降,第二次注射后热度亦未下降。

initially [iˈniʃəli] *ad.* 最初,开始

A body of research initially had an apparently limited aim.

一批研究工作开始就有一个明显有限的目标。

initiate [iˈniʃieit] *v.* 开始,创始;启动

Depression is not diagnosed if an organic factor initiated or maintained the depression.

如果有一器质性因素引起或维持抑郁,则不作抑郁症诊断。

If the connection limit is reached, the server does not initiate new connections until the number of current connections decreases.

如果达到连接限制,则服务器要等到当前连接数减少后才会启动新的连接。

initiation [iˌniʃiˈeiʃən] *n.* 开始,创始

Two weeks after the initiation of hormonal therapy, the patient improved.

开始激素治疗法两周后,患者好转了。

initiative [iˈniʃiətiv] *n.* 首创精神,主动性

For full rehabilitation, it is important to encourage the patient's initiative.

为了全面康复,鼓励发挥病人的主动性是很重要的。

In treating the patient, the initiatives of the doctors and nurses were brought into full play.

在治疗病人时,充分发挥了医生和护士们的主观能动作用。

initiator [iˈniʃieitə] *n.* 创造人,发起者,传授者,教导者

The initiator of this program is a young doctor, a doctorate graduate from a medical university.

这个计划的发起人是一位青年医师,是一所医科大学的博士毕业生。

It has been found that initiator, plasticizer, stabilizer, crosslinking agent and composition of blends influence significantly the crosslinking reaction.

研究发现引发剂、塑化剂、稳定剂、交联剂以及混合剂中的组成都显著影响交联反应。

inject [inˈdʒekt] *v.* 注入,注射

Before the operation, the surgeon injected a drug (potassium citrate) into the heart of the patient.

手术前,外科医生给病人的心脏注射了一种药(枸橼酸钾)。

Sanamycin (Actinomycin C) should only be injected intravenously.

萨纳霉素(放线菌素 C)仅作静脉注射用。

injection [inˈdʒekʃən] *n.* 注射

A new typhoid vaccine given by a single injection protects against typhoid fever for at least 17 months.

一种新的伤寒疫苗,注射一次,至少可以预防伤寒 17 个月。

Injection can take the place of oral administration.

注射可代替药物口服。

injudicious [ˌindʒuˈdiʃəs] *a.* 判断欠妥的,不慎重的

Traumatic rupture of the uterus may occur as a result of the injudicious use of oxytocin.

催产素在使用不当时也可引起损伤性子宫破裂。

injudiciously [indʒuːdiʃəsli] *ad.* 欠考虑地

Chloramphenicol, when used injudiciously, may cause gray syndrome in the newborn.

当使用氯霉素不当时也可引起新生儿的灰婴综合征。

injure [ˈindʒə] *v.* 损伤,损害

You will injure your health by smoking too much.

当你吸烟过多时它将损伤你的身体。

injurious [inˈdʒuəriəs] *a.* 有害的,致伤的

Acute inflammation is the immediate and early response of the organism to an injurious agent.

急性炎症是机体对有害因子的立即和早期反应。

Cold is much less injurious to cells than heat.

与高温相比,寒冷对细胞的损害作用要小得多。

injury [ˈindʒəri] *n.* 伤害,损害

If the injury is severe, there may also be death of tissue cells.

如果损伤严重,组织的细胞也可出现坏死。

Surgery has brought back sight to people with more and more extreme eye injuries.

手术给眼睛受伤越来越严重的人们带来了复明的机会。

innate [iˈneit] *a.* 先天的,天生的

Innate defects are conditions or characteristics that are present in an individual at birth and are inherited from his parents.

先天性缺陷是某个人生来就具有的,是由父母遗传来的某种疾患或特征。

Chomsky believes that language is universal and innate.

乔姆斯基认为,语言是普遍存在的并且是与生俱来的。

innervate [ˈinəːveit] *v.* 促使…活动;使受神经支配

The nervous system innervates the muscles and also controls the functions of many of the internal organs.

神经系统不仅促使肌肉活动,而且还控制许多内脏器官的功能。

Smooth muscle, like cardiac muscle, is innervated by the autonomic nervous system.

平滑肌与心肌一样受自主神经系统支配。

innervation [inəːˈveiʃən] *n.* 神经支配,神经分布

The nervous innervation here has been changed.

此处神经分布已被改变。

innocent [ˈinəsnt] *a.* 良性的,无害的,单纯的

If the tumor is confined to a local area and does not spread, it is called a benign, or innocent, tumor.

如果肿瘤限于一局部区域而不扩散,那就叫做良性肿瘤。

Of course, some innocent tumors can be anything but innocent in their effect.

当然某些良性肿瘤有不好的后果,但其本身作用是无害的。

Associated hyperventilation can cause innocent changes in the T waves and ST segments, which can be confused with coronary artery disease.

相关的过度通气可引起单纯的T波和ST段改变,这可能与冠状动脉病变相混淆。

innocuous [iˈnɔkjuəs] *a.* 无害的

Abdominal amniocentesis is totally innocuous.

腹壁羊膜穿刺术是完全无害的。

A study in Britain warns that antacids may not be as innocuous as they are thought to be.

英国的一项研究警示:抗酸药可能不是人们所想的那样对人体无害。

innovation [inəuˈveiʃən] *n.* 革新,创新,新方法

More innovations are on the horizon.

不久将会有更多创新。

innovative [ˈinəuveitiv] *a.* 革新的,创新的

This technique is still regarded as an innovative approach.

这一技术现在仍被看作是一种创新方法。

inoculate [iˈnɔkjuleit] *v.* 接种,注入

Thin shavings are inoculated into culture media such as Mycose agar or dermal trichophyton media(DTM).

将薄刮屑接种在海藻糖琼脂培养基内或皮肤癣菌试验培养基内。

Mosquitoes, during a blood meal, inoculate sporozoites that rapidly enter liver parenchymal cells.

蚊子吸人血时就将类孢子虫注入人体，该类孢子虫很快进入肝实质细胞内。

inoculation [iˌnɔkjuˈleiʃən] *n.* 接种，预防注射

All the children have been given inoculation against small-pox.

所有这些儿童均已进行了接种以预防天花。

Later, actual inoculation with a drop of pus from a smallpox victim was made available.

后来人们用天花患者的一滴脓液进行了真正的接种。

inoperable [inˈɔpərəbl] *a.* 不宜手术的；不能手术的

Metastasis has rendered the tumor inoperable.

癌细胞的转移使得这一肿瘤不宜手术。

If you leave it long enough, the cancer may have spread so that it is inoperable.

如果你搁置时间很长，癌细胞可能已经扩散，以致不能手术。

inorganic [ˌinɔːˈgænik] *a.* 无机的

Substances can be classified into organic and inorganic.

物质可分类为有机的和无机的。

The ions are dissolved in the cell water, and they provide inorganic chemicals for cellular reactions.

离子溶于细胞内水液，并为细胞反应提供无机化学物质。

inotropic [ˌinəuˈtrɔpik] *a.* 影响(肌)收缩力的，变力的，正性肌力的

Long-term use of inotropic agents can adversely affect survival in patients with heart failure.

长期使用正性肌力药物能对心衰病人生存产生不利影响。

Calcium antagonists have negative inotropic effects and should be used cautiously if left ventricle dysfunction is present.

钙拮抗剂有负性肌力作用，当左心室出现功能不全时应慎用。

The term "inotropic" is commonly used in discussing changes in myocardial contractility.

变力性一词通常用来描述心肌收缩性的变化。

inpatient [ˈinˌpeiʃənt] *n.* 住院病人

This hospital receives more than 1000 outpatients every day in addition to the 600 inpatients.

这家医院除600名住院病人外，每天要接纳1000多名门诊病人。

The seriously wounded worker has been sent to the operating room of the inpatient department.

那位严重受伤的工人已被送到住院部手术室去了。

Initially, it must be decided whether inpatient or outpatient treatment is needed.

首先必须确定是需要住院治疗还是需要门诊治疗。

inquest [ˈinkwest] *n.* 验尸

Inquest is carried out when the death is sudden or take place under suspicious circumstances.

当死亡是突然发生的或在可疑情况下发生时，就需要做尸体检验。

inquire [inˈkwaiə] *v.* 询问，调查

A special group will be appointed by the hospital to inquire into the matter.

关于此事医院将指定一个专门小组来进行调查。

inquiry [inˈkwaiəri] *n.* 询问，查询，调查

History should include inquiry about fever, abdominal pain, nausea and vomiting.

应当询问患者有无发热、腹痛、恶心和呕吐的病史。

In answer to your recent inquiry, the book you mention is not in stock.

答复您最近的查询，您所提及的书现在无货。

Gastrointestinal diseases have been the subject of genetic inquiry.

胃肠道疾病现在已成为遗传研究的课题。

insanity [inˈsæniti] *n.* 精神错乱

Insanity is a general term for unsoundness of mind or any mental disorder.
"精神错乱"是表示精神不健康或任何思维异常时的一个通用术语。

insect [in'sekt] *n.* 昆虫

Some insects establish themselves on the skin as parasites, others inject poison, and still others transmit disease.
一些昆虫常寄生在皮肤上成为寄生虫,另一些会注入毒物,还有一些甚至会传播疾病。

insecticide [in'sektisaid] *n.* 杀虫剂

The great majority of chlorinated insecticides such as DDT and DDD are harmful to man.
大多数氯化杀虫剂如 DDT 和 DDD 对人都有害。
Some of these threats are becoming more serious with the emergence of insecticide-resistant vectors.
随着抗杀虫剂病媒的出现,有些疾病的威胁越来越严重。

insemination [inˌsemi'neiʃn] *n.* 授精

Artificial insemination means introduction of viable sperm into the vagina, cervical canal or uterus by artificial means.
人工授精是指采用人工方法把活力好的精子输送至阴道、宫颈管或子宫内。
Artificial insemination is timed to coincide with the day on which the woman is expected to ovulate.
人工授精时间安排应与妇女预期排卵日相符。

insensible [in'sensəbl] *a.* 无感觉的,麻木的;不省人事的

This is also true in the presence of increased insensible water loss, as with fever or elevated environmental temperatures.
在发热时或在环境温度升高时,人们常常感觉不到水分的丢失已在增加。

insensitive [in'sensitiv] *a.* 不敏感的,感觉迟钝的

Apart from being insensitive to pain, the patients are normal in other physiological functions.
除了对疼痛不敏感外,患者的其他生理功能都是正常的。

insensitivity [inˌsensi'tiviti] *n.* 不敏感性

Insensitivity or indifference to pain is not the common human experience.
对疼痛感觉迟钝或淡漠,是人类很少见的现象。

insert [in'səːt] *v.* 插入,嵌入

This catheter can easily be inserted into the bladder without significant discomfort.
这个导管能容易地插入膀胱而没有明显的不舒服感觉。

insertion [in'səːʃən] *n.* 插入

Percutaneous insertion of a cardiac catheter is usually through a peripheral blood vessel into the chambers of the heart under X-ray control.
经皮肤插入心导管通常是在 X 线控制下经外周血管而进入心腔。

insidious [in'sidiəs] *a.* 隐性的

Bleeding from hiatus hernia and gastric carcinoma is usually insidious(but not always).
裂孔疝和胃癌出血常常是隐性的(但不总是如此)。
The onset of pulmonary tuberculosis is insidious.
肺结核起病隐袭。

insidiously [in'sidiəsli] *ad.* 隐袭地

Simple mechanical obstruction of the colon may develop insidiously.
结肠的单纯性机械性梗阻的起病可能是隐袭性的。
The deafness came on insidiously, followed by chronic right sided headache.
耳聋的出现为隐袭性的,以后即出现慢性右侧偏头痛。

insight ['insait] *n.* 自知力

The term insight is often applied to a patient's recognition that he has psychological problems.

自知力一词常用来指病人对自己有无精神性疾病的认知。

insignificant [insigˈnifikənt] *a.* 无意义的，无关紧要的

The mouth and rectum are, in general, insignificant sites of absorption of environmental chemicals.

一般情况下，口腔和直肠是环境化学物的不太重要的吸收部位。

The detachment of fragments of infected blood clot accounts for the septic emboli which may complicate a relatively insignificant abscess.

受感染的血块碎片的脱落可以造成败血性栓塞，从而使比较轻微的脓肿变得复杂起来。

insist(on) [inˈsist] *v.* 坚持

The doctor insisted that the leprosy patient should be isolated.

医生坚持麻风病人需要隔离。

There may be cyanosis of the lips and nail beds and sinus tachycardia, and the patient may insist on sitting upright.

可能出现在嘴唇和甲床等部位的发绀以及发生窦性心动过速，此时病人会要求采取坐位。

in situ [inˈsaitju] *ad.* 原位

Carcinoma in situ means the lesion is non-invasive.

原位癌意味着病变是非浸润性的。

Cervical carcinoma in situ does not definitely progress to invasive carcinoma.

宫颈原位癌并不一定会进展为浸润癌。

insoluble [inˈsɔljubl] *a.* 不可溶的

This process of changing insolube and non-diffusible substances into soluble and diffusible substances is called digestion.

把不溶性和非扩散性物质变成可溶性和扩散性物质的过程叫做消化。

insomnia [inˈsɔmniə] *n.* 失眠(症)

Insomnia is not a disease but may be the symptom of many diseases.

失眠并不是一种疾病，而可能是很多疾病的一种症状。

The most frequent causes of insomnia are anxiety and pain.

失眠最常见的原因是焦虑和疼痛。

Decreased appetite, weight loss, and insomnia commonly occur in bereavement.

丧亲之痛通常使人食欲不振，体重减轻，并且失眠。

inspect [inˈspekt] *v.* 检查，视察

Inspect the iris before evaluating the pupillary size and response.

在评估瞳孔大小和反应以前应该检查虹膜。

inspection [inˈspekʃən] *n.* 检查，检验；望诊

The exposed position of the eye leads itself readily to external inspection.

眼睛处于暴露地位便于外部检查。

It should be an absolute rule that inspection of the part to be examined should always come first.

在需要检查的部位首先进行望诊，这应该是一项绝对的规则。

inspiration [ˌinspəˈreiʃn] *n.* 吸气

Inspiration may be costal or abdominal, the latter being deeper.

吸气可采用胸式或腹式的方法，腹式吸气较深。

During inspiration, expansion of the chest occurs and air enters the lungs, all portion of the tracheobronchi become enlarged.

在吸气时，胸部扩张，此时空气进入肺内，气管支气管树的所有部位都扩大。

inspire [inˈspaiə] *v.* 吸入

Palpation is best performed with patients lying to the right and inspiring deeply.

在病人右侧卧位深吸气时最易进行触诊。

inspissate [inˈspiseit] *v.* (使)浓缩

A large collection of pus, unless discharged, may eventually become inspissated and then calcified.
大量蓄积的脓液,除非将其排出,否则最终可被浓缩,并被钙化。

instability [ˌinstəˈbiliti] *n.* 不稳定性
The infants of diabetic mothers tend to have general instability of glucose control.
糖尿病母亲的婴儿一般倾向有血糖调节不稳(的现象)。
Explosive personality disorder is characterized by instability of mood with liability to intemperate outbursts of anger, hate, violence or affection.
暴发性人格障碍以无控制的勃然大怒、憎恨、暴力行为和情感等不稳定为特征。

install [inˈstɔːl] *v.* 安装,设置
The tiny intraocular lenses are permanently installed inside the eye.
微型人工晶体(眼球内透镜)可永久性地植入眼内。
It is also a necessity to install smoke detectors to keep your child safe from burn injuries.
安装烟雾探测器让孩子免受烧伤也是必要的。

installation [ˌinstəˈleiʃən] *n.* 装置,设备
The operation for the installation of such a tube is called a tracheostomy.
装置这种管子的手术被称作气管造口术。

instance [ˈinstəns] *n.* 例子,实例,情况
In rare instances, infectious hepatitis may pursue a very rapid course and prove fatal.
在少有的情况下,传染性肝炎的病程进展迅速,并证明是致命的。
In most instances the clinical syndrome of rheumatic fever follows an infection due to streptococcus group A.
大多数病例中,在 A 组链球菌感染后出现风湿热的临床症候群。
Tumors may be elevated or deepseated, and in some instances are pedunculated(fibromas).
肿瘤可高出皮面或位于皮下,而且有的有蒂(如纤维瘤)。

instant [ˈinstənt] *a.* 立即的,直接的
The operation gives the patient instant vision.
手术使病人马上就能恢复视力。

instantly [ˈinstəntli] *ad.* 立即,即刻
A surgical team was instantly sent out to the spot of the accident by an ambulance.
外科医疗队已用救护车立刻送往出事地点。
In sensitive individuals, symptoms appear instantly.
过敏的患者症状立即出现。

instill [inˈstil] *v.* 逐渐灌输,注入,输入
If the stomach contents had a pH of 3.5 or less, 60 ml of antacid was instilled.
如果胃内容物的 pH 值为 3.5 或更低,则需输入 60ml 抗酸剂。

instinct [ˈinstiŋkt] *n.* 本能;天性
The role that instinct plays in human behavior is not yet clear.
本能在人的行为中所起到的作用至今尚未明了。

institute [ˈinstitjuːt] *v.* 实施,采取
Once the shock becomes progressive, the person will usually die unless strong measures of treatment are instituted.
一旦休克变成进行性加重,除非实施强有力的治疗,否则患者通常将会死亡。
After a disease is documented, it is necessary to establish the etiologic diagnosis in order to institute appropriate therapy.
当一种疾病得到证实以后,还必须明确病因诊断,以便采取适当的治疗措施。

institution [ˌinstiˈtjuːʃən] *n.* 机构
Hepatitis may occur in epidemic outbreaks in camps, schools, and institutions for children.

肝炎可能在军营、学校和儿童机构暴发流行。

institutional [ˌinstiˈtjuːʃənəl] *a.* 社会福利事业的,慈善机构的

Institutional care will remain necessary for some people, especially those who are severely disabled or live alone.

社会福利机构提供的照顾将仍是必需的,尤其是对那些严重残疾或独居的人们。

The death rate among institutional epileptics is four times that of the general population.

(医院、孤儿院等)慈善机构中的癫痫病死亡率是一般人群中的四倍。

instruction [inˈstrʌkʃən] *n.* 教育;指导;指令

The new DNA molecule functions with new instructions and begins to reproduce itself.

新的 DNA 分子按新的指令运作,并开始复制自己。

We now know that one gene carries the instructions for the synthesis of one enzyme that does a particular job.

我们现在知道一个基因带有合成一种能完成特定作用的酶的指令。

instructive [inˈstrʌktiv] *a.* 有教益的

The books and magazines in the reading room are very instructive.

阅览室里的那些书和杂志都是很有教益的。

instrument [ˈinstrumənt] *n.* 仪器,器械,工具

Movement of the echoes is traced on an electronic instrument called an oscilloscope, and record on film.

反射波的移动在叫做示波器的电子仪器上被描绘下来并记录在薄片上。

Those surgical instruments which were made in China are excellent.

那些中国制造的手术器械好极了。

The safety and capability of this instrument in providing adequate samples for histologic studies were first confirmed in dogs.

在为组织学研究提供足够的样本方面,这种工具的安全性和有效性最初是在狗身上得到证实的。

instrumentation [ˌinstrumenˈteiʃən] *n.* 器械;器械检查术

Medical instrumentation is growing in precision.

医学仪器精密化程度正在日益增长。

Occasionally, endocarditis may follow instrumentation in the gastrointestinal tract.

偶尔心内膜炎可发生于胃肠道器械检查术后。

insufficiency [insəˈfiʃənsi] *n.* 闭锁不全;功能不全

Pyelonephritis is the leading cause of renal insufficiency.

肾盂肾炎是肾功能不全的首要原因。

In rare cases, an early diastolic murmur of pulmonary insufficiency may be heard.

在少数病例中能听到肺动脉瓣闭锁不全的舒张早期杂音。

insufficient [insəˈfiʃənt] *a.* 不足的,不充分的

Our future approach will have to take into account the insufficient results.

我们未来的探索一定要考虑到这种不充分的结果。

insufflation [ˌinsʌˈfleiʃn] *n.* 吹入(法),吹入器

Insufflation is an act of blowing a vapor or powder into a cavity, as the lungs.

吹入(法)是把蒸气或粉末吹进体腔(如肺)。

A new kind of mouth-to-mouth insufflation is widely used in urgent resuscitation.

一种新型的嘴对嘴吹入器正被广泛用于紧急复苏。

insula [ˈinsjulə] *n.* 岛,脑岛

Insula is a triangular area of the cerbral cortex lying in the floor of the lateral fissure.

脑岛位于大脑皮层外侧裂底部的在三角区内。

insulate [ˈinsjuleit] *v.* 隔离,使绝缘

The separate nerve fibers are insulated from each other by Schwann cells.
各种神经纤维通过许旺氏细胞彼此间相互隔离。

insulation [ˌinsjuˈleiʃən] *n.* 隔离,绝缘材料

The fat in this sheet of tissue serves as insulation as well as a reserve store for energy.
这层组织中的脂肪既起着绝缘作用,又可作能量贮备。

insulin [ˈinsjulin] *n.* 胰岛素

The clinical picture of diabetes is due to diminished availability or effectiveness of insulin.
糖尿病的临床表现是由于胰岛素的可利用性或有效性降低造成的。

Insulin preparations are either fast acting, intermediate acting, or long acting.
胰岛素有短效、中效和长效制剂。

When the supply of glucose fails, as in insulin hypoglycaemia, grave consequences follow.
当葡萄糖供应不足时,如胰岛素性低血糖,会出现严重的后果。

insulinoma [ˌinsjuliˈnəumə] *n.* 胰岛素瘤

Insulinoma causes obesity from increased energy intake secondary to recurrent hypoglycemia.
胰岛素瘤病人由于反复发作低血糖使摄食增加导致肥胖。

insult [ˈinsʌlt] *n.* 损害

Most brain insults are accompanied by raised intracranial pressure.
大多数脑损伤都伴有颅内压的升高。

insurance [inˈʃuərəns] *n.* 保险,保险费

When her husband died, she received 50 000 pounds in insurance.
当她丈夫去世时,她得到了 5 万英镑的保险金。

Long-term medical insurance provides only 5% of the cost in some countries.
在某些国家,长期医疗保险仅提供 5% 的费用。

intact [inˈtækt] *a.* 未受损的

In the intact cell, the enzymes concerned are restricted to specific organelles.
在未受损伤的细胞内,这些酶被限制在特殊的细胞器内。

If there is delay, the membranes should be ruptured if they are intact.
如进展延缓,胎膜完整时应行破膜。

intake [ˈinteik] *n.* 摄取(量)

Volunteers were supplied with an extra 1000 kilocalories above normal energy intake.
志愿人员被提供多于正常 1 千卡的能量摄取。

Excessive intake can result also from taking very large amounts of calcium by mouth.
口服大量钙也能引起过度吸收。

integral [ˈintigrəl] *a.* 组成的;完整的; 不可或缺的

Identification of the agent involved should be an integral part of the treatment of the poisoned patient.
鉴别所用的化学剂应作为对中毒病人治疗的一个组成部分。

All nonpathogens, pathogens and spores must be destroyed in order to achieve integral asepsis.
所有的非病原体、病原体和孢子都要被消灭以达到完全无菌。

The adrenal gland plays an integral part in this process.
肾上腺在此过程中起重要作用。

The use of a comparator group that is of the highest possible quality is integral to the proper interpretation for the analysis of outcomes in clinical trial.
使用尽可能高质量的参比组对临床试验结果分析的恰当解释是不可或缺的。

integrase [ˈintigreis] *n.* 整合酶

HIV-1 integrase (IN) integrates viral DNA into host cells through two steps metal ions-dependent reactions.
HIV-1 整合酶(IN)通过两步依赖金属离子的反应将病毒 DNA 整合到宿主细胞中。

Integrase is one of the three enzymes of the virus that is required for viral replication.
整合酶是病毒复制所需要的三种酶之一。

integrate [ˈintigreit] *v.* 使成整体

Some viruses are able to become integrated into the cell's genetic content.
有些病毒能整合到细胞的遗传物质中去。

The stem cells not only formed new lung tissues but was also able to integrate into the existing lung tissues.
干细胞不仅可形成新的肺组织，而且能结合进现存的肺组织。

integration [ˌintiˈgreiʃən] *n.* 结合，综合，整合

Some viruses may persist indefinitely by the integration of their DNA with that of the host cell.
有些病毒通过其 DNA 与宿主细胞 DNA 的结合可以无限期地存留下来。

integrin [ˈintigrin] *n.* 黏合素分子，整合素

The second phase of tight adhesion is mediated by adhesion molecules of the integrin family.
紧密连接的第二步由黏合素分子介导。

The integrin family comprises over 20 different heterodimers.
整合素家族包括 20 多种不同的异二聚体。

Studies indicate that certain integrins can exist on the surface of a cell in an inactive conformation.
研究表明某些整合素能以无活性构象存在于细胞表面。

integrity [inˈtegriti] *n.* 完整，完全

This procedure may preserve the integrity of normal tissues.
本方法能完全地保存正常组织的完整性。

Numerous diseases are related to alteration in or loss of integrity of pharmacologic receptors.
许多疾病的治疗效果与其对药物受体的改变或缺损有关。

integument [inˈtegjumənt] *n.* 体被，皮；包膜

A severe burn presents two distinct problems, the shock and the local damage to the integument.
严重的烧伤出现两个明显的问题，即休克和皮肤的局部损伤。

intellectual [ˌintiˈlektjuəl] *a.* 智力的

Developmental speech disorder is not explicable in terms of general intellectual retardation.
发育性言语障碍是不能按一般智能发育延缓来解释的。

Intellectual functions tend to be relatively preserved but can be affected when the chronic encephalopathy is severe.
思维功能常能相对保留，但当慢性脑病严重时也会受到影响。

intelligence [inˈtelidʒəns] *n.* 智力，才智

The prognosis is generally poor and related most closely to the level of intelligence.
预后往往不良，且与智力水平的关系极为密切。

It is doubtful that using a single test to estimate the intelligence of persons from different social, racial, cultural, or economic backgrounds is reliable.
仅用一种测验方法来评估各种社会、种族、文化、经济背景的人们的才智，其可靠性是非常可疑的。

intelligible [inˈtelidʒəbl] *a.* 易于理解的

A muddled explanation was scarcely intelligible.
混乱的解释是难以被理解的。

intemperate [inˈtempərit] *a.* 无节制的

His intemperate (ie thoughtlessly angry or rude) remarks got him into trouble.
他那不加克制（即一味地怒气冲冲或粗鲁）的讲话使他陷入了困境。

intended [inˈtendid] *a.* 计划的，有意向的

The reason for using an intended population rather than the whole accessible population for the clinical study is simply a matter of convenience and practicality.

临床研究中用计划人群而不是整个可获得人群的理由仅仅是考虑到方便和实际可行性。

intense [in'tens] *a.* 强烈的，紧张的

In spite of intense research the etiology of leukemia remains unknown at present.

尽管做了认真的研究，白血病的病因至今仍未明了。

In recent years the miscellaneous group of conditions primarily involving the musculo-skeletal structures has been the subject of intense study.

近几年来，主要累及人体肌肉、骨骼组织的各种疾病已经成为深入研究的课题。

The patient's skin rash is most intense over the face and back.

这个病人的皮疹在整个脸上和背上极多。

intensify [in'tensifai] *v.* 加强，加剧

Pregnancy appears to intensify the severity of diabetes mellitus.

妊娠会加重糖尿病的严重程度。

We aimed to determine the efficacy and safety of giving intensified antiplatelet therapy for patients undergoing percutaneous coronary intervention.

我们的目的是要确定对接受经皮冠状动脉介入治疗的患者进行强化抗血小板治疗的疗效和安全性。

intensity [in'tensiti] *n.* 强度；强烈

Increased pulmonary artery pressure leads to an increased intensity of the second heart sound.

肺动脉压增加导致第二心音强度的增强。

The intensity of the physical exercise needed to reduce your risk of heart disease depends on your individual fitness level.

降低患心脏病危险所需的体育锻炼的强度取决于个人身体的健康水平。

intensive [in'tensiv] *a.* 加强的，增强的；深入细致的

Under intensive care, the patient is getting better day by day.

在重点监护下，这病人一天天好起来了。

Large general hospitals now usually have a variety of specialized intensive care units.

大的综合性医院现在通常都有各种专门化的监护室（加强护理病房）。

intent [in'tent] *n.* 意图

The presence of the intent to learn is, then, a prime requisite for effective learning.

那么，具有学习的意图就是有效学习所最必需的东西。

a. 专一的，专注的

I was so intent(up) on my work that I didn't notice the time.

我专心于我的工作，没有注意到时间。

intention [in'tenʃən] *n.* 愈合，意向

The healing of a clean, uninfected surgical incision approximated by surgical sutures is referred to as healing by first intention.

干净、无感染的外科切口经缝合后的愈合称为一期愈合。

Healing by second intention refers to the healing of the wounds that create large defects on the skin surface, causing extensive loss of cells and tissue.

二期愈合是指皮肤表面缺损较大的伤口的愈合，这种伤口细胞和组织的坏死较广泛。

intentional [in'tenʃənl] *a.* 有意的，故意的

Acute poisoning can be described as either accidental or intentional.

急性中毒可分为意外中毒和有意中毒两类。

The intentional or accidental ingestion of corrosives causes a severe chemical gastritis.

有意或无意摄入了具有腐蚀性的东西时可引起严重的化学性胃炎。

intentionally [in'tenʃənəli] *ad.* 有意(识)地，故意地

These surgical fields are left out quite intentionally in this book.

本书中有意地省略了外科领域(问题)。

interact(with) [ˌintəˈrækt] *v.* 互相作用

Numerous drugs exert their effects or side effects by interacting with enzymes.

许多药物通过与酶相互作用而发挥其药理作用或副作用。

interaction [ˌintəˈrækʃən] *n.* 相互作用,交互作用

The interaction of a drug with a specific receptor site is characterized by at least three factors.

药物与特异性受体的相互作用至少有三个因素。

intercellular [ˌintəˈseljulə] *a.* (细)胞间的

The plasma membranes of adjacent cells are separated by an intercellular space.

邻近细胞的浆膜被细胞间隙分隔开。

At this stage,the capillary endothelial intercellular junctions have widened and allow passage of macromolecules into the interstices.

在这个阶段,毛细血管内皮细胞间连接扩大,使得大分子得以进入细胞间质。

interchange [ˌintə(ː)ˈtʃeindʒ] *n.* ,v. 交换,互换

The blood is in fact an active carrier of oxygen and an important medium of gaseous interchange in the body.

事实上,血是一种具有活力的运输氧气的载体,同时也是体内气体交换的一个重要媒介。

interchangeable [ˌintəˈtʃeindʒəbl] *a.* 可交换地,可互换地

Fat and carbohydrates are interchangeable in their use in the body to a certain degree.

脂肪和糖在体内利用时,在一定程度上是可以互相交换的。

interchangeably [ˌintəˈtʃeindʒəbli] *ad.* 可互换地,可交换地

The following terms are often used erroneously and sometimes interchangeably.

下列术语常被误用,有时相互替换。

interchromosomal [ˌintəˌkrəuməˈsəuməl] *a.* 染色体间的

Interchromosomal translocations are most easily detected by spectral karyotyping.

检测染色体间易位最简单的方法是光谱核型分析。

Studies from diverse organisms show that distinct interchromosomal interactions are associated with many developmental events.

在多种生物中的研究显示各种染色体间的相互作用与许多发育过程相关。

intercommunication [ˈintəːkəˌmjuniˈkeiʃən] *a.* 相互联系,相互交流

There is regular intercommunication between the surgical specialists utilizing microsugery.

采用显微外科的专家们之间,有定期的相互交流(活动)。

intercostal [ˌintəˈkɔstəl] *a.* 肋间的

Intercostal nerve blocks are useful for postoperative pain relief.

肋间神经阻滞有助于缓解术后疼痛。

The intercostal and abdominal muscles contract,and the pressure in the lungs increases.

肋间肌和腹肌收缩,肺内压升高。

intercourse [ˈintəkɔːs] *n.* 交际;性交

Intercourse may cause bleeding from carcinoma or an adenomatous polyp of the cervix.

性交可使宫颈癌或宫颈腺瘤性息肉出血。

intercurrent [ˌintəˈkʌrənt] *a.* 在过程中发生的;间发的,介入的

Intercurrent infection is common in diabetic patients,particularly of the urinary tract and skin.

糖尿病人常发生感染,特别是尿路和皮肤(感染)。

Intercurrent infection must always be considered and treated.

必须经常考虑到反复感染的可能及其相应治疗。

interdependence [ˌintədiˈpendəns] *n.* 相互依赖,相互依存

There is a greater interdependence of the different organ systems than has been suspected.

在不同的器官系统之间存在着比以往觉察到的更大的相互依赖关系。

interdependent [intədiˈpendənt] *a.* 互相依存的

Medical and nursing practices have become more interdependent and the boundaries between them less clear.

医护工作变得更加相互依存,二者之间的界限不太清楚。

interdigitate [ˌintəˈdidʒiteit] *vi.* (如双手十指叉握似地)相间错杂,互相交叉; vt. 使交合

Interdigitating dendritic cells sarcoma is a form of malignant histiocytosis affecting dendritic cells.

并指状树突状细胞肉瘤是一种影响树突状细胞的恶性组织细胞增多症。

interface [ˈintəfeis] *n.* 界面,接口

Interface hepatitis refers to the lytic necrosis that involves the hepatocytes around the limiting plate at the peripheral of the lobules.

界面性肝炎是指发生在小叶周边界板处肝细胞的溶解坏死。

Interface hepatitis can occur in acute and chronic hepatitis.

界面性肝炎可发生于急性和慢性肝炎。

interfere(with) [ˌintəˈfiə] *v.* 干扰

Certain drugs also interfere with vitamin D metabolism.

某些药物也干扰维生素 D 的代谢。

The nasal obstruction often interferes seriously with the child' s nursing.

鼻阻塞常严重地妨碍婴儿喂奶。

Retention of sputum in the tracheobronchial tree may interfere with the ability of the lung to resist infection.

痰液在气管支气管树中积蓄会降低肺抵抗感染的能力。

SMZ does not interfere with the metabolism of mammalian cells.

SMZ 对于哺乳动物细胞的代谢并无影响。

interference [ˌintəˈfiərəns] *n.* 干扰,阻碍

Any interference with cardiac blood supply will result in damage to the heart muscle.

心肌血液供应的任何阻碍都会导致心肌损害。

In megaloblastic anemia interference with normal cellular maturation increases intramedullary cell death.

巨幼红细胞性贫血对正常细胞成熟过程的干扰增加了骨髓内细胞的死亡。

interferon [ˌintəˈfiərɔn] *n.* 干扰素

Interferon is a kind of hormone like substance.

干扰素是一种激素样物质。

At the very least, interferon will serve as a useful supplement to existing therapies for some cancers.

至少,干扰素对于某些癌症的现有疗法将起着有益的辅助作用。

intergenic [ˌintəˈdʒenik] *a.* 基因间的

RNA Pol Ⅱ recruitment to the target gene TATA box is not required for the intergenic transcription.

基因间转录不需要募集 RNA 聚合酶Ⅱ至靶基因 TATA 盒。

The intragenic and intergenic recombination frequencies observed varied considerably from experiment to experiment.

不同实验中基因内和基因间的重组频率很不相同。

interindividual [intəˌindiˈvidjuəl] *a.* 个体间的

The causes of this variability often may be related to interindividual differences in drug metabolism, drug interactions, or bone marrow reserves.

这种变异性的原因通常可能与药物代谢、药物相互作用或骨髓储备的个体间差异有关。

interior [inˈtiəriə] *a.* 内面的,内部的

The external, epithelial, and mucosal barriers protect the interior environment.
外部、上皮和黏膜屏障可以保护内环境。

interleukin(IL) [ˌintəˈljuːkin] *n.* 白(细胞)介素

Both estrogen and androgen suppress the production of IL-b.
雌激素和雄激素二者都可抑制白(细胞)介素-b 的生成。

Cytokines include traditional hormones, colony-stimulating factors and interleukins.
细胞因子包括传统的激素、集落刺激因子以及白介素。

intermediary [ˌintəˈmiːdjəri] *a.* 中间的

The liver is one of the internal organs especially adapted for intermediary metabolism and storage.
肝脏是特别适宜于中间代谢和储存的内脏器官之一。

intermediate [ˌintə(ː)ˈmiːdjət] *a.* 中间的

The host in which the larval stages of parasite develop are called the intermediate hosts.
寄生虫发育中的幼虫阶段的所在的宿主叫做中间宿主。

n. 中间体,媒介物

The manifestation of character neurosis are intermediate between normal character traits and neurotic symptoms.
性格神经症的表现是正常性格特征与神经症状之间的中间体。

intermittent [ˌintəˈmitənt] *a.* 间歇的,断断续续的

Colic is usually intermittent, and the interval of freedom from pain may at times be helpful.
绞痛通常是间歇的,疼痛间歇期有时也有参考价值。

Hydralazine is a long acting drug which should be administered by intermittent injection rather than continuous infusion.
肼苯哒嗪是一种长效药物,应做间断性注射而不宜连续滴注。

internal [inˈtəːnl] *a.* 内的,内部的,体内的

The complexity of the body's internal clock is becoming increasingly clear to researchers.
研究者们越来越清楚地认识到人体内部生物钟的复杂性。

The bleeding must be coming from an internal injury.
此出血一定来自身体内部的损伤。

Internal medicine is a branch of medicine dealing with the diagnosis and medical treatment of disease of internal structure of the human body.
内科是医学的一个分支,涉及人体内部结构疾病的诊断和药物治疗。

internalization [inˌtəːnəlaiˈzeiʃən] *n.* 内化;内化作用

This increased accumulation and penetration of the drug can be attributed to the efficient internalization of the drug-containing micelles by the endocytotic mechanism.
药物蓄积和渗透的增加归因于含药胶束经细胞内饮机制而被有效内化的结果。

Confocal microscopy confirmed the internalization of the drug into the tumor cells.
共聚焦显微镜检证实药物通过内化作用进入肿瘤细胞。

internalize [inˈtəːnəlaiz] *v.* 内化,内吞

The phagocytic cells internalize microorganisms and then kill them.
吞噬细胞内化微生物并杀灭它们。

interne [ˈintəːn] *n.* [法] 实习医师

The interne assisted the surgeon in performing the operation.
实习医生协助外科医生做手术。

interneuron [ˌintəˈnjuərɔn] *n.* 中间神经元

Interneuron acts as a link between the different neurones in a reflex arc.
中间神经元在反射弧中不同神经元之间起联系作用。

internist [inˈtəːnist] *n.* 内科医师

An anesthesiologist should follow the patient closely in conjunction with the internist.
麻醉医生应当会同内科医生严密地观察病人的表现。

interoceptor [ˌintərəu'septə] *n.* 内感受器
Interoceptor is composed of sensory nerve cells that respond to and monitor changes within the body.
内感受器由感觉神经细胞组成，能监测体内变化并对其变化作出反应。

interoperability [ˌintərˌɔpərə'biliti] *n.* 互用性，共享
Achieving interoperability between electronic health records (EHRs) and registries will be increasingly important as adoption of EHRs and the use of patient registries for many purposes both grow significantly.
由于为多种目的而采用电子健康档案（EHRs）和使用病例登记都在显著增加，实现电子健康档案和病例登记的共享将越来越重要。
Greenway understands the importance of healthcare interoperability.
林荫道（一医疗服务公司名---译者注）理解医疗保健互用性的重要。

interphase ['intəfeiz] *n.* 分裂间期
Interphase is characterized by growth of the cell and duplication of its chromosomes.
分裂间期以细胞生长及其染色体复制为特征。
In some cells duplication of the chromosomes occurs during interphase; in others, during early prophase or late telophase.
有些细胞中染色体的复制发生在分裂间期，在另一些细胞中则发生在早前期或晚末期。

interpose [inter'pəuz] *v.* （使）插入，（使）干预
The tricuspid and the mitral valves are interposed between the ventricles and atria on the right and left sides of heart respectively.
三尖瓣和二尖瓣分别插在右侧和左侧心脏的心房和心室之间。

interpret [in'təːprit] *v.* 口译，解释，翻译
Will you please interpret for me?
请你为我翻译一下好吗？
All laboratory tests must be interpreted in the light of the clinical picture.
一切实验室化验必须从临床的角度来加以解释。
The presence of blood in the cerebrospinal fluid must be taken into account when interpreting the cell count and protein level.
在解释细胞计数和蛋白水平时，必须考虑到脑脊液内存在血液的情况。

interpretable [in'təːpretəbl] *a.* 可解释的
These reported medical data may not be interpretable.
这些报道的医学数据可能无法解释。

interpretation [inˌtəpri'teiʃən] *n.* 解释，阐明
The cause of this disease may be given several interpretations.
此病病因有几种解释。

interrelation [ˌintəri'leiʃən] *n.* 相互关系，相互联系
Parasitology is the science of parasitism to study the interrelation between parasite and host under certain environmental conditions.
寄生虫学是一门研究在一定环境条件下寄生虫和宿主之间相互关系的科学。

interrogation [inˌtərə'geiʃən] *n.* 讯问，质问
This article introduces the most fundamental skills necessary for the medical investigation—interrogation and examination.
该文介绍医疗检查上所需的两种最基本的技能——问诊和检查。

interrupt [intə'rʌpt] *v.* 中断，打扰
Therapeutic vaccine may well help multiple sclerosis sufferers by interrupting the progress of the

disease.

治疗性疫苗通过中断病情进展的方式可以有效地解除多发性硬化症患者的痛苦。

The therapy must not be interrupted until a satisfactory clinical and hematologic remission occurs.

不到临床表现和血象开始好转的时候,就不能停止治疗。

interscapular [ˌintə(ː)ˈskæpjulə] *a.* 肩胛间的

Tearing interscapular pain suggests dissecting aneurysm.

肩胛间撕裂样疼痛提示有夹层动脉瘤的存在。

intersex [ˈintəseks] *n.* 雌雄间性,间性

An individual with both male and female sex characteristics is called intersex.

具有男性和女性特征的个体被称为间性。

interspace [ˈintəspeis] *n.* 间隙

Electron microscopic histochemical studies have shown that this interspace contains glycoproteins and lipids which are thought to contribute to cellular cohesion.

电镜组织化学的研究显示此细胞间隙内会有糖蛋白和类脂质,它们被认为有助于细胞的内聚力。

interspecific [ˌintəspiˈsifik] *a.* 物种之间的,种间的

The notion that interspecific hybrids are rare is ill-founded.

认为种间杂交是罕见的这一观念是无根据的。

A major barrier to interspecific hybridization is sterility in the F1 progeny.

种间杂交的主要障碍是 F1 代的不育性。

intersperse [ˌintəˈspəːs] *v.* 散布,点缀

The LINE family represents a class of interspersed repetitive sequences.

LINE 家族是一类分散重复序列。

He interspersed the text with explanatory diagrams.

他在文本中穿插了解释性图表。

interstitial [ˌintəˈstiʃəl] *a.* 间质的

As a result of endothelial damage to capillaries, fluids is lost across capillaries and venules into interstitial spaces.

由于毛细血管内壁的损伤,体液便通过毛细血管和小静脉进入间质空隙而流失。

Interstitial nephritis and renal papillary necrosis are caused by both phenacetin and acetaminophen.

非那西汀和醋氨酚都可引起间质性肾炎和肾乳头坏死。

The protein concentration of the interstitial fluid in the brain is low.

脑内间隙液的蛋白质浓度低。

interstitium [ˌintə(ː)ˈstiʃiəm] *n.* 间质组织,小间隙

At high magnification, many neutrophils are seen in the tubules and interstitium in a case of acute pyelonephritis.

高倍镜下,见急性肾盂肾炎的肾小管和肾间质中有许多中性粒细胞。

interval [ˈintəvəl] *n.* 间隔,间距

Treatment consists of keeping the patient flat in bed for a 24-hour interval, then allowing him to be up so long as he does not experience headache again.

治疗包括病人在床上平卧 24 小时(的间隔),然后只要他不再感到头痛就允许起床活动。

This medicine must be taken at intervals of 6 hours.

此药应每 6 小时服用一次。

The patient should be followed at regular intervals with careful repeat examination.

对这位病人应进行定期随访,作仔细的复查。

intervene [ˌintəˈviːn] *v.* 干预,介入

The number of hours that have intervened between the accident and operation is a crucial factor.
事故与手术之间插入时间的长短是一个决定性因素。

To intervene manually in a routine and cause the computer to execute a jump instruction。
在程序运行过程中,进行人工中断或干预,使计算机执行一条转移指令。

Alcoholic addicts do not know that they have a problem and thus it is necessary for friends and family members to intervene.
酗酒成瘾者并不知道他们自己的问题,因此有必要让其朋友和家人对此进行干预。

intervention [ˌintəˈvenʃən] *n.* 干涉,介入

Surgical intervention is indicated in case the hemorrhage is beyond control.
万一出血无法控制就需要进行外科手术。

The extent of a malignant disease should be ascertained for effective therapeutic intervention.
为了采用有效的治疗方法,应查明恶性病的严重程度。

interventional [ˌintəˈvenʃənəl] *a.* 干涉的,介入的

The surgeon watches the operation on a video monitor which displays images obtained by interventional magnetic resonance imaging.
外科医生从视频监视器上观察手术操作,该监视器可将介入的磁共振成像所获得的图像显示出来。

Interventional radiology is a clinical subspecialty that uses fluoroscopy, CT, and ultrasound to guide percutaneous procedures such as inserting catheters, or dilating or stenting narrowed ducts or vessels.
介入放射学是临床上的一个亚专科,它利用荧光屏检查、计算机断层摄影和超声来指导经皮操作如插入导管,或对狭窄的管道或血管进行扩张或提供支持装置。

intervertebral [ˌintəˈvəːtibrəl] *a.* 椎(骨)间的

Between the articulating vertebral bodies is the intervertebral disc.
两个椎体之间连接处是椎间盘。

The intervertebral discs account for one quarter of the total length of the backbone.
所有椎间盘占脊柱总长度的四分之一。

interview [ˈintəvjuː] *n.* 会见,访问,面试

During this interview, the physician should inquire about the previous health care.
在访谈过程中,医生应当询问患者既往的保健情况。

Applicants will be called for interview in due course.
求职者将在适当时间应邀参加面试。

intervillous [ˌintəˈviləs] *a.* 绒毛间的

There may be calcification of the decidual plate, but the intervillous circulation is not impaired by this.
也许胎盘蜕膜板已有钙化,但绒毛间的循环并未因此受损。

intestinal [inˈtestinəl] *a.* 肠的

In addition to intestinal symptoms, a severe toxemia may occur.
除肠道症状外,还可发生严重的毒血症。

intestine [inˈtestin] *n.* 肠

The small intestine is much longer than the large intestine.
小肠比大肠长得多。

intima [ˈintimə] (pl. intimae [ˈintimiː]) *n.* 内膜

Arterial thrombi are much more commonly associated with atherosclerosis—a chronic disease of the intima of the arteries.
动脉血栓通常多伴有动脉粥样硬化——一种慢性的动脉内膜的疾病。

intimate [ˈintimit] *a.* 亲密的,深切(了解)的

During hospitalization these two patients have become intimate friends.

住院期间,这两位病人变成了亲密的朋友。

Professor Huang has an intimate knowledge of the theory of genome.

黄教授对基因组的理论有较深的了解。

intimately [ˈintimitli] *ad.* 亲密地,内部地

The uptake of transmitters is also intimately linked with functions of the nervous system.

递质的再摄取也同样与神经系统的功能密切相关。

intolerance [inˈtɔlərəns] *n.* 不容忍,不耐受

If intolerance is noted, either reduction of carbohydrate content or its exclusion must be carried out.

如已发现不耐受情况,必须减少或取消碳水化合物含量。

Some patients with heat intolerance due to thyrotoxicosis do not recognize this as abnormal.

有些由于甲状腺毒症而缺乏对热的耐受力的病人,没有认识到这种现象是不正常的。

intolerant [inˈtɔlərənt] *a.* 不容忍的,不能耐受的

People who were lactose intolerant could still consume lactose-reduced milk, low-fat hard cheese and yogurt.

不能耐乳糖的人仍能摄入低乳糖牛奶,低脂肪硬奶酪和酸奶。

intonation [ˌintəˈneiʃən] *n.* 音调,语调

In English, some questions have a rising intonation.

在英语(会话)中,有些问句常用升调。

intoxicate [inˈtɔksikeit] *v.* 使醉,使中毒

He had been in the bar all night and was thoroughly intoxicated.

他已在酒吧内泡了一整夜,并喝得烂醉。

A small number of patients are hypersensitive to the drug, and became intoxicated with the usual doses.

少数病人对药物过敏,甚至在常规用量下也会中毒。

intoxication [inˌtɔksiˈkeiʃən] *n.* 中毒

Initially, morphine stimulates the vomiting center, and emesis occurs early in intoxication.

开始时吗啡可兴奋呕吐中枢,故中毒时呕吐最早出现。

There is no known antidote for antihistamine intoxication.

现在还不知有抗组胺药物中毒的解毒剂。

intraabdominal [intrəæbˈdɔminəl] *a.* 腹内的

Intra-abdominal abscess is the most frequent serious complication of peritonitis.

腹内脓肿是腹膜炎最常见的严重并发症。

Noninvasive diagnosis of intraabdominal arterial disease will not be covered here.

在此将不叙述对腹内动脉疾病的非损伤性诊断。

intraalveolar [ˈintrəælˈviələ] *a.* 肺泡内的

The transplant was consolidated due to massive intraalveolar exudate.

植入的肺因肺泡内有大量渗出物而变硬。

The latter increases intraalveolar pressure and therefore reduces transudation of fluid from the alveolar capillaries.

后者使肺泡内压力增加,因此减少由肺泡毛细血管来的漏出液。

intraaortic [ˌintrəeiˈɔːtik] *a.* 主动脉内的

Intraaortic balloon counterpulsation augments cardiac output by reducing afterload, increases coronary blood flow and may decrease myocardial oxygen consumption.

主动脉内气囊反搏术通过减少后负荷来增加心输出量,并且能增加冠状动脉内的血流,也可减少心肌耗氧量。

intraarterial [ˌintrəɑːˈtiəriəl] *a.* 动脉内的

If it does not delay treatment unduly, recording pulmonary vascular pressure and intraarterial

pressure directly is advisable.
如果不会不恰当地耽误治疗，建议直接监测肺血管内压力和动脉内压力。

intraarticular [ˌintrəuɑːˈtikjulə] *a.* 关节内的
In osteoarthritis, corticosteroids are given by intraarticular injection.
患有骨关节炎时，皮质激素可作关节腔内注射。

intrabronchial [ˌintrəˈbrɔŋkiəl] *a.* 支气管内的
Atelectasis from obstruction of a major airway may require intrabronchial suction through an endoscope.
大气道阻塞引起的肺不张可能要经内镜行支气管内抽吸。

intracardiac [ˌintrəˈkɑːdiæk] *a.* 心内的
The use of acupuncture anesthesia has been extended to more complicated operation such as intracardiac direct vision surgery with the aid of extracorporeal circulation.
针刺麻醉已能用于更加复杂的外科手术，如在体外循环的条件下进行心内直视手术。
The use of intracardiac electrophysiologic techniques with programmed stimulation can be helpful in detecting cardiac rhythm abnormalities.
使用心脏内电生理程序性刺激技术有助于监测心脏的节律异常。

intracellular [ˌintrəˈseljulə] *a.* 细胞内的
Viruses are obligate intracellular parasites.
病毒是一种专性细胞内寄生物。
About 56 percent of an adult human body is fluid. Some of this fluid is inside the cell and is called intracellular fluid.
成年人身体约 56% 是液体，有些液体在细胞内，称为细胞内液。

intracerebral [ˌintrəˈseribrəl] *a.* 脑内的
The mice have been given intracerebral injections of the pathogenic strain.
这些鼠脑内已注射了各种致病菌。

intracordally [ˌintrəˈkɔːdli] *ad.* 心内地
Epinephrine or isoproterenol may be administered intracordally in cardiac arrest.
在心脏骤停时可向心内注射肾上腺素或异丙肾上腺素。

intracranial [ˌintrəˈkreiniəl] *a.* 颅内的
The unexpected death of this person was caused by an intracranial hemorrhage.
这人的意外死亡是由于颅内出血。
The child's skull x-ray shows diffuse intracranial calcifications.
这小儿头颅 X 线片显示颅内广泛钙化。

intractability [inˌtræktəˈbiləti] *n.* 难治，顽固
The discovery of a duodenal ulcer without the complications of bleeding, obstruction, perforation, or intractability to medical therapy calls for a trial of medical management.
十二指肠溃疡如无出血、梗阻、穿孔等合并症或属非难治性的均可用内科治疗。

intractable [inˈtræktəbl] *a.* 难治的，顽固的
The doctor is treating a diabetic patient with intractable angina.
医生正在治疗一个伴有难治的心绞痛的糖尿病患者。
A 15-year-old girl presented with a 4-year history of intractable asthma.
一个 15 岁的女孩有 4 年顽固性哮喘的病史。

intracytoplasmic [ˌintrəˌsaitəuˈplæzmik] *a.* 细胞浆内的
Intracytoplasmic sperm injection is an in vitro fertilization procedure in which a single sperm is injected directly into an egg.
卵细胞浆内单精子注射是单个精子注射到卵子中的体外受精方式。

intradermal [ˌintrəˈdəːməl] *a.* 皮内的
An intradermal (i. d.) injection delivers antigen into the dermis of the skin.

皮内注射将抗原注入皮肤组织的真皮层。

Definitie diagnosis is made with the use of intradermal skin tests.

通过皮内试验确定诊断。

intraepithelial [ˌintrəˌepiˈθiːliəl] *a.* 上皮内的

Complications include cervical intraepithelial neoplasia and pelvic inflammatory disease.

并发症包括子宫颈上皮内肿瘤形成和盆腔感染。

Cervical intraepithelial neoplasia is divided into 3 grades.

宫颈上皮内瘤变分为 3 级。

High grade intraepithelial neoplasia includes carcinoma in situ, which may progress to invasive carcinoma.

高级别上皮内瘤变包括原位癌,可能进展为浸润癌。

intragenic [ˌintrəˈdʒenik] *a.* [遗] 基因内的

In humans, expansion of intragenic triplet repeats is associated with various diseases.

在人类,基因内的三联重复序列扩增与多种疾病有关。

More than 75% of all genes with long intragenic tandem repeats encode cell-surface proteins.

含基因内长串联重复序列的基因中,超过 75% 都编码细胞表面蛋白。

intrahepatic [ˌintrəhiˈpætik] *a.* 肝内的

Intrahepatic hypertension acts as a potent stimulus for renal Na^+ retention.

肝内(血管)高压对肾脏钠潴留是一个重要的刺激因子。

The main diagnostic problem is to distinguish between an intrahepatic and extrahepatic cause.

诊断的主要问题是区别肝内和肝外的病因。

intraject [ˈintrəˈdʒekt] *n.* 皮内注射器

The new intraject consists of an actuator and a glass cartridge containing the medication.

新型的皮内注射器由一个促动装置和一个装有药物的玻璃筒组成。

intralipid [ˌintrəˈlipid] *n.* 脂肪乳剂

The proposal is to establish the hyperlipemic mouse model by long-term gastric perfusion of intralipid or intralipid plus glucose.

建议采用脂肪乳剂或脂肪乳剂加葡萄糖长期灌胃来建立小鼠高脂血症模型。

Studies on the stability of intralipid must be done.

必须进行脂肪乳剂的稳定性的研究。

intraluminal [ˌintrəˈljuːminəl] *a.* 管腔内的

The detail of intraluminal mucosa demonstrated on modern air-contrast barium examinations far exceeds that available by other, more sophisticated diagnostic imaging examinations.

气-钡双重造影术比其他更复杂的影像学检查能更清楚地显示管腔内的黏膜。

intramural [ˌintrəˈmjuərəl] *a.* (器官)壁内的

All fibromyomata begin as intramural growths, which are commonly of small or moderate size.

所有纤维肌瘤开始时均为肌壁间肌瘤,通常为小或中等大小肿瘤。

intramuscular [ˌintrəˈmʌskjulə] *a.* 肌内的

The route of administration may be intramuscular or intravenous.

给药方法可肌内注射,亦可静脉注射。

Penicillin G procaine suspension is designed for deep intramuscular injection.

普鲁卡因青霉素 G 混悬液是专为深部肌内注射而设计的。

intramuscularly [ˌintrəˈmʌskjuləli] *ad.* 肌内地

Injections should be given intramuscularly within five days after exposure to measle patients.

与麻疹病人接触后应在 5 天内做肌内注射。

intranasal [ˌintrəˈneizəl] *a.* 鼻内的

Differing from cocaine mainly in their longer duration of action, the amphetamine are rapidly absorbed after oral and intranasal administration(peak blood level is 30 minutes to 3 hours).

口服和鼻腔吸入安非他明能快速吸收(血药浓度可在 30 分钟至 3 小时达到峰值),而给予可卡因的特点是作用持续时间长。

intranuclear [ˌintrəˈnjuːkliə] *a.* 核内的

Intranuclear inclusion bodies can be demonstrated in the bronchial mucosa in the case of adenoviruses.

在腺病毒病例中的支气管黏膜可看到核包涵体。

intraocular [ˌintrəˈɔkjulə] *a.* 眼内的,眼球内的

An estimate of intraocular pressure can be obtained by palpation of the globe through the lids.

眼压可以在眼睑上对眼球触诊来估计。

The intraocular lenses have basically made these people normal again.

人工晶体(眼球内透镜)使这些人基本上恢复了正常视力。

intraoperative [ˌintrəˈɔpərətiv] *a.* 外科手术中的

Long-standing pulmonary hypertension or recurrent pulmonary infarction may result in irreversible pulmonary hypertension leading to intraoperative death.

长期肺血管高压或反复发生的肺梗死会引起不可逆的肺动脉高压,导致手术中死亡。

intrapericardial [ˌintrəˌperiˈkɑːdiəl] *a.* 心包内的

The venous pressure varies with the intrapericardial pressure.

静脉压随着心包内压而变化。

intraperitoneal [ˌintrəˌperitəuˈniːəl] *a.* 腹膜内的

Peritoneal dialysis in ARF is effected through a temporary intraperitoneal catheter.

急性肾衰(ARF)时,腹膜透析是通过一根临时置入腹膜腔内的管子进行的。

However, in toxicologic studies, such special routes as intraperitoneal, intramuscular, and subcutaneous injections are often used.

然而,在毒理学研究中,特殊途径如腹腔注射、肌内注射和皮下注射常被采用。

intrapleural [ˌintrəˈpluərəl] *a.* 胸膜内的

It has been proposed that large negative intrapleural pressures during acute severe asthma may be associated with the development of interstitial edema.

有人提出急性重症哮喘时较大的胸膜内负压可能与间质水肿的形成有关。

intrastromal [ˈintrəˈstrəuməl] *a.* 基质内的

An implant known as an intrastromal corneal ring(ICR) has been designed by Keravision of Santa Clara in California.

一种称为基质内角膜环(ICR)的植入物已由加州圣克拉拉的 Keravision 公司设计出来。

intrathecal [ˌintrəˈθiːkəl] *a.* 鞘内的

Spinal anesthesia is achieved by injecting a local anesthetic into the lumbar intrathecal space.

将局麻药注射到腰部鞘内间隙可获得脊髓麻醉。

intrathoracic [ˌintrəθɔːˈræsik] *a.* 胸内的

The trachea is normally in the midline position. A shift of the trachea from its midline position is indicative of intrathoracic disease.

正常的气管处于中线位置,若气管从其中线位置移位则表明胸腔内有了疾病。

intrauterine [ˌintrəˈjuːtərain] *a.* 子宫内的

The longer the membranes are ruptured the greater the likelihood of intrauterine infection.

胎膜破裂的时间越长,宫内感染发生的可能性越大。

intravascular [ˌintrəˈvæskjulə] *a.* 脉管内的,血管内的

Sepsis was a well-known underlying cause of disseminated intravascular coagulation.

众所周知败血症是扩散性血管内凝血的根本原因。

intravenous [ˌintrəˈviːnəs] *a.* 静脉内的

The route of administration may be intramuscular or intravenous.

给药方法可肌内注射,亦可静脉注射。

Actinomycin D used in some diseases is designed for intravenous injection only.
治疗某些疾病用的放线菌素 D 只能作静脉注射。

intravenously [ˌintrəˈviːnəsli] *ad.* 由静脉内

In case of collapse, normal salt solution should be given intravenously.
如果出现虚脱,应该静脉注射生理盐水。

intraventricular [ˌintrəvenˈtrikjulə] *a.* 心室内的

Intraventricular hemorrhage usually occurs as a result of extension from an intraparenchymal or a subarachnoid site.
室内出血通常是由于在实质脏器内或者是蛛网膜下腔内出血后再蔓延的结果。

intravesical [ˌintrəˈvesikəl] *a.* 膀胱内的

Two patients required both intravenous and intravesical administration of amphotericin B.
2 例病人需要在静脉内和在膀胱内注入两性霉素 B。

intravital [ˌintrəˈvaitəl] *a.* 活体的

The macrophages were demonstrated by intravital staining.
巨噬细胞通过活体染色来显示。

We have developed novel laboratory tools and protocols for intravital imaging acquisition of the thymus.
我们已经开发出新颖的实验室设备和操作规程,用于胸腺的活体图像采集。

intricacy [ˈintrikəsi] *n.* 错综,复杂;(*pl.*)错综复杂的事物

The developments in electron microscope techniques have made it possible to reveal the tremendous intricacies of intracellular organization.
电子显微镜技术的发展已使显示细胞内细胞器的极其复杂的结构成为可能。

intricate [ˈintrikit] *a.* 复杂的

But hypothermia cannot be used safely in long and intricate surgery.
但是,低温法不能安全地使用于时间长的复杂手术。

The respiratory system is an intricate arrangement of spaces and passageways which serve to conduct air into the lungs.
呼吸系统是由许多空腔和管道错综复杂地组合在一起的,其作用是引导空气进入肺部。

intriguing [inˈtriɡiŋ] *a.* 引起兴趣的

The most intriguing details of thermoregulation are emerging from studies of hibernation.
有关温床调节的最引起兴趣的详情来自对冬眠的研究。

The motion of bacteria was so intriguing that Leeuwenhock recorded the activity in the classic illustration.
细菌的运动十分有趣,促使李文霍克用标准的图解记录下了它们的活动。

intrinsic [inˈtrinsik] *a.* 内在的;内部的

Vitamin B_{12} is present in liver and requires intrinsic factors for absorption.
维生素 B_{12}存在于肝内,并需要内源因素以助吸收。

Intrinsic activity implies that drug binds to the receptor and results in pharmacologic actions.
内在活性意指药物与受体结合并产生药理作用。

introduce [ˌintrəˈdjuːs] *v.* 引进;转入,传入;采用;介绍;插入,导入

The professor introduced the interns to each other.
教授介绍实习医生们相互认识。

When Gruntzig introduced a dilating balloon catheter in 1974, it was a significant improvement.
1974 年 Gruntzig 推出了一种扩张球囊导管,这是一个非常显著的进步。

Through this spot the needle of a hypodermic containing 2 percent procaine or mepivacaine solution is introduced.
通过此点皮下进针后注入 2% 普鲁卡因或甲哌卡因溶液。

introduction [ˌintrəˈdʌkʃən] *n.* 介绍;采用;引进;传入;导言

With the introduction of potent modern drugs, the possibility now exists that we ourselves may be in part responsible for the state of the treated patient.
当推荐各种强力新药时，我们本身就对受治病人的使用后果负有了一部分责任。
I have used discretion however in the introduction of new material.
我对新资料的采用一直持谨慎态度。
One must part the labia before introduction of the speculum so that the orifices are exposed.
在阴道镜插入之前，应分开阴唇以暴露尿道外口和阴道口。

introductory [intrəˈdʌktəri] *a.* 介绍的；导言的；初步的
An introductory course in medicine is given by some schools in the latter half of the second year.
某些学校在第二年的下学期开设医学绪论课。
There are always introductory remarks on the first page of many medical books.
许多医学书籍的第一页常有一个绪言。

intron [ˈintrɔn] *n.* 内含子
Introns are not expressed.
内含子是不表达的。
The collagen gene has 50 introns.
胶原基因有 50 个内含子。

introspection [ˌintrəuˈspekʃən] *n.* 内省，判断法
Some psychologists tried to contrast retrospection and introspection.
一些心理学家试图对比回顾与内省。
When compared to global introspection, there is a great improvement in the consistency of ratings among reviewers.
与综合判断法相比较，各评估者间评估等级的一致性有很大改进。

intubate [ˈintjubeit] *v.* 插管
This allows the trachea to be intubated within 60 ~ 90 seconds.
这样能在 60 ~ 90 秒钟内行气管插管。

intubation [ˌintjuˈbeiʃən] *n.* 插管(法)
Oxygen is usually given by mask beforehand to allow maximum time for intubation.
通常事先给予面罩吸氧，使有最大限度的时间可用以插管。
Obstruction of respiratory tract may be caused by secretions resulting from chronic obstructive pulmonary disease, intubation, or anesthetic agents.
呼吸道的阻塞可由慢性阻塞性肺部疾病、插管或麻醉剂产生的分泌物引起。

intussusception [ˌintəsəˈsepʃən] *n.* 套叠，肠套叠
Small bowel intussusception is an uncommon cause of early postoperative obstruction in adults.
小肠套叠不是成年人早期术后肠梗阻常见的原因。
90% of postoperative intussusceptions occur during the first 2 postoperative weeks.
90% 的术后肠套叠发生于手术后的头两周。

invade [inˈveid] *v.* 入侵，侵犯
The micro-organisms invade the body successfully where they grow and reproduce in sufficient numbers to produce the clinical features of a disease.
微生物侵入人体，在体内生长并大量繁殖以致产生疾病的临床症状。
Scientists have recently witnessed live how aggressive cells from the immune system invade brain tissue and cause considerable brain damage.
科学家们最近现场目睹了免疫系统的激进细胞如何入侵脑组织并引起大量脑损伤。

invalid[1] [ˈinvæliːd] *n.* 伤病员，病弱者
It really revolutionized eye care for these patients, because they used to be invalids.
对这些病人的眼睛治疗确实是一个革命，因为他们过去只能是残疾人。
a. 有病的

The invalid boy is confined to a wheel chair.
这个体弱多病的男孩只能坐在轮椅里活动。

invalid[2] [in'vælid] *a.* 无效的

A prescription is invalid without the signature of a medical doctor.
处方没有医生的签名是无效的。

invalidate [in'vælideit] *v.* 使无效，使无力

The side reaction does not invalidate its use.
此药即使有副作用也不要取消其使用。

invalidism ['invəlidizəm] *n.* 病弱，伤残

On the other hand, it should not be allowed to become an excuse for invalidism.
另一方面，不应使它成为导致病残的借口。

invaluable [in'væljuəbl] *a.* 非常宝贵的，无价的

Invasive hemodynamic monitoring is invaluable for guiding therapy in complicated patients.
对病情复杂的病人而言，非创伤性血流动力学监测对指导治疗是极有价值的。

invariable [in'vɛəriəbl] *a.* 不变的，恒定的，一律的

Pallor is invariable in syncope whereas cyanosis may occur in seizure.
发生晕厥时病人总是面色苍白而癫痫发作时可出现发绀。

In hereditary spherocytosis splenomegaly is almost invariable and, rarely, may cause abdominal discomfort.
遗传性球形红细胞增多症几乎都有脾肿大，但很少引起腹部不适。

invariably [in'vɛəriəbli] *ad.* 不变地，总是

Anemia is almost invariably associated with lower erythrocyte count.
贫血几乎总是伴有红细胞计数较少的情况。

Necrosis is invariably a pathological consequence of cell damage.
坏死必然是细胞损伤的病理性结果。

invariant [in'vɛəriənt] *a.* 不变的，不变量，不变式

The T-cell receptor complex is made up of antigen-recognition proteins and invariant signaling proteins.
T 细胞受体复合物由抗原识别蛋白和恒定信号蛋白组成。

invasion [in'veiʒən] *n.* 侵入 ，侵害，侵袭

A number of major pathogens cause disease without further invasion of host tissues.
有一些严重的致病菌不需深层地侵入人体组织就可致病。

Inflammation is the body' s reaction to invasion by an infectious agent, antigen challenge or even just physical damage.
炎症是机体对感染物的入侵、抗原的刺激、或只是物理性损伤所作出的反应。

invasive [in'veisiv] *a.* 侵入的，侵害的

More information should be obtained to strengthen the case for or against the performance of invasive studies.
应获取更多信息，以确定此病例是否应进行损伤性检查。

In the present case, it appears that invasive lung cancer caused local consumption coagulopathy.
此病例似乎是由侵入性肺癌引起了局部消耗性血凝病。

inverse [in'vəːs] *a.* 倒转的，相反的

There is a general inverse correlation between the latent period and the severity of symptoms.
潜伏期长短与病状的严重程度之间一般呈相反的关系。

inversely [in'vəːsli] *ad.* 相反地

The incidence of coronary heart disease is inversely related to the level of high density lipoproteins.
冠心病的发生率与高密度脂蛋白的浓度值成反比关系。

The blood cholesterol level tends to change inversely with thyroid function.
血胆固醇水平常倾向和甲状腺的功能成反比变化。

inversion [inˈvəːʃən] *n.* 倒位(染色体畸变)；反向；转化

Inversion is the structural abnormality characterized by reversal of a segment with the chromosome.
倒位是以染色体片段颠倒为特征的结构异常。

Inversion is applied to the state to the womb after childbirth when its upper part is pulled through the cervical canal.
内翻用于描述产后子宫上部经宫颈管道牵拉出来时的状态。

invert [inˈvəːt] *v.* 倒置

The QRS-complex is prolonged and slurred with a small Q-, an upright tall R-wave and an inverted T-wave in S1.
S1 导联表现为 QRS 综合波群时间延长和小的 Q 波，高耸直立的 R 波和倒置的 T 波。

invertebrate [inˈvəːtibrit] *n.* 无脊椎动物

Any animal that has no spinal column is called invertebrate.
任何没有脊柱的动物叫无脊椎动物。

inverted [inˈvəːtid] *a.* 内生性的

Inverted papilloma usually occurs in the bladder and nasal cavity.
内生性乳头状瘤常发生于膀胱和鼻腔。

If not adequately excised, inverted papilloma has a high rate of recurrence.
如果切除不充分，内生性乳头状瘤很容易复发。

investigate [inˈvestigeit] *v.* 调查，调查研究

Some bioengineers have taken the lead in investigating the effects of this technological innovation.
有些生物工程学家已带头对这项技术革新的效果进行调查。

We should investigate whether some genes coding for products are related to the disease.
我们应该研究某些基因编码的产物是否与这种疾病有关。

investigation [inˌvestiˈgeiʃən] *n.* 调查，调查研究

The important laboratory investigation is to search for tubercle bacilli.
重要的化验检查是寻找结核菌。

investment [inˈvestmənt] *n.* 投资

For various reasons, including the high costs of vaccine development and the prospect of much higher profitability from investments in other products, the number of vaccine manufacturers had declined.
由于各种原因，包括生产疫苗成本高以及投资其他产业收益更高的前景，生产疫苗的厂家已减少。

invisible [inˈvizəbl] *a.* 看不见的，无形的

Germs are invisible to the naked eye.
细菌是肉眼看不见的。

X-rays, gamma-rays, and other radiations from radioactive sources are invisible and can injure a person seriously.
X 线、γ 射线及其他来自放射源的辐射线是肉眼看不见的，并能严重损害人体。

in vitro [inˈvaitrəu] *ad.* [拉] 在试管中，在体外，离体

In vitro means the studies performed outside a living organism such as in a laboratory.
离体是指在活体以外(如在实验室)进行的研究，

Unfortunately, the in vitro work does not help us.
遗憾的是体外的研究对我们没有什么帮助。

in vivo [inˈviːvəu] *ad.* [拉] 在活的机体内，在体

In vivo means the studies carried out in living organisms.
在体是指在活体内进行的研究。
A mutagenicity program consisting of four in vitro and two in vivo studies has been carried out.
有关致突变性的研究也已经开展,包含四个体外研究和两个体内研究。

involuntary [inˈvɔləntəri] *a.* 不随意的
Muscles are divided into two great classes: the voluntary and the involuntary muscles.
肌肉分成两大类:随意肌和不随意肌。

involute [ˈinvəluːt] *v.* 退化
The mammalian thymus involutes with age.
哺乳动物的胸腺随着年龄的增加而逐年退化。

involution [ˌinvəˈluːʃən] *n.* 退化
Cortisol produces eosinophilia and causes involution of lymphoid tissues.
应用氢化可的松之后可引起嗜酸性粒细胞增多症和淋巴组织的退化。

involve [inˈvɔlv] *v.* 累及,牵涉;包含
Paralysis most frequently involves the legs, although any muscle group can be involved.
尽管任何肌肉群均可受累,但麻痹最常累及到腿部。
Endometriosis occasionally involves the bladder.
子宫内膜异位偶尔侵及膀胱。
In carcinoma involving the gastrointestinal tract, blood loss is the most common cause of anemia.
胃肠道有癌肿时,失血是贫血最常见的原因。
Sleep apnea disorder involves two major symptoms.
睡眠呼吸暂停疾病包括两种主要症状。

involvement [inˈvɔlvmənt] *n.* 累及,牵连;病
Involvement of the cranial nerves when present may result in strabismus and deafness.
当出现波及脑神经的情况时,可导致斜视及耳聋。
Arthritis may refer to dozens of different types of joint involvement.
关节炎可以涉及几十种不同类型的关节疾患。
Cytomegalovirus might cause more subtle yet clinically significant forms of neurological involvement.
巨细胞病毒可能引起更加细微的但有明显临床表现的神经系统疾病。

iodide [ˈaiədaid] *n.* 碘化物
Dietary sources of iodine are sea food and vegetables grown in soil containing iodide and also iodized table salt.
碘的食物来源是海产品类食物、生长在含碘土壤的蔬菜以及加碘后的食盐。
It is stored in fat and may provide excess iodides for months after the discontinuation of therapy.
在停止治疗后数月,沉积于脂肪组织内的碘化物还会释放出多余的部分。

iodine [ˈaiədiːn] *n.* 碘
After 60 sec, the dye is washed off and the smear is flooded with an iodine solution.
60 秒钟后洗去染料,涂片用碘液漫过。

iodization [ˌaiəudaiˈzeiʃən] *n.* 碘化
Discontinuation of salt iodization was associated with a rapid return of thyroid dysfunction in school-age children.
中止食盐加碘与学龄儿童甲状腺功能不全的快速反弹联系在一起。
The government must encourage and ensure that all salt producers and/or processors abide by government rules and regulations, and that the iodization program is effective in eliminating iodine deficiency disorders.
政府必须鼓励和确保所有食盐生产者和(或)加工者遵守政府规章制度,并且确保碘化方案对消除碘缺乏病有效。

iodohippurate [ˈaiədəuˈhipjuːreit] *n.* 碘马尿酸钠

In this paper HPLC is applied to study radiochemical purity and chemical purity of ^{131}I-sodium iodohippurate.

本文用高效液相色谱法研究了碘^{131}马尿酸钠 I 注射液的放化纯度和化学纯度。

We want to know the crystal and molecular structures of iodohippurate.

我们想了解碘马尿酸钠的晶体和分子结构。

ion [aiən] *n.* 离子

The kidneys regulate the concentrations of most of the ions in the body fluids.

肾脏调节体液中大多数离子的浓度。

The haemoglobin removes hydrogen ions in the capillaries as above and carries them to the lungs.

如上所述,血红蛋白清除毛细血管的氢离子,并将其带到肺部。

ionic [aiˈɔnik] *a.* 离子的

In ionic bonds, electrons are tranferred from one atom to another.

在离子键中,电子从一个原子传递给另一个原子。

Ionic detergent is an ionic surface active agent.

离子去垢剂是一种离子表面活性剂。

ionizable [ˈaiənaizəbl] *a.* 离子化的

Most bell shaped pH curves are interpreted to suggest two or more ionizable groups involved in catalytic activity.

大多数钟形 pH 曲线,被解释为表示有两个或更多的离子化基团,且与催化活性有关。

ionization [ˌaiənaiˈzeiʃən] *n.* 电离,离子化

The extent of ionization of weak organic acids and bases depends on the *PH* of the medium.

弱有机酸和弱有机碱的电离度取决于介质的酸碱度。

X-ray ionization effect is the basic principle of X-ray protection.

X 线的电离效应是 X 线防护的基本原理。

ionize [ˈaiənaiz] *v.* (使)电离,离子化

The hydrogen ions are partially derived from the ionized histidyls in the β-chains.

氢离子部分来源于 β 链中离子化的组氨酰残基。

ionizing [ˈaiəˌnaiziŋ] *n.* 离子化的,电离的

The immune system is extremely sensitive to ionizing radiation.

免疫系统对电离辐射极其敏感。

Medical ionizing radiation plays most part in artificial radiation application.

在人工辐射应用上,医用电离辐射起着最重要的作用。

ionophore [aiˈɔnəfɔː] *n.* 离子载体

Neutrophils activated with a calcium ionophore released huge amounts of active proteases.

钙离子载体激活的中性粒细胞释放了大量的活性蛋白酶。

The membranes containing the ionophores were evaluated.

包含离子载体的膜已被评估。

iontophoresis [ai,ɔntəufəˈriːsis] *n.* 离子透入(疗法)

Iontophoresis is a novel drug delivery system designed to improve the delivery rate of compounds.

离子导入是一种旨在提高药物传递速率的新型药物传递系统。

Iontophoresis enhances drug delivery across the skin by electrorepulsion and electroosmosis.

离子导入可通过电子斥力和电渗增强药物的透皮转运。

ipratropium [iprəˈtrəupiəm] *n.* 异丙托溴铵

Anticholinergic medicines such as ipratropium block this effect, allowing the airways to open.

抗胆碱能药如异丙托溴铵可以阻断这种效应,使气道开放。

The clinical result of inhaled salbutamol, ipratropium bromide and budesonide in the treatment of bronchiolitis was satisfactory.

吸入沙丁胺醇、异丙托溴铵和布地奈德来治疗细支气管炎的临床结果令人满意。

ipsilateral [ˌipsiˈlætərəl] *a.* 同侧的

Commonly involvement of the seventh cranial nerve will be associated with ipsilateral loss of taste.

通常第七脑神经受累将伴有同侧的味觉丧失。

IQ(intelligence quotient) *n.* 智力商数

In childhood and adult life IQ represents intellectual ability relative to the rest of the population.

在儿童和成人的生活中,智商是与人群中其他人的智能相比较得出的。

iridectomy [iriˈdektəmi] *n.* 虹膜切除术

Iridectomy is one of the most outstanding achievements in ophthalmic surgery.

虹膜切除术是眼科手术最杰出的成就之一。

iridocyclitis [ˌiridɔsaiˈklaitis] *n.* 虹膜睫状体炎

Inflammation of the iris and ciliary body of the eye is called iridocyclitis.

眼内虹膜和睫状体的炎症被称为虹膜睫状体炎。

iris [ˈaiəris] *n.* 虹膜

The purpose of the iris is to regulate the amount of light entering the eye.

虹膜的作用是调节进入眼睛的光线。

The muscle of the ciliary body is similar in direction and method of action to the radial muscle of the iris.

睫状体肌肉在活动的方向和方式上与虹膜的辐射状肌肉相似。

iritis [aiəˈraitis] *n.* 虹膜炎

Iritis may cause pain in or around the eye usually with blurring of vision.

虹膜炎可引起眼内或眼周疼痛,通常伴有视力模糊。

Iritis is uncommon in rheumatoid arthritis and systemic lupus erythematosus.

虹膜炎不常见于类风湿关节炎和系统性红斑狼疮等疾病。

iron [ˈaiən] *n.* 铁

A deficiency of iron may lead to anemia.

铁缺乏可导致贫血。

Daily iron requirements vary depending on age, sex, and physiological status.

每日铁需求量因年龄、性别和生理状况而异。

Sideroblastic anemia may be caused after excessive iron administration.

服用过多的铁后可引起铁粒幼红细胞性贫血。

irradiate [iˈreidieit] *v.* 照射

The irradiated lymphoma may be melting away in the course of a week.

被照射的淋巴瘤可在一周疗程中消失。

Surgical wounds in heavily irradiated tissues may heal slowly or may break down in the presence of infection.

手术伤口在大剂量照射组织时愈合缓慢,或在感染时发生破裂。

irradiation [iˌreidiˈeiʃən] *n.* 照射

The ovaries may be affected by pelvic irradiation for malignant disease.

卵巢可因对恶性肿瘤的盆腔照射而受到影响。

In certain patients in whom medical conditions contraindicate surgery, irradiation therapy is performed.

不允许行外科手术的某些内科疾病患者,宜行放射疗法。

irrational [iˈræʃənəl] *a.* 无理性的,不合理的

The news of serious illness drives some patients to irrational and destructive behavior, others handle it sensibly.

知道患上了严重的疾病,使有些病人做出无理性的和危害性的行为,而另一些人却能处之

泰然。

irregular [iˈregjulə] *a.* 不规则的

The patient has an irregular pulse.

病人脉搏不规则。

irregularity [iˌregjuˈlæriti] *n.* 不规则，无规律

Such irregularities may be considered indicative of mental defects.

可把这些不正常现象看成是智力不健全的指征。

Some arrhythmia are regular irregularity.

有些心律不齐是有规律的不规则。

irrelevant [iˈreləvənt] *a.* 不相关的，离题的

What you say is irrelevant to the subject.

你说的话并不切题。

irreparable [iˈrepərəbl] *a.* 不能修复的；无可挽回的

Normally, his vision would be declared an irreparable loss, and doctors would not attempt treatment.

一般情况下，他的视力会被宣布为不可挽回的损失，医生也不会去试图治疗。

irresistible [ˌiriˈzistəbl] *a.* 不可抵抗的

Bulimia is characterized by an irresistible urge to consume large quantities of food.

贪食癖表现为一种不可抵抗的吃光大量食物的强烈欲望。

irrespective [ˌirisˈpektiv] *a.* 不考虑的；不问的；无关的

The term "immunity" is used here as the state of resistance to infective disease, irrespective of how this is brought about.

这里所说的术语"免疫力"，只是对传染性疾病的抵抗力而言，且不考虑它是怎样产生的。

Appendicitis should be suspected in all patients who have abdominal pain, irrespective of age.

凡有腹痛的病人，不问其年龄大小都应考虑到有无阑尾炎的可能性。

Chronic renal disease advances in a programmed course, irrespective of the primary nephropathy.

慢性肾脏疾病按固定的过程发展，与原发肾脏疾病无关。

irresponsibility [ˈirisˌpɔnsəˈbiliti] *n.* 不负责任

The irresponsibility spreads this infectious disease.

不负责任的行为导致了这种传染病的蔓延。

irreversible [ˌiriˈvəːsibl] *a.* 不可逆的，不可反转的

Septic shock is usually recognized after irreversible changes have taken place.

败血症休克往往在出现了不可逆转的变化后才被发现。

Irreversible shock does not respond to adequate treatment and death is inevitable.

不可逆休克对适当的处理无反应，因而死亡是不可避免的。

irrigate [ˈirigeit] *v.* 冲洗

This could be demonstrated by washing epithelial cells from the surface of the colon mucosa utilizing a dental irrigating machine.

此点可用牙科冲洗器从结肠黏膜的表面冲洗上皮细胞加以证实。

irrigation [ˌiriˈgeiʃən] *n.* 灌溉；冲洗法

Give the patient colonic irrigation.

给病人做结肠灌洗。

irritability [ˌiritəˈbiliti] *n.* 应激性，兴奋性

Irritability is shown by nerve cells, which can generate and transmit electrical impulses when stimulated appropriately.

显示应激性的为神经细胞，当其受到适当刺激时能产生并传导电冲动。

Irritabililty of the bladder is a condition in which the presence of a small amount of urine in the bladder produces a desire to urinate.

膀胱易激惹性(或过敏)是膀胱内尿量少时可产生尿意的一种情况。

irritable [ˈiritəbl] *a.* 烦躁的,易激怒的

While recovery is taking place, the child may remain weak and irritable until fully recovered.

在恢复阶段直至完全康复之前,病儿依然虚弱和烦躁。

The patient with peptic ulcer is usually restless and irritable.

患有消化性溃疡的病人往往烦躁不安,易于激动。

irritant [ˈiritənt] *a.* 刺激(性)的

Traces of irritant chemicals will remain in the eye despite 10 minutes of irrigation.

即使经 10 分钟的冲洗,少量刺激性化学物仍会残存于眼内。

n. 刺激物

Care must be taken to get rid of possible irritants such as smoking, fumes and excessive cold air.

必须注意消除可能的刺激物如吸烟、烟雾和过冷的空气。

These acute exacerbations frequently follow a bad cold, exposure to smoke, or their irritants.

这些急性病情加重常发生在重感冒、受烟雾或其他刺激物的刺激之后。

irritate [ˈiriteit] *v.* 刺激,使兴奋

This medicine will irritate the skin.

这药会刺激皮肤。

The lotion is irritating to the eyes.

这种洗液对眼睛是有刺激性的。

The vomiting relieves him considerably, for it removes the irritating substance.

呕吐使他感到缓解了许多,因为呕吐除去了刺激性物质。

irritation [iriˈteiʃən] *n.* 刺激;激怒

This mononuclear cell reaction may represent response to local irritation by the tumor.

这单核细胞的反应可能是肿瘤对局部刺激的反映。

The broad spectrum penicillins such as ampicillin and amoxicillin may cause gastrointestinal irritation.

广谱青霉素诸如氨苄青霉素和羟氨苄青霉素可引起胃肠道刺激症状。

irritative [ˈiriteitiv] *a.* 刺激的

In chronic intestinal obstruction an irritative diarrhoea may result from the secretion of fluid behind a partial obstruction.

在慢性肠梗阻时,由于不全梗阻部位以下部分的液体分泌,可引起刺激性腹泻。

ischemia [isˈkiːmiə] *n.* 局部缺血(=ischaemia)

Myocardial ischemia may be confused if the site of the pain is high.

如果疼痛部位较高,可能被误诊为心肌缺血。

Glomeruli injured by chronic ischaemia become converted to hyaline balls.

由于慢性缺血而受损的肾小球可转变为玻璃样小球。

ischemic [isˈkiːmik] *a.* 局部缺血的

In some infarcts, plasma exudes from the ischemic blood vessels.

在某些梗死时,血浆从局部缺血的血管内渗出。

ischialgia [ˌiskiˈældʒiə] *n.* 坐骨神经痛

Ischialgia is a type of pain felt in tissues innervated by the sciatic nerve and its roots.

坐骨神经痛是受坐骨神经及其根部神经支配的组织的疼痛。

He developed an exacerbation of LBP and ischialgia on the left side, but now conservative treatment failed.

他的左侧腰痛和左侧坐骨神经痛加重了,但是现在保守治疗无效。

island [ˈailənd] *n.* 岛

Hypermethylation of CpG islands is a common epigenetic alteration associated with cancer.

CpG 岛过甲基化是一种与癌有关的常见表观遗传改变。

Cities are particularly vulnerable to climate change because of a phenomenon known as the urban heat island effect.

由于一种被称为城市热岛效应的现象，城市特别容易受到气候变化的危害。

islet [ˈailit] *n.* 小岛；胰岛

The pancreas was of particular interest；it showed a striking increase in number and size of islets.

特别有趣的是胰腺，其胰岛的数目和大小显著增加。

isoagglutinin [ˌaisɔəgˈluːtinin] *n.* 同种凝集素

Isoagglutinin is one of the antibodies occurring naturally in the plasma that cause agglutination of red blood cells of a different group.

同种凝集素是血浆中自然存在的一种抗体，它可使不同血型的红细胞发生凝集。

isoantibody [ˌaisəuˈæntibɔdi] *n.* 同种抗体

Isoantibody is an antibody that occurs naturally against the components of foreign tissues from an individual of the same species.

同种抗体是自然存在的一种抗体，能对抗同种内不同个体的组织成分。

isochromosome [ˌaisəuˈkrəuməsəum] *n.* ［遗］等臂染色体

An isochromosome is a chromosome in which one arm is missing and the other duplicated in a mirror-image fashion.

等臂染色体是指染色体的一条臂缺失而另一条臂以镜像形式重复。

A person with 46 chromosomes carrying an isochromosome，therefore，has a single copy of the genetic material of one arm and three copies of the genetic material of the other arm.

一个人的 46 条染色体中若有 1 条等臂染色体，则该人仅含有单倍量的该染色体一条臂上的遗传物质，而含有三倍量的另一条臂上的遗传物质。

isoelectric [ˌaisəuiˈlektrik] *a.* 等电的，等电势的

Isoelectric focusing electrophoresis can be used to screen abnormal hemoglobin.

等电聚焦电泳（的技术）可用来筛选异常的血红蛋白。

isoenzyme [ˌaisəuˈenzaim] *n.* 同工酶

Various enzymes having the same mechanism but with different chemical，physical or immunological characteristics are termed isoenzymes.

具有相同作用机制，但其化学、物理或免疫学特征不同的各种酶，统称为同工酶。

Isoenzymes catalyse the same type of reaction but have slight physical and immunological differences.

同工酶能催化同一形式的化学反应，但有某些轻微的物理学和免疫学的差异。

isoferritin [ˌaisəuˈferitin] *n.* 同功铁蛋白

Ferritin is an Fe-storage glycoprotein known to exist as tissue-specific isoferritins and measuable in the serum by radioimmunometric methods.

铁蛋白是一种储铁的糖蛋白，已知其以组织特异性的同功铁蛋白的形式存在，并可用放射免疫方法检测血清来测定。

isoform [ˈaisəfɔːm] *n.* 异构型，同种型，同等型，同工型

A protein isoform is any of several different forms of the same protein.

蛋白异构体就是同一种蛋白的几种不同形式之一。

isogeneic [ˌaisəudʒiˈniːik] *a.* 同系的，同基因的

That never seemed possible before the days of transplantation in isogeneic inbred animals.

这在同系近亲繁殖动物间进行移植术之前的时代，似乎绝不可能。

isograft [ˈaisəgrɑːft] *n.* 同种移植，同基因移植

An isograft is a graft of tissue between two individuals who are genetically identical such as monozygotic twins.

同种移植是指在两个遗传基因上相同的人之间的组织移植，如同卵双胎。

The expression of ADAR1 mRNA in the allograft group was significantly higher than that in the isograft group.

异种移植组中 ADAR1 mRNAde 的表达明显高于同种移植组。

isointensity [ˌaisəuin'tensiti] *n.* 等信号

A few lesions showed isointensity signal peripheral enhancement with centripetal filling in on FL2D sequences.

有些病变在 FL 2D 序列扫描时呈等信号周围增强并向中间充填。

The comparatively typical features of MRI were a large accompanying soft tissue mass, slight periosteal reaction, and isointensity on T2WI with significant enhancement.

MRI 的相对典型特征是一个大的伴随性软组织块、轻微的骨膜反应和 T2WI 等信号并有明显增强。

isolate ['aisəleit] *v.* 隔离,孤立;分离

Isolate patients who are sputum positive for first fortnight of treatment.

对痰阳性患者隔离治疗两周。

Presumably, the majority of the listed agents are capable of causing isolated acute viral laryngitis.

据推测,列举的因素中大多数可以引起孤立的(单一的)急性病毒性喉炎。

Isolated hematuria, either gross or microscopic, may be found at initial presentation in about 26% patients.

约 26% 的患者在最初表现中可单独出现肉眼或镜下血尿。

Andrew Schally isolated and synthesized LH-RH, a chemical capable of being an oral contraceptive.

安德鲁・沙利氏分离并合成了一种能作为口服避孕药的化合物 LH-RH。

isolation [ˌaisəu'leiʃən] *n.* 分离;隔离

Special precautions must be taken for isolation and growth of these bacteria.

应采用特殊的保护措施来分离和培养这些细菌。

Isolation of a virus does not necessarily establish its etiological role in the myocardial disease.

分离出一种病毒也未必能确定是心肌病的病因。

isoleucine [ˌaisəu'ljuːsiːn] *n.* 异亮氨酸

It is usually confirmed by amino acid analysis showing marked elevations in plasma levels of leucine, isoleucine, valine, and alloisoleucine.

常常通过氨基酸分析来确诊,氨基酸分析常显示血浆中亮氨酸、异亮氨酸、缬氨酸和别异亮氨酸水平明显升高。

Rice is low in isoleucine.

米饭中异亮氨酸含量低。

isomer ['aisəumə] *n.* (同分)异构体,同质异能素

Isomers often have very different chemical properties.

同分异构体的化学性质常有很大差别。

Isomers are compunds with identical chemical formulas but different arrangements of atoms.

同分异构体是化学式相同而原子排列不同的化合物。

isomerase [ai'sɔməreis] *n.* 异构酶

Isomerase catalyze structural or geometric changes in a molecule.

同分异构酶可以催化一个效应分子在结构上或几何形状上的改变。

isometric [ˌaisəu'metrik] *a.* 等长的;非等渗的

When possible, a few minutes of isometric exercise can help prevent the loss of muscle mass.

如果可能的话,数分钟的等长运动可有助于预防肌肉萎缩。

isoniazid [ˌaisəu'naiəzid] *n.* 异烟肼

Isoniazid is used in the treatment of tuberculosis.

异烟肼可用于治疗结核病。

Prophylaxis with isoniazid is recommended for household contacts of patients with active tuberculosis.

对接触活动性结核病人的家庭成员，可推荐预防性服用异烟肼。

isoprenaline [ˌaisəu'prenəli(ː)n] *n.* 异丙肾上腺素

If the patient presents with asystole, atropine and isoprenaline may help to maintain the circulation.

对于心跳停止的病人，可给予阿托品和异丙肾上腺素维持循环。

isopropanol [ˌaisəu'prəupənɔl] *n.* 异丙醇

When an unstable hemoglobin is suspected, the isopropanol denaturation test may be useful.

当怀疑不稳定型血红蛋白时，可用异丙醇变性试验来检测。

The predominant symptoms of isopropanol ingestion are gastrointestinal and neurologic, which develop soon after ingestion.

当误食异丙醇后不久其突出的表现是出现胃肠道和神经系统的症状。

isoproterenol [ˌaisəuˌprəutə'riːnɔl] *n.* 异丙肾上腺素

Isoproterenol is a beta-adrenergic receptor agonist.

异丙肾上腺素是一种 β-肾上腺素受体的激动剂。

Long-term administration of various drugs (e. g. isoproterenol, atropine, epinephrine) for bradyrhythmias is no longer necessary.

对心动过缓再也没有必要长期服用像异丙肾上腺素、阿托品、肾上腺素等类药物了。

isotonic [ˌaisəu'tɔnik] *a.* 等渗的，等张的，等压的

The solution is isotonic with blood.

这溶液与血液是等渗的。

Isotonic saline is ideal for subcutaneous administration.

等张盐水是皮下注射的理想溶液。

isotope ['aisəutəup] *n.* 同位素

A chemical element having the same atomic number as another but possessing a different atomic mass is called isotope.

一化学元素和另一(元素)有相同的原子数，但原子质量不同即称为同位素。

Radioactive isotopes decay into other isotopes or elements, emitting alpha, beta or gamma radiation.

放射性同位素可以衰变成其他种类同位素或元素，放射出 α，β 或 γ 射线。

Antigens may be labeled in various means, as with dyes or isotopes.

抗原可以用不同手段予以标记，如用染料或同位素等。

isotopic [ˌaisəu'tɔpik] *a.* 同位素的

Being a noble gas, Xe resists chemical bonding with other elements and is thus easy to purify for isotopic analysis.

由于氙是惰性的，不易与其他元素产生化学键，因此很容易纯化以进行同位素分析。

Evidence from isotopic dating suggests that the greenstone belts vary considerably in age.

来自同位素年龄鉴定的证据指出，绿岩带在年龄上彼此差异相当大。

isotype ['aisəutaip] *n.* 同型，同种型

The isotype of an immunoglobulin chain is determined by the type of consistant (C) region it has.

免疫球蛋白链的同种型取决于其恒定区(C 区)类型。

isovist ['aisəuvist] *n.* 伊索显

This paper reports a randomized double-blind clinical trial of two kinds of X-ray contrast media, Isovist 280 (30 cases) and Omnipaque 300 (28 cases), for cerebral angiography in 58 patients.

本文报告两种 X 线造影剂伊索显 280(30 例)与欧乃派克 300(28 例)在 58 例病人脑血管造影中的随机双盲临床试验。

isozyme [ˈaisəuzaim] *n.* 同工酶

There may be several types of enzyme that catalyze the same reaction; these are known as isoenzymes or isozymes.

可以催化相同反应的各种类型的酶统称为同工酶。

Isozymes of dehydrogenases, oxidases, transaminases, phosphatases, and proteolytic enzymes are known to exist.

已知下列的酶都有同工酶:如脱氢酶、氧化酶、转氨酶、磷酸酶以及蛋白水解酶。

issue [ˈisjuː, ˈiʃjuː] *v.* (流,涌,发)出

The spinal nerves issue from the spinal cord, to the right and to the left of it, between each pair of corresponding vertebrae.

脊神经从脊髓出来,到脊髓的左右两边,在每一对对应的脊椎之间。

Black smoke issuing from the chimney is harmful to people' s health.

烟囱里涌出的黑烟对人们的健康有害。

n. 问题;发行

The key issue in the evaluation of the patient with chest discomfort is to distinguish potentially life-threatening conditions from other causes of chest discomfort.

在对胸部不适的病人进行诊断时,一个重要的问题是将可能威胁生命的疾病与其他引起胸部不适的疾病区分开来。

The issue of a new edition of this dictionary is oncoming.

这本字典新版本的发行即将开始。

isthmus [ˈisməs] *n.* 峡部

The uterine isthmus is the inferior-posterior part of uterus, on its cervical end — here the uterine muscle is narrower and thinner.

子宫峡部位于子宫体下后方,即宫颈末端;该处的子宫较窄、肌层较薄。

itch [itʃ] *n.* 痒

Itch is local discomfort or irritation of the skin, prompting the sufferer to scratch or rub the affected area.

痒是皮肤产生局部不适或受到刺激,它迫使患者去抓或去搔局部痒处。

v. 痒,瘙痒

Are your mosquito bites still itching?

你身上蚊子咬过的地方现在仍然痒吗?

Cholestatic jaundice usually itches severely.

胆汁淤积性黄疸常有严重的瘙痒。

itching [ˈitʃiŋ] *n.* 痒,瘙痒

Skin manifestations include itching, patchy erythema, cyanosis and oedema.

皮肤的表现为瘙痒、红斑、发绀和水肿。

The patient has a very bad itching of his eyes from time to time.

这个病人常常觉得眼睛痒得很。

itchy [ˈitʃi] *a.* 发痒的

This bumpy, itchy rash induces scratching that can in turn cause skin infections.

这种痒疹疙瘩诱使患者搔痒,随后可能引发皮肤感染。

item [ˈaitəm] *n.* 条,项目

Diet is an important item in treatment.

在治疗中饮食是一个重要的项目。

iteration [ˌitəˈreiʃən] *n.* 反复,(计算机)循环,迭代

This medical question evolved from experience with the database and multiple iterations of exploratory analyses.

这一医学问题是从数据库的经历和多次反复的探索性分析中发展而来。

An iteration procedure can be used to determine the eigenvalue.
迭代方法可用来确定特征值。
Multiple test cycles are executed during the iteration.
在一个迭代期间要执行多个测试周期。

iterative [ˈitərətiv] *a.* 迭代的
The analysis becomes an iterative process.
这一分析计算工作实际上是一个逐次迭代的过程。
The iterative methodology improves on the spiral methodology.
迭代方法是在螺旋型方法的基础上发展而来的。

ixodiasis [ˌiksəuˈdaiəsis] *n.* 蜱病
Tick bites can cause ixodiasis.
蜱叮咬能引起蜱病。

J

jaundice [ˈdʒɔːndis] *n.* 黄疸

The level of jaundice may fluctuate, and is initially usually mild.

黄疸的水平可有波动，初期一般很轻。

The results of the physical examination fit in with the description of jaundice.

体检的结果和有关黄疸病的记述相符。

jaw [dʒɔː] *n.* 颚，颌，颌骨

The permanent teeth are 32 in number, 16 each in the upper and lower jaws.

恒牙的数目为 32 个，上下颚各 16 个。

An older child complained of pain behind the angle of his jaws.

一较大儿童主诉其两下颌骨角后方疼痛。

jejunal [dʒiˈdʒuːnəl] *a.* 空肠的

Jejunal diverticulosis is an uncommon acquired condition.

空肠憩室病是一种少见的获得性疾病。

jejunoileostomy [dʒiˌdʒuːnɔˈiliəstəmi] *n.* 空肠回肠吻合术

Jejunoileostomy is usually performed for intestinal disease (e. g. Crohn's disease) but sometimes for the treatment of obesity.

通常在治疗小肠疾病（如克罗恩氏病）时常做空肠回肠吻合术，但有时也是为了治疗肥胖症。

jejunum [dʒiˈdʒuːnəm] *n.* 空肠

The small intestine is divided into three parts: the duodenum, jejunum and ileum.

小肠分为三部分：十二指肠、空肠和回肠。

The chyme leaves the stomach, and is slowly carried down the duodenum into the jejunum, or second portion of the small intestine.

食糜离开胃，缓慢下行到十二指肠并进入空肠，即小肠的第二部分。

jeopardize [ˈdʒepədaiz] *v.* 危及

The incapacitation of the microbe thus effected may or may not jeopardize its survival as a species.

使微生物丧失能力的这种作用，可能危及也可能不危及其作为物种的生存。

jerk [dʒəːk] *n.* 急跳；反射

Progressive neurological disorders in infancy may be associated with massive myoclonic jerks affecting the whole body.

婴儿进行性的神经系统疾患可伴有累及全身的大量肌阵挛性抽动。

jet [dʒet] *v.* 喷射，喷注

Poststenotic dilation of the pulmonary artery is due to injury of the wall by "jetting" blood in pulmonary stenosis.

肺动脉狭窄后的扩张是由于肺动脉狭窄形成的喷射状血流对管壁的损伤而造成的。

n. 喷射，喷注

The ejection of blood through narrowed stenotic valves can produce high speed "jets" of blood that injure the endocardium.

血流通过狭窄的瓣膜喷出可产生高速的血液喷注而损伤心内膜。

jog [dʒɔg] *v.* 慢跑；蹒跚行进

Not everyone loves to jog or go to the gym.
不是每个人都喜欢慢跑或去健身房。
Jogging after meal is good for the health.
饭后慢步走有益于身体健康。
n. 轻推;慢跑
Jogging is a kind of repetitive endurance activities.
慢跑是一种重复性的耐力运动。

joint [dʒɔint] *n.* 关节;接头
The primary function of a joint is to provide motion and flexibility to the human frame.
关节的主要功能是使人体能够活动和屈曲。
The doctor prescribed a new medicine for the pain in my joints.
医生给我开了一种治关节痛的新药。
Can you see the joints?
你能看出接头的地方吗?
You can make these short pipes into one long pipe if you use some joints.
如果使用一些接头,你就可以把这些短管子接成一根长管子。

jointly [ˈdʒɔintli] *ad.* 共同地,联合地
They took care of that problem jointly.
他们共同处理那个问题。

journal [ˈdʒəːnl] *n.* 杂志
This young doctor reads regularly quite a few famous medical journals in English.
这位青年医生经常阅读一些英文的著名医学杂志。
I would like to suggest you to submit your thesis to the journal of Environmental Health and Preventive Medicine.
我想建议你把你的论文向《环境卫生与预防医学》杂志投稿。

judge [dʒʌdʒ] *v.* 判断,认为,评价
I judged him to be about 50.
我判断他大约 50 岁。
As far as I can judge, they are all to blame.
依我看来,他们都应承担责任。
Fluorescence of a spirochete on the slide is judged to be a positive result.
载玻片上螺旋体的荧光特性被判定为阳性结果。

judgement [ˈdʒʌdʒmənt] *n.* 判断,判断力
He lacks sound judgement.
他缺乏正确的判断力。
This judgement requires assessing the effects of risky behavior on the health status.
这一判断需要评估高危行为对健康状况的影响。

judicious [dʒuːˈdiʃəs] *a.* 明智的,慎重的
Some investigators report that their judicious use to support respiratory drive is beneficial.
有些研究人员指出,慎重使用这类药物对维持呼吸动力有益。

jugular [ˈdʒʌgjulə] *a.* 颈的,颈静脉的
Jugular venous distention develops in right-sided heart failure.
右心衰竭可出现颈静脉扩张。
Jugular venous pulsation normally falls with inspiration but may rise in constrictive pericarditis.
正常的颈静脉搏动随吸气减弱但缩窄性心包炎时的颈静脉搏动随吸气增强。

juice [dʒuːs] *n.* 果汁,体液
Drinking various kinds of fruit juice is helpful to health.
饮用各种果汁对健康是有益的。

Phenytoin is insoluble at the normal pH of the gastric juice.
苯妥英钠在胃液的正常 pH 值时是不溶解的。

junction [ˈdʒʌŋkʃən] *n.* 连接
The synapse is the junction between two neurons.
突触是两个神经元之间的接头。
The rash is first seen at the back of the ears and at the junction of the forehead and the hair.
皮疹最早见于耳后及头发与前额交接处。

junctional [ˈdʒʌŋkʃənəl] *a.* 交叉的,连接的
The diversity of lymphocyte receptors is further amplified by junctional diversity.
淋巴细胞受体的多样性进一步被其连接的多样性所扩大。
A clear junctional zone was found on the supracondylar humerus.
肱骨髁上区可见明显的交界区。

juncture [ˈdʒʌŋktʃə] *n.* 交界处
Fissures are painful because of their location below the mucocutaneous juncture.
由于裂伤位于黏膜皮肤交接处以下,因而疼痛。

junior [ˈdʒuːniə] *a.* 年幼的;(职位或等级)较低的
He is junior to me by five years.
他比我小 5 岁。
They are students of a junior high school nearby.
他们是附近一所初中的学生。
n. 年幼者;(大学)三年级学生
He is her junior by three years.
他比她小 3 岁。
They are juniors of this university.
他们是这所大学的三年级学生。

junk [dʒʌŋk] *n.* 垃圾
It is sad that children are now heavily exposed to junk food and lacking adequate exercise.
可悲的是,如今孩子们过多地食用垃圾食品,而且缺乏足够的体育锻炼。
Junk DNA means noncoding regions of DNA that have no apparent function.
垃圾 DNA 是 DNA 的非编码区,没有明显的功能。

justifiable [ˈdʒʌstifaiəbl] *a.* 正当的,无可非议的
Induction is often justifiable in cases of postmaturity in which the menstrual history is certain.
在月经史明确的过期妊娠病例,引产是恰当的。

justification [ˌdʒʌstifiˈkeiʃən] *n.* 证明为正当,理由是…
The justification is that any delay in treatment may increase the possibility of permanent sequelae or death occurring.
理由是在治疗上的任何延误都可增加持久性后遗症的可能性或导致死亡。

justify [ˈdʒʌstifai] *v.* 证明…为正当
You can hardly justify such conduct.
你很难证明此种行为是正当的。
If there is a serious maternal or fetal diagnostic problem, X-ray examination is still sometimes justified.
如果存在严重的母婴诊断问题,X 线检查有时仍可应用。
In few patients with rheumatoid arthritis can long-term corticosteroid therapy be justified.
很少类风湿关节炎病人被认为有理由应用长疗程的皮质激素治疗。

juvenile [ˈdʒuːvinail] *a.* 青少年的;幼稚的
A mild to moderate anemia is common in juvenile rheumatoid arthritis.
幼年型类风湿性关节炎常有轻度至中度贫血。

Interest in juvenile bipolar disorders has waxed and waned over the years.
多年来,对于青少年的双相疾病的兴趣时高时低。

juxtacortical [ˌdʒʌkstəˈkɔːtikəl] *a.* 近皮质的

Chondromas arising on the surface of bone are called subperiosteal or juxtacortical chondromas.
发生于骨表面的软骨瘤称为骨膜下或皮质旁软骨瘤。

Chondrosarcoma is subclassified according to site as central (intramedullary) and peripheral (juxtacortical and surface).
软骨肉瘤根据部位再分为中央型(髓内)和外周型(皮质旁和骨表面)。

juxtaglomerular [ˌdʒʌkstəgləuˈmerjulə] *a.* 近肾小球的

Renin is secreted by the juxtaglomerular cells of the kidney in response to fall in blood pressure.
肾素是由肾脏肾小球旁细胞分泌,以对应血压下降。

The juxtaglomerular apparatus is a microscopic structure in the kidney, which regulates the function of each nephron.
肾小球旁器是肾脏的显微结构,可以调节每个肾单位的功能。

K

kala-azar ['Kɑːlɑːɑː'zɑː] *n.* 黑热病

Kala-azar is a highly fatal infectious disease endemic in the tropics and subtropics.

黑热病是在热带及亚热带传播的死亡率高的传染病。

Early diagnosis and treatment of kala-azar reduces its reservoir and controls its epidemic in India.

在印度，通过对黑热病的早期诊断和对病人的早期治疗可减少传染贮源，控制黑热病的流行。

kalium ['keiliəm] *n.* 钾(19 号元素)

A proper balance between sodium, kalium, and calcium in the blood plasma is necessary for proper cardiac function.

血浆内钠、钾和钙的适当平衡对于维持适当的心功能是必需的。

kaliuresis [ˌkeilijuə'riːsis] *n.* 尿钾排泄

As a consequence of increased delivery of sodium to the distal nephron, sodium-potassium ion exchange is enhanced, and kaliuresis results.

作为运送到远端肾单位的钠增多的后果，钠-钾离子交换增加，导致尿钾排泄。

kallikrein [ˌkæli'kriːin] *n.* 激肽释放酶

The local injection of kallikrein itself can increase the permeability of small blood vessels by releasing kinin.

局部注射激肽释放酶可以通过释放激肽增加小血管的通透性。

Kallmann ['kɑːlmɑːn] *n.* 卡尔曼综合征

In Kallmann syndrome, the sense of smell is either diminished (hyposmia) or completely absent (anosmia).

卡尔曼综合征患者嗅觉减退或者缺失。

Kallmann syndrome is a condition characterized by delayed or absent puberty and an impaired sense of smell.

卡尔曼综合征以青春发育延迟或缺失，并伴嗅觉受损为特征。

kanamycin [ˌkænə'maisin] *n.* 卡那霉素

Kanamycin is now considered the drug of choice in Escherichia coli infections.

如今卡那霉素被认为是治疗大肠杆菌感染最好的药物。

kaolin ['keiəlin] *n.* 白陶土

Kaolin-type is a clay mineral, part of the group of industrial minerals, with the chemical composition $Al_2Si_2O_5(OH)_4$.

白陶土型黏土是一种黏土矿物，它是工业矿物的一种，其化学成分为 $Al_2Si_2O_5(OH)_4$。

Kaolin is used in ceramics, medicine, coated paper, as a food additive in toothpaste and so on.

白陶土可用于陶瓷、医药、铜版纸、作为牙膏中的食品添加剂等。

karyogamy [ˌkæri'ɔgəmi] *n.* 核融合

Karyogamy is the fusion of pronuclei of two cells, as part of syngamy, fertilization, or fungus conjugation.

核融合是两个细胞原核的融合，如两性生殖、受精或真菌接合。

The total duration from germination of pollen grains on the stigma to the completion of karyogamy is about 25 ~ 28 hours.

从花粉在柱头上萌发开始至完成雌雄性核融合的总持续时间为 25 ~ 28 小时。

karyokinesis [ˌkæriɔkaiˈniːsis] *n.* (间接)核分裂,有丝分裂

Karyokinesis occurs during cell division before division of the cytoplasm(cytokinesis).

有丝分裂发生在细胞浆分裂(细胞质变动)之前的细胞分裂期间。

karyolysis [ˌkæriˈɔlisis] *n.* 核溶解

Karyolysis refers to the fade of basophilia of the chromatin.

核溶解是指染色质的嗜碱性消失。

Karyolysis reflects loss of DNA because of enzymatic degradation by endonucleases.

核溶解反映出由于核酸内切酶的降解作用造成的 DNA 的丢失。

karyon [ˈkæriɔn] *n.* 细胞核

60% cancer karyon, cytoplasm display positive signal of staphylococcus aureus L-form DNA.

60% 癌细胞核和胞浆内显示金葡菌 L 型 DNA 阳性信号。

20 cases of expression of L-form DNA of staphylococcus aureus in laryngocarcinoma karyon were detected with nucleic acid in situ hybridization.

应用原位核酸杂交技术检测 20 例喉癌细胞核内金葡菌 L 型 DNA 的表达。

karyopyknosis [ˌkæriəupikˈnəusis] *n.* 核固缩

Karypyknosis is characterized by nuclear shrinkage and increased basophilia.

核固缩表现为细胞核收缩,嗜碱性增强。

Karypyknosis is both seen in apoptotic cell death and necrosis.

核固缩可见于凋亡性细胞死亡和坏死。

karyorrhexis [ˌkæriəuˈreksis] *n.* 核碎裂

Karyorrhexis means that the pyknotic nucleus undergoes fragmentation.

核碎裂是指固缩的细胞核发生碎片化。

Nuclear changes are the most important morphology of necrosis, which appear in three patterns, including karyopyknosis, karyorrhexis and karyolysis.

细胞核的改变是坏死最重要的形态学表现,它有三种形式,包括核固缩、核碎裂和核溶解。

karyotype [ˈkæriətaip] *n.* 染色体组型,核型

When photographed, cut out, and arranged systematically in pairs 1 to 23, they constitute the karyotype.

将染色体成像、剪切,然后按由第 1 对至 23 对的顺序排列起来就构成了染色体组。

keloid [ˈkiːlɔid] *n.* 瘢痕疙瘩

Keloid is an overgrowth of granulation tissue, sometimes producing a lump many times larger than the original scar.

瘢痕疙瘩是肉芽组织的过度增生,有时可形成比原有瘢痕大许多倍的肿块。

Keloids are fibrotic tumors characterized by relatively acellular centers with excessive deposition of extracellular matrix component, such as collagen type Ⅰ.

瘢痕疙瘩是一种纤维性肿块,其特征是中央相对细胞稀少,伴有过量的细胞外基质沉积,如 I 型胶原。

Kelvin [ˈkelvin] *n.* 开尔文(英物理学家)

A temperature in Kelvin is equal to a Calsius temperature plus 273.15. Symbol: K.

开尔文温度等于摄氏温度加 273.15。符号为:"K"。

keratin [ˈkerətin] *n.* 角蛋白,角质

Keratin is the principal constituent of epidermis, hair, nails, horny tissues, and the organic matrix of the enamel of the teeth.

角蛋白是组成表皮、毛发、指甲、角化组织及牙釉质有机基质的主要成分。

The keratinocyte is a cell of ectodermal origin which has the specialized function of producing keratin.

角质细胞是来自外胚叶的细胞,具有合成角蛋白的特殊功能。

keratinase [ˈkerətineis] *n.* 角蛋白酶

A keratinase-producing gram-positive bacterium, isolated from feather waste, was identified as Bacillus subtilis YYW-1.
从羽毛废物中分离出的产角蛋白酶的革兰氏阳性细菌，经鉴定为枯草芽孢杆菌 YYW-1。
The keratinase was purified to homogeneity by three-step chromatography.
经过三步层析纯化，得到同质的角蛋白酶。

keratinization [ˌkerətinaiˈzeiʃən] *n.* 角(质)化
Excessive keratinization of epidermis is called hyperkeratinization.
表皮过多的角质化称为过度角化症。
When the formation of keratin cells is rapid or the process of normal keratinization is interfered with, pathologic exfoliation results, producing scales.
当角质细胞迅速形成时，或当正常的角化过程受到干扰时，则引起病理性的表皮剥脱，产生皮屑。

keratinocyte [kəˈrætinəsait] *n.* 角质形成细胞，角化细胞
Keratinocyte is an epidermal cell that produces keratin.
角化细胞是一种能产生角蛋白的表皮细胞。
The keratinocyte, or squamous cell, is the principal cell of the epidermis.
角质形成细胞，或称鳞状细胞，是表皮的主要细胞。

keratitis [ˌkerəˈtaitis] *n.* 角膜炎
Some kinds of keratitis—dendritic keratitis, for example—may follow symptoms of upper respiratory tract infection, such as fever.
有些种类的角膜炎，例如树突状角膜炎，可伴随上呼吸道感染的症状，如发热等(同时出现)。
Measles usually is a self-limited disease, but a number of complications such as bronchitis, keratitis, hepatitis and bacterial pneumonia may ensue.
麻疹通常是一种自限性疾病，但是也会继发出现一些并发症，如支气管炎、角膜炎、肝炎和细菌性肺炎。

keratoderma [ˌkerətəuˈdəːmə] *n.* 皮肤角化病
Keratoderma may be inherited (hereditary) or, more commonly, acquired.
皮肤角化病可以是遗传性的，但后天获得者更为常见。
Keratoderma is a skin condition where the skin appears "horny".
皮肤角化病是一种皮肤病，该处皮肤呈"角状"。

keratoma [ˌkerəˈtəumə] *n.* 角化病
Seborrhoeic keratoma (or warts) are yellow or brown oval spots with clearly marked perimeters and raised surfaces.
脂溢性角化病(或疣)是黄色或棕色的卵圆形斑块，周边清楚，高出皮面。

keratomalacia [ˌkerətəuməˈleiʃiə] *n.* 角膜软化
Keratomalacia is a frequent cause of blindness among Indians.
印度人主要的致盲原因是角膜软化病。
Keratomalacia is a progressive disease of the eye due to vitamin A deficiency.
角膜软化是一种因维生素 A 缺乏所导致的眼睛的进行性疾患。

keratosis [ˌkerəˈtəusis] (*pl.* keratoses [ˌkerəˈtəusiːz]) *n.* 角化病
Solar keratosis are pre-malignant, though only a few turn into squamous cell carcinomas.
光化性角化病尽管仅少部分可转化为鳞状细胞癌，但仍然属癌前病变。
The seborrheic keratosis is a common example of such a benign pigmented epithelial neoplasm.
脂溢性角化病是一个良性着色性上皮瘤常见的例子。

kernicterus [kəˈniktərəs] *n.* [德] 核黄疸(通常是重症新生儿黄疸的后遗症，亦称胆红素脑病)
Kernicterus is seen most often in premature infants in whom several abnormalities are simultane-

ously present.
核黄疸病最常出现于早产儿,且患儿同时存在有多种异常。

ketoacidosis [ˌkiːtəuˌæsiˈdəusis] *n.* 酮症酸中毒
Acidosis resulting from the presence of increaed ketone bodies is termed ketoacidosis.
酮体增多引起的酸中毒被称为酮症酸中毒。
Diabetic ketoacidosis must be treated with insulin.
糖尿病酮症酸中毒必须用胰岛素治疗。

ketoconazole [ˌkiːtəuˈkɔnəzəul] *n.* 酮康唑,酮哌咪唑
Ketoconazole is well tolerated at doses of 400mg or less.
酮康唑的服用剂量为400mg 及以下时,病人能很好地耐受。
Ketoconazole appeared to be the least effective treatment of uncomplicated funguria.
酮康唑对于无并发症的霉菌尿的效果似乎最差。

ketone [ˈkiːtəun] *n.* 酮; 甲酮
Ketone bodies are a group of three related substances: acetone, acetoacetic acid, and β-hydroxybutyric acid.
酮体是三种相关的一组物质:丙酮、乙酰乙酸和 β-羟丁酸。
The breath may smell of ketones in patients with ketoacidosis.
酮症酸中毒病人的呼气中可有酮味。

ketonemia [ˌkiːtəuˈniːmiə] *n.* 酮血症
Ketonemia is a condition in which there is an increased concentration of ketones in the blood.
酮血症就是血液中酮的浓度增高。

ketonuria [ˌkiːtɔˈnjuəriə] *n.* 酮尿(症)
Ketonuria may occur in diabetes mellitus, starvation, or after persistent vomiting and results from the partial oxidation of fats.
酮尿可发生于糖尿病、饥饿或持续性呕吐以及脂肪不完全氧化时。

ketosis [kiːˈtəusis] *n.* 酮病
Ketosis is the combination of increased ketones in both the blood and the urine.
酮病是指在血液和尿液两者中的酮同时增高。
Ketosis may result in severe acidosis.
酮病可导致严重的酸中毒。

keystone [ˈkiːstəun] *n.* 要旨,基本原理
Accurate diagnosis is now and always will be the keystone of rational treatment.
疾病的确诊不但现在是而且永远是合理治疗的基石。

kidney [ˈkidni] *n.* 肾
A nephritis patient should learn to care for his kidneys.
肾炎患者应该学会保护自己的肾的方法。
The surgeons have successfully transplanted an artificial kidney for this patient.
外科医生们成功地给这个病人做了人工肾脏移植手术。

killer [ˈkilə] *n.* 杀人者,灭…的东西
He told us about his experience with acupuncture as a pain killer.
他对我们讲述了他应用针刺术作为止痛手段的经验。

kilobase [ˈkiləubeis] *n.* 千碱基(核酸链长度单位)
A common glutathione-S-transferase M1 (*GSTM1*) polymorphism is caused by a 50-kilobase (kb) germline deletion.
一种常见的谷胱甘肽-S-转移酶 M1 (*GSTM1*) 多态性是由于 50 千碱基(kb)种系缺失所致。

kilocalorie [ˈkiləuˌkæləri] *n.* 千卡(热量单位)
Kilocalorie is the amount of heat required to raise 1kg of water 1℃.

千卡是指将 1 千克水的温度升高 1℃所需的热量。

kilovoltage [ˌkiləuˈvəultidʒ] *n.* 千伏电压

Reducing kilovoltage and mAs and other parameters can effectively reduce the radiation dose.

降低千伏电压和毫安秒等参数能够有效地减少照射剂量。

Gemstone spectral CT can realize instantaneous 80 to140 kilovoltage switching, which is the physical basis of single energy imaging.

宝石能谱 CT 可以实现瞬时 80 至 140 千伏电压切换,这是其单能量成像的物理基础。

kinase [ˈkaineis] *n.* 激酶

The protein kinase is the same protein kinase which phosphorylates glycogen synthetase.

蛋白激酶与那种可以使糖原合成酶进行磷酸化的蛋白激酶实际为同一种酶。

The level of creatinine kinase may be elevated, with predominant elevated fraction from skeletal muscles.

肌酸酐激酶水平可上升,其主要升高的部分来源于骨骼肌(的代谢)。

kinesthesia [ˌkinisˈθiːʒiə] *n.* 运动觉;肌肉运动知觉

Short-term programs that incorporate kinesthesia, balance and agility techniques may result in more rapid symptom relief and functional improvements。

合并运动觉、平衡和灵活性技术的短期项目可以更迅速的缓解症状和改善功能。

The addition of kinesthesia and balance exercises to strength training has more benefits over strength training alone.

力量训练时增加运动觉和平衡运动较之单独的力量训练益处更大。

kinetic [kaiˈnetik, kiˈnetik] *a.* 动(力)学的,(活)动的

Each subject's dose was individually determined by predictive kinetic studies.

每个受试者的剂量均由预见性动力学研究分别确定。

The kinetic nature of competitive antagonist is that the agonist can produce the same maximum effect in the presence of it.

竞争性拮抗剂的动力学特性是在它存在的情况下激动剂可产生同样的最大效应。

kinetism [ˈkainitizəm] *n.* (肌肉)运动能力

We want to know factors influencing fat metabolism and relations with kinetism.

我们想了解影响脂肪代谢的因素及其与运动能力的关系。

Research on the kinetism of rats in different air conditions was done.

我们对在不同气体环境下大鼠运动能力进行了研究。

kinetochore [kiˈnetəkɔː] *n.* [遗] 动粒,着丝粒

The kinetochore links the chromosome to microtubule polymers from the mitotic spindle during mitosis and meiosis.

在有丝分裂和减数分裂过程中,动粒将染色体与有丝分裂纺锤体发出的微管聚合物相连。

The kinetochore is the protein structure on chromatids where the spindle fibers attach during cell division.

动粒是细胞分裂时染色单体上的蛋白质结构,与纺锤丝相连。

kingdom [ˈkiŋdəm] *n.* 界;领域;王国

It was the first time to discover so many hemolysin genes encoded by one chromosome in microbial kingdom.

如此多的溶血素基因编码于同一个染色体,这在微生物界是首次发现。

British, Australian and Latin American textbooks describe all living things as five kingdoms.

英国、澳大利亚和拉丁美洲的教科书将所有生物分为五界。

kinin [ˈkainin] *n.* 激肽

The actions of kinin in inflammation include increased vascular permeability, smooth muscle contraction, vasodilation and pain.

在炎症中,激肽的作用包括增加血管通透性、收缩平滑肌、扩张血管和引起疼痛。

Researches have found that the blood pressure in body is controlled by the renin-angiotensin system (RAS) and kallikrein-kinin system (KKS).
研究发现,机体的血压是由体内肾素-血管紧张素系统(RAS)和激肽释放酶-激肽系统(KKS)控制的。

kininase [ˈkainineis] *n.* 激肽酶
The action of bradykinin is short-lived, because it is quickly inactivated by an enzyme called kininase.
缓激肽作用非常短暂,因为它很快被一种称激肽酶的物质灭活。
Kininase Ⅱ is also known as angiotensin-converting enzyme Ⅱ.
激肽酶Ⅱ也被称作是血管紧张素转化酶Ⅱ。

kininogen [kaiˈninədʒin] *n.* 激肽原
Kallikrein cleaves a plasma glycoprotein precursor kininogen to produce bradykinin.
激肽释放酶裂解血浆中糖蛋白前体物质激肽原而产生缓激肽。
In the cardiovascular system, the kininogen-kallikrein-kinin system exerts a fine control of vascular smooth muscle tone and arterial blood pressure.
在心血管系统,激肽原-激肽释放酶-激肽系统能精确调节血管平滑肌的张力和动脉血压。

kinking [ˈkiŋkiŋ] *n.* 扭结;缠线
Kinking of endotracheal tube (ETT) is not an infrequent problem during general anesthesia.
在全身麻醉中,气管内导管弯折并非是少见的问题。
Early detection and immediate management of the ETT kinking may reduce the possibility of morbidity and mortality in anesthesia.
早期发现和及时处理气管内管弯折可以降低麻醉所致并发症和死亡率。

kit [kit] *n.* 试剂盒,用具包,工具箱
First-aid kit is very useful in the urgent situation.
急救箱在紧急情况下非常有用。
Using commercial kit is more convenient but expensive for the experiments.
在实验中使用商家的试剂盒要方便但昂贵些。

klebsiella [ˌklebziˈelə] *n.* 克雷伯氏杆菌
Klebsiella can also attach to the urinary tract and infect the kidneys.
克雷伯氏菌还能侵入尿道和感染肾脏。
The bacterium, known as Klebsiella pneumoniae, is often found in hospitals, where it can cause pneumonia and other life-threatening infections.
这种被称为肺炎克雷伯氏菌的细菌经常发现于医院,可引起肺炎和其他威胁生命的感染。

knee [niː] *n.* 膝
The knee jerk is an example of a spinal reflex.
膝反射是脊髓反射的一个例子。
All patients with unstable knees due to trauma should be considered for angiography.
外伤后膝关节不稳固的患者应考虑进行血管造影术。

knit [nit] *v.* 编结; 皱起; 接合(断骨等); (使)紧密结合
By using this method, it takes one -third less time for the bones to knit and only half the time for function to be restored.
采用这种方法,骨愈合缩短了三分之一的时间,恢复功能只需一半的时间。

knockout [ˈnɔkaut] *n.* 基因敲除
In β7 gene knockout mice, the formation of GALT is drastically impaired.
在β7基因敲除的小鼠体内,GALT的形成受到强烈的伤害。
(注:GALT=galactose-1-p-uridyltransferase 半乳糖-1-对-脲嘧啶核苷酸,转移酶)
Knockout means deactivation of specific genes, which is used in laboratory organisms to study gene function.

基因敲除是指使特定基因失活,用于研究实验生物基因的功能。

knowledgeable [ˈnɔlidʒəbl] *a.* 有知识的,有见识的

Medical investigator should be sufficiently knowledgeable about the Privacy Rule.

医学研究者应充分知晓隐私规则。

kochia [ˈkɔkiə] *n.* 地肤子

Kochia acoparia-alcohol extract has significant effects of antipruritic.

地肤子醇提取物起着显著的止痒剂的作用。

The results showed that kochia acoparia differed from the substitutes in utricle, trichome, stoma and shape of seed under SEM.

结果显示扫描电镜下地肤子与其他替代药材的胞果、毛茸、气孔和种子形态特征有区别。

koilocyte [ˈkɔiləusait] *n.* 凹空细胞

Koilocyte is the characteristic change of HPV infected cervical epithelium.

凹空细胞是 HPV 感染的宫颈上皮的特征性改变。

In condylomata acuminate, koilocytes are characterized by nuclear enlargement and atypia.

在尖锐湿疣中,凹空细胞具有核增大和异型的特征。

kwashiorkor [ˌkwaːʃiˈɔːkə] *n.* 恶性营养不良病

Kwashiorkor is a clinical syndrome which results form a severe deficiency of protein with adequate caloric intake.

恶性营养不良病是一种临床综合征,它由于摄入适当的热量但严重缺乏蛋白质所引起的。

kyphoscoliosis [ˈkaifəu, skɔliˈəusis] *n.* 脊柱后侧凸

When it comes to a case combined with kyphoscoliosis, it is not easy to suture the meningocele through a posterior laminectomy.

当遇到脑膜膨出并发脊柱后侧凸病例时,通过后侧椎板切除术缝合脊膜膨出是不容易的。

A 46-year-old man has a lateral thoracic meningocele associated with kyphoscoliosis of the thoracic spine upon medical examination.

一位 46 岁男性在体检时发现患有侧向胸段脊膜膨出,伴发胸段脊柱后侧凸。

kyphosis [kaiˈfəusis] *n.* 驼背,脊柱后凸

Kyphosis frequently develops in elderly persons because of degenerative osteoarthritis of thoracic spine.

驼背常常发生于老年人,这是因为胸部脊柱出现了退行性骨关节炎之故。

Patients lose height with compression fractures and may develop kyphosis of the dorsal spine.

脊柱压缩性骨折可使病人身高变矮并且会出现脊柱后凸的现象。

kyphotic [kaiˈfɔtik] *a.* 驼背的;脊柱后凸的

The time from trauma to operation and the severity of kyphotic deformity were inversely correlated with postoperative correction rates.

从受伤到手术的时间长短和驼背畸形的严重程度与手术后矫正率之间呈负相关。

Extension of the ankylosed kyphotic cervical spine during conventional immobilization or for radiologic procedures resulted in neurologic deficits.

在常规制动或影像学检查过程中,僵硬后凸的颈椎过伸导致神经功能受损。

L

label [ˈleibl] *n.* 标签，瓶签；标记

All the bottles on the shelf have special labels.

架上所有的药瓶都贴有专门的标签。

Can you read the label on this bottle?

你会认这个药瓶上的标签吗？

v. 贴标签，做标记；把…列为

The bottle was labeled poison.

瓶上已标明为毒药。

We now suspect that many diseases once labeled psychological may be caused by chemical alterations.

现在我们怀疑许多曾经列为心理学上的疾病可能是由化学变化引起的。

labetalol [ləˈbetələul] *n.* 柳胺心定（抗高血压药）

Labetalol is effective in the emergent treatment of hypertension.

柳胺心定可有效治疗高血压急症。

labile [ˈleibail] *a.* 易变化的，不稳定的

Proteins are labile structure, easily disrupted.

蛋白质结构不稳定，容易解体。

The high-energy phosphate bond is very labile.

高能磷酸键很不稳定。

lability [ləˈbiliti] *n.* 易变性，不稳定性

The acid lability (pH 3) of rhinoviruses is probably the reason for their absence from the intestine.

鼻病毒对酸敏感（pH 3）可能是它们不存在于肠道的原因。

laboratory [ləˈbɔrətəri, ˈlæbərətəri] *n.* 实验室，检验室，化验室，药厂

However, many clinical laboratories report values in traditional units.

但是，许多临床检验室仍采用传统的单位报告检测值。

The fact that viruses multiply in certain tissue cultures and in living chick embryos makes possible laboratory study of these substances.

病毒能在特定的组织培养中以及在活的雏鸡胚胎中繁殖的事实使得在实验室里研究这些物质成为可能。

At times a complete history and laboratory examinations, including a biopsy, are essential to arrive at a diagnosis.

有时一个完整的病史及包括活检在内的许多化验检查对作出诊断是必不可少的。

Cordarone which is used in treating angina pectoris is produced by the Laboratories Labaz of France.

治疗心绞痛的乙胺碘呋酮是由法国拉巴兹制药厂生产的。

labour [ˈleibə] *n.* 分娩

The other important observations which must be made during labour relate to fetus.

分娩期应同时重视对胎儿的观察。

No labour is certainly normal until the third stage is safely concluded.

第三产程未安全结束前，不能肯定分娩是正常的。

labyrinth [ˈlæbərinθ] *n.* 迷宫，迷路

Fluid in the bony labyrinth is a transudate of plasma.

骨迷路内的液体是由血浆渗出来的。

lacerate [ˈlæsəreit] *v.* 撕裂，划破（软组织）

The heart may be bruised or lacerated either by blunt or penetrating trauma.

心脏可以由于钝创伤或穿透性创伤而被碰伤或撕裂。

When fatty tissue is lacerated, a large amount of fat enters the circulation.

当脂肪组织撕裂时，大量的脂肪进入血液循环。

laceration [ˌlæsəˈreiʃən] *n.* 撕裂，划破，裂伤

A laceration is a tear or disruption of the continuity of tissue produced by stretching.

撕裂是由于伸展（过度）致使连续性的组织被撕开或破裂。

One of other factors is laceration by a sharp foreign body.

其他因素之一是锐利异物的割裂。

Lachnospira [ˌlæknəuˈspirə] *n.* 毛螺菌属

Lachnospira is a genus of weakly gram-positive, anaerobic bacteria of uncertain affiliation.

毛螺菌属的细菌呈革兰染色弱阳性，厌氧，归属未定。

Lachnospira are motile, curved rods that ferment glucose and are found in the rumen of bovine animals.

毛螺菌能运动，菌体弯曲杆状，发酵葡萄糖，存在于牛的肠腔。

lacrimal [ˈlækriməl] *a.* 泪的

Proliferation of lymphocytes in lacrimal and salivary glands may cause bilateral painless enlargement.

泪腺和唾液腺淋巴细胞增生，可引起两侧腺体无痛性肿大。

lacrimation [ˌlækriˈmeiʃən] *n.* 流泪

Stimulation of the eye by foreign bodies may bring forth lacrimation.

异物刺激眼睛可引起流泪。

lactase [ˈlækteis] *n.* 乳糖酶

Lactase deficiency is by far the most common defect of nutrient assimilation in the world.

乳糖酶缺乏是世界上最常见的营养吸收缺陷疾病。

lactate [ˈlækteit] *n.* 乳酸

There is an increase in the blood lactate, with a corresponding metabolic acidosis.

血液中乳酸增多可引起代谢性酸中毒。

Determination of lactate levels in cerebrospinal fluid is used in the diagnosis and management of meningitis.

脑脊液中乳酸水平的测定用于脑膜炎的诊断和处理。

v. 分泌乳汁，授乳

Prolactin deficiency is manifested as an inability to lactate.

催乳素缺乏表现为不能分泌乳汁。

lactation [lækˈteiʃən] *n.* 泌乳；哺乳

During lactation prolactin is secreted in large amounts by the anterior lobe of the pituitary gland.

哺乳期间垂体前叶分泌大量生乳素。

Pregnancy and lactation increase the need for rest.

怀孕期和哺乳期需要更多的休息。

lacteal [ˈlæktiəl] *n.* 乳糜管

Each villus contains a capillary network and a lymph vessel called a lacteal.

每个绒毛内都有一个毛细血管网和一条叫做乳糜管的淋巴管。

lactic [ˈlæktik] *a.* 乳（酸）的

Adrenaline breaks down liver glycogen and muscle glycogen to lactic acid.

肾上腺素把肝糖原和肌糖原分解成乳酸。

These reactions illustrate why alcoholics sometimes suffer from lactic acidosis.

这些反应说明为什么酒精中毒者有时会发生乳酸酸中毒。

lactobacillus [ˌlæktəubəˈsiləs] (*pl.* lactobacilli [ˌlæktəubəˈsilai]) *n.* 乳(酸)杆菌

In breast-fed children, the intestine contains large numbers of lactic acid streptococci and lactobacilli.

母乳喂养的小孩,其肠道内容物含有大量的乳酸链球菌和乳酸杆菌。

The species Lactobacillus acidophilus is found in milk and is associated with dental caries.

嗜酸性乳杆菌常可见于牛乳中,并与龋齿(的生成)有关。

lactose [ˈlæktəus] *n.* 乳糖

Galactose is a constituent of lactose.

半乳糖是乳糖的一个组成成分。

lacuna [ləˈkjuːnə] *n.* 腔隙,陷窝

The dead bone is recognized by its empty lacunae.

识别死骨可以通过空空的骨陷窝。

In hypertensive cerebrovascular disease, the development of single or multiple, small, cavitary infarcts is known as lacunae.

在高血压性脑血管疾病中,单个或多个小的空隙样梗死被称为腔隙。

lacunar [ləˈkjuːnəː] *a.* 腔隙性的

The effects of hypertension on the brain include lacunar infarcts, slit hemorrhages, hypertensive encephalopathy, and massive intracerebral hemorrhage.

高血压对脑的影响包括腔隙性梗死、裂隙性出血、高血压脑病和大片脑出血。

On microscopic examination lacunar infarcts consist of areas of tissue loss with scattered lipid-laden macrophages and surrounding gliosis.

显微镜下,腔隙性梗死包括组织缺失区,散在含脂质的巨噬细胞和周围增生的胶质细胞。

Lagovirus [ˌlægəˈvaiərəs] *n.* 兔病毒属

The Lagovirus genus consists of two species: rabbit hemorrhagic disease virus and European brown hare syndrome virus.

兔病毒属有两个种:兔出血病病毒和欧洲粽野兔综合征病毒。

Phylogenetic analysis of the entire viral genome revealed a new member of the genus Lagovirus within the family Caliciviridae.

经病毒全基因组进化树分析,揭示了杯状病毒科兔病毒属中一个新的成员。

lamina [ˈlæminə] (*pl.* laminae [ˈlæminiː]) *n.* 板,层

Arterial thrombi are pale or show alternating laminae of pale and dark red material, without an obvious distinction between "head" and "tail".

动脉血栓呈苍白色,或显示出苍白与暗红色物质的间隔层,其头尾之间并无明显区别。

laminectomy [ˌlæmiˈnektəmi] *n.* 椎板切除术

Pressure upon the spinal cord can be removed surgically by laminectomy.

脊髓受压可经外科椎板切除术解除。

languor [ˈlæŋgə] *n.* 疲倦,乏力

The symptoms of acute bronchitis are partly general, that is, fever, headache, malaise, languor, and various general pains.

急性支气管炎的症状部分属于全身性的,有发热、头痛、不舒服、乏力以及各种全身性的疼痛。

lanolin [ˈlænəlin] *n.* 羊毛脂

Lanolin is a natural moisturizer with powerful emollient and protective properties.

羊毛脂是一种天然的具有强大润肤和保护性能的湿润剂。

Lanolin keeps skin soft and supple in the same way that it protects the sheep.

羊毛脂以保护绵羊的相同方式来保持皮肤的柔软。

laparoscopy [ˌlæpəˈrɔskəpi] *n.* 腹腔镜检查

An early diagnosis can be achieved in most instances by laparoscopy.

大多数病例能用腹腔镜检查达到早期诊断的目的。

laparotomy [ˌlæpəˈrɔtəmi] *n.* 剖腹术

In that case laparotomy should be performed without delay.

如果是那种情况就应该立即做剖腹术。

If there is any doubt about the diagnosis, laparotomy is indicated.

假若诊断可疑,可做剖腹术。

largely [ˈlɑːdʒli] *ad.* 大量地; 大部分; 主要

The results seem to depend largely upon a bloodless field and the thoroughness of the removal of all infected tissue.

效果似乎大部分取决于缺血区以及对所有受感染组织的彻底清除。

Hypertension is more common in women than men, largely owing to the longer survival of women.

高血压在女性中较男性更为常见,其主要原因是由于女性的寿命较男性更长。

larva [ˈlɑːvə] (*pl.* larvae [ˈlɑːviː]) *n.* [拉] 幼虫,蚴

The passage of larvae through the lungs may result in pneumonitis.

蛔蚴通过肺部可引起肺炎。

larval [ˈlɑːvəl] *a.* 幼虫的,蚴的

The first type is that the development of both larval and adult stages must take place in the host.

第一种类型是幼虫和成虫两个阶段的成长必须在宿主内进行。

laryngalgia [ˌlærinˈgældʒiə] *n.* 喉痛

Pain in the larynx is called laryngalgia.

喉部疼痛称为喉痛。

An inflammation of the nerves of the larynx can also cause laryngalgia.

喉神经的炎症也可引起喉痛。

laryngeal [ləˈrindʒiəl] *a.* 喉的

Laryngeal cancer has recently become more common in women.

喉癌成为近来妇女中较常见的一种疾病。

Laryngeal examination usually shows a mass or ulceration at the tumor site in patients with laryngalgia.

喉痛病人的喉部检查常显示有硬块或肿块处有溃疡。

Laryngeal reflex can be induced by irritating the larynx.

喉反射可用刺激喉的方法来诱发。

laryngectomy [ˌlærinˈdʒektəmi] *n.* 喉切除术

Surgical removal of the whole or a part of the larynx is called laryngectomy, as in the treatment of laryngeal carcinoma.

切除全部或部分喉的外科手术叫作喉切除术,用来治疗喉癌。

Total laryngectomy is required for many advanced larynx cancers.

许多晚期喉癌患者需作全喉切除术。

laryngitis [ˌlærinˈdʒaitis] *n.* 喉炎

A veteran physician cured him of chronic laryngitis.

一位老练的医生治愈了他的慢性喉炎。

A laryngitis patient feels dryness and soreness of throat, and may have hoarseness, cough and dysphagia.

喉炎病人常感觉喉部干燥和疼痛,也可有声音嘶哑、咳嗽和吞咽困难。

laryngoscope [ləˈriŋgɔskəup] *n.* 喉镜

Laryngoscope is an instrument for examining the larynx.

喉镜是一种用来检查喉部的器械。

laryngoscopic [ˌlæriŋgəuˈskɔpik] *a.* 喉镜检查的

Direct laryngoscopic examinations reveal the presence of a foreign body in the larynx.

直接喉镜检查可显示喉部异物的存在。

laryngoscopy [ˌlæriŋˈgɔskəpi] *n.* 喉镜检查

Direct laryngoscopy will confirm the diagnosis of a foreign body.

直接喉镜检查可证实对异物的诊断。

Small benign tumors of the vocal cord producing hoarseness may be locally excised under direct or indirect laryngoscopy.

造成嘶哑的良性小声带肿瘤在直接或间接的喉镜检查下可以进行局部切除。

laryngostomy [ˌlærinˈgɔstəmi] *n.* 喉造口术

Anything that obstructs the flow of air from the nose to the larynx may call for a laryngostomy.

任何东西阻塞从鼻腔到喉部的气流时,则要求做喉造口术。

laryngotomy [ˌlæriŋˈgɔtəmi] *n.* 喉切开术

Inferior laryngotomy is a life-saving operation when there is obstruction to breathing at or above the larynx.

喉下部切开术是在喉或喉以上部位发生呼吸阻塞时施行的急救手术。

larynx [ˈlæriŋks] *n.* 喉

The walls of the larynx are formed of cartilage.

喉壁系由软骨构成。

As a rule, interference with flow of air in or above the larynx will produce inspiratory dyspnea.

通常,喉内和喉上部的气流障碍将引起呼吸困难。

laser [ˈleizə] *n.* 激光,激光器

Medical advances have made possible the use of laser in eye surgery.

医学进展使激光应用于眼睛手术成为可能。

Laser is a device for generating, amplifying and concentrating light waves into an intense beam in one specific direction.

激光是将产生和扩大光波聚成强烈光柱的一种装置。

(注:laser 系 light amplification by stimulated emission of radiation 的首字母缩略词。)

latency [ˈleitənsi] *n.* 潜伏期,潜隐期

Latency means that a disease agent may initiate pathogenesis that does not manifest overt disease for many years or even decades.

潜伏期系指某致病因子可能引起发病机制,但几年甚至几十年都不表现出明显的疾病。

A number of diseases have latency periods when no “markers” are present.

很多疾病具有潜伏期,在此期间无症状出现。

latent [ˈleitənt] *a.* 潜伏的,隐性的

There is a general inverse correlation between the latent period and the severity of symptoms.

潜伏期与病状的严重性之间一般呈相反的关系。

Latent period is seemingly inactive period as that between exposure of tissue to an injurious agent and the manifestation of response.

潜伏期是表面上的不活动期,即组织接触损伤性刺激物和表现出反应之间的时期。

lateral [ˈlætərəl] *a.* 侧的,外侧的

The kidneys are lateral to the vertebral column.

肾脏位于脊柱两侧。

lattice [ˈlætis] *n.* 格子,晶格,网络

Immune-complex lattice size is influenced by many factors.

免疫复合物晶格的大小受到很多因素的影响。

laurocapram [ˌlɔːrəˈkæpræm] *n.* 月桂氮䓬酮

Laurocapram and its derivatives have not been widely accepted for pharmaceutical use.
月桂氮䓬酮及其衍生物在药物制剂中的应用还未被广泛接受。
Laurocapram is used as the penetration enhancer in cosmetic preparations.
月桂氮䓬酮在化妆品中用作渗透增强剂。

lavage [ləˈvɑːʒ] *n.* [法] 灌洗
Peritoneal lavage should be performed.
应该施行腹腔灌洗。
The nurse gave the patient a gastric lavage.
护士给病人洗胃。

lax [læks] *a.* 松弛的
The articular capsule of these joints is thin and lax but the bones are joined by strong collateral ligaments.
这些关节的关节囊又薄又松弛,但是关节的骨骼有很强的侧副韧带相联结。

laxative [ˈlæksətiv] *a.* 轻泻的
The doctor advised the patient to take this medicine for laxative purpose.
医生建议病人服用此药以达到轻泻的目的。
n. 轻泻药
If a person has appendicitis, a laxative could cause the appendix to rupture.
假如一个人患了阑尾炎,服用泻药很可能造成阑尾穿孔。
Prolonged use of strong laxatives leads to severe hypokalemic alkalosis.
长期使用强烈的泻药可导致严重的低血钾性碱中毒。

lead[1] [liːd] *a.* 领导的;最重要的
Lead researcher Dr. Argenziano said that the success rate proved we can do this surgery in a closed chest approach.
首席研究员阿基兹安鲁博士说这样的成功率证明我们能用不开胸的方法进行手术。
A lead editorial appearing in today's newspaper calls on people of the country to carry out an anti-epidemic health movement.
今天报纸发表的重要社论号召全国人民开展防止流行病的卫生运动。

lead[2] [liːd] *n.* 导联
The clinical examination of all cardiac patients is incomplete without the recording of a 12-lead ECG.
所有心脏病人的临床检查如果没有 12 导联心电图的记录将是不完整的。

lead[3] [led] *n.* 铅
Lead is a natural element with thousands of uses.
铅是一种自然元素,具有许许多多的用途。
Even continuous low-level exposure causes lead to accumulate in the body and cause damage。
与铅的长期微量接触也可使其在体内积聚并造成损害。

leak [liːk] *v.* 漏,渗
Ascitic fluid may leak through the diaphragm to create a pleural effusion.
腹水可以漏过横膈膜造成胸腔积液。
The leaking of the heart is due to serious valve lesions.
心脏漏血是由于严重的瓣膜损伤引起的。

leakage [ˈliːkidʒ] *n.* 泄漏,漏出
The leakage of toxic waste is reaching alarming proportions.
有毒废物的泄漏已达到令人震惊的程度。
A leakage of blood through the valve is known as incompetence of the valve.
血液漏过瓣膜,被称为瓣膜闭锁不全。

lean [liːn] *a.* 瘦的,贫弱的

This patient is also at risk for substantial reduction in lean body mass due to disuse of muscles.
由于肌肉不经常使用,这种病人常瘦弱且体质下降到危险的程度。

lecithine [ˈlesiθiːn] *n.* 卵磷脂

Lecithine is a pure, natural product that is obtained from plant oils, mainly soya oils.
卵磷脂是从植物油,主要是大豆油中获得的纯天然产物。

Lecithine is used to stabilize intravenous fat emulsions.
卵磷脂用来稳定静脉脂肪乳剂。

lectin [ˈlektin] *n.* 植物凝集素,外源凝集素

Lectin is a special class of proteins.
植物血凝素是一类特殊的蛋白质。

Lectin molecules contain two or more sugar-binding sites.
植物血凝素分子具有两个或更多的糖结合位点。

Lecythophora [ˌlesiˈθɔfərə] *n.* 烧瓶状霉属

Two cases of endocarditis patients have been reported becoming infected with Lecythophora.
有两例心肌炎患者发生烧瓶状霉菌感染的报道。

The genus Lecythophora is a mold that lacks a known sexual state.
烧瓶状霉属是一种缺乏已知的性生殖性状的霉菌。

leflunomide [leˈflʌnəmaid] *n.* 来氟米特

In this paper, the clinical applications of leflunomide were discussed.
本文对来氟米特的临床应用进行了讨论。

Is leflunomide a new oral agent in the treatment of acute pancreatitis?
来氟米特是治疗急性胰腺炎的一种新型口服药吗?

Legionella [ˈliːdʒəˈnelə] *n.* 军团菌

Legionellosis is the illness caused by exposure to the bacterial pathogen Legionella.
军团菌病是感染军团菌病原体引起的疾病。

Man-made water systems sometimes provide environments that let Legionella bacteria increase to large numbers.
人工供水系统有时为军团菌的大量繁殖提供了环境基础。

legionellosis [ˌliːdʒəneˈləusis] *n.* 军团(杆)菌病

Legionellosis has a broad range of manifestations from a mild grippe to a fulminant multisystem disease.
军团菌病表现多样化,从轻微流感型到暴发性多系统疾病。

Studies on the pathogenesis of legionellosis are limited.
关于军团(杆)菌病的发病机制的研究很有限。

legionnaires' disease [ˌliːdʒənˈnɛəs diˈziːz] *n.* 军团病

Legionnaires' disease is a bacterial infection of the lungs. Symptoms appear after an incubation period of about seven days.
军团病是一种肺部的细菌性感染,大约在 7 天潜伏期之后便会出现症状。

legislation [ˌledʒisˈleiʃn] *n.* 立法

Legislation will be difficult and take time.
立法并不容易而且需要时间。

The legislation includes specific provisions for women in active labor who risk delivering during transport.
法规还包括了对临产产妇在运送过程中面临分娩风险的特殊条款。

legitimate [liˈdʒitimeit] *a.* 合法的

The rules and regulations described here are for the protection of patients, not to prevent legitimate medical research.
在此提及的规章制度都旨在保护患者,而非阻止合法的医学研究。

legume [ˈlegjuːm] *n.* 豆,(豆)荚

Foods high in amino acids include meats, eggs, milk, grains and legumes.

富含氨基酸的食物包括肉、蛋、奶、谷类和豆类。

leiomyoma [ˌlaiəumaiˈəumə] *n.* 平滑肌瘤

Uterine leiomyomas are benign smooth muscle neoplasms that may occur singly, but most often are multiple.

子宫平滑肌瘤是平滑肌的良性肿瘤,可单发,但通常多发。

Leiomyomas are sharply circumscribed, discrete, round, firm, gray-white tumors varying in size from small, barely visible nodules to massive tumors.

平滑肌瘤是边界清楚、独立、圆形、质实的灰白色肿块,大小不一,可小到几乎肉眼看不见,也可大到巨块状。

Dysphagia is one of the manifestations of the patients with esophageal leiomyoma.

吞咽困难是食管平滑肌瘤患者的症状之一。

leiomyosarcoma [ˈlaiəuˌmaiəusɑːˈkəumə] *n.* 平滑肌肉瘤

Leiomyosarcomas are equally common before and after menopause, and have a peak incidence at 40 to 60 years of age.

平滑肌肉瘤在绝经前后同样常见,高峰年龄在 40 ~ 60 岁。

Leiomyosarcoma is a relatively rare form of cancer, and accounts for 5-10% of soft tissue sarcomas, which are in themselves relatively rare.

子宫平滑肌肉瘤是一种相对罕见的癌症,占原本就相对少见的软组织肉瘤的 5% ~ 10%。

leishmaniasis [ˌliːʃməˈnaiəsis] *n.* 利什曼病

After recovery dermal leishmaniasis sometimes develops.

疾病恢复后有时却会发生皮肤利什曼病。

leisure [ˈleʒə] *n.* 空闲,闲暇

We have been working all week without a moment's leisure.

我们整整干了一周,无一刻闲暇。

length [leŋθ] *n.* 长短,长度

Pension depends on length of service with the company.

养老金的多少取决于为公司服务时间的长短。

By the end of the first month the embryo will have reached a length of only 1/8 inch, but it will consist of millions of cells.

到第一个月末,胚胎将只达到 1/8 英寸长,但它却是由数百万个细胞组成。

lengthen [ˈleŋθən] *v.* (使)延长,(使)伸长

Some think it is possible that nursing the infant may lengthen the period of this immunity.

有人认为,用母乳哺育婴儿有可能延长这种免疫作用的时效。

These appearances are also seen in the elderly with normal blood pressure, and are caused by lengthening and hardening of the arteries.

这些现象也见于血压正常的老年人,它是由动脉伸长和硬化引起的。

lens [lenz] *n.* 透镜,镜片;晶体,晶状体

The development of contact lenses has opened a new world of sight for many people who have vision problems.

隐形镜片(又称隐形眼镜)的应用为许多有视力毛病的人们开创了一个视力新世界。

Intraocular lens implants have given back the sight of numerous elderly people which they had before their vision was dimmed or lost to cataracts.

眼内晶体植入使无数中老年人由于白内障而变得模糊或完全丧失的视力得到恢复。

Specialists are designing soft contact lenses which can deliver medication to the eyes instead of eye drops.

医学专家正在设计能代替滴眼液将药物送到眼内的软质隐形镜片。

lentigo [len'taigəu] *n.* 着色斑，雀斑（复数 lentigines）

The term lentigo refers to a common benign localized hyperplasia of melanocytes occurring at all ages, but often initiated in infancy and childhood.

雀斑一词是指黑色素细胞常见的良性局限性增生，可以发生在任何年龄，但通常开始于婴幼年期。

The histologic feature of a lentigo is linear melanocytic hyperplasia restricted to the cell layer immediately above the basement membrane.

雀斑的组织学特征是黑色素细胞的线样增生，局限于刚好在基底膜上的一层细胞。

lentivirus [ˌlenti'vaiərəs] *n.* 慢病毒

Lentiviruses are a group of retroviruses that include the human immunodeficiency virus, HIV-1. They cause disease after a long incubation period.

慢病毒是一组包含人类免疫缺陷病毒在内的逆转录病毒，它们经过一段长的潜伏期后导致疾病。

The result of cell long-term proliferation assay demonstrated that cell growth was inhibited by lentivirus.

细胞长期增殖实验的结果表明细胞生长受慢病毒的抑制。

leonurine [liəu'njuːrin] *n.* 益母草碱

There was small amount of leonurine during the early stages of blooming, and then it gradually increased.

开花初期时存在微量的益母草碱，然后含量逐渐增高。

Pharmacokinetics of leonurine in rats is essential.

益母草碱在大鼠体内的药动学研究是必要的。

leonurus [liəu'njuːrəs] *n.* 益母草

You must establish the fingerprints method of capillary electrophoresis for leonurus injection.

你必须建立益母草注射液的毛细管电泳指纹图谱。

We will set out to study the cultivation technique of GAP of Leonurus.

我们将要开始研究益母草 GAP 栽培技术。

leprosy ['leprəsi] *n.* 麻风病

Mycobacterium are the agents of tuberculosis and leprosy.

结核病和麻风病的病原体属于分枝杆菌属。

leptin ['leptin] *n.* 瘦素

Previous studies suggest a possible link between leptin and hepatic inflammation.

此前的研究表明瘦素和肝炎之间可能有联系。

The mutation that affect signaling by leptin was hypothesized to contribute to human obesity.

已假设影响瘦素信号传递的突变与人体肥胖有关。

leptospira [ˌleptə'spaiərə] *n.* 钩端螺旋体属（=leptospire）

The mechanism by which leptospira organisms cause damage to tissues is obscure.

钩端螺旋体造成组织损伤的机制尚不清楚。

All pathogenic leptospirae are harbored by animal hosts and are communicated via water and soil.

全部致病性钩端螺旋体都聚藏在动物宿主内，且可通过水及土壤传播。

leptospiral [ˌleptə'spaiərəl] *a.* 钩端螺旋体的

There are few sequelae of leptospiral infections.

钩端螺旋体感染很少有后遗症。

leptospirosis [ˌleptəspaiə'rəusis] *n.* 钩端螺旋体病

Leptospirosis is being reported more frequently.

钩端螺旋体病正在被更为频繁地报道出来。

The laboratory diagnosis of laptospirosis depends on isolation of the organisms by bacteriologic methods or serologic tests.

钩端螺旋体病的实验室诊断依靠细菌学方法分离病原体或血清学试验。

leptospiruria [ˌleptəuspiˈrjuəriə] *n.* 钩端螺旋体尿

Leptospiruria is usually limited to two to four weeks, but sometimes persists for months.

尿排出钩端螺旋体多在 2 周到 4 周内，有时可持续数月。

leptotene [ˈleptəutiːn] *n.* （细胞分裂中的）细线期

At leptotene stage, the two sister chromatids of each chromosome are so closely aligned that they cannot be distinguished.

在细线期，每条染色体的两个姐妹染色单体紧密排列在一起而不能区分。

Prophase may be divided into successive stages leptotene, zygotene, pachytene , diplotene , and diakinesis .

前期可被分为连续的阶段：细线期、偶线期、粗线期、双线期和终变期。

lesion [ˈliːʒən] *n.* 损害，损伤

The influence of environmental factors may result in lesions.

环境因素的影响可引起损害。

No lesions other than preexisting pancreatitis were found at laparotomy.

除既往存在的胰腺炎外，剖腹术未发现其他病变。

Not all mass-like lesions of the lung are due to carcinoma.

肺的肿块样病灶并非都是由癌所致。

Many rectal lesions can be demonstrated by barium enema.

许多直肠疾病可由钡灌肠检出。

lethal [ˈliːθəl] *a.* 致死的，致命的

The amount of a drug which may be sufficient enough to cause death is called a lethal dose.

足够引起死亡的药物量称为致死剂量。

Lethal changes have occurred elsewhere in the cell.

细胞的其他部位已发生了致死性改变。

Leukemia and cystic fibrosis are lethal diseases.

白血病和囊性纤维变性是致命的疾病。

lethargic [leˈθɑːdʒik] *a.* 昏睡的，冷淡的

The patient appears acutely ill with a dull, expressionless, lethargic face.

患者的病势更显严重：面容呆钝、淡漠而且呈倦睡神态。

lethargy [ˈleθədʒi] *n.* 嗜睡症

Early clinical evidence of protein malnutrition is vague and includes lethargy, apathy, or irritability.

蛋白缺乏性营养不良的早期临床迹象是不明显的，它包括嗜睡、情感淡漠和烦躁。

The rural inhabitants claim that their ability to work is severely reduced as a result of the weakness and lethargy caused by schistosomiasis.

农村居民声称由于血吸虫引起的虚弱和嗜睡，他们的劳动能力被大大地降低了。

leucine [ˈluːsin] *n.* 亮氨酸

The changes in transport activity closely correspond to similar changes in the levels of the leucine-binding proteins.

转运活性的变化与亮氨酸结合蛋白水平的类似变化非常相符。

There is a direct relationship between the level of leucine in the medium and the level of the leucine binding protein.

媒介中亮氨酸水平和亮氨酸结合蛋白水平有直接关系。

leucoplakia [ˌljuːkəˈpleikiə] *n.* 白斑病

In the leucoplakia group, complete response was achieved in four out of five treated patients.

在白斑病组，完全有效的占接受治疗患者的五分之四。

The clinicopathology of laryngeal leucoplakia was studied in 9 cases.

对 9 例喉白斑病进行了临床病理分析。

leucorrhoea [ˌljuːkəˈriːə] *n.* 白带

The term leucorrhoea, which is now infrequently used, should be confined to an increase in the physiological secretion.

白带一词目前不常用,应限于生理性分泌增加。

In the third month, sixth month and twelfth month after placement of IUD (intrauterine device), three side-effects including blood dripping, menorrhagia and leucorrhea were found.

在放置宫内节育器后 3 个月、6 个月和 12 个月时,出现淋漓出血、月经量增多和白带增多三种副作用。

leukemia [ljuːˈkiːmiə] *n.* 白血病

Lymph node enlargement occurs early in chronic lymphocytic leukemia.

慢性淋巴性白血病出现淋巴结肿大较早。

Radiologists and others working near radiation have a high incidence of leukemia and skin and bone cancer.

放射科医生和其他接近辐射的人员,白血病、皮肤癌和骨癌的发病率高。

leukemic [ljuːˈkiːmik] *a.* 白血病的

Leukemic infiltrates are frequently seen on histologic examination.

做组织学检查时,常见有白血病浸润。

leukemogenic [ljuːˌkiːməuˈdʒenik] *a.* 致白血病的

The alkylating agents are highly leukemogenic.

烷化剂有很强的致白血病作用。

leukemoid [ljuːˈkiːmɔid] *a.* 白血病样的,类白血病的

Leukemoid reactions, in the absence of infection, are associated with gastric, lung, and pancreatic carcinomas.

如果在没有感染时出现了类白血病反应,则应考虑它与胃癌、肺癌和胰腺癌等症有关。

leukocidin [ljuːˈkɔsidin] *n.* 杀白细胞素

Panton-Valentine leukocidin gene (PVL gene) from the isolates of Staphylococcus aureus was detected by using multiple PCR technique.

应用多重 PCR 技术从金黄色葡萄球菌分离物中检测出 P-V 杀白细胞素(PVL)基因。

Necrotizing pneumonia and arthritis took place due to Staphylococcus-aureus-producing P-V leukocidin in a 10-year-old boy.

一名 10 岁男孩因金黄色葡萄菌产生的 P-V 杀白细胞素发生了坏死性肺炎和关节炎。

leukocyte [ˈljuːkəsait] *n.* 白细胞(=leucocyte)

The leukocyte count varies from 5000 to 9000 per cubic millimeter.

白细胞计数每立方毫米为 5000 ~ 9000 不等。

Phagocytosis by leucocytes has been shown to be more efficient in the presence of specific antibody.

在有特异性抗体时,白细胞的吞噬作用更大。

Another important set of leucocytes is the lymphocytes.

另一批重要的白细胞是淋巴细胞。

leukocytic [ˌljuːkəˈsitik] *a.* 白细胞的

The substance liberated from cells in this situation is termed leukocytic pyrogen.

在此条件下,由细胞分泌出来的这种物质被命名为白细胞致热原。

leukocytosis [ˌljuːkəsaiˈtəusis] *n.* 白细胞增多

Leukocytosis is a universal hematologic feature of chronic leukemias.

白细胞增多是慢性白血病的一种普遍性血液学特征。

The third category includes fever, leukocytosis, and general humoral or adaptive responses to injury of any kind.

第三类包括发热、白细胞增多和对任何损伤的全身体液反应或适应性反应。

leukoencephalopathy [ˌljuːkəˌensefəˈlɔpəθi] *n.* 白质脑病

Leukoencephalopathy refers to the destruction of the myelin sheaths that cover nerve fibers.
白质脑病是指包绕神经纤维的髓鞘遭到了破坏。

Progressive multifocal leukoencephalopathy is a serious viral infection of the brain that strikes people with HIV and AIDS.
进行性多灶性白质脑病是脑内一种严重的病毒感染，常侵犯 HIV 感染的人和艾滋病病人。

leukopenia [ˌljuːkəuˈpiːniə] *n.* 白细胞减少

Occurrence of leukopenia and thrombocytopenia seems to suggest leukemia.
出现白细胞减少和血小板减少似乎提示有白血病。

In megaloblastic anemia, because all cell lines are affected, leukopenia and thrombocytopenia may occur with anemia.
在巨幼红细胞性贫血时，由于所有细胞系均受到影响，白细胞减少和血小板减少的现象可与贫血同时出现。

leukoplakia [ˌljuːkəuˈpleikiə] *n.* 黏膜白斑

Leukoplakia of the oral cavity, vulva, and penis is a kind of precancerous conditions because of the association with cancer.
口腔、外阴和阴茎的黏膜白斑是一种癌前状态，因为它们与癌症的发生有关。

Leukoplakia of the vulva is a heterogeneous group of lesions presents as white, plaquelike mucosal thickening that may produce itching and scaling.
外阴的黏膜白斑是一组异质性的病变，可表现为白色的斑块状的黏膜增厚，并引起瘙痒和脱屑。

leukopoietin [ˌljuːkəupɔiˈiːtin] *n.* 白细胞生成素；粒细胞生成素

Leukopoietin is a substance serving as the humoral regulator of leukopoiesis.
白细胞生成素是充当白细胞生成的体液调节剂的一种物质。

leukotriene [ˌljuːkəuˈtraiiːn] *n.* 白三烯，白细胞三烯

Some of leukotrienes stimulate the movement leukocytes.
有些白三烯可以促进白细胞的运动。

Leukotriene receptor antagonist is a new drug to treat allergic rhinitis.
白三烯受体拮抗剂是治疗变应性鼻炎的一种新药。

Arachidonic acid is the starting material from which potent inflammatory compounds such as leukotrienes are made.
花生四烯酸是合成强力炎症化合物如白三烯的起始原料。

levamisole [leˈvæːmisəul] *n.* 左旋咪唑

The aim is to understand the use of levamisole as immunoregulation in clinic.
目的就是了解左旋咪唑作为免疫调节药在临床的使用情况。

levodopa [ˌliːvəuˈdəupə] *n.* 左旋多巴

Levodopa competes with tyrosine and tryptophan at the blood-brain barrier.
左旋多巴在血脑屏障与酪氨酸和色氨酸竞争。

We investigate the consequences of levodopa therapy.
我们研究左旋多巴治疗的结果。

levorphanol [leˈvɔːfənəul] *n.* 左旋吗喃

Levorphanol is a synthetic narcotic.
左旋吗喃是一种合成的麻醉镇痛药。

levothyroxine [ˌliːvəuθaiˈrɔksiːn] *n.* 左旋甲状腺素

Celiac disease in patients with hypothyroidism requires elevated levothyroxine doses.
甲状腺功能减低症患者的脂肪泻需要增加左旋甲状腺素的剂量。

If hypothyroidism has been diagnosed, substitution with levothyroxine should be initiated.
如果诊断出甲状腺功能减低症,左旋甲状腺素的替代治疗就必须立即开始。

levulose [ˈlevjuləus] *n.* 左旋糖

Hyperglycemia enhances the formation of advanced glycation end products (AGEs) that result from the auto-oxidation of glucose and levulose.
高血糖促进了由葡萄糖和左旋糖自氧化作用引起的晚期糖基化终末产物的形成。

The infusion of levulose was unable to change the NPY secretory pattern during insulin-induced hypoglycemia
输入左旋糖不能改变胰岛素诱导的低血糖期间神经肽的分泌模式。

leydig [ˈleidig] *n.* 间质

Gynecomastia may occur with cirrhosis of liver, leydig cell tumors of testis, or with drugs.
男性乳腺发育可由肝硬化、睾丸间质细胞瘤或药物引起。

The article reviews the interaction and regulation of sertoli cells and leydig cells in testis.
本文综述了睾丸支持细胞与间质细胞之间的相互作用与调节。

liability [laiəˈbiliti] *n.* 倾向,易于,易患

With the increased liability to infection, hypostatic pneumonia may occur.
随着易感性增加,可能发生坠积性肺炎。

liable [ˈlaiəbl] *a.* 倾向的,易于的

Man is not liable to suffer from many bacterial diseases which affect animals.
人是不容易患能侵袭动物的许多细菌性疾病的。

liberate [ˈlibəreit] *v.* 释放,放出

The blood platelets liberate a special ferment, which causes the clotting of blood.
血小板释放出一种特殊的酶,这种酶能引起血液凝固。

When the amount of oxygen in the plasma is reduced, the hemoglobin immediately begins liberating oxygen into the plasma.
当血浆内氧的含量减少时,血红蛋白便立即开始将氧释放到血浆内。

liberation [ˌlibəˈreiʃən] *n.* 释放(作用)

Here liberation refers to the release of the drug from whatever form in which it has been administered.
在这里"释放作用"是指药物从给药时的剂型中释放出来。

This may be attributed to hydrolysis of the nucleoprotein, with liberation of nucleic acid which stains densely with basic dyes.
这可归因于核蛋白的水解作用,释放出核酸,核酸可被碱性染料浓染。

libido [liˈbiːdəu] (*pl.* libidines [liˈbidiniːz]) *n.* 性欲

Amenorrhea, loss of libido, GI complaints and sometimes jaundice and splenomegaly can occur in the presence of severe anemia.
严重贫血时可能出现闭经、性欲丧失、胃肠不适,有时甚至出现黄疸和脾肿大。

library [ˈlaibrəri] *n.* 文库

This collection of cDNA clones is referred to as a cDNA library.
cDNA 克隆的集合体称为 cDNA 文库。

license [ˈlaisəns] *v.* 许可,特许

Vaccines must be administered by the licensed route to ensure immunogenicity and safety.
应通过发放许可证途径管理疫苗的使用,以保证其免疫原性和安全性。

This drug store is licensed for the sale of non-prescription drugs and prescription drugs as well.
这家药房获准出售非处方药以及处方药。

n. 执照

A doctor who opens a private clinic must have a license issued by the bureau of health.
医生开设私人诊所必须有卫生局颁发的执照。

lichen [ˈlaikən] *n.* 苔藓

Skin was negative except for a few lesions on both elbows and knees consistent with lichen nitidus.

除两肘和两膝部有少许光泽苔藓样皮损外,其余皮肤无异常。

Manifestations of chronic graft-versus-host disease are lichen sclerosus and eosinophilic fasciitis.

慢性移植物抗宿主病表现为硬化性苔藓和嗜酸性筋膜炎。

lid [lid] *n.* 盖子;眼睑

Keep the lid on the kettle before the water boils.

水煮沸之前不要揭开水壶的盖子。

The upper lid closes over the eye like a curtain.

上眼睑紧靠眼睛就像窗帘一样。

lidocaine [ˈlaidəukein] *n.* 利多卡因

The patient was treated with lidocaine.

此病人用利多卡因治疗过。

lie [lai] *n.* 平卧;产式

By abdominal examination it is possible to ascertain the lie, presentation and attitude of the fetus.

通过腹部检查可查明胎产式、胎先露和胎儿姿势。

life-expectancy [ˈlaif-iksˈpektənsi] *n.* 预期寿命

The result from the current use of drugs for improving life-expectancy in patients with lipid disorders is disappointing.

现行用药物治疗改善脂类紊乱患者的预期寿命的效果,是令人失望的。

lifeless [ˈlaiflis] *a.* 无生命的; 单调的;没有生气的

The child was delivered, but lifeless. As the obstetrician gazed at the still form a shiver of horror passed over her.

孩子虽然生下来了,但却是死的。产科医生看到静止不动的孩子的时候,一阵恐惧的颤抖贯穿了她的全身。

lifelong [ˈlaiflɔŋ] *a.* 毕生的,终身的

One attack of measles usually confers a lifelong immunity, though second attack does occur.

麻疹一次得病通常可终身免疫,但的确也可再次得病。

lifespan [ˈlaifˈspæn] *n.* 使用期;有效期;寿命期限

The lifespan of inflammatory macrophages varies with the causal agent.

炎性巨噬细胞的寿命随病因因子而异。

The lifespan of an erythrocyte has been estimated at 90 to 125 days.

红细胞的生命期估计在 90 ~ 125 天之间。

It is also helpful to plan for the entire lifespan of a patient registry, including how and when the registry will end and any plans for transition at that time.

对患者登记的整个使用期作出计划也是很有用的,包括登记将何时结束、如何结束以及结束时的任何过渡计划。

life-threatening [ˈlaifˈθretəniŋ] *a.* 威胁生命的

Anaphylaxis is a life-threatening allergic reaction that can occur quickly.

过敏是一种威胁生命的变态反应,能够很快地发生。

Not all medical emergencies listed below are life-threatening.

不是所有列在下面的急诊都会危及生命。

lifetime [ˈlaiftaim] *n.* 一生; 终身

A good scientist spends his lifetime carrying on experiments to find new truths.

一位优秀的科学家往往毕生不停地做实验以求发现新的原理。

Depression and anxiety disorders are common public health problems, with 10 to 20% lifetime prevalence.

抑郁症和焦虑症是常见的公共卫生问题,终生患病率为 10% ~20% 。

ligament ['ligəmənt] *n.* 韧带

Relaxation of ligaments aids in producing deformities.

韧带松弛会助长畸形发展。

ligamentous [ˌligə'mentəs] *a.* 韧带的

The ligamentous structures in a child are stronger than the growth plates of the bones.

儿童的韧带组织比其骨骼的生长板要牢固。

ligand ['laigənd] *n.* 配体

This model gives a rigid picture of the enzyme and cannot account for the effects of allosteric ligands.

这种模型描述酶为固定的图形,因而不能解释变构配体的效应。

Interaction of CTLA-4 with these same ligands now induces down regulation of T cell functions.

CTLA-4 与其相应的配体之间的相互作用可使 T 细胞的功能下调。

ligase ['ligeis, 'lai-] *n.* 连接酶

Ligase is an enzyme that can catalyze the joining of two large molecules by forming a new chemical bond.

连接酶是一种通过形成新的化学键促使两个大分子连接起来的酶。

DNA ligase can also join two blunt ends together without any need for compatibility of single-stranded overhangs.

DNA 连接酶也能将两个平末端连接在一起而不需要有互补的突出单链。

ligate ['laigeit] *v.* 结扎

An indirect hernia sac should be anatomically isolated, dissected to its origin from the peritoneum, and ligated.

斜疝疝囊应根据解剖分离到腹膜的起点后才予以结扎。

ligation [lai'geiʃən] *n.* 结扎,(结)扎法

Repair can usually be limited to high ligation.

修复手术通常限于高位结扎。

In animals, ligation of the cystic duct alone does not produce acute cholecystitis.

仅仅结扎动物的胆囊管并不会引起急性胆囊炎。

ligature ['ligətʃə] *n.* 结扎线

The long ends of blood vessels that project beyond a ligature should be removed.

突出在结扎线外的血管的长端应当割掉。

lightheaded ['lait'hedid] *a.* 头昏眼花的

If you begin to breathe too fast or feel lightheaded, slow your breathing.

如果你开始呼吸速度过快或感到有些头昏,减慢你的呼吸。

In general, syncope is defined by a brief loss of consciousness (fainting) or by dimmed vision and feeling uncoordinated, confused, and lightheaded.

一般说来,晕厥的定义是意识的短暂丧失(晕倒)或两眼发黑,并感到共济失调、意识迷糊或头昏眼花。

likelihood ['laiklihud] *n.* 可能(性)

Renal disease increases the likelihood that patient will develop toxemia.

肾病增加病人产生毒血症的可能。

There appears to be a 10% likelihood that diabetic pregnancy will result in a major malformation.

约 10% 的糖尿病妊娠将有导致巨大畸形的可能性。

likely ['laikli] *a.* 有可能的

The more severe the headache, the more likely it is to be associated with nausea.

头痛越严重,越有可能引起恶心。

Illnesses accompanying recurrent infections with a given virus are usually less severe and are more likely to involve the upper respiratory tract.

伴有某种病毒反复感染的疾病通常不严重，而且多累及上呼吸道。

likeness [ˈlaiknis] *n.* 相似，类似

It has recently been discovered that these likenesses are carried in the centre part of nucleus of the cell.

最近发现这些相似之处在细胞核的中心部分。

likewise [ˈlaikwaiz] *ad.* 同样地，也，又

Likewise, IgA is the most abundant antibody in the organism.

同样地，IgA 是机体中量最多的抗体。

I am going to do some gymnastic exercise and you would be well advised to do likewise.

我打算去做做体操，也劝你照样做。

The nails likewise may be involved, either from local inflammation due to the treponema from suppuration, or from constitutional derangement.

指（趾）甲同样可被累及，或由于螺旋体引起的局部发炎化脓所致，或由于全身紊乱所致。

limbic [ˈlimbik] *a.* 边缘的

Vasopressin is a peptide hormone in the blood, but the brain uses it as a neurotransmitter, particularly in the limbic system.

血管加压素是血液中的一种肽类激素，但是脑用它来作神经递质，特别是在边缘系统中。

limit [ˈlimit] *v.* 限制，限定

The clearance is said to be perfusion rate limited.

清除率是受灌注率所限制的。

I shall limit myself to three aspects of the subject.

我将仅就三方面探讨这一问题。

n. 界限，范围

The vital signs of the patient are within normal limits.

此患者的生命迹象在正常范围内。

Most drugs have a safe upper limit of dosage.

多数药物有安全剂量上限。

limitation [ˌlimiˈteiʃən] *n.* 限界，限制，限度，局限

Limitation of joint movements may be temporary or permanent due to joint adhesions.

由于关节的粘连，关节的运动可能暂时或永久性受限。

lincomycin [ˌliŋkəuˈmaisin] *n.* 林可霉素

Lincomycin hydrochloride is a white or practically white, crystalline powder and is odorless or has a faint odor.

盐酸林可霉素是一种白色或几乎白色的结晶性粉末，无味或有微弱的气味。

Lincomycin shares many of the pharmacologic, toxicologic, and antibacterial properties of erythromycin.

林可霉素与红霉素具有很多相同的药理学、毒理学和抗菌特性。

line [lain] *v.* 给…装衬里

A sheet of tissue which lines the surface of an organ is called a membrane.

一层薄的组织衬贴在器官的内侧表面叫做膜。

lineage [ˈliniidʒ] *n.* 血统，家系，世系

They suspect it may be a new lineage of the Kashmiri bee virus, but it could be something completely novel.

他们怀疑这是克什米尔蜜蜂病毒的一个新变种，但也可能是某种新病毒。

linear [ˈliniə] *a.* 直线的；线形的，线性的

Localized scleroderma, a term which includes morphea and linear scleroderma, involves the skin

exclusively.
局部性硬皮病包括硬斑病及线形硬皮病，仅限于皮肤受累。
There was a linear relationship between total placental protein and weight.
全胎盘蛋白与重量之间有着直线的关系。
The flow velocities showed a strong positive linear correlation with age.
流速与年龄有很强的正线性相关。

linearly [ˈliniəli] *ad.* (直)线地；线性地
Imipramine and desipramine levels were linearly correlated with clinical response to the drug.
丙咪嗪和去郁敏(去甲丙咪嗪)水平与对药物的临床反应呈线性相关。

linen [ˈlinin] *n.* 床单
Its infective agent survives long in clothes, bed linen, toys or furniture, and may be carried by a third person.
其有传染性的病原长期存活在衣服、床单、玩具和家具上，并可由第三者传染。

linezolid [liˈnezəulid] *n.* 利奈唑胺
Clinical data of 13 elderly patients with lung infection who were treated with linezolid were analyzed retrospectively.
回顾性分析了 13 例应用利奈唑胺治疗的老年肺部感染患者的临床资料。

liniment [ˈlinimənt] *n.* 搽剂
In general, salves and liniments are used to heal acute inflammations.
药膏和搽剂常用于治疗急性炎症。
Zhongtong Caji, a kind of liniment, is a traditional Chinese medicinal formula that is widely used for clinical treatment of inflammation and sprains.
肿痛擦剂是一种传统的中药剂型，广泛应用于炎症和扭伤的临床治疗。

lining [ˈlainiŋ] *n.* 内面，内壁，内膜
The over production of bile acids may irritate the lining of the colon and trigger abnormal cell growth.
胆汁酸的过度分泌可能会刺激结肠的内壁细胞，引起其异常生长。

link [liŋk] *v.* 连接，联系
Some scientists think that viruses may be linked to some kinds of cancer.
有些科学家认为病毒也可能与某些癌症有关。
It is not clear how the various peptide chains are linked together.
各种肽链是如何连接在一起的还不清楚。
n. 联系
The link between the hypothalamus and the posterior lobe of the pituitary gland is provided by the circulating blood and by nerve fibres.
下丘脑和脑垂体后叶间的联系是依赖循环血液和神经纤维来实现的。

linkage [ˈliŋkidʒ] *n.* 键；连接；连锁
Linkage study is an approach to identifying the genetic factors in diseases.
连锁分析是确定疾病的遗传因素的一种方法。
The phenomenon of sex-linkage is the same in humans as was observed in Drosophila.
人类的性连锁现象与已在果蝇中观察到的相同。

linked [liŋkt] *a.* 连接的；连锁的
Genes located on the sex chromosomes are termed sex-linked genes.
位于性染色体上的基因称为性连锁基因。
Father and mother both can pass X-linked genes to a daughter.
父母双方均可将 X-连锁的基因传给女儿。

linoleic [ˌlinəˈliːik] *n.* 亚麻油酸，亚油酸
Linoleic is one of polyunsaturated acids.

亚油酸是多不饱和脂肪酸中的一种。
Conjugated linoleic acid should be taken every day.
共轭亚油酸应该每天服用。

liparoid [ˈliːpərɔid] *a.* 脂肪的,脂肪样的
The drug has significantly curative effect in treating liparoid liver.
这种药物对脂肪肝具有显著的疗效。
B-ultrasound shows that the improvement of liparoid liver in this group is superior to that of the control group.
B 超显示这组的脂肪肝改善程度优于对照组。

lipase [ˈlaipeis] *n.* 脂酶
When the retinal esters are ingested, they are hydrolyzed in the intestine by pancreatic lipase.
视黄醛醇酯经摄入后在小肠被胰脂酶水解。

lipid [ˈliːpid] *n.* 脂质,脂类
Lipid is a major energy producing foodstuff.
脂类是主要的产能食物。
Cell wall lipids are uncommon in Gram positive bacteria.
在革兰阳性菌中不常见到细胞壁脂质。

lipid-insoluble [ˈlipidinˈsɔljubl] *a.* 非脂溶性的
The absorption of large lipid-insoluble substances is accomplished by specialized transport processes.
非脂溶性的大分子物质的吸收系由特殊的转运机制来完成。

lipidome [ˈlipidəum] *n.* 脂组
The lipidome refers to the totality of lipids in cells.
脂组意指细胞的全部脂质。
Research suggests that the lipidome of an individual may be able to indicate cancer risks associated with dietary fats.
研究提示,一个个体的脂组有可能显示与脂肪饮食有关的癌症风险。

lipidosis [ˌlipiˈdəusis] *n.* 脂沉积症
In particular, the increase in triglyceride content was remarkable, indicating that myocardial lipidosis may be induced by aging.
尤其值得注意的是甘油三酯含量的显著增加提示心肌细胞脂沉积症可由衰老引起。
Glucosylceramide lipidosis results from a defective lysosomal degradation of this glycolipid.
葡糖神经酰胺脂沉积症可由对糖脂溶酶体的降解缺陷引起。

lipid-soluble [ˈlipidˈsɔljubl] *a.* 脂溶的
The lipid-soluble substances are able to traverse the membrane by dissolving in the lipoid phase.
脂溶性物质溶于脂相才能透过质膜。

lipoblast [ˈlipəblæst] *n.* 脂肪母细胞
Lipoblasts are indicative of fatty differentiation and helpful for diagnosis.
脂肪母细胞表示脂肪分化,有助于诊断。
Lipoblasts contain round clear cytoplasmic lipid vacuoles that scallop the nucleus.
脂肪母细胞胞质内含有圆形、境界清楚的脂质空泡,可以将细胞核压成扇贝状。

lipocyte [ˈlipəsait] *n.* 脂细胞
Lipocytes may also contribute to collagen formation in other fibrotic liver disease, such as alcoholic cirrhosis.
在其他纤维性肝病(如酒精性肝硬化)中,脂肪细胞也可促进胶原形成。

lipodystrophy [ˌlipəuˈdistrəfi] *n.* 脂肪代谢障碍;脂肪营养不良
The results showed that the secretion of growth hormone decreased in patients with lipodystrophy in various degrees.

结果表明,在脂肪营养不良患者体内生长激素分泌存在以不同程度的减少。

Lipodystrophy is a kind of idiopathic disease of adipose tissue atrophy.

脂肪营养不良是一种先天性脂肪组织萎缩性疾病。

lipofuscin [ˌlipəuˈfʌsin] *n.* 脂褐质

This drug can effectively decrease the lipofuscin in keratinized cell.

这种药物能有效降低角质化细胞脂褐素含量。

Taurine can prevent the increase of lipofuscin and lipid peroxidation level of myocardium and cerebral cortex in rats after exercise.

牛磺酸可防止大鼠在运动后其心肌和大脑皮质的脂褐素和脂质过氧化水平的增加。

lipogenesis [ˌlipəuˈdʒenisis] *n.* 脂肪生成

De novo lipogenesis is involved in fatty acid biosynthesis.

脂肪重新生成涉及脂肪酸生物合成。

Retinoic acid upregulates preadipocyte genes to block lipogenesis.

维 A 酸上调前脂肪细胞基因来阻止脂肪生成。

lipogenic [ˌlipəuˈdʒenik] *a.* 脂肪生成的

These are lipogenic genes.

这些是生成脂肪的基因。

There is a renewed interest in the ultimate role of fatty acid synthase (FASN) —a key lipogenic enzyme catalysing the terminal steps in the denovo biogenesis of fatty acids — in cancer pathogenesis.

最近,大家对脂肪酸合酶在肿瘤发病机制中的根本作用兴趣重燃。FASN 作为一种关键的脂肪生成酶,可以催化脂肪酸从头合成的最终步骤。

lipoid [ˈlipɔid] *a.* 脂样的,类脂的

Lipoid pneumonia has been reported in debilitated infants.

关于体弱婴儿的脂质性肺炎已经有过报道。

lipolysis [liˈpɔlisis] *n.* 脂(肪分)解

Myocardial lipolysis also increase early in ischemia, apparently through a catecholamine-dependent mechanism.

在心肌缺血的早期,通过儿茶酚胺依赖性机制,心肌的脂肪分解也会增加。

Diabetes often leads to fatty liver because of increased lipolysis due to insulin deficiency.

糖尿病患者由于缺乏胰岛素引起脂肪分解加快,常出现脂肪肝。

lipolytic [ˌlipəuˈlitik] *a.* 分解脂肪的

These are lipolytic genes.

这些是分解脂肪的基因。

We analyze the association between lipogenic and lipolytic genes.

我们研究生成脂肪的基因和分解脂肪的基因之间的联系。

lipoma [liˈpəumə] *n.* 脂瘤

Lipomas are more common than leiomyomas or hemangiomas in the small intestine.

小肠内脂瘤比平滑肌瘤或血管瘤常见。

lipomatosis [ˌlipəuməˈtəusis] *a.* 脂(肪)过多症

Solid masses of fat density indicate benign lipomatosis, which occurs with obesity, Cushing's syndrome, and steroid therapy.

发现脂肪密度的实质性肿块提示良性脂肪过多症,它常发生于肥胖、库欣综合征和类固醇治疗时。

lipophilic [ˌlipəˈfilik] *a.* 亲脂的

Thiopental is a lipophilic substance that diffuses easily into both muscle and brain.

硫喷妥为亲脂性药物,易扩散到肌肉和大脑。

lipopolysaccharide [ˌlipəuˌpɔliˈsækəraid] *n.* 脂多糖

Lipopolysaccharide is a complex and unique glycolipid consisting of three distinct but covalently linked regions.
脂多糖是一种复杂而独特的糖脂,它由三个不同部分以共价键(的方式)连接而成。
In addition, the lipopolysaccharide molecule itself appears to have direct cytotoxic effects.
此外,脂多糖分子自身也有直接的细胞毒作用。

lipoprotein [ˌlipəu'prəutiːn] *n.* 脂蛋白
Lipoproteins contain bound cholesterol.
脂蛋白含有结合的胆固醇。
HDL is abbreviated from high-density lipoprotein.
HDL 是英文高密度脂蛋白的缩写。

liposarcoma [ˌlipəusɑː'kəumə] *n.* 脂肉瘤
Liposarcomas are more common in patients over the age of 40.
脂肉瘤多见于 40 岁以上的病人。

liposome ['lipəusəum] *n.* 脂质体
Liposomes as drug carriers targeting to lymphatic metastatic tumors had been intensively studied.
脂质体作为靶向淋巴转移性肿瘤的药物载体已被着重研究.
Liposomes possess unique properties owing to the amphiphilic character of the lipids.
脂类的两亲性特征使脂质体具有独特的性质。

lipotropin [li'pɔtrəpin] *n.* 脂肪酸
The endorphins are segments of β-lipotropin, and the enkephalins are segments of the endorphins.
内啡肽是 β-脂肪酸释放激素的片段,而脑啡肽又是内啡肽的片段。

liquefaction [ˌlikwi'fækʃən] *n.* 液化(作用)
This is an important factor in the liquefaction of pus.
这是脓汁液化的重要因素。
Non-liquefaction of semen is one of the familiar reasons resulting in male infertility.
精液不液化是引起男性不育的常见原因之一。

liquefy ['likwifai] *v.* (使)溶化,(使)液化
Air is liquefied by subjecting it to a high pressure at a low temperature.
空气处于高压低温的环境下可以液化。

listeriosis [lisˌtiəri'əusis] *n.* 李斯特菌病,李斯特菌感染
Listeriosis is an infection caused by the gram-positive motile bacterium *Listeriamonocytogenes*.
李斯特菌病是一种由李斯特单胞菌引起的感染,这种细菌革兰阳性,能运动。
Listeriosis is relatively rare and occurs primarily in newborn infants, elderly patients, and patients who are immunocompromised.
李斯特菌感染相对少见,主要发生于新生儿、老年人以及免疫功能不全的病人。

lithium ['liθiəm] *n.* 锂
Lithium inhibits both thyroid hormone synthesis and release.
锂既可以抑制甲状腺素的合成又可抑制其释放。
Lithium carbonate has proved to be the best means of controlling mania and of preventing recurrent attacks.
已证明碳酸锂是控制躁狂症和预防其复发的最好方法。
In general, a lithium battery may last 10 to 12 years in most clinical circumstances.
在大多数临床情况下,锂电池一般可用 10 ~ 12 年。

lithotomy [li'θɔtəmi] *n.* 切(开取)石术,截石
For the remainder of the internal examination, the patient remains in the lithotomy position.
为继续进行(盆腔内)其余的检查,病人仍取截石位。

lithotripsy ['liθəˌtripsi] *n.* 碎石术

At this time, gallstone lithotripsy appears promising but the benefits of this therapeutic modality have yet to be established.
目前来看,胆结石碎石术有其发展前景,但这种治疗方法的优点还没有确定下来。

lithotripter [ˈliθəˌtriptə] *n.* 碎石器
Extracorporal lithotripter is an instrument for crushing calculi in the urinary bladder.
体外碎石器是一种用来打碎膀胱结石的器械。

liver [ˈlivə] *n.* 肝(脏)
The stomach lies between the liver and the spleen.
胃位于肝和脾之间。
The liver is an important site of metabolism of carbohydrates, proteins, and fats.
肝脏是进行碳水化合物、蛋白质和脂肪代谢的一个主要部位。

load [ləud] *n.* 负载,负荷
The overburdened heart may be carrying an extra pressure or volume load.
负荷过重的心脏可能是承担额外的压力负荷或容量负荷。

lobar [ˈləubə] *a.* 叶的
Chest X-ray shows consolidation in lobar distribution.
胸部 X 线检查见有呈大叶性分布的实质阴影。
Lobar pneumonia, a type of pneumococcal pneumonia, is an acute infectious disease.
大叶性肺炎——一种肺炎球菌性肺炎,属于急性传染病。

lobe [ləub] *n.* 叶
Chronic abscess in the upper lobe is greatly similar to tuberculosis.
慢性上叶肺脓肿非常类似于肺结核。
Chest roentgenogram showed right middle lobe and lingula infiltrates.
胸部 X 线片显示右肺中叶及舌叶有浸润。

lobectomy [ləuˈbektəmi] *n.* 叶切除术
Rarely, emergency lobectomy may be required for massive hemoptysis.
偶尔由于大量咯血而需行紧急肺叶切除。
Lobectomy is used in patients with smaller or more peripheral tumors.
肺叶切除术适用于肿瘤较小或较典型的周围型肺肿瘤患者。

lobelia [ləuˈbiːljə] *n.* 半边莲属
Are there any plants or flowers of the genus Lobelia?
这里种植有半边莲属的植物或花吗?
Lobelia species plants subordinate to Campanulaceae.
半边莲属的植物归属于桔梗科。

lobomycosis [ˌləubəumaiˈkəusis] *n.* 洛博芽生菌病
Lobomycosis is a chronic fungal infection of the skin, endemic in rural regions in South America and Central America.
洛博芽生菌病是一种皮肤的慢性真菌感染,是南美和中美洲农村地区特有的疾病。
Lobomycosis has been found in humans and dolphins and is restricted to the Amazon Valley in Brasil.
洛博芽生菌病见于人和海豚,但仅局限于巴西亚马逊河流域。

lobular [ˈlɔbjulə] *a.* 小叶的
The lobular architecture is preserved and there is little or no necrosis or fibrosis.
小叶结构仍保持完整,极少或没有坏死和纤维化。

lobulated [ˈlɔbjuˌleitid] *a.* 分成小叶的
The physician palpated an abdominal mass, mostly in the left flank, and it was thought to be firm and lobulated.
医生于患者腹部触到一个包块,它主要位于腹部左侧,包块坚实而呈分叶状。

local [ˈləukəl] *a.* 局部的

It's an outpatient procedure that requires only local anesthetic.

它是一种只需采用局部麻醉的门诊手术。

localization [ˌləukəlaiˈzeiʃən] *n.* 定位

Films taken of the patient in the prone position aid in localization of the obstruction in the small or large intestine.

病人俯卧摄片有助于小肠或大肠梗阻的定位。

Cerebral localization refers to the determination of the situation of the various centers of the brain.

大脑定位是指脑的各种中枢位置的确定。

localize [ˈləukəlaiz] *v.* 使限制于局部;定位

Hot applications localize the infection.

热敷使感染局限化。

Any suspected localized areas of infection should likewise be cultured.

任何有怀疑的局部感染同样应作培养。

X-rays of the abdomen may localize the site of the tumour.

腹部 X 线片可以确定肿瘤的位置。

locally [ˈləukəli] *ad.* 局部地

This drug is applied locally to the skin and mucous membranes.

这药可局部应用于皮肤和黏膜。

locate [ləuˈkeit] *v.* 位于,确定…的位置

The pulmonary semilunar valve is located between the right ventricle and the pulmonary artery.

肺动脉半月瓣位于右心室和肺动脉之间。

As a rule, an infection causes the death of many of the tissue cells located at the point of infection.

一般说来,感染引起感染部位的许多组织细胞死亡。

The optic disc should be located if necessary by following a branch of the retinal artery to its source.

如有必要,应沿着视网膜动脉的一个分支追溯到其发源处,找出视神经盘的位置。

location [ləuˈkeiʃən] *n.* 定位,位置

The location of the nerve receptors which transmit hunger impulses is still uncertain.

传送饥饿冲动的神经感受器位置仍然不能确定。

The leads of EKG showing the change most clearly depend upon the location of the infarction.

哪个心电图导联显示改变最清楚,取决于梗死的部位。

lochia [ˈləukiə] *n.* 恶露,经血

Normally blood clot is dissolved by plasmin as it is formed in the cavity of the uterus, so that the lochia remains fluid.

正常情况下,血块在子宫腔内形成时即被纤维蛋白酶溶解,故经血保持流体。

locomotion [ˌləukəˈməuʃən] *n.* 运动

The foot is concerned mainly with support and locomotion of the body.

足主要担负对身体的支持和运动。

locus [ˈləukəs] *n.* 部位,位置;位点

The drug should not disappear too rapidly from the locus of action.

药物不应从作用部位消失过快。

lodge [lɔdʒ] *v.* 住宿;嵌(射)入;停留

The bullet(was) lodged in his brain.

子弹射进了他的脑部。

In some cases the bolus of food is firmly lodged in a position where it can be neither seen nor

felt.
在某些病例中食物团块牢固地嵌在一个既看不到又感觉不到的位置上。
Haematuria can result from systemic arterial emboli in the kidney but these fragments can lodge in any part of the body.
体循环中的动脉栓子出现在肾脏引起血尿,但这些栓子的断片可停留在身体任何部位。

lodgment [ˈlɔdʒmənt] *n.* 沉积处,存放处
The air passages of children are frequent sites for the lodgment of foreign bodies.
儿童的呼吸道常是异物停留的部位。

loin [lɔin] *n.* 腰
In the classical glomerulonephritis the child wakes with malaise, headache and loin pain; there may be slight fever.
患典型的肾小球性肾炎时,孩子常因感觉不适、头痛和腰痛而惊醒,并可能有微热。

longevity [lɔnˈdʒeviti] *n.* 长寿;寿命
It's well known that longevity is hereditary.
众所周知,长寿是有遗传性的。
Certain biological differences also contribute to the greater longevity of women.
某些生物学上的差异也能使妇女的寿命更长。

longitudinal [ˌlɔndʒiˈtjuːdinəl] *a.* 经度的;纵(向)的
If the lie is transverse, the height of the fundus may be a little lower than with a longitudinal lie.
如是横产式,子宫底高度较纵产式略低。
Longitudinal research involves conducting a study over a period of time, sometimes for months or even years.
纵向研究指进行一项研究需要跨越一段时间,有时要数月或甚至数年。

long-term [ˈlɔŋtəːm] *a.* 长期的
Inorganic arsenic may cause a distal axonopathy after long-term lower-level exposures.
长期低剂量接触无机砷能引起远端轴突病。
Half of all long-term medical-care financing is private pay, by individual patients.
所有长期医疗费用中有一半由病人自己支付。
Long-term cooking destroys folic acid.
长时间烹煮会破坏叶酸。

loop [luːp] *n.* 襻,环
The major loop diuretics are furosemide(Lasix) and ethacrynic acid(Edecrin).
主要的肾小管襻利尿剂有速尿和利尿酸两种。
This is a classic endocrine feedback loop.
这是一个典型的内分泌反馈环路。

loose [luːs] *a.* 松散的
There are a few loose stools composed mostly of blood and mucus.
仅有的几次稀便内主要的是血和黏液。

loperamide [ləuˈperəmaid] *n.* 洛哌丁胺(商品名:Imodium)
A doctor told me that diarrhea can be treated with anti-diarrhea agents such as loperamide(Imodium).
有位医生告诉我腹泻可用抗腹泻药治疗,如洛哌丁胺。

lordosis [lɔːˈdəusis] *n.* 脊柱前凸
Lordosis of the lumbar region may be seen in the erect position.
在直立位时,可见其腰部的脊柱向前凸出。

lotion [ˈləuʃən] *n.* 润肤乳;洗液,洗剂
Lotion is a liquid medicinal or cosmetic preparation applied to the skin.
润肤乳;是用于皮肤的液体药剂或美容剂。

louse [laus] (*pl.* lice [lais]) *n.* 虱

Lice infect hair, clothes, feeding on blood daily.

虱子常寄生于毛发、衣物,并以吸血为生。

lubricant ['luːbrikənt] *n.* 润滑剂

Magnesium stearate is by far the most extensively used tableting lubricant.

硬脂酸镁是目前应用最广泛的片剂润滑剂。

A wide range of lubricants are available for pharmaceutical applications.

多种润滑剂都可用于制药。

lubricate ['luːbrikeit] *v.* 使润滑

Water also lubricates our joints.

水同样也可对关节起润滑作用。

Vaginal discharge is a fluid that is produced by glands in the vaginal wall and the cervix, and it plays a vital role in keeping the vagina clean and lubricated.

阴道分泌物(白带)是由阴道壁和宫颈的腺体产生的液体,在保持阴道洁净和润滑中起着重要作用。

lucency ['ljuːsənsi] *n.* 透明;光亮

Radiographic findings include patchy areas of lucency and sclerosis as well as bony collapse at articular surfaces.

射线照相术结果包括密度不均的斑片状影和骨质硬化以及关节面的骨质塌陷。

lumbago [lʌm'beigəu] *n.* 腰痛

Severe lumbago, of sudden onset while bending or lifting, can be due either to a slipped disc or to a strained muscle or ligament.

在弯腰或提物时突然发作的严重腰痛,可能是由于椎间盘脱出或者肌肉或韧带的拉伤所致。

lumbar ['lʌmbə] *a.* 腰的

Lumbar puncture is contraindicated in this case.

此病例应禁忌腰穿刺。

The usual course of lumbar strain is spontaneous remission with time.

腰部劳损的通常病程是随时间而自行缓解。

lumen ['luːmin] (*pl.* lumens 或 lumina ['luːminə]) *n.* 腔,管腔

The lumen of the coronary artery is greatly narrowed by atherosclerotic thickening of the inner coat.

冠状动脉管腔由于内层的动脉粥样硬化增厚而显著变窄。

When the lumen of appendix is obstructed, the pain becomes colicky in character.

阑尾管腔受梗阻时,疼痛转为绞痛性的。

luminal ['luːminəl] *a.* 管腔的

A relatively slight alteration in coronary luminal diameter can produce a large decrease in coronary flow.

冠状动脉血管直径相对轻微的改变可使冠状动脉血流量明显降低。

lump [lʌmp] *n.* 块,肿块

The patient with breast cancer usually presents with a lump in the breast.

乳癌患者常常表现为乳房内有肿块。

lunar ['ljuːnə] *a.* (与)月亮(有关)的;阴历的

A lunar eclipse is an eclipse of the moon.

月食是月亮被遮掩。

At the end of the second lunar month of pregnancy the uterus is as large as a goose egg.

妊娠的第二个月末时,子宫像鹅蛋一样大。

The Lunar New Year will come soon.

阴历新年即将到来。

lupus [ˈluːpəs] *n.* 狼疮

Steroids are used for lupus erythematosus and in acute benign pericarditis if it is severe.

对于红斑性狼疮以及严重的急性良性心包炎，可用类固醇治疗。

lustreless [ˈlʌstəlis] *a.* 无光泽的

The necrotic area may become swollen, firm, dull and lustreless.

坏死区可能变得肿胀、坚硬、混浊而且无光泽。

luteal [ˈluːtiəl] *a.* 黄体的

The results of follicular development are follicular atresia, follicular stasis and ovulation of non-maturating follicles with luteal phase inadequacy.

当黄体期功能不全时，卵泡发育结果为卵泡闭锁、卵泡发育停滞或未成熟卵泡排卵。

There are 57 cases having anovulation or luteal phase inadequacy in the group of polycystic ovary syndrom.

多囊卵巢综合征组中有 57 例无排卵或者黄体功能不全。

luteinization [ˌluːtiinaiˈzeiʃən] *n.* 黄体(素)化

With a dose of 2mg/kg administered in vivo, the induced ovulation was completely inhibited while the process of granulosa cell luteinization and the synthesis and secretion of progesterone remained unaffected.

以每公斤两毫克剂量体内用药可完全抑制排卵，而不影响颗粒细胞黄体化及孕酮的合成和分泌。

luteinize [ˈljuːtiːnaiz] *v.* 黄体化

For example, luteinizing hormone(LH) receptors are almost exclusively in the gonads.

例如，黄体生成素受体几乎全部分布在性腺器官。

The objective of this study was to determine the incidence and recurrence rate of luteinized unruptured follicle syndrome in women with unexplained infertility.

这项研究的目的是为了确定不明原因不孕妇女黄素化卵泡未破裂综合征的发病率和复发率。

luteum [ˈluːtiəm] [拉] *a.* 黄的，黄色的

After ovulation the corpus luteum secretes both oestrogen and progesterone, and these bring about progestational changes in the endometrium.

排卵后黄体分泌雌激素和孕酮，它们使子宫内膜发生孕前的变化。

luxurious [lʌgˈzjuəriəs] *a.* 奢侈的，舒适的

He is living in luxurious surroundings.

他生活在非常舒适的环境。

lyme [laim] *n.* 莱姆病

Lyme disease is a multisystemic illness with dermatologic, rheumatic, neurologic, and cardiac features.

莱姆病是一种有皮肤、风湿、神经和心脏多种表现的多系统疾病。

lymph [limf] *n.* 淋巴

Lymph is usually a clear, transparent, watery fluid.

淋巴液通常为清亮而透明的水状液体。

The combination of a focus with regional lymph node involvement is called the primary complex.

病灶连同局部淋巴结侵犯一起称为“原发性综合病变”。

lymphadenectomy [limˌfædiˈnektəmi] *n.* 淋巴结切除术

It is not necessary to perform pelvic lymphadenectomy for stage I case because of low incidence of positive node.

I 期患者无需施行骨盆的淋巴结切除术，因为淋巴结阳性率较低。

Inguinofemoral lymphadenectomy can only detect less than 30% of early stage vulvar cancer patients, but may cause complications in most patients.

进行腹股沟淋巴结清扫仅能在不到 30% 的早期外阴癌患者检测到阳性淋巴结,而且大多数患者会出现并发症。

lymphadenitis [ˌlimfædiˈnaitis] *n.* 淋巴结炎

The woman patient is ill with lymphadenitis.

这妇女患淋巴结炎。

The toxin may cause lymphadenitis, arthritis, synovitis, and nephritis.

此毒素可引起淋巴腺炎、关节炎、滑膜炎和肾炎。

lymphadenoma [ˌlimfædiˈnəumə] *n.* 淋巴组织瘤

Severe cases of lymphadenoma frequently do not respond to sanamycin alone.

对严重型的淋巴组织瘤单独使用放线菌素 C 往往不起作用。

lymphadenopathy [limˌfædiˈnɔpəθi] *n.* 淋巴结病

The inguinal region should be palpated to detect hernias and lymphadenopathy.

应在腹股沟区触诊以探查疝气或淋巴结病变。

In chronic myelocytic leukemia, lymphadenopathy is an unusual manifestation.

在慢性粒细胞性白血病中,淋巴结肿大并不常见。

lymphangiography [limˌfændʒiˈɔgrəfi] *n.* 淋巴管造影术

Positive lymphangiography predicts for disease in other intraabdominal sites, such as portal lymph nodes and spleen.

淋巴管造影结果呈阳性提示在腹腔内的其他部位如门静脉淋巴结和脾脏等处发生病变。

lymphangioma [limˌfændʒiˈəumə] *n.* 淋巴管瘤

Lymphangiomas are benign tumors of the heart, virtually always recognized only at autopsy.

淋巴管瘤是心脏的良性肿瘤,它往往只在尸检时才被发现。

lymphangitis [ˌlimfænˈdʒaitis] *n.* 淋巴管炎

Occasionally, one may encounter a patient with recurrent lymphangitis in whom there is no apparent anatomic reason for the disease.

医生偶尔会遇到反复发作淋巴管炎的病人,但该病人却没有任何明显的解剖结构异常。

lymphatic [limˈfætik] *a.* 淋巴的

The infection spreads by way of lymphatic vessels.

感染沿着淋巴管扩散。

n. 淋巴管

The cancer cells may spread by lymphatics to the lymph nodes in the chest.

癌细胞可经淋巴管扩散到胸部的淋巴结。

lymphedema [ˌlimfiˈdiːmə] *n.* 淋巴水肿

Once lymphedema is diagnosed, treatment should begin immediately.

淋巴水肿一经诊断,应该立即予以治疗。

Radiation, sports injuries, tattooing and any physical insult to the lymphatic pathways can also cause lymphedema.

放射、运动损伤、文身和任何其他对淋巴通路的创伤也会导致淋巴水肿。

lymphoblast [ˈlimfəblæst] *n.* 成淋巴细胞,原始淋巴细胞

Lymphoblasts may or may not be present in the peripheral blood but are always present in the bone marrow.

原始淋巴细胞可以出现也可以不出现在周围血液中,但在骨髓中总是存在的。

lymphocyte [ˈlimfəsait] *n.* 淋巴细胞

The average lymphocyte count is 2100/cu. mm.

平均淋巴细胞计数是 2100/立方毫米。

The small lymphocyte is the heart of the immune system.

小小的淋巴细胞是免疫系统的核心。

lymphocytic [ˌlimfəˈsitik] *a.* 淋巴细胞的

Lymph node enlargement occurs early in chronic lymphocytic leukemia.

慢性淋巴细胞性白血病出现淋巴结肿大较早。

lymphocytosis [ˌlimfəusaiˈtəusis] *n.* 淋巴细胞增多(症)

In this case, the white blood cell count tends to be low, with a relative lymphocytosis.

在这一病例中,白细胞计数偏低,伴有淋巴细胞相对增多。

lymphogranuloma [ˌlimfəu,grænjuˈləumə] *n.* 淋巴肉芽肿

Lymphogranuloma venereum is a sexually transmitted infection.

性病淋巴肉芽肿是一种性传播性感染。

Clinical data of 24 eosinophilic lymphogranuloma cases were retrospectively studied.

回顾性研究了 24 例嗜酸性淋巴肉芽肿的临床资料。

lymphoid [ˈlimfɔid] *a.* 淋巴的,淋巴样的

The spleen is a highly vascular, lymphoid organ.

脾脏是个血管和淋巴极为丰富的器官。

Lymphoid tissue in the lung is concentrated in regional lymph nodes in the hilar structures.

肺内的淋巴样组织多聚集在肺门部位的淋巴结内。

lymphokine [ˈlimfəkain] *n.* 淋巴因子,淋巴激活素

The low molecular weight substances liberated are vasoactive peptides, histamine and lymphokines.

释放出的低分子量物质有作用于血管的肽、组织胺及淋巴因子。

lymphoma [limˈfəumə] *n.* 淋巴瘤

Localized lymphoma may be treated with radiotherapy followed by drugs.

局限性淋巴瘤可用放射治疗后再加药物治疗。

Lymphomas are currently divided into Hodgkin's and non-Hodgkin's types.

淋巴瘤目前被分为霍奇金淋巴瘤和非霍奇金淋巴瘤两种类型。

lymphopoiesis [ˌlimfəupɔiˈiːsis] *n.* 淋巴生成,淋巴细胞生成,淋巴组织生成

The formation of lymphocytes or lymphatic tissue is called lymphopoiesis.

淋巴细胞或淋巴组织的形成称为淋巴生成。

lymphosarcoma [ˌlimfəsɑːˈkəumə] *n.* 淋巴肉瘤

I do remember seeing many cases that were called "mediastinal lymphosarcoma" invading the lung.

我的确记得看到许多入侵肺部的称为纵隔淋巴肉瘤的病例。

lymphoscintigraphy [ˌlimfəusinˈtigrəfi] *n.* 淋巴显像,淋巴系闪烁造影

Investigation by dynamic lymphoscintigraphy showed no or diminished activity of lymph vessels in the lower extremities.

动态淋巴显像研究显示下肢淋巴管的活动缺乏或减弱。

Lymphoscintigraphy is a technique that is used to determine the sentinel lymph node.

淋巴系闪烁造影是用于确定前哨淋巴结的一种技术。

lymphotoxin [ˌlimfəuˈtɔksin] *n.* 淋巴毒素

The 20-100μg/ml CMP could stimulate human spleen cells to produce lymphotoxin.

20 ~ 100 微克/毫升的磷酸胞苷能刺激人体脾细胞产生淋巴毒素。

There is no association between the gene polymorphisms of lymphotoxin αNco Ⅰ and Helicobacter pylori infection in Chinese patients with gastroduodenal diseases.

在中国的胃十二指肠疾病患者中,没有发现淋巴毒素 αNco Ⅰ基因多态性与幽门螺杆菌感染之间的关联。

lyophilic [ˌlaiəˈfilik] *a.* 亲液的

Lyophilic colloids are highly solvated as well as charged.

亲液胶体经过高度溶剂化并带电。

The particles in a lyophilic system have a great affinity for the solvent, and are readily solvated.
亲液体系中的粒子与溶剂有极高亲和力且易被溶剂化。

lyophilization [laiˌɔfiliˈzeiʃən] *n.* 冻干法，冰冻干燥

In the process of lyophilization, organisms are subjected to extreme dehydration in the frozen state.
冰冻干燥过程是将微生物在冰冻状态下进行高度脱水。

lyophobic [ˌlaiəuˈfəubik] *a.* 疏液的

In a lyophobic system the particles resist solvation and dispersion in the solvent.
在疏液体系中，粒子可抵抗溶剂中的自身溶解和分散。

Lyophobic colloids have no affinity for the dispersing medium and are not solvated.
疏液胶体对分散介质没有亲和力且不被溶剂化。

lyse [laiz] *v.* 溶解，溶化

Gramicidin inhibits growth but does not lyse bacteria.
短杆菌肽可抑制细菌的生长但不能溶解细菌。

lysine [ˈlaisiːn] *n.* 赖氨酸

Large amounts of lysine are excreted.
大量的赖氨酸被排出。

Iron, lysine and vitamin C supplements are recommended.
建议补充铁、赖氨酸和维生素 C。

lysis [ˈlaisis] *n.* 溶解

Passive immunity utilizes antibodies to mediate tumor cell lysis and other biological effect or function.
被动免疫法是利用抗体介导肿瘤细胞溶解和产生其他生物学作用来进行免疫。

lysogeny [laiˈsɔdʒini] *n.* 溶原性

Lysogeny state takes place when a bacteriophage infects certain types of bacteria.
当一种噬菌体感染某些细菌时，溶原状态就会发生。

This paper is related to the screening of lactic acid bacteria lysogeny strain.
这篇文章涉及乳酸菌溶原性菌株的筛选。

lysosomal [ˌlaisəˈsəuməl] *a.* 溶酶体的

There is an increase in the hepatic lysosomal copper concentration.
肝细胞溶酶体内的铜浓度增加。

lysosome [ˈlaisəsəum] *n.* 溶酶体

Lysosomes are membrane bound structures containing numerous hydrolytic enzymes.
溶酶体是由膜包绕的结构，含多种水解酶。

Foreign particles(e. g. bacteria) taken into the cell are broken down by the enzymes of the lysosomes.
异物(如细菌)被摄入细胞后，便被溶酶体的酶所分解。

lysozyme [ˈlaisəzaim] *n.* 溶菌酶

Lysozyme can catalyze the breakdown of some bacterial cell walls.
溶菌酶能催化某些细菌细胞壁的崩解。

lytic [ˈlitik] *a.* 溶解性的

Lytic necrosis is a special liquefactive necrosis that only involves the parenchymal cells.
溶解坏死是一种特殊的液化性坏死，只累及实质细胞。

Lytic necrosis in the hepatitis is shown as a focus of the inflammatory cell infiltration in the parenchyma.
溶解坏死在肝炎中表现为肝实质内炎细胞浸润灶。

M

maceration [ˌmæsəˈreiʃən] *n.* 浸渍,衰弱

Maceration is widely employed for the extraction of nonvolatile plant compounds used in pharmaceutical products.

浸渍被广泛应用于医药产品中非挥发性植物化合物的提取。

The solvent used for maceration, percolation, and soxhlet extraction was 50% ethanol.

用于浸渍、渗滤、索氏提取的溶剂均为50%的乙醇。

macroautophagy [ˌmækrəuɔːˈtɔfədʒi] *n.* 大自噬

Inhibition of macroautophagy triggers apoptosis.

抑制大自噬可引发凋亡。

Enhancing macroautophagy protects against ischemia/reperfusion injury in cardiac myocytes.

增强大自噬可保护心肌细胞缺血/再灌注损伤。

macrocytic [ˌmækrəuˈsitik] *a.* 大红细胞的,巨红细胞的

The red cells are macrocytic and the WBCs have multilobed nuclei.

其血片上的红细胞呈大细胞性,白细胞核呈多分叶状。

macrocytosis [ˌmækrəusaiˈtəusis] *n.* 巨红细胞症

Macrocytosis is common in alcoholic persons, and in fact its presence in an otherwise healthy person raises the possibility of occult alcohol abuse.

巨红细胞症常见于嗜酒者,健康人若出现巨红细胞症,其潜在酗酒的几率便会增加。

macroglobulinemia [ˌmækrəuˌglɔbjuliˈniːmiə] *n.* 巨球蛋白血症

DFPP is a safe and effective method in a short period of time for the treatment of Waldenstrom macroglobulinemia.

双重血浆置换是一种短期内治疗 Waldenstrom 巨球蛋白血症安全有效的方法。

Waldenstrom's macroglobulinemia is a result of a condition called lymphoplasmacytic lymphoma.

Waldenstrom 巨球蛋白血症是由称作淋巴浆细胞性淋巴瘤的病症所导致。

macromolecule [ˌmækrəuˈmɔlikjuːl] *n.* 大分子

The protein, polysaccharides, lipids, and nucleic acids are macromolecules.

蛋白质、多糖、脂类和核酸是大分子。

Hydrolytic enzymes can digest macromolecules.

水解酶能消化大分子。

Molecular genetics is the study of macromolecules important in biological inheritance.

分子遗传学是研究对生物的遗传起重要作用的大分子的一门学科。

macronutrient [ˌmækrəˈnjuːtrient] *n.* 宏量营养素

These compounds are foodlike and are usually intended to replace or substitute for normal macronutrients, such as fat, protein, and /or carbohydrate.

这些食物样的化合物常常用来取代或代用作宏量营养素,如脂肪、蛋白质和(或)碳水化合物。

macrophage [ˈmækrəufeidʒ] *n.* 巨噬细胞

Macrophages are a family of phagocytic cells located throughout the body.

巨噬细胞是一种遍布全身的吞噬细胞系。

Macrophage bind to microorganisms, internalize them and then kill them.

巨噬细胞结合微生物,将其内在化后杀灭它们。

macroscopic [ˌmækrəu'skɔpik] *a.* 肉眼可见的;宏观的

The cells are microscopic, while the tissues are macroscopic.

细胞是肉眼看不见的,而组织是肉眼可见的。

Macroscopic features of chronic inflammation are extremely variable.

慢性炎症的肉眼特征极不一致。

macrosomatia [ˌmækrəusə'meiʃiə] *n.* 巨体

Hyperinsulinism plus an abundant glucose supply is probably the major cause for macrosomatia in infants of the diabetic mothers.

有高胰岛素症再加上丰富的糖类的供应可能是糖尿病母亲所生的婴儿成为巨大婴儿的主要原因。

maculopapular [ˌmækjuləu'pæpjuːlə] *a.* 斑丘疹的

This 7-year-old girl, at 17 months of age, developed sudden onset of intermittent high fever, maculopapular skin rash and abdominal pain.

该 7 岁女孩在 17 个月时突然发生间歇高热、皮肤斑丘疹及腹痛。

magenta [mə'dʒentə] *n.* 品红

A process for treating basic magenta waste water by composite-coagulation adsorption is proposed.

人们提出了复合混凝吸附的方法处理碱性品红废水。

Some yellow, magenta, cyan and black liquid dyes for inks were manufactured and purified by membrane separation.

采用膜分离技术制备和提纯了黄、红、青、黑色墨水用液体染料。

magnesium [mæg'niːzjəm] *n.* 镁

Magnesium sulfate is the treatment of choice for impending eclampsia.

子痫发生前可选用硫酸镁治疗。

Magnesium trisilicate possesses antacid and absorptive properties to enchance effectiveness.

三矽酸镁具有制酸和吸附作用,能增强药效。

magnet ['mægnit] *n.* 磁铁;[电磁] 磁体;磁石

Magnet system is comprised of main magnet, gradient system and RF system.

磁体系统由主磁体、梯度系统和射频系统组成。

Magnet includes permanent magnet, conventional magnet, namely resistive magnets and superconducting magnet.

磁体包括三种:永磁体、常导磁体(阻抗磁体)和超导磁体。

magnetic [mæg'netik] *a.* 磁的,有磁性的

Magnetic resonance imaging scans are so sensitive that they often reveal anatomic abnormalities that are clinically meaningless.

磁共振成像扫描十分灵敏,它们可以显示临床不注意的解剖异常。

A new technique uses magnetic beads coated with specific antibodies.

一种新的技术是用特异性抗体包被的磁珠。

magnetism ['mægnitizm] *n.* 磁力现象,磁性

The Faraday effect was the first demonstration of a connection between magnetism and light.

法拉第效应是磁力与光被联系在一起的首次证明。

magnification [ˌmægnifi'keiʃən] *n.* 放大

Nearly all human cells are invisible without high magnification.

几乎所有人的细胞只能在高倍放大下才可以被看见。

With the help of magnification, the surgeon could see details and detect problems that would escape the naked eyes.

借助放大镜,外科医生可看到细节并能查出肉眼觉察不到的问题。

magnify ['mægnifai] *v.* 放大,扩大

Numerous agents acting at two or more receptor sites may magnify each other's effects.
许多作用在两个或两个以上受体部位的药物,可增加彼此的效应。
A microscope is an instrument which is used for magnifying objects.
显微镜是用来放大物体的一种仪器。

magnitude [ˈmægnitjuːd] *n.* 重要性;大小;量
The magnitude and duration of bleeding vary considerably among patients.
出血的程度与持续时间在病人中有很大差异。

magnolia [mægˈnəuliə] *n.* 辛夷
A TLC identification method of magnoliae has been established.
我们建立了辛夷的薄层层析鉴别法。
He studies the essential oils of magnoliae specifically.
他专门研究辛夷香精油。

magnolol [ˈmægnəulɔl] *n.* 厚朴酚
My tutor adopted HPLC method for determination of honokiol and magnolol content in Huoxiang Zhengqi liquid.
我导师采用高效液相色谱法测定藿香正气水中和厚朴酚与厚朴酚的含量。
The average recovery rates of magnolol and honokiol were respectively 100.92% (RSD = 1.79%) and 101.23% (RSD=1.79%).
厚朴酚与和厚朴酚的平均回收率分别是100.92%(RSD=1.79%),101.23%(RSD=1.79%)。

mainstay [ˈmeinstei] *n.* 主要依据;骨干
Sublingual glyceryl trinitrate(0.5mg) remains the mainstay of therapy.
舌下含服硝酸甘油片(0.5mg)仍然是主要的治疗方法。

maintenance [ˈmeintənəns] *n.* 保持,维修
Nuclei are necessary for the maintenance and continuation of life.
细胞核对于保持和延续生命是必需的。
The reflex action has to do with the maintenance of the posture or muscle tone.
这种反射动作与保持体态和肌肉的紧张度有关。

majority [məˈdʒɔriti] *n.* 大多数
In the majority of animals, no genes are incorporated.
在大多数动物身上,没有基因是紧密结合的。
The majority of patients with severe lower gastrointestinal bleeding will stop bleeding spontaneously.
大多数严重下消化道出血的病人可自行停止出血。

makeup [ˈmeikʌp] *n.* 组成,体格,编排
Molecular biology is the study of the structure, function, and makeup of biologically important molecules.
分子生物学是研究生物体重要分子的结构、功能和组成的一门学科。
He used to have a stout makeup, but now he suffers from a stomach ailment.
过去他身体一直很强壮,但他现在却患有胃病。
That book is welcome to the readers because of its good makeup.
那本书由于版面编排得好很受读者欢迎。

malabsorption [ˌmæləbˈsɔːpʃən] *n.* 吸收不良
Most cases of vitamin D deficiency, however, are a result of diseases causing fat malabsorption or severe liver and kidney diseases.
然而,维生素D缺乏的大多数情况,是由于引起脂肪吸收不良的疾患或严重的肝肾疾患所致。

malady [ˈmælədi] *n.* 病,痼疾

His mother suffers from a chronic malady.
他母亲患有慢性痼疾。

malaise [mæˈleiz] *n.* 不适，欠爽

General malaise may appear in many diseases.
许多疾病可出现全身不适。
In many infectious diseases there are early manifestations such as fever, malaise, sore throat, and headache.
许多传染病都有像发热、不适、咽痛和头痛等这类的早期表现。

malaria [məˈlɛəriə] *n.* 疟疾

Malaria is an infectious disease caused by a minute parasite transmitted by mosquitoes.
疟疾是由蚊子传播的小寄生虫所引起的一种传染病。
Acute malaria in children rarely presents a classic clinical picture.
儿童患急性疟疾很少有典型的临床表现。

maldigestion [ˌmældiˈdʒestʃən] *n.* 消化不良

Pancreatic insufficiency in cystic fibrosis may lead to maldigestion and malabsorption of nutrients.
囊性纤维化时的胰腺功能障碍可引起消化不良和营养吸收障碍。

male [meil] *a.* 男性的，雄性的

On the average, male babies weigh more at birth than female ones.
一般来说，男性婴儿出生时比女性婴儿要重。
Male animals are often larger than the females.
雄性动物往往比雌性动物要大一些。
n. 男性，男子，雄性生物
The human male has the genotype XY.
人类男性的基因型为 XY。
Males are afflicted in somewhat greater numbers than females.
男性病人略多于女性病人。

malformation [ˌmælfɔːˈmeiʃən] *n.* 畸形，变形

Congenital malformations occur twice as often among twins as among singleton pregnancies.
先天畸形常发生于双胎，是单胎妊娠时的两倍。

malfunction [mælˈfʌŋkʃən] *n.* 功能障碍，功能不良

Physiological malfunction of mental origin does not involve tissue damage and is usually mediated through the automatic nervous system.
精神源性的生理功能障碍不涉及组织损伤，而通常是通过自主神经系统来传递。
The artificial pacemaker needs care, and complications or malfunctions may occasionally occur.
使用人工起搏器需要细心，因为偶尔会发生并发症或功能失常。

malignancy [məˈlignənsi] *n.* 恶性、恶性肿瘤；癌

In view of the malignancy of the lesion we cannot but resort to radical incision.
鉴于病变是恶性的，我们不得不采取根治切除术。
The difficult cases are those in younger patients with ovarian tumours of doubtful malignancy.
困难的病例是那些年轻妇女怀疑为卵巢恶性肿瘤者。
Breast cancer is the most common malignancy in women in most of countries.
乳腺癌是当今大多数国家妇女最常见的恶性肿瘤。
Small-cell lung cancer (SCLC) is an aggressive malignancy with a tendency of early distant metastases.
小细胞肺癌是一种恶性程度较高的肿瘤，具有早期发生远处转移的倾向。

malignant [məˈlignənt] *a.* 有害的；恶性的

Lung cancer is a malignant disease.

肺癌是一种恶性疾病。
Examples of this are seen in the arteriolar lesions of malignant hypertension.
这种例子还见于恶性高血压的小动脉病变。
Ascites fluid should be examined for bacterial and malignant cells.
腹水应送细菌学检查及寻找恶性细胞。

malnutrition [ˌmælnjuːˈtriːʃən] *n.* 营养不良
The study of the effects of malnutrition in the human is of value.
对人体营养不良后果的研究是有价值的。
It is now generally accepted that malnutrition per se is not a cause of cirrhosis in man.
目前普遍认为营养不良本身并不是人类肝硬化的原因。

malodorous [mæˈləudərəs] *a.* 恶臭的
Their urine often becomes grossly cloudy, malodorous, and, in about 50 percent of cases, bloody.
他们的尿通常是混浊的、有恶臭，约半数患者有血尿。

malondialdehyde [ˈmæləunˈdaiˈældihaid] *n.* 丙二醛
Malondialdehyde is a highly reactive compound that is not typically observed in pure form.
丙二醛是一种高活性化合物，一般不以纯化合物形式存在。

malposition [ˌmælpɔˈziʃən] *n.* 错位，异位
Malpresentations and malpositions should be detected at an early stage of labour.
分娩早期就应发现先露异常和胎位不正。

malpractice [mælˈpræktis] *n.* 治疗不当，医疗差错
No other issue has received more attention in recent years than malpractice.
近年来，没有任何其他问题比医疗差错更引起大家注意。

maltitol [ˈmɔːltitəl] *n.* 麦芽糖醇
Maltitol is made by the hydrogenation of maltose which is obtained from starch.
麦芽糖醇是从淀粉中获得的麦芽糖经过氢化作用产生的。
Maltitol is about 90% as sweet as sugar, non-cariogenic, and significantly reduced in calories.
麦芽糖醇的甜度大约是糖的90%，不产生龋齿，而且可明显降低热量。

mammalian [mæˈmeiljən] *a.* 哺乳动物的
The mammalian red blood cell is originally nucleated.
哺乳动物的红细胞起初是有核的。
The intact, functioning, mammalian host has a remarkable series of defense mechanisms against injury.
健康的、各项功能正常的哺乳动物宿主，有一系列有效的、对付损伤的防御机制。

mammogram [ˈmæməgræm] *n.* 乳房X线照片
Before any replacement therapy is recommended, a mammogram should be obtained to rule out an occult lesion.
在推荐使用替代疗法之前，一定要做乳腺影像学检查以便排除看不见的损伤。

mammography [mæˈmɔgrəfi] *n.* 乳房X线照相术
Because mammography has about a 10% rate of false-negativity, biopsies should be done on all palpable lesions in the absence of evidence that the mass is benign.
因为乳房X线照片大约有10%的假阴性率，所以在无法确定肿块是良性时应进行活检。

manage [ˈmænidʒ] *v.* 处理，管理；设法（对付）
The headache associated with malignant hypertension is managed by antihypertensive agents.
恶性高血压引起的头痛用抗高血压药治疗。
There are also more unique, alternative ways to manage the pain without resorting to conventional medicine, such as acupuncture, exercise and mindfulness meditation.
也有一些更独特的可选择的方法来对付疼痛，而不用求助常规医学，如：针刺、运动，意念冥想等。

management ['mænidʒmənt] *n.* 治疗；处理

Nitroglycerin for the management of patients with angina pectoris is given sublingually.
硝酸甘油治疗心绞痛是舌下给药。

Its greatest value is in the management of acidosis.
其最大的价值是对酸中毒的处理。

mandatory ['mændətəri] *a.* 强制性的，义务的，命令的

Early recognition and prompt management of the hypotensive shock are rewarding and mandatory.
早期诊断和及时治疗低血压休克既有好处也很必要。

Adequate intrapartum monitoring is mandatory in both spontaneous and induced labor.
在自然临产或引产时，必须做严密的产程监测。

mandible ['mændibl] *n.* 下颌骨

There was some difficulty in opening the mouth because the mandible was underdeveloped.
由于下颌骨发育不良，患者张口有些困难。

maneuver [mə'nuːvə] *n.* 手法，操作法

A number of simple maneuvers produce characteristic changes depending on cause of murmur.
因为杂音形成的原因不同，所以用一些简单的方法可使杂音发生特征性的变化。

manganese [mæŋgə'niːz, 'mæŋgəniːz,] *n.* 锰

An acute syndrome occurs after exposure to high levels of manganese.
接触高浓度的锰后会出现急性症状。

mania ['meiniə] *n.* 躁狂；癖好

Mania is a state of mind characterized by excessive cheerfulness and increased activity.
躁狂症是以患者过度欢欣和活跃为特征的一种精神状态。

Cow mania is also called bovine spongiform encephalopathy, and it may be transmitted to human beings.
疯牛病也称作牛海绵状脑病，它可以传染给人类。

The old man has a mania for collecting stamps.
那位老人是个集邮迷。

manic ['meinik] *a.* 躁狂的

The initial episode in bipolar disorders is often manic.
双相疾病的初次发作常为躁狂性。

Contrary to popular belief, all manics are not necessarily happy.
与通常的看法相反，并非所有躁狂病人都感觉愉快。

manifest ['mænifest] *v.* 表现，显示，证明

Some patients may manifest cerebellar signs.
有些患者可能出现小脑征候。

Total renal failure is manifested by oliguria.
完全性肾功能衰竭的表现为无尿。

When a person's immune system is weakened perhaps due to stress or sickness. varicella virus will be reactivated that manifests as shingles.
当人的免疫系统由于压力或疾病被削弱时，水痘病毒就会重新激活，表现为带状疱疹。

a. 明白的，明显的

This principle should be manifest to all of them.
这条原则应是他们全体都明白的。

Acute placental failure may become manifest during labour when the uterine contractions interfere with blood flow.
急性胎盘功能衰竭可能在分娩期子宫收缩阻断血流时更为明显。

manifestation [ˌmænifes'teiʃən] *n.* 表示，表现

Digitalis toxicity has several manifestations.

洋地黄中毒有多种表现。

clinical manifestations include chest pain, hypotension, and cardiac dysrhythmias.

临床表现为胸痛、低血压和心律失常。

manifold [ˈmænifəuld] *a.* 各式各样的

TIA occur in patients with atherosclerotic narrowing, occlusion, or emboli to the major arteries of the brain, and the symptoms are manifold.

TIA 见于脑部主要动脉粥样硬化性狭窄、闭塞或血栓形成的病人，症状多种多样。

manipulate [məˈnipjuleit] *v.* 操作；处理；操纵

Such portable X-ray equipment is easy to manipulate.

这种手提式 X 线设备操作简便。

Her face remains relaxed as the doctor cuts through the skin, saws through the bone, manipulates her heart and starts the repair.

当医生切开皮肤，锯开胸部骨头后，处理她的心脏并开始修补时，她的面部表情一直保持平静。

mankind [mæˈkaind] *n.* 人类

Although the development of antibiotics has been of incalculable benefit to mankind, it has also given rise to serious complications.

虽然抗生素的发展给人类带来了无法估量的好处，但是也引起了一些的严重麻烦。

This subject—heredity—has fascinated mankind for thousands of years.

遗传这一问题，千百年来强烈地吸引着人们。

mannan [ˈmænæn] *n.* ［生化］甘露聚糖

Mannan-binding lectin is a member of collectin family and plays an important role in innate immune defense.

甘露聚糖结合凝集素（MBL）系胶原凝集素家族成员，是天然免疫系统中的重要分子。

mannan-oligosaccharides [ˌɔligəuˈsækəraid] *n.* 甘露低聚糖

This article introduces the research development of modification of some functional oligosaccharides, such as mannan-oligosaccharides, chitosan, isomaltoligosaccharide and so on.

该文介绍了甘露低聚糖、壳低聚糖、异麦芽低聚糖等几种功能性低聚糖的改性研究进展。

mannitol [ˈmænitɔl] *n.* 甘露醇

The use of mannitol or furosemide has been controversial in the treatment of acute tubular necrosis.

甘露醇或速尿用于治疗急性肾小管坏死是有争议的。

If oliguria develops, furosemide or an infusion of mannitol may forestall renal failure.

如出现少尿，用呋塞米或输注甘露醇可预防肾功能衰竭。

mannose [ˈmænəuz] *n.* 甘露糖

Mannose is the most important representative of monosaccharides.

甘露糖是一种最主要的单糖。

The most important representatives of monosaccharides are glucose, arabinose, galactose, mannose, ribose, and fructose.

单糖中最具代表性的有葡萄糖、阿拉伯糖、半乳糖、甘露糖、核糖和果糖。

manometer [məˈnɔmitə] *n.* 测压计；（液体）压力计

A manometer often consists of a U-tube containing mercury, water, or other liquid, open at one end and exposed to the gas under pressure at the other end.

测压计常为一 U 形管，内充有水银、水或其他液体，其一端开口，而另一端则与受压气体相连接。

Once the cerebrospinal fluid drips from the needle, immediately attach the manometer.

一旦脑脊液从针孔滴出，就要立即接上测压计。

manometry [məˈnɔmitri] *n.* 测压法

Esophageal manometry remains the gold standard for the assessment of esophageal motor activity.
食管测压仍然是食管运动功能评估的金标准。
Esophageal manometry is a test used to measure the function of the lower esophageal sphincter and the muscles of the esophagus.
食管测压是用于测量食管下端括约肌和食管肌肉功能的一种检查。

manual [ˈmænjuəl] *a.* 手工的,手动的
It allows younger people to maintain an active lifestyle, including weight-lifting and manual work.
它能够使年轻人继续保持一种积极的生活方式,例如举重,手工劳动等。
All applications should have manual save controls.
所有的应用程序都应该有手工保存控件。

mapping [ˈmæpiŋ] *n.* 作图;定位
Gene mapping before 1950 was essentially limited to the X chromosome.
1950 年以前,基因作图仅限于 X 染色体。

marasmus [məˈræzməs] *n.* 消瘦,衰弱
Marasmus can be confused with dehydration, and very often children suffer both.
消瘦与脱水很难区分,两者常常同时出现在儿童身上。
Nutritional marasmus is the most frequent form of PEM in cases of prolonged food shortage.
消瘦型营养不良是 PEM(蛋白质能量营养不良)中最常见的形式,由于长期食物匮乏所引发。

margin [ˈmɑːdʒin] *n.* (边)缘,界限
About 95 per cent of patients with acute cholecystitis have tenderness just below the right costal margin.
约 95% 的急性胆囊炎患者在右肋缘正下方有压痛。
A significant margin of safety between the effective and toxic dose is claimed.
主张有效量和中毒量之间应该有较大的安全界限。

marijuana [ˌmæriˈwɑːnə] *n.* 大麻(=marihuana)
Among 1986 high school seniors, 51% had used marijuana at some time.
(美国)1986 年中学高年级学生中有 51% 的人曾使用过大麻。

marital [ˈmæritl] *a.* 婚姻的
Chronic marital distress and conflict can lead to acute and chronic health changes.
婚姻问题上的长期折磨和冲突会引起急性和慢性的健康变化。

marked [mɑːkt] *a.* 显著的
There is a marked difference between an ordinary wound and an infected wound.
一般伤口与感染伤口显然不同。

marker [ˈmɑːkə] *n.* 标记,标志
Such EEG changes might be useful as a marker of a past episode of depression.
这些脑电图改变可以用作以往抑郁发作的标志。

marrow [ˈmærəu] *n.* 髓
Carcinoma of the lung metastasizes to bone marrow(15%).
肺癌转移到骨髓(15%)。
Platelets are formed in the bone marrow.
血小板是在骨髓中形成的。

masculinization [ˌmæskjulinaiˈzeiʃən] *n.* 男性化
Masculinization means the abnormal development of male sexual characteristics in a female usually as the result of hormone therapies or adrenal malfunction.
男性化指女性异常出现男性体征,常由于激素治疗或者肾上腺功能紊乱引起。
Patients with polycystic ovary syndrome accompanied by hyperandrogenism may show signs of masculinization.
伴有高雄激素的多囊卵巢综合征患者会出现男性化体征。

masculinize [ˈmæskjulinaiz] *v.* 男性化(指女子)

Removal of the ovarian tumor is followed by regression of masculinizing phenomena.

卵巢肿瘤切除后男性化现象会逐渐消退。

mask [mɑːsk] *n.* 面罩；口鼻罩；面具

Doctors and nurses wear masks during a surgical operation to protect against infection.

医生和护士在外科手术时戴有口罩(口鼻罩)以防感染。

v. 伪装,掩盖

Inadequate treatment may mask the symptoms.

不适当的治疗可能掩盖症状。

The first heart sound is soft as the valve does not close properly and may be completely masked by the systolic murmur.

由于瓣膜不能完全关闭,第一心音柔和,有时可完全被收缩期杂音掩盖。

mass [mæs] *n.* 质量;块;肿块

This mass contains a collection of pus.

这个肿块中有脓存积。

massage [ˈmæsɑːʒ] *n.* 按摩,推拿

His attempt to bring the patient back to life by cardiac massage has proved successful.

他设法用心脏按摩来抢救病人,终于获得成功。

After discharge, the patient should come regularly for the massage.

出院以后,病人应定期来院进行按摩。

v. 按摩,推拿

The infants who were massaged were discharged from the hospital an average of six days earlier than premature infants who were not massaged.

经过按摩的婴儿比没有接受按摩的早产婴儿平均提前6天出院。

massive [ˈmæsiv] *a.* 大范围的;大量的

Acute massive necrosis is an extremely rare complication but invariably fatal.

急性大片坏死是一种极少见的并发症,常不可避免死亡。

Abnormal accumulation of fluid in the pleural space may be massive or slight.

胸膜腔内异常积液可多可少。

Massive bleeding must be brought under control immediately, otherwise an operation is indicated.

大出血必须及时加以控制,否则就需进行手术。

mast cell [mæst] *n.* 肥大细胞

Although baseline gene expression of ET-1 and ETA was slightly higher in mast cell-deficient rat hearts, the differences were not significant (Table 1).

虽然肥大细胞缺陷大鼠心脏中ET-1和ETA基因的基础表达水平略高,但差异无显著性(见表1)。

mastectomy [mæsˈtektəmi] *n.* 乳房切除术

If the operation is to combat breast cancer a radical mastectomy is performed.

如果用手术治疗乳腺癌,就需要做乳房根治术。

Prophylaxis of breast cancer is performed with simple mastectomy and reconstruction rather than subcutaneous mastectomy.

预防乳腺癌的方法是施行单纯乳腺切除术和乳房再造,而不是皮下乳腺切除术。

masticate [ˈmæstikeit] *v.* 咀嚼

When the food is sufficiently masticated and thoroughly mixed with saliva, it is thrust into the back part of the mouth and there swallowed as a ball or bolus.

当食物被充分咀嚼并与唾液充分混合时,就被推送至口腔的后部(咽后壁),呈球状或团块状的食团被吞咽。

mastication [ˌmæstiˈkeiʃən] *n.* 咀嚼

Proper mastication is very important to digestion.
充分的咀嚼对于食物的消化是很重要的。

mastitis [mæsˈtaitis] *n.* 乳腺炎
Mastitis usually caused by bacterial infection through damaged nipples.
乳腺炎通常是通过已受损的乳头受细菌感染引起的。
Mastitis is characterized by the painful, nonerythematous swelling of one or both breasts.
乳腺炎以一侧或双侧乳腺有疼痛性、非红斑性肿胀为特征。

mastocyte [ˈmæstəsait] *n.* 肥大细胞
Basophils are functionally similar to mastocyte but are circulating.
嗜碱性粒细胞在功能上类似于肥大细胞，但它是循环中的细胞。

mastocytosis [ˌmæstəusaiˈtəusis] *n.* 肥大细胞(贮积)病，着色荨麻疹
The systemic release of PGD2 together with histamine in patients with mastocytosis causes flushing, rhinorrhea and severe hypotension.
患肥大细胞贮积病的病人出现全身性 PGD2 和组织胺的释放，这会引起面色潮红、流涕和严重低血压。

mastoidectomy [ˌmæstɔiˈdektəmi] *n.* 乳突切除术
Usually the infection of mastoid responds to antibiotics, but mastoidectomy may be required in severe cases.
通常乳突感染用抗生素治疗有效，但重症者需要做乳突切除术。

mastoiditis [ˌmæstɔiˈdaitis] *n.* 乳突炎
Mastoiditis is a suppurative infection of the mastoid air cells.
乳突炎是乳突气室的化脓性感染。
Before the days of the antibiotics, uncontrolled middle-ear infection was the major cause of mastoiditis.
在抗生素问世之前，未控制的中耳感染是乳突炎的主要起因。

match [mætʃ] *v.* 比得过，和…相配
Subsequent rates of pregnancy and pain relief have matched or exceeded the averages achieved through major surgery.
随后的受孕率和疼痛缓解情况，都比得上和超过了通过大手术所取得的平均值。
In bone marrow transplants human leucocyte antigen (HLA) and natural killer (NK) receptors must be matched to ensure success.
骨髓移植中人类白细胞抗原与天然杀伤细胞受体必须相配以保证成功。

matching [ˈmætʃiŋ] *n.* 配合
Matching of blood between donor and recipient provides a more reliable measure of compatibility.
供血者和受血者之间的配血是提供相容性可靠的方法。

materially [məˈtiəriəli] *ad.* 实质上；大大地
All these factors materially increase a person's predisposition to coronary artery thrombosis.
这一切因素实质上使人更加易患冠状动脉血栓形成。

maternal [məˈtəːnl] *a.* 母亲的，母方的
The fetus is unaffected by this maternal disease.
胎儿不受这种母体疾病的影响。
My maternal grandmother devoted herself to women's higher education.
我的外祖母曾献身于妇女高等教育事业。
The maternal mortality rate from all causes is increased about tenfold in patients with hypertension.
所有原因引致的产妇死亡率在高血压患者大约增加 10 倍。

maternity [məˈtəːniti] *n.* 母性；产院
Maternity and child welfare programmes are the shopwindow on a nation's health services.

妇幼保健福利规划是一个国家卫生事业的窗口。

Now more and more women in rural areas give birth to their children in maternity centers.

现在越来越多的农村妇女在妇产院生小孩。

mathematical [ˌmæθiˈmætikəl] *a.* 数学的

Computers make mathematical computations in much less time than a person can.

计算机比一个人用少得多的时间进行数学演算。

Mathematical models for outcome in ARF in critically ill patients are not reliably predictive.

预测病情严重病人发生急性肾衰(ARF)后的预后情况所使用的数学模型并不可靠。

mathematically [ˌmæθəˈmætikli] *ad.* 数学地

She is not mathematically inclined.

她对数学并不感兴趣。

mathematics [ˌmæθəˈmætiks] *n.* 数学

Mathematics is his strongest subject.

数学是他学习得最好的科目。

matrix [ˈmeitriks](*pl.* matrixes 或 matrices [ˈmeitrisiːz]) *n.* [拉] 基层,基质,母质; 床;型片(牙)

Embedded in the matrix of the cytoplasm are found variable numbers of mitochondria.

可以发现数目不同的线粒体包埋在细胞质的基质中。

These amorphous matrix densities are found in irreversibly injured cells in other systems.

这些不定形的基质致密物,也可见于其他系统的不可逆性损害的细胞内。

A three-step hypothesis has been proposed describing the sequence of biochemical events during tumor cell invasion of the extracellular matrix.

关于肿瘤细胞侵入细胞外基质这一生化过程已有一种三步式假说。

maturation [ˌmætjuˈreiʃən] *n.* 成熟

In each case development is related to biological maturation but it is also influenced by nonbiological factors.

在各种情况下,发育与生物学的成熟有关,但也受非生物学因素的影响。

The lymphatic organs are those organs in which maturation, differentiation, and proliferation of lymphocytes take place.

淋巴器官是淋巴细胞经历成熟、分化和增生过程的场所。

mature [məˈtjuə] *a.* 成熟的

These monocytes are mature.

这些单核细胞已成熟了。

The mature corpus luteum may measure from 1 to 3 mm. in diameter.

成熟黄体的直径可为 1 ~3 毫米。

maturity [məˈtjuəriti] *n.* 成熟,成熟期

You should consider gestational age and maturity, but an accurate gestational age is not always known in the emergency department.

你必须推测孕龄和胎儿成熟度,但是在急诊室往往不能准确判断孕龄。

maxillary [ˈmæksiləri] *a.* 上颌骨的,上颌的

The most common complication of upper respiratory disease in adults is maxillary sinusitis.

成人中上呼吸道疾病的最常见的并发症是上颌窦炎。

mean [miːn] *a.* 中间的;平均的

There were 98 men and 75 women with a mean age of 50 ± 6 years (standard deviation) (range:32-63 years).

有 98 名男性和 75 名女性,他们的平均年龄是 50 岁± 6 岁(标准差)(范围是 32-63 岁)。

The control group consists of 10 healthy volunteers from 22 to 49, and the mean age was 32.6±10.8 years old.

对照组由 10 名健康自愿者组成，年龄从 22 岁到 49 岁，平均 32.6 岁±10.8 岁。

n. 均数

This province has 500,000 medical workers, above the national mean.

该省有 50 万医务工作者，超过了全国平均数。

measles [ˈmiːzlz] *n.* 麻疹

Measles is a disease of cosmopolitan distribution, endemic in all but isolated populations.

麻疹分布于世界各地，除隔离的人群外，各地均可流行。

Measles must be differentiated from other disorders accompanied by an eruption.

麻疹应与伴有发疹的其他疾病相鉴别。

measurable [ˈmeʒərəbl] *a.* 可计量的，适度的

By this time, measurable amounts were detected in some patients.

此时在某些患者中，检查出了可测的量。

Measurable effects on body chemical processes occur only after prolonged malnutrition.

只有长时期营养不良才明显影响人体化学变化的过程。

measurably [ˈmeʒərəbli] *ad.* 适度地；显著地

The cancer patient has improved measurably.

那位癌症病人已显著好转。

Free erythrocyte protoporphyrin (FEP) is measurably increased in circumstances of altered heme synthesis.

在血红素合成有改变的情况下，游离红细胞原卟啉有一定程度的增加。

measure [ˈmeʒə] *n.* 测量；度量法；措施

The pH scale is a measure of the concentration of hydrogen ions in the blood.

pH 标度是血液中氢离子浓度的测定计量。

v. 测量；量

The spinal cord measures some 18 inches in length and is about as thick as the little finger.

脊髓大约为 18 英寸长，小指般粗。

mebendazole [miˈbendəzəul] *n.* 甲苯达唑

Doctors can treat ascariasis successfully with mebendazole.

医生使用甲苯达唑可有效地治疗蛔虫病。

mechanical [miˈkænikəl] *a.* 机械的

Mechanical trauma such as crushing may cause direct disruption of cells.

机械性创伤，例如挤压伤，可直接使细胞破裂。

mechanism [ˈmekənizm] *n.* 机制，机理

The mechanism of these changes is incompletely understood.

对这些变化的机制尚不完全了解。

Electrolyte concentrations are regulated by various mechanisms.

电解质浓度可受不同机制的调节。

mechlorethamine [ˌmeklɔːˈeθəmiːn] *n.* 二氯甲基二乙胺，氮芥

Severe local reactions of exposed tissues necessitate rapid intravenous injection of mechlorethamine for most clinical uses.

被暴露的组织局部反应严重，大多数临床使用中需要快速静脉注射二氯甲基二乙胺。

meconium [miˈkəuniəm] *n.* 胎粪

Children with cystic fibrosis and with meconium ileus may be missed.

有囊性纤维症和胎粪性肠梗阻的儿童可能被漏掉。

The efficacy of pulmonary surfactant replacement therapy for meconium aspiration syndrome remains controversial.

肺表面活性物质治疗胎粪吸入综合征的作用还存在争议。

medial [ˈmiːdjəl] *a.* 内侧的，中间的

Sensation may be diminished over the medial calf.
小腿内侧感觉减退。

medially [ˈmiːdiəli] *ad.* 中间地

The middle rectal artery runs medially to the rectum.
直肠中动脉行向直肠中部。

median [ˈmiːdjən] *a.* 中央的,正中的

In the adult three quarters of the liver lie to the right of the median line.
成人肝脏的四分之三位于正中线之右。

The median survival time of the 287 patients was 9 months (8-10 months).
287 名患者的中位生存时间为 9 个月(8 ~ 10 个月)。

Of 404 Ross operations done before November 2004,60 were young patients with a median age of 12 years (ranging from 1 to 20 years).
在2004 年11 月以前所做的404 例 Ross 手术中,60 例是平均年龄为12 岁(1 ~20 岁)的年轻患者。

n. 中位数,正中部

The average follow-up time was 22.1 months and the median was 15.5 months.
平均随访时间是22.1 个月,中位数是15.5 个月。

In addition, cyclophosphamide methotrexate and 5-fluorouracil (CMF) therapy produced prolonged amenorrhea in 39% of the menstruating patients for a median of ten months.
此外,环磷酸酰胺甲氨蝶呤 5-氟尿嘧啶联合疗法使行经期妇女中的 39% 长期闭经平均约十个月。

mediastinal [ˌmiːdiæsˈtainəl] *a.* 纵隔的

Carcinoma of the lung metastasizes to the mediastinal and hilar lymph nodes.
肺癌转移到纵隔及肺门淋巴结。

mediastinoscope [ˌmiːdiəˈstainəskəup] *n.* 纵隔镜

The invention of mediastinoscopes provides a new useful tool for detecting diseases of the mediastinum.
纵隔镜的发明为纵隔疾病的诊断提供了新的有用的工具。

Mediastinoscopes play an important role in the therapeutics of mediastinum diseases.
纵隔镜在纵隔疾病的治疗学上扮演了重要角色。

mediastinoscopy [ˌmiːdiˌæstiˈnɔskəpi] *n.* 纵隔镜检查

Mediastinoscopy is performed under general anesthesia in the operating room.
纵隔镜检查必须在手术室全身麻醉的情况下进行。

mediastinotomy [ˌmiːdiˌæstiˈnɔtəmi] *n.* 纵隔切开术

Anterior mediastinotomy has its main use in the staging of left upper lobe lesions.
前纵隔切开术主要用于左上肺叶病变。

mediastinum [ˌmiːdiæsˈtainəm] (*pl.* mediastina [ˌmiːdiæsˈtainə]) *n.* 纵隔

Between the lungs is a space called the mediastinum,containing the heart and other organs.
两肺之间有一间隙,称为纵隔,内有心脏和其他器官。

Symptoms arise from local compression in the neck and superior mediastinum.
症状起自颈部与上纵隔处的局部压迫。

mediate [ˈmiːdieit] *v.* 作为引起…的媒介;处于中间

Such diseases are essentially mediated by an abnormal gene or by deletion of a gene.
这种疾病实质上是由一个异常基因或一个基因缺失所致。

The adhesion and aggregation of platelets is mediated through release of ADP(adenosine diphosphate).
血小板的黏附和聚集是二磷酸腺甙的释放所介导的。

mediator [ˈmidieitə] *n.* 介体;介质

Endotoxin activation of these mediators occur in a matter of minutes.
这些介质的内毒素激活可在几分钟内完成。
Some of these potential mediators are of importance in particular types of inflammation.
这些潜在介质中有些在各种类型的炎症中是重要的。

medicaid [ˈmedikeid] *n.* [美] 医疗补助方案(或制度)
Medicaid, which provides short-term care for many poor, is the primary source for long-term institutional care of the elderly.
为贫民提供短期医疗照顾的医疗补助制度,现在是对老年人长期社会福利照顾的主要来源。
Forty percent is provided by medicaid, a medical assistance program for those demonstrating financial need.
那些确实有经济困难的人,其40%是由医疗救助方案提供帮助。

medically [ˈmedikəli] *ad.* 用内科方法,在医疗上
Of all the patients 35 were treated surgically and 29 medically.
在全部病人中,35 人用手术治疗,29 人用药物治疗。
These alloys are used medically in prostheses and in the production of tungsten carbide cutting and drilling components.
这些合金在医疗上主要用于假肢以及生产碳化钨切割刀具和钻头的组件。

medicare [ˈmedikεə] *n.* (老年)保健医疗制度
Medicare is US government scheme providing medical care, especiallg for old people.
保健医疗是美国政府执行的一种医疗制度,尤指为老年人提供的医疗保健。

medication [ˌmediˈkeiʃən] *n.* 药疗法;药物
Usually the symptoms of urticaria are very brief, nonbothersome, and do not require medication.
荨麻疹的症状通常很短暂,无甚影响,且不需要药物治疗。
Thiazide diuretics are used in conjunction with antihypertensive medications.
噻嗪类利尿剂可与抗高血压药联合应用。
This type of medications may mask symptomatology and assessment of clinical severity.
此型药物可能掩盖症状及妨碍对临床严重度的评价。

medicolegal [ˌmedikəuˈliːgəl] *a.* 法医学的
It may be of great medicolegal importance to establish accurately the time at which death occurred.
准确地确定死亡发生的时间可能具有重要的法医学意义。
Some practical applications of blood groups for medicolegal purposes include disputed paternity cases.
血型在法医学上的一些实际应用包括解决有争议的亲子关系案件。

mediocre [ˈmiːdiəukə, miːdiˈəukə] *a.* 普通的,平庸的
The development or lack of development of these skills differentiates the top-flight clinician from the mediocre.
能否掌握这些技能,是一流医师和普通医师区别所在。

meditation [ˌmediˈteiʃən] *n.* 沉思;反省
Along with regular exercise, he practiced stress reduction technique, including meditation.
除了经常锻炼外,他还做一些包括沉思在内的减少紧张心情的活动。

medium [ˈmiːdjəm] *n.* 媒质,介质
Some drugs such as acetylsalicylic acid are best absorbed from an acidic medium.
有些药物如乙酰水杨酸在酸性环境中吸收最好。
a. 中等的,中间的
His hair has small amounts of copper, large amounts of zinc and medium amounts of sodium.
他的毛发含铜量低,含锌量大,含钠量中等。

MEDLARS [ˈmed,lɑːz] *abbr.* (美)医学文献分析与检索系统(Medical Literature Analysis and Retrieval System)

MEDLARS is a computerised biomedical bibliographic retrieval system.

MEDLARS 是一种计算机生物医学文献检索系统。

Today, through the Internet and World Wide Web, MEDLARS search services are available around the world without charge.

现在通过互联网,全世界可以免费使用 MEDLARS 检索服务。

MEDLINE [ˈmedˌlain] *n.* (美)联机医学文献分析和检索系统(等于 on-line MEDLARS)

MEDLINE is the best known of NLM's databases.

MEDLINE 是最著名的美国国立医学图书馆数据库。

MEDLINE contains journal citations and abstracts for biomedical literature from around the world.

MEDLINE 包括全世界生物医学文献的期刊引文和摘要。

medulla [meˈdʌlə] *n.* 髓(质)

Small doses have a stimulating effect upon various centers in the medulla oblongata region of the brain.

小剂量(的尼古丁)对脑延髓各个中枢具有兴奋作用。

The secretory cells of the medulla are not charged with lipoid and fat.

髓质的分泌细胞里没有类脂质和脂肪。

medullary [meˈdʌləri] *a.* 髓的

Morphine depresses the cerebral cortex, the hypothalamus, and the medullary centers.

吗啡抑制大脑皮质、下丘脑和延髓中枢。

medulloblastoma [meˌdʌləublæsˈtəumə] *n.* 成神经管细胞瘤

Medulloblastoma is a childhood disease but can show up as late as the sixth decade of life.

成神经管细胞瘤多发于儿童,但也可晚至 60 岁发病。

meet [miːt] *v.* 适应;支持;达到;遵守

They had to change the original plan so as to meet the new situation.

他们不得不改变原计划以适应新形势。

When a worker is hospitalized, all expenses are met by the state.

工人住院时,所有费用都由国家承担。

The results of the medical research have met advanced world standards.

这项医学研究的成果已达到世界先进水平。

The basic principles relating to nursing care must be strictly met.

必须严格遵守有关护理的基本原则。

(注:动词 meet 的一些基本词义如遇见、会见、满足、符合等,在四级词汇已有。)

megacolon [ˌmegəˈkəulən] *n.* 巨结肠

Colonic perforation is a rare complication during toxic megacolon.

即使在中毒性巨结肠时,结肠并发症穿孔也很少见。

Tap water enemas are contraindicated in congenital megacolon because of the danger of excessive water absorption.

在先天性巨结肠病人中,因为有水吸收过量的危险,禁用自来水灌肠。

megakaryocyte [ˌmegəˈkæriəsait] *n.* 巨核细胞

There is a profound deficiency of circulating platelets despite adequate numbers of megakaryocytes in the marrow.

尽管骨髓中仍有足够数量的巨核细胞,但循环系统中的血小板仍极度缺乏。

megaloblast [ˈmegələuˌblæst] *n.* 巨成红细胞,巨幼细胞

Megaloblasts are present in the marrow which is hypercellular, evidence that anemia is in part due to suppression of the release.

骨髓中出现巨成红细胞且计数增高，证明这种贫血部分是细胞释放受抑制所致。

megaloblastic [ˌmegələuˈblæstik] *a.* 巨成红细胞的

Megaloblastic cells may appear in the bone marrow.

骨髓中可能出现巨成红细胞。

meiosis [maiˈəusis] (*pl.* meioses [maiˈəusiːz]) *n.* [希] 减数分裂，成熟分裂

After meiosis I, each progeny cell has 46 chromosomes.

在减数分裂的第一阶段完成后，每个子代细胞都有 46 个染色体。

In meiosis the chromosome content is changed from diploid to haploid.

在减数分裂中，所含染色体从二倍体变为单倍体。

meiotic [maiˈɔtik] *a.* 减数分裂的，成熟分裂的

The first and second meiotic divisions are the two divisions occurring during meiosis.

第一次减数分裂和第二次减数分裂是减数分裂过程中的两次分裂。

During the prophase of the first meiotic division the chromosomes shorten and thicken.

在第一次减数分裂前期染色体缩短变粗。

melamine [ˈmeləmiːn] *n.* 三聚氰胺

The toxicity of melamine and its analogue in man and animals has been reported widely.

三聚氰胺及其类似物对人类和动物的毒性已经广泛报道。

Melamine can be present at low levels in food.

食物中可以含有低浓度的三聚氰胺。

melancholia [ˌmelənˈkəuljə] *n.* 忧郁症

Melancholia is a term used to denote generally the depressive syndrome until the end of the 19th century.

忧郁症这个术语，一直到 19 世纪末，还被用来泛指抑郁综合征。

These symptoms of melancholia are most likely to respond to antidepressants.

忧郁症的这些症状最可能对抗抑郁剂起反应（即药物有效）。

melanin [ˈmelənin] *n.* 黑（色）素

The melanin synthesized by the melanocyte population of the epidermis absorbs radiant energy and protects the skin from the harmful effects of ultraviolet light.

表皮黑色素细胞合成的黑色素能吸收放射能，保护皮肤使其不受紫外线的伤害。

melanocortin [ˌmelænəuˈkɔːtin] *n.* 黑皮素

Classical neurotransmitter systems, such as dopamine and serotonin, as well as the neuropeptide melanocortin, are receiving the most attention.

经典神经递质系统，如多巴胺和血清素，以及神经肽黑皮素，正在受到最大关注。

The gene for the melanocortin-1 receptor (MC1R) plays a role in the presence of freckles; individuals with the dominant variant of MC1R have freckles.

负责深色的黑皮素受体-1（MC1R）的基因会使得雀斑产生，那些 MC1R 呈现显性的人会有雀斑。

melanocyte [ˈmelənəuˌsait] *n.* 黑素细胞

The melanocyte is actually a dendritic cell, a feature rarely appreciated at the light-microscope level.

黑素细胞实际上为一种树枝状细胞，在光学显微镜下难以观察到这种特征。

The racial differences in pigmentation are due to differences in the packaging of melanin by the melanocytes, rather than to differences in numbers of melanocytes.

各人种间肤色的差异是由于黑素细胞对黑色素的包裹程度不同，而不是黑素细胞数量的多少不同。

melanoma [ˌmeləˈnəumə] *n.* 黑素瘤

Melanoma usually occur in the skin but are also found in the eye and the mucous membranes.

黑素瘤通常发生在皮肤上，但也可见于眼部或黏膜。

In metastatic melanoma a generalized darkening of the skin may occur.
在转移性黑素瘤中可发生全身性皮肤黑变。

melanosis [ˌmeləˈnəusis] *n.* 黑变病，黑素沉着病

Generalized melanosis is a diffuse darkening of the skin that imparts a reddish-gray color seen in association with lymphoma, hepatoma, and melanoma.
全身性黑素沉着病病人全身皮肤变黑且透出灰红色，常与淋巴瘤、肝细胞瘤和黑色素瘤有关。

melatonin [ˌmeləˈtəunin] *n.* 褪黑激素；N-乙酰-5-甲氧基色胺

As nights shorten in spring, the brain 's release of melatonin goes down .
在春季，黑夜时间缩短，大脑释放的褪黑素也随之减少。

In response to these signals, the pineal gland modulates its secretion of melatonin, dubbed the sleep hormone because it is released only in dim light or the dark.
由于褪黑素只在弱光或黑暗中才会释出，所以也叫睡眠激素，当接收到这些讯号之后，松果体会调节褪黑素的分泌。

melena [miˈliːnə] *n.* 黑便

Melena as a presenting symptom suggests less severe bleeding than hematemesis.
出血表现为黑便者比表现为呕血者程度要轻。

Bleeding occurs from ileal ulcers and may present as melena or bright red blood in stools.
出血来自回肠溃疡，粪便中可出现黑便或鲜血。

memantine [meˈmæntiːn] *n.* 美金刚胺

Memantine can reduce pain.
美金刚胺可减轻疼痛。

Memantine hydrochloride is used for moderate and severe Alzheimer's disease.
盐酸美金刚胺可用于治疗中度或重度的阿尔茨海默氏病。

membrane [ˈmembrein] *n.* 膜

The chromosomes are surrounded by a nuclear envelope consisting of two membrane layers.
染色体由双层膜组成的核膜围绕着。

membranous [ˈmembrənəs, memˈbreinəs] *a.* 膜的

Membranous nephropathy is a common cause of the nephrotic syndrome in adults.
膜性肾病是成人肾病综合征的常见原因。

Membranous nephropathy is characterized by diffuse thickening of the glomerular capillary wall.
膜性肾病的特征性病变是肾小球毛细血管壁的弥漫性增厚。

memory [ˈmeməri] *n.* 记忆，存储

Memory cells have the ability to recall previous contact with a particular antigen, such that subsequent exposure leads to a more rapid and larger production of antibody.
记忆细胞有能力记住以前曾接触过的特异性抗原，若以后再接触（抗原）便可导致更快更多地产生抗体。

menace [ˈmenəs] *n.* 威胁

Thousands of cases of cholera in Latin America have focused public attention on the menace of contaminated food and water.
拉丁美洲所发生的数以千计的霍乱病例引起公众对污染的水和食物威胁的关注。

menarche [miˈnɑːki] *n.* 月经初潮

Menarche occurs at a mean age of 12. 8 years in the United States, and 97% of American girls experience menarche by 14. 6 years.
美国女性月经初潮的平均年龄为 12. 8 岁，97% 的美国女孩在 14. 6 岁之前便已经来月经。

In order to investigate the menarche age and psychosexual behavior of girls, a health-education questionnaire was adopted for the 2447 girl students in the middle schools of seven cities.
为了解中学女生月经初潮年龄和性心理行为状况，采用“健康教育问卷”对 7 市中学 2447

名女生进行了调查。

Mendelian [menˈdiːliən] *a.* 孟德尔的，孟德尔法则的，遗传的

Today the subject has four main subdivisions—Mendelian genetics，population genetics，cytogenetics，and molecular genetics.

现在，该学科主要包括四大部分—孟德尔遗传学、种群遗传学、细胞遗传学以及分子遗传学。

One way that we can gain an understanding of the functional effects of various types of genomic variations is to survey the mutations that have been associated with human Mendelian disease.

阐明不同类型基因组变异的功能效应的一种方法是检测与人类遗传疾病有关的基因突变。

meninges [miˈnindʒiːz] *n.* [希] 脑(脊)膜

The term "lumbar puncture" means hollow-needle puncture of the meninges of the lumbar subarachnoid space.

腰椎穿刺一词意指以中空的针穿刺腰蛛网膜下腔的脑脊膜。

meningioma [miˌnindʒiˈəumə] *n.* 脑(脊)膜瘤

Successful resection of meningiomas is common and incomplete resection or recurrence is treated with focal irradiation.

脑膜瘤大多可以成功地切除，若切除不彻底或复发则需进行局部放疗。

Meningiomas account for about one sixth of all primary neoplasms of the central nervous system.

脑膜瘤约占所有中枢神经系统原发肿瘤的六分之一。

Meningioma tumours are more common in older people and in women.

脑膜瘤在老年人和女性中较常见。

meningismus [ˌmeninˈdʒisməs] *n.* 假性脑(脊)膜炎

In deep coma，meningismus may be absent，despite the presence of bacterial or chemical meningitis.

在深度昏迷状态下，尽管可出现细菌性或化学性脑膜炎，但不太可能出现假性脑膜炎。

meningitis [ˌmeninˈdʒaitis] *n.* 脑膜炎

Aseptic meningitis was thought to be a specific disease，but it is now known that most cases are caused by virus.

无菌脑膜炎曾被认为是一种特异疾病，现在已知大多数此病是由病毒引起的。

The sugar content is usually low in bacterial meningitis and normal in viral infections.

患细菌性脑膜炎时脑脊液中的糖含量通常较低，而患病毒性感染时糖含量正常。

meningococcal [məˌniŋgəuˈkɔkəl] *a.* 脑膜炎球菌的

Meningococcal infections may occur sporadically or as epidemic.

脑膜炎球菌感染的发生，可呈散发性亦可为流行性。

Patients with meningococcal disease are usually more dehydrated than they appear.

脑膜炎球菌病人脱水通常比他们所表现出来的要严重。

meningococcemia [məˌniŋgəukɔkˈsiːmiə] *n.* 脑膜炎球菌血症

Most patients with uncomplicated meningococcemia defervescence within the first 24 hours of antibiotic therapy.

大多数无并发症的脑膜炎球菌菌血症病人在开始抗生素治疗 24 小时内退热。

About 20 percent of patients with meningococcal disease have meningococcemia without meningitis.

约 20% 的脑膜炎球菌病病人只有脑膜炎球菌菌血症而无脑膜炎。

meningococcus [məˌniŋgəuˈkɔkəs] (*pl.* meningococci [məˌniŋgəuˈkɔksai]) *n.* 脑膜炎球菌

Meningococci are spread from person to person by airborne droplets of infected nasopharyngeal secretions.

受感染患者的鼻咽部分泌物可形成飘浮于空气中的飞沫将脑膜炎球菌传给他人。

meningoencephalitis [miˈniŋgəuən,sefəˈlaitis] *n.* 脑膜脑炎

Meningoencephalitis combines inflammatory process of the leptomeninges with inflammation of the brain parenchyma.

脑膜脑炎是指软脑膜的炎症合并脑实质的炎症。

A variety of viral agents cause aseptic meningitis or meningoencephalitis.

各种病毒性因子可引起无菌性脑膜炎或脑膜脑炎。

menometrorrhagia [ˌmenəuˌmetrəˈreidʒiə] *n.* 月经过多

Menometrorrhagia is a condition in which prolonged or excessive uterine bleeding occurs irregularly and more frequently than normal.

月经过多是指经期与正常相比,时间延长或子宫出血过多,不规律或者更加频繁。

menopausal [ˌmenəˈpɔːzəl] *a.* 绝经(期)的

Not every patient suffers the menopausal syndrome to the same degree.

不是所有的患者都患有同样程度的绝经期综合征。

Menopausal syndrome is a common disease and affects the life of the women.

绝经期综合征是绝经期妇女的常见病,影响妇女的生活。

menopause [ˈmenəpɔːz] *n.* 绝经(期)

Retention of normal ovaries in women after the menopause is still a matter of contention.

绝经期后妇女的正常卵巢是否保留仍然是个争论的问题。

Menstruation ends at the menopause between the ages of 47 to 53.

月经在 47 ~ 53 岁间的绝经期中止。

menorrhagia [ˌmenəˈreidʒiə] *n.* 经血过多

Menorrhagia for a few periods after the menarche is not uncommon.

月经初潮后少数几个周期出现月经过多并非少见。

menotropin [ˌmenəˈtrəupin] *n.* 促生育素;(绝经期)促性腺激素

Human urinary-derived menotropin preparations are exposed to the theoretical risk of infection from menopausal donors of urine.

人尿源性促生育素理论上有被绝经患者捐赠的尿液感染的风险。

Menotropin consists of gonadotropins that are extracted from the urine of postmenopausal women, which usually include luteinizing hormone and follicle-stimulating hormone.

促生育素是从绝经妇女尿液中提取的促性腺激素,通常包括黄体生成素和卵泡刺激素。

mensis [ˈmensis] (*pl.* menses [ˈmensiːz]) *n.* 月经

In the description of vaginal discharge, the relation to menses and coitus and the response to therapy should be noted.

在描述阴道分泌物时应记录与月经及性交的关系,以及对治疗的反应。

menstrual [ˈmenstruəl] *a.* 月经的

The patient complains of menstrual disorder.

病人主诉月经失调。

menstruate [ˈmenstrueit] *v.* 行经

The term primary amenorrhoea refers to a patient of any age who has never menstruated.

原发性闭经一词是指任何年龄未曾行经的患者。

menstruation [ˌmenstruˈeiʃən] *n.* 月经,行经

Menstruation is the most striking outward manifestation of the cycle.

月经是此周期中最显著的外在表现。

Normal menstruation depends upon the integrated action of the endocrine and nervous system.

正常的月经依赖于内分泌作用和神经系统作用的整合。

mental [ˈmentl] *a.* 心理的,精神的,智力的,脑力的

This medical college offers "Mental Hygiene" as an elective course.

这所医学院开设"心理卫生学"作为一门选修课。

Additional causes include mental health problems and reproductive disorders.
其他的原因包括有精神健康问题和生殖系统疾病。
As shock supervenes, restlessness, mental obtundation, and coma may follow in rapid succession.
随着休克的发生,烦躁不安、神志迟钝及昏迷相继迅速出现。
Dementia or partial or complete lack of mental development is characteristic of congenital syphilis.
痴呆或部分或全部智力发育不全是先天梅毒的特点。
Serious mental deterioration is not a normal part of aging.
脑力严重衰退并不是年老的正常情况。

mentally [ˈmentli] *ad.* 精神上,智力上
Thus far, most patients described have been mentally retarded.
到现在,所述大多数的病人是智力迟钝的。

mental-status [ˈmentlˈsteitəs] *n.* 精神状态
The mental-status examination is a description of a person' s mental-status at one point in time.
精神状态检查是对一个人在某一时刻的精神状态的描述。

meperidine [məˈperidin] *n.* 哌替啶
The duration of action of meperidine is extremely short.
哌替啶的作用时间非常短。

mephenytoin [məˈfenitɔin] *n.* 美芬妥英
CYP2C19 , historically termed mephenytoin hydroxylase, that displays penetrant pharmacogenetic variability, with just a few SNPs accounting for the majority of the deficient, poor metabolizer phenotype.
CYP2C19,历史上曾称为美芬妥英羟化酶,呈现强烈的遗传药理学变异性,其中仅仅几个SNPs可以解释大部分缺陷的、弱代谢表型。

meprobamate [miˈprəubəmeit] *n.* 氨甲丙二酯; 眠尔通
Minor tranquillizers, such as the benzodiazepines and meprobamate, are used to treat neuroses and to relieve anxiety and tension due to various causes.
弱安定药,例如苯[并]二氮䓬类和眠尔通,用于治疗神经官能症和减轻由于各种原因引起的焦虑和紧张。

mercaptopurine [məˌkæptəuˈpjuəriːn] *n.* 巯嘌呤(尤指6-巯基嘌呤,用以治疗急性白血病)
Concomitant medications at the commencement of adalimumab were corticosteroids (38%), azathioprine/6-mercaptopurine (41%), and methotrexate (23%).
在开始服用阿达木单抗时,合并用药为类固醇(38%)、硫唑嘌呤/6-巯基嘌呤(41%)和甲氨蝶呤(23%)。
All maintenance therapy utilizes low-dose 6-mercaptopurine (6MP) and methotrexate (MTX), while maintenance in APL primarily consists of all-trans-retinoic acid (ATRA).
所有的维持疗法都使用低剂量的6-巯基嘌呤(6MP)和甲氨蝶呤(MTX),在急性髓细胞白血病(APL)初期的维持治疗中还要联合使用全反式维甲酸(ATRA)。

mercurial [məːˈkjuəriə] *n.* 汞剂
Mercurials are now seldom used since the newer agents are more effective.
现在很少使用汞剂,因为新一代的制剂更有效。

mercury [ˈməːkjuri] *n.* 汞,水银
The death of this patient was not connected with mercury poisoning.
这个病人的死亡与汞中毒无关。
Toxic symptoms of mercury poisoning may occur with 0.1gm, and 0.5gm is almost always fatal unless immediate treatment is given.
0.1克汞即可出现汞中毒的毒性症状,0.5克汞几乎总是致死性的,除非立即进行治疗。

mercy [ˈməːsi] *n.* 慈悲,仁慈;宽容

They were treated with mercy.
他们受到仁慈的待遇。
They are planning to introduce a bill which would authorize the mercy killing.
他们正计划提出一个提案,使安乐死合法化。

merge [məːdʒ] *v.* (使)合并,(使)结合
Bilateral involvement of the salivary or parotid glands occur, which may merge with the cervical adenopathy.
双侧唾液腺或腮腺受累可与肿大的颈部淋巴结融合。

meridian [məˈridiən] *n.* 经,经脉;子午线,经线
The theory of meridians and collaterals was systematized by the acient Chinese people in their prolonged clinical practice.
经络理论是古代中国人在长期临床实践中总结出来的。

merozoite [ˌmerəˈzəuait] *n.* 裂殖子
Rupture of the schizont releases more merozoites into the blood and causes fever.
裂殖体破裂时释放出更多的裂殖子进入血液使患者发烧。

mesangial [meˈsændʒiəl] *a.* (肾小球)系膜的
The entire glomerular tuft is supported by mesangial cells lying between the capillaries.
整个肾小球毛细血管丛由毛细血管间的系膜细胞支撑。
The normal mesangium contains about 2 to 4 mesangial cells, which have a macrophage-like function.
正常系膜含有 2 ~4 个具有巨噬细胞样功能的系膜细胞。

mesenchymal [mesˈeŋkiməl] *a.* 间质的
Mesenchymal cells such as fibroblasts and smooth muscle are quiescent cells.
间质细胞如成纤维细胞和平滑肌是静止的细胞。
Uterine sarcomas are a rare form of uterine malignancy that arise from uterine mesenchymal elements (ie, smooth muscle and connective tissue).
子宫肉瘤是一种来源于子宫间质(即:平滑肌和结缔组织)的罕见的子宫恶性肿瘤。

mesenteric [ˌmesənˈterik] *a.* 肠系膜的
The largest tributary of the portal tube is the superior mesenteric vein.
汇入门脉的最大分支是肠系膜上静脉。
Mesenteric lymphadenopathy may cause abdominal pain.
肠系膜淋巴结病变可引起腹部疼痛。

mesentery [ˈmesəntəri] *n.* 肠系膜
The small intestine is attached to the abdominal wall by its mesentery.
小肠通过系膜连接于腹壁。

mesial [ˈmiːsiəl] *a.* 近中的,中间的,中央的
EEG recordings showed epileptiform paroxysms in the left mesial frontal region.
脑电图记录显示癫痫样发作在左侧中央额部。
The mesial prefrontal cortex is thought to be important to social behavior.
中央前额皮质被认为与社交行为关系密切。

mesoderm [ˈmesəudəːm] *n.* 中胚层
Muscles are formed by the mesoderm.
肌肉由中胚层形成。
The ectoderm, mesoderm, and endoderm form everything that is in the body.
外胚层、中胚层和内胚层形成身体所有的一切。

mesoendemic [ˌmesəuenˈdemik] *a.* 中度流行的
In mesoendemic areas malaria is frequent but only seasonal.
疟疾在中度流行区经常可以见到,但有季节性。

mesomer [ˈmiːsəuməː] *n.* 内消旋体

Although the two rings are joined by a formal double bond, contributions from the aromatic mesomer reduce its bond order substantially.

尽管这两个环以正规的双键链接，但是芳香族的内消旋体实际上降低了它的键级。

It was shown that γ-cyclodextrin influences the equilibrium between mitomycin C and its zwitterion mesomer.

研究显示 γ 环糊精影响了丝裂霉素 C 与其两性离子内消旋体之间的平衡。

mesothelial [ˌmesəuˈθiːliəl] *a.* 间皮的

Lymphocytes predominate in the cell count, and mesothelial cells are rare.

淋巴细胞占大多数，而间皮细胞很少。

mesothelioma [ˌmesəuˌθiːliˈəumə] (*pl.* mesotheliomas 或 mesotheliomata [ˌmesəuˌθiːliˈəumətə]) *n.* 间皮瘤

Most people with mesothelioma, a cancer of the chest lining, die within one or two years.

间皮瘤是一种胸膜恶性肿瘤，大多数患者在一两年内就会死去。

The incidence of mesotheliomas is rising and it is estimated that there may be as many as 3000 cases by the year 2000.

间皮瘤的发病率正逐年增加，有人估计 2000 年可能达到 3000 例之多。

mesothelium [ˌmesəuˈθiːliəmˌˌmez-] *n.* 间皮

Malignant mesothelioma is a mesothelium-derived carcinoma with high malignancy.

恶性间皮瘤是一种起源于间皮细胞的高度恶性肿瘤。

There were significant changes in diaphragmatic peritoneal mesothelium and lymphatic capillaries.

膈腹膜间皮和膈毛细淋巴管均发生了明显的变化。

message [ˈmesidʒ] *n.* 信息

Some messages about the outside world (e. g. heat, cold) come to us through the skin.

外部世界的一些信息（如冷、热）可经过皮肤传给我们。

Spinal nerves are those that carry messages to and from the spinal cord.

脊神经是那些把信息输入和输出脊髓的神经。

messenger [ˈmesindʒə] *n.* 送信者，使者

Hormones are chemical messengers which stimulate particular organs or tissues to function.

激素是化学使者，能使特定的器官或组织兴奋而发挥作用。

meta-analysis [ˌmetəəˈnælisis] *n.* 荟萃分析；元分析

Meta-analysis has been defined as "the statistical analysis of a collection of analytic results for the purpose of integrating the findings".

荟萃分析定义为"以合并研究结果为目的，收集分析结果的一种统计学方法"。

In statistics, a meta-analysis combines the results of several studies that address a set of related research hypotheses.

在统计学中，元分析是对多项具有相关研究假设的结果进行的综合性分析。

metabolic [ˌmetəˈbɔlik] *a.* 新陈代谢的

Chills are accompanied by an increase in metabolic activity as measured by oxygen consumption.

通过测定氧气的消耗发现寒战伴有代谢活动的增强。

The patient should not take anything when coming for the basal metabolic test.

来做基础代谢测验时患者不应该吃任何东西。

metabolically [ˌmetəˈbɔlikəli] *ad.* 代谢上的

A differentiated cell is metabolically active.

已分化的细胞其代谢活性高。

metabolism [meˈtæbəlizəm] *n.* 代谢，新陈代谢

The exact function of L-ascorbic acid in cell metabolism is still far from understood.

L-抗坏血酸在细胞代谢中确切的功能还很不清楚。

Vitamin B_{12} is thought to influence nuclear structure by affecting folate metabolism.

据认为维生素 B_{12}是通过干扰叶酸代谢来影响核的结构的。

metabolite [me'tæbəlait] *n.* 代谢产物

Often the concentration of metabolite far exceeds the concentration of drug.

代谢产物的浓度常远超过药物的浓度。

The thromboxanes are metabolized extensively, and the metabolites appear in the urine.

血小板凝集素广泛地被代谢,其代谢产物经尿排出。

metabolize [me'tæbəlaiz] *v.* 产生代谢变化,引起代谢

Neostigmine itself is metabolized by plasma acetylcholinesterase.

新斯的明本身被血浆乙酰胆碱酯酶所代谢。

If these agents are given orally, they will be metabolized to inactive compounds by nitrate reductase in the liver.

如果口服,这些药物会被肝脏的硝酸盐还原酶代谢成无活性的化合物。

metabolome [mi'tæbələum] *n.* 代谢组

The metabolome represents the collection of all metabolites in a biological cell, tissue, organ or organism.

代谢组是指一个生物细胞、组织、器官或机体内所有代谢物的总和。

Metabolome can give an instantaneous snapshot of the physiology of a cell.

代谢组能够给出一个细胞的生理学即时“快照”。

metabolomics [ˌmetəbə'lɔmiks] *n.* 代谢组学

Historically, the metabolomics approach was one of the first methods to apply the scope of systems biology to studies of metabolism.

从历史上看,代谢组学是在系统生物学领域研究代谢作用的最早的一种方法。

In the post-genomic era, genomics, transcriptomics, proteomics and metabolomics provide great opportunity for the development of metabolic engineering.

后基因组学时代的基因组学、转录组学、蛋白质组学和代谢组学为代谢工程的发展提供了极好的机遇。

metabonomics [miˌtæbəu'nɔmiks] *n.* 代谢组学

Following on the heels of genomics and proteomics, metabonomics may lead to more efficient drug discovery and individualized patient treatment with drugs.

紧随基因组学和蛋白组学之后,代谢组学可能引起更有效的药物发现和个体化的病人药物治疗。

Metabonomics is the study of metabolic responses to drugs, environmental changes and diseases.

代谢组学是研究对药物、环境变化和疾病的代谢反应。

metacarpophalangeal [ˌmetəˌkɑːpəufə'lændʒiəl] *a.* 掌指的

The chronic disease may produce fixed deformities and ulnar deviation at the metacarpophalangeal joints.

慢性病变可导致关节固定畸形,在掌骨和指骨关节处向尺侧偏斜。

metacentric [ˌmetə'sentrik] *a.* 定倾中心的,中央着丝粒的

A metacentric chromosome has two arms with approximately equal length.

中央着丝粒染色体两臂长度相似。

Y chromosome has two types of polymorphism: metacentric (or submetacentric) and acrocentric chromosomes.

Y 染色体有二种类型的多态性,即中间着丝粒(或亚中间着丝粒)和近端着丝粒染色体。

metacercaria [ˌmetəsəː'kɛəriə] (*pl.* metacercariae [ˌmetəsəː'kɛəriiː]) *n.* 囊蚴

After ingestion of the contaminated fish, the metacercariae excyst in the duodenum.

进食被污染的鱼后,囊蚴便在十二指肠脱囊。

metagenomics [ˌmetədʒiˈnɔmiks] *n.* 宏基因组学,元基因组学

In metagenomics, the power of genomic analysis is applied to entire communities of microbes, bypassing the need to isolate and culture individual microbial species.

宏基因组研究的重要作用是分析一个宿主的全部微生物种群的基因,不必分离培养某一种微生物。

The emerging field of metagenomics offers a new way of exploring the microbial world.

宏基因组学的诞生为微生物领域的研究开辟了新的途径。

metal [ˈmetl] *n.* 金属

Soil heavy metal pollution is an important aspect of soil pollution.

土壤重金属污染是土壤污染的一个重要方面。

Arsenic is the most common cause of acute heavy metal poisoning in adults

砷是引起成人急性重金属中毒的最常见原因。

metalloenzyme [meˌtæləuˈenzaim] *n.* 金属(结合)酶,含金属酶

Zinc has been found to be an integral part of many metalloenzymes.

人们已发现锌是许多含金属酶的一个组成成分。

metalloid [ˈmetəːlɔid] *n.* 类金属,非金属

Metals and metalloids exert their toxic effects in biological system through many different mechanisms.

金属和类金属通过多种不同的机制而对生物系统发挥有毒的效应。

metalloprotein [miˌtæləuˈprəutiːn] *n.* 金属蛋白

In the metalloproteins some metal ion is attached directly to the protein.

在金属蛋白中,某些金属离子直接结合在蛋白质上。

metaphase [ˈmetəfeiz] *n.* (细胞分裂)中期

In the second stage, or metaphase, of mitosis, the chromosomes align on the equator of the spindle fibers.

在有丝分裂的第二个时期即中期,染色体排列在纺锤丝的赤道上。

metaplasia [ˌmetəˈpleizjə] *n.* (组织)转化,化生,组织变形

Squamous metaplasia is a common reaction of the bronchial mucosa to various injuries and may progress to squamous carcinoma.

支气管黏膜对各种损伤的常见反应是鳞状上皮化生,而且可能发展成为鳞状上皮癌。

metaplastic [ˌmetəˈplæstik] *a.* 化生性的

In a metaplastic change, the precursor cells existing in normal tissues differentiate along a new pathway.

在化生性改变中,存在于正常组织中的前体细胞沿着新的方向分化。

Squamous cell carcinomas in the respiratory tract arise from metaplastic squamous cells transformed by the normal columnar epithelium.

呼吸道鳞状细胞癌发生于正常柱状上皮转化的化生的鳞状上皮。

metaproteome [ˌmetəˈprəutiəum] *n.* 宏蛋白组

The study of proteins expressed by indigenous microbiota, metaproteome, may provide insights into the functioning of the microbial ecosystems.

对土著微生物群落表达的蛋白的研究(宏蛋白组学)可揭示微生物生态系的功能。

Study on metaproteome of microbiota will be important to understanding the relationship between intestinal flora and host.

研究微生物群落宏蛋白组对理解肠道菌群和宿主的关系是很重要的。

metastable [ˌmetəˈsteibl] *a.* 亚稳的

Additives can be used to obtain the metastable form of pharmaceutical compounds.

添加剂可用于形成制剂的亚稳形式。

Milling of griseofulvin produced an increased metastable solubility.

灰黄霉素研磨成粉可以增加其亚稳溶解度。

metastasis [meˈtæstəsis] (*pl.* metastases [meˈtæstəsiːz]) *n.* 转移

Metastasis through blood vessels is the common route for sarcomas.

血管是肉瘤常见的转移途径。

All these tumours are capable of metastasis by lymphatics and blood vessels.

所有这些肿瘤都能通过淋巴管和血管转移。

metastasize [miˈtæstəsaiz] *v.* 转移,迁徙

Cancer from other sites may metastasize to the ovaries.

其他部位的癌可能转移至卵巢。

Some malignant teratomas metastasize with multiple elements.

有些恶性畸胎瘤可带着多种组织成分转移。

metastatic [ˌmetəˈstætik] *a.* 转移性的

If there are multiple cancerous nodules in an organ, they are probably metastatic.

如果一个器官有多个癌结节,则可能为转移瘤。

Metastatic calcification occurs especially in the walls of arteries and in the kidneys.

转移性钙化主要发生于动脉壁和肾脏。

This investigation was undertaken to define the value of laparoscopy in the staging of patients with colorectal carcinoma metastatic to the liver.

本研究的目的是要确定腹腔镜检对结肠直肠癌转移至肝脏患者进行分期中的作用。

metatarsophalangeal [ˌmetəˌtɑːsəufəˈlændʒiəl] *a.* 跖趾的

The metatarsophalangeal joints of the feet may also be tender on pressure.

脚上的跖趾关节也可有压痛。

methacholine [ˌmeθəˈkəuliːn] *n.* 乙酰甲胆碱

The cardiovascular effects of methacholine are more pronounced than those of acetylcholine.

乙酰甲胆碱的心血管作用比乙酰胆碱更为明显。

methadone [ˈmeθədɔn] *n.* 美沙酮,美散痛

Tolerance to methadone is acquired very slowly.

对美沙酮的耐受作用产生很慢。

methane [ˈmiːθein] *n.* 甲烷

Among the toxic gases are sulfur dioxide, methane, the oxide of nitrogen, ammonia, hydrogen sulfide, and hydrogen cyanide.

常见的有毒气体中有二氧化硫、甲烷、氧化氮、氨、硫化氢以及氰化氢。

methanol [ˈmeθənɔl] *n.* 甲醇

Methanol poisoning can be treated with ethanol.

甲醇中毒可用乙醇来处理。

methemoglobin [metˌhiːməuˈgləubin] *n.* 正铁血红蛋白,高铁血红蛋白

Cyanosis due to the formation of methemoglobin in red cells is more common but not dangerous.

更常见的是由于红细胞内形成正铁血红蛋白,因而发生发绀,但无危险。

Methemoglobin has such high oxygen affinity that virtually no oxygen is delivered to tissues.

高的血红蛋白与氧有很强的亲和力,所以实际上没有氧气被释放到组织中去。

methemoglobinemia [ˌmeθiməuˌgləubiˈniːmiə] *n.* 高铁血红蛋白血症

While methemoglobinemia clears spontaneously over several hours, hemolytic anemia may take several weeks to resolve.

高铁血红蛋白症会在几个小时后自动消失,而溶血性贫血需要几个星期才能纠正。

It is well known that the nitrate from environment is causally related to infant methemoglobinemia and esophageal cancer.

环境中的硝酸盐与婴儿高铁血红蛋白血症及食管癌的病因关联已为人们所熟知。

methenamine [meˈθiːnəmiːn] *n.* 环六亚甲基四胺,乌洛托品(尿道抗菌药)

Methenamine is used as a urinary suppressant in patients with recurrent bacteriuria and urinary tract infections but is not used for acute infections.

乌托洛品是一种尿道抑菌剂，常用于复发性菌尿和尿路感染，但不用于急性感染。

methicillin [meθiˈsilin] *n.* 二甲氧基苯青霉素钠，新青霉素 I

Methicillin in a dosage of 250 to 300mg/kg/day should be administered parenterally.

可用二甲氧基苯青霉素 250～300mg/kg/d 非经肠道给药（即肌注或静脉内滴注）。

methionine [meˈθaiəniːn] *n.* 蛋氨酸，甲硫氨酸（肝胆疾病辅助用药）

A methionine-free diet improves the findings of mental retardation, diarrhea, and convulsions.

饮食中缺乏蛋氨酸会引起反应迟钝、腹泻和痉挛。

That's ture lack of methionine in the milk .

牛奶中确实缺乏蛋氨酸。

The consensus that diets low in methionine and devoid of choline and folate are sufficient to independently induce tumor formation.

食物中蛋氨酸低并缺乏胆碱和叶酸可足以独立地诱发肿瘤，这已经成为共识。

methodologically [ˌmeθədəˈlɔdʒikəli] *ad.* 方法学地，方法论地

Methodologically well- done prospective studies are lacking.

目前缺少运用良好方法学的前瞻性研究。

methodology [meθəˈdɔlədʒi] *n.* 一套方法，方法论

A new cardiopulmonary resuscitation methodology has been developed recently.

最近研究出一种新的心肺复苏术。

Despite the present surgical methodology as well as medical treatment, the prognosis of extrahepatic biliary atresia remains poor.

尽管除药物治疗外还有现行的外科方法，肝外胆道闭锁的预后仍然很差。

methotrexate [ˌmeθəˈtrekseit] *n.* 甲氨蝶呤

The therapeutic success was related to achieving targeted methotrexate concentrations in plasma during high-dose therapy for pediatric acute lymphoblastic leukemia (ALL).

大剂量甲氨蝶呤治疗儿童急性淋巴细胞性白血病的成功与达到该药所需血浆浓度有关。

methyl [ˈmeθil] *n.* 甲基

The predominant form of vitamin B_{12} in serum is methyl B_{12}.

血清中维生素 B_{12} 的主要类型是甲基 B_{12}。

Besides producing all the CNS (central nervous system) effects, methyl alcohol causes acidosis and blindness.

甲醇除了产生全部的中枢神经系统作用外，还引起酸中毒和失明。

methylate [ˈmeθileit] *v.* 甲基化，加甲基

The adrenal medulla is the only organ having the capacity to methylate norepinephrine to form epinephrine.

肾上腺髓质是唯一有能力使去甲肾上腺素再甲基化而形成肾上腺素的器官。

methylation [ˌmeθiˈleiʃənt] *n.* 甲基化

As expected, tumor cells showed the highest methylation levels.

正如所预料的，肿瘤细胞呈高度甲基化。

It was also brought to light that nutrition and drugs can influence DNA methylation patterns.

也有人报道了营养和药物可以影响 DNA 甲基化模式。

methyldopa [ˌmeθilˈdəupə] *n.* 甲基多巴，2-甲基二羟苯丙氨酸（口服降压药）

Methyldopa inhibits central sympathetic outflow. Its side effects include sedation, dry mouth, hepatitis, fever and positive Coombs' test.

甲基多巴抑制中枢交感神经输出，其副作用有镇静、口干、肝炎、发热和 Coombs 试验阳性。

methylenetetrahydrofolate [ˌmeθiliːn, tetrə, haidrəuˈfəuleit] *n.* 亚甲基四氢叶酸

Complete inactivation *via* rare point mutations in methylenetetrahydrofolate reductase (MTHFR)

causes severe mental retardation, cardiovascular disease, and a shortened lifespan.
亚甲基四氢叶酸还原酶(MTHFR)的罕见点突变造成该酶完全失活,引起严重智力发育迟缓、心血管疾病及预期寿命缩短。

methylmalonic acidemia [ˌmeθilməˌlɔnikˌæsiˈdiːmiə] *n.* 甲基丙二酸血症

Dialysis immediately before liver transplantation for patients with methylmalonic academia is considered to be necessary.
甲基丙二酸血症病人在肝移植前必须立即进行透析。

Hyperglycemia is an exceptional manifestation of methylmalonic acidemia.
高血糖是甲基丙二酸血症的一个特殊表现。

methylmalonic aciduria [ˌmeθilməˌlɔnikˌæsiˈdjuəriə] *n.* 甲基丙二酸尿症

Recurrent, life-threatening metabolic decompensations often occur in patients with methylmalonic aciduria.
反复的威胁生命的代谢失代偿经常发生于甲基丙二酸尿症病人。

Methylmalonic aciduria is a common inherited autosomal recessive disorder.
甲基丙二酸尿症是一种常见的常染色体隐性遗传病。

methylmercury [ˈmeθilˈməːkjuri] *n.* 甲基汞

Methylmercury was produced directly and indirectly as part of many industrial processes.
许多工业生产过程会直接或间接产生甲基汞。

Minamata disease is the name of a disorder caused by methylmercury poisoning that was first described in the inhabitants of Minamata Bay and resulted from their eating fish contaminated with mercury industrial waste.
水俣病是甲基汞中毒引起的一种疾病,首次发生于居住在日本水俣湾的居民中,是由食用了含汞工业废水污染的鱼所致。

methylphenidate [ˌmeθilˈfenideit] *n.* 哌甲酯,利他灵

Methylphenidate is used in the treatment of attention deficit hyperactivity disorder.
哌甲酯用于 治疗注意力缺陷多动障碍综合征。

This study aims at determining the effects of methylphenidate administration on behavioral inhibition in adult rats.
本研究的目的是要确定利他灵对成年大鼠的行为抑制作用。

methylprednisolone [ˌmeθilpredˈnisələun] *n.* 甲基去氢氢化可的松,甲基泼尼松龙,甲基氢化泼尼松

Intravenous corticosteroids such as methylprednisolone, 20 to 100mg, should be administered and may need to be repeated every 2 to 4 hours.
应由静脉给予皮质激素如甲基强的松龙 20 ~ 100 毫克,每 2 ~ 4 小时重复一次。

methyltestosterone [ˌmeθiltesˈtɔstərəun] *n.* 甲基睾丸酮

Methyltestosterone is used to suppress lactation, to treat menstrual and menopausal disorder, and to treat breast cancer in women.
甲基睾丸酮常用来抑制乳汁分泌,治疗月经和绝经时的疾病,并可治疗妇女的乳腺癌。

meticulous [miˈtikjuləs] *a.* 过细的,细致的,精确的

Owing to the absence of specific symptoms and signs, making the diagnosis requires meticulous care on the part of the physician.
由于缺乏明显的症状和体征,要求医生在作出诊断时特别谨慎小心。

The meticulous removal of any fragments of nail or cuticle under a magnifying glass is important.
重要的是要在放大镜下仔细清除所有甲碎片或甲小皮。

In this setting, a detailed and meticulous history of the behavior of the pain is the cornerstone of the evaluation.
在这种情况下,有关疼痛的详细的、准确的病史是诊断的基础。

meticulously [miˈtikjuləsli] *ad.* 过细地,谨慎地

Only through meticulously conducted clinical studies will the true value of this procedure be fully clarified.
只有通过严谨的临床研究,这一方法的真实价值才会完全清楚。

metoclopramide [ˌmetəˈkləuprəmaid] *n.* 胃复安
They found that metoclopramide worked faster to quell symptoms of nausea and vomiting than droperidol.
他们发现胃复安比达哌啶醇能更快速地减轻呕吐和恶心的症状。
HD metoclopramide combining with other drugs can get a satisfactory effect in the prevention of vomiting.
大剂量胃复安结合其他药物对呕吐的预防起到满意的效果。

metrology [miˈtrɔlədʒi] *n.* 度量衡学
Metrology is the science of measurement.
度量衡学是一门测量的学科。

metronidazole [ˌmiːtrəˈnaidəzəul] *n.* 灭滴灵,甲硝唑(口服抗滴虫及阿米巴药)
Metronidazole has very good antimicrobial activity against most anaerobic microorganisms.
甲硝唑对大多数厌氧微生物有很好的抗菌作用。

metropolitan [ˌmetrəˈpɔlitən] *a.* 大城市的;主要都市的
Nearly all the intensive care units were in large metropolitan hospitals.
几乎所有重症监护室过去都设在大城市的医院中。

metrorrhagia [ˌmiːtrəˈreidʒiə] *n.* 子宫出血
Metrorrhagia is most likely due to organic pathology, such as endometrial or cervical polyps or carcinomas.
子宫不规则出血最易因器质性病变如子宫内膜、子宫颈的息肉或癌引起。

micelle [maiˈsel] *n.* 微胶粒,胶囊
Solubilization of cyclosporin A by using sodium cholate/lecithin mixed micelles has been demonstrated.
胆酸钠/卵磷脂混合微胶粒对环孢素 A 的增溶作用已被证实。
The use of micelles in pharmacy is an important tool that finds numerous applications.
在药剂学中胶囊是一种重要工具,被发现具有多种用途。
Polymeric micelles are nanosized particles that are made up of polymer chains.
聚合物胶囊是由高分子链组成的纳米级微粒。

miconazole [maiˈkɔnəzəul] *n.* 咪康唑
Four small, uncontrolled studies have been published using miconazole bladder irrigation.
四篇有关使用咪康唑进行膀胱冲洗的无对照的小型研究已经发表。

microangiopathy [ˌmaikrəuˌændʒiˈɔpəθi] *n.* 微血管病
Diabetic microangiopathy affects two sites preferentially: the retina and the kidney.
糖尿病性微血管病首先影响两个部位,即:视网膜和肾脏。

microarray [ˌmaikrəuəˈrei] *n.* 微排列,微阵列
DNA microarrays have many potential uses in addition to providing a visual portrait of gene expression.
除了可提供基因表达的可视图像外,DNA 微阵列还有许多潜在的用途。

microautophagy [ˌmaikrəuɔːˈtɔfədʒi] *n.* 微自噬
Microautophagy is the continuous internalization of the cytosol into the vesicular system.
微自噬是指细胞溶质持续的内化到囊泡系统中。
In microautophagy, cytoplasmic components are engulfed by an invaginated vacuolar membrane.
在微自噬过程中,细胞质成分被一个内陷的泡膜所吞噬。

microbe [ˈmaikrəub] *n.* 微生物
Microbes include bacteria, some fungi, mycoplasmas, protozoa, rickettsiae, and viruses.

微生物包括细菌、某些真菌、支原体、原生动物、立克次体和病毒。

Although microbes cannot fly, the dust of the air is alive with them.

微生物尽管不会飞,但是空气中的灰尘却充满着微生物。

The skin is the first line of defense against microbes and other infective organisms.

皮肤是防御微生物和其他传染性生物体的第一道防线。

microbial [maiˈkrəubiəl] *a.* 微生物的

Simple organisms constitute the microbial world.

简单生物组成了微生物世界。

Microbial growth is further abetted by the prevalence of dirt and the lack of sunlight.

污物遍布,阳光不足,也会进一步促使微生物生长。

microbicide [maiˈkrəubisaid] *n.* 杀微生物剂

Germicide (microbicide) is an agent that kills the growthing microbes but not necessarily the resistant spore forms of germs.

杀菌剂(杀微生物剂)是一种能杀死正在生长的微生物,但未必能杀死具有抵抗力的细菌的芽孢。

microbiologic(al) [ˌmaikrəubaiəˈlɔdʒik(əl)] *a.* 微生物学的

A sterile object, in the microbiological sense, is free of living microorganisms.

从微生物学的观点来看,一个无菌的物体就是没有活的微生物的物体。

microbiology [ˌmaikrəubaiˈɔlədʒi] *n.* 微生物学

Medical microbiology includes the study of many types of cells.

医学微生物学包括了对多种细胞类型的研究。

microbiome [ˌmaikrəuˈbaiəum] *n.* 微生物组

Our knowledge of species and functional composition of the human gut microbiome is rapidly increasing.

我们对人体肠道微生物组的种类及其功能组成的了解正在快速地增多。

Human microbiome research has become one of the most exciting fields in biology, prebiotics, and probiotics.

人体微生物组的研究已成为在生物学、益菌生和益生菌研究中最令人振奋的领域之一。

microbiota [ˌmaikrəubaiˈəutə] *n.* 微生物区系

The activity of the microbiota is proportionately much greater in laboratory animals than it is in humans.

实验室动物中微生物区系群落的活力比人体内的成比例地大得多。

Gut microbiota is a potential new territory for drug targeting.

肠道微生物区系是一个潜在的药物研究靶的新领域。

microcapsule [ˌmaikrəuˈkæpsjuːl] *n.* 微囊,微囊剂

Microcapsules have been applied in medicine and pharmacy for a long time.

微囊已经在医学和药学中应用了很长时间。

The microcapsules were obtained by evaporating the solvent at elevated temperatures.

微囊通过高温下溶剂挥发制得。

microcephaly [ˌmaikrəuˈsefəli] *n.* 小头

Physical examination at 2.5 months revealed a large, floppy, retarded infant with mild microcephaly.

两个半月时的体格检查显示为一身子大、皮肤松软、发育迟缓的婴儿,有轻微小头畸形。

microchimerism [ˌmaikrəukaiˈmerizəm] *n.* 微嵌合状态,微嵌合性

Microchimerism refers to a small population of cells or DNA in one individual that derives from another genetically distinct individual.

微嵌合状态是指一个个体内存在一小群细胞或 DNA,后者来源于另一个遗传上不同的个体。

Blood transfusion is a newly recognized cause of microchimerism, it seems to be common in severe traumatic injuries.

输血是近年来被认为引起微嵌合体的原因之一,在严重外伤者似乎很常见。

microcirculation [ˌmaikrəusəːkjuˈleiʃən] *n.* 微循环

Microcirculation refers to the flow of blood in the entire system of finer vessels of the body.

微循环是指身体的微细血管完整系统内的血液流动。

Stasis within the microcirculation has many results.

微循环的郁滞会产生许多后果。

The 7th World Congress for Microcirculation was held at the Sydney Convention Center of Australia.

第 7 届世界微循环会议是在澳大利亚的悉尼会议中心举行的。

microcirculatory [ˌmaikrəuˈsəːkjulətəri] *a.* 微循环的

There may actually be transient intravascular microcirculatory thrombosis.

实际上,还可能有暂时的微循环血管内血栓形成。

microclimate [ˈmaikrəuklaimit] *n.* 微小气候

Microclimate characteristics of the two valleys were complex and diversified.

两河谷局部微小气候均呈现复杂性、多样性特征。

This creates a microclimate which surrounds the building, creating relaxation outdoor spaces.

这样的处理在建筑周围形成了微小气候,创建了适合休闲的室外空间。

microcommunity [ˌmaikrəukəˈmjuːniti] *n.* 微(生物)群落

In the human body, there are many microcommunities which normally benefit the host health.

人体内有许多微生物群落,正常情况下它们对人体健康有益。

In the microbial world microcommunities refer to different populations of microbes normally living in nature and inside the body.

在微生物界,微群落指正常生活在大自然和机体内的不同种类的微生物群体。

microculture [ˌmaikrəuˈkʌltʃə] *n.* 微量(细胞)培养

Harvesting of each microculture is accomplished with an automatic cell harvester, and incorporation of [3H] TdR is determined in a β-scintillation counter.

每一微量(细胞)培养的收获由一个自动细胞收集器来完成,其 [3H] 脱氧胸苷的掺入量则用 β-闪烁计数器来测定。

microcystin [ˌmaikrəuˈsistin] *n.* 微囊藻毒素

Microcystins are extremely stable in water because of their chemical structure.

微囊藻毒素因其化学结构而在水中十分稳定。

Microcystins are cyanobacterial toxins that represent a serious threat to drinking water.

微囊藻毒素是对饮用水有严重威胁的蓝藻毒素。

microdeletion [ˌmaikrəudiˈliːʃən] *n.* 微缺失

Y chromosome microdeletions are specifically associated with severe spermatogenic failure.

Y 染色体微缺失与严重生精功能障碍尤其相关。

Male infertility can be induced by many factors, and extensive studies have strongly indicated that Y chromosome microdeletions are closely related to male reproductive dysfunction.

男性不育原因多样,大量研究表明 Y 染色体微缺失与男性不育的关系密切。

microdissection [ˌmaikrəudiˈsekʃən] *n.* 微切技术

Individual hepatocyte was isolated from cryostat tissue section using laser microdissection technique.

应用激光微切技术从冰冻组织切片上将单个肝细胞分离出来。

microembolus [ˌmaikrəuˈembələs] *n.* 微栓子

This article provides an overview about the current state of technical and clinical aspects of microembolus detection.

本文概括了目前微栓子检测的技术和临床情况。

A 17-year-old adolescent boy with localized osteosarcoma developed a single pulmonary tumor microembolus after surgical resection.

一名 17 岁患有局限性骨肉瘤的青春期男孩在手术切除肿块后发生了单个肺部的肿瘤微栓子。

microemulsion [ˌmaikrəui'mʌlʃən] *n.* 微乳

Microemulsions are becoming more widely used in the cosmetic and chemical industries.

微乳在化妆品和化学工业中的应用越来越广泛。

Various o/w microemulsions were prepared by the spontaneous emulsification method.

通过自发乳化方法可以制备多种水包油型微乳。

microencapsulation [ˌmaikrəuinˌkæpsju'leiʃən] *n.* 微粒包裹技术

The other prospect for new therapies is based on cell microencapsulation.

另一种有发展前景的新治疗方法建立在细胞微粒包裹技术基础上。

microenvironment [ˌmaikrəuin'vaiərənmənt] *n.* 微环境

Moreover, the microenvironment of cancer cell is more complex, so the activin Nrf2 is of great importance for the resistance to cancer cells and growth.

而且,癌细胞的微环境更加复杂,因此激活素 Nrf2 对抗癌细胞的生长有重要意义。

microfilaria [ˌmaikrəufi'lɛəriə] *n.* 微丝蚴

In 1956, microfilaria rate in crowd was 15.13% and main vector was Culex pipiens pallens.

在 1956 年,人群微丝蚴感染率为 15.13%,主要传播媒介为淡色库蚊。

Microfilaria is a term used to describe the juvenile stage of any parasite that lives in the host's circulatory system.

微丝蚴此术语用于描述生活在宿主循环系统的某种寄生虫的幼年期。

microflora [ˌmaikrəu'flɔːrə] *n.* 微生物群落(区系)

We found that this incubation substantially reduced the gram-negative microflora.

我们发现那种孵化方式大量减少了革兰氏阴性菌落。

Mouth is in direct contact with the outside world of the body and therefore abundant with microflora sets there already in childhood.

口腔是我们身体与外界直接接触,因此在儿童时期就有大量的菌落生长于此。

microglia [mai'krɔgliə] *n.* 小神经胶质,小神经胶质细胞

Microglias are the mononuclear phagocytes residenting in the brain and spinal cord.

小胶质细胞是定居于大脑和脊髓中的单核吞噬细胞。

Microglia which acts as police of CNS will be changed by any small changes of CNS.

小胶质细胞是中枢神经系统的“警察”,中枢神经系统的任何微小改变都会引起它的变化。

microgram ['maikrəugræm] *n.* 微克

For this case, clear-cut results are generally seen after a total dose of 5000 micrograms.

对这一病例,通常是在使用总量达 5 000 微克后可以见到明显效果。

micrometer [mai'krɔmitə] *n.* 测微计

Routine training is given in the use of other instruments such as micro cell absorption meter, titrimeter, spectrophotometer, and micrometer syringe burette.

也用其他器材作常规训练,如微量细胞吸收计、滴定计、分光光度计以及微量注射滴定计。

micron ['maikrɔn] *n.* 微米

A millimetre may be divided into a thousand parts, each known as one micron.

一毫米可以分为一千份,每份称为一微米。

micronise ['maikrənaiz] *v.* 微粉化

Micronized progesterone for oral administration became available in the 1980s.

在 20 世纪 80 年代,出现了口服微粉化黄体酮。

Two methods to micronise the HGH were used — spray drying and zinc precipitation.

使用了两种人类生长激素微粉化方法—喷雾干燥法和锌沉淀法。

micronucleus [ˌmaikrəuˈnjuːkliəs] *n.* 小核，微核

Micronuclei are chromosome fragments that are not incorporated into the nucleus at cell division.

微核是指在细胞分裂过程中没有进入细胞核中的染色体片段。

micronutrient [ˌmaikrəuˈnjuːtriənt] *n.* 微量营养素，微量养料

Minerals and vitamins, the so-called micronutrients, have no caloric value but are essential for life.

矿物质和维生素，即常说的微量营养素，虽然没有热能，但也是生命所必需的。

Deficiency of certain dietary substrates (so called micronutrients) may be linked to heightened cancer risk.

饮食中某些物质（即微量营养素）的缺乏可能与患癌症的危险性增加有关。

microorganism [ˌmaikrəuˈɔːgənizm] *n.* 微生物

Louis Pasteur was convinced that microorganisms caused disease.

路易・巴斯德确信微生物可以引起疾病。

micropenis [ˌmaikrəuˈpiːnis] *n.* 小阴茎

This is a case of 19 years male who presented with micropenis.

这是一个表现为小阴茎的 19 岁男性病例。

Presence of micropenis reflects intrauterine hypogonadotrophic hypogonadism.

出现小阴茎可反映子宫内促性腺素分泌不足性腺功能减退。

microRNA (or miRNA) *n.* 微 RNA，微小 RNA

An important class of noncoding RNA genes are known as microRNA.

有一类重要的非编码 RNA 基因被称为微小 RNA。

MiRNAs are short 22-nucleotide-long noncoding RNAs.

微小 RNA 是一类短的、仅 22 个核苷酸长的非编码 RNA。

microsatellite [ˌmaikrəuˈsætəlait] *n.* 微卫星

This class of polymorphisms is often referred to as "microsatellites".

这类多态性常称为微卫星。

microscope [ˈmaikrəskəup] *n.* 显微镜

Microscope is a useful instrument for producing a greatly magnified image of an object, which may be so small as to be invisible to the naked eye.

显微镜是一种可将肉眼看不见的微小物体变成极大的放大图像的有用仪器。

The body consists of millions of cells which can only be seen with the aid of a microscope.

身体是由数以百万计的细胞组成的，而细胞只有借助显微镜才能看到。

With special staining techniques Golgi body can be detected under the optical microscope.

采用特殊的染色技术，在光学显微镜下就能看到高尔基体。

microscopic(al) [ˌmaikrəˈskɔpik(əl)] *a.* 显微镜的；用显微镜可见的；微观的；显微的

Cells are tiny microscopical units.

细胞是显微镜下才能看到的微小单元。

Anything invisible is said to be microscopic.

任何（用肉眼）看不见的东西都被说成是微观的。

The microscopic appearance can best be studied in the highly specialized cells of the convoluted tubule of the kidney.

肾曲小管高度特异性细胞的微观形态可加以充分研究。

microscopically [ˌmaikrəsˈkɔpikəli] *ad.* 用显微镜

Damage to the genetic apparatus more gross than that described above can sometimes be seen microscopically.

比上述更显著的遗传结构的损伤有时在显微镜下可见。

microscopy [maiˈkrɔskəpi] *n.* 显微镜检查（法）

Material resistant to digestion sometimes forms one variety of residual body seen on electron microscopy.
不能消化的物质有时形成电镜下可见到的某一种形式的残留体。
All methods of microscopy have two functions.
所有的显微镜检查法都有两种功能。

microsection [ˌmaikrəuˈsekʃən] *n.* 薄切片，显微切片
Microsections of the tumor are obtained at autopsy.
尸检时可获取此肿瘤的显微切片。
The researcher can perform histochemical stains, immunohistochemical stains, in situ hybridization, and tissue microsection.
研究人员能够做组织化学染色、免疫组织化学染色、原位杂交和组织显微切片。
These tissues underwent the standard histologic processing of fixation, embedding in paraffin, and microsection.
这些组织经过了固定、石蜡包埋和薄切片等标准组织学处理过程。

microsleep [ˌmaicrəˈsliːp] *n.* 微睡眠
The sleep-deprived mind is prone to microsleep.
缺少睡眠使人倾向于意识的多次“短暂休眠”。
Quantifying microsleep is helpful in assessing subjective sleepiness.
量化微睡眠可帮助评估主观的嗜睡度。

microsomal [ˌmaikrəuˈsəuməl] *a.* 微粒体的
Ethanol is not metabolized by the microsomal drug metabolizing system.
乙醇不是通过微粒体药物代谢酶系统而被代谢的。
A key to these complex relationship eventually may be found through a detailed study of the compounds on the microsomal enzymes of different species.
这些复杂关系的关键，可通过详细研究该化合物对不同种属微粒体酶的效应而最终予以阐明。

microsome [ˈmaikrəusəum] *n.* 微粒体
Cytochrome P450 2D6 (CYP2D6) is an important microsome enzyme in liver which metabolizes about 20% ~25% of drugs used in clinic.
细胞色素 P450 2D6(CYP2D6)是一种重要的肝微粒体酶，代谢约 20% ~25% 的临床用药。
Microsomes are a valuable tool for investigating the metabolism of compounds and for examining drug-drug interactions by in vitro-research.
微粒体是体外研究化合物代谢和检测药物与药物相互作用的一种重要工具。

microsphere [ˈmaikrəsfiə(r)] *n.* 微球
Microspheres are small spherical particles, with diameters in the micrometer range (typically 1 μm to 1000μm).
微球体是很小的球形颗粒，其直径为微米级(通常从 1 微米到 1000 微米)。
Cancer microsphere technology is the latest trend in cancer therapy.
癌微球技术是癌症治疗的最新趋势。
Delivering drugs through biodegradable microspheres has numerous advantages compared to conventional delivery systems.
与传统递送系统相比，通过生物可降解性微球来递送药物有着众多优势。

microsurgery [ˌmaikrəˈsəːdʒəri] *n.* 显微外科，显微手术
Microsurgery is basically a technique for expanding the visual horizon of the surgeon.
显微外科主要是一种扩大外科医生视野的技术。
Microsurgery emerges as a result of the advances of precision optical instruments.
由于精密光学仪器的进展产生了显微外科学。
Microsurgery has proved to be not only effective but also less traumatic.

显微手术表明不仅有效，而且造成的创伤也较小。

microtiter [ˌmaikrəu'taitə] *n.* 微量滴定

The intensity of the color was measured by microtiter reader at 405nM, and results were expressed by optical densities(OD).

颜色的强度用微量滴定读数器于 405nM 波长处进行测定，其结果以光密度的读数来表示。

microtubule [ˌmaikrəu'tjuːbjuːl] *n.* 微管

There are two basic types of cytoskeletal elements, termed microtubules and microfilaments.

细胞骨架的成分有两种基本类型，即微管和微丝。

Microtubules may cause a cell to elongate.

微管可使细胞伸长。

microvillus [ˌmaikrəu'viləs]（*pl.* microvilli [maikrəu'vilai]）*n.* 微绒毛，微小突起物

Each microvillus is a very thin, finger-like process.

每根微绒毛都是十分细小的指状突起。

Microvilli are only visible in the electron microscope.

微绒毛只能在电子显微镜下才能看见。

microwave ['maikrəuweiv] *n.* 微波

Microwave ovens have effects on the food heated or cooked and on the people who ingest microwaved foods.

微波炉对加热或烹调的食物以及微波食物食用者都会产生影响。

Microwaves are radio waves with wavelengths ranging from as long as one meter to as short as one millimeter, or equivalently, with frequencies between 300MHz (0.3GHz) and 300GHz.

微波是波长范围从 1 米到 1 毫米，相当于频率在 300 兆赫(0.3 千兆赫)与 300 千兆赫之间的无线电波。

micturition [ˌmiktju'riʃən] *n.* 排尿

Emptying of the bladder through the urethra is called micturition.

通过尿道排空膀胱称为排尿。

The patient has frequent micturition.

病人排尿频繁。

midway ['midwei] *n.* 中途

The uterine fundus reached midway between the symphysis and the umbilicus.

子宫底达到耻骨联合与脐的中间。

This figure stands midway between the incidence in Asia and U. S. A.

这个数字位于亚洲和美国两者发病率之间。

midwife ['midwaif]（*pl.* midwives ['midwaivz]）*n.* 助产士，接生员

Midwives are trained in modern delivery methods.

助产士接受新法接生的训练。

The work of domiciliary midwives is mainly concerned with antenatal and postnatal care, and in some cases conducting deliveries in community hospitals.

家庭助产士主要是做产前和产后护理，有时在社区医院接生。

midwifery ['midwifəri] *n.* 助产学，接生法

Modern midwifery has been extensively adopted in rural areas as well as in cities.

农村地区和城市一样已广泛采用了现代接生法。

migraine ['maigrein] *n.* 偏头痛

This 42-year-old female patient has suffered migraine headache since her ninth year.

这位 42 岁的女病人自 9 岁起患偏头痛至今。

migrate [mai'greit] *v.* 游走，移行

Virgin lymphocytes migrate from the thymus and bone marrow to the secondary lymphoid tissues.

未接触抗原的淋巴细胞从胸腺和骨髓迁移至(外周)第二级淋巴组织。

Monocytes migrate from the venules in inflammatory lesions.

单核细胞从炎症灶的小静脉游出。

Granulocytes and mononuclear phagocytes migrate simultaneously from blood to the site of inflammation.

粒细胞和单核吞噬细胞同时从血流中涌到炎症部位。

The stone may have originated in the kidney and then migrated into the bladder.

结石可能原发于肾脏,然后移动到膀胱内。

The gonococci migrate rapidly up to the vas deferens and soon reach the epididymis, causing gonorrheal epididymitis.

淋球菌会迅速播散到输精管并立即到达附睾,引起淋病性附睾炎。

migration [mai'greiʃən] *n.* 迁移,移动,游走

Radiolabelled cells are used for quantitative measurements of cell migration.

放射性标记的细胞可用于细胞迁移的定量测定。

Internally, traumatic damage may happen during migration of larval stages of hookworm and ascaris.

在体内,创伤性损伤可能发生在钩虫和蛔虫的幼虫游移时期。

migratory ['maigrətəri] *a.* 迁移的,移行的,游走的

Acute rheumatic fever causes migratory arthritis.

急性风湿热引起游走性关节炎。

The migratory larval flukes tunnel into the lung at the periphery.

移行的吸虫幼虫在肺的外周掘隧道以图进入。

mild [maild] *a.* 温和的,轻度的

When you exercise vigorously, waste products which act as mild poisons to the nervous system are formed.

当你剧烈运动时,体内产生废物,这些物质对于神经系统具有轻度的毒性。

mildew ['mildjuː] *n.* 霉

The fungi are frequently apparent as the "mildew" on cloths, food, and leather goods during damp weather.

在天气潮湿(的季节里),真菌常以"发霉"的形式出现在衣服、食物及皮革制品上。

mildly ['maildli] *ad.* 温和地,轻度地

The mildly ill patient will do well on sodium salicylate.

病情轻的患者用水杨酸钠治疗可收到良好效果。

milestone ['mailstəun] *n.* 里程碑,重大事件

Koch's discovery of the bacillus of tuberculosis is a milestone along the long road still lying ahead.

柯霍关于结核杆菌的发现是仍在延续的长征途中的一个里程碑。

Harold Gillie's book "Plastic Surgery of the Face", which was published in 1920, is a milestone in this branch of surgery.

哈鲁德 · 格里于 1920 年出版的《面部矫形外科学》一书是外科该领域的一个里程碑。

miliary ['miliəri] *a.* 粟粒状的

Corticosteroids may be used in miliary tuberculosis.

皮质类固醇可用于粟粒性结核病。

milieu [mi'ljuː] *n.* 周围,环境

None had improved after 2 to 6 weeks of comprehensive milieu therapy.

在 2 至 6 周综合性环境治疗之后,无人出现病情好转。

military ['militəri] *a.* 军事的

Influenza B outbreaks are most common in schools and military camps.

乙型流感最常在学校和军营里暴发。

A history of the geographic areas in which the patient has lived and a travel history should include locations during military service.

病人的居住史和旅行史应包括入伍后的驻地。

milliliter [ˈmiliˌliːtə] *n.* 毫升

The blood cell count falls below 2000 per cubic milliliter.

每毫升血细胞计数降低至 2000 以下。

millimeter [ˈmiliˌmiːtə] *n.* 毫米

Blood pressure is measured in millimeters of mercury.

血压是以毫米汞柱计算的。

They may range in size from a few millimeters to several centimeters.

它们的大小变化可在数毫米至数厘米之间。

mimic [ˈmimik] *v.* 模仿;酷似

You have to mimic the body's environment and then the cells grow normally.

必须善于模拟身体的环境,然后细胞才能正常生长发育。

Intestinal obstruction or peritoneal infection may mimic an attack of colic.

肠梗阻或腹膜炎可有类似绞痛的发作。

The electrocardiogram of this patient mimics myocardial infarction.

此病人的心电图类似心肌梗死。

mineral [ˈminərəl] *a.* 矿物质的,无机的

Numerous studies have examined vitamin and mineral nutriture in the elderly.

许多研究已调查了老年人中维生素和矿物质的营养状况。

The essentials of the diet include: carbohydrates, proteins, fats, vitamins, mineral salts, water and roughage.

饮食的主要部分包括:糖类、蛋白质、脂肪、维生素、无机盐、水和粗糙食物。

n. 矿物质,无机物

It is already known that vast amounts of minerals exist in the ocean.

现已知大量的矿物质存在于海洋中。

This can result directly from not having enough of these minerals in the diet.

这可能直接由于膳食中缺乏此类无机物所致。

mineralization [ˌminərəlaiˈzeiʃən] *n.* 矿质化,盐沉积;钙化作用

Furthermore, the high levels of serum calcium and phosphate increase the rate of bone mineralization.

而且高水平血清钙和磷可加快骨盐沉积的速率。

Appropriate concentrations of calcium and phosphorus in serum are essential for mineralization of osteoid.

血清中钙和磷保持适当的含量对骨样组织的钙化作用是必需的。

minidose [ˈminidəus] *n.* 小剂量

Patients receiving aspirin or minidose heparin have a slightly higher risk of developing wound hematoma.

正在接受阿司匹林或小剂量肝素治疗的病人发生伤口血肿的危险性稍高。

minimal [ˈminiməl] *a.* 最低限度的

The remaining two thirds of the population would show only minimal benefit, and for some very low fat diets would be harmful.

其余三分之二的人群受益极少,而过低脂肪饮食对某些人会有害处。

minimally [ˈminiməli] *ad.* 最低限度地

Aspirin minimally prolongs the bleeding times of normal subjects.

阿司匹林能够最低程度延长正常受试者的出血时间。

minimization [ˌminimaiˈzeiʃən] *n.* 最小化

Minimization of risks also requires a precise determination of what information is necessary.

风险的最小化还要求精确确定什么信息是必需的。

minimize [ˈminimaiz] *v.* 使减到最少,使降到最低

It is very important to minimize the risk of introducing infection into the genital tract during labour.

分娩期间尽量减少将感染带进生殖道的危险是非常重要的。

Adequate caloric intake as carbohydrate or fat helps to minimize protein requirements.

进食含有适当热量的食物如碳水化合物或脂肪,可减少蛋白质的需要量至最低限度。

minimum [ˈminiməm] *n.* 最小(量),最低(量)

This patient will need a minimum of two weeks to get recovered.

这个病人最少需要两周才能复原。

The temperatue of the sick child was at its minimum this morning.

这个病儿的体温今天早晨处于最低状态。

a. 最小的,最低的

Minimum amount of water in the human body is 50%.

在人体中,水至少占50%。

minisatellite [miniˈsætəlait] *n.* 小卫星

Another class of indel polymorphisms results from the insertion, in tandem, of varying numbers (usually in the hundreds to thousands) of copies of a DNA sequence 10 to 100 base pairs in length, known as a minisatellite.

另一类插缺多态性源自长 10 ~ 100 碱基对的 DNA 序列的重复串联插入,重复次数通常为几百 ~ 几千次,称为小卫星。

"Minisatellites" consist of repetitive, generally GC-rich, variant repeats that range in length from 10 to over 100 bp.

"小卫星"包括反复的、通常富含 GC 的不同的重复序列,重复序列长度从 10 到 100 碱基对不等。

minor [ˈmainə] *a.* 较少的,不重要的

Minor amounts of aspiration are frequent during surgery and are apparently well tolerated.

在手术期间少量肺吸入是常见的,而且显然耐受良好。

He got minor injuries.

他受了一些轻伤。

Hypertension is not a minor disease.

高血压不是一种小病。

n. 未成年人;副修科目

A minor is a person under the age of 18.

未成年人是指 18 岁以下的人。

Medical education is his minor in the study of clinical medicine.

医学教育是他学习临床医学过程中的副修项目。

minority [maiˈnɔrəti] *n.* 少数; 少数民族

A minority of about 15 percent lack a red cell protein called the Rh factor and are said to be Rh negative.

大约 15% 的少数人缺乏一种叫做 Rh 因子的红细胞蛋白质,被称为是 Rh 阴性。

A minority of ATP is from breakdown of substances in the absence of oxygen.

少量 ATP 是在无氧条件下的物质分解产生的。

Lack of adequate health insurance is a major problem for many women, especially minority women.

缺乏充足的健康保险对许多妇女来说是一个主要问题,尤其是少数民族妇女。

minute [maiˈnjuːt] *a.* 微小的，精密的

Living things consist of minute structure called cells.

生物由被称为细胞的微小结构组成。

Water containing minute quantities of lead may be hazardous after long-term drinking.

长期饮用含有微量铅的水是危险的。

A magnifying lens is of inestimable value in examing minute lesions.

在检查微小的损害时，用放大镜有无法估量的意义。

miosis [maiˈəusis] *n.* 瞳孔缩小，缩瞳

Pilocarpine causes miosis, reduces intraocular pressure, and is used in wide-angle glaucoma.

毛果芸香碱具有缩瞳和降低眼内压作用，用于开角性青光眼。

miotic [maiˈɔtik] *a.* 缩瞳的 *n.* 缩瞳药

The miotic effects of carbachol and bethanechol are greater than those produced by acetylcholine.

氨甲酰胆碱和氨甲酰甲胆碱的缩瞳作用大于乙酰胆碱。

mirabilite [miˈræbilait] *n.* 芒硝

There was a long history in the distinction between saltpetre and mirabilite in ancient China.

中国古代辨别硝石与芒硝的历史很悠久。

The development process of mining technology for calcium mirabilite mines was introduced in the conference.

在会议上介绍了钙芒硝矿开采技术的发展过程。

miracidium [ˌmairəˈsidiəm] (*pl.* miracidia [mairəˈsidiə]) *n.* 毛蚴，纤毛幼虫

Eggs that are excreted in the urine and feces and that reach fresh water hatch into ciliated miracidia.

虫卵由尿液和粪便中排出，再次进入淡水中，孵化成毛蚴。

Once mature, miracidia have a mean lifespan of 11 to 12 days.

毛蚴一旦成熟，其平均寿命为 11～12 天。

miraculous [miˈrækjuləs] *a.* 奇迹般的，令人惊叹的

For patients and eye doctors alike, these developments have been nothing short of miraculous.

不论对病人还是对眼科医生来说，这些发展简直是个奇迹。

The speed with which sulfa drugs cure many cases of pneumonia seems almost miraculous.

磺胺类药物治疗许多肺炎病例收效之快简直是难以想象的。

miraculously [miˈrækjuləsli] *ad.* 不可思议地，令人惊喜地

After reviewing the data, the doctor informed the patient that his heart was miraculously fit.

医生在查看了检查数据后告知病人说他的心脏出奇地健康。

misattribute [misəˈtribjut] *v.* 错误地归因于

Depressed patients misattribute personal success and failure.

抑郁症患者对个人成功和失败的原因有错误的认识。

miscalculation [ˈmiskælkjuˈleiʃən] *v.* 算错(数量等)

Many pregnancies are considered prolonged due to miscalculation of the expected date of delivery.

许多妊娠由于预产期计算错误被认为是过期。

miscarriage [ˈmisˈkæridʒ] *n.* 流产，小产

Smoking affects women's reproductive health, increasing the risks of earlier menopause, miscarriage and low birthweight babies.

吸烟影响妇女的生殖健康，从而增加了过早停经、流产和娩出低体重儿的危险性。

Scientists have found a way of determining the blood type of unborn babies without taking examples from the child so eliminating the risk of miscarriage.

科学家们发现了一种不需取胎儿血样的方法来检测胎儿血型，从而消除流产的风险。

miscellaneous [ˌmisiˈleinjəs] *a.* 混杂的，多种多样的

In addition, other miscellaneous causes are able to produce nasal airway obstruction.

此外,其他多种病因也可引起鼻道堵塞。

miscode [ˈmiskəud] *v.* 给…错误编码

It is not known whether this type of hereditary agammaglobulinemia is due to an enzyme defect or a structural protein which is miscoded.

这种类型的遗传性无丙种球蛋白血症是由于一种酶的缺陷,还是由于一种结构蛋白的编码错误所致,尚不清楚。

misdiagnose [ˌmisˈdaiəgnəuz] *v.* 误诊

Every year the neurosurgeon see many patients who have been misdiagnosed with Alzheimer's disease.

每年这位神经外科医生都看到许多病人被误诊为阿尔茨海默氏病。

misdiagnosis [ˌmisˌdaiəgˈnəusis] *n.* 误诊

We do not deny that misdiagnosis does occur occasionally.

我们并不否认偶尔确有误诊。

misinterpret [ˌmisinˈtəːprit] *v.* 误解;误译

The patient misinterpreted the doctor's advice.

病人误解了医生的劝告。

Hearing impairment or visual loss may produce confusion and disorientation misinterpreted as dementia.

听觉受损或视觉丧失可引起意识模糊和定向力障碍,从而被误认为痴呆。

mismatch [misˈmætʃ] *n.* 失配,失谐

In the absence of inhalational injury, pulmonary changes following a burn can include decreased compliance and ventilation-perfusion mismatch.

在没有吸入性损伤的情况下,烧伤后的肺部功能的改变有肺顺应性的下降和通气-血流的比例失调。

mispair [ˌmisˈpɛə] *v.* 错配

The covalent binding of chemicals to DNA causes nucleotide mispairing during replication.

共价结合到 DNA 上的化学物能导致复制过程中核苷酸错配。

miss [mis] *v.* 错过; 漏掉;想念

If you miss this chance of operation, you will receive chemotherapy for several courses.

如果你错过了这次手术机会,你就得做好几个疗程的化疗。

Many children who are sick are now missed, because they can have normal IgA and IgG levels, yet they still have poor antibody responses and get the same bacteria and viruses again and again.

现在很多生病的孩子都被忽视了,因为他们的免疫球蛋白 A 和免疫球蛋白 G 的水平正常,但是他们的抗体反应依然很差,从而反复地感染同样的病毒和细菌。

These doctors and nurses had served me very well during my hospitalization, and I would miss them always.

这些医生和护士在我住院期间都做得很好,我会常常想念他们。

missense [ˈmisˌsens] *n.* ,*a.* 错义(的)

The most common missense mutation in the β-globin gene leads to sickle cell anemia in the homozygote.

β-珠蛋白基因中最常见的错义突变可引起纯合子中的镰形细胞贫血症。

mistakenly [misˈteikənli] *ad.* 错误地

Others believe mistakenly that they have insomnia.

其他一些人误认为自己患有失眠症。

mistreat [ˌmisˈtriːt] *v.* 虐待

Some parents with affective disorders have at times mistreated or neglected their children.

有些患感情障碍的父母有时虐待或不重视自己的子女。

misunderstand [ˌmisˌʌndəˈstænd] *v.* 误会，误解

The patient misunderstood the dosage stated in the drug instructions.

这位病人误解了药品说明书中所陈述的用法剂量。

The stomach, so often abused and misunderstood, is a combination storage pouch and churn.

常常被过度使用和误解的胃既是一个贮藏袋，又是一个搅拌器。

misunderstanding [ˌmisˌʌndəˈstændiŋ] *n.* 误会，误解

The doctor has made his intentions very clear, hoping there will be no misunderstanding of them.

医生把他的打算已说得很清楚了，希望不致产生任何误会。

mite [mait] *n.* 螨

Dust mite sensitivity is a common cause of allergic rhinitis.

对尘螨敏感是引起过敏性鼻炎的一个常见原因。

mithramycin [ˌmiθrəˈmaisin] *n.* 光辉霉素，光神霉素

The mechanism of action of mithramycin is similar to that of dactinomycin.

光辉霉素的作用机制与放线菌素 D 类似。

mitigation [ˌmitiˈgeiʃən] *n.* 减轻；缓和

FDA established an enforceable new framework for risk management of drug with known safety concerns, called Risk Evaluation and Mitigation Strategies.

FDA 建立了一个强制性的新框架，用于已知安全问题的药物的风险管理，称作风险评估和风险降低策略。

mitochondrial [ˌmaitəˈkɔndriəl] *a.* 线粒体的

Mitochondrial DNA differs from nuclear DNA.

线粒体 DNA 不同于核 DNA。

Mitochondrial DNA codes for 13 proteins, as well as 2 rRNAs and 22 tRNAs.

线粒体脱氧核糖核酸为 13 种蛋白质、2 种核糖体核糖核酸和 22 种转移核糖核酸编码。

mitochondrion [ˌmaitəˈkɔndriɔn] (*pl.* mitochondria [ˌmaitəˈkɔndriə]) *n.* 线粒体

Mitochondria are distinctively shaped organells.

线粒体是具有特殊形态的细胞器。

Anoxia and many poisons cause reversible osmotic swelling of mitochondria.

缺氧和许多中毒可使线粒体发生可逆性渗透性肿胀。

mitogen [ˈmaitədʒən] *n.* 有丝分裂原，分裂素，促细胞分裂剂

Mitogens such as platelet-derived growth factor may result in proliferation of smooth muscle cells.

促细胞分裂剂如血小板衍生的生长因子可引起平滑肌细胞增殖。

These mitogens, such as hepatocyte growth factors (HGF), are especially important in tissue repair.

这些有丝分裂原，如肝细胞生长因子，对组织修复来说特别重要。

mitomycin [ˌmaitəuˈmaisin] *n.* 丝裂霉素

Mitomycin C may cause cell clumping, which may interfere with accurate quantification and dispensing, or may decrease the yield of treated cells.

丝裂霉素 C 可引起细胞结块而干扰准确的定量和调剂，或者降低被处理细胞的产生率。

mitosis [maiˈtəusis] (*pl.* mitoses [maiˈtəusiːz]) *n.* (间接)核分裂，有丝分裂

A tumor cell undergoes mitosis to become two.

一个肿瘤细胞通过核分裂变成两个。

When a complete set of new chromosomes has been formed, the cell then divides into new daughter cells which is the process of cell mitosis.

当整套新的染色体形成后，细胞就分裂成为两个新的子细胞，此过程称为细胞有丝分裂。

mitotic [maiˈtɔtik] *a.* 核分裂的，有丝分裂的

There are indications that growth controlling or regulatory mechanisms influence mitotic activity of neoplastic cells.

有迹象表明,生长的控制或调节机制可影响肿瘤细胞核分裂。

There is no nuclear membrane or mitotic apparatus in procaryotic cells.

原核生物细胞无核膜或有丝分裂器。

mitral [ˈmaitrəl] *a.* 二尖瓣的

Thirty per cent of patients with mitral stenosis give no history of rheumatic fever.

约30%二尖瓣狭窄的患者无风湿热病史。

With active myocarditis, the heart dilates and there is relative mitral insufficiency and regurgitation.

活动性心肌炎时心脏会扩大,二尖瓣会相对(关闭)不全,还有返流现象。

mix [miks] *v.* 混合,配制

You should mix these ingredients together.

你应当将这些成分进行混合。

The chemist mixed up some medicine for me.

药剂师给我配制了一些药。

mixture [ˈmikstʃə] *n.* 合剂,混合物

Air is a mixture of many kinds of gases.

空气是许多气体的一种混合物。

The medicine for stopping coughing is usually in the dosage form of mixture.

止咳药通常采用合剂的剂型。

The mixture of gastric juice and food is known as chyme.

胃液和食物的混合物叫做食糜。

mobile [ˈməubail] *a.* 运动的,活动的

The emergency mobile resuscitation equipment is now available.

移动式急救复苏设备现在可供使用。

mobility [məuˈbiliti] *n.* 可动性,移动性

The joint mobility is limited with severe hydrops.

因为严重积水,关节活动能力受限。

Mobility performance and capacity as well as the effects of mobility on health status should be assessed routinely in all elderly patients.

应常规性地评估所有老年病人的活动状况和能力以及活动对健康状态的影响。

mobilization [ˌməubilaiˈzeiʃən] *n.* 活动

Decubitus ulcers and mobilization of calcium stores with formation of renal calculi may also be seen.

褥疮性溃疡和伴随肾结石形成的钙堆积活动均可见到。

mobilize [ˈməubilaiz] *v.* 动员;使活动

When a person becomes infected with disease germs, the body mobilizes all kinds of defensive functions to combat them.

当一个人受到致病菌感染时,身体则动员所有的防御功能与细菌抗争。

The physiological stress of pregnancy can mobilize lead from maternal bone and the free lead can cross the placental barrier.

妊娠的生理应激能够将铅由母体的骨骼中动员出来,而游离的铅可能穿过胎盘屏障。

modality [məuˈdæliti] *n.* 方式;用药程式

The choice of therapeutic modality (or modalities) will depend on the specific circumstances of each case.

治疗方式的选择以每个病例特殊情况为依据。

All modalities of treatment have not changed the prognosis of neonatal hepatitis.

所有的治疗方法都未曾改变新生儿肝炎的预后。

model [ˈmɔdəl] *n.* 模型

In a logistic regression model, the association between exposure and outcome is measured by using the odds ratio (OR).
在罗吉斯回归模型中，暴露与结局的关联程度通过比值比(OR)来衡量。
Therefore, these factors were included in the model.
因此，这些因素都包括进了模型。

modeling [ˈmɔdliŋ] *n.* 模仿法，模拟法
Modeling is the use of statistical analysis, computer analysis, or model organisms to predict outcomes of research.
模拟法是采用统计分析、计算机分析或模式生物来预测研究成果的方法。

modem [ˈməudem] *n.* 调制解调器
Does your computer have a modem?
你的电脑有调制解调器吗？
Typically, the modem is connected to one of the serial ports on the computer.
通常，调制解调器连接到计算机上的其中一个串行端口。

moderate [ˈmɔdərit] *a.* 中等的；适度的；温和的
At the time of the accident, the bus was driving at a moderate speed.
事故发生时，汽车正以中速行驶。
Renal biopsy is often necessary in moderate to severe cases of renal disease.
中度到重度肾病疾患常需做肾活检。
v. [ˈmɔdərət] 使和缓；减轻；节制
These newly built hospitals will moderate the increasing demands for better health care.
这些新建的医院将可缓和对更好医疗日益增长的需求。
People should eat a balanced and varied diet and moderate their consumption of fried and fatty foods.
人们应吃平衡和多样化的饮食，节制对煎炸和油腻食物的食用。

moderately [ˈmɔdəritli] *ad.* 中等，适度地
Children with moderately severe rickets are late in standing and walking.
患有中度佝偻病的儿童站立和行走往往推迟。
The examination for professional title of doctors this year was moderately difficult.
今年的医师职称考试有点难。

modification [ˌmɔdifiˈkeiʃən] *n.* 更改，改变；缓和
Modification of the structure of acetylcholine alters its pharmacologic properties dramatically.
乙酰胆碱结构的改变可使该药的药理学特性发生巨大变化。
A few simple modifications to this plan would greatly improve it.
这计划作几处简单的修改，就会大有改善。
Asepsis is absolute; there is no compromise or modification.
无菌是绝对的，不存在任何折中或权宜之计。

modifier [ˈmɔdifaiə] *n.* 修饰基因
Modifier polymorphisms are important for the de novo risk of some events and for the risk of drug-induced events.
修饰基因多态性对某些事件的初发风险和药物诱发事件的风险都很重要。

modify [ˈmɔdifai] *v.* 缓和；减轻；修改
The modified procedure is not simpler than the original one.
改良的方法并不比原来简单。
Other pharmacologic agents such as chlorpromazine also modify nucleic acid synthesis.
其他药物如氯丙嗪也可改变核酸的合成。
The general manage scheme for premature rupture of membranes is modified depending on the gestational age of the patient.

胎膜早破一般处理方案根据患者的孕龄而有所变化。

There is no convincing evidence that administration of corticosteroids modifies the duration of the acute disease.

使用皮质类固醇类药物影响急性患者的病期,是没有确实证据的。

modulate [ˈmɔdjuleit] *v.* 调节

Taken together, our results suggest that RTN3 could bind with Bcl-2 and mediate its accumulation in mitochondria, which modulate the anti-apoptotic activity of Bcl-2.

总之,我们的结果表明 RTN3 能与 Bcl-2 结合,介导其在线粒体的聚积,从而调节 Bcl-2 的抗凋亡活性。

modulation [ˌmɔdjuˈleiʃən] *n.* 调变,调幅,调节,调整,调制

Immune modulation refers to medical intervention to alter the body's immune response when it is not performing properly.

免疫调节就是指当机体免疫反应不能正常进行时通过医学干预来改变机体的免疫反应。

Immune modulation is the deliberate attempt to change the course of an immune response.

免疫调节是改变免疫应答过程的精细步骤。

modulator [ˈmɔdjuˌleitə] *n.* 调节者,调节剂

This implications estrogens as modulators of gene transcription.

这意味着雌激素是基因转录的调节者。

Immune modulators are the substances that control the expression of the immune response.

免疫调节剂是控制免疫反应表达的物质。

moiety [ˈmɔiəti] *n.* 组成部分,成分

The glycerin moiety of fat can be turned into sugar.

脂肪的甘油分子能转化成糖。

It is also important to note that cell walls contain several unique chemical moieties.

还应着重指出细胞壁含有一些独特的化学成分。

moist [mɔist] *a.* 湿性的

Rhonchi or scattered moist rales may be present as a manifestation of bronchitis.

干啰音或散在湿性啰音的出现是支气管炎的症候。

Dry heat is not such a powerful bactericidal agent as moist heat owing to its lower power of penetration.

由于干热的穿透力较低,所以它不是一种像湿热那样的有效的杀菌方法。

moisten [ˈmɔisn] *v.* 弄湿,变潮湿

You must keep this medicine from being moistened.

你不要让这药受潮。

The nasal epithelial cells produce a secretion which also traps particles and moistens the air.

鼻上皮细胞产生一种可以黏附微粒和使空气湿润的分泌物。

moisture [ˈmɔistʃə(r)] *n.* 湿气,潮湿

Humidity is a measure of moisture in the atmosphere.

湿度是测量大气中湿气含量的单位。

Bacteria live in an environment of moisture and food materials.

细菌生长在潮湿和有营养物的环境里。

molar [ˈməulə] *n.* 磨牙

Only by obtaining material from the back molars, could Leeuwenhoek satisfy himself of the vitality of his animalcules.

只有从后磨牙取牙垢时,列文赫克才对其口腔微生物的活力感到满意。

molarity [məuˈlæriti] *n.* 摩尔浓度

The molarity of ethanol droplet test is a popular rapid method for assessing soil water repellency under field and laboratory conditions.

乙醇微滴摩尔浓度测试是在田野和实验室条件下评价土壤斥水性的常用快速方法。

The effect of mobile phase buffer molarity on the sensitivity of fluorescence detection and resolution of porphyrin isomers was investigated.

研究了流动相缓冲液摩尔浓度对卟啉同分异构体荧光检测敏感性和分辨率的影响。

mold [məuld] *n.* 霉,霉菌

Flemming found that there were no bacteria in the area close to the mold.

弗莱明发现在霉的邻近部位无细菌。

Most antibacterial agents are derived from molds.

大多数抗菌药是从霉菌分离出来的。

mole [məul] *n.* 胎块;痣

Abortion of cystic mole usually occurs at about five months' gestation or earlier.

葡萄胎流产通常发生在妊娠 5 个月左右或更早。

Invasive moles can develop both before and after the treatment by curettage.

侵蚀性葡萄胎可能发生于诊刮前后。

molecular [mə'lekjulə] *a.* 分子的

Molecular biology is a discipline of the study of the molecules that are associated with living organisms, especially proteins and nucleic acid.

分子生物学是一门研究与活的生物体分子特别是蛋白和核酸有关的学科。

Because of their high molecular weight and tendency to form colloidal solutions, proteins do not readily pass through body membranes.

由于蛋白质分子量大且倾向于形成胶体溶液,故不易通过机体内的膜。

A fuller understanding of cardiac function and dysfunction will ultimately require studies at the cellular, molecular, and genetic levels.

较深入的了解心脏功能及功能障碍最终需要在细胞、分子和遗传水平上进行研究。

molecule ['mɔlikjuːl] *n.* 分子,微小颗粒

Protein molecules are too large to pass through capillary walls.

蛋白质分子过大,以至于不能通过毛细血管壁。

In gene splicing, scientists use special enzymes to break a DNA molecule apart at specific places between genes.

在基因拼接过程中,科学家们运用特定的酶在基因之间的特定位点切断 DNA 分子。

molluscacide [mɔ'lʌskəsaid] *n.* 灭螺剂,软体动物杀灭剂

The most active molluscacide is N-trityl-morpholine, which is used at 0.1 to 0.5 ppm/hr.

最速效的灭螺剂是三苯甲基吗啡,应用浓度为每小时 0.1 ~ 0.5ppm。

monilia [mə'niliə] *n.* 念珠菌

Rarely, the patient may develop a secondary infection with monilia or bacteria.

在很少情况下,患者可能发生继发性念珠菌或细菌感染。

Monilia is the common name for a type of yeast-like fungus that is part of the body's normal flora and commonly found in the mouth, skin, intestinal tract and vagina.

念珠菌是一种酵母样真菌的常用名,它是身体正常菌群的一部分,常见于口腔、皮肤、肠道和阴道。

monitor ['mɔnitə] *v.* 监视,监测,监控

As for these patients, the initial response to therapy should be closely monitored.

对于这些病人,应密切监测治疗初期的反应。

All infants of the diabetic mothers should have hourly blood sugar monitoring during the first 4-6 hours after birth.

所有糖尿病母亲的婴儿,应在出生后 4 ~ 6 小时内每小时进行一次血糖监测。

n. [计算机] 显示器,监视器

The printer is the most commonly used output device after the monitor.

打印机是除显示器外最常用的输出设备。

Otherwise the video can be connected through the VCR first and then out to the monitor.

视频也可以先通过 VCR 连接,然后输出到监视器上。

monkshood [ˈmʌŋkshud] *n.* 附子;乌头

First aid and nursing care for a patient with intoxication of kusnezoff monkshood root are important.

附子中毒的急救和护理很重要。

Extract of monkshood root could increase content of endotoxin in rat.

附子提取物可以提高大鼠的内毒素。

monoamine [ˌmɔnəuəˈmiːn] *n.* 一元胺,单胺

These drugs seem to increase the efficiency of monoamine neurotransmitter in the brain.

这些药物看来可增加大脑中的单胺神经递质的效力。

Physical examination of the patient with a monoamine oxidase inhibitor overdose is variable and often normal initially.

服用单胺氧化酶抑制剂过量的病人,其体检结果不一而且往往开始都是正常的。

monoclonal [ˌmɔnəuˈkləunəl] *a.* 单克隆的

Monoclonal Abs(mAbs)can be made in large quantities and against virtually every Ag.

单克隆抗体能被大量的制造并有效地对抗每一种抗原.

The use of monoclonal antibodies has greatly increased the specificity for many such antigenic probes.

单克隆抗体的应用大大增加了这类抗原探针的特异性。

monocular [məˈnɔkjulə] *a.* 单眼的

Ordinarily any defect in vision that is monocular is attributable to a lesion in the eye, retina, or optic nerve on that side.

一般而言,单眼的任何视力缺损均归因于该侧眼睛、视网膜或视神经的病变。

monocyte [ˈmɔnəsait] *n.* 单核细胞

Chronic inflammations consist of lymphocytes, monocytes, and plasma cells.

慢性炎症中有淋巴细胞、单核细胞和浆细胞。

On entering the tissues, the monocytes swell to extremely large size and are then called macrophages.

单核细胞进入组织后即膨胀得很大,此时称为巨噬细胞。

monoethanolamine [ˈmɔnəuˌeθənəˈlæmiːn] *n.* 乙醇胺,单乙醇胺

Monoethanolamine is a compound that can be readily derived from cell membranes.

乙醇胺是一种易从细胞膜中分离得到的化合物。

Capillary zone electrophoresis in the presence of monoethanolamine was used in a micropreparative mode.

含乙醇胺的毛细管区带电泳被用于微量制备模式。

monofunctional [ˌmɔnəuˈfʌŋkʃənəl] *a.* 单功能的

The monofunctional methylating agents (procarbazine, temozolomide) have greater capacity for mutagenesis and carcinogenesis.

单功能甲基化药物(甲基苄肼、替莫唑胺)有更强致突变和致癌的能力。

monolayer [ˈmɔnəˌleiə] *n.* 单层,单分子层

The lipid component of the cell membrane cannot in fact be a monolayer.

事实上,细胞膜的脂质成分不可能是单分子层。

monomer [ˈmɔnəmə] *n.* 单体,单分子物

The monomers that make up proteins are the 20 amino acids.

组成蛋白质的单体是 20 种氨基酸。

Fimbriae originate in the cytoplasmic membrane and are composed of self-aggregating protein

monomers.
菌毛来源于胞浆膜，是由自凝蛋白单体构成的。

monomeric [ˌmɔnəˈmerik] *a.* 单体的
Nucleotides are the monomeric units of the nucleic acid macromolecule.
核苷酸是核酸大分子的单体单元。

mononuclear [ˌmɔnəˈnjuːkliə] *a.* 单核的
Granulocytes and mononuclear phagocytes migrate simultaneously from blood to the site of inflammation.
粒细胞和单核吞噬细胞同时从血液中涌到炎症部位。
The parenchyma adjacent to involved bronchi may be necrotic and there is a mononuclear infiltrate.
与受累支气管毗邻的肺实质可能有坏死，且有单核浸润。

mononucleosis [ˌmɔnəˌnjuːkliˈəusis] *n.* 单核细胞增多症
Hepatitis, pneumonia and mononucleosis are also caused by viruses.
肝炎、肺炎和单核细胞增多症也是由病毒引起的。
Infectious mononucleosis is usually mild, terminating spontaneously after a few weeks.
传染性单核细胞增多症通常病情轻，数周后自然消失。

monoplegia [ˌmɔnəuˈpliːdʒiə] *n.* 单瘫
Lower motor neuron monoplegia may result from purely motor conditions involving the anterior horn cells.
单纯的包括前角细胞在内的运动神经疾病可引起下运动神经元单瘫。

monosaccharide [ˌmɔnəuˈsækəraid] *n.* 单糖
Carbohydrates are broken down to monosaccharides and absorbed as such into the portal blood stream.
碳水化合物分解成单糖并以这种形式被吸收进门脉血流。

monosodium [ˈmɔnəusəudium] *n.* 谷氨酸钠，味精
Monosodium glutamate, a salt of glutamic acid, is commonly used as flavor enhancer in China and Japan.
味精是一种在中国和日本广泛用于增加鲜味的谷氨酸盐。
Monosodium glutamate is the inducer of oxidative stress.
味精是氧化应激反应的诱导剂。

monosomy [ˌmɔnəˈsəumi] *n.* 单体性
Monosomy for any autosome is lethal early in embryogenesis.
任何常染色体单体性在胚胎形成早期是致命的。

monoxide [mɔˈnɔksaid] *n.* 一氧化物
Carbon monoxide destroys the oxygen-carrying ability of the blood if you breathe it.
如果人吸入一氧化碳，血液携带氧的功能就受到破坏。
Just a small amount of carbon monoxide will kill a person.
只要少量的一氧化碳就能使人致命。

mood [muːd] *n.* 心情，情绪
All of us have been in a "bad mood" or have had the "blues" at one time or another.
我们大家时而都有心情不好或闷闷不乐的情况。
Some patients find it difficult to describe their mood in terms of anxiety or depression.
一些病人认为他们的情绪很难用焦虑或抑郁来表达。

morbid [ˈmɔːbid] *a.* 疾病的，病态的
Morbid obesity also produces mechanical and physical stresses that predispose to hypertension.
病态的肥胖也可增加身体的力学和运动负担，易导致高血压。

morbidity [mɔːˈbiditi] *n.* 发病率；病态

Coronary arteriography has a small morbidity and mortality.
冠状动脉造影引起的并发症及死亡率甚小。
The reasons for this higher morbidity from all causes are not fully understood.
对于各种原因造成的这种较高的发病率，人们还不能完全理解其缘由。
The morbidity rate is the number of cases of a disease found to occur in a stated number of the population, usually given as cases per 100,000 or per million.
患病率是在规定的人口数中所发现的某病病例数，通常以每十万人口或百万人口中的患病人数表示。

morgue [mɔːg] *n.* 陈尸所，停尸间
The liver cancer patient who died just 10 minutes ago has been sent to the morgue of the hospital.
10 分钟前死亡的那位肝癌患者已被送往医院的停尸间。

Morinda [ˈmɔːrində] *n.* 巴戟天属
Different kinds of life elements have been found in Morinda officinalis.
巴戟天含有多种生命元素。
We study the effect of various organic fertilizers on the growth and active constituents of Morinda officinalis.
我们考察各种有机肥料对巴戟天的生长和有效成分的影响。

morphea [mɔːˈfiə] *n.* 硬斑病
Localized scleroderma, a term which includes morphea and linear scleroderma, involves the skin exclusively.
局部性硬皮病，包括硬斑病和线形硬皮病，仅限于皮肤受累。

morphine [ˈmɔːfiːn] *n.* 吗啡
The physician found it necessary to give the patient morphine by injection.
内科医生认为有必要给病人注射吗啡。
Morphine is mainly used to relieve pain for certain patients in time of need.
吗啡主要是在某些病人需要时用来止痛。

morphogenesis [ˌmɔːfəuˈdʒenisis] *n.* 形态发生，形态建成
Morphogenesis depends on cell locomotion and change in shape.
形态建成依赖于细胞的运动和形状改变。

morphologic [ˌmɔːfəˈlɔdʒik] *a.* 形态学的
Not both diseases are defined in morphologic terms.
两种疾病不都是根据形态学来下定义的。
The tumors were considered adenoma on morphologic grounds.
根据形态学考虑，这些肿瘤为腺瘤。

morphologically [ˌmɔːfəˈlɔdʒikəli] *ad.* 形态学上
Morphologically, protozoa exibit a wide variety of shapes and sizes.
在形态学上，原虫的形态与大小是多种多样的。

morphology [mɔːˈfɔlədʒi] *n.* 形态学
These cells are irregular in morphology.
这些细胞在形态上不规则。

mortality [mɔːˈtæliti] *n.* 死亡率
Acute toxic dilatation of the colon with bleeding and perforation still has a high mortality.
伴有出血和穿孔的急性中毒性结肠扩张，死亡率仍很高。
Overall mortality rates for postoperative pneumonia vary from 20-40%.
手术后肺炎总死亡率为 20% ~40%。

morula [ˈmɔːr(j)ulə] *n.* 桑葚胚
The morula is produced by embryonic cleavage, the rapid division of the zygote.

桑葚胚由胚胎卵裂，即受精卵快速分裂形成。

The studies were performed on the cryopreservation of mouse morula by vitrification, embryo splitting and embryo transfer.

对小鼠桑椹胚的玻璃化冷冻保存、胚胎分割及胚胎移植技术进行了系统的研究。

mosaic [məˈzeiik] *a.* 镶嵌的，马赛克式的

If the fluid mosaic model is correct, it must explain the three types of movement across membranes.

假如液体镶嵌模型是正确的，就必然能够解释通过细胞膜的三种类型的跨膜运动。

mosaicism [məuˈzeiisizəm] *n.* 镶嵌性，嵌合现象

Mosaicism is the presence of two or more cell lines with different karyotypes in a single individual.

镶嵌性是指在一个个体内存在由不同核型组成的两种或两种以上细胞系的状态。

Mosaicism for trisomy 21 occurs in some patients.

有些病人出现 21 三体性嵌合现象。

motif [məuˈtiːf] *n.* 基序；主旨，（文学，绘画）作品的主题；基本花纹

Study of protein motifs may reveal answers to many important biological questions.

对蛋白质基序的研究可揭示许多生物学上重大问题的答案。

The motif of the picture is about peace.

这幅画的主题是和平.

There are four helix-loop-helix motifs in calmodulin, two at each end of the molecule, which has a dumbbell shape.

钙调蛋白有四个螺旋-环-螺旋基本结构，分子的两个末端各 2 个，呈哑铃状。

motile [ˈməutail] *a.* 有自动力的，能动的

A bacterium is considered motile only if it seems to be moving in a definite direction.

只有细菌向一定方向运动时，才能认为该菌有自动力。

motilin [ˈməutilin] *n.* 胃动素；蠕动素

The changes of concentration of serum motilin and gastrin in critical newborn were observed.

对危重病新生儿的血清胃动素和胃泌素浓度的变化进行了观察。

They have observed the changes of gastrin content, the motilin content and the intestinal propulsion caused by the three prescriptions.

他们观察了三组药物对血浆胃动素、胃泌素含量及小肠推进的影响。

motility [məuˈtiliti] *n.* 活动性，运动力

Some algae have a plant's characteristic photosynthetic capabilities combined with an animal's motility.

有些藻类既具有植物特有的光合作用能力，也具有动物的活动性。

The motility of the fallopian tube is also under the control of estrogen.

输卵管的能动性也在雌激素控制下。

motion [ˈməuʃn] *n.* 运动

It is this molecular motion that we call heat.

就是这种分子运动我们称之为热。

Kinetic energy is the energy arising from motion.

动能就是由于运动而产生的能量。

motor [ˈməutə] *a.* 运动的

The most common form of adult motor neuron disease is amyotrophic lateral sclerosis.

成人运动神经疾病最常见的为肌萎缩性侧束硬化症。

The most severe injury to the spinal cord, producing absence of all motor and sensory function below the injury level, is a complete spinal cord injury.

脊柱最严重的损伤是完全性脊柱损伤，它会引起损伤部位以下所有的运动和感觉功能丧失。

mottling [ˈmɔtliŋ] *n.* 斑点，斑纹

One reason for mottling is the color of the drug which differs from that of the tablet excipient.
药物形成斑点的一个原因是药的颜色与片剂赋形剂颜色不同。
Mottling was reduced initially by increasing granule strength.
斑点减少最初是通过增加颗粒强度实现的。

mount [maunt] *v.* 增长，上升
Evidence is mounting which supports a relationship between maternal diabetes and an increased incidence of congenital malformations.
支持母亲糖尿病和先天畸形发生之间相关的证据正在增多。
n. 载(玻)片
Wet mounts of bacteria are usually prepared by placing a drop of a liquid culture on a glass slide and covering it with a cover slip.
细菌湿片的制成通常是在玻片上滴一滴细菌的液体培养液，再盖上盖玻片。

mourning [ˈmɔːniŋ] *n.* 悲伤，哀悼
Mourning is a psychological process set in motion by loss of a loved object.
悲伤是一种因爱的对象丧失而引起的心理过程。

mouse [maus] *n.* 【电脑】鼠标器，鼠标
I prefer a mouse over a touchpad.
相较于触摸板，我更喜欢用鼠标。
A trackball is essentially an upside-down mouse.
轨迹球鼠标实际就是倒置的普通鼠标。

moxibustion [ˌmɔksiˈbʌstʃən] *n.* 灸法，艾灸，艾灸疗法
The science of acupuncture and moxibustion is an important part of traditional Chinese medicine.
针灸学是中医学的一个重要组成部分。
Moxibustion is a type of Chinese medicine which involves burning a herb close to the skin.
艾灸是一种中医方式，它是用艾草靠近皮肤处燃烧来进行治疗。
Moxibustion has been used to correct a breech presentation.
艾灸已被用来纠正臀先露。

mucilage [ˈmjuːsilidʒ] *n.* 胶浆剂；黏液
Mucilages are most commonly used as adjuvant in pharmaceutical preparations.
胶浆剂是药物制剂中最常用的辅料。
Mucilage and gums have been known since ancient times for their medicinal uses.
人们自古代就已经知道黏液和树胶可作药用。

mucin [ˈmjuːsin] *n.* 黏蛋白
The microsections revealed a mucin negative cancer.
显微切片证实这是一个黏蛋白阴性癌。

mucinous [ˈmjuːsinəs] *a.* 黏蛋白(状)的
About 10 per cent of ovarian cancer is classified as mucinous.
约10%的卵巢癌归入黏液性。

mucocele [ˈmjuːkəsiːl] *n.* 黏液囊肿
Mucoceles are the most common type of inflammatory salivary gland lesion.
黏液囊肿是涎腺炎症性病变最常见的类型。
Mucoceles demonstrate a cystlike space that is lined by inflammatory granulation tissue or by fibrous connective tissue.
黏液囊肿表现为囊样的腔隙，囊壁为炎性肉芽组织或纤维结缔组织。

mucociliary [ˌmjuːkəuˈsiliəri] *a.* 黏膜纤毛的
The mucociliary transport mechanism is damaged by endotracheal intubation.
气管内置管使黏膜纤毛转运机制受损。

mucocutaneous [ˌmjuːkəukjuˈteinjəs] *a.* 黏膜皮肤的

For mucocutaneous infections acyclovir has been the mainstay of therapy.
阿昔洛韦是治疗黏膜皮肤感染的主要药物。
Patients usually present with mucocutaneous lesions or lymph node involvement.
病人常有皮肤黏膜损害或淋巴结受累。

mucoid [ˈmjuːkɔid] *a.* 黏液样的
Of more specific symptoms, the most common is cough often with mucoid sputum.
较特异的症状以咳嗽最为常见，常咯黏痰。
There is a heavy mucoid discharge coming from the nose.
鼻部有稠的黏液样分泌物。

mucolytic [ˌmjuːkəuˈlitik] *a.* 黏液溶解的
Bronchodilators and mucolytic agents given by nebulizer may help in patients with severe chronic obstructive pulmonary disease.
经雾化器给予支气管扩张剂和黏液溶解剂，对伴有严重慢性阻塞性肺部疾患的病人是有帮助的。

mucopolysaccharide [ˌmjuːkəuˌpɔliˈsækəraid] *n.* 黏多糖；黏多糖体
The renal tubular cells appear foamy because of the accumulation of neutral fats and mucopolysaccharides.
因为中性脂肪和黏多糖堆积，肾小管细胞呈泡沫样。
Mucopolysaccharides are gelatinous, slimy, or sticky molecules composed of units or that are related to hexoses.
黏多糖是一种胶质黏稠的分子，由单体分子或与己糖有关的分子构成。

mucopolysaccharidosis [ˌmjuːkəupɔliˌsækəraiˈdəusiːs] (*pl.* -ses) *n.* 黏多糖病
Mucopolysaccharidoses are inheritable disorders caused by a deficiency of lysosomal enzymes needed for the degradation of glycosaminoglycans.
黏多糖病是由于降解黏多糖的溶酶体酶缺乏所致的遗传性疾病。
Mucopolysaccharidosis I is a severe progressive disorder.
I 型黏多糖病是一种严重的进行性疾病。

mucormycosis [ˌmjuːkəmaiˈkəusis] *n.* 毛霉菌病
Pulmonary mucormycosis is a progressive severe pneumonia, accompanied by high fever and toxicity.
肺毛霉菌病是一种进行性的重症肺炎，伴有高热和中毒症状。

mucosa [mjuˈkəusə] *n.* 黏膜
A small area of gastric or duodenal mucosa is injured.
胃或十二指肠一小片区域的黏膜受到损伤。

mucosal [ˌmjuːkəusəl] *a.* 黏膜的
Laryngeal lesions include mucosal hyperemia and thickening, nodules, and ulcerations.
喉部的病变包括黏膜充血及增厚、出现结节和溃疡。
Dysentery usually refers to an inflammation of the mucosal lining, although deeper tissue also may be affected.
痢疾通常指肠黏膜层发炎，虽然有时也可涉及深层组织。

mucositis [ˌmjuːkəuˈsaitis] *n.* 黏膜炎
The acute toxicities of the conditioning regimen for bone marrow transplantation include severe mucositis of the mouth and, at times, of the esophagus.
骨髓移植的治疗方案引起的急性毒性反应为严重的口腔黏膜炎，有时为食管黏膜炎。

mucous [ˈmjuːkəs] *a.* 黏液的
Epithelial membranes include mucous membranes and serous membranes.
上皮膜包括黏膜和浆膜。

mucus [ˈmjuːkəs] *n.* 黏液

Mucus is a conjugated protein.
黏液是一种结合蛋白。
Most bacteria are well protected from mouthwash under thick layers of mucus.
大多数细菌由于受到厚厚的黏液层的保护而不被漱口剂冲走。
When you have a cold, however, your nasal passages are clogged with mucus.
然而，当你伤风时，鼻腔通道被黏液堵塞。

multiallelism [ˌmʌltiˈælelizəm] *n.* 复等位基因现象，复等位基因性
The A, B and O alleles at this locus are a classic example of multiallelism.
该基因座上的 A、B 和 O 等位基因是复等位基因的典型例子。
Microsatellite markers generate a large number of alleles, which is known as multiallelism.
微卫星标记可以产生大量等位基因，就是所谓的复等位基因现象。

multidetector [ˌmʌltidiˈtektə] *a.* 多探测器的
Multislice CT and multidetector CT actually mean the same machine.
多层 CT 和多排 CT 实际上指的是同一种机器。

multidomain [ˌmʌltidəuˈmein] *n.* 多域
The domains of a multidomain protein are often interconnected by a segment of the polypeptide chain lacking regular secondary structure.
多域蛋白质的域常由缺乏规则二级结构的多肽链的节段相互连接。

multidrug [ˈmʌltiˌdrʌg] *n.* 多药
The multidrug resistance associated protein, MRP2, has a large number of nonsynonymous cSNPs.
多药耐受相关蛋白(MRP2)有大量非同义的 cSNPs(基因编码区单核苷酸多态性)。

multifactor [ˈmʌltiˌfæktə] *a.* 多因子的，多种因素的
Crohn's disease is a complex multifactor disease.
克罗恩病是一种复杂的多因子疾病。
The interactions between MMR genes were evaluated using multifactor approach.
可用多种因素的方法评估麻腮风混合疫苗基因之间的相互作用。
n. 复因子，多种因素
Cervical spondylotic myelopathy is a serious degenerative disease of cervical spine, of which the mechanism results from multifactor.
脊髓型颈椎病是一种严重的退行性疾病，其发生机制是多种因素作用的结果。

multifactorial [ˌmʌltifækˈtɔːriəl] *a.* 多因子的，多因素的
We think of coronary artery disease as having multifactorial etiology.
我们认为冠状动脉疾病具有多因素病因。
Since the development of infections is multifactorial, designing control measures is complex.
因为传染的发生受多种因素影响，故策划控制措施也很复杂。

multifold [ˈmʌltifəuld] *a.* 多种的；多倍的
Micro-electromechanical System is an amalgamation of multifold subjects and it can find broad applications in various fields.
微电子机械系统(MEMS)是多种学科的交叉融合，应用领域极为广泛。
The integrated mechanism of lung ischemia reperfusion injury is multifold.
肺部缺血再灌注损伤的整体机制是多方面的。

multiformat [ˈmʌltiˈfɔːmæt] *a.* 多幅的，多规格的
Multiformat laser camera application played an essential role in the development of CT.
多幅激光相机的应用在 CT 的发展过程中发挥了必不可少的作用。

multifunctional [ˌmʌltiˈfʌŋkʃənl] *a.* 多功能的
In multifunctional proteins, the different domains can each perform a different task.
多功能蛋白质内不同区域可执行不同的任务。

multigenic [ˌmʌlti ˈdʒenik] *a.* 多基因的

The vast majority of genetic polymorphisms, having a modest impact on the affected genes, are part of a large array of multigenic factors that impact on drug effect.

绝大多数基因多态性只是大批影响药效的多基因因子中的一部分，对所影响的基因只有轻度的作用。

multimedia [ˌmʌltiˈmiːdiə] *a.* 多媒体的；使用多媒体的

We bought a multimedia encyclopedia.

我们买了一套多媒体百科全书。

Network teaching needs multimedia database.

网络教学需要多媒体素材库的支持。

multimodality [ˌmʌltimɔˈdæliti] *n.* 多模式；多峰性

Determining the stage of colorectal cancer often requires a multimodality, multistep imaging approach.

确定结直肠癌的分期通常需要多形式、多步骤的影像手段。

Multimodality treatment is the general trend in cancer management, and is the inevitable result of the development in clinical oncology as well.

综合治疗模式是肿瘤治疗的根本趋势，也是临床肿瘤学发展的必然结果。

multipara [mʌlˈtip(ə)rə] *n.* 经产妇

The clinical data of 21 patients with ante or post partum cardiomyopathy are reported in this article, which includs 10 cases of primipara (47.6%) and 11 cases of multipara (52.4%).

本文报告分娩前后心肌病 21 例，其中初产妇 10 例(47.6%)，经产妇 11 例(52.4%)。

There was no significant difference between primipara and multipara, except its detection rate by CT that was decreased with increase of age.

除 CT 的检出率随年龄增长而下降外，初产妇与经产妇无显著差异。

multiphase [ˈmʌltifeiz] *n.* 多相；*a.* 多相的

A restore is a multiphase process.

还原是一个多阶段过程。

Carcinogenic risk escalates with multiphase acquisition in a single CT study, and with multiple individual CT tests.

在单一的 CT 研究和多个独立 CT 检验中，随着扫描部位的增加，致癌风险升高。

multiplanar [ˌmʌltiˈpleinə] *a.* 多平面的

The objective of this article is to evaluate the diagnostic value of MSCT 3D and multiplanar reconstruction (MPR) for trauma of bones and joints.

本文的目的是探讨 MSCT 三维重建技术和多平面重建(MPR)技术在骨关节创伤中的诊断价值。

Regarding the detection of the embolus, multiplanar volume reconstruction (MPVR) was better than maximum intensity projection (MIP) and volume rendering (VR).

对于栓子的检测，多层面容积重建(MPVR)优于最大密度投影(MIP)和容积再现(VR)。

multiple [ˈmʌltipl] *a.* 多数的；多重的

There are numerous examples of multiple primary tumours arising in a particular field.

有许多关于多发性原发瘤起源于特殊部位的例子。

A tendency to multiple pregnancy is inherited, and it occurs more frequently in certain families.

多胎妊娠有遗传倾向，在某些家族发生较频繁。

multiplication [ˈmʌltipliˈkeiʃən] *n.* 倍增；繁殖

The vaginal fluid is acid(pH 4) and this prevents multiplication of most pathogenic organisms.

阴道液呈酸性(pH 4)，可防止大多数致病菌的繁殖。

multiplicity [ˌmʌltiˈplisiti] *n.* 多样；众多；复杂

Medical microbiology is so directly concerned with this multiplicity of different cell types and

their interactions.
医学微生物学直接涉及众多不同类型的细胞和它们之间的相互作用。

multiply [ˈmʌltiplai] *v.* 增加;繁殖;乘
Bacteria multiply very fast when they have proper material to feed on.
在能够得到适当养料的时候,细菌繁殖得很快。
If the wound is sutured and stapled too soon it can create an environment deprived of oxygen that causes the flesh-eating bacteria to multiply and spread deep within the tissues.
如果伤口过早缝合和订合,就会创建一个缺氧环境,让嗜肉细菌繁殖并扩散到组织深部。

multiprogrammable [ˌmʌltiˌprəuˈgræməbl] *a.* 多程序的
In the past few years, multiprogrammable pacemakers have been introduced in clinical medicine.
过去几年中,临床医学已引进多程序起搏器。

multislice [ˌmʌltiˈslais] *a.* 多层面的
Multislice CT provides a reliable and rapid diagnosis even in the haemodynamically unstable patient and should not be delayed for management of the fracture.
即使对于血流动力学不稳的患者,多层螺旋 CT 亦能够做出可靠和快速的诊断,不应因处置骨折而延误检查。
The development of multislice CT technology, combined with increased computing power and synchronized power injectors, has added a new dimension to CT.
多层面 CT 成像技术的发展,结合计算功能和同步化功能提高的注射器,扩展了 CT 用途的新方向。

multitude [ˈmʌltitjuːd] *n.* 大批;大量
During a lifetime, man is exposed to a multitude of pain inducing injury and diseases.
人在一生中要遭受到许许多多导致疼痛的损伤和疾病的折磨。

multivalent [mʌltiˈveilənt] *a.* 多价的
Precipitation reactions occur upon mixing, at the right proportions, of soluble multivalent antigen and (at least) divalent antibodies.
按适当比例混合可溶性多价抗原和(至少)二价抗体时则可发生沉淀反应。

multivariate [ˌmʌltiˈvɛərieit] *a.* 多变量的,多元的
The propensity scores were used to create matched comparison groups in multivariate risk modeling.
使用倾向分数建立多变量风险模型中的匹配对照组。
In this study, we used multivariate analysis to determine which genetic polymorphisms in alcohol metabolizing enzymes were independently associated with the development of alcoholic cirrhosis.
在本研究中,我们采用多元分析来确定哪些乙醇代谢酶基因多态性能独立影响酒精性肝硬化发展。

mumps [mʌmps] *n.* 流行性腮腺炎
Mumps is an acute contagious viral infection.
流行性腮腺炎是一种急性接触性病毒传染病。
Mumps vaccine does not provide absolute protection against mumps.
流行性腮腺炎疫苗并不能绝对预防流行性腮腺炎的发生。

mural [ˈmjuərəl] *a.* (墙)壁的,壁内的
This thrombus on the wall of a ventricle (mural thrombus) may then break off.
心室壁的血栓(壁内血栓)可能脱落。
Lesions of the mural endocardium also may occur in rheumatic fever.
风湿热时也可发生壁性心内膜病变。

murmur [ˈməːmə] *n.* 杂音
Murmurs of mitral regurgitation may be heard in a case of mitral valve insufficiency.

在二尖瓣闭锁不全的病例中可听到二尖瓣回流杂音。

The tighter the stenosis, the higher the atrial pressure and the longer the murmur.

狭窄越严重,则心房压越高,杂音也就越长。

muscle [ˈmʌsl] *n.* 肌肉

Muscles possess mechanisms for converting energy derived from chemical reactions into mechanical energy.

肌肉具有把化学反应所产生的能量转变为机械能的机制。

Our skeletal muscles endow us with the ability to move.

我们的骨骼肌赋予我们行动的能力。

Tendon reflexes are preserved in weak muscles.

肌无力时腱反射仍可存在。

muscular [ˈmʌskjulə] *a.* 肌的,肌肉的

Disease of the neuromuscular junction is not associated with muscular atrophy.

神经肌肉接头的疾病不伴有肌萎缩。

Muscular dystrophies are intrinsic diseases of the muscle fiber.

肌营养不良是肌纤维的内在疾病。

A feeling of generalized muscular weakness is common in the absence of neurological disease.

全身肌无力的感觉,在没有神经疾患时是常见的。

muscularis [ˌmʌskjuˈlæris] [拉] *a.* 肌的

The tunica muscularis is composed mainly of smooth muscles, the thickest part of which is in the isthmus.

肌层主要由平滑肌组成,峡部达到最厚。

n. 肌层

Endoscopic ultrasound miniprobe image showed a tumor invading into the muscularis propria.

超声内镜微型探针检查显示肿瘤侵犯到固有肌层。

musculature [ˈmʌskjulətʃə] *n.* 肌肉系统

The musculature overlying the forehead—the frontalis and corrugator is almost never involved.

覆盖在前额的肌肉——额肌和皱眉肌几乎从不受累。

musculoaponeurotic [ˌmʌskjuləuˌæpəunjuˈrɔtik] *a.* 肌腱膜的

The musculoaponeurotic layer of the nose consists of intertwined fibrous and muscular tissue.

鼻部的肌腱膜层由环形缠绕的纤维和肌肉组织构成。

Previous anatomic studies have demonstrated that the lymphatic drainage system is also located superficial to the musculoaponeurotic layer.

以往的解剖学研究已证实淋巴引流系统也位于肌腱膜的浅层。

musculoskeletal [ˌmʌskjuləuˈskelitəl] *a.* 肌(与)骨骼的

Occupational stress is obviously associated with musculoskeletal disorders in the lower extremities.

职业压力与下肢肌肉骨骼疾病有明显的联系。

mutagen [ˈmjuːtədʒən] *n.* 致突变剂

As many mutations cause cancer, mutagens are therefore also very likely to be carcinogens.

由于多次突变可致癌,因此致突变剂也很可能是致癌物。

A mutagen is a natural or human-made agent which can alter the structure or sequence of DNA.

致突变剂是能改变 DNA 结构或序列的一种天然或人造药剂。

mutagenesis [ˌmjuːtəˈdʒenisis] *n.* 诱变,引起突变

The purpose of the present study was to explore the relationship between inflammatory leukocyte activation and mutagenesis using co-culture systems.

本研究的目的是用共培养系统来揭示炎性白细胞活化和诱发突变之间的联系。

mutagenic [ˌmjuːtəˈdʒenik] *a.* 诱变的,致突变的

These metals are mutagenic by virtue of their ability to induce reactive oxygen intermediates in cells.

这些金属有致突变的作用,依赖其自身的能力能诱发细胞内产生活性氧中间产物。

Many strains of microorganism have been improved by processes involving radiation or mutagenic agents.

许多微生物品系通过包括辐射或诱变剂在内的处理而已有改善。

mutagenicity [ˌmjuːtədʒəˈnisəti] *n.* 诱变,致突变性

This notice contains the Guidelines for Mutagenicity Risk Assessment.

本通告包含诱变风险评估指南。

The mutagenicity of physical agents (e. g. ,radiation) is not addressed here.

在此未列出物理诱变剂(如辐射)。

mutant [ˈmjuːtənt] *n.* 突变体,突变株

X-rays have been widely employed experimentally to produce microbial mutants.

X 线已广泛应用于实验性地诱生微生物的突变株。

mutate [mjuˈteit] *v.* 变异;突变

A rapidly mutating SARS virus could complicate work toward a vaccine and reliable diagnostic tests.

SARS 病毒的迅速变异给疫苗研究和可靠诊断测试的工作带来困难。

The hepatitis B virus can cause liver cells to mutate and eventually lead to the development of liver cancer.

乙肝病毒能引起肝细胞的突变而最终导致肝癌的发生。

mutation [mjuːˈteiʃən] *n.* 变化,变异;突变

Viruses cause cell mutation by injecting themselves into the DNA or RNA of a cell.

病毒通过将自身整合入细胞的脱氧核糖核酸和核糖核酸而引起细胞突变。

Similar but not identical genetic disease may result from mutations.

相似但不完全相同的遗传病可由突变造成。

mutational [mjuːˈteiʃənəl] *a.* 突变的

This slow process can encourage stepwise mutational change to resistance in the bacterial cells.

这一缓慢过程促进针对病菌细胞抵抗力的逐步突变。

mutism [ˈmjuːtizəm] *n.* 哑症,缄默症

Paralysis, blindness, and mutism are the most common conversion symptoms.

瘫痪、失明和哑症都是最常见的转换症状。

Many cases of school refusal or elective mutism might be included in the disturbance of emotions specific to childhood.

许多拒绝上学和有选择的缄默症也可包括在童年特有的情绪障碍之中。

mutural [ˈmjuːtʃərəl] *a.* 相互的

There is mutural aid and benefit in different species of organism.

不同生物之间存在互助互利的关系。

myalgia [maiˈældʒiə] *n.* 肌痛

Muscle tenderness may be marked in the presence of severe myalgia.

在出现严重肌痛时,肌肉压痛可以很显著。

Patients develop sepsis 1-3d after abortion occasionally, with fever, chills, severe myalgias and abdominal pain.

偶尔病人在流产后 1~3 天出现败血症,表现为发热、寒战、剧烈肌痛和腹痛。

myasthenia [ˌmaiæsˈθiːniə] *n.* 肌无力,肌衰弱

Myasthenia gravis is associated with antibody to the acetylcholine receptors on motor endplates of muscles and lead to muscle weakness of all striated muscle groups.

重症肌无力是由于抗体与肌肉运动终板上的乙酰胆碱受体相结合导致了所有横纹肌群软

弱无力。

mycelial [mai'siːliəl] *a.* 菌丝体的

Mycelial forms are commonly called molds.

菌丝体形态通常被称为霉。

Actinomycetes form fairly extensive mycelial structure.

这些放线菌形成相当宽阔的丝状结构。

mycelium [mai'siːliəm] *n.* 菌丝体

The fungi usually grow as branched filaments known as a mycelium.

真菌通常以分支丝状物，即所谓菌丝体形式生长。

Fungal colonies composed of mycelia are found in soil and on or within many other substances.

由菌丝体组成的真菌菌落存在于土壤中和其他许多物体的表面或内部。

Mycelium is the vegetative part of a fungus, consisting of a mass of branching, thread-like hyphae.

菌丝体是真菌的植物性生长方式，由一团分枝线状的菌丝组成。

mycobacterium [ˌmaikəubæk'tiəriəm] (*pl.* mycobacteria [maikəubæk'tiəriə]) *n.* 分枝杆菌

Mycobacteria have a very hydrophobic surface.

分枝杆菌的表面呈极端疏水性。

Paraaminosalicylic acid had bacteriostatic activity against mycobacterium tuberculosis.

对氨基水杨酸对结核分枝杆菌有抑制作用。

mycophenolate [maikəu'fiːnəleit] *n.* 骁悉（商品名：cellcept）

Mycophenolate, belonging to immunosuppressive agents, is used to prevent rejection of heart or kidney transplants.

骁悉属于免疫抑制剂，用于防止心肾移植物的排斥作用。

mycoplasma [ˌmaikəu'plæzmə] (*pl.* mycoplasmas 或 mycoplasmata [maikəu'plæzmətə]) *n.* 支原体

The mycoplasmas lack cell walls, and, as a result, the cells lack any defined shape.

支原体没有细胞壁，因此无一定的细胞形态。

Mycoplasma pneumoniae may cause pneumonia, and it is the only mycoplasma definitely pathogenic to man.

肺炎支原体可引起肺炎，它是能使人致病的惟一支原体。

mycosis [mai'kəusis] *n.* 真菌病，霉菌病（复数 mycoses）

Systemic mycoses due to opportunistic pathogens are infections of patients with immune deficiencies who would otherwise not be infected.

由条件致病菌导致的全身真菌病发生于免疫缺陷的患者，免疫功能正常者不会被感染。

Mycoses often start in the lungs or on the skin due to the inhalation of fungal spores or localized colonization of the skin.

由于真菌孢子吸入或在皮肤局部繁殖，真菌病常开始于肺部或皮肤。

mycotic [mai'kɔtik] *a.* 真菌病的，霉菌病的

Diseases caused by fungi are called mycotic infections.

真菌引起的疾病叫做真菌感染。

The mycotic aneurysms most commonly occur in the brain and they may rupture.

霉菌性动脉瘤最常发生于大脑并可破裂。

mycotoxin [ˌmaikəu'tɔksin] *n.* 霉菌毒素

Many moulds on grains, fruit and oilseeds produce mycotoxins, some of which have been shown to cause liver cancer in animals.

粮食、水果以及油料种子上的许多霉菌都可产生霉菌毒素，其中有些已显示可引起动物肝癌。

mydriasis [mi'draiəsis] *n.* 瞳孔散大，瞳孔扩大

Meperidine does not produce miosis and may even cause mydriasis.
哌替啶不引起缩瞳,甚至有扩瞳作用。

myelitis [maiə'laitis] *n.* 脊髓炎

The most usual myelitis(transverse myelitis) most often occurs during the development of multiple sclerosis.
最常见的脊髓炎(横贯性脊髓炎)最常发生在多发性硬化症的发展过程中。

Myelitis can occur either with or without associated encephalitis.
脊髓炎出现时,可伴有或不伴有脑炎。

myeloblast ['maiələuˌblæst] *n.* 成髓细胞,原始粒细胞

The diagnosis is made on finding myeloblast cells in the peripheral blood or the marrow.
诊断依据是在周围血象或骨髓内发现原始粒细胞。

myelocyte ['maiələusait] *n.* 中幼粒细胞

Myelocyte is normally found in the bloodforming tissue of the bone marrow, but may appear in the blood in a variety of disease, such as infections.
正常情况下,中幼粒细胞常见于骨髓的造血组织中,但也可出现在患有某种疾病(例如感染)的病人血液中。

These then become myelocytes, with primary and secondary granules.
这些细胞再转化成带有原始颗粒和次级颗粒的髓细胞。

myelocytic [ˌmaiələu'sitik] *a.* 粒细胞性的

In chronic myelocytic leukemia, lymphadenopathy is an unusual manifestation.
在慢性粒细胞性白血病中,淋巴肿大并不常见。

myelodysplasia [ˌmaiələudis'pleiziə] *n.* 脊髓发育不良

Patients with myelodysplasia present with symptoms of anemia, with bleeding and bruising due to either decreased or dysfunctional platelets or with infection.
患有脊髓发育不良的病人可表现为贫血,由于血小板功能障碍或血小板减少引起的出血和青紫以及感染。

myelofibrosis [ˌmaiələufai'brəusis] *n.* 骨髓纤维变性,骨髓纤维化

The therapy for myelofibrosis is directed at control of symptoms.
骨髓纤维化的治疗目的在于控制该病的症状。

myelography [ˌmaiə'lɔgrəfi] *n.* 脊髓(X 线)造影术,脊髓照相术

Myelography is invasive. Potential complications include headache, seizures and meningitis.
脊髓 X 线造影术是侵入性的,潜在的并发症有头痛、癫痫发作和脑膜炎。

When it is probable that myelography will be indicated, the lumbar puncture can often delayed until this procedure is done.
如有可能和有必要作脊髓造影,则腰穿常可延长到脊髓造影后进行。

myeloid ['maiələid] *a.* 脊髓的,髓系的,髓样的

The components of the hematopoietic system have been traditionally divided into the myeloid tissues and the lymphoid tissues.
传统上,造血系统分为髓系组织和淋巴组织。

Myeloid neoplasms arise from early hematopoietic progenitors, including acute myeloid leukemias, myelodysplastic syndromes and chronic myeloproliferative disorders.
髓系肿瘤起源于早期造血前体细胞,包括急性髓系白血病、骨髓增生异常综合征和慢性骨髓增生性疾病。

myeloma [ˌmaiə'ləumə] (*pl.* myelomas or myelomata [ˌmaiə'ləumətə]) *n.* 骨髓瘤

Plasma protein electrophoresis will usually show a myeloma band in the gamma region.
血浆蛋白电泳常在 γ 区显示有一骨髓瘤带。

Cold urticaria with cryoglobulinemia is seen in multiple myeloma.
有冷球蛋白血症的冷性荨麻疹可见于多发性骨髓瘤。

Radiotherapy of the whole body is also used in the primary treatment of myeloma.
全身的放射疗法也可作为骨髓瘤的初期治疗。

myelomatosis [ˌmaiələuməˈtəusis] *n.* 骨髓瘤(病),多发性骨髓瘤

Multiple myelomatosis occurs usually after the age of 50 years.
多发性骨髓瘤一般在 50 岁以后发病。

myelopathy [ˌmaiəˈlɔpəθi] *n.* 脊髓病;骨髓病

Thoracic and lumbar compressions cause myelopathy and a spinal stenosis syndrome.
胸腰部脊椎受压时可引起脊髓病和脊髓狭窄综合征。

myelophthisis [ˌmaiəˈlɔfθisis] *n.* 脊髓痨,骨髓痨,全骨髓萎缩

Bone marrow aspiration and biopsy is helpful when leukemia or myelophthisis is suspected.
当怀疑为白血病或骨髓痨时抽取骨髓做活检是有帮助的。

The mechanisms of normochromic-normocytic anemias involved are hypoproliferation, hypoplasia and myelophthisis.
正色正常红细胞性贫血的机制为增生不足,再生不良和全骨髓萎缩。

myelosclerosis [ˌmaiələuˌskliəˈrəusis] *n.* 骨髓硬化,脊髓硬化

A rare case of acute myelosclerosis has been described in a 20-year-old man.
已经报道过一例 20 岁男性患者急性骨髓硬化症的罕见病例。

Three cases of myelosclerosis associated with systemic lupus erythematosus are described.
论文报道了 3 例系统性红斑狼疮相关性骨髓硬化症。

myelosuppression [ˌmaiələusəˈpreʃən] *n.* 骨髓抑制

5-Fluorouracil causes myelosuppression and mucositis.
5-氟尿嘧啶可引起骨髓抑制和黏膜炎。

myocardial [maiəuˈkɑːdiəl] *a.* 心肌的

During myocardial ischemia, the blood vessels are dilated fully.
在心肌缺血期间,血管充分扩张。

The outstanding characteristic of acute myocardial infarction is severe, prolonged pain.
急性心肌梗死的突出特征是严重而持久的疼痛。

myocarditis [ˌmaiəukɑːˈdaitis] *n.* 心肌炎

Acute myocarditis may cause heart failure and arrythmia.
急性心肌炎可引起心衰和心律不齐。

Myocarditis may develop in patients with human immunodeficiency virus (HIV) infection.
心肌炎可出现于人类免疫缺陷病毒感染的病人。

The clinical diagnosis of myocarditis, even in fatal cases, is often not made.
心肌炎的临床诊断往往甚至在致死的病例中也未作出。

myocardium [ˌmaiəuˈkɑːdiəm] *n.* 心肌

Myocarditis is the inflammation of the myocardium most commonly due to acute viral infection.
心肌炎是心肌的炎症,大多是由于急性病毒感染。

Ischemia (lack of oxygen) of the myocardium is heralded by such pain.
心肌缺血(缺氧)有这种先兆疼痛。

myoclonic [maiəuˈklɔnik] *a.* 肌阵挛的

For a child with myoclonic epilepsy clonazepam or nitrazepam can be given in slowly increasing doses.
对肌阵挛癫痫的患儿可按缓慢增加剂量的方式给予氯硝西泮或硝基泮。

myoclonus [maiˈɔklənəs] *n.* 肌阵挛

The progressive myoclonic ataxias are characterized by active myoclonus and progressive cerebellar ataxia.
进行性肌阵挛性共济失调以活动性肌阵挛和进行性小脑性肌阵挛为其特征。

myocyte [ˈmaiəsait] *n.* 肌细胞;肌丝层

The myocyte diameter and cross section were reduced progressively along with the duration of muscle denervation.

肌细胞直径及横截面积随失神经支配时间延长呈进行性下降。

From a diagnostic standpoint, the aim is to try and develop biomarkers that identify patients with ACS, even when there is no evidence of myocyte necrosis.

从诊断的角度来看，其目标是尝试和研发一些生物指标，用这些指标能在没有证据表明肌细胞坏死的情况下鉴定患急性冠状动脉综合征（ACS）的病人。

myocytolysis [ˌmaiəusaiˈtɔlisis] *n.* 液化性肌溶解

Vacuolar degeneration or myocytolysis may be seen in the margins of myocardial infarcts.

空泡变性和液化性肌溶解可见于心肌梗死的边缘。

Subendocardial vacuolization and myocytolysis are indicative of sublethal ischemic change of myocardium.

心内膜下空泡变性和液化性肌溶解是心肌亚致死性缺血性改变的一种表现。

myofibroblast [ˌmaiəuˈfaibrəblæst] *n.* 肌纤维母细胞

In nodular fasciitis, plump, immature-appearing fibroblasts and myofibroblasts are arranged randomly or in short intersecting fascicles.

在结节性筋膜炎，肥胖的不成熟样的成纤维细胞和肌纤维母细胞随机排列或呈相互交织的短束状。

The proliferation of hepatic satellite cells and their activation into myofibroblasts play an important role in the pathogenesis of liver cirrhosis.

肝星状细胞的增生以及活化转变为肌纤维母细胞在肝硬化的发生中起重要作用。

myofibrosis [ˌmaiəufaiˈbrəusis] *n.* 肌纤维化；肌纤维变性

Strong evidence implicates that the infiltration of inflammatory cells is a critical part of the process resulting in cardiac myofibrosis.

有力的证据表明炎性细胞浸润是心肌纤维化过程中的关键部分。

Myofibrosis can be caused by continued damage such as inflammatory and ischemia, etc.

持续的损伤因素如炎症、缺血等可引起肌纤维变性。

myoglobin [maiəuˈgləubin] *n.* 肌红蛋白

The protein myoglobin is composed of a single polypeptide chain and contains no quaternary structure.

肌红蛋白由一条多肽单链组成，无四级结构。

myoglobinuria [ˌmaiəuˌgləubiˈnjuəriə] *n.* 肌红蛋白尿

Myoglobinuria presents special problems to the electrically burned patient.

电击伤患者的特殊表现是出现肌红蛋白尿。

myoma [maiˈəumə] (*pl.* myomas 或 myomata [maiˈəumətə]) *n.* 肌瘤

Large myomas are likely to be irregular, whereas a pregnant uterus is normally symmetric.

大的肌瘤可能形状不规则，而妊娠子宫为正常对称的。

Ovarian tumors can be distinguished from the uterus by palpation, and myomas are part of the uterus.

卵巢肿瘤能够通过触诊与子宫区别开来，而子宫肌瘤则位于子宫。

myomectomy [ˌmaiəuˈmektəmi] *n.* 肌瘤切除术

For a younger woman myomectomy is to be preferred because it leaves the possibility of childbearing.

对较年轻妇女以肌瘤切除术为好，因为这样可保留生育的可能性。

myometrium [ˌmaiəuˈmiːtriəm] *n.* 子宫肌层

The myometrium may also show some hyperplasia.

子宫肌层也可能有些增生。

myonecrosis [ˌmaiəuneˈkrəusis] *n.* 肌坏死

Hyperbaric oxygen has been used in patients with the gangrene syndromes and clostridial myonecrosis.
高压氧治疗已用于患有坏疽综合征及梭状芽胞杆菌感染肌坏死的病人。

myopathy [maiˈɔpəθi] *n.* 肌病
Muscle pain induced by exercise, is often indicative of myopathy, particularly metabolic ones.
由运动诱发的肌痛常提示肌病，尤其是代谢性肌病。

myopia [maiˈəupjə] *n.* 近视
Myopia is corrected by wearing spectacles with concave lenses.
配戴凹透镜可矫正近视眼。
Myopia is called near-sightedness because the myope can see objects near him with complete clarity.
近视眼之所以称为近视，是由于近视患者可完全清晰地看见靠近他的物体。

myositis [ˌmaiəuˈsaitis] *n.* 肌炎
Myositis can arise spontaneously or after penetrating trauma.
肌炎可自发出现或在穿通伤之后发生。
Focal myositis is characterized by a rapidly progressive lump in muscle.
局灶性肌炎是以迅速增大的肌肉肿块为其特征。
MRI can be used to detect active myositis noninvasively.
肌炎活动期可以用无创性的磁共振检查进行识别。

myostatin [ˌmaiəuˈstætin] *n.* 肌骨素；肌肉生长抑素
This paper investigated the expression of myostatin gene in different tissues of rats.
该文章研究了大鼠不同组织中肌肉生长抑制素基因的表达情况。
The potential medicine is designed to inhibit the myostatin protein, which limits muscle growth.
该药物潜在作用是抑制肌肉生长抑制素蛋白来限制肌肉生长。

myotonia [ˌmaiəuˈtəuniə] *n.* 肌强直
Myotonia is the persistent contraction of a muscle after cessation of voluntary contraction or in response to a mechanical or electrical stimulus.
肌强直是肌肉在自主收缩停止后或机械性以及电刺激后发生的持续性收缩。

myriad [ˈmiriəd] *a.* 无数的，繁多的
The myriad species of bacteria inhabit almost every environmental niche on the Earth.
地球上每一个角落几乎都寄居着种类繁多的细菌。
These bacteria exclude myriad organisms of fascinating shapes and metabolic capabilities.
这些细菌还未包括那些千姿百态、代谢各异的无数微生物。

myristate [miˈristeit] *n.* 豆蔻酸
1% of carbomer 940 and 67% of ethanol and isopropyl myristate were the optimum matrix.
以 1% 卡波姆 940 和 67% 的乙醇以及肉豆蔻酸异丙酯为最佳配方。
We selected Tween80, Span80, ethanol, isopropyl myristate, Jojoba oil, Vitamin E oil, and distilled water as ingredient.
我们选择 Tween80、Span80、乙醇、肉豆蔻酸异丙酯、霍霍巴油、维生素 E 油、蒸馏水为原料。

myrj [maidʒ] *n.* 卖泽
The surfactants tested in this study including Tween-80, Myrj-52.
这项研究测试的表面活性剂包括：吐温-80 和卖泽-52.
Myrj-52 is a polyoxyethylene stearate.
卖泽-52 是一种脂肪酸聚氧乙烯酯。

myrrh [məː] *n.* 没药
They are frankincense and myrrh.
它们是乳香和没药。

The gift of myrrh is a prophecy of the death and burial of the earthly body of Christ.
没药作为礼物代表基督尘世身体的死亡和埋葬的一个预言。

myxedema [ˌmiksiˈdiːmə] *n.* 黏液(性)水肿

In both myxedema and hyperthyroidism amenorrhoea occurs in severe cases.
黏液性水肿和甲状腺功能亢进的严重病例均可发生闭经。

myxoma [mikˈsəumə] (*pl.* myxomas or myxomata [mikˈsəumətə]) *n.* 黏液瘤

Myxomas occur mostly (75%) in women, becoming clinically manifest between the ages of 35 and 60.
黏液瘤多发生于女性(75%),在 35 岁至 60 岁之间出现临床症状。

N

nadir [ˈneiˌdiə] *n.* 最低点

Most alkylating agents cause acute myelosuppression, with a nadir of the peripheral blood granulocyte count at 6 to 10 days and recovery in 14 to 21 days.

大部分烷化剂都引发急性骨髓抑制,外周血粒细胞计数最低出现在 6 ~ 10 天,在 14 ~ 21 天得以恢复。

nafcillin [næfˈsilin] *n.* 乙氧萘青霉素;萘夫西林;新青霉素Ⅲ

Nafcillin is an inducer of the cytochrome P450 3A4 isoenzyme.

萘夫西林是细胞色素 P450 3A4 同工酶的诱导剂。

Nafcillin sodium is a narrow-spectrum beta-lactam antibiotic of the penicillin class.

萘夫西林钠是一种窄谱的青霉素族 β 内酰胺类抗生素。

nail [neil] *n.* 甲,爪;钉

Our finger nails need cutting now and then.

我们的指甲需要经常修剪。

Various nail dystrophies should also be kept in mind.

各种指甲的营养不良也应当考虑到。

naked [ˈneikid] *a.* 裸露的

Microbes are too small to be seen by the naked eye.

微生物太小,肉眼看不见。

Because of the inclusion of the carbon particles in the antigen, flocculation can be determined with the naked eye.

由于抗原中包含碳颗粒,所以用肉眼即可测定絮状沉淀。

naloxone [ˈnæləksəun] *n.* 纳洛酮

Naloxone should be available in case respiratory depression occurs.

纳洛酮应当用于呼吸受到抑制的病人。

In these cases naloxone should be given by slow intravenous injection.

对于这些病人应给予纳洛酮缓慢静脉注射。

nanocapsule [ˌnænəˈkæpsjuːl] *n.* 毫超微囊剂,纳米囊

The prepared nanocapsules were used for controlling drug release of anticancer agents.

制备的纳米囊用于控制抗癌药剂的药物释放。

They avoid the use of surfactants in parenteral formulations of nanocapsules.

他们避免在纳米囊肠外制剂中使用表面活性剂。

nanogenerator [ˈnænəuˈdʒenəreitə] *n.* 纳米调控器

The author injected the nanogenerators into mice, and reported reduced tumor growth and increased survival time.

作者报道将纳米调控器注入大鼠体内,肿瘤生长减缓,生存时间延长。

nanomaterial [ˌnænəˌməˈtiəriəl] *n.* 纳米材料

With the development of nanotechnology, a growing number of people are expected to be exposed to nanomaterials.

随着纳米技术的发展,越来越多的人正有待接触纳米材料。

Nanomaterials with proven beneficial effects are on the market.

已证明有益的纳米材料正在上市销售。

Carbon nanotubes have become a research topic of nanomaterial domain because of the unique structure and properties.
碳纳米管因其独特的结构和性能而成为纳米材料领域的一个研究主题。

nanomedicine [ˌnænəu'medisin] *n.* 纳米医学
Nanomedicine is based on molecular nanotechnology and molecular manufacturing.
纳米医学是建立在分子纳米技术和分子制作技术基础上的。

nanoparticle [ˌnænə'pɑːtikl] *n.* 纳米颗粒,纳米粒
Nanoparticle is a collective name for nanospheres and nanocapsules.
纳米粒是纳米球和纳米囊的统称。
Nanoparticles are used in nanomedical research and other biotechnological applications.
纳米粒应用于纳米医学研究和其他生物技术。
Nanomedicine enabled the development of nanoparticle therapeutic carriers.
纳米医学促进了纳米颗粒治疗性载体的研发。

nanopharmaceutical [ˌnænəuˌfɑːmə'suːtikəl] *n.* 纳米药物制剂
Nanopharmaceutical has been defined as a pharmaceutical product to control human biological systems at the molecular level, using engineered nanotechnology.
纳米药物制剂定义为以纳米工程技术制备在分子水平调控人体系统的产品。

nanorobot ['nænəu'rəubɔt] *n.* 纳米机器人
Such nanorobot may destroy all viruses and complete the necessary replication in an hour.
这样的纳米机器人可以毁灭所有的病毒颗粒,并在一小时内完成所需要的修复。

nanosphere ['nænəsfiə] *n.* 毫微球,纳米球
Nanospheres have been used for gene delivery applications.
纳米球已被用于基因传递。
Lipid nanospheres are used for the passive targeting of cosmetic agents to skin.
脂质纳米球可用于制备被动靶向的皮肤化妆品。
Cellulose derivatives have been used to prepare nanospheres entrapping 5-fluorouracil.
纤维素衍生物已用于制备包裹 5-氟尿嘧啶的纳米球。

nanotechnology ['nænəuˌtek'nɔlədʒi] *n.* 纳米技术
Nanotechnology includes positional assembly and self-replication.
纳米技术包括定位组装和自我复制。

nap [næp] *n.* 小睡(尤指白天)
He usually takes a quick nap after lunch.
他常在午饭后小睡一会儿。
In some cultures, sleep may be divided into a midafternoon nap and a shortened night sleep.
在某些国家中,睡眠可以分为午睡和缩短的夜间睡觉。
v. 小睡(尤指白天)
About 60 percent of American adults nap when given the opportunity during the daytime.
约有 60% 的美国成年人只要有机会白天随时打个盹。

narcolepsy ['nɑːkəlepsi] *n.* 嗜眠病,发作性睡病
Narcolepsy is an illness that causes sudden, uncontrollable attacks of sleep.
嗜眠病是一种引起突然的、无法控制的睡眠侵袭。
Genetic susceptibility to narcolepsy is closely linked to a specific region of the major histocompatibility complex on chromosome 6.
发作性睡病的遗传易感性与第 6 号染色体上主要组织相容性复合体上的一个特定区域密切相关。
Narcolepsy is characterized by excessive daytime sleepiness.
发作性睡病具有白天嗜睡过多的特征。

narcosis [nɑː'kəusis] *n.* 麻醉

Although solvents may cause narcosis if inhaled or ingested, the injury that solvents and oils have produced most commonly is chemical pneumonitis, following their ingestion and aspiration.

虽然吸入或摄入溶剂可导致麻醉，但摄入或吸入溶剂和油类以后产生的最常见的损伤是化学性肺炎。

Medullary narcosis is produced by injection of a local anesthetic into the medullary subarachnoid space.

脊髓麻醉是通过用局部麻醉药注射到脊髓蛛网膜下腔而产生的。

narcotic [nɑːˈkɔtik] *a.* 麻醉的

Narcotic alkaloids are divided into naturally occurring, semisynthetic, and synthetic derivatives.

麻醉性生物碱分为天然、半合成和合成衍生物。

n. 麻醉剂

Morphine is still the best narcotic for pain relief.

吗啡仍为效果最好的麻醉性镇痛药。

Narcotics should be used cautiously in patients with pulmonary insufficiency, emphysema, and asthma.

对肺功能不全、肺气肿和气喘病人，使用麻醉剂时必须慎重。

naris [ˈneiris] (*pl.* nares [ˈnɛəriːz]) *n.* 鼻孔

The two external(or anterior) nares are the nostrils, leading from the nasal cavity to the outside.

两个外鼻孔（鼻前孔）是鼻腔与外界相通的孔窍。

There are approximately five small vesicular lesions 2mm in diameter on the cheek and nares.

在面颊和两侧鼻孔处约有五个直径为 2mm 的疱疹性损害。

nasal [ˈneizəl] *a.* 鼻的

During asthma, often, too, there is marked nasal congestion.

哮喘时也常有明显的鼻充血。

On many occasions, stained nasal smears will reveal significant numbers of eosinophils in allergic rhinitis.

在许多情况下，染色的鼻涂片可揭示出过敏性鼻炎嗜酸性细胞的有效数字。

nasogastric [ˌneizəuˈgæstrik] *a.* 鼻胃的

After initial assessment ensuring airway, breathing, and circulatory resuscitation, place a nasogastric tube for gastric decompression.

在保证气道通畅、呼吸和循环系统复苏之后，再上一根鼻胃管进行胃部减压。

nasopharynx [ˌneizəuˈfæriŋks] *n.* 鼻咽

Respiratory difficulty is due to obstruction to the nasopharynx by secretions and vomitus.

呼吸困难是由于鼻咽被分泌物和呕吐物所阻塞。

The areas affected in order of frequency are the nasopharynx, nose and tonsil.

侵犯部位，按照其频率，依次为鼻咽部、鼻和扁桃腺。

nasotracheal [ˌneizəutrəˈkiəl] *a.* 鼻气管的

Treatment of atelectasis consists of clearing the airway by chest percussion, coughing, or nasotracheal suction.

对肺不张的处理包括胸部叩击，咳嗽或经鼻气管吸引使气道畅通。

The nasotracheal intubation is more comfortable than the orotracheal intubation, but the latter is technically easier to insert.

经鼻气管插管比经口气管插管要舒服些，但是后者在技术上插入容易些。

natriuresis [ˌneitrijuəˈriːsis] *n.* 尿钠排泄；利钠作用

Most patients are prescribed loop diuretics rather than thiazides due to the higher efficiency of induced diuresis and natriuresis.

由于髓袢利尿剂具有较高的利尿和利钠效果，大多数病人被建议使用该药而非噻嗪类利尿剂。

Adrenomedullin, a bioactive peptide, has been intensively studied in the last decade. It has several biological actions, such as vasodilation, natriuresis, diuresis, etc.
近十年,人们对肾上腺髓质素(一种生物活性肽)进行了深入研究,发现它有诸如舒张血管、利钠、利尿等多种生物作用。

natriuretic [ˌneitrijuəˈretik] *a.* 促钠尿排泄的,利钠的
One of the spectacular advances in the past 40 years in the treatment of cardiac failure has been the development of natriuretic agents.
过去四十年心衰治疗的突出进展之一是排钠利尿剂的发展。
Atrial natriuretic peptide is synthesized in cardiac atrial muscle.
心房利钠肽是在心房肌中合成的。
Most diuretics are natriuretics that promote the excretion of sodium salts in the urine.
大多数利尿剂是能促使尿中钠盐排泄的促尿钠排泄药。

naturally [ˈnætʃərəli] *ad.* 自然地,天然地
Immunity can be acquired naturally or artificially.
免疫能自然获得或人工获得。
Radioactive elements may occur naturally, as is the case with such very heavy isotopes as radium and uranium.
放射性元素可以是天然存在的,如镭和铀一类很重的同位素就是如此。
Naturally a traumatic hole in the artery is an uncontrolled leak and lowers arterial pressure.
当然,动脉创伤口是一个控制不了的漏洞,且能降低动脉压。

nature [ˈneitʃə(r)] *n.* 大自然;性质;本质
Man is engaged in a constant struggle with nature.
人类在不断地与大自然作斗争。
Chemists study the nature of gases.
化学家研究气体的性质。
Many important questions in immunology have centred on the nature of the receptor on T cells that mediates specific antigen recognition.
许多免疫学的重要问题都集中在能介导特异性抗原识别的 T 细胞受体的性质上。
Visceral pain is described as dull and aching in nature.
内脏痛本质上是一种模糊不清的疼痛。

nausea [ˈnɔːsiə] *n.* 恶心
Varying degrees of nausea and vomiting are common.
各种程度不同的恶心和呕吐是常见的现象。
The symptoms of the disease include nausea, vomiting and diarrhea as well as acute abdominal pain or colic.
此病的症状有恶心、呕吐、腹泻及急性腹痛或绞痛。

nearsightedness [ˌniəˈsaitidnis] *n.* 近视,眼光短浅
Nearsightedness is a condition in which the eyeball is too long from front to back.
近视是眼球前后距离过长的一种病态。
The implantable lenses can be designed to correct farsightedness or nearsightedness.
可植入的人工晶体经过设计可以矫正远视或近视。

nebulizer [ˈnebjuːlaizə] *n.* 喷雾器,雾化器
Nebulizer is an instrument used for applying a liquid in the form of a fine spray.
喷雾器是一种把液体变成细小雾滴的器械。
Bronchodilators and mucolytic agents given by nebulizer may help in patients with severe chronic obstructive pulmonary disease.
经雾化器给予支气管扩张剂和溶解黏液的药物,对患有严重慢性阻塞性肺部疾患者可能有帮助。

necessarily [ˈnesisərili] *ad.* 必定,必然

It should be borne is mind that fracture is not necessarily the consequence of an unusual external stress.

应当记住,骨折并非一定是外界异常压力作用的结果。

necessitate [niˈsesiteit] *v.* 使成为必需,需要

The small capacity of the stomach necessitates small frequent feedings.

小容量的胃必须少食多餐。

The prevention and cure of a series of diseases necessitated organ grafting at the beginning.

一系列疾病的预防和治疗一开始就需要器官移植。

necessity [niˈsesəti] *n.* 需要;必要性

These specialists ensure that they will always come in cases of extreme necessity.

这些专家保证在特别需要的时候他们一定会来。

When confronted with dyspeptic symptoms of recent origin in a patient over 40 years, the first necessity is to exclude gastric cancer.

每当 40 岁以上病人具有近期消化不良症状时,首先必须排除胃癌。

necrobiosis [ˌnekrəubaiˈəusis] *n.* 渐进性坏死

Necrobiosis lipoidica (with or without diabetes) presents as bilateral, well-defined plaques with a smooth, glistening surface and yellow color.

脂性渐进性坏死(伴或不伴有糖尿病),表现为对称的、境界清楚的斑块,表面黄色,光滑发亮。

Necrobiosis lipoidica is a necrotizing skin condition that usually occurs in patients with diabetes.

类脂质渐进性坏死是一种常见于糖尿病患者中的慢性皮肤疾病。

necropsy [ˈnekrɔpsi] *n.* 尸体剖检,验尸

Necropsy revealed gross cardiomegaly with severe coronary artery disease.

尸检发现明显心脏肥大,伴有严重冠心病。

What has been found by necropsy is of utmost importance.

尸检所发现的(情况)是极其重要的。

necrose [neˈkrəus] *v.* 发生坏死

The tissue becomes necrosed.

此处组织发生坏死。

necrosis [neˈkrəusis] (*pl.* necroses [neˈkrəusiːz]) *n.* 坏死

Acute massive necrosis is an extremely rare complication but invariably fatal.

急性大片坏死是一种极少见的并发症,常不可避免地引起死亡。

Severe nuclear damage is customarily taken as evidence of cell necrosis.

严重核损伤通常被认为是细胞坏死的证据。

necrospermia [ˌnekrə(u)ˈspəːmiə] *n.* 死精子症

Further, the zinc levels of seminal plasma in the necrospermia group were lower than those in the control group.

进而,死精症组精浆锌含量低于正常对照组。

necrotic [neˈkrɔtik] *a.* 坏死的

The cells have become necrotic.

这些细胞已经坏死。

On examination, the throat was found full of necrotic materials.

检查发现,咽部充满了坏死物质。

necrotizing [ˈnekrətaiziŋ] *a.* 坏死性的

The lesions are those of a bronchopneumonia accompanied by hemorrhage and necrotizing bronchitis.

病变表现为支气管肺炎,伴有出血性和坏死性支气管炎。

needle ['niːdl] *n.* 针;穿刺针

Hollow needles are used to inject substances into the body, to obtain specimens of tissue, or to withdraw fluid from a cavity.

空心针头用于向体内注射药物,获取组织标本,或从腔室中抽出液体。

The needle should be aligned in the direction of the vein when performing a venipuncture.

作静脉穿刺时,穿刺针应与静脉走向一致。

After the biopsy needle is inserted, a small amount(preferably<0. 5ml) of marrow is aspirated into a syringe.

在活检用的穿刺针插入后,少量骨髓(最好<0. 5ml)可吸入注射器内。

negate [ni'geit] *v.* 否定,否认

However, this study does not negate the fact that certain viruses can and do produce congenital malformation.

然而,这个研究不能否定下列事实,即某些病毒能够而且实际上引起先天畸形。

negative ['negətiv] *a.* 阴性的

Sputum cultures are usually negative.

痰培养通常为阴性。

Positive findings have much more significance than negative ones.

阳性结果比阴性结果有更大的意义。

negligent ['neglidʒənt] *a.* 疏忽

He was negligent of his duties.

他玩忽职守。

negligible ['neglidʒəbl] *a.* 可以忽略的,微不足道的

With the introduction of rifampin, TB has decreased in mortality to a negligible low.

采用利福平之后,结核病的死亡率已降至微不足道的低点。

The complications of this operation are not negligible.

这种手术的合并症是不可忽视的。

This is statistically negligible.

这一点在统计学上是可忽略不计的。

Neisseria [nai'siəriə] *n.* 奈瑟菌属

Meningococcal infections are caused by Neisseria meningitidis.

脑膜炎球菌感染由脑膜炎奈瑟菌引起。

neoadjuvant [ˌniːəu'ædjuvənt] *n.* 新佐剂 *a.* 新辅助的

In all these patients, surgery should be the treatment of choice, and neoadjuvant chemotherapy is advisable.

对所有这些病人来说,手术应该是首选治疗,辅助化疗也是可取的。

Evaluate the safety of neoadjuvant chemoradiation with 5-fluorouracil in rectal cancer.

评价用5-氟尿嘧啶作为直肠癌辅助化疗的安全性。

neocentromere [niəu'sentrəmiə] *n.* 新着丝粒

Some marker chromosomes lack identifiable centromeric DNA sequences, but contain neocentromeres.

有些标记染色体没有明确的着丝粒 DNA 序列,但含有新着丝粒。

These marker chromosomes containing neocentromeres represent small fragments of chromosome arms that have somehow acquired centromere activity.

这些含有新着丝粒的标记染色体来自染色体臂片段,具有一些着丝粒活性。

neomycin [ˌniəu'maisin] *n.* 新霉素

Neomycin is soluble but is not absorbed from the gastrointestinal tract.

新霉素是水溶性的,但不被胃肠道吸收。

This is commonly done for the preoperative "sterilization" of the bowel by drugs such as neomy-

cin.
用新霉素这类药进行手术前肠道消毒是常有的事。

neonatal [ˌniəuˈneitl] *a.* 新生(期)的

Patients with moderate-to-large ventricular septal defects usually do not exhibit cardiac murmurs in the early neonatal period.
具有中型到大型室间隔缺损的患者在新生儿早期经常不出现心脏杂音。

neonate [ˈniəuneit] *n.* 新生儿 *a.* 新生的

Meningitis has the worst prognosis in the neonate.
新生儿患脑膜炎的预后最为不良。
An additional 3-30% of neonates may be infected at the time of delivery because of exposure to infected cervical secretions or breast milk.
此外,3%～30%新生儿由于接触已有感染的宫颈分泌物或母乳,可在分娩时受到感染。

neoplasia [ˌni(ː)əuˈpleiziə] *n.* 瘤形成

Because of the nature and complexity of neoplasia, it is difficult to compose a simple definition that will characterize or be appropriate for all tumors.
由于肿瘤形成的性质和复杂性,很难下一个表示所有肿瘤特征的或适用于所有肿瘤的简单定义。

neoplasm [ˈniəuplæzm] *n.* 新生物,(肿)瘤

Neoplasm means a new and abnormal growth: any benign or malignant tumour.
新生物指新的和异常的生长物:可以是任何良性或恶性肿瘤。
There are numerous varieties of ovarian neoplasms and cysts.
卵巢肿瘤和囊肿的种类很多。
The suffix "-oma" is usually reserved for neoplasm.
"-oma"这一后缀通常只用于表示肿瘤。

neoplastic [niəuˈplæstik] *a.* 赘生物的,瘤的

Examination of the sputum for neoplastic cells may establish the diagnosis in some cases.
检查痰中肿瘤细胞,可对某些病例作出诊断。

neostigmine [ˌniəuˈstigmin] *n.* 新斯的明

Neostigmine, unable to penetrate the blood-brain barrier, does not cause CNS toxicities.
新斯的明不能透过血脑屏障,因而不引起中枢神经系统中毒。

neovascularization [ˈniːəuˌvæskjuləraiˈzeiʃən] *n.* 新生血管形成

By 5 to 7 days after injury, granulation tissue fills the wound area and neovascularization is maximal.
损伤后5～7天,肉芽组织填补缺损,新生血管形成达到高峰。
Neovascularization refers to the blood vessel formation in adults and involves the branching and extension of adjacent pre-existing vessels.
新生血管形成是指在成人体内血管的形成,涉及已存在血管的分支和延长。

nephrectomy [neˈfrektəmi] *n.* 肾切除术

A left nephrectomy with excision of a retroperitoneal mass was carried out.
施行了左肾切除术并摘除了一腹膜后肿块。
Partial nephrectomy may be performed for carcinoma of a solitary kidney or tumor involving both kidneys.
单肾肿瘤或双肾肿瘤均可作部分肾切除术。

nephritic [niˈfritik] *a.* 肾炎的

The manifestations of nephritic syndrome include grossly visible hematuria, mild to moderate proteinuria, edema and hypertension.
肾炎综合征的临床表现包括肉眼血尿、轻至中度蛋白尿、水肿和高血压。
Nephritic syndrome is the classic presentation of acute poststreptococcal glomerulonephritis.

肾炎综合征是急性链球菌感染后肾小球肾炎的典型表现。

nephritis [neˈfraitis] *n.* 肾炎

The prognosis of patients with acute nephritis is usually favourable.

患急性肾炎病人的预后通常是良好的。

Chronic nephritis is a disease hard to get rid of.

慢性肾炎是一种难以根治的疾病。

nephroblastoma [ˌnefrəublæˈstəumə] *n.* 肾母细胞瘤

The results suggested that the genesis of nephroblastoma is relevant to the retarded differentiation of fetal kidney.

结果显示肾母细胞瘤的发生与胚胎肾分化停滞有关。

MVC is an indicator of the prognosis of patients with nephroblastoma.

MVC 是判断肾母细胞瘤患者预后的指标。

nephrogenic [ˌnefrəˈdʒenik] *a.* 肾源性的

Nephrogenic adenoma is an unusual lesion that in the past was believed to represent metaplasia of the urothelium in response to injury.

肾源性腺瘤是一种不常见的病变,过去认为是代表尿路上皮损伤后的化生。

Nephrogenic adenoma is typically less than a centimeter, but may be sizable, and may resemble cancer clinically.

典型的肾源性腺瘤小于 1cm,但也可以相当大,临床上类似于癌。

nephrolithiasis [ˌnefrəuliˈθaiəsis] *n.* 肾结石,肾石病

These abscesses generally arise from an initial urinary tract infection, often in association with nephrolithiasis.

这些脓肿来源于原发的尿路感染,后者多与肾结石有关。

nephrolithotomy [ˌnefrəuliˈθɔtəmi] *n.* 肾石切除术

Nephrolithotomy is normally performed in combination with an incision into the renal pelvis.

肾石切除术通常与肾盂的切开同时进行。

nephrologist [neˈfrɔlədʒist] *n.* 肾病学专家

Nephrologists have attempted for years to find a solution to the problem.

肾病学家们多年来试图找出解决此问题的方法。

nephron [ˈnefrɔn] *n.* 肾单位

The functional unit of the kidneys is the nephron.

肾脏的功能单位为肾单位。

As more and more nephrons are destroyed, the kidney shrinks in size, and its efficiency is gradually decreased.

由于肾单位的损坏越来越多,肾脏常皱缩变小,其功能也逐渐减退。

nephropathy [niˈfrɔpəθi] *n.* 肾病

IgA nephropathy is characterized by the presence of prominent IgA deposits in the mesangial regions, detected by immunofluorescence microscopy.

IgA 肾病的特征是 IgA 显著沉积于系膜区,可通过免疫荧光显微镜检测。

IgA nephropathy is a frequent cause of recurrent gross or microscopic hematuria and is probably the most common type of glomerulonephritis worldwide.

IgA 肾病是复发性肉眼或镜下血尿的常见原因,它可能是世界上最常见的肾小球肾炎。

nephropexy [ˈnefrəˌpeksi] *n.* 肾固定术

Nephropexy is the surgical fixation of a floating or mobile kidney.

肾固定术是用外科手术固定浮动或游走肾。

The aim of the study was to design an experimental model for more reliable nephropexy.

这项研究的目的是设计一个更可靠肾固定术的实验模型。

nephroptosis [ˌnefrɔpˈtəusis] *n.* 肾下垂

If this action fails to work normally, such prolapses as gastroptosis, nephroptosis, hysteroptosis will be brought about.

如果该功能不能正常运行,则会出现诸如胃下垂、肾下垂、子宫下垂等病状。

The kidney fixation was used to treat nephroptosis by means of the pedicled muscle psoas major with muscle film petal.

肾下垂常采用带蒂腰大肌肌膜瓣的肾固定术来治疗。

nephrosclerosis [ˌnefrəuskliəˈrəusis] *n.* 肾硬化

Microscopic sections showed minimal interstitial nephritis and nephrosclerosis.

显微切片表明有极轻微的间质性肾炎和肾硬化。

nephrosis [neˈfrəusis] *n.* 肾病

The term nephrosis is sometimes used loosely for the nephrotic syndrome.

肾病一词有时用来泛指肾病综合征。

Nephrosis is characterized by a group of symptoms resulting from kidney tissue damage and impaired nephric function.

肾病以一组因肾组织损伤和肾功能受损而导致的症状为特征。

nephrostomy [neˈfrɔstəmi] *n.* 肾造口术

Long-term urine drainage by nephrostomy may be complicated by the attendant problems of infection.

肾造口术所致的长期尿引流可能并发随之而来的感染问题。

Obstruction of the upper urinary tract can be treated by insertion of a catheter into the renal pelvis under ultrasound guidance(percutaneous nephrostomy).

上尿路梗阻可以通过在超声引导下插管至肾盂来治疗(经皮肾造口术)。

nephrotic [neˈfrɔtik] *a.* 肾病的

Children with nephrotic syndrome generally have minor glomerular changes on renal biopsy.

肾病综合征患儿经肾组织活检通常可见有轻微的肾小球改变。

nephrotoxicity [ˌnefrəutɔkˈsisiti] *n.* 肾中毒

Infrequent nephrotoxicity does occur with some cephalosporins.

某些头孢菌素类的确偶尔可引起肾脏中毒。

nerve [nəːv] *n.* 神经

The basic unit of nervous system is the individual nerve cell.

神经系统的基本单位是单个神经细胞。

Some nerve axon are several feet long.

有些神经轴突长达数英尺。

nestin [ˈnestin] *n.* 巢蛋白

Nestin was originally described as a neuronal stem cell marker during central nervous system development.

巢蛋白最初被认为是中枢神经系统发育过程中的一种神经元干细胞的标记。

Nestin is an intermediate filament protein expressed transiently by neural progenitor cells and reactivated glial cells and is involved in cell survival and repair.

巢蛋白是短暂表达于神经元前体细胞和活化胶质细胞的一种中间丝蛋白,参与细胞存活和修复。

net [net] *a.* 纯净的 *n.* 净值

The result is a net intraluminal secretion of water and electrolytes.

其结果是一种单纯的水及电解质的肠腔内分泌。

network [ˈnetwəːk] *n.* 网,网状结构;网络

The capillary network forms an efficient arrangement for gas exchange.

毛细血管网为气体交换形成了有效的安排。

You can plug into the national computer network.

你可以接通全国计算机网络。

neural [ˈnjuərəl] *a.* 神经的

Breathnach believes the Merkel cell to be of neural crest origin rather than of either ectodermal or mesenchymal origin.

Breathnach 认为梅克尔细胞源于神经嵴而不是源于外胚叶或间质。

The melanocyte, derived from the neural crest, is the pigment-producing cell of the epidermis.

源于神经嵴的黑素细胞是表皮内产生色素的细胞。

neuralgia [njuəˈrældʒiə] *n.* 神经痛

The current hypothesis as to etiology suggests that the neuralgia is most commonly caused by compression of the nerve roots.

目前对于神经痛病因的假说认为神经痛多由于神经根受压引起。

Trigeminal neuralgia is an excruciating, sharp pain experienced in one of the divisions of the trigeminal nerve.

三叉神经痛是一种发生于三叉神经某一分支内的剧烈锐痛。

neuraminidase [ˌnjuərəˈminideiz] *n.* 神经氨酸酶

Neuraminidase enzymes are glycoside hydrolase enzymes that cleave the glycosidic linkages of neuraminic acids.

神经氨酸酶是分解神经氨酸糖苷键的糖苷水解酶。

The best-known neuraminidase is the viral neuraminidase, a drug target for the prevention of the spread of influenza infection.

最有名的神经氨酸酶是病毒神经氨酸酶,它是阻止流感传播的一个药物靶点。

neurasthenia [ˌnjuərəsˈθiːniə] *n.* 神经衰弱

Neurasthenia can be caused by organic damage, such as a head injury, or it can be due to neurosis.

神经衰弱的病因可为器质性损伤,如头部损伤,亦可为神经官能症。

Neurathenia is a neurotic disorder characterized by fatigue, irritability, headache, depression, insomnia, and difficulty in concentration.

神经衰弱是以疲乏、易激惹、头痛、抑郁、失眠和注意力难以集中为特征的一种神经症性疾病。

neurilemma [ˌnjuəriˈlemə] *n.* 神经膜

The brain and the spinal cord have no neurilemma.

脑和脊髓没有神经膜。

Neurilemma is a part of the mechanism by which the peripheral nerves repair themselves when damaged.

神经膜是周围神经受损伤时自我修复机制的一部分。

neurinosarcoma [ˌnjuərinəusɑːˈkəumə] *n.* 神经鞘肉瘤

Of particular significance is the observation of uterine-vaginal neurinosarcomas(all grossly detected), which are rarely observed in the historical controls.

对子宫阴道神经鞘肉瘤的观察(全部肉眼检查),具有特殊的意义,在历史的对照(标本)中,这种肉瘤非常少见。

neuritis [njuːˈraitis] *n.* 神经炎

Neuritis is a disease of the peripheral nerves showing the pathological changes of inflammation.

神经炎是具有炎症性病理变化的周围神经病变。

Alcoholic neuritis is due to thiamine deficiency in chronic alcoholism.

酒精性神经炎是由于慢性酒精中毒时硫胺(维生素 B_1)缺乏所致。

neurobiology [ˌnjuərəubaiˈɔlədʒi] *n.* 神经生物学

This review summarizes recent research in sirtuin neurobiology.

这篇综述概述了长寿蛋白神经生物学的近期研究。

The neurobiology of Alzheimer disease was defined by neuroimaging.
阿尔茨海默病的神经生物学系由神经影像学来界定。

neuroblastoma [ˌnjuərəublæs'təumə] *n.* 成神经细胞瘤

Bone marrow metastasis occurs early in neuroblastoma and with high frequency.
在成神经细胞瘤中骨髓转移发生较早，发生率亦高。

neurocutaneous [ˌnjuərəukju'teiniəs] *a.* 皮神经的

An increased incidence of certain intracranial neoplasms is seen in the neurocutaneous syndromes.
在皮肤神经综合征的患者可以看到某些颅内肿瘤的发病率也不断增加。

neurocytoma [ˌnjuərəsai'təumə] *n.* 神经细胞瘤

Composed of small round cells with neuronal differentiation, neurocytoma has a particularly favorable prognosis.
神经细胞瘤由伴有神经元分化的小圆形细胞构成，预后相当好。

The cellular origin of central neurocytoma and the molecular events leading to tumorigenesis have been largely unknown.
中枢神经细胞瘤的细胞起源和导致肿瘤发生的分子机制在很大程度上还是未知的。

neurodegenerative [ˌnjuːrəudi'dʒenərətiv] *a.* 神经变性的

Alzheimer disease is one of neurodegenerative diseases.
阿尔茨海默病是神经变性性疾病之一。

Parkinson's disease is the second most common neurodegenerative disorder.
帕金森氏病是第二最常见的神经变性性疾病。

neurodevelopmental [ˌnjuərəudiˌveləp'mentəl] *a.* 神经发育的

Minor physical anomalies may provide important clues to understanding schizophrenia spectrum disorders from a neurodevelopmental perspective.
从神经发育学的角度，微小躯体异常可以为理解精神分裂症谱系疾病提供重要的线索。

Our results provided direct evidence that ADHD is a neurodevelopmental disorder.
我们的研究结果给出了 ADHD（多动症）是一种神经发育性疾病的直接证据。

neuroendocrine [ˌnjuərəu'endəkrain] *n.* 神经内分泌

The bronchial mucosa contains a population of neuroendocrine cells that have neurosecretory-type granules.
支气管黏膜包含神经内分泌细胞群，细胞内有神经内分泌颗粒。

All small cell carcinomas are high grade and poorly differentiated neuroendocrine carcinoma.
所以小细胞癌都是高级别低分化的神经内分泌癌。

neurofibrillary [ˌnjuərəu'faibriləri] *a.* 神经原纤维的

These findings may have implications for therapeutic strategies aiming at prevention of neurofibrillary degeneration and cognitive decline, and identify potential new targets for drug development.
这些发现可能蕴含着阻止神经原纤维变性和认知减退的治疗策略，并且有可能找出药物开发的新靶点。

neurofibroma [ˌnjuərəufai'brəumə] *n.* 神经纤维瘤

Diffuse neurofibroma occurs most commonly among children and young adults, typically involving the skin and subcutaneous tissues of the head and neck.
弥漫性神经纤维瘤最常见于儿童和青年人，典型发生于头颈部的皮肤和皮下组织。

Diffuse neurofibroma is a poorly defined lesion in the subcutaneous fat that spreads along connective tissue septa and surrounds rather than destroys adjacent normal structures.
弥漫性神经纤维瘤是一种皮下脂肪内的边界不清的病变，沿着结缔组织间隔蔓延，包绕而不是破坏周围正常结构。

neurofibromatosis [ˌnjuərəufiˌbrəumə'təusis] *n.* 神经纤维瘤病

Neurofibromatosis type 2 is an autosomal-dominant inherited tumor predisposition syndrome caused by mutations in the NF2 gene on chromosome 22.

2 型神经纤维瘤病是一种常染色体显性的遗传综合征，具有肿瘤易患性，由 22 号染色体上的 NF2 基因突变导致。

Patients with neurofibromatosis type I have an associated increased risk of certain malignancies.

I 型神经纤维瘤病的患者发生某种恶性肿瘤的危险性明显增加。

neurogenesis [ˌnjuərə ˈdʒenisis] *n.* 神经发生

These findings suggest that the behavioral effects of chronic antidepressants may be mediated by the stimulation of neurogenesis in the hippocampus.

这些发现表明，慢性抗抑郁药的行为影响可能是通过刺激海马神经发生来介导。

neurohumoral [ˌnjuərəuˈhjuːmərəl] *a.* 神经递质的，神经体液的

Congestive heart failure is also characterized by a complex series of neurohumoral adjustment.

充血性心力衰竭也有一系列复杂的神经体液调节过程。

There is accumulating evidence suggesting that neurohumoral activation reduces life expectancy in patients with heart failure.

越来越多的证据表明神经体液激活能减少心衰病人的预期寿命。

neuroleptic [ˌnjuərəuˈleptik] *a.* 抑制精神的 *n.* 精神抑制药，安定药

Agranulocytosis is an infrequent but potentially fatal side effect of neuroleptic drugs.

粒细胞缺乏症是精神抑制药的一种不常见但可能致命的副作用。

Neuroleptic medications are the primary treatment for these disorders.

精神抑制药治疗是这些疾病的主要治疗方式。

neurologic [ˌnjuərəˈlɔdʒik] *a.* 神经的

The neurologic symptoms noted with botulism help differentiate it from staphylococcal food poisoning.

由肉毒中毒而产生的神经系统症状，有助于与葡萄球菌性食物中毒相鉴别。

It often takes many months of hospitalization to recover from neurologic dysfunction.

神经功能障碍常需住院好几个月才能痊愈。

neurological [ˌnjuərəˈlɔdʒikəl] *a.* 神经病学的

Neurological signs are uncommon in delirium.

谵妄不常出现神经病学体征。

These genes may represent a promising target for the therapeutic drug development for Alzheimer's disease (AD) and other neurological disorders.

这些基因可能代表着阿尔茨海默病(AD)和其他神经疾病治疗性药物开发的一个有希望的靶位。

neurology [njuəˈrɔlədʒi] *n.* 神经学，神经病学

Detection of the presence and nature of facial paresis is a common exercise in neurology.

检查面神经麻痹及其性质是神经病学常用的方法。

neuroma [njuəˈrəumə] (*pl.* neuromas or neuromata [njuəˈrəumətə]) *n.* 神经瘤

The symptoms of Morton's neuroma are usually pain and numbness of adjacent toes.

Morton 神经瘤的症状常有邻近的足趾出现麻木和疼痛。

Rarely, a neuroma in the wound can be responsible for focal pain and tenderness late in the postoperative course.

罕见的是伤口内神经瘤能在术后很久引起病灶区的疼痛及压痛。

neuromuscular [ˌnjuərəuˈmʌskjulə] *a.* 神经肌肉的

ACTH (adrenocorticotropic hormone) has been advocated for the treatment of certain neuromuscular illnesses.

促肾上腺皮质激素已被提倡用来治疗某些神经肌肉疾病。

neuromyelitis [ˌnjuərəˈmaiəˈlaitis] *n.* 神经脊髓炎

Neuromyelitis optica is an inflammatory, demyelinating disease of the central nervous system.
视神经脊髓炎是一种炎症性的、中枢神经脱髓鞘的病变。

The term neuromyelitis optica refers to the co-occurrence of optic neuritis and myelitis.
视神经脊髓炎这一术语指的是视神经炎和脊髓炎共存。

neuron [ˈnjuərɔn] *n.* 神经元

The sensory or afferent fibers of cranial nerves arise from neurons outside the brain.
脑神经的感觉纤维或传入纤维起自脑外的神经元。

neuronal [ˈnjuərənəl] *a.* 神经元的

In this respect any drugs which stabilize the normal neuronal membrane can be expected to be of benefit.
在这方面，任何稳定正常神经元膜的药物都可预期有良好疗效。

neuronophagia [ˌnjuərənəuˈfeidʒiə] *n.* 噬神经细胞现象

This is an example of neuronophagia in which a dying neuron is surrounded by microglial cells.
这是噬神经细胞现象的一个实例，一个垂死的神经元被小胶质细胞包绕。

Pathologic examination reveals perivascular mononuclear infiltrates and neuronophagia.
病理检查显示血管周单核细胞浸润和噬神经细胞现象。

neuropathogenesis [ˌnjuərəuˌpæθəˈdʒenisis] *n.* 神经病发病机制，神经病发生

That may contribute to our knowledge of VZV neuropathogenesis.
这可能有助于我们理解水痘带状疱疹病毒的神经发病机制。

These are critical in HIV neuropathogenesis.
这些对 HIV 的神经发病机制很是关键。

neuropathy [njuəˈrɔpəθi] *n.* 神经病

Any disease of the peripheral nerves, usually causing weakness and numbness, is termed neuropathy.
外周神经的疾病叫神经病，常引起无力和麻木。

Acute ischemic optic neuropathy can produce pale swelling of the optic disc.
急性缺血性视神经病能引起视盘的苍白色水肿。

neuropeptide [ˌnjuərəˈpeptaid] *n.* 神经肽

The immunohistochemical method was used to show the neuropeptide expressions in situ.
利用免疫组织化学方法在组织原位显示(胸腺内的)神经肽的表达。

Neuropeptide Y is an important sympathetic vasoconstrictive neurotransmitter, and plays roles with norepinephrine together.
神经肽 Y 是一种重要的交感缩血管神经递质，与去甲肾上腺素共同发挥作用。

neuropharmacology [ˌnjuərəuˌfɑːməˈkɔlədʒi] *n.* 神经药理学

Neuropharmacology may be defined as the study of drugs that affect the nervous system and its neuronal components.
神经药理学是对影响神经系统及其神经元成分的药物进行研究的科学。

neuropil [ˈnjuərəpil] *n.* 神经毡

Glioneuronal tumor with neuropil-like islands is considered a rare variant of astrocytoma, characterized by discrete neuronal differentiated cells with a GFAP-positive glial background.
伴有神经毡样岛的胶质神经元肿瘤被认为是星形细胞瘤的一种少见变异，其特征是在 GFAP 阳性的胶质背景中散在神经元分化的细胞。

Embryonal tumor with abundant neuropil and true rosettes is an increasingly recognized entity that belongs to the family of embryonal tumors of the CNS.
伴有丰富神经毡和真菊形团的胚胎性肿瘤是一种逐渐被认识的疾病，属于 CNS 中胚胎性肿瘤家族。

neuropsychology [ˌnjuərəusaiˈkɔlədʒi] *n.* 神经心理学

Research in child neuropsychology has relied on the study of children who suffer from developmental disorders.
对儿童神经心理学的研究依赖于对发育障碍患儿的研究。

neuroscience [ˌnjuərəu'saiəns] *n.* 神经系统科学
The word "neuroscience" is young.
"Neuroscience"这个词语出现还不久。
The Society for Neuroscience was founded as recently as 1970.
神经系统科学学会创立于 1970 年。

neurosis [njuə'rəusis]（*pl.* neuroses [njuə'rəusiːz] ）*n.* 神经官能症
The patient with neurosis avoided the doctor' s questions.
那个神经官能症患者对医生的提问避而不答。
In the so-called cardiac neurosis, precordial distress is brought on by exertion or excitement.
在所谓的心脏神经官能症中，劳累或兴奋会引起心前区不适。

neurosurgeon [ˌnjuərəu'səːdʒən] *n.* 神经外科医生
I' ve been a neurosurgeon for 40 years.
我已当了 40 年的神经外科医生。

neurosurgery [ˌnjuərə'səːdʒəri] *n.* 神经外科(学)
Separate intensive care units are established for neurosurgery.
神经外科建立了单独的重症监护室。
He is a chief physician in the department of neurosurgery of Union Hospital.
他是协和医院神经外科的一位主任医师。

neurosurgical [ˌnjuərəu'səːdʒikəl] *a.* 神经外科的
In advanced cases, neurosurgical measures may be required for the relief of intractable pain.
对于晚期病人，需要通过神经外科措施来缓解病人顽固性疼痛。

neurotensin [ˌnjuərəu'tensin] *n.* 神经降压素
Neurotensin's influence, they found, depends on biochemical signaling pathways inside the cell.
他们发现神经降压素的影响依赖于细胞内生物化学信号途径。
This article deals with the changes of neuropeptide Y（NPY）and neurotensin（NT）in platelet extract and in plasma during hemodialysis（HD）.
本文探讨血液透析(HD)过程血小板提取液和等离子体中神经肽 Y(NPY)与神经降压素(NT)的含量变化。

neurotoxicity [ˌnjuərəutɔk'sisəti] *n.* 神经毒性
Neurotoxicity is the most common adverse drug reaction seen in clinic.
神经毒性是临床上最常见的药物不良反应。
A number of reports have appeared implicating neurotoxicity of local anesthetics as a possible cause of neurologic complications after spinal anesthesia.
一些报道已经显示局麻药的潜在神经毒性是脊髓麻醉后神经并发症的一个可能原因。

neurotoxicology [njuərəˌtɔksi'kɔlədʒi] *n.* 神经毒理学
The International Neurotoxicology Association is an organization of scientists working in the field of neurotoxicology.
国际神经毒理学协会是一个在神经毒理学领域工作的科学家组织。
Neurotoxicology is defined as the science that deals with the adverse effects of naturally occurring and synthetic chemical agents on the structure or function of the nervous system.
神经毒理学是一门科学，它研究天然和合成化学药剂对神经系统结构或功能的不良反应。

neurotransmitter [ˌnjuərəutræns'mitə] *n.* 神经递质
Neurotransmitters are the chemical agents of communication between the neurons of brain.
神经递质是大脑神经元之间信息交流的化学物质。

neurotropism [njuə'rɔtrəpizəm] *n.* 向神经性，亲神经性，神经趋向性

The severity of inner ear infection was correlated with the CNS lesions, confirming the neurotropism of CMV.

内耳感染的严重性与中枢神经系统的损害有关,证实巨细胞病毒的亲神经性。

Our study is to investigate the neurotropism of varicella zoster virus.

我们在研究水痘带状疱疹病毒的神经趋向性。

neurovirulence [ˌnjuərəu'viruləns] *n.* 神经毒力(指病原体侵害神经的能力)

Investigating pathogenic mechanisms that contribute to CMV neurovirulence is difficult.

研究巨细胞病毒产生神经毒力的发病机制是困难的。

neutral ['njuːtrəl] *a.* 中立的,中性的

Organic anions combine with organic cations to form a neutral complex.

有机的阴离子与阳离子结合形成一个中性复合物。

In a neutral environment, the metabolic rate of humans consistently produces more heat than is necessary to maintain the core body temperature at 37℃.

在正常情况下,人体代谢所产生的热量一般较保持核心体温于37℃所必需的热量多。

neutralize ['njuːtrəlaiz] *v.* 中和;(使)成为无效

Initially, the presence of food neutralized excess acid in the stomach.

在起始时,食物的存在中和了过多的胃酸。

Several types of antibodies neutralize the adverse effects of the parasite multiplication.

有几种类型的抗体可消除寄生虫繁殖产生的有害作用。

neutrino [njuː'triːnəu] 中微子

The physical characteristics of the neutrino are remarkable.

中微子的物理特征非同寻常。

There is a lepton which is neutral, called a neutrino.

中性的轻子叫做中微子。

neutron ['njuːtrɔn] *n.* 中子

Carbon-14 contains eight neutrons.

14C 含有 8 个中子。

A neutron having an energy level exceeding 105 electron volts is called fast neutron.

一个中子的能级超过 105 电子伏称作快中子。

neutropenia [ˌnjuːtrəu'piːniə] *n.* 中性白细胞减少(症)

Neutropenia is a reduction below normal of the numbers of circulating neutrophils.

中性粒细胞减少症是循环血中的中性粒细胞计数减少至正常以下的一种病症。

neutrophil ['njutrəfil] *n.* 嗜中性白细胞

The leukocytes are almost entirely neutrophils in purulent meningitis.

患化脓性脑膜炎时,白细胞几乎完全是嗜中性细胞。

Phagocytosis of bacteria by neutrophils is an imperfect process.

嗜中性白细胞对细菌的吞噬作用是一个不完整的过程。

neutrophilia [ˌnjuːtrəu'filiə] *n.* 中性粒细胞增多(症)

Neutrophilia in adults is defined as an absolute blood neutrophil count of more than 7500 cells/mm^3.

成人的中性粒细胞增多症是指血液中的中性粒细胞绝对值超过 7500 细胞/mm^3。

nevertheless [ˌnevəðə'les] *conj.* 然而

Nevertheless, when confronted with dyspeptic symptoms of recent origin in a patient over 40 years the first necessity is to exclude gastric cancer.

然而每当 40 岁以上病人出现近期消化不良症状时,首先必须排除胃癌。

The epididymal tumor becomes smaller; nevertheless almost always a residual inflammation remains.

附睾肿块变小,但几乎总有残余炎症发生。

nevus [ˈniːvəs] (*pl.* nevi [ˈniːvai]) *n.* 痣

There was a capillary flame nevus on the forehead.

前额有一毛细血管火焰状痣。

Darkening may be due to inflammation, nevi, lentigines, melasma, etc.

颜色加深可能是由于炎症、痣、着色斑、黄褐斑等所致。

newborn [ˈnjuːbɔːn] *n.* 新生儿

Retrolental fibroplasia(RLF) may appear after the use of oxygen in the newborn.

给新生儿氧气后可能出现晶状体后纤维组织形成。

a. 新生的

A newborn child comes equipped with a finely-tuned pair of ears, but he doesn't know how to use them.

新生小孩一出世就有一对听力很好的耳朵，但他不知道如何使用它们。

niacin [ˈnaiəsin] *n.* 尼克酸，抗糙皮病维生素，维生素 PP

Niacin is found in meats, poultry, fish and brewer's yeast.

维生素 PP 存在于肉、家禽、鱼和啤酒酵母中。

Niacin, for example, can readily be converted to nicotinamide adenine dinucleotide(NAD).

尼克酸很容易转变为尼克酰胺腺嘌呤二核苷酸。

niclosamide [niˈkləusəmaid] *n.* 氯硝柳胺

Niclosamide appears to be the best molluscacide and has an excellent record in some countries.

氯硝柳胺似乎是最好的灭螺剂，在一些国家其应用效果非常良好。

nicotinamide [ˌnikɔˈtinəmaid] *n.* 烟酰胺

Good sources of nicotinamide are meat, yeast extracts, and some cereals. A deficiency of the vitamin leads to pellagra.

烟酰胺的极好来源是肉、酵母浸出物和某些谷类。缺乏此种维生素可引起糙皮病。

nicotine [ˈnikətin] *n.* 尼古丁

Nicotine induces vasospasm and may aggravate preexisting angina pectoris.

尼古丁可引起血管痉挛，并能使原来就有的心绞痛加重。

Nicotine is a very poisonous colorless. soluble fluid alkaloid obtained from tobacco or produced synthetically.

尼古丁(烟碱)是毒性很强的无色的可溶性液体生物碱，可以从烟草中得到或由人工合成产生。

nicotinic [ˌnikəˈtinik] *a.* 烟碱的

Nicotinic acid is thought to inhibit release of VLDL from the liver.

烟酸被认为可抑制肝脏释放 VLDL(超低密度脂蛋白)。

Deficiency of nicotinic acid is associated with sun-exposed skin rash, glossitis, and angular stomatitis.

烟碱酸缺乏表现为日晒后出现皮疹、舌炎和口角炎。

nidus [ˈnaidəs] *n.* 巢，核，滋生地

The nidus of an osteoid osteoma consists of an interlacing network of osteoid and bony trabeculae.

骨样骨瘤的骨巢由相互交错的骨样组织和骨小梁构成。

Bacteria or bile pigment may serve as a nidus for crystal formation.

细菌或胆色素可作为结晶形成的滋生地。

nifedipine [naiˈfedipiːn] *n.* 硝苯吡啶，利心平，心痛定

Calcium channel blockers such as nifedipine are useful for Raynaud's phenomenon.

钙通道阻滞剂如心痛定对雷诺氏现象(的治疗)有效。

nigrosin [ˈnaigrəsiːn] *n.* 苯胺黑

Dyes such as congo red or nigrosin can be used for negative staining.

刚果红或苯氨黑等染料可用作负染剂。

nimodipine [niˈmɔdipiːn] *n.* 尼莫地平

The administration of nimodipine reduces the morbidity from vascular spasm.

服用尼莫地平可减少血管痉挛的发病率。

niosome [ˈnaiəsəum] *n.* 类脂质体，泡囊

Preparation of niosomes was optimized for highest percent drug entrapment.

优化类脂质体制备以达最高的药物包封率。

The niosome diameter is between 100 and 180 nm.

类脂质体的直径在 100 ~ 180 纳米之间。

nipagin [ˈniːpədʒin,ˈnai-] *n.* 尼泊金，对羟基苯甲酸甲酯(防腐剂)

Nipagin M is an inert substance, and has good compatibility with various chemicals.

尼泊金甲酯是一种惰性物质，它与多种化学药品具有良好的相容性。

Nipagin was not detected in two commercial soy sauces by this method.

用这种方法在售卖的两种酱油中未检测出尼泊金。

nitrate [ˈnaitreit] *n.* 硝酸盐

Food additives, such as nitrates in bacon and other meats, have been linked to gastrointestinal cancer.

食品添加剂，如薰猪肉和其他肉类食品中的硝酸盐，与胃肠道癌症有关。

nitrite [ˈnaitrait] *n.* 亚硝酸盐

Nitroglycerin and other nitrites are not given orally in the management of angina pectoris.

硝酸甘油和其他亚硝酸盐类在治疗心绞痛时都不口服给药。

nitrobenzene [ˌnaitrəuˈbenziːn] *n.* 硝基苯

Another drawback is that nitrobenzene is both poisonous and explosive.

另一个缺点是硝基苯既有毒又易爆炸。

In this report, advances on nitrobenzene wastewater treatment in recent years are reviewed.

该报告对近年来硝基苯废水处理的进展进行了综述。

nitrocellulose [ˌnaitrəuˈseljuləus] *n.* 硝化纤维素，火棉

Nitrocellulose is a highly flammable compound formed by nitrating cellulose through exposure to nitric acid or another powerful nitrating agent.

火棉是一种高度易燃的化合物，它是由硝化纤维素与硝酸或另一种强大的硝化试剂反应产生。

Nitrocellulose was used as the first flexible film base, beginning with Eastman Kodak products in August, 1889.

硝化纤维素作为首个弹性片基，于 1889 年 8 月开始用于伊士曼柯达公司产品。

nitrofurazone [ˌnaitrəufəˈræzəun] *n.* 硝基糠腙，呋喃西林

Nitrofurazone is bactericidal for many gram-positive and gram-negative bacteria causing diseases.

呋喃西林是一种杀菌剂，可以治疗革兰氏阳性和阴性菌引起的疾病。

Topical nitrofurazone may cause allergic skin reaction.

局部用呋喃西林可能引起皮肤过敏反应。

nitrogen [ˈnaitridʒən] *n.* 氮

All proteins contain carbon, hydrogen, oxygen, nitrogen, and sulfur.

所有的蛋白质都含有碳、氢、氧、氮和硫。

nitrogenous [naiˈtrɔdʒinəs] *a.* 含氮的

Nucleotide is constructed of three compounds: deoxyribose, phosphate, and nitrogenous base.

核苷酸由脱氧核糖、磷酸和含氮的碱基三种化合物构成。

There are four nitrogenous bases in DNA.

DNA 中有四种含氮的碱基。

nitroglycerin [ˌnaitrəˈglisərin] *n.* 硝酸甘油(三硝酸甘油酯)

The use of nitroglycerin may give relief to the anginal pain at the time of its occurrence.
心绞痛发作时，使用硝酸甘油可以使其缓解。

Nitroglycerin should never be administered to a patient with acute myocardial infarction.
硝酸甘油绝不能给急性心肌梗死的病人服用。

nitrosamine [ˌnaitrəusəˈmiːn] *n.* 亚硝胺

Nitrosamines are chemical compounds that have carcinogenic properties.
亚硝胺是具有致癌特性的化合物。

Tobacco-specific nitrosamines (TSNA) are found only in tobacco products, and are highly carcinogenic.
烟草特有亚硝胺(TSNA)仅存在于烟草产品中，具有高度的致癌性。

nitrosourea [naiˌtrəusəuˈjuəriə] *n.* 亚硝脲

The nitrosoureas have an important role in the treatment of brain tumors.
亚硝脲在脑肿瘤治疗中具有重要作用。

nocardiosis [nəukɑːdiˈəusis] *n.* 诺卡(放线)菌病

In 50% of cases of pulmonary nocardiosis, disease is disseminated outside the lungs.
在患肺部放线菌病的病例中有50%播散到肺外器官。

nociceptive [ˌnəusiˈseptiv] *adj.* 疼痛的；有疼痛反应的

Endogenous descending inhibitory system plays an important role in the modulation of nociceptive transmission.
内源性下行抑制系统在痛觉传递的调节中起重要作用。

Nociceptive pain may be relieved by morphine and non-steroidal anti-inflammatory drugs.
吗啡和非甾体类抗炎药可以缓解伤害性疼痛。

nociceptor [ˌnəusiˈseptə] *n.* 伤害感受器

The nociceptor releases signaling molecules called neurotransmitters that activate neurons in the dorsal horn, prompting them to transmit the alarm message up to the brain.
伤害感受器的神经末梢会释放称为神经递质的信号分子，后者活化背角的神经元，促使它们将警报上传至脑部。

Visceral pain is caused by stimulation of visceral nociceptors by inflammation, distention, or ischemia.
内脏痛是由炎症、腹胀或缺血刺激内脏感受器而产生的。

nocturia [nɔkˈtjuəriə] *n.* 夜尿症

Nocturia is a valuable sign of heart failure.
夜间多尿是心力衰竭一个重要的症状。

nocturnal [nɔkˈtəːnl] *a.* 夜间的，夜间发生的

Approximately 80 percent of patients with chronic obstructive lung diseases have nocturnal oxygen desaturation during sleep.
大概有80%的慢阻肺患者，夜间睡眠时有氧饱和不足现象。

node [nəud] *n.* 结，结节

The sinus node is organized around a central sinus node artery.
窦房结是在一中央窦房结动脉周围形成的。

In most people the primary lesion and the associated lymph node lesion heal and calcify.
绝大多数患者的原发性损害和其局部淋巴结病变都可痊愈和钙化。

nodosum [nəuˈdəusəm] *n.* 结节

Erythema nodosum does occur in pulmonary tuberculosis.
结节性红斑的确可以出现于肺结核。

nodular [ˈnɔdjulə] *a.* 结节状的；有结节的

Focal nodular hyperplasia of liver is sometimes difficult to differentiate from primary hepatic carcinoma.

肝脏局灶性结节样增生有时不易与原发性肝癌鉴别。

Caution must be exercised in the case of hypersensitivity to iodinated contrast media, latent hyperthyroidism and bland nodular goitre.

对碘造影剂过敏、隐匿性甲状腺亢进和轻微结节性甲状腺肿的病例,应慎重。

nodule ['nɔdjuːl] *n.* 结,小结

The hard nodules may eventually break down and form ulcers.

硬结最后可溃破,形成溃疡。

If rheumatic nodules are present, rheumatic infection is active and severe.

如出现风湿性结节,则表明风湿性感染正在活动并且是严重的。

noggin ['nɔgin] *n.* 头蛋白

Noggin was initially found in Xenopus embryo and shown to be essential for head development.

头蛋白最初是在非洲蟾的胚胎中发现的,并显示它对蟾头部的发育是必不可少的。

noise [nɔiz] *n.* 噪声

Our second concern is with shot noise.

我们的第二个顾虑是散粒噪声。

In common use, the word noise means any unwanted sound.

噪声一词常用来指任何不希望听到的声音。

nomenclature [nəu'menklətʃə] *n.* 命名法

The first part offers a concise summary of the nomenclature, chemistry formulations, and the uses of the compound.

第一部分简述该化合物的命名、化学方程式和用途。

noncoding [nɔn'kəudiŋ] *a.* 非编码的

Polymorphisms in noncoding regions of genes may occur in the 3' and 5' untranslated regions, in promoter or enhancer regions, in intronic regions, or in large regions between genes.

非编码区的基因多态性可发生在 3' 和 5' 非翻译区、启动子或增强子区、内含子区、或基因间的大区域内。

nondepolarizer [nʌndiː'pəuləraizə] *n.* 非去极化型肌松药

Rocuronium is the most frequently used nondepolarizer for emergency intubations.

罗库溴铵是紧急插管时最常使用的非去极化型肌松药。

Vecuronium is a nondepolarizer most widely studied for gender differences in its effect.

维库溴铵是一种非去极化型肌松药,最常用于研究性别差异的效应。

nondifferential [ˌnɔndifə'renʃəl] *a.* 无差异性的

Nondifferential underascertainment of drug use will weaken observed associations.

无差异性低估药物使用会低估观察到的关联性。

nondiscrimination ['nɔndiskrimi'neiʃən] *n.* 反歧视

The Genetic Information Nondiscrimination Act (GINA) was signed into law in 2008.

遗传信息反歧视法案(GINA) 签署于 2008 年。

nondisjunction [ˌnɔndis'dʒʌŋkʃən] *n.* 不分离,不离开

Failure of chromosomes to separate normally during cell division is termed nondisjunction.

细胞分裂过程中染色体没有正常分开称为不离开。

The failure of any process in meiosis can result in chromosomal nondisjunction.

减数分裂任何一个环节的错误都能导致染色体的不分离。

nonfatal [nɔn'feitl] *a.* 非致命的

Most benign tumors are nonfatal.

大多数良性肿瘤是不致命的。

The ratio of nonfatal to fatal cases of poisoning is approximately 7 to 1.

中毒的非致命病例与致命病例的比率大约是 7 : 1。

non-genetic [nɔn-dʒi 'netik] *a.* 非遗传性的

The goal of this research was the assessment of non-genetic and genetic risk factors of renal lesions in children after heart transplants.
这项研究的目标是评价儿童心脏移植后肾脏损害的非遗传性和遗传性危险因子。

non-genotoxic [nɔnˌdʒenəuˈtɔksik] *a.* 非遗传毒性的
A number of both genotoxic and non-genotoxic carcinogens can induce cholangiocarcinoma in rats.
许多遗传毒性和非遗传毒性致癌物都能引起大鼠胆管癌。
Rodent liver is highly susceptible for the induction of tumors by non-genotoxic chemicals.
啮齿类动物肝脏对非遗传毒性化学药品诱导的肿瘤有高度的易感性。

nonhereditary [nɔnhiˈreditəri] *a.* 非遗传的
As a result nonhereditary cases are of later onset than hereditary ones.
结果,非遗传型的发病较遗传型的发病要晚。

nonhomogeneous [ˌnɔnhəuməˈdʒiniəs] *a.* 不均匀的
Important features of hepatic carcinoma in CT enhancement are the nonhomogeneous enhancement in arterial phase and low density in delay phase .
肝癌 CT 增强的重要特征是动脉期表现为不均匀强化和延迟期呈低密度。

noninfectious [ˌnɔninˈfekʃəs] *a.* 非传染性的
Noninfectious disease is not spread by contact,inhalation etc.
非传染性疾病是不会通过接触、吸入等而蔓延的。
This is a single condition model of prevention of noninfectious disease.
这是非传染性疾病预防的单一条件模式。

noninvasive [ˌnɔninˈveisiv] *a.* 非侵害的
Thus,tests that are noninvasive and simple to perform are desired.
因此,无损伤性的和易操作的检验方法是人们所期望的。
A low serum-ferritin concentration(<12ng/ml)identifies Fe deficiency and currently represents the best noninvasive test of Fe status.
低血清铁蛋白浓度(<12ng/ml)表明缺铁,是当前表示铁量最好的非损伤性检查。

nonionized [nɔnˈaiənaizd] *a.* 非电离的,非离子化的
Nonionized lipid-soluble drugs are resorbed and not eliminated.
非电离的脂溶性药物可以被再吸收,但却不被排泄。

non-ionizing [nɔnˈaiənaizi] *a.* 非电离的
Non-ionizing radiation is described as a series of energy waves composed of oscillating electric and magnetic fields traveling at the speed of light
非电离辐射被描述为由振荡电磁场组成的、以光速传播的一系列能量波。
Near ultraviolet, visible light, infrared, microwave, radio waves, and low-frequency RF (longwave) are all examples of non-ionizing radiation.
近紫外、可见光、红外、微波、无线电波,以及低频射频(长波)都是非电离辐射的例子。

nonoperative [ˌnɔnˈɔpərətiv] *a.* 非手术的
Nonoperative management is appropriate for the majority of proximal humerus fractures.
非手术治疗适用于大多数的肱骨近端骨折。
Unlike available nonoperative therapy,this approach offers an excellent means of symptomatic palliation and local disease control.
与已使用的非手术疗法不同,该疗法能极为有效地减轻症状并控制局部病灶。

nonparalytic [ˌnɔnpærəˈlitik] *a.* 非麻痹的,非瘫痪的
The nonparalytic form of the disease is identical with the aseptic meningitis syndrome.
该病的非瘫痪形式与非细菌性脑膜炎综合征相同。

nonparenchymal [ˌnɔnpəˈreŋkiməl] *a.* 非实质的
Overproduction of the extracellular matrix is controlled by cytokines produced by nonparenchymal cells.

细胞外基质的过度产生是由非实质细胞所分泌的细胞因子控制的。

nonpathogenic [ˈnɔnˌpæθəˈdʒenik] *a.* 非病源的，不致病的

Some bacteria are harmless or even distinctly beneficial to the body and are called nonpathogenic.

某些细菌是无害的，甚至对人体明显有益，所以就称为非病原菌。

A few nonpathogenic saprophytes will also produce alkalinization.

少数非致病性的腐物寄生菌也会产生碱化作用。

nonpolar [ˈnɔnˈpəulə] *a.* 非极性的

However, a significant number of nonpolar residus will remain on the surface exposed to the water solvent.

但是，一定量的非极性残基仍强留接触水溶剂的表面上。

nonproductive [ˈnɔnprəˈdʌktiv] *a.* 不产生痰的

About two thirds of the patients have a nonproductive cough, and epistaxis occurs in about 10 per cent.

约 2/3 患者有干咳，而鼻出血则约占 10%。

nonproprietary [ˌnɔnprəuˈpraiətəri] *a.* 非专利的

In addition to the nonproprietary name of a particular compound, I will list here its common name, trade name and code designation.

某一化合物除了其非专利名称外，这里我还要列举它的通用名、商品名和代号。

nonseminoma [ˈnɔnˌsemiˈnəumə] *n.* 非精原细胞瘤

Histopathologically, testicular germ cell tumors are divided into two major groups: pure seminoma and nonseminoma.

按照组织病理学，睾丸生殖细胞肿瘤分为两大类：纯精原细胞瘤和非精原细胞瘤。

Among patients with late relapse, pure seminoma was revealed in 14 patients, and nonseminoma in 15 patients.

晚期复发的患者中有 14 例纯精原细胞瘤，15 例非精原细胞瘤。

nonsense [ˈnɔnsəns] *n.* 无义

Base pair substitutions that lead to a stop codon are termed nonsense mutations.

碱基对的置换导致终止密码子的出现，称作无义突变。

nonsterile [nɔnˈsterail] *a.* 有菌的，未消毒的

An object or substance is sterile or nonsterile; it can never be semisterile or almost sterile.

一个物体或物质要么是消毒的，或是未消毒的，绝不可能是半消毒的或者几乎是消毒的。

non-suppurative [ˈnɔnˈsʌpjuərətiv] *a.* 非化脓性的

Tuberculous pericarditis is very rare and non-suppurative.

结核性心包炎极罕见，并且是非化脓性的。

nonsurgical [nɔnˈsəːdʒikəl] *a.* 非外科的

Nonsurgical disorders frequently increase the risk of surgical procedures.

非外科疾病常常增加外科手术的危险性。

Recently there appears the first nonsurgical method of sterilizing women to end their childbearing years.

最近出现了第一种非手术方法使妇女绝育，结束她们的生育年代。

nonsynonymous [nɔnsiˈnɔniməs] *n.* 非同义

cSNPs are further classified as nonsynonymous (or *missense*) or synonymous (or *sense*) .

cSNPs(基因编码区单核苷酸多态性)可进一步分类为：非同义(或错义)多态性和同义(或有义)多态性。

nontoxic [ˌnɔnˈtɔksik] *a.* 无毒的

Under usual conditions penicillin is nontoxic.

在通常情况下，青霉素是无毒的。

nonverbal [nɔnˈvəːbəl] *a.* 不用语言的

Unilateral temporal lobe surgery produced mild to moderate amnesia for either verbal or nonverbal material.
单侧颞叶手术可导致轻到中度有关语言或非语言内容的失忆。

nonvirulent [nɔn'virjulənt] *a.* 无毒力的,无致病力的
Many bacteriophages are nonvirulent on entering a host cell.
很多噬菌体在进入寄生细胞时是无致病力的。

noradrenaline [ˌnɔːrə'drenəliːn] *n.* 去甲肾上腺素
Noradrenaline is also secreted by the adrenal medulla.
去甲肾上腺素也由肾上腺髓质分泌。

noradrenergic [nɔːˌædrə'nəːdʒik] *a.* 去甲肾上腺素激活的,产生去甲肾上腺素的
It is a nonstimulant, highly selective inhibitor of the noradrenergic transporter.
它是一种非兴奋性、高度选择性的去甲肾上腺素转运蛋白抑制剂。
This study demonstrated a marked loss of noradrenergic and sensory nerve fibers.
该研究显示去甲肾上腺素能和感觉神经纤维明显减少。

norepinephrine [ˌnɔːrəpi'nefrin] *n.* 去甲肾上腺素
Norepinephrine may be used in patients who are refractory to dopamine.
如果患者用多巴胺升压无效,可给予去甲肾上腺素。
With equivalent doses, norepinephrine has a weaker constrictor action on skin vessels than does epinephrine.
在剂量相同的情况下,去甲肾上腺素具有的收缩皮肤血管的作用比肾上腺素要弱些。

norfloxacin [nɔː'flɔksəsin] *n.* 诺氟沙星;氟哌酸
Our results showed that effect of ciprofloxacin on acute bacterial dysentery was better than that of norfloxacin.
我们的结果显示环丙沙星对急性细菌性痢疾的疗效优于诺氟沙星。
Norfloxacin is not suitable for everyone and some people should never use it.
诺氟沙星不是对每个人都适合,有些人就不应该使用它。

norm [nɔːm] *n.* 标准,准则
In conduct disorders, the major feature is violation of the rights of others or of age-group norms.
在行为障碍中,主要特征是侵犯他人权利并违犯某一年龄段的行为准则。
Because serum Ig. concentrations may vary with age, ethnic group, and environmental factors, appropriate norms must be used with any type of population assessment.
因为血清 Ig 的浓度可能随年龄、种族和环境因素而变化,所以合适的标准必须能适用于对任何群体进行评价。

normality [nɔː'mæliti] *n.* 当量浓度;正态性;常态
The normality of a solution is the gram equivalent weight of a solute per liter of solution.
溶液的当量浓度是每升溶液中所含溶质的克当量数。
The normality of the data was examined with a Kolmogorov-Smirnov test.
使用柯尔莫哥罗夫-斯米尔诺夫试验来检测数据的正态性。

normoblast ['nɔːmə'blæst] *n.* 幼红细胞
Basophilic stippling was seen as well as normoblasts.
可见嗜碱性颗粒及正常幼红细胞。
If hemorrhage was massive and acute, occasional normoblasts and immature WBCs may be seen.
如果出血量大而且急,间或可见幼红细胞和未成熟的白细胞。

normocytic [nɔːmə'sitik] *a.* 正常红细胞的
Decreased RBC production, termed bone-marrow failure, results in normochromic-normocytic anemias.
被称为骨髓衰竭的红细胞生成减少导致正色正常红细胞性贫血。

normotensive [ˌnɔːmə'tensiv] *a.* 正常血压的

In both normotensive and hypertensive subjects, this change is observed most commonly in arterioles in the spleen.

无论是正常血压或高血压者,这种病变均最常见于脾细动脉。

A normotensive subject has a systolic pressure below 140mmHg and a diastolic pressure below 90mmHg.

一个血压正常的人其收缩压应在 140 毫米汞柱以下,舒张压在 90 毫米汞柱以下。

norovirus [ˌnɔːrə'vaiərəs] *n.* 诺如病毒

Pigs are susceptible to infection and mild diarrheal disease when experimentally challenged with related human norovirus strains.

在人类的诺如病毒感染实验中猪易于被感染,引起轻微腹泻。

Norovirus is an RNA virus that causes approximately 90% of epidemic non-bacterial outbreaks of gastroenteritis around the world.

诺如病毒是一种 RNA 病毒,引起全球近 90% 的非细菌性胃肠炎。

nosebleed ['nəuzbliːd] *n.* 鼻出血;衄血

The most common clinical manifestation is spontaneous and recurrent nosebleeds beginning on average at age 12 years.

最常见的临床表现是在平均 12 岁左右时出现自发性和反复出现的鼻出血。

The objective of this article is to study the clinical features of the nosebleed patients during the same periods in the differential altitudes and provide references against nosebleed.

本文的目的是研究同一时期不同海拔地区鼻出血的临床特点,为开展鼻出血预防提供依据。

nosocomial [ˌnɔsə'kəumiəl] *a.* 医院的

Nosocomial infections are infections acquired during or as a result of hospitalization, generally those manifesting after 48h of hospitalization.

院内感染指在住院期间获得的感染,通常在入院 48 小时后有临床表现。

Hamory et al identified Candida albicans as a cause of 11% of all nosocomial urinary tract infections.

Hamory 等人证实,11% 的医院内泌尿系感染由白色念珠菌引起。

nostril ['nɔstril] *n.* 鼻孔

The nostrils communicate with the mouth by way of the nasopharynx.

鼻孔通过鼻咽部与口相通。

notable ['nəutəbl] *a.* 著名的

There were two notable publications which discussed the relationship between the fields of heredity and cytology.

曾有两份著名的出版物讨论了遗传与细胞学领域之间的关系。

A notable example is the reduction of prontosil to sulfanilamide.

典型的例子是百浪多息还原成氨苯磺胺。

noteworthy ['nəntˌwəːði] *a.* 值得注意的,显著的

It is noteworthy that T. tonsurans alone affects adults(chiefly women) regularly; the other endothrix types are almost always confined to children.

值得注意的是仅断发癣菌有规律性地感染成人(主要是妇女),而其他的如发内癣菌几乎总是感染儿童。

noticeable ['nəutisəbl] *a.* 显而易见的;重要的

Artery damage may be present for years without causing any noticeable symptoms.

动脉损伤可存在多年而无明显症状。

notoriously [nəu'tɔːriəsli] *ad.* (尤指因坏事)著名地

Although identification of growth retarded infant at birth is easy, the diagnosis of affected fetus

during pregnancy has been notoriously difficult.
尽管生长迟缓婴儿出生后很容易鉴别,但在妊娠期对受影响胎儿的诊断是非常困难的。

nourish [ˈnʌriʃ] *v.* 提供营养,养育

We need good food to nourish our bodies.
我们需要好的食物来营养我们的身体。
Any good food nourishes the brain cells along with all the other cells of the body.
任何一种好的食品能滋养脑细胞,同时也能滋养身体其他细胞。

nourishment [ˈnʌriʃmənt] *n.* 营养物,滋养品

Each cell takes in nourishment and uses it as fuel to perform work.
每个细胞摄取营养,用其作为燃料来工作。

novartis [ˈnəuvətis] *n.* 诺华

Novartis was created in 1996 from the merger of Ciba-Geigy and Sandoz Laboratories, both Swiss companies with long histories.
诺华公司创建于 1996 年,由 Ciba-Geigy 和 Sandoz 两家具有悠久历史的瑞士公司合并而成。
Novartis International AG is a multinational pharmaceutical company based in Basel, Switzerland, ranking number two in sales (46.806 billion US $) among the world-wide industry in 2010.
诺华国际公司是一家跨国制药公司,总部设在瑞士巴塞尔,在 2010 年全球范围内的行业中销售(468.06 亿美元)排名第二。

novel [ˈnɔvəl] *a.* 新的,新颖的,新奇的

It has been found that cases of severe acute respiratory syndrome (SARS) are caused by a novel coronavirus.
最近已发现严重急性呼吸系统综合征病例是由一种新型的冠状病毒引起的。
The best-remembered moments were those that were exciting, unusual, or novel.
记得最清楚的时刻,通常是一些令人激动的、不寻常的或新奇的时刻。

noxious [ˈnɔkʃəs] *a.* 有害的,有毒的

Noxious gases are dangerous to health.
毒气对于健康有害。

nuclear [ˈnjuːkliə] *a.* 核的,核心的

The nucleus is bounded by a nuclear membrane.
细胞核被核膜包围。
Often, the nuclear pores are plugged by a granular material.
通常情况下,核膜孔被颗粒状物质所填充。
The functions of the nuclear envelope are diverse.
核膜的功能是多种多样的。
Significant nuclear incidents are rare but very devastating.
重大的核事故是很少见的,可是一旦发生则是毁灭性的。

nuclear-powered [ˈnjuːkliəˈpauəd] *a.* 核动力的

The nuclear-powered pacemaker was introduced about 10 to 15 years ago in clinical medicine.
大约 10～15 年前,核动力起搏器开始用于临床。

nucleate [ˈnjuːklieit, ˈnjuːkliit] *v.* 使成核;a. 有核的

The class I genes (HLA-A, HLA-B, and HLA-C) encode proteins that are an integral part of the plasma membrane of all nucleated cells.
I 类基因(HLA-A、HLA-B、HLA-C)编码所有有核细胞质膜上的一些必不可少的蛋白。
Nucleated red blood cells can be seen in peripheral blood in regenerative anemia.
在再生障碍性贫血症的外周血中能够见到有核红细胞。

nucleic [njuːˈkliːik] *a.* 核的

Two types of nucleic acid occur in cells: deoxyribonucleic acid and ribonucleic acid.
细胞中有两种核酸:脱氧核糖核酸和核糖核酸。

Nucleic acid macromolecules act as the repository for the genetic information.
核酸大分子可充作遗传信息的储藏所。

Many drugs bring about effects or side effects by interacting with enzymes and nucleic acids.
许多药物与酶和核酸相互作用,可以产生药理作用和副作用。

nucleolus [nju:'kli:ələs] *n.* 核仁

The nucleus contains a dense body called the nucleolus.
细胞核中含有致密体称为核仁。

Ribosomes are manufactured in the nucleolus.
核糖体在核仁中形成。

nucleophile ['nju:kliəfail] *n.* 亲核物质,亲核体

All molecules or ions with a free pair of electrons can act as nucleophiles.
凡具有自由电子对的所有分子或离子都能充当亲核体。

The oxygen atom in the water molecule has two lone pairs of electrons, so water can act as a nucleophile.
水分子中的氧原子有 2 个孤对电子,因此水能充当亲核体。

nucleophilic [ˌnju:kliəu'filik] *a.* 亲核的

Some carcinogens react with nucleophilic biomacromolecules to form adducts.
一些致癌物与亲核的生物大分子反应从而形成加合物。

nucleoprotein [ˌnju:kliəu'prəuti:n] *n.* 核蛋白

Nucleoproteins are essential for cell division and reproduction.
核蛋白是细胞分裂和增生所必需的。

Ribosomes are nucleoproteins containing RNA; chromosomes are nucleoproteins containing DNA.
核糖体是含有 RNA 的核蛋白;而染色体是含有 DNA 的核蛋白。

In the nucleoproteins, the protein is associated with chains of deoxyribonucleic acids.
在核蛋白中,蛋白质与脱氧核糖核酸链相连。

nucleoside ['nju:kliəsaid] *n.* 核苷

The nucleotide base-sugar combination without the phosphate group is a nucleoside.
不带磷酸基团的核苷酸碱基-糖的复合物称作核苷。

Nucleoside comprises adenosine, guanosine, cytidine, thymidine, and uracil.
核苷包括腺苷、鸟苷、胞嘧啶、胸腺嘧啶和尿嘧啶。

nucleosome ['nju:kliəsəum] *n* [细胞] [生化] 核小体

Nucleosomes are the basic unit of DNA packaging in eukaryotes, consisting of a segment of DNA wound around a histone protein core.
核小体是真核细胞中 DNA 包装的基本单位,包含缠绕在组蛋白核心周围的一段 DNA。

The nucleosome core particle consists of about 146 bp of DNA wrapped in 1.67 left-handed superhelical turns around the histone octamer.
核小体核心颗粒包含大约 146bp 的 DNA,后者在组蛋白八聚体上呈左手螺旋缠绕 1.67 圈。

nucleotide ['nju:kliətaid] *n.* 核苷酸

Many individual carbohydrates, lipids, and nucleotides are encountered in all animal and plant forms.
多种碳水化合物、脂类和核苷酸单体可见于所有动植物。

Each DNA molecule is composed of a long sequence of hundreds to thousands of nucleotides.
每个 DNA 分子都是由数百个乃至数千个核苷酸组成的长序列构成的。

nucleus ['nju:kliəs] (*pl.* nuclei ['nju:kliai]) *n.* 细胞核;核

The nucleus encloses the cell's genetic information, which is in the form of deoxyribonucleic acid arranged in chromosomes.

核包封着细胞的遗传信息,后者以脱氧核糖核酸的形式排列于染色体中。

The nuclei are larger than normal but contain less than optimal amounts of DNA for cell division.

核比正常增大,但其 DNA 含量少于适合于细胞分裂的最佳量。

nuisance [ˈnjuːsns] *n.* 讨厌;损害

Some people find eyeglasses unsightly or a nuisance.

有些人觉得传统眼镜不雅观或讨厌。

null [nʌl] *a.* 无效的;零位的

The results of the first experiments to prove the value of the new drug were null.

为证明这种新药价值所做的首批试验的结果无效。

Null cells are early population of lymphocytes bearing neither T-cell nor B-cell differentiation antigens.

裸细胞是既没带有 T 细胞鉴别抗原也没带有 B 细胞鉴别抗原的早期的淋巴细胞群。

nulliparous [nʌˈliperəs] *a.* 未经产的

Fibromyomata are more often found in nulliparous women or in women who have not been pregnant for some time.

纤维肌瘤较常见于未产妇女或有一段时间未曾怀孕的妇女。

Nulliparous women are at greater risk for breast cancer.

未经产的妇女患乳腺癌的危险较大些。

numb [nʌm] *a.* 麻木的,无感觉的

The injured arm easily goes numb.

受伤的臂容易麻木。

numbness [ˈnʌmnis] *n.* 麻木,无感觉

Negative phenomena result from loss of sensory function and are characterized by numbness.

由于感觉功能丧失引起的阴性现象以麻木为特征。

The subjective symptoms consist of pruritus(itching), sensations of heat(burning), cold(tingling), prickling, biting, formication, pain and numbness.

主观症状有瘙痒、热觉(烧灼感)、冷觉(麻刺感)、针刺感、(咬)痛、蚁行感、疼痛和麻木。

numerator [ˈnjuːməreitə] *n.* 分数的分子

Registries with systematic data collection provide both numerators and denominators for assessment of drug safety events.

使用系统性数据收集的注册登记为药物安全事件的评估提供了分子和分母。

numerical [njuːˈmerikəl] *a.* 数字的;数值的

Relatedness among a large number of organisms can be estimated by a numerical analysis.

通过数据分析,可估计出多种微生物的相关性。

numerous [ˈnjuːmərəs] *a.* 为数众多的

Complications of H. influenzae meningitis are numerous.

流感嗜血杆菌脑膜炎的并发症是很多的。

The white corpuscles are about one third larger but less numerous than the red corpuscles.

白细胞比红细胞大约大 1/3,但数量要少得多。

nursery [ˈnəːsəri] *n.* 婴儿室; 托儿所

In addition, nurseries and kindergartens have been established all over the country.

此外,托儿所、幼儿园已在全国各地普遍地建立起来。

nutmeg [ˈnʌtmeg] *n.* 槟榔

Nutmeg liver is the liver with chronic passive congestion and hemorrhagic necrosis.

槟榔肝是肝脏慢性淤血伴出血性坏死。

Central areas are red and slightly depressed compared with the surrounding tan viable parenchyma, forming a " nutmeg liver" pattern.

与周围棕褐色、相对正常的肝组织相比，中央区呈红色，并稍显凹陷，二者形成“槟榔肝”的形态。

nutraceutical [ˌnjuːtrəˈsjuːtikəl] *n.* 营养药品；保健食品

Nutraceuticals today are often taken as food additives in the hope that they will be beneficial diet additives.

今天的营养药品常常作为食品添加剂来使之成为有益的饮食辅助。

In the US and Europe, nutraceuticals exist in a regulatory twilight zone.

在美国和欧洲，保健食品处于受控制的边缘区域。

nutrient [ˈnjuːtriənt] *n.* 营养品，营养素

Food that are rich in one nutrient may also contain other nutrients.

富于一种营养的食物，也可能含有其他营养。

Nutrients include carbohydrates, fats, proteins, minerals and vitamins.

营养素包括碳水化合物、脂肪、蛋白质、矿物质和维生素。

nutrition [njuːˈtriʃən] *n.* 营养

The kilocalorie is the standard heat unit used in the science of nutrition.

千卡是营养学上使用的标准热量单位。

The well-being of each individual cell is dependent on the adequacy of its environment to furnish nutrition and carry away metabolites.

每个细胞的健康都取决于其周围环境是否能提供充足的营养物质并运走其代谢产物。

nutritional [njuˈtriʃənl] *a.* 营养的

Nutritional deficiency may occur as a consequence of many factors other than primary lack of a nutrient in the diet.

营养缺乏除原发于食物中营养素缺少外，尚可继发于多种其他因素。

No mention is made of a nutritional disturbance.

没有提到营养障碍。

nutritive [ˈnjuːtritiv] *a.* 有营养的

It is very convenient to observe the reproduction of cells by the method of making cultures of living matter in a nutritive medium.

通过在培养基中对活质的培养，观察细胞的繁殖是非常方便的。

nyctalopia [ˌniktəˈləupiə] *n.* 夜盲症

Lack of vitamin A in the diet is one cause of nyctalopia.

饮食中缺乏维生素 A 是夜盲症的原因之一。

Retinal fatigue from exposure to very bright light is a cause of nyctalopia.

强光下暴露过久引起的视网膜疲劳是夜盲症的原因之一。

nystagmus [nisˈtægməs] *n.* 眼球震颤

Vestibular nystagmus and vertigo result from sudden interruption of vestibular input.

前庭神经的输入突然中断可引起前庭性眼球震颤和眩晕。

Although nystagmus is a complex subject, some general rules, although not absolute, can be followed.

虽然眼球震颤是一个复杂的问题，但有些一般性规律（虽非绝对性的）仍可遵循。

nystatin [ˈnistətin] *n.* 制霉菌素

Localised disease may be treated at first with relatively inexpensive drugs such as nystatin, or clotrimazole.

局限性疾病可以首先使用相对便宜的药物，如制霉菌素或克霉唑。

The results of drug sensitivity showed that amphotericin and nystatin were the most sensitive and flucytosine (5-Fc) was the most resistant.

药敏结果显示，最敏感的是两性霉素和制霉菌素，最耐药的是 5-氟胞嘧啶。

O

obese [əu'biːs] *a.* 过度肥胖的，肥大的

A fifth of men and a third of women are obese.

有五分之一的男性和三分之一的女性是过度肥胖。

Researchers announced they had isolated a gene in mice that makes the animals obese.

研究人员宣称他们已从小鼠体内分离出一种可使小鼠发胖的基因。

obesity [əu'biːsiti] *n.* 过度肥胖

Diabetes is associated with obesity and inactivity.

糖尿病与过度肥胖和缺少运动有关。

Obesity causes high blood pressure, heart attack and diabetes.

肥胖可导致高血压、心脏病发作和糖尿病。

Obesity is a chronic disease that is increasing in prevalence.

肥胖是一种慢性疾病，患病率逐渐增高。

objective [əb'dʒektiv] *n.* 目标，目的

The primary therapeutic objectives should be to prevent and to cure disease.

治疗的主要目的应是预防和治愈疾病。

The prime objective of follow-up is detection of recurrence.

随访最重要的目的是发现复发病例。

a. 客观的

No one can argue he is wholly objective about anything.

谁也不敢说他对什么事情都持客观态度。

Also recorded are objective and subjective symptoms obtained from the nursing history.

从护理病史获得的客观和主观症状也要都记录下来。

obligate ['ɔbligeit] *v.* 使有责任

The principle of beneficence ethically obligates researchers to minimize potential harms to the individuals.

善行原则从伦理上要求研究者尽量减少对个人的潜在危害。

a. 专性的

An obligate anaerobe can survive only in the absence of oxygen.

专性厌氧性生物只能在无氧条件下生存。

obligation [ˌɔbli'geiʃən] *n.* 义务；责任

In this case, the anesthetist's obligation is to ensure an open airway at all times.

在这种情况下，麻醉师的责任就是要一直保持呼吸道通畅。

obligatory [ɔ'bligətəri] *a.* 强制性的，必须履行的

Fluid and electrolyte replacement is obligatory and particularly so prior to surgery.

应进行强制性的补充液体和电解质，特别是在外科手术以前更应补足。

In this condition, combinations of drugs or sympathectomy are virtually obligatory.

在此情况下，药物的合并使用或交感神经切除术几乎是同样必要的。

oblique [ə'bliːk] *a.* 斜的，倾斜的

When due to indirect violence, the fracture is situated at a distance from the point of impact, and is usually oblique or spiral.

当由间接暴力造成时，骨折位于撞击点的远处，而且常常是斜形的或螺旋形的。

obliquely [ə'bliːkli] *ad.* 斜地，倾斜地；成四十五度角

More commonly the thrombus will be cut obliquely or transversely so that islands or strands of granular material will be seen.

常常须斜切或横切这种血栓，才能看到颗粒物质呈岛状或束状分布。

obliquimeter [ˌɔbli'kwimitə] *n.* 骨盆斜度计

Obliquimeter is an apparatus for determining the angle of the pelvic brim with the upright body.

骨盆斜度计这一仪器是用来测量直立体位时骨盆上口的角度的。

Orthopaedic surgeon usually uses obliquimeter to examine patients.

骨外科医生经常用骨盆斜度计来检查患者。

obliteration [ɔˌblitə'reiʃən] *n.* 消灭

The ultimate objective is complete expansion of the lung and obliteration of the empyema space.

最终目的是肺完全扩张，消灭脓腔。

obscure [əb'skjuə] *a.* 不清楚的

The causation of the lesion is obscure.

该病变的原因不明。

The mechanism of the vasoconstriction in heart failure has remained obscure.

心力衰竭时的血管收缩机制仍然不清楚。

v. 隐藏；遮掩

Jaundice is frequently obscured in individuals with dark skin or edema.

皮肤黝黑或有水肿的病人其黄疸常被遮掩。

Another cause of erroneous diagnosis is the dominance of extracardiac problems which may obscure the cardiac lesion.

误诊的另一原因是心外的临床表现占优势，它可掩盖心脏的损害。

observable [əb'zəːvəbl] *a.* 可观察到的，显著的

In an organic disease, there are observable gross or microscopic changes in an organ.

在器质性疾病中，有可能观察到某一器官显著或微小的变化。

observation [ˌɔbzə'veiʃən] *n.* 观察，监视

Observation of exudates and secretions for odor, color, and consistency may be helpful.

观察患者的渗出物与分泌物的气味、颜色和黏稠度对诊治是很有帮助的。

obsession [əb'seʃən, ɔb-] *n.* 强迫症；强迫观念

There are different theories that have different perspectives in the causation of obsession.

不同的理论对强迫症的成因有不同的看法。

The obsessions of obsessive-compulsive patients are unrealistic, but are frightening.

强迫症患者的强迫观念是不真实的，但是令人害怕的。

obsolete ['ɔbsəliːt] *a.* 作废的，过时的

The more traumatic approach will gradually become obsolete.

造成较多创伤的方法将逐渐被废除。

Many old medical terms are obsolete .

许多旧的医学术语已废弃不用了。

obstetrician [ˌɔbste'triʃən] *n.* 产科医生

The obstetrician has dealt with two cases of puerperal fever today.

产科医生今天处理了两例产褥热病人。

obstetrics [ɔb'stetriks] *n.* 产科学

The place of radiological examination in obstetrics is diminishing.

放射学检查在产科的地位正在减弱。

Shortages of doctors are severe in rural areas and in certain specialities, such as surgery, pediatrics and obstetrics.

医生的严重缺乏表现在农村地区或是某些专业上，比如外科、儿科和产科。

obstinate [ˈɔbstinit] *a.* 顽固的

The obstinate old man refused to go to hospital.

那位倔强的老人不肯去医院看病。

obstruct [əbˈstrʌkt] *v.* 阻塞

There may be sufficient inflammatory swelling to obstruct the airway.

可能存在严重的炎性肿胀而阻塞气道。

Unlike the earlens, Spindel's hearing aid would not obstruct the normal hearing pathway.

与鼓膜接触传感器不同,史平德尔的助听器不会阻碍正常的听道。

obstruction [əbˈstrʌkʃən] *n.* 阻塞

Bronchial obstruction by endotracheal or tracheostomy tubes often occurs.

气管插管及气管切开插管常可发生支气管阻塞。

This swelling in turn causes obstruction of the bile duct.

这种肿胀又引起胆管阻塞。

obstructive [əbˈstrʌktiv] *a.* 引起阻塞的;妨碍的

The pathogenesis of atelectasis involves obstructive and nonobstructive factors.

肺不张的发病机制包括阻塞性和非阻塞性因素。

Occassionally the disease begins with the features of acute obstructive laryngitis.

偶尔在疾病开始时表现为急性阻塞性喉炎的特征。

obtainable [əbˈteinəbl] *a.* 可获得的,可取得的

But oxygen and nutrients are obtainable only from the external environment.

但氧和营养物只能从外部环境中获得。

This apparatus, commonly known as Wood's light, is obtainable commercially.

这种仪器,通称为伍氏灯,在市场上可以买到。

obviate [ˈɔbvieit] *v.* 排除,避免

Dose reduction obviates the possibility of side effects.

减少用药量可避免副作用的可能性。

occasion [əˈkeiʒən] *v.* 为…而引起

This is occasioned by an excess urinary excretion of nitrogen.

这是由尿液排出的氮质过量所引起的。

occasional [əˈkeiʒənəl] *a.* 偶然的

In subacute intestinal obstruction distension is more marked, vomiting is only occasional and the bowel may act at times.

在亚急性肠梗阻时,腹胀很明显,呕吐偶尔发生,肠管时而活动。

occasionally [əˈkeiʒənəli] *ad.* 偶然,间或

Corticosteroids occasionally are used if hemolysis is very severe.

如果溶血很严重,间或用皮质类固醇。

Occasionally, the metabolites are toxicologically more potent.

偶尔有些代谢产物的毒性更大。

occipital [ɔkˈsipitəl] *n.* 枕骨 *a.* 枕部的

The experiment demonstrates the safety and feasibility of fMRI studies with simultaneous occipital nerve stimulation in a subject with externalized electrodes.

本实验证明了脑功能磁共振成像同时经受来源于体表电极的枕神经刺激的研究的安全性和可行性。

occlude [ɔˈkluːd] *v.* 堵塞

Capillaries may also be occluded in vasculitis which affects particularly the small vessels.

在主要累及小血管的脉管炎中毛细血管也可被堵塞。

In this condition the lumen of the intestine is occluded, but its blood supply is intact.

患本病时肠腔闭塞,但肠的血液供应是完好的。

occlusal [ɔ'kluːsəl] *a.* 咬合(面)的

It is now possible to study, outside the mouth, the interaction of the occlusal surfaces of the teeth with the temporomandibular joint.

现在可在口腔外研究牙的咬合面与颞下颌关节之间的相互作用。

occlusion [ɔ'kluːʒən] *n.* 堵塞;咬合

It may be primarily due to vascular occlusion.

它主要是由于血管阻塞所致。

Complete occlusion of an artery of the heart, usually results from progressive atherosclerosis, but rarely from embolism.

心脏动脉的完全堵塞通常是因渐进性粥样硬化,很少是因栓塞所致。

Occlusion is the key to oral function and subsequently the key to restorative oral diagnosis.

咬合是口腔功能的关键,因而也是口腔修复诊断的关键。

occlusive [ɔ'kluːsiv] *a.* 堵塞的

Occlusive venous thrombi are usually formed mainly of soft red thrombus which contracts well.

阻塞性静脉血栓一般主要由软的收缩良好的红色血栓组成。

The diagnosis for this patient is occlusive coronary artery disease.

对这个病人的诊断是闭塞性冠状动脉病。

occult [ɔ'kʌlt] *a.* 隐秘的;玄奥的

The feces are examined for occult blood.

检查大便以找出有无潜血。

Sensitization to chemicals and drugs may occur at any age and may be occult.

对化学物质和药物过敏可在任何年龄发生,而且可能是潜在的。

occupation [ˌɔkju'peiʃən] *n.* 职业

The name, age and occupation of every patient must be recorded in the case history.

每个病人的姓名、年龄和职业需在病史中记录下来。

In a study of 340000 individuals, clear inverse gradients were found in mortality by education, income, and occupation for white and nonwhite.

一项对 340000 人进行的研究发现,白人和非白人的死亡率与受教育程度、收入、职业呈明显的相反梯度曲线。

occupational [ˌɔkju'peiʃənl] *a.* 职业的

A number of conditions are classified as "occupational diseases".

有一些疾病被列为"职业性疾病"。

The incidence of occupational diseases is lessening each year owing to the safety and health measures adopted in all the industries.

由于整个工业系统实行了劳动保护和保健措施,职业病的发病率正在逐年降低。

occurrence [ə'kʌrəns] *n.* 发生;出现

It appears that cancer must depend for its occurrence on certain very special etiologic factors.

看来癌症的发生依赖于某些非常特别的病因学因素。

octamer ['ɔktəmə] *n.* [高分子] 八聚物

The nucleosome core particle consists of about 146-bp of DNA wrapped in 1.67 left-handed superhelical turns around the histone octamer.

核小体核心颗粒包含大约 146bp 的 DNA 左手超螺旋缠绕在组蛋白八聚体上 1.67 圈。

A histone octamer is at the center of a nucleosome core particle.

组蛋白八聚体位于核小体核心颗粒中心。

octapeptide [ɔktə'peptaid] *n.* 八肽

The hormone oxytocin is an octapeptide.

激素催产素是一种八肽。

octreotide ['ɔktriətaid] *n.* 奥曲肽

Somatostatin analogs, such as octreotide, successfully control hormone hypersecretion in patients with acromegaly, islet cell tumors, carcinoids.

生长抑素类似物如奥曲肽在肢端肥大症、胰岛细胞瘤、良性肿瘤患者中能成功地控制激素的高分泌。

The synthesis technique of octreotide was optimized.

优化了奥曲肽的合成技术。

ocular [ˈɔkjulə] *a.* 眼的

Frequently no ocular cause can be found and the headache must be ascribed to overuse of the frontalis muscle.

有些头痛常不能从眼睛找到原因,而要归因于使用额肌过度。

Diplopia may arise from disorders of the ocular motor nerves(Ⅲ, Ⅳ, Ⅵ).

当眼球运动神经(第Ⅲ、Ⅳ、Ⅵ对脑神经)产生功能障碍时可以出现复视。

ocularmucocutaneous [ˈɔkjulə ˌmjukəukju ˈteiniəs] *a.* 眼-黏膜-皮肤的

The mid-1970s saw the discovery of the ocularmucocutaneous syndrome caused by practolol.

20 世纪 70 年代中期发现了由普拉洛尔所引起的眼-黏膜-皮肤综合征。

odds [ɔdz] *n.* 几率;机会;可能性

While there has been a recent emphasis on biomarkers and genes that might be linked to cancer survival, the health habits can increase the odds for cancer survival.

尽管一直强调生物标记和基因可能与癌症生存有关,但有些好的卫生习惯可增加癌症生存的概率。

The odds are heavily in favor of my providing him with serviceable vision as long as he lives.

只要他还活着,我就可以找到有利时机为他提供必要的视力。

odor [ˈəudə] *n.* 气味,香气,臭气(= odour)

Triggers of vasomotor rhinitis include temperature changes and strong odors.

气温变化和强烈的气味可以触发血管运动性鼻炎。

The nose contains an array of sensors, tuned to pick up the odours from growing bacteria.

鼻有一批可调整到接收生长中细菌气味的传感器。

odorless [ˈəudəles] *a.* 没有气味的

New cleanser will keep bathroom clean and odorless.

新型清洁剂会使洗澡间保持清洁,没有臭气。

Methocillin-S occurs as a white, almost odorless crystalline powder.

邻氯青霉素钠是一种白色、几乎无任何气味的结晶状粉末。

odorous [ˈəudərəs] *a.* 有气味的,臭的

An odorous breath may result from improper oral hygiene and pyorrhea or from chronic infection of the tonsils, adenoid or nasal mucosa.

口臭是由口腔卫生不好和脓溢或者是由扁桃体、增殖腺以及鼻腔黏膜的慢性感染所引起。

offend [əˈfend] *v.* 违反,冒犯;使…不舒服;触怒

A patient mustn't offend against the doctor's advices.

病人不应违反医生的指导。

Treatment should include removal of any offending antibiotics.

治疗措施应包括停用所有使人不舒服的抗生素。

She was offended by the medical malpractice.

她被医疗事故所激怒。

offender [əˈfendə] *n.* 冒犯者;犯规的人

Smoking is inhibited here; offenders will be fined five dollars.

此处禁止吸烟,违者罚款 5 美元。

These drugs include almost all the sleeping pills, the principal offenders being the barbiturates, heroin, morphine, and other narcotics.

这些毒品几乎包括所有的催眠药，主要违规药品有巴比妥类、海洛因、吗啡及其他麻醉药。

offensive [ɔ'fensiv] *a.* 讨厌的

She finds tobacco smoke offensive.

她感到烟草的烟很难闻。

offer ['ɔfə] *v.* 提供，提议

The mother offered her son a kidney for organ transplantation.

母亲提供给儿子一个肾脏作器官移植。

Professor Li offered to give a lecture on AIDS for freshman students.

李教授提议给一年级学生作关于艾滋病的讲座。

official [ə'fiʃəl] *a.* 官方的，根据药典配制的

This is an official medicine.

这是一种根据药典配制的药物。

n. 官员，公务员

Urban officials want the census to be as accurate and complete as possible.

城市的官员们希望人口普查尽可能地准确和完整。

offset ['ɔfset] *v.* 抵消

Will exercise help offset Parkinson's Disease?

运动有助于减缓帕金森氏病吗？

Fruit and veggie diet may offset genetic risk for heart disease.

水果和全素饮食可以减少心脏病的遗传危险性。

offspring ['ɔfspriŋ] *n.* 子孙，儿女，后代

Approximately 50% of these women will transmit the organism to their offspring.

这些妇女约50%将此病原体传给出生婴儿。

Milks produced by the various mammals are uniquely adapted to the needs of offspring of the particular species.

各种哺乳动物的乳汁专门适应于本类动物后代的需要。

Genes are units of heredity passed from parents to offspring and are contained in a person's cells.

基因是可从亲代传递给子代的遗传单位，它们存在于人的细胞中。

ofloxacin [ə'flɔksəsin] *n.* 奥氟沙星

Ofloxacin also is used for lower respiratory tract infection, skin and soft tissue infection.

奥氟沙星也可用于下呼吸道、皮肤和软组织感染。

oilimmersion [ɔili'məːʃən] *n.* 油浸法

Under an oilimmersion lens the treponemata appear as motile white corkscrew-shaped organisms against the dark background.

在油镜下，以暗视野为背景，密螺旋体表现为活动的白色螺旋形生物体。

ointment ['ɔintmənt] *n.* 软膏，软膏剂

The ointment is used externally for healing such burns.

此软膏外用可使这类灼伤愈合。

As for the efficacy of penicillin ointment, there can be no question.

关于青霉素软膏的效能，那是不容置疑的。

Emulsifying ointment is used to treat dry skin conditions, such as eczema and dermatitis.

乳化软膏剂可用于治疗皮肤干燥病如湿疹、皮炎等。

olfactory [ɔl'fæktəri] *a.* 嗅的，嗅觉的

Olfactory neuroblastoma often arise superiorly and laterally in the nose from the neuroendocrine cells dispersed in the olfactory mucosa.

嗅神经母细胞瘤常发生于鼻腔的顶部和侧壁，起源于嗅黏膜内散在的神经内分泌细胞。

Dr. Axel works on how olfactory information is handled in the cortex, the highest level of human

and mouse brains.
阿克塞尔博士致力于嗅觉信息在大脑皮层——人和鼠脑最高级中枢内的处理。

oligergastic [ˌɔlidʒəˈgæstik] *a.* 精神薄弱的

Certain oligergastic reaction forms will be considered in the psychiatric examination of a child.
我们在儿童精神检查中应该考虑到某些精神薄弱的反应形式。

An oligergastic individual may become depressed easily.
一个精神薄弱的人容易变得抑郁。

oligoadenylate [ˌɔligəuəˈdenileit] *n.* 寡腺苷酸

Oligoadenylate synthetase is an enzyme produced in response to interferon stimulation of cells.
寡腺苷酸合成酶是细胞受干扰素刺激后产生的一种酶。

oligoasthenoteratospermia [ˌɔligəuˈæsθənəuˌterətəˈspəːmiə] *n.* 少弱畸精症

Oligoasthenoteratospermia, a reduction in motility and number of spermatozoa and a change in their morphology, is one of the most relevant causes of infertility in men.
少弱畸精症,即精子活力降低、数目减少、形态改变,是男性不育最多的原因之一。

oligodendroglioma [ˌɔligəuˌdendrəuglaiˈəumə] *n.* 少突胶质细胞瘤

The differential diagnosis for oligodendroglioma may be difficult when an oligodendroglioma-like component occupies most of the pilocytic astrocytoma.
当少突胶质细胞瘤样成分占据毛细胞性星形细胞瘤的大部分时少突胶质细胞瘤的鉴别诊断会比较困难。

Our previous study confirmed that oligodendrogliomas had higher frequency of chromosome 1p/19q deletion.
我们以往的研究证实少突胶质细胞瘤染色体 1p/19q 缺失发生的频率较高。

oligohydramnios [ˌɔligəuhaiˈdræmniɔs] *n.* 羊水过少

If oligohydramnios is present, the uterus feels tight around the baby.
如果出现羊水过少,子宫壁就会紧包着胎儿。

Oligohydramnios is a condition in which the amount of amniotic fluid bathing a fetus during pregnancy is abnormally small.
羊水过少是妊娠期间浸泡胎儿的羊水量异常少的一种情况。

oligomenorrhea [ˌɔligəuˌmenɔːˈriːə] *n.* 月经稀发

Women with polycystic ovary syndrome (PCOS) are likely to suffer from oligomenorrhea.
多囊卵巢综合征女性有可能出现月经稀发。

Eating disorders can also result in oligomenorrhea.
饮食紊乱也会产生月经稀发。

oligonucleotide [ˌɔligəuˈnjuːkliəutaid] *n.* 低(聚)核苷酸,寡核苷酸

Oligonucleotide synthesis is the chemical synthesis of relatively short fragments of nucleic acids with defined chemical structure (sequence).
寡核苷酸合成是指化学合成相对短片段的、有明确化学结构(序列)的核苷酸。

oligoovulation [ˌɔligəuˌəuvjuːˈleiʃən] *n.* 稀发排卵

Oligoovulation is seen in women with irregular cycles, or very long cycles (more than 50 days).
稀发排卵出现在月经不规律或月经周期较长(大于 50 天)的女性中。

oligosaccharide [ˌɔligəuˈsækəraid] *n.* 低聚糖

Oligosaccharides are carbohydrates that have recently gotten attention for their health benefits.
低聚糖是因有益健康而近来受到关注的碳水化合物。

Important oligosaccharide carbohydrates are raffinose and stachyose.
重要的低聚糖碳水化合物有棉籽糖和水苏糖。

Oligosaccharide is a carbohydrate that consists of a relatively small number of monosaccharides.
低聚糖是由相对数量较少的单糖构成的碳水化合物。

oligospermia [ˌɔligəuˈspəːmiə] *n.* 少精子症

The diagnosis of oligospermia is based on one low count in a semen analysis performed on two occasions.
少精子症的诊断建立在两次精液常规分析显示精子数目降低的基础上。
Both of abnormal chromosome karyotype and Y-chromosome microdeletion are important to cause azoospermia and severe oligospermia.
染色体核型异常和 Y 染色体微缺失均是无精子症和严重少精子症的重要原因。
Klinefelter syndrome is relatively common among infertile males or males with oligospermia or azoospermia.
Klinefelter 综合征在不育男性中及少精或无精症男性中比较常见。

oligozoospermia [ˌɔligəuzəuə' spə:miə] *n.* 精子减少,少精子症
Oligospermia, also oligozoospermia, refers to semen with a low concentration of sperm and is a common finding in male infertility.
少精子症,也称精子减少,是指精液中精子密度的降低,常见于男性不育。

oliguria [ˌɔli'gjuəriə] *n.* 尿过少,少尿
Dysfunction may result in dysuria, oliguria and edema.
功能障碍可导致排尿困难、少尿和水肿。
Oliguria refers to the excretion of an abnormally small amount of urine, less than 500ml/24hr.
少尿是指排泄的尿量异常的少,少于 500 毫升/24 小时。

oliguric [ˌɔli'gjurik] *a.* 少尿的
Treatment in the oliguric phase is the same as for acute renal failure.
少尿期的治疗与急性肾功能衰竭相同。

omasum [əu'meisəm] *n.* 瓣胃
The omasum is the third compartment of the stomach in ruminants.
瓣胃是反刍动物的第三胃。
The result indicates that the proventricul volume (except for omasum) of the goats fed on green grass is the largest, that of the goat grazed is the medium and that of the goats fed on hay is the smallest.
结果表明:前胃(瘤胃、网胃、瓣胃)容积(除瓣胃外)表现为青草羊最大,其次为放牧羊,干草羊最小。

omental [əu'mentəl] *a.* 网膜的
Diffuse peritoneal and omental seeding are well-known forms of dissemination of metastatic carcinoma.
腹膜和网膜广泛种植转移是癌症扩散的主要形式。

omentin [əu'mentin] *n.* 网膜素,一种由网膜脂肪组织分泌的细胞因子
Human omentin is an adipocyte-derived protein that counteracts obesity and related insulin resistance.
人类的网膜素是一种由脂肪细胞分泌的蛋白质,具有抗肥胖及相关胰岛素抵抗的作用。
Differences in omentin expression have been noted in adipose tissue from normals and patients with inflammatory bowel disease although its significance is unknown.
已发现正常人与炎症性肠病患者的脂肪组织中网膜素的表达有差异,但其意义尚不清楚。

omentum [əu'mentəm] *n.* 网膜,大网膜
Bowel or omentum may herniate alongside the drain.
肠管或网膜可能沿引流道疝出。
These greater omentum lesions appeared as characteristics of thickened, shifted and peculiar echo.
大网膜病变(在超声检查下)显示出有增厚、改变和回声异常的特点。

omics ['əumiks] *n.* 组学
Technologies that are collectively called *omics* have made it feasible to measure an enormous number of molecules within a tissue or cell.

总称为“组学”的技术使得测定一种组织或一个细胞的大量分子成为可能。

Researchers are rapidly taking up omes and omics, as shown by the explosion of the use of these terms in PubMed since the mid '90s.

自 20 世纪 90 年代中期以来,研究人员正快速从事“组”和“组学”研究,表现为 PubMed 上这些术语的爆炸性使用。

Metabonomics is a new branch of “omics” science in post-gene time.

代谢组学是后基因时代出现的一门新兴“组学”学科。

omission [əu'miʃən] *n.* 遗漏,省略

These friends have saved me from many omissions and errors in my medical paper, and their help is gratefully acknowledged.

这些朋友帮助我减少了医学论文中许多遗漏和错误,对他们的帮助谨致以衷心的感谢。

omit [ə'mit] *v.* 省略;遗漏,忽略

The following morning, breakfast is omitted and the drug is administered.

第二天早晨不要吃早饭,要服药。

Few doctors will omit to feel pulse and to take temperature.

几乎没有医生会忽略摸脉和量体温。

omphalocele ['ɔmfələusiːl] *n.* 脐疝;脐突出

In abdominal wall malformations such as gastroschisis and omphalocele, the heart may be shifted to the left as well.

有腹裂和脐疝等腹壁畸形患者也可能存在心脏左移。

Therefore, an omphalocele should be carefully sought if holoprosencephaly is found.

因此,如果发现前脑无裂畸形,就要仔细检查有无脐疝。

oncogene ['ɔŋkədʒiːn] *n.* 癌基因,致癌基因

Some viruses carry oncogenes.

有些病毒携带着致癌基因。

Many oncogenes have been shown to be associated with specific chromosomal breakpoints or translocations.

许多致癌基因与特殊的染色体断裂点或易位有关。

oncogenesis [ˌɔŋkəu'dʒenisis] *n.* 肿瘤发生

High oncogenic risk HPVs are currently considered to be the most important factor in cervical oncogenesis.

高危型 HPVs 目前被认为是宫颈癌发生的最重要的危险因素。

Research on retroviruses has provided important insights into mechanisms of oncogenesis in humans, including the discovery of viral oncogenes and cellular proto-oncogenes.

有关逆转录病毒的研究为人类肿瘤发生的机制提供了重要信息,包括病毒癌基因和细胞原癌基因的发现。

oncogenic [ˌɔŋkəu'dʒenik] *adj.* 致瘤的;瘤源性的

Researchers now have begun to make connections between the development of certain types of cancer and specific viral, bacterial, and parasitic infections. These infections are referred to as oncogenic, or tumor-producing, infections.

目前,研究人员已经将某些类型的癌的发生与特定的病毒、细菌和寄生虫的感染联系起来,这类感染被称为致瘤感染。

Oncogenic signals involve activation of kinases.

致瘤信号涉及激酶的活化。

oncology [ɔŋ'kɔlədʒi] *n.* 肿瘤学

Dr. Li has been working in the Department of Oncology for more than ten years.

李医生在肿瘤科工作已有十多年了。

oncoprotein [ˌɔŋkəu'prəutin] *n.* 原癌基因,癌[基因]蛋白质

Ras is one of the first oncoproteins ever identified.
Ras 是已确认的最早发现的原癌基因之一。

oneirophobia [əuˌnaiərəu'fəubiə] *n.* 恐梦症
Oneirophobia is a fear of dreams.
恐梦症是对做梦的恐惧。

online ['ɔn'lain] *a.* 联机的，联线的，网络的
The research appears in the June 24 online issue of Nature Cell Biology.
这项研究发表在 6 月 24 日网络版的 Nature Cell Biology 杂志上。
ad. 联机地，联线地
People who are interested in donating an organ can contact the United Network for Organ Sharing (UNOS) at 804-782-4920 or go online at www. unos. org to obtain more information and to locate the nearest transplant center.
对捐献器官感兴趣的人，可与器官共享联盟网(UNOS)联系，电话是 804-782-4920，或通过联线网站 www. unos. org 以获得更多的信息，并找到最近的移植中心。

onset ['ɔnset] *n.* 开始；发作
The time of onset of pain has diagnostic importance.
疼痛发作时间具有诊断意义。
The onset is usually gradual, following upon bronchitis.
(本病)发病往往缓慢，继发于支气管炎。

ontogeny [ɔn'tɔdʒəni] *n.* 个体发生；个体发育
The differences in gene dosage and ontogeny of the α- and β-globins are important to an understanding of the pathogenesis of many hemoglobinopathies.
α 和 β 珠蛋白基因剂量和个体发生的差异对于理解多种血红蛋白病的发病机制非常重要。
So ontogeny is not only the result of the interaction of heredity and environment, but it is also influenced greatly by the initial structure and substantive motility.
所以，个体发育不单是遗传和环境相互作用的结果，还要受其原有结构和主观能动性的巨大影响。

oocyte ['əuəsait] *n.* 卵母细胞；卵囊
Primary oocyte is a diploid.
初级卵母细胞是二倍体。
Oocytes are quite hardy, they can exist outside the body for at least a year in warm moist soil.
卵囊很坚硬，在体外温湿的土壤中至少可活一年。

oogenesis [ˌəuə'dʒenisis] *n.* 卵子发生
Oogenesis differs in several important ways from spermatogenesis.
卵子发生在几个方面不同于精子发生。
Much of oogenesis occurs during fetal life.
卵子发生很多是在胎儿时期。

oogonia [ˌəuə'gəuniə] (oogonium 的复数形式) *n.* 卵原细胞
The ova develop from oogonia, cells in the ovarian.
卵细胞由卵巢内的卵原细胞发育而来。
There was no typical Golgi complex in oogonia, but there were some Golgi vesicles.
卵原细胞内无典型的高尔基复合体，但有高尔基囊泡。

oophorectomy [ˌəuɔfə'rektəmi] *n.* 卵巢切除术
Bilateral oophorectomy will bring about permanent arrest of the disease.
两侧卵巢切除术将永久性阻止此病发生。

ooze [uːz] *v.* 渗出，冒出
Hemorrhage is a frequent sign, varying from a slight oozing of blood to a copious flooding that may

prove fatal.
出血是一个常见体征，其程度从轻微渗血直至可能导致死亡的大量流血。
A large quantity of blood oozes out of the blood vessels following serious burns.
严重烧伤后，大量血液从血管渗出。

opacification [əuˌpæsifiˈkeiʃən] *n.* 浑浊化，不透明
Recently, the study on the mechanisms of lens opacification is widely carried out.
近来，对晶状体浑浊化机制的研究正在广泛进行。
We reviewed the effect of designing intraocular lens on posterior capsule opacification.
我们综述了人工晶状体设计对后囊混浊的影响。

opacity [əuˈpæsəti] *n.* 混浊，不透明
Eye changes include chronic iridocyclitis, corneal band opacity and complicated cataract.
眼部改变包括慢性虹膜睫状体炎、角膜带状混浊并可合并白内障。
Occasionally, when a bronchus is obstructed by tenacious mucus, there is an opacity caused by lober or segmental collapse.
当支气管偶尔被黏液阻塞，就会因肺叶或肺段萎陷而形成一个不透光区。

opalescent [ˌəupəˈlesənt] *adj.* 乳白色的
Lipid within the ascitic fluid will cause it to appear opalescent, ranging from cloudy to completely opaque and chylous.
腹水会因其中的脂质而呈现为乳白色，从浑浊至完全的不透明及乳糜状。
The doctor tried to relieve and even eliminate the pain of pulpitis in opalescent teeth with the sterilized eugenol cottonball after the blockade of the pulp devitalizer.
医生试图在用牙髓失活剂阻断后，用消毒过的丁香酚棉球置于乳白色牙齿上来减轻甚至消除牙髓炎所致的疼痛。

opaque [əuˈpeik] *a.* 不透光的，不透明的
An opaque foreign body in the neck will be clearly demonstrated on a lateral roentgenogram.
颈部的不透光异物可在 X 线侧位片上清楚地显现出来。
An artificial lens was installed inside the eye to replace the opaque natural lens removed in cataract surgery.
一个人工晶体被植入眼内代替在白内障手术中被摘除的混浊的自然晶体。

open [ˈəupən] *v.* 开，开口
The cells forming simple tubular glands form a single tube which opens directly on to the free surface.
构成单管腺的细胞形成一个单管直接开口于游离面。
When the left ventricle goes into contraction, the aortic similunar valve opens.
当左心室收缩时，主动脉半月瓣开放。
a. 开的，畅通的
You must keep your bowels open.
你必须保持大便通畅。
A nurse's open communication with the patient about test procedures makes possible increased trust on the part of the patient.
护士就检查程序与病人进行坦率的交谈可以增加病人（对医务人员）的信任。

opening [ˈəupəniŋ] *n.* 孔，穴；开口
The Y-U operation permits judgement of the size of the opening of the pylorus that remains.
Y-U 型幽门成形术允许按需要决定所保留幽门的开口大小。

operability [ˌɔpərəˈbiliti] *n.* 可手术性
The decision should be made about the operability of the lesion.
必须就病灶手术的可能性作出决定。

operant [ˈɔperənt] *n.* 自发反应

In psychology, operant refers to any response which is not elicited by external stimuli.
心理学上，自发反应是指不是外界刺激引起的反应。
a. 自发反应的
Operant responses are frequently referred to as voluntary behavior.
自发反应常被称为自主行为。

operate [ˈɔpəreit] *v.* 起作用，奏效
This law operates universally.
这个规律是普遍起作用的。
The medicine gradually operated.
这药慢慢奏效了。
Several factors may then operate to prevent excessive redistribution of blood into the lung.
于是几个因素可能起作用以制止血液过多地重新分配至肺部。

operation [ˌɔpeiˈreiʃən] *n.* 手术
The surgical operation on him admits of no delay.
对他施行外科手术刻不容缓。
This case history reminded me of that major operation which was performed last year.
这份病史使我想起去年做的那个大手术。
Radical operation is an extensive resection of tissue for the complete extirpation of disease.
根治手术是为了完全消除疾病的一种广泛组织切除。

operative [ˈɔpərətiv] *a.* 运转的，有效的，手术的
The phenomenon of fever has been operative for hundreds of millions of years.
发热现象的处理已有了千万年。
Many old regulations which are irrelevant to the modern medical services are still operative.
许多不适合当今医疗的旧规章仍在沿用中。
Treatment of this acute disease requires operative measures.
治疗这种急性病需要施行手术。

operon [ˈɔpərən] *n.* 操纵子
The operon codes for single messenger RNA molecules and acts as a unit of genetic transcription and genetic regulation.
操纵子为单个信使 RNA 指定遗传编码，是基因转录和调节的功能单位。

ophthalmic [ɔfˈθælmik] *a.* 眼的
Needle-like crystals may form in ophthalmic solutions and, if present, the solution must not be used.
滴眼液里可能形成针状结晶体，如有，此溶液不应使用。

ophthalmologic(al) [ˌɔfθælməˈlɔdʒik(əl)] *a.* 眼科学的
Ophthalmologic examination of this baby at 6 months was normal.
这个婴儿 6 个月时眼科学检查正常。

ophthalmologist [ɔfθælˈmɔlədʒist] *n.* 眼科学家，眼科医生
Filatov was the most eminent ophthalmologist of the former Soviet Union.
费拉托夫是前苏联最杰出的眼科学家。

ophthalmology [ɔfθælˈmɔlədʒi] *n.* 眼科学
Ophthalmology is a branch of medicine dealing with the eye, its anatomy, physiology, pathology and clinical practice, etc.
眼科学是医学的一个分科，涉及眼的解剖学、生理学、病理学和临床实践等。

ophthalmoplegia [ɔfˌθælməˈpliːdʒiə] *n.* 眼肌麻痹
Chronic progressive external ophthalmoplegia is a disorder characterized by slowly progressive paralysis of the extraocular muscles.
慢性进行性眼外肌麻痹是一种以眼外肌慢性进行性麻痹为特征的疾病。

Ophthalmoplegia may be congenital or acquired.
眼肌麻痹可能是先天的或获得性的。

ophthalmoscope [ɔfˈθælməskəup] *n.* 检眼镜,眼底镜

The ophthalmologist thoroughly examines the retina and the interior part of the eye with an instrument called ophthalmoscope.
这位眼科专家用一种称作检眼镜的仪器详尽地检查视网膜和眼的内部。

The direct ophthalmoscope enables a fine beam of light to be directed into the eye and at the same time allows the examiner to see the spot where the beam falls inside the eye.
直接检眼镜能使一细小光束直接照射到眼内,同时使检查者可以观察到光束照射到的眼内的部位。

opiate [ˈəupieit] *n.* 鸦片制剂,麻醉剂,镇静剂

Fentanyl is in a class of medications called opiate analgesics.
芬太尼是属于鸦片止痛剂类的药物。

Heroin is an opiate drug that is synthesized from morphine.
海洛因是一种从吗啡合成的鸦片类药物。

opioid [ˈəupiɔid] *a.* 阿片类的

Results showed higher levels of opioid receptors in the brains of rats whose mothers had eaten junk food during pregnancy.
结果显示在怀孕期间食用垃圾食品的母鼠其后代的脑部阿片受体水平更高。

Fear of abuse and dependence is a major factor limiting access to opioid analgesics.
担心滥用和依赖是阿片类止痛药使用受到限制的一个主要因素。

opisthotonos [ˌɔpisˈθɔtənəs] *n.* 角弓反张

Physical examination reveals hypertonicity and muscular rigidity with severe opisthotonos.
体格检查发现张力过高和肌肉僵硬,伴有严重的角弓反张。

Auditory stimuli provokes the patient convulsions with opisthotonos.
听觉刺激诱使病人出现惊厥和角弓反张。

opium [ˈəupiəm] *n.* 阿片,鸦片

Opium has analgesic and narcotic action due to its content of morphine.
阿片由于含有吗啡,所以具有止痛和麻醉作用。

Opium has the same uses and side-effects as morphine and prolonged use may lead to dependence.
阿片与吗啡具有相同的用途和副作用,长期使用可导致依赖性。

Morphine, opium, and codeine are the only natural(opium-derived)opioids.
天然的阿片类(阿片衍生物)仅有吗啡、鸦片和可待因(三种)。

opponent [əˈpəunənt] *a.* 对立的,对抗的

Contractive muscles and extensors are opponent muscles.
收缩肌和伸肌是对抗肌肉。

opportunistic [ˌɔpətjuːˈnistik] *a.* 机会性的;机会致病性的,条件致病性的

Azidothymidine increases survival and prevents development of recurrent opportunistic infections.
叠氮胸苷能提高病人生存率,防止机会感染再发生。

Infection, often with opportunistic organisms, must be treated energetically.
感染常常是由条件致病菌引起,必须给予强效治疗。

oppose [əˈpəuz] *v.* 反对;相对,对抗

One among the five surgeons would oppose this operation program.
五位外科医生中有一人将反对这一手术方案。

Drug eruptions are often somewhat pruritic, as opposed to secondary syphilis.
与二期梅毒相反,药物疹常有一点痒感。

opposite [ˈɔpəzit] *a.* 对面的;相反的

Opponens brings the digits opposite to other digits.
对掌肌可使手指向其他各指的反向运动。

Conversely, those drug treatments are relatively or absolutely contraindicated in the opposite situations.
在相反的情况下，这些药物疗法是相对或绝对禁忌的。

prep. 在…的对面

In the human, the upper pole of each kidney lies opposite the 12th thoracic vertebra, and the lower pole lies opposite the third lumbar vertebra.
人体每个肾脏的上极正对第十二胸椎，下极正对第三腰椎。

opsonin ['ɔpsənin] *n.* 调理素

Molecules such as antibody, complement and C-reactive protein that promote phagocytosis are said to act as opsonins.
促进吞噬作用的分子如抗体、补体和 C 反应蛋白统称为调理素。

Opsonin is a substance, usually antibody or complement in component, which coats a bacterium and enhances phagocytosis by phagocytic cells.
调理素是一种物质，通常是抗体或补体成分，它包绕在细菌外，可增强吞噬细胞的吞噬作用。

opsonization [ˌɔpsənai'zeiʃən] *n.* 调理素化，调理素作用

The process of coating a particle, such as a microbe, to target it for ingestion (phagocytosis) is called opsonization.
将微生物包被一种颗粒，使其易于被消化(吞噬)的过程被称为调理素化。

Coating of bacteria with antibodies or the complement protein C3b (opsonization) normally results in phagocytosis of bacteria by macrophages.
用抗体或补体蛋白 C3b 包被细菌(调理素化)正常情况下会导致细菌被巨噬细胞吞噬。

optic ['ɔptik] *a.* 眼的；视力的

Tissue therapy was thought effective in atrophy of optic nerve.
用组织疗法治疗视神经萎缩，曾被认为有效。

The optic disc should be located if necessary by following a branch of the retinal artery to its source.
如必要，应沿着视网膜动脉的一个分支追溯到其起源处，找出视神经盘的位置。

optical ['ɔptikəl] *a.* 光学的；视觉的

Nowadays the optical microscope was greatly improved.
至今光学显微镜已经有了很大改进。

Now many people know that the mirage is an optical phenomenon.
现在许多人都知道海市蜃楼是一种视觉现象。

optimal ['ɔptiməl] *a.* 最适宜的，最好的

This pH is the one at which enzyme activity is optimal.
这个 pH 值就是酶活性处于最适宜状态时的 pH。

The optimal inspiratory to expiratory time ratio is 1 : 2 to 1 : 3.
最好的吸气/呼气时间比例是 1 : 2 至 1 : 3。

optimization [ˌɔptimai'zeiʃən] *n.* 最优化

The FDA Center for Drug Evaluation and Research (CDER) is aware of a steadily increasing number of carcinogenicity studies in progress employing some form of dietary restriction or optimization.
(美国)食品药品管理局的药品评价与研究中心(CDER)发觉应用膳食限制或膳食最优化的某种形式进行致癌性研究的数量正在稳定地增加。

optimize ['ɔptimaiz] *v.* 使尽可能完善；使优化

Radiologists are expected to "optimize" radiation doses by exposing patients only to enough radi-

ation to get a clear image.
希望放射学家优化放射剂量使病人仅接受能获得清晰图像的最低辐射。

optimum [ˈɔptiməm] *n.* 最适度,最适条件
The optimum pH can also be viewed as a consequence of the protein nature of enzymes.
最适 pH 也可视为酶的蛋白质本质的一种结果。

option [ˈɔpʃən] *n.* 选择
What options are now available to the physician with a patient in severe intractable heart failure?
面对一个严重的顽固性心衰病人,现在有什么方法可供内科医生选择呢?
Spinal fusion has been shown to be an effective option to treat lumbar degenerative spondylolisthesis.
脊椎融合术已被证明是治疗退行性腰椎滑脱有效的选择。

optional [ˈɔpʃnənl] *a.* 可任意选择的;随意的
Molecular genetics is an optional subject at the college.
分子遗传学是该校的一门选修课。

oral [ˈɔːrəl] *a.* 口的;口头的
The soft palate forms the back of the roof of the oral cavity.
口腔后顶部是软腭。
Oral Fe is safer than parenteral Fe; the rate of response is the same with either route.
经口服用铁比不经胃肠道用铁安全,而见效的速度却相同。

orally [ˈɔrəli] *ad.* 口头地;口服地
Penicillin may be given orally.
青霉素可以口服。

orange [ˈɔrindʒ] *n.* 橙
Acridine orange is a nucleic acid selective fluorescent cationic dye useful for cell cycle determination.
吖啶橙是一种核酸选择性荧光阳离子染料,对测定细胞周期有用。
The cell-permeant SYTO 82 orange fluorescent nucleic acid stain exhibits bright, orange fluorescence upon binding to nucleic acids.
细胞渗透性 SYTO 82 橙色荧光核酸染料在结合到核酸上时显示出明亮的橙色荧光。

orbit [ˈɔːbit] *n.* 眼眶
In the orbit the maxillary nerve passes through the infraorbital groove and canal in the floor of the orbit.
在眶内,上颌神经经过眶下沟和眶下管。

orbital [ˈɔːbitəl] *a.* (眼)眶的,眼窝的
Orbital cellulitis often results from contiguous spread from infected sinuses.
眼眶蜂窝织炎常发生于被感染鼻窦的邻近扩散。
CT should be used to rule out an orbital abscess, especially in patients with decreased eye movement.
应进行 CT 检查以排除眼窝脓肿,尤其是对眼球运动减少的病人。

orbitography [ˌɔːbiˈtɔgrəfi] *n.* 眶造影术
Orbitography and orbital venography provide complementary diagnostic information for us.
眶造影术和眶静脉造影术为我们提供了辅助诊断的信息。
The simulations were achieved under geometrical configurations corresponding to actual MERIS observations after using its proper orbitography.
运用合适的眶造影术后,几何构型与实际的 MERIS 观察相一致,这样仿真就完成了

orbitomeatal [ˌɔːbitəmiˈeitəl] *a.* 听眶的
Orbitomeatal line, also called orbitocanthal line, is the positioning line of head CT .
听眶线也叫听眦线,是头部 CT 的定位线。

orbivirus [ˌɔːbiˈvaiərəs] *n.* 环状病毒

The only orbiviruses believed to infect humans are the tick-borne Kemerovo viruses of Siberia.

被认为唯一能感染人的那些环状病毒是西北利亚蜱传播的克莫罗弗病毒。

Orbiviruses can infect and replicate within a wide range of arthropod and vertebrate hosts.

环状病毒可广泛感染节肢动物和脊椎动物并在其体内复制。

orchidectomy [ˌɔːkiˈdektəmi] *n.* 睾丸切除术

Surgical removal of a testis is called orchidectomy, usually to treat such diseases as seminoma (a malignant tumour of the testis).

切除睾丸的外科手术叫睾丸切除术,通常用于治疗精原细胞瘤(睾丸的恶性肿瘤)这类疾病。

Removal of the action of androgen can be achieved by administration of estrogens or gonadotrophin-releasing hormone analogues, or by orchidectomy.

通过给予雌激素或促性腺激素释放激素类似物,或者通过睾丸切除可去除雄激素的作用。

orchidopexy [ˈɔːkidəuˌpeksi] *n.* 睾丸固定术

In order to save testicle, early surgical exploration orchidopexy may be mandatory to avoid recurrence.

为挽救睾丸功能,必须早期施行手术探查并行睾丸固定术以避免隐睾复发。

Orchidopexy is a surgery to move an undescended testicle into the scrotum and permanently fix it there.

睾丸固定术是将隐睾移至阴囊内并将其永久固定的手术。

orchitis [ɔːˈkaitis] *n.* 睾丸炎

Orchitis usually manifests as testicular swelling and tenderness over 2 to 3 days.

睾丸炎常表现为 2 到 3 天以上的睾丸肿胀和压痛。

Orchitis can be relieved by prednisolone (40mg daily for 4 days).

睾丸炎的缓解可采用泼尼松,每日 40mg,共用 4 天。

orderly [ˈɔːdəli] *n.* 护理员;勤杂员

Nurses, nursing aides, orderlies, and inhalation therapists may participate in patient care in the intensive care units.

护士、助理护士、护理员、气雾师均可参与重症监护室的病人护理工作。

organ [ˈɔːgən] *n.* 器官

Each system is made up of organs, and each organ has its share in the work of the system.

每个系统由一些器官组成,而每个器官在系统中都有自己的作用。

Each organ is made up of units called cells.

每个器官由称之为细胞的单位组成。

Most organs contain a number of different kinds of tissue.

多数器官含有若干不同的组织。

organelle [ˌɔːgəˈnel] *n.* 细胞器

Each cell contains many highly organized physical structures called organelles.

每个细胞都含有许多称为细胞器的高度组织化的身体结构。

organic [ɔːˈgænik] *a.* 器官的;器质性的;有机的,有机物的

Diseases in which structural changes are demonstrable are known as organic diseases.

呈现结构变化的疾病就叫作器质性疾病。

Our products are certified 'organic', meaning they are free of: Genetically Modified Organisms (GMO), chemical fertilisers and pesticides, they have not been irradiated, etc.

我们的产品被证实为"有机的",意味着它们不含转基因、化肥和农药,没有受过辐射等。

Volatile organic compounds (VOCs) are found in everything from paints and coatings to underarm deodorant and cleaning fluids.

挥发性有机化合物(VOCs)无处不在,从油漆和涂料到腋下除臭剂和清洗液。

organism [ˈɔːgənizm] *n.* 生物(体),微生物,细菌;机体

Bacteria are very small,unicellular organisms.

细菌是极小的单细胞生物。

Physiology means the science of function in living organisms.

生理学是有关生物体功能的科学。

Metabolism means the chemical reactions that occur in the animal organism.

新陈代谢是指动物机体内发生的化学反应。

If the resistence of the body is high,the imprisoned organisms may eventually die.

如果人体的抵抗力强,被困的细菌可最终死亡。

organization [ˌɔːgənaiˈzeiʃən] *n.* 机构;机化

Research regarding cancer is being carried on by many organizations in our country.

我国许多机构正在进行着癌症的研究。

The removal of the thrombus takes place mainly by organizations.

这种血栓的清除主要是通过机化来进行的。

organize [ˈɔːgənaiz] *v.* 使机化

The infarcted tissue is slowly organized to leave a depressed scar.

梗死的组织被缓慢机化,遗留一个凹陷的瘢痕。

organochlorine [ˌɔːgənəuˈklɔːriːn] *n.* 有机氯

The largest application of organochlorine chemistry is the production of vinyl chloride.

有机氯化学的最大应用是生产氯乙烯。

Chlorinated hydrocarbon (organochlorine) insecticides,solvents,and fumigants are widely used around the world

氯化烃(有机氯)杀虫剂、溶剂和熏剂在全世界被广泛应用。

organogenesis [ˌɔːgənəuˈdʒenisis] *n.* 器官发生

Once gastrulation is complete,organogenesis begins.

一旦原肠胚形成,器官发生就开始。

organophosphate [ˌɔːgənəˈfɔsfeit] *n.* 有机磷酸盐

Atropine is the treatment for organophosphate toxicity.

在有机磷中毒时可用阿托品解救。

orient [ˈɔːriənt] *v.* 定向,定位

Most teachers are academically oriented.

大多数教师侧重于学术。

orientation [ˌɔːrienˈteiʃən] *n.* 方向,定向

To serve the people is the fundamental orientation of public health work in China.

为人民服务是中国公共卫生工作的根本方向。

What is chiefly required is a re-orientation of general practitioners towards a preventive,rather than curative,role.

首要的要求是重新把全科医师的责任由治疗转向预防。

orifice [ˈɔrifis] *n.* 孔;口,管口

Identification of the ectopic orifice establishes the diagnosis.

确认异位外口才能确诊。

In all cases the hernial orifices should be examined and the rectum palpated.

对全部病例都必须检查其疝气管口,并对直肠作触诊。

origin [ˈɔridʒin] *n.* 起源,起因

Epigastric discomfort or pain is a common symptom and is most frequently of intra-abdominal origin.

上腹部不适或疼痛是一种常见的症状,其产生原因多在腹内。

original [əˈridʒənəl] *a.* 原始的,最初的

Such scar tissue may be stronger than the original tissue.
这样的瘢痕组织会比原来的组织更坚固一些。
The recurrence of infectious hepatitis may be much worse than the original attack.
复发的传染性肝炎可能比初发的严重得多。

originate [ə'ridʒineit] *v.* 发源;发生
Each nerve originates from the spinal cord by two roots—the anterior and the posterior.
每条脊神经通过前根和后根起始于脊髓。
The majority of brain tumors originate from the neuroglia and are called gliomas.
大多数脑肿瘤来源于神经胶质,称为神经胶质瘤。

ornithine ['ɔːniθiːn] *n.* 鸟氨酸
L-ornithine is a kind of mesostate essential in the metabolism, an amino acid which is not made of protein.
L-鸟氨酸是人体代谢中必不可少的中间代谢产物,它是一种不参与蛋白组成的氨基酸。
Large amount of cystine as well as arginine, lysine and ornithine was excreted in the urine.
大量的胱氨酸、精氨酸、赖氨酸以及鸟氨酸从尿中排出。

oropharyngeal [ˌɔːrəu'færiŋgiəl] *a.* 口咽的
Aspiration of oropharyngeal and gastric contents is normally prevented by the gastroesophageal and pharyngoesophageal sphincters.
正常情况下,胃食管(贲门)和咽食管括约肌可防止口咽和胃内容物的吸入。

oropharynx [ˌɔːrəu'færiŋks] *n.* 口咽
Aspiration of bacteria from the oropharynx may follow dental anaesthesia.
自口咽吸入细菌可在牙科麻醉时发生。

orthopedic [ˌɔːθəu'piːdik] *a.* 矫形外科的
He devised a new orthopedic apparatus for the non-surgical treatment.
他设计了一种非手术治疗的新的矫形外科用具。

orthopedics [ˌɔːθəu'piːdiks] *n.* 矫形外科学
Mr. Brown specializes in orthopedics.
布朗先生专长矫形外科学。

orthopnea [ˌɔːθɔ'pniːə] *n.* 端坐呼吸
Orthopnea is a sign of severe left ventricular failure.
端坐呼吸是严重左心室衰竭的一种体征。
Patients with dyspnea due to both cardiac and pulmonary diseases may report orthopnea.
患者由于心肺疾病引起的呼吸困难都可表现为端坐呼吸。

orthosis [ɔː'θəusis] *n.* 矫正器
An orthosis is an appliance used to correct deformities or to improve the function of movable parts of the body.
矫正器是用于矫正畸形或改善身体活动部位功能的一种器具。

orthostatic [ˌɔːθə'stætik] *a.* 直立的,直体的
Orthostatic hypotension is a fall in blood pressure associated with dizziness, syncope and blurred vision occuring upon standing.
直立性低血压是站立时出现血压下降并伴有头昏、晕厥以及视力模糊。

orthotopic [ˌɔːθeu'tɔpik] *a.* 常位的,正位的
The aim of this study is to determine the frequency of hyperuricemia in children following orthotopic liver transplantation.
本研究的目的是确定原位肝移植后儿童患高尿酸血症的频度。
This article summarizes the outcomes and clinical experience of orthotopic heart transplantations in Shanghai Zhongshan Hospital.
本文总结了上海中山医院原位心脏移植治疗的效果及临床经验。

os calcis [ɔs-ˈkælsis] [拉] *n.* 跟骨

We assessed the bone mechanical properties in os calcis of that patient.

我们评估了那位患者的跟骨机械性能。

oscillate [ˈɔsileit] *v.* 使振动，摆动

Currents associated with the muscular action of the heart cause the spot of light to oscillate and thus trace a typical curve on the light-sensitive chart.

伴随心肌活动的电流使光点摆动，因而在光敏图纸上绘出一条典型的曲线。

oscillation [ɔsiˈleiʃən] *n.* 摆动

Bradykinetic oscillation is seen in epidemic encephalitis.

缓慢性摆动见于流行性脑炎。

Periodic breathing results from oscillation of the feedback control mechanisms regulating respiration.

周期性呼吸是由于调节呼吸的反馈控制机制波动的结果。

oscillograph [ɔˈsiləgraːf] *n.* 示波器

Oscillograph is an instrument for recording electric oscillation.

示波器是一种记录电振荡的仪器。

oscillopsia [ˌɔsiˈlɔpsiə] *n* 振动幻觉

Oscillopsia may be caused by the loss of vestibulo-ocular reflex, or involuntary eye movements.

振动幻觉可能由前庭眼球反射缺失或眼球不自主运动所致。

osmolarity [ˌɔzməuˈlæriti] *n.* 渗透性

The release of vasopressin is enhanced by stress and increased osmolarity of the blood.

紧张和血液渗透压的升高可增强加压素的释放。

osmotic [ɔzˈmɔtik] *a.* 渗透的

The pressure built up within the cell as a result of this water intake is termed osmotic pressure.

由于水渗入细胞内而形成的压力称为渗透压。

The osmotic diuretic effects of glucose cause polyuria and polydipsia.

葡萄糖的渗透性利尿作用引起多尿和烦渴。

osseous [ˈɔsiəs] *a.* 骨的，骨性的

After several months of vitamin D deficiency osseous changes of rickets can be recognized.

在维生素 D 缺乏几个月以后就能见到佝偻病的骨骼变化。

Bone, or osseous tissue, is a rigid form of connective tissue that forms most of the skeleton.

骨或骨组织为硬型结缔组织，它组成骨骼的大部分。

ossific [ɔˈsifik] *a.* 骨化的，成骨的

Attempts to estimate fetal maturity by radiological examination of the ossific centres have not proved to be reliable.

企图用放射学方法检查成骨中心来估计胎儿成熟度已证实不可靠。

ossification [ˌɔsifiˈkeiʃən] *n.* 骨化

The formation of bone or of a bony substance is called ossification.

骨或骨质的形成称为骨化。

osteitis [ˌɔstiˈaitis] *n.* 骨炎

Osteitis is characterized by inflammatory infiltrate, osteoneogenesis, and bony sclerosis with remodeling.

骨炎的特征是炎细胞浸润、新骨形成和骨硬化，伴有结构重塑。

Sternal osteitis, a potential consequence of cardiac surgery, remains rare.

胸骨骨炎是心外科手术潜在的后果，但很少发生。

osteoarthritis [ˌɔstiəuɑːˈθraitis] *n.* 骨关节炎

Osteoarthritis is a degenerative disease in old people.

骨关节炎是老年人的一种退行性疾病。

Joint arthroplasty has revolutionized the management of severe and disabling osteoarthritis.
关节成形术使严重和可致残的骨关节炎的处理明显改善。

osteoarthropathy [ˌɔstiəuɑːˈθrəupəθi] *n.* 骨关节病

Hypertrophic osteoarthropathy is a disabling condition that may occur secondarily to primary lung cancer.
肥大性骨关节病是一种致残性疾病，可继发于原发性肺癌。

Charcot neuro-osteoarthropathy is a devastating condition affecting most commonly the foot/ankle joint in diabetic patients and may lead to severe deformities and amputation.
夏科神经性骨关节病是一种破坏性疾病，最常累及糖尿病患者的足和踝关节，可导致严重的畸形和截肢。

osteoblast [ˈɔstiəˌblæst] *n.* 成骨细胞

Osteoblasts produce and secrete proteins that constitute the bone matrix. The matrix is subsequently mineralized under the control of the same cells.
成骨细胞产生和分泌组成骨基质的蛋白质，随后基质在成骨细胞（同一细胞）的控制下矿质化。

osteoblastoma [ˌɔstiəublæsˈtəumə] *n.* 骨母细胞瘤

Osteoblastoma is larger than 2 cm and involves the spine more frequently.
骨母细胞瘤大于2cm，更多累及脊柱。

Spinal osteoblastomas are considered benign tumors but can be locally aggressive.
脊柱骨母细胞瘤被认为是良性肿瘤，但可能具有局部侵袭力。

osteocalcin [ˌɔstiəuˈkælsin] *n.* 骨钙蛋白，骨钙素

Osteoblast synthesize a number of proteins that are incorporated into the bone matrix, including osteocalcin.
成骨细胞合成许多蛋白质，包括骨钙蛋白，渗合到骨基质中。

osteochondritis [ˌɔstiəuˌkɔnˈdraitis] *n.* 骨软骨炎

The placental-fetal transmission of treponemes leads to congenital syphilis, and then causes severe fetal osteochondritis and periostitis that leads to multiple bony lesions.
螺旋体经胎盘-胎儿传播途径可导致先天性梅毒，进而引起严重的胎儿骨软骨炎和骨膜炎，导致多骨性病变。

Osteochondritis dissecans is a joint disorder that affects the articular cartilage and subchondral bone, most commonly at the knee.
分离性骨软骨炎是一种关节病，累及关节软骨和软骨下骨组织，最常发生于膝关节。

osteochondroma [ˌɔstiəkɔnˈdrəumə] *n.* 骨软骨瘤

Osteochondromas usually stop growing at the time of growth plate closure.
骨软骨瘤通常在骺板闭合后停止生长。

The lump was excised and histologically confirmed to be a soft-tissue osteochondroma.
肿块切除后组织学证实是软组织的骨软骨瘤。

osteoclast [ˈɔstiəˌklæst] *n.* 破骨细胞；折骨器

Mature osteoclasts are usually larger (50 to 100μm diameter) multinucleate cells with abundant mitochondria, numerous lysosomes, and free ribosomes.
成熟的破骨细胞常常是较大的（直径 50 ~ 100 微米）多核细胞，有丰富的线粒体，为数甚多的溶酶体和游离的核糖体。

Osteoclast is an instrument for use in surgical refracture of bone.
折骨器是用于外科骨再折术的器械。

osteoclastoma [ˌɔstiɔklæsˈtəumə] *n.* 破骨细胞瘤

Osteoclastoma is a rare tumour of bone, caused by proliferation of osteoclast cells.
破骨细胞瘤是罕见的骨肿瘤，由破骨细胞增生引起。

osteochondrosis [ˌɔstiəukɔnˈdrəusis] *n.* 骨软骨病

Children with osteochondrosis generally have diffuse joint pain and swelling.
患骨软骨病的儿童常有弥漫性关节疼痛和肿胀。

osteogenesis [ˌɔstiəu'dʒenisis] *n.* 骨生成；骨发生

Marrow stromal cells have the capacity of osteogenesis.
骨髓基质细胞具有成骨能力。

An ideal bone-grafting material should be able to produce bone by osteogenesis, osteoinduction, and osteoconduction.
理想的植骨材料应当具备骨生成性、骨诱导性和骨传导性。

osteoid ['ɔstiɔid] *a.* 骨样的

Osteoid osteoma and osteoblastoma are benign bone tumors that have identical histologic features but differ in size, sites of origin, and symptoms.
骨样骨瘤和骨母细胞瘤都是良性骨肿瘤，它们具有相同的组织学结构，但大小、发生部位和临床症状不一样。

Osteoid osteoma and osteoblastoma histologically resemble each other, with characteristically increased osteoid tissue formation surrounded by vascular fibrous stroma.
骨样骨瘤和骨母细胞瘤组织学特征类似，均伴有增多的骨样组织形成，骨样组织周围为纤维血管间质。

osteolytic [ˌɔstiəu'litik] *a.* 溶骨的

Bone X-rays may show typical multiple osteolytic areas.
骨骼 X 线片可显示出典型的多发性溶骨区域。

osteomalacia [ˌɔstiəumə'leiʃiə] *n.* 骨软化症，软骨病

Vitamin D deficiency produces osteomalacia in nongrowing bone.
非生长期的骨骼缺乏维生素 D 则可引起软骨病。

When calcium is removed from the bones and they lose some of their hardness, a disorder osteomalacia results.
当钙自骨中丢失使骨失去其某些硬度时，就会发生软骨病。

osteomyelitis [ˌɔstiəumaiə'laitis] *n.* 骨髓炎

The duration of therapy for osteomyelitis may have to be extended.
治疗骨髓炎的持续时间可能不得不予以延长。

osteopathia [ˌɔstiə'pæθiə] *n.* 骨病

He is a specialist in osteopathia.
他是一位骨病专家。

osteopathy [ˌɔsti'ɔpəθi] *n.* 整骨术

Students study in detail osteopathy.
学生们详细地学习了整骨术。

osteophyte ['ɔstiəˌfait] *n.* 骨赘

Spondylosis produces a characteristic appearance on X-ray, including narrowing of the space occupied by the disc and the presence of osteophytes.
脊柱关节强直在 X 线片上具有典型的表象，包括有椎间盘所占的空间变窄以及出现骨赘。

osteopoikilosis [ˌɔstiəuˌpɔiki'ləusis] *n.* 脆弱性骨硬化

The imaging features of osteopoikilosis are typical.
脆弱性骨硬化的影像学表现是非常典型的。

Eight cases of osteopoikilosis verified by clinic and radiology were retrospectively analyzed.
对由临床及影像学所确诊的 8 个脆弱性骨硬化病例进行了回顾性分析。

osteoporosis [ˌɔstiəupə'rəusis] *n.* 骨质疏松（症）

Prolonged immobilization also favours the development of osteoporosis.
长期（卧床）不动也会促使形成骨质疏松。

This osteomalacia is easily distinguishable from the more common osteoporosis.
这种骨软化症很容易与更为常见的骨质疏松症相鉴别。

osteoprotegerin [ˌɔstiəuprəuˈtedʒərin] *n.* 骨保护素

Genetic and treatment studies in mice suggest that osteoprotegerin may protect against vascular calcification.
对小鼠的基因研究和治疗研究提示骨保护素可能有保护血管避免钙化的作用。

Some data support a role for osteoprotegerin in the vasculature as an inhibitor of calcification and a marker, rather than a mediator, of atherosclerosis.
一些资料支持骨保护素具有抑制血管钙化的作用,并且是动脉粥样硬化的标志物,而非介质。

osteosarcoma [ˌɔstiɔsɑːˈkəumə] *n.* 骨肉瘤

Osteosarcoma, a malignant bone tumour, is usually seen in children and adolescents but can occur in adults of all ages.
骨肉瘤是恶性骨肿瘤,多见于儿童和青少年,也可发生于任何年龄的成年人。

osteosclerosis [ˌɔstiəuskliəˈrəusis] *n.* 骨硬化

Idiopathic osteosclerosis can be defined as developmental variations of normal bony architecture, which are unrelated to local stimuli.
特发性骨硬化被定义为正常骨性结构发育过程中的变异,与局部刺激无关。

This report aims to clarify the difference in terminology and presentation of Worth syndrome and Van Buchem disease known to produce mandibular osteosclerosis.
该报道旨在明确 Worth 综合征和 Van Buchem 病在命名和临床表现上的不同,这两种疾病均可导致下颌骨硬化。

osteotomy [ˌɔstiˈɔtəmi] *n.* 截骨术,骨切开术

Persons in the fifth and sixth decades may benefit from osteotomy.
截骨术对 50 ~ 60 岁的人有益。

Block osteotomy is a kind of operation in which a section of bone is removed.
大块骨切骨术是一部分骨被切除的一种手术。

otherwise [ˈʌðəwaiz] *ad.* 另外;在其他方面

You think this severely burned patient cannot be cured, but he thinks otherwise.
你认为这个严重烧伤的病人不能治好,但他的看法不同。

The principal method of giving drugs is by mouth, and doses which are not otherwise specified are assumed to be oral doses.
用药的主要方法是口服,各种药物剂量如果未经另外专门指定,一概设想为口服剂量。

The patient should be considered to have carcinoma of the stomach until proved otherwise.
在得到否定证据之前,应认为病人患的是胃癌。

He is short-sighted, but otherwise he is in good health.
他虽近视,但在其他方面倒是十分健康的。

Certainly, some babies have been salvaged who otherwise would have died.
的确,一些本来认为要死掉的婴儿已经得救了。

otitis [əuˈtaitis] *n.* 耳炎

The child was evaluated and found to have bilateral otitis media.
对病儿作了检查,发现他有双侧中耳炎。

otolaryngology [ˌəutəˌlæriŋˈgɔlədʒi] *n.* 耳鼻喉科学

Otolaryngology is among the first to utilize the microscope.
耳鼻喉科是最早使用显微镜的学科之一。

otosclerosis [ˌəutəuskliəˈrəusis] *n.* 耳硬化症

Auditory hallucinations occur in alcohol hallucinosis and otosclerosis.
酒精幻觉症和耳硬化症可引起听幻觉(幻听)。

otoscope [ˈəutɔskəup] *n.* 耳镜

Otoscope consists of a funnel speculum, a light, and lenses, used for examining the eardrum and the external meatus.

耳镜由漏斗形窥镜、灯和透镜等组成，用于检查鼓膜及外耳道。

outbreak [ˈautbreik] *n.* 暴发

Hepatitis may occur in epidemic outbreaks in camps, schools, and institutions for children.

肝炎可能在兵营、学校和儿童机构暴发流行。

outburst [ˈautbəːst] *n.* 暴发

The outbursts cannot readily be controlled by the affected person, who is not otherwise prone to antisocial behaviour.

这类暴发(文中指情绪)不能很快地得到患者的控制，但患者在其他方面并没有对抗社会的行为。

outcome [ˈautkʌm] *n.* 结果，后果，成果，效果

The outcome of our experiment will be published soon.

我们的实验结果即将发表。

The present study aims to evaluate the outcome of stroke unit care in the subjects.

本研究的目的是在测试人群中评价卒中单元护理的效果。

One study reported that 8 of 20 such children had poor neurological outcomes.

一份研究报道说，20 例这类儿童中有 8 例神经系统预后不良。

outgrow [autˈgrəu] *v.* 生长速度超过

Many patients either "outgrow" their endometriosis or become pregnant and remain asymptomatic indefinitely.

很多病人或随着年龄的增长，子宫内膜异位症不再发展，或因妊娠可维持长短不一的无症状时期。

outline [ˈautlain] *v.* 概括，概述

The results of the various tests of immunologic function are outlined in the section on Laboratory Data.

各种免疫学功能试验的结果在"实验室化验数据"部分作了概括介绍。

The treatment of pulmonary edema due to congestive heart failure is outlined below.

充血性心力衰竭引起的肺水肿的治疗简述如下。

outlook [ˈautluk] *n.* 展望，前景；观点；眼界

Contact lenses brighten our outlook.

隐形眼镜使我们前景光明。

Since the use of antitoxin has become universal, the outlook in diphtheria is very favorable.

因为抗毒素的使用已很普遍，这对治疗白喉的前景十分有利。

outnumber [autˈnʌmbə] *v.* 在数量上超过

Subclinical cases outnumber clinically evident cases of brucellosis by 12 to 1.

布氏杆菌病的亚临床病例已超过了临床病例，其比例为 12 : 1。

outpatient [ˈautˌpeiʃənt] *n.* 门诊病人

Depressed-children treated as outpatients reported a negative view of the future in one study.

一项研究中报道，接受门诊治疗的抑郁症患儿对未来持消极看法。

He is receiving physical therapy in the outpatient department of this hospital.

他现在正在这个医院的门诊部接受理疗。

output [ˈautput] *n.* 输出

The essential physiological defect in shock is a marked reduction of cardiac output.

在休克时生理学上的主要缺陷是心输出量显著减少。

The reduced cardiac output can only be compensated for by an increase in heart rate.

心输出量减低时，只能通过心率加速来代偿。

outright [aut'rait] *ad.* 彻底地;立即

Chemotherapy medications work by killing cancer cells outright, preventing them from multiplying, or by halting the spread of a tumour.

化疗药物可通过立即杀死癌细胞,防止它们扩增,或停止肿瘤的扩散而起作用。

outstanding [aut'stændiŋ] *a.* 杰出的,突出的

His father was considered one of the most outstanding surgeons of the twentieth century.

他的父亲被认为是20世纪最杰出的外科医生之一。

The outstanding features of bacillary dysentery in children are dehydration and acidosis.

儿童患菌痢时的突出特征是脱水和酸中毒。

ovarian [əu'vεəriən] *a.* 卵巢的

There are many ovarian follicles in various stages of maturation in the ovary.

在卵巢中有许多不同成熟时期的卵泡。

Primary amenorrhoea occurs with ovarian dysgenesis.

原发性闭经发生于卵巢发育不全。

ovary ['əuvəri] *n.* 卵巢

There was a pelvic mass separate from the right ovary in a female patient.

一位女患者有一个和右侧卵巢相分离的盆腔内肿块。

The ovary is the favorite site for endometriosis.

卵巢是子宫内膜异位症的好发部位。

A normal ovary may be felt in a thin woman by the examiner.

检查者可扪及到消瘦妇女的正常卵巢。

overactive [ˌəuvər'æktiv] *a.* 活动过度的

For various reasons the thyroid gland may become either underactive or overactive.

由于不同的原因,甲状腺的功能既可低下也可能过高。

overactivity [əuvəræk'tiviti] *n.* 活动过度,过度活跃

The clinical manifestations of shock may be due to the intense sympathetic and adrenal medullary overactivity.

休克的临床表现可能是由于交感神经兴奋和肾上腺髓质过度活跃。

overall ['əuvərɔːl] *a.* 全面的;综合的; 总的

The overall clinical picture was compatible with pernicious anemia.

总的临床表现与恶性贫血相符。

Overall mortality rates for postoperative pneumonia vary from 20% - 40%.

手术后肺炎的总死亡率约为20% ~40%。

overcome [ˌəuvə'kʌm] *v.* 战胜,克服,压倒

This "prozone" phenomenon will be overcome by diluting the serum.

稀释血清可以克服这一前区现象。

During the course of the disease antibodies are produced in sufficient numbers to overcome the microorganisms and the person recovers.

在患此病过程中,产生大量抗体,战胜微生物,个体便恢复健康。

The competitive antogonism of medicines can be overcome by increasing the concentration of the agonist.

药物的竞争性拮抗作用可通过增加激动剂的浓度消除。

overdiagnosis ['əuvədaiəg'nəusis] *n.* 滥诊

Judging from these reports, overdiagnosis was one of the main problems at that time.

从这些报告判断,滥诊成为当时的主要问题之一。

overdistension [ˌəuvədis'tenʃən] *n.* 过度扩张

Uterine action in labour may be inefficient because of the overdistension of the uterus.

由于子宫过度膨胀,分娩时可出现子宫收缩乏力。

overdosage [ˌəuvəˈdəusidʒ] *n.* 超剂量

In humans, overdosage of morphine causes respiratory arrest and death.

对人来说,过大剂量吗啡可引起呼吸骤停和死亡。

Constipation may be aggravated by overdosage with oral preparations of iron.

便秘可因过量服用铁剂而加重。

overdose [əuvəˈdəus] *n.* 用药过量

An overdose of any drug can lead to problems.

任何药物用量过多都会引起问题。

overdue [ˈəuvəˈdjuː] *a.* 过期的

The fetus is two weeks overdue, ie still not born two weeks after the expected date of birth.

那胎儿已超过预产期两周了,即超过预产期两周还未出生。

Detailed research into the laugh mechanism is long overdue.

对笑的机制早该进行详尽的研究了。

overestimate [ˌəuvəˈestimeit] *v.* 过高估计,过高评价

I think you are overestimating her ability.

我想你过高地估计了她的能力。

The importance of these discoveries cannot be overestimated, and this inaugurates a new era in cancer immunotherapy.

对这些发现的重要性怎么估计也不算过高,而且这一切开创了癌症免疫疗法的新纪元。

overestimation [ˌəuvəˌestiˈmeiʃən] *n.* 估计过高

Workers in the petroleum industry may smoke less than average, resulting in an overestimation of expected kidney cancer deaths and a reduction in the standardized mortality ratio(SMR).

石油工业工人吸烟量可能低于平均数,导致对预期肾癌死亡数的估计过高,以及标准化死亡率的降低。

overexposure [ˌəuvəriksˈpəuʒə] *n.* 曝光过度

Overexposure to ultraviolet rays can cause skin cancer and may contribute to premature aging of the skin.

对紫外线暴露过度能引发皮肤癌,还可能引起过早的皮肤老化。

overexpress [ˈəuvəikˈspres] *v.* (基因等)过表达

Mice that overexpress human heat shock protein 27 have increased renal injury following ischemia reperfusion.

过表达人热休克蛋白 27 的小鼠在缺血再灌注后肾脏损害增加。

We generated a transgenic mouse overexpressing full-length non-mutant HSF1.

我们制造了一种转基因小鼠可以过表达全长野生型 HSF1 基因。

overhaul [ˌəuvəˈhɔːl] *n.* 变革,检修

Until such an overhaul could be accomplished, the Committee of Institute of Medicine called upon HHS to revise the Privacy Rule and associated guidance.

在这一大变革实现前,医学研究所委员会要求卫生福利部修订隐私规则和相关指南。

The instruments for medical examination need a complete overhaul.

这些医疗体检仪器需要彻底检修。

overhydration [ˌəuvəhaiˈdreiʃən] *n.* (体内)水分过多

The patient must be carefully monitored for overhydration.

必须密切注意监测患者是否有体内水分过多的现象。

Overhydration means an excess of water in the interstitium; dehydration is the contrary. Hypervolemia and hypovolemia refer only to abnormal changes in blood volume and are not synonymous with overhydration and dehydration.

水分过多是组织间隙水分过多,脱水则相反。血量过多和血量过少仅指血容量的异常变化,和水分过多以及脱水两词不是同义的。

overlap [ˈəuvəlæp] *n.* 重叠,交错;部分一致

There is considerable overlap between the various personality disorders.

在各种人格障碍中有相当多的重叠现象。

v. 重叠,部分相同

The clinical features of the two conditions may overlap, differentiation being possible only on the basis of the microscopic findings.

这两种疾病的临床特征有可能相似,而两者的鉴别只能根据显微镜的观察。

overlie [ˌəuvəˈlai] *v.* 覆在…上面

The node is firm but not tender and there is no erythema of the overlying skin.

该结节硬但无触痛,其表面皮肤无红斑。

overload [ˌəuvəˈləud] *v.* 使超载

Cells are overloaded with these substances.

细胞中这些物质的含量过多。

n. 超载,负担过重

Elevated serum-ferritin levels occur in Fe-overload states.

血清铁蛋白水平升高的现象出现于铁负荷过高状态。

overlook [ˌəuvəˈluk] *v.* 忽略

It is unfortunate that this information is so frequently overlooked.

不幸的是,这类信息常被忽略。

Since these drugs are taken for long periods of time, the possibility of poisoning should not be overlooked.

由于这些药物长期服用,中毒的可能性绝对不能忽视。

overproduce [ˌəuvəˈprɔdjuːs] *n.* 过量生产,过量合成

Overproduce of IGF-Ⅱ can cause hypoglycemia because of inappropriate stimulation of insulin receptors by IGF-Ⅱ.

胰岛素样生长因子Ⅱ的过量合成因其不适当激活胰岛素受体而导致低血糖。

overrate [əuvəˈreit] *v.* 对…估计(或估价)过高

Physicians need to find out whether aroma therapy and relaxation therapies are overrated and expensive fads for patients with advanced cancer.

医生们需要查明芳香疗法和松弛疗法对晚期癌症病人的作用是否被过高估计而只是一些花钱的时尚。

overrepresent [ˈəuvəˌrepriˈzent] *v.* 使有过多的代表

Transitions are overrepresented among single base pair substitutions causing genetic disease.

在单碱基替换导致的遗传病中,转换占大多数。

overriding [ˈəuvəˈraidiŋ] *a.* 压倒一切的,高于其他的

All these factors are subject to the overriding requirements of medical safety.

所有这些因素应服从于压倒一切的医疗安全的需要。

oversea(s) [ˈəuvəˈsiː(z)] *ad.* 在国外

More than 40 per cent of their research staff are located overseas.

他们(的研究机构中)有40%以上的研究人员在国外工作。

oversight [ˈəuvəsait] *n.* 疏忽;监督;失察

Many cases of malpractice are caused by oversight.

许多医疗事故是因疏忽造成的。

We will further improve health oversight in this area.

我们将进一步改善这一区域的卫生监督。

The doctor was responsible for the oversight of this medical project.

这位医师的职责是监督这一项医学工程。

overuse [ˈəuvəˈjuːz] *v.* 把…过度(久)使用

Frequently no ocular cause can be found and the frontal headache must be ascribed to overuse of the frontalis muscle or to anxiety.
有些前额的疼痛常常不能从眼睛找到原因，而必须从过度使用额肌或从焦虑来找原因。

overwhelming [ˌəuvəˈwelmiŋ] *a.* 压倒一切的；极大的
There is overwhelming evidence that the sun's ultraviolent rays are the prime cause of skin cancer.
充分有力的证据表明太阳的紫外线是皮肤癌的主要原因。
Prof. Smith has achieved an overwhelming success in the field of microsurgery.
史密斯教授在显微外科领域取得了极大的成功。

overwhelmingly [ˌəuvəˈwelmiŋli] *ad.* 势不可挡地；极大地
The data from proper statistical studies overwhelmingly favor this type of treatment.
正确的统计学研究数据有力地支持这种类型的治疗。
Tubal pregnancy is overwhelmingly the most common form of ectopic gestation.
输卵管妊娠显然是宫外孕中最常见的一型。

oviduct [ˈəuvidʌkt] *n.* 输卵管
The vast majority of ectopic pregnancies occur in the oviduct.
绝大多数异位妊娠发生在输卵管。

ovulate [ˈəuvjuleit] *v.* 排卵
By measuring estrogen levels in a women's breath, aroma scan could tell her when she's ovulating.
通过测量妇女呼吸中的雌激素水平，香味检测器可告诉她排卵的时间。
One of the main reasons why people become infertile is that the woman may be unable to ovulate.
人们不育的一个主要原因是女性不能排卵。

ovulation [ˌəuvjuˈleiʃən] *n.* 排卵
The temperature drops with ovulation and rises with menstruation.
排卵时体温下降，而行经时则升高。
Even with regular menstrual cycles of normal length, the date of ovulation is only approximately known.
即使月经周期规则而且正常的妇女，其排卵日期也只能大概知道。

ovulatory [ˈəuvjulətəri] *a.* 排卵的
Ovulatory dysfunction is abnormal, irregular, or absent ovulation. Menses are often irregular or absent.
排卵功能障碍是指异常排卵、不规律排卵或者无排卵。月经也常不规律或者不来。
There are varying causes for ovulatory dysfunction; the most frequent one is polycystic ovarian syndrome.
排卵功能障碍有各种各样的原因，最常见的是多囊卵巢综合征。

ovum [ˈəuvəm] *n.* 卵，卵子
In fact, an ovum is not even discharged from the ovary until after the completion of oogenesis.
事实上直至卵发生完成，卵子才从卵巢排出。
After a menstrual period the endometrium proliferates in preparation for the reception of a fertilized ovum.
月经期后子宫内膜增生，准备接受受精卵。

oxacillin [ˌɔksəˈsilin] *n.* 苯唑青霉素；新青霉素 Ⅱ
Your doctor has prescribed oxacillin, an antibiotic, to help treat your infection.
你的医生已经开了一种抗生素苯唑西林，用来帮助治疗你的感染。
Other work in our lab has shown that honey can make MRSA more sensitive to antibiotics such as oxacillin-effectively reversing antibiotic resistance.
我们实验室的其他研究已经显示蜂蜜能使 MRSA 对苯唑西林等抗生素更敏感，有效地逆

转抗生素耐药性。

oxalate [ˈɔksəleit] *n.* 草酸盐

Oxalate stone in the urinary bladder may produce pain by mechanical and chemical irritation.

膀胱中的草酸盐结石可通过机械和化学刺激引起疼痛。

oxidant [ˈɔksidənt] *n.* 氧化剂

Experimental and clinical studies support the pivotal role played by reactive oxidant species in the mechanism of platelet activation.

实验及临床研究均支持活性氧在血小板活化机制中发挥关键作用。

Oxidant stress might mediate the effects of TGF-β1 and promote airway remodeling in children with severe asthma.

氧化应激介导了 TGF-β1 的作用,促进了重症哮喘儿童的气道重塑。

oxidase [ˈɔksideis] *n.* 氧化酶

Cyanide inhibits the activity of cytochrome oxidase.

氰化物能抑制细胞色素氧化酶的活性。

oxidation [ˌɔksiˈdeiʃən] *n.* 氧化(作用)

The oxidation of each molecule of NADH therefore generates three molecules of ATP.

氧化每分子 NADH 可产生三分子 ATP。

Most biological oxidations are accomplished by the removal of a pair of hydrogen atoms from a molecule.

大多数生物氧化是通过从一个分子上脱掉一对氢原子来完成的。

oxidative [ˈɔksideitiv] *a.* 氧化的

The brain is peculiarly susceptible to oxidative damage.

大脑对氧化损伤特别敏感。

Oral supplementation with antioxidants may improve sperm quality by reducing oxidative stress.

口服抗氧化剂可通过减少氧化应激而改善精子质量。

oxide [ˈɔksaid] *n.* 氧化物

Automobile exhaust contains another dangerous pollutant called nitrogen oxide.

汽车排出的废气中含有另一种危险的污染环境的物质,称之为氧化氮。

oxidize [ˈɔksidaiz] *v.* 氧化

Ascorbic acid can be reversely oxidized to dehydroascorbic acid.

抗坏血酸能可逆地氧化为脱氢抗坏血酸。

Vitamin C is readily oxidized outside the body hence should be protected from exposure.

维生素 C 在体外易于被氧化,因此决不可暴露于空气中。

oxidoreductase [ˈɔksidəuriˈdʌkteis] *n.* 氧化还原酶

Azoreductase belongs to the family of oxidoreductases.

偶氮还原酶属于氧化还原酶家族。

oxycodone [ˌɔksiˈkəudəun] *n.* 氧可酮;羟考酮

We will get to assess the efficacy and safety of oxycodone tablets (Tylox) for the treatment of pain.

我们将要评估氧可酮片(泰勒宁片)的镇痛效果及其安全性。

We should investigate the progress of clinical application of controlled-release oxycodone.

我们应该调查控释羟考酮的临床应用进展。

oxygen [ˈɔksidʒən] *n.* 氧,氧气

Jogging and other aerobic exercise can increase the body 's oxygen consumption, promote metabolism.

慢跑和其他有氧运动能增加机体的耗氧量,促进新陈代谢。

The oxygen uptake (VO_2) of an athlete is the amount of oxygen which the body uses in a minute.

运动员的摄氧量(VO_2)是指其机体在一分钟内使用的氧气量。

oxygenate [ɔk'sidʒineit] *v.* 氧合,氧化

The small pulmonary veins collect the oxygenated blood from the capillary bed.

小肺静脉从毛细血管床采集氧合血液。

Arteries carry oxygenated blood that had received oxygen from the lungs to all parts of the body.

动脉将含氧血(从肺部获得氧气的血液)输送到身体各部。

oxygenation [ˌɔksidʒi'neiʃən] *n.* 氧合(作用),充氧(作用)

Adequate oxygenation was maintained by oxyhood until the evening of the fifth hospital day.

用氧气罩维持充足的给氧状态直到住院第 5 日晚。

The patient should be provided with adequate oxygenation and precise fluid and electrolyte replacement.

该病人应充分给氧和精确地补充水和电解质。

This lack of oxygenation causes a bluish color in the child suffering a severe attack of asthma.

缺乏氧合作用使得患有哮喘的重症患儿的肤色发青。

oxyhemoglobin [ˌɔksiˌhiːməu'gləubin] *n.* 氧合血红蛋白

Hemoglobin, when admixed with cerebrospinal fluid, is converted to the pigments- oxyhemoglobin and bilirubin.

血红蛋白在与脑脊液混合时转变为色素氧合血红蛋白和胆红素。

oxyphil ['ɔksifil] *adj.* 嗜酸性的

Up to date, five cell types have been identified in normal parathyroid tissues; chief cells, vacuolated chief cells, dark chief cells, oxyphil cells and transitional oxyphil cells.

到目前为止,正常甲状旁腺中被证实有 5 种细胞:主细胞、空泡状主细胞、暗主细胞、嗜酸性细胞和过渡性嗜酸性细胞。

Oxyphil cell adeomas of the lacrimal gland are rare tumors. We report the first documented case in Nigeria.

泪腺的嗜酸细胞腺瘤非常少见。我们首先报道了发生在尼日利亚的一个病例。

oxytocic [ɔksi'təusik] *a.* 催产的

Posterior pituitary injection contains the pressor and oxytocic principles.

垂体后叶注射液含有加压的和催产的成分。

n. 催产药

The agents that stimulate the smooth muscles of the uterus are called oxytocics.

兴奋子宫平滑肌的药物称为催产药。

oxytocin [ˌɔksi'təusin] *n.* 催产素

Labor should be initiated by an intravenous infusion of oxytocin in this case.

对这一病例,应使用静脉滴注催产素使其临产。

Oxytocin infusion will often bring about evacuation of the uterus, but prostaglandins are more effective.

催产素静脉滴注通常可使子宫排空,但前列腺素更有效。

ozonation ['əuzəˌneiʃən] *n.* 臭氧化

pH has been found to increase very slightly because of ozonation.

臭氧化可使 pH 值轻微增加。

Ozonation is very effective for destroying or inactivating viruses and bacteria, as well as Cryptosporidium and Giardia.

臭氧处理对杀死或灭活病毒和细菌、以及隐孢子虫和贾第虫非常有效。

ozone ['əuzəun] *n.* 臭氧

Many chemicals, such as sulphur dioxide and ozone, act as irritants to the bronchial tubes of the lung.

许多化学物质,如二氧化硫和臭氧,对肺支气管具有刺激作用。

P

pace [peis] *n.* 步;速度

The pace of the anemia determines the degree of symptoms.

贫血进展的速度决定症状的严重程度。

pacemaker [ˈpeismeikə] *n.* 起搏器;起搏点

The artificial cardiac pacemaker functions in a manner very similar to the natural pacemaker.

人工心脏起搏器的作用在方式上与自然起搏点相似。

Many people whose hearts cannot beat effectively alone have been saved by pacemakers.

起搏器已经拯救了许多心脏不能独自有效跳动的病人。

pachytene [ˈpækətiːn] *n.* 粗线,粗线期(等于 pachynema);*a.* 粗线的,粗线期的

Druring pachytene stage,the chromosomes become much more tightly coiled.

在粗线期,染色体盘绕的更加紧密。

In meiosis,the association of four homologous chromatids can be seen during the pachytene stage of prophase.

在减数分裂前期的粗线期,可以看到四个同源的染色单体的联结。

pacing [ˈpeisiŋ] *n.* 调整速率,定速度

Artificial cardiac pacing has a very important role because drug therapy alone is usually ineffective.

人工心脏起搏具有重要作用,因为单靠药物治疗常常无效。

packed [ˈpækt] *a.* 大量的,成堆的;压缩的

Hypovolemia caused by hemorrhage is ideally corrected with packed red blood cells.

出血引起的低血容量最好用大量红细胞加以纠正。

If anemia produces cardiopulmonary symptoms,packed RBC transfusions may be necessary.

如贫血产生心肺症状,可能需要输给浓缩的红细胞。

The packed cell volume(PCV)or hematocrit of male is 40% ~54%.

男性红细胞压积是 40% ~54%。

paclitaxel [pækliˈtæksəl] *n.* 紫杉醇(抗肿瘤药)

This study was to define the maximal tolerant dose of paclitaxel in weekly paclitaxel with concurrent intensity-modulated radiotherapy for local-regionally advanced NPC.

本研究旨在确定紫杉醇每周 1 次与调强放射治疗同期使用治疗局部晚期鼻咽癌患者时紫杉醇的最大耐受剂量。

PACS(picture archiving communication system) [ˈpiktʃə ˈɑːkəviŋ kəˌmjuːniˈkeiʃən ˈsistəm] *n.* 图像存储与传输系统

Reasonable storage of PACS is an essential step in hospital digitization.

合理的 PACS 存储是医院信息化建设的必要步骤。

paeoniflorin [ˌpiəniˈflɔːrin] *n.* 芍药苷

The contents of paeoniflorin were different in the peonies growing in different fertility of soil.

不同土壤条件下生长的芍药中其芍药苷的含量不同。

The average recovery rate of paeoniflorin was 100.61% (n=6,RSD=0.89%).

芍药苷的平均回收率为 100.61%,RSD= 0.89%(n=6)。

pagophagia [peigəuˈfeidʒiə] *n.* 食冰癖

Pica and especially pagophagia only suggest Fe lack as the mechanism in the diagnosis of hypo-

chromic-microcytic states.
异食癖，特别是食冰癖，在低色素小红细胞状态的诊断中只能提示其产生机制是缺铁。

painkiller [pein'kilə] *n.* 止痛剂
She is taking painkiller.
她在服用止痛剂。
Researchers in California have found that certain painkillers provide greater and longer-lasting relief for women than they do for men.
加利福尼亚州的研究人员已发现某些止痛药可提供女性比男性更强和持续时间更长的止痛作用。

paint [peint] *n.* 涂布剂
Flaky metal powders commonly used as paint and pigments, are generally produced by grinding in ball mills or vibration mills.
常用于涂料和颜料的片状金属粉末一般是采用球磨机或者震动磨碎机捻磨而成。
Best results were obtained with propoxur in standard acrylic emulsion paint.
残杀威在标准丙烯酸乳胶涂料中得到了最好的结果。

pair [pɛə] *v.* 配对，成对
Homologous chromosomes pair during the prophase of the first meiotic division.
同源染色体配对发生在第一次减数分裂前期。
Adenine is always paired with thymine.
腺嘌呤总是和胸腺嘧啶配对。

palate ['pælit] *n.* 腭
The uvula is a part of the soft palate.
悬雍垂是软腭的一部分。
The tonsils are red and swollen, as are the fauces and soft palate.
扁桃体是红肿的，咽门、软腭同样如此。

palilalia [ˌpæli'leiljə] *n.* 言语重复
Palilalia is defined as a verbal tic that results in "an involuntary repetition of words, phrases, and sentences".
言语重复被定义为一种语言痉挛，表现为单词、短语和句子无意识的重复。
We reported a case of palilalia in a 71-year-old patient.
我们曾报道过一例 71 岁的言语重复症患者。

palindrome ['pælindrəum] *n.* 回文
When read 5' to 3', the palindrome sequence is the same on both strands.
从 5 末端读向 3 末端，回文序列在两条链是一样的。
The restriction enzyme EcoRI recognizes the specific palindromic six-base pair sequence 5'-GAATTC-3' wherever it occurs in a double-stranded DNA molecule.
限制性内切酶 EcoRI 可识别特异的六碱基回文序列 5'-GAATTC-3'，无论它在双链 DNA 分子的什么位置。

palindromic [ˌpælin'drɔmik] *a.* 复发的
Palindromic rheumatism is characterized by recurrent episodes of acute arthritis with periarticular inflammation.
复发性风湿症以复发性急性关节炎伴随关节周围炎为特征。
The symptoms of palindromic rheumatism can be similar to those of many other forms of arthritis or other auto-immune diseases.
复发性风湿病的症状与其他很多类型的关节炎或其他自身免疫性疾病的症状相似。

palliate ['pæliːˌeit] *v.* 减轻
The objective of our study was to palliate sufferings of patients and to enhance the success rate of esophagus electrode insertion.

本研究的目的是要减少病人痛苦,提高植入食管电极的成功率。

Unfortunately, the majority of patients will not qualify for either option, and therefore, photodynamic therapy and palliate stenting are the second modalities to follow.

不幸的是,大多数患者不适合上述任何一种治疗方法,因此,光动力学疗法和缓解性支架可作为第二类治疗模式。

palliation [ˌpæli'eiʃən] *n.* 缓和,减轻

Prevention of obstruction or bleeding in intestinal cancer patient may offer palliation for long periods.

防止肠道癌肿病人出现梗阻或流血可获得较长时间的姑息疗效。

palliative ['pæliətiv] *a.* 缓和的,姑息的

Usually only palliative treatment is possible once symptoms have appeared.

一旦症状出现通常只有采用姑息疗法。

Radiation therapy plays an important role as a palliative measure in relieving the pain.

放射疗法作为一种姑息措施在减轻疼痛上起着重要作用。

pallidotomy [ˌpæli'dɔtəmi] *n.* 苍白球切开术

Pallidotomy with staged procedure is recommended for the treatment of Meige syndrome in patients on whom deep brain stimulation could not be performed.

对不能进行深部脑刺激的美格综合征的病人建议用阶段性的苍白球切开手术来治疗。

pallor ['pælə] *n.* 苍白

Pallor is the most important due to iron deficiency.

面色苍白是缺铁最重要的症状。

Some patients with obvious pallor, anemia, and shortness of breath fail to report the presence of blood in their stools.

有些有明显苍白、贫血、气短的病人未能向医生报告大便带血的现象。

palmar ['pælmə] *a.* 掌的

Why does the palmar heart desquamate? Is it due to lack of a certain vitamin?

为什么手掌心会脱皮? 是缺维生素吗?

The two ligaments were composed of three parts: dorsal part, palmar part and proximal part.

这两个韧带由三部分组成:即背侧部、掌侧部和近心部。

palpable ['pælpəbl] *a.* 可触知的

Nerve involvement occurs early, and nerves may be palpable.

神经损害发生较早,且神经常可触摸到。

Palpable purpura is a raised lesion that is due to inflammation of the vessel wall with subsequent hemorrhage.

可触知的紫癜是由于血管壁炎症引起出血所致的隆起性病损。

palpate ['pælpeit] *v.* 触诊

It is not uncommon to be able to palpate hard, fixed supraclavicular nodes in patients with advanced esophageal cancer.

在晚期食管癌患者,常可触到硬而固定的锁骨上淋巴结。

palpation [pæl'peiʃən] *n.* 触诊,扪诊

The diagnosis of this disease may be aided by abdominal palpation.

本病的诊断可借助于腹部触诊。

Palpation for evidence of thickening in this area should be attempted.

证实这一部位有无增厚的触诊,是应该尝试的。

palpitation [ˌpælpi'teiʃən] *n.* 心悸

Palpitation may occur during mild exertion.

轻度劳累时可发生心悸。

Usually the patient is unaware of palpitations, and recovery following an episode is prompt and

complete without residual neurologic or cardiac sequelae.
通常病人未感觉到心悸,而且发作后很快地完全恢复,不遗留神经或心脏后遗症。

palsy ['pɔːlzi] *n.* 麻痹,瘫痪

Head trauma, with or without skull fracture, is also a major cause of the third cranial nerve palsy.
有或没有颅骨骨折的头部外伤也是第三颅神经麻痹的主要原因。

Cranial nerve palsies such as eighth nerve deafness and eye changes may also occur in meningovascular neurosyphilis.
脑膜血管性神经梅毒也可出现脑神经瘫痪如第 8 对神经性耳聋和眼的变化。

pamphlet ['pæmflit] *n.* 小册子

This is the book, or pamphlet, which has been recommended for every physician.
这就是推荐给每个医生阅读的书,或者说是小册子吧。

panacea [pænə'siə] *n.* 万应药,万灵药

No drug or operation is a panacea for all pain.
无任何药物或手术可作为治疗疼痛的万应药。

Steroids are not, however, a panacea for inflammatory disorders.
然而,类固醇并不是治疗炎症疾病的万灵药。

pancarditis [ˌpænkɑː'daitis] *n.* 全心炎

Patients with acute rheumatic fever may develop varying degrees of pancarditis with associated valve disease, heart failure.
急性风湿热的患者可能发生不同程度的全心炎及其相关的心瓣膜病和心力衰竭。

Some parasites may directly or indirectly affect various anatomical structures of the heart, with infections manifested as myocarditis, pericarditis, pancarditis, or pulmonary hypertension.
有些寄生虫可直接或间接侵入心脏的不同解剖部位,造成的感染表现为心肌炎、心外膜炎、全心炎或肺动脉高压。

pancolitis [ˌpænkə'laitis] *n.* 全结肠炎

This case reports a patient with chronic diarrhea and pancolitis caused by coinfection of paracoccidioidomycosis and histoplasmosis.
该病例报道了一名慢性腹泻和全结肠炎的患者,由南美芽生菌病和组织胞浆菌病共同感染引起。

Pancolitis affects approximately 20% to 40% of the total ulcerative colitis population and remains a therapeutic challenge for clinicians.
全结肠炎大约发生于 20% 至 40% 的溃疡性结肠炎患者,其治疗对临床医生仍具挑战性。

pancreas ['pæŋkriəs] *n.* 胰腺

One function of the pancreas is to secrete enzymes.
胰腺的功能之一是分泌酶。

Carcinoma of the head and body of the pancreas is usually fatal within one year.
胰头和胰体癌一般在 1 年内使病人死亡。

pancreatectomy [ˌpæŋkriə'tektəmi] *n.* 胰切除术

Total pancreatectomy (Whipple's operation) involves the entire gland and part of the duodenum.
胰腺全切术(惠普尔氏手术)是指切除全部胰腺及部分十二指肠。

pancreatic [ˌpæŋkri'ætik] *a.* 胰(腺)的

The Ascaris adults may perforate a suture line or cause a bile or pancreatic duct obstruction.
蛔虫成虫可穿破缝合线,或引起胆管或胰腺管阻塞。

pancreatin ['pæŋkriətin] *n.* 胰酶

Pancreatin is administered for conditions in which pancreatic secretion is deficient; for example, in pancreatitis.
胰酶(药物)用于胰腺分泌物不足的情况,例如,胰腺炎。

pancreatitis [ˌpæŋkriə'taitis] *n.* 胰腺炎

Pancreatitis is more common in alcoholics and occurs occasionally in mumps.
胰腺炎常易发生于嗜酒者,偶见于腮腺炎时。
These clinical signs are far from being proof of the presence of pancreatitis.
这些临床体征远远不能证明胰腺炎的存在。
Severe upper abdominal pain is the outstanding symptom of acute pancreatitis.
剧烈的上腹部疼痛是急性胰腺炎的突出症状。

pancytopenia [ˌpænsaitəu'piːniə] *n.* 全血细胞减少
If pancytopenia is present, a bone marrow aspirate and biopsy are required to diagnose.
当出现全血细胞减少时,需要通过骨髓穿刺和活检来诊断。
Signs of aplastic anemia vary with the severity of the pancytopenia.
患再生障碍性贫血时的体征因全血细胞减少的严重程度而异。

pandemic [pæn'demik] *n.* 大流行(病)
Global epidemics or pandemics of influenza have occurred approximately every 10 to 15 years since the 1918-1919 pandemic.
自 1918 ~ 1919 年的流感大流行以来,全球性流行或大流行几乎每 10 ~ 15 年就要发生一次。
Influenza virus periodically emerges in a new antigenic version capable of causing a global pandemic.
流感病毒周期性地以新的抗原变体出现,能引起全球性大流行。

panel ['pænl] *n.* 方案
The simplest screen to be included in the core panel is a white blood cell count and differential that should be performed on all individuals being evaluated for change in immune status.
核心方案中最简单的筛选项目是白细胞的计数和分类,这是对评估所有个体免疫状况的变化而应当完成的。

pangenesis [pæn'dʒenisis] *n.* 泛生论
Pangenesis is one of the early theories of hereditary.
泛生论是早期的遗传学理论之一。

panniculitis [pəˌnikju'laitis] *n.* 脂膜炎
Panniculitis can be the initial presentation of both alpha-1 antitrypsin deficiency and pancreatic disease.
脂膜炎可以是 α1 抗胰蛋白酶缺乏和胰腺疾病的首发症状。
Panniculitis refers to disorders with inflammation of the subcutaneous fat. Such inflammation can be primary or can be a reaction pattern induced by a systemic process.
脂膜炎是指皮下脂肪组织的炎症性疾病,这种炎症可以原发也可以是全身性疾病的反应。

pantothenic [ˌpæntə'θenik] *a.* 泛酸的
Pantothenic acid is the precursor of coenzyme A.
泛酸是辅酶 A 的前体。
Pantothenic acid plays an important role in the transfer of acetyl group in the body.
泛酸在人体内对乙酰基的转移起着重要的作用。

papain [pə'peiin] *n.* 木瓜蛋白酶
Papain also can be made into detergent, laundry powder and hands wash.
木瓜蛋白酶也可用于制作洗涤剂、洗衣粉、洗手液等洗涤品。
This text summarizes the configuration and composing of the papain and the use in foodstuff, medicine and industry.
本文对木瓜蛋白酶的结构、组成以及在食品、医药、工业中的用途进行了综述。

papillary [pə'piləri] *a.* 乳头(状)的
At autopsy, a small 0.5cm papillary renal cortical adenoma was identified.
在尸检中,发现一个 0.5cm 的小乳头状肾皮质腺瘤。

papilledema [ˌpæpiliˈdiːmə] *n.* 视神经乳头水肿

Papilledema is not always symmetrically present.

乳头水肿并不总是对称性出现的。

Papilledema is the painless, passive bilateral disk swelling that is associated with increased intracranial pressure.

视神经乳头水肿由颅内压增高所致，表现为无痛性、被动性、双侧性视盘肿胀。

papillitis [ˌpæpiˈlaitis] *n.* 视神经乳头炎；乳头炎

Papillitis is the inflammation of the first part of the optic nerve where the nerve leaves the eyeball.

视神经乳头炎是离开眼球起始部分的视神经炎症。

Diabetics are also likely to develop necrotizing renal papillitis.

糖尿病患者也容易发生坏死性肾乳头炎。

papilloma [ˌpæpiˈləumə] *n.* 乳头(状)瘤

Aromatic amines produce papillomas and bladder cancer.

芳香类胺可导致乳头瘤和膀胱癌。

papillomatosis [ˌpæpiˌləuməˈtəusis] *n.* 乳头状瘤病

Diffuse papillomatosis refers to the formation of multiple papillomas.

弥漫性乳头状瘤病系指多发性乳头状瘤的形成。

As a mildly contagious disease, papillomatosis is transmitted by both direct and indirect contact.

乳头状瘤病为一种轻度的接触性传染病，可由直接或间接接触而传播。

papule [ˈpæpjuːl] *n.* 丘疹

Nodules are a form of papules, but larger and deeper.

结节是丘疹的一种形式，但更大和更深。

The eruption in the early stages shows erythema, swelling, papules, and vesicles.

早期皮疹表现为红斑、肿胀、丘疹和水疱。

para-aminosalicylic [ˌpærəˌæminəuˌsæliˈsilik] *a.* 对氨基水杨酸的

Para-aminosalicylic acid is an antituberculosis medication.

对氨基水杨酸是一种抗结核药。

Para-aminosalicylic acid(PAS) is administered by mouth and commonly causes nausea, vomiting, diarrhoea, and rashes.

口服对氨水杨酸常引起恶心、呕吐、腹泻和皮疹。

para-articular [ˌpærə-ɑːˈtikjulə] *a.* 关节旁的

X-rays of joints show that the patient has para-articular osteoporosis and soft tissue swelling.

关节的 X 线检查显示此病人有关节旁骨质疏松及软组织肿胀。

paracentesis [ˌpærəsenˈtiːsis] *n.* (放液)穿刺术

Paracentesis is the process of drawing off excess fluid from a part of the body through a hollow needle or cannula.

穿刺术是通过空心针或插管把身体某部位过量液体抽出来的方法。

Diagnostic paracentesis(50 to 100 ml) should be part of the routine evaluation of the patient with ascites.

有腹水的患者应按常规进行诊断性腹腔穿刺(50～100ml)。

paracetamol [pəˌræsiˈtæmɔl] *n.* 对乙酰氨基酚；醋氨酚；扑热息痛

Paracetamol is used to treat mild or moderate pain, such as headache, toothache, and rheumatism.

对乙酰氨基酚用于解除轻度或中度疼痛，如头痛、牙痛和风湿病。

Paracetamol toxicity is the most frequent cause of liver damage in the United Kingdom.

在联合王国，最常见引起肝损伤的原因是醋氨酚的毒性作用。

Paracetamol treatment can significantly enhance the activity of telomerase.

扑热息痛治疗能明显增强端粒酶的活性。

paracolic [ˌpærəˈkɔlik] *a.* 结肠旁的

Paracolic sulci are lateral depressions of the peritoneum nesting the cecum.

结肠旁沟是腹膜侧方围绕盲肠的凹陷部位。

Various lengths of intestine may herniate posterior to the right colon into the right paracolic gutter.

不同长度的肠管可从右结肠后方疝入右侧结肠旁沟。

paracortex [pærəˈkɔːteks] *n.* 副皮质区

The paracortical area, or paracotex, is the T-cell area of lymph nodes, lying just below the follicular cortex, which is primarily composed of B cells.

副皮质区就是淋巴结中的 T 细胞区,位于主要由 B 细胞组成的滤泡皮质的正下面。

paracrine [ˈpærəkrin] *n.* 旁分泌

Another meaning of paracrine is the secretion of a hormone by an organ other than an endocrine gland.

旁分泌的另一含义是激素系由某一器官而不是由某一内分泌腺分泌。

These so called autocrine and paracrine systems are used commonly during development and by most growth factors.

通常在发育时大多数生长因子采用所谓的自分泌和旁分泌系统发挥作用。

paradigm [ˈpærədaim] *n.* 范例

It has provided important paradigms for how receptors activate intracellular signalling cascade.

这为细胞受体如何激活细胞内信号级联反应提供了重要的范例。

paradoxically [ˌpærəˈdɔksikəli] *ad.* 反论地,自相矛盾地

Paradoxically, fluid retention can sometimes be eliminated by drinking more water, not less.

相反,液体的滞留有时只能通过多喝水的方法来消除,而不是少喝水。

Although iron is the most available element on this planet, paradoxically anemia resulting from its deficiency is very common.

虽然铁是地球上最容易得到的元素,但令人费解的是由于铁缺乏所致的贫血却甚为常见。

paraffin [ˈpærəfin] *n.* 石蜡

Liquid paraffin is a mineral oil, which has been used as a laxative.

液体石蜡是一种矿物质油,用作轻泻剂。

The liquid paraffin is best dispensed from a plastic oil dropper.

液体石蜡最好用塑料油滴管滴入。

paraganglioma [ˌpærəgæŋgliˈəumə] *n.* 副神经节瘤

A paraganglioma is a rare neuroendocrine neoplasm that may develop at various body sites.

副神经节瘤是一种少见的神经内分泌肿瘤,可发生于身体的多个部位。

Only about 60% of bladder paragangliomas presented with hematuria, and most of them were microscopic hematuria.

只有大约 60% 的膀胱副节瘤表现为血尿,而且多数为镜下血尿。

paragonimiasis [ˌpærəˌgɔniˈmaiəsis] *n.* 并殖吸虫病,肺吸虫病

Children with cerebral paragonimiasis are usually mentally retarded.

有脑并殖吸虫病的儿童往往智力发育迟缓。

parainfluenza [ˌpærəinfluˈenzə] *n.* 副流感

Parainfluenza viruses are associated with upper respiratory tract infections.

副流感病毒可引起上呼吸道感染。

Serologic tests are also available for the diagnosis of adenovirus, respiratory syncytial and parainfluenza virus infection.

血清学试验仍然是诊断腺病毒、呼吸道合胞病毒以及副流感病毒感染的可用方法。

parakeratosis [ˌpærəˌkerəˈtəusis] *n.* 角化不全症

Pathological changes of condyloma are characterized as proliferation, especially dysplasia, hyperkeratosis and parakeratosis.

湿疣的病理变化以增生为主,尤以异型增生、角化过度和角化不全为特征。

Granular parakeratosis(GP) is an uncommon, benign cutaneous eruption of intertriginous areas that represents a distinctive clinicopathologic entity.

颗粒性角化不全是一种少见、良性的、长在擦烂部位的皮疹,表现出一种特殊的临床病理变化。

parallel [ˈpærəlel] *v.* 与…相似;与…平行

The concentration of parathyroid hormone roughly parallels the fetal calcium requirements.

甲状旁腺激素的浓度,与胎儿的需钙量大致平行。

The deep veins tend to parallel arteries and usually have the same names as the corresponding arteries.

深静脉常与动脉平行,并与相应的动脉同名。

paralysis [pəˈrælisis] (*pl.* paralyses [pəˈrælisiːz]) *n.* 麻痹,瘫痪

Paralysis may be due to affection of lower motor neurones or due to disorder of upper motor neurones.

瘫痪可由于下运动神经元受损或由于上运动神经元的疾患引起。

Diaphragmatic paralysis may call for prolonged artificial respiration.

膈肌麻痹病例需要长时间的人工呼吸。

paralytic [ˌpærəˈlitik] *a.* 麻痹的,瘫痪的

Paralytic shellfish poisoning is primarily a neurologic poisoning.

麻痹性贝类中毒主要是一种神经性中毒。

Paralytic ileus starts with nausea and vomiting, associated with hyperactivity of the bowel and then with gross distension and absence of bowel sounds.

麻痹性肠梗阻首先出现恶心和呕吐,伴有肠道功能亢进,然后出现明显的膨胀和肠鸣音消失。

paralyze [ˈpærəlaiz] *v.* 使麻痹

Many signs of anesthesia are absent in the paralyzed patient.

许多麻醉征象不出现于麻痹病人中。

A recent study indicates that it is possible for paralyzed patients to someday control the use of robotic arms just by mere thought.

一个近期的研究表明瘫痪的病人将有可能全凭意念来操纵机器臂。

parameter [pəˈræmitə] *n.* 参数

Different drugs differ in their parameters of drug actions.

不同的药物具有不同的作用参数。

The evaluation of the clinical status of the mother can be monitored by standard parameters.

母体临床状态的估计可通过标准参数来监护。

Other parameters include allergic type symptoms in other organs such as the nose, gastrointestinal tract, and skin.

其他指标包括其他器官(如鼻、胃肠道和皮肤)的变态反应型症状。

parametrium [ˌpærəˈmiːtriəm] (*pl.* parametria) *n.* 子宫旁组织

Palpation of parametria is requisite to clinical staging of carcinoma of the cervix.

宫旁组织的触诊对宫颈癌的临床分期必不可少。

paramount [ˈpærəmaunt] *a.* 至上的,首要的

Maintaining the airway clear of secretions is paramount in the prevention of postoperative pneumonia.

持续清除气道内的分泌物对预防手术后肺炎是至关重要的。

Under such circumstances, disinfection may be a measure of paramount importance in disease

prevention.
在这种情况下,消毒可能是预防疾病的首要措施。

paranasal [pærə'neizəl] *a.* 鼻旁的,鼻侧的

In the US,38 million people suffer chronic inflammation of the nasal cavity and paranasal sinuses.
在美国有 3800 万人的鼻腔和副鼻窦患有慢性炎症。

paraneoplastic [ˌpærəˌniːəu'plæstik] *a.* 副肿瘤性的

Tumor hypoglycemia is one of several "paraneoplastic syndromes" in which the tumor produces no insulin,but induces hypoglycemia by releasing a substance.
肿瘤低血糖是几个"副肿瘤性综合征"的一种,该肿瘤并不产生胰岛素而是释放一种物质诱发低血糖。

paranoia [ˌpærə'nɔiə] *n.* 妄想狂,偏执狂

Paranoia is more frequent in women.
偏执狂多见于女性。
Paranoia must be of at least six months duration.
偏执狂至少应有 6 个月的发病持续时间。

paranoid ['pærənɔid] *a.* 类妄想狂的,类偏执狂的

Duration distinguishes paranoia from paranoid disorder.
持续时间(长短)可区别偏执狂和类偏执狂疾病。
For a diagnosis of acute paranoid disorder,the duration of the illness must be at least one week.
发病时间必须至少一星期,方可作出急性类偏执狂的诊断。

paraplegia [ˌpærə'pliːdʒiə] *n.* 截瘫,下身麻痹

Loss of sensation and of motion in the lower part of the body is called paraplegia.
身体下部感觉和运动的丧失叫做截瘫。
Paralysis of the lower portion of the body is called paraplegia.
躯体下部的瘫痪称为截瘫。

paraplegics [ˌpærə'pliːdʒiks] *n.* 截瘫患者

There are computer-controlled devices that help paraplegics move by giving electrode signals to leg muscles.
电脑控制的装置可通过将电刺激信号传至腿部肌肉的方法帮助截瘫患者移动。

parapophysis [ˌpærə'pɔfisis] *n.* 椎体横突

A special spinal tractor was put on parapophysis of T12-L3 vertebrae.
将特制的脊柱牵引器放置在 T12 ~ L3 椎体横突上。

paraproteinemia [ˌpærəprəutiː'niːmiə] *n.* 异常蛋白血(症),病变蛋白血(症)

Multiple myelomatosis is one of the paraproteinemias.
多发性骨髓瘤是一种异常蛋白血症。

parasite ['pærəsait] *n.* 寄生物,寄生虫

Viruses are obligate intracellular parasites.
病毒为细胞内专性寄生物。
Traumatic damage occurs when the parasite invades the skin.
寄生虫侵犯皮肤时便发生外伤性损伤。

parasitemia [ˌpærəsai'tiːmiə] *n.* 寄生物血症(尤指血内疟原虫)

The degree of malarial parasitemia is reflected in the percentage of red blood cells infected.
疟原虫血症的程度可通过红细胞受感染的百分比来反映。
The prognosis is poor if diagnosis is late,parasitemia is high or organs are failing.
如诊断延误,出现高寄生物血症或器官衰竭,则预后差。

parasitic [ˌpærə'sitik] *a.* 寄生的,寄生物的

Many species of worms are parasitic by nature and select the human organism as their host.

许多蠕虫是寄生性质的，而且选择人体作为宿主。

Most parasitic infections primarily affect populations in poor developing countries.

大多数寄生虫感染主要影响到贫穷发展中国家。

parasiticide [ˌpærəˈsitisaid] *n.* 杀寄生虫药

Parasiticide is an agent used to destroy parasites(excluding bacteria and fungi).

杀寄生虫药是用于杀灭寄生虫(不包括细菌与霉菌)的药剂。

parasitism [ˈpærəˌsaitizəm] *n.* 寄生虫感染;寄生(生活)

Thus, the whole course of parasitism is a continuous and dynamic process of interaction between the parasite and host.

因此，寄生虫感染的整个过程是寄生虫与宿主之间持续相互作用的动态过程。

Parasitism, on the contrary, denotes this kind of association in which man(animal or plant), the host, is to some degree injured through the activities of the other animal, the parasite.

相反，寄生生活表示这样一种关系：人(动物或植物)，即宿主，由于其他动物如寄生虫的活动而在某种程度上受到损害。

parasitize [ˈpærəsaitaiz] *v.* 寄生于，侵害

The amoeba can parasitize man when he swims in infected water.

阿米巴可侵害在污染的水中游泳的人。

parasitology [ˌpærəsaiˈtɔlədʒi] *n.* 寄生虫学

Parasitology is the branch of medical science concerned with the study of parasites.

寄生虫学是关于研究寄生虫的医学科学分支。

Medical parasitology deals primarily with the animal parasites of man and their medical significance, as well as their importance in human communities.

医学寄生虫学主要是研究人体的动物寄生虫，及其在医学上的意义，同时还研究它们在人类社会中的重要性。

parasitosis [ˌpærəsaiˈtəusis] (*pl.* parasitoses [ˌpærəsaiˈtəusiːz]) *n.* 寄生虫病，寄生物病

Under certain conditions and invariably in some parasitoses, the damage is considerable, resulting in varying degrees of disease.

在某些情况下，而且总是在患某些寄生虫病时，损伤是严重的，可引起不同程度疾病。

parasomnia [ˌpærəˈsɔmniːə] *n.* 深度睡眠状态

Nocturnal arousal disorders, or parasomnia, can occur in adoledcents secondary to attention deficit disorders.

夜间觉醒障碍或深度睡眠可以继发于青少年的注意力缺陷症。

parasympathetic [ˌpærəˌsimpəˈθetik] *a.* 副交感(神经)的

The sinus node is richly supplied with autonomic nerves, both sympathetic and parasympathetic.

窦房结分布有丰富的自主神经(包括交感和副交感神经)支配。

parathormone [ˌpærəˈθɔːməun] *n.* 甲状旁腺素

Parathormone's formal name: Parathyroid Hormone.

甲状旁腺素的正式名称是甲状旁腺激素。

Parathormone, substance produced and secreted by the parathyroid glands that regulates serum calcium concentration.

甲状旁腺素是甲状旁腺产生和分泌的物质，可调节血清钙浓度。

parathyroid [ˌpærəˈθairɔid] *a.* 甲状旁腺的

There is no evidence that gonadal or parathyroid hormones participate in the metabolic responses to infection.

没有证据表明性激素或甲状旁腺激素参与了对感染的代谢反应。

n. 甲状旁腺

The functions of the thyroid gland and the parathyroid are quite dissimilar to each other.

甲状腺与甲状旁腺的功能完全不同。

parathyroidectomy [ˌpærəˌθairɔiˈdektəmi] *n.* 甲状旁腺切除术

Parathyroidectomy is the surgical removal of one or more parathyroid glands.

甲状旁腺切除术是指手术切除一个或多个甲状旁腺。

Hypocalcemia is a common problem after parathyroidectomy or thyroidectomy.

低钙血症是甲状旁腺切除术或甲状腺切除术后的一个共同问题。

paratyphoid [ˌpærəˈtaifɔid] *n.* 副伤寒

The paratyphoid fever mimics typhoid in all respects, but are usually milder.

副伤寒在各方面都酷似伤寒,但病情常常轻些。

pardanthus [pəˈdænθəs] *n.* 射干

Black seeds of Pardanthus look like blackberries.

射干的黑种子看起来像黑莓。

Pardanthus can detoxicate and eliminate phlegm.

射干能够解毒和祛痰。

parenchyma [pəˈreŋkimə] *n.* 实质,主质

Leukemic infiltrates of the renal parenchyma may occur alone or may be associated with nephromegaly.

肾实质白血病浸润可单独发生或伴有肾肥大。

Frequently the viral infection will involve the mucous membranes of the upper respiratory passage prior to involvement of the lung parenchyma.

病毒感染常在涉及肺实质前先累及上呼吸道黏膜。

parenchymal [pəˈreŋkiməl] *a.* 实质的,主质的

Lung parenchymal involvement is both interstitial and alveolar.

肺实质受累指肺间质及肺泡两者均受累。

A chest X-ray usually shows localized parenchymal consolidation of lobar pneumonia.

胸部 X 线片通常可显示大叶性肺炎的局限性实变。

parent [ˈpɛərənt] *a.* 作为来源的

The metastasis may be either more or less differentiated than the parent tumor.

转移瘤比原发瘤分化的程度可能高一些或低一些。

The oxidation products of other drugs are more toxic than the parent substances.

另一些药物的氧化产物却比原来的药物毒性更大。

parenteral [pæˈrentərəl] *a.* 肠道外的,不经肠的

Parenteral administration of folate will overcome these deficiencies.

肠道外给予叶酸治疗可纠正这些缺乏症。

Total parenteral nutrition is not needed in the acute illness, but has an integral role in intractable or persistent diarrhea.

全肠外营养在急性期不需要,但在难治性或持续性腹泻中起重要作用。

parenterally [pæˈrentərəli] *ad.* 非肠道地

Administered drugs, whether given orally or parenterally, become distributed nonuniformly throughout the body.

无论是口服还是非肠道给药,全身药物的分布都是不均匀的。

In an emergency case, this drug should be administered parenterally rather than orally.

在急诊时,此药应进行注射而不采用口服。

paresthesia [ˌpærisˈθiːziə] *n.* 感觉异常

A complaint of paresthesias at or near the site of viral inoculation is present in 50%-80% of patients in the prodromal stage.

前驱期有 50% ~80% 的病人主诉病毒入侵处或附近的感觉异常。

At the onset of rabies there may be insidious fever and a return of pain or paresthesia at the site of the bite.

狂犬病发病时可能有不知不觉的逐渐发热,以及咬伤部位再次出现疼痛或感觉异常。

paresthesial [ˌpæris'θiːziəl] *n.* 感觉异常

The neuropathy may cause pain and paresthesials of the lower extremities, marked sensitivity to touch, and a "burning" feeling.

神经病可能引起疼痛和下肢感觉异常,对触摸极为敏感,并有灼痛感。

parietal [pə'raiitəl] *a.* 壁的

The parietal pleura is supplied by somatic nerves.

壁胸膜分布有躯体神经。

parity ['pæriti] *n.* 产次

The condition of the external os of the cervix may indicate parity.

宫颈外口可提示经产情况。

parkinsonism ['pɑːkinsənizəm] *n.* 帕金森综合征

The two important features of Parkinsoism are tremor of digital muscles and muscular rigidity, each feature may occur alone, the tremor is worse at rest.

帕金森综合征的两个重要特征是手指肌肉震颤和肌肉强直,每种特征可单独出现,在休息时震颤加重。

parotid [pə'rɔtid] *n.* 腮腺(=parotid gland)

The parotid gland is the largest of the paired salivary glands.

腮腺是成对唾液腺中的最大者。

a. 腮腺的

Parotid swelling is usually painful, but not necessarily.

腮腺肿胀一般为疼痛性的,但不一定都是如此。

parotitis [ˌpærə'taitis] *n.* 腮腺炎

Parotitis due to mumps virus usually produces swelling of the parotid gland above and below the angle of the jaw.

流行性腮腺炎病毒所致的腮腺炎通常引起下颌角上、下方的腮腺肿胀。

parous ['pærəs] *a.* 经产的

Woman having given birth to one or more children is a parous woman.

分娩过一个或多个婴儿的妇女为经产妇。

In parous women these changes are exaggerated.

在经产妇此种变化加重。

paroxysm ['pærəksizm] *n.* 发作,阵发

A sudden recurrence or intensification of symptoms is called paroxysm such as spasm or convulsion.

症状突然再发或加剧称为发作,如痉挛或抽搐。

If paroxysm of coughing are exhausting, postural drainage is often a useful adjunct.

如果阵发性的剧烈咳嗽使患者筋疲力尽,体位引流常常是有效的辅助治疗。

paroxysmal [ˌpærək'sizməl] *a.* 阵发性的

This patient had an attack of paroxysmal abdominal pain of intestinal origin last night.

这个病人昨晚发作了肠源性的阵发性腹痛。

Paroxysmal nocturnal dyspnea is a valuable sign of left ventricular failure.

阵发性夜间呼吸困难是左心室衰竭的重要症状。

parthenogenesis [ˌpɑːθinəu'dʒenisis] *n.* 单性生殖,孤雌生殖

Insects can carry out parthenogenesis.

昆虫能进行单性生殖。

Parthenogenesis occurs in some plants and invertebrates, especially arthropods.

单性生殖发生在某些植物和无脊椎动物,特别是节肢动物。

partial ['pɑːʃəl] *a.* 部分的,不完全的

The pulse rate may serve as a partial guide for the person who must take thyroid extract.
脉搏速率可作为病人必须服用甲状腺浸膏的部分依据。

Because of insufficient treatment the chancre may relapse after partial disappearance.
由于治疗不充分，下疳部分消退后可再复发。

Partial thromboplastine time(PTT) examines the integrity of the intrinsic system mainly.
部分凝血酶原时间主要检测内源性凝血系统的完整性。

partially [ˈpɑːʃəli] *ad.* 部分地，不完全地

The victim simply chokes on too large a piece of food which he could not swallow and which partially or completely blocks his air intake.
受害者单纯因吞食大块的食物而噎塞，这样就会部分或完全阻断空气的吸入。

Keeping the patient at rest and partially suppressing cough may help the bleeding to subside.
使病人保持安静并部分抑制咳嗽有助于流血停止。

participant [pɑːˈtisipənt] *n.* 参加的人，参与者

All the participants in the conference on clinical pathology may have an opportunity to speak.
所有参加临床病理会议的人都有机会发言。

The mast cell is an active participant in several neoplastic or proliferative disorders.
肥大细胞积极参与一些肿瘤和增殖性的疾病。

participate [pɑːˈtisipeit] *v.* 参与，分享

Eosinophils, basophils, mast cells and platelets participate in the inflammatory response.
嗜酸性粒细胞、嗜碱性粒细胞、肥大细胞和血小板都参与炎症反应。

Immunoglobulins participate in cell-mediated immunity by promoting the antibody-dependent cellular cytotoxicity functions of certain T lymphocytes.
免疫球蛋白通过促进某些 T 细胞的抗体依赖性细胞毒作用而参与细胞介导的免疫。

participation [pɑːˌtisiˈpeiʃən] *n.* 参与

To bring about all these reactions requires the absolute participation of the nervous system.
要引起所有这些反应就绝对需要神经系统的参与。

particle [ˈpɑːtikl] *n.* 颗粒

A virus particle consists of nucleic acid enclosed in a protein coat.
病毒颗粒由核酸和包绕在其外的蛋白质外壳构成。

Don't use absorbent cotten on an open burn—it will leave particles of cotton in the wound.
不要将脱脂棉用于开放性烧伤创面，因为会在伤口上留下棉花的碎屑。

particulate [pɑːˈtikjulit] *n.* 微粒，颗粒

Particulates, the tiny particles produced mainly by the burning of diesel fuel, are the most dangerous.
微粒，主要由燃烧柴油产生的微小粒子，是最危险的。

partition [pɑːˈtiʃən] *n.* 隔开物

The interventricular septum is a partition between the right and left ventricles.
室间隔为左、右心室之间的间隔。

partogram [ˈpɑːtəgræm] *n.* 产程图

All events during labour are noted on a partogram — a most useful graphical record of the course of labour.
在产程图上记录分娩情况是一种最有用的分娩过程的图表式记录。

parturition [ˌpɑːtjuəˈriʃn] *n.* 分娩

Parturition usually starts spontaneously about 280 days after conception, but it may be started by artificail means.
分娩通常于怀孕后约 280 天时自动开始，但可用人工方法起动。

Parturition has usually a striking effect on pre-eclampsia — blood pressure falls, edema disappears and proteinuria clears, generally after a few days.

分娩对先兆子痫孕妇常有显著的作用,如血压下降、水肿消失和蛋白尿消除,通常发生在分娩之后几天。

passage [ˈpæsidʒ] *n.* 通过;通道;排便

The passage of the blood from the right ventricle to the left auricle is called small, or pulmonary, circuit of the circulatory system.

血液从右心室到左心房的流程叫做(循环系统中的)小循环,即肺循环。

The passage of a small stone along the ureter causes one of the most excruciating pains known to man.

小块结石通过输尿管会引起一种人们最难忍受的疼痛。

Smoking irritates the throat and respiratory passages.

吸烟刺激喉咙和呼吸道。

An evacuation of the bowels is called passage.

肠道的排空称作排便。

Diarrhea may be defined as the frequent passage of loose or watery stools.

可以给腹泻下定义为频繁地排出稀的或水样粪便。

passive [ˈpæsiv] *a.* 消极的,被动的

Passive exposure to tobacco smoke results in chronic pulmonary disease as well as lung cancer for some adults.

被动吸烟对某些人可引起慢性肺部疾病以及肺癌。

Immunity acquired by transfer of antibodies or lymphocytes from an immune donor is named passive immunity.

通过转移免疫供者的抗体或淋巴细胞而获得的免疫力称为被动免疫。

paste [peist] *n.* 糊剂

A paste is typically a highly filled suspension of solid particles in a liquid phase.

糊剂是一种固体颗粒高度填充于液相中的典型混悬剂。

The paste can also be used as an external application to reduce pain or inflammation.

糊剂也可以外用以减轻疼痛和炎症。

pasteurization [ˌpæstəraiˈzeiʃən] *n.* 巴氏消毒法

Pasteurization is the process of killing bacteria in the milk by heating.

巴氏消毒法是通过加热杀灭牛奶中细菌的过程。

pasteurize [ˈpæstəraiz] *v.* 用巴氏法对…消毒

The milk is pasteurized.

此牛奶用巴氏法消了毒。

patch [pætʃ] *n.* 斑

The lesions may be rounded patches of necrotizing pneumonia that break down, giving rise to abscesses.

病变表现为圆形的坏死性肺炎斑块,斑块崩解则形成脓肿。

Peyer's patches are oval elevated areas of lymphoid tissue on the mucosa of small intestine.

派伊尔氏结是小肠黏膜上卵圆形的淋巴组织隆起区。

patchy [ˈpætʃi] *a.* 斑状的

The lesions in small arteries tend to be more patchy.

小动脉的病变往往呈斑块状。

The classic radiographic appearance of viral pneumonia is one of a patchy bronchopneumonia.

病毒性肺炎的典型 X 线片上的形状是斑片状支气管肺炎的一种。

patella [pəˈtelə] *n.* 髌骨

The anterior subcutaneous location of the patella makes it vulnerable to direct trauma.

髌骨位于机体的前方及皮下,易于受到直接创伤。

patellar [pəˈtelə] *a.* 髌骨的

The patellar apprehension test is useful when a spontaneously reduced patellar dislocation is suspected.

当怀疑已复位的髌骨自发脱位时，髌骨恐惧试验（对诊断）是有用的。

patency ['peitənsi] *n.* 开放，未闭

Treatment of aspiration involves reestablishing patency of the airway and preventing further damage to the lung.

对吸入的处理包括使气道重新通畅并防止进一步损害肺。

patent ['peitənt] *a.* 开放的，不闭的；专利的

The trachea is kept patent by a serie of C-shaped bars of cartilage.

一系列的 C 形软骨片使气管管腔保持通畅。

The patient suffers from pulmonary artery stenosis associated with patent ductus arteriosus.

这个病人患肺动脉狭窄，合并有动脉导管未闭。

n. 专利（权）

Edison held the patent on the early phonograph.

爱迪生拥有早期留声机的专利权。

v. 为…取得专利权

How long does it take to patent this newly developed medicine?

这种新研制的药物取得专利需多长时间？

When a new drug is manufactured and patented, three names are involved: the chemical, the generic and the trade-mark names.

当一种新药投产和授予专利权时，应包括三个名称：即化学名、通用名和商标名。

pathogen ['pæθədʒin] *n.* 病原体，病原菌

The pathogen is sensitive to not many chemicals.

这种病原体对少数化学药物敏感。

The purpose of this section is only to introduce the reader to the names and general properties of the major pathogens.

本节的目的仅在于给读者介绍主要病原体的名称及其一般性质。

pathogenesis [ˌpæθə'dʒenisis] *n.* 发病机制

These substances are believed to be of importance in the pathogenesis of malignant hypertension.

这些物质被认为在恶性高血压发病机制中有重要意义。

Thus, in our model of pathogenesis, hypotension would develop in the phagocytic phase of endotoxemia.

因此，在我们的发病机制模型中，内毒素血症的吞噬阶段可出现低血压。

The role of bacteria in the pathogenosis of acute cholecystitis is not clear.

细菌在急性胆囊炎的发病机制中所起的作用还不太清楚。

pathogenetic [ˌpæθədʒi'netik] *a.* 发病的，致病的

Endotoxin is considered the important pathogenetic factor in the illness.

内毒素被认为是该病的重要发病因素。

Pathogenetic factors in functional dyspepsia are genetic predisposition, inflammation, and psychosocial factors.

功能性消化不良的发病因素有遗传易感性、炎症和社会心理因素。

pathogenic [ˌpæθə'dʒenik] *a.* 致病的

Two types of amoebae are pathogenic for man.

对人类有致病作用的阿米巴有两型。

Of the fungi only yeasts and molds include pathogenic types.

在真菌中，只有酵母和霉菌有致病型。

pathogenicity [ˌpæθədʒi'nisəti] *n.* 致病性，病源性

The pathogenicity of an agent describes its ability to cause disease.

病原体的致病性是指它的致病能力。
An organism with high pathogenicity is the smallpox virus.
天花病毒是致病性高的微生物。

pathognomonic [pəˌθɔgnəˈmɔnik] *a.* 特殊(病征)的,能确定诊断的
Cataplexy is a pathognomonic symptom of narcolepsy.
昏倒是发作性嗜睡病的一个确诊性的症状。
It is a pathognomonic sonographic marker of Crisponi syndrome.
这是 Crisponi 综合征的确诊性超声诊断标志。

pathological [ˌpæθəˈlɔdʒikəl] *a.* 病理(学)的
Cirrhosis is a pathological diagnosis and therefore implies liver biopsy in all suspected cases.
肝硬化是一病理诊断,因而意味着对所有拟诊病例需进行肝脏活体组织检查。
For this reason, pathological significance can be attached to its finding.
由于这个原因,其检查结果才具有病理学意义。

pathologist [pəˈθɔlədʒist] *n.* 病理学家
Pathologists are often faced with the problem of differential diagnosis.
病理学家经常碰到鉴别诊断的问题。
Different pathologists will reach different conclusions.
不同的病理学家可能得出不同的结论。

pathology [pəˈθɔlədʒi] *n.* 病理学
No recognizable hypersensitivity reactions contribute to the pathology of amoebiasis.
在阿米巴病的病理学中未见过敏反应参与。

pathomechanism [ˌpæθeuˈmekənizəm] *n.* 病理机制
Our findings support the hypothesis of an underlying autoimmune pathomechanism in this rare disease.
我们的研究结果支持自身免疫病理机制参与该罕见疾病的假说。

pathophysiologic [pæθəuˌfiziəˈlɔdʒik] *a.* 病理生理的
Acute intrarenal vasoconstriction is an important pathophysiologic event in acute renal failure.
急性肾内血管收缩在急性肾衰中是一个重要的病理生理过程。

pathway [ˈpɑːθwei] *n.* 小路,旁道
Preexcitation syndrome may be caused by accessory pathways between the atria and the ventricle.
预激综合征是由于心房和心室间存在有附加旁道所致。

patient-centered [ˈpeiʃənt-ˈsentəd] *a.* 以病人为中心的
The nursing staff should provide a patient-centered plan for meeting the unique needs of each patient.
护理部应制订一份以病人为中心的计划来满足每个病人的独特需要。

pauciarthritis [ˌpɔːsiɑːˈθraitis] *n.* 少关节炎
Pauciarthritis involving the small joints of the hands and feet may be seen in psoriatic arthritis.
累及手和脚小关节的少关节炎可在银屑病性关节炎中见到。

peak [piːk] *n.* 顶点,顶峰
The action of this insulin reaches its peak in about four hours and passes off within eight hours.
这种胰岛素的作用在四小时左右达到顶点,在八小时内消失。
a. 高峰的;最高的
Measles is prevalent during the first 6 months of the year with a peak incidence in March.
麻疹在一年的前六个月流行,发病率高峰在三月份。

peanutagglutinin [ˌpiænətəˈgluːtinin] *n.* 花生凝集素
Peanutagglutinin activity is inhibited by lactose and galactose which compete for the binding site.
乳糖和半乳糖通过竞争结合位点而抑制花生凝集素的活性。
Peanutagglutinin binds to carbohydrates on the membranes of normal keratinocytes.

花生凝集素与正常角质细胞膜上的碳水化合物结合。

pecten [ˈpekten] *n.* 梳膜;梳状突起

The distribution of lymphatic vessels in anal pecten of rats' rectum is similar to that in cutis.

大鼠直肠肛梳区的淋巴管分布与皮肤的相似。

pectin [ˈpektin] *n.* 果胶

Pectin is a natural part of human diet, but does not contribute significantly to nutrition.

果胶是人类饮食中的天然组分,但没有明显的营养价值。

The main use for pectin is as a gelling agent, thickening agent and stabilizer in food.

果胶的主要用途是作为食品胶凝剂、增稠剂和稳定剂。

peculiar [piˈkjuːljə] *a.* 特有的,特殊的;怪僻的

Lesions may be few or numerous, and in arrangement they may be discrete or may coalesce to form patches of peculiar configuration.

损害可能很少或很多,其排列形式可有散在性的,也可以相互融合并形成特殊形态的斑片。

pediatric [ˌpiːdiˈætrik] *a.* 小儿科的

A pediatric ward is for sick children only.

小儿科病房只供患病儿童使用。

Treatment of pediatric cholera is difficult in respect to initiating and maintaining intravenous fluids.

治疗儿童霍乱难在确定开始时及维持时所需的静脉输液量。

pediatrician [ˌpiːdiəˈtriʃən] *n.* 儿科医生,儿科专家

A skilled pediatrian should be available for neonatal management at the time of delivery.

分娩时应有技术熟练的儿科医生到场,进行新生儿的处理。

pediatrics [ˌpiːdiˈætriks] *n.* 儿科学

Pediatrics mainly deals with the diagnosis and treatment of the diseases of children.

儿科学主要研究儿童疾病的诊断和治疗。

Intrauterine growth retardation continues to be a clinical problem even in the face of recent advances in obstetrics and pediatrics.

即使产科学和儿科学有很多最新进展,宫内生长迟缓仍是个临床难题。

pedigree [ˈpedigriː] *n.* 家谱,谱系

Then the geneticist prepared a pedigree chart or family tree.

然后遗传学家作出家谱图或叫家族树。

Pedigree is a list of an individual' s ancestor, used in human genetics in the analysis of inheritance.

家谱是一个人祖先的名单,用于人类遗传学中分析遗传特征。

pedunculated [piˈdʌŋkjuleitid] *a.* 有脚的,有蒂的

Subserous tumours tend to grow up into the abdomen, and may become pedunculated.

浆膜下肿瘤有生长到腹腔内的倾向,可能变为带蒂肿瘤。

peeling [ˈpiːliŋ] *n.* 剥皮,剥离,脱皮

Side effects of Retin-A may include peeling, dryness, burning, stinging, or itching.

全反维生素 A 酸的副作用包括脱皮、干燥、灼热、刺痛或发痒。

We do not recommend peeling the scab.

我们不建议剥离此痂。

peer [piə] *n.* 同等地位的人;同行;同龄人 a. 同等的

However, the surgical professor and his peers persist that a complicated operation will save the life of this patient.

不过,这位外科教授和他的同事们都坚持,一次复杂的手术可以挽救这个病人的生命。

Young people should be encouraged to communicate with their peers and develop their interpersonal skills.

应该鼓励年轻人和他们的同龄人交往，发展他们的交际能力。

Peer review is commonly accepted as an essential part of scientific publication.

同行评议通常被认为是科学文章发表的必要环节。

A peer-to-peer(abbreviated to P2P) computer network is one in which each computer in the network can act as a client or server for the other computers in the network.

对等(P2P)计算机网络是指该网络内的每一台计算机能够充当该网络内其他计算机的客户端或服务器。

pellagra [pəˈleigrə] *n.* 糙皮病，玉米红斑病

A severe lack of niacin can lead to pellagra.

严重缺乏烟酸(维生素 PP)能导致糙皮病。

Vitamin deficiency diseases such as pellagra and beriberi are rarely seen in the United States except in alcoholics.

除了酗酒者，维生素缺乏性疾病如糙皮病和脚气病在美国很少见到。

pellet [ˈpelit] *n.* 小丸，小药丸

Pellets offer many additional features compared to conventional tablets.

与传统片剂相比，小丸剂具有很多其他特性。

Pellets have been used in the pharmaceutical industry for more than four decades.

小丸用于制药行业已经超过四十年了。

pellucida [peˈljuːsidə] *n.* 透明区

Our objective is to investigate the empty zona pellucida as the storage carrier in the cryopreservation of human sperm.

我们的目的是探讨空卵透明带作为冷冻保存人类精子的贮存载体。

Human empty zona pellucida is an efficient vehicle for single spermatozoa cryopreservation.

人透明带空腔是一种有效的冻存单个精子的载体。

pelvic [ˈpelvik] *a.* 骨盆的

It is easier to palpate the pelvic organs if the patient's rectum is empty.

如能使直肠保持排空状态，则可较容易地触及盆腔脏器。

Pelvic congestion is common with pelvic inflammatory disease.

盆腔充血常见于盆腔炎性疾病。

pelvis [ˈpelvis] *n.* 骨盆；盂；肾盂

Femoral hernias occur more commonly in females because of the wider female pelvis.

股疝较常发生于女性，因女性的骨盆较宽。

The tube begins with the pelvis of the kidney and empties into the base of the bladder.

管道从肾盂开始，通入膀胱的底部。

pelvospondylitis [ˈpelvəuˌspɔndiˈlaitis] *n.* 骨盆脊椎炎

Pelvospondylitis is a kind of inflammation of the pelvic portion of the spine.

骨盆脊椎炎是一种脊柱骨盆部分的炎症。

These medical conditions or symptoms may be relevant to medical information for pelvospondylitis.

这些医学状况或症状可能与骨盆脊椎炎相关。

pemetrexed [ˈpemitrekst] *n.* 培美曲塞

Pemetrexed disodium is the only agent for the treatment of malignant pleural mesothelioma (MPM).

培美曲塞二钠是唯一治疗恶性胸膜间皮瘤(MPM)的药物。

The treated group received 500 mg·$(m^2)^{-1}$ of pemetrexed and 120mg·$(m^2)^{-1}$ of oxaliplatin by intravenous infusion on the first day, and repeated for every 3 weeks.

治疗组第1天静脉滴注培美曲塞500 mg·$(m^2)^{-1}$和奥沙利铂120 mg·$(m^2)^{-1}$，并每3周重复应用。

pending [ˈpendiŋ] *a.* 悬而未决的

Pending culture results therapy active against both gram-positive and gram-negative bacteria should be given.

在培养结果出来之前，应积极给予抗革兰氏阳性菌和革兰氏阴性菌（药物）的治疗。

penetrance [ˈpenitrəns] *n.* 穿透性；（遗传特征）外显率

We have examined this family and suggest that it has an autosomal dominant trait with incomplete penetrance.

我们研究了这个家庭，认为它有一种常染色体显性不完全外显。

Penetrance ranges from more than 75% to 100% in different families when relatives are studied with electrocardiography and echocardiography.

对亲属进行心电图和超声心动图的检查时发现不同家族的外显率超过 75%，甚至达到 100%。

penetrate [ˈpenitreit] *v.* 贯穿；透过

In time the hole may penetrate the whole thickness of the wall of the stomach.

最后空洞可以穿透胃壁全层。

The organisms are incapable of penetrating through the unbroken skin.

微生物不能穿过未破裂的皮肤。

penetrating [ˈpenitreitiŋ] *a.* 穿透的；渗透的

Penetrating injuries carry a greater risk of infection than is the case with blunt injuries.

穿透性损伤比钝挫性损伤有更大可能性引起感染。

penetration [ˌpeniˈtreiʃən] *n.* 穿透，穿入

Penetration of host cells is an essential step in the pathogenesis of viral infections.

病毒穿入宿主细胞是病毒感染发生过程中的一个关键步骤。

penicillamine [ˌpenisiˈlæmiːn] *n.* 青霉胺（抗风湿性关节炎药）

Proteinuria or nephrotic syndrome may complicate treatment with penicillamine and gold.

用青霉胺和金综合治疗时可并发蛋白尿或肾病综合征。

penicillin [ˌpeniˈsilin] *n.* 青霉素

Penicillin is a polar substance that does not enter brain at all.

青霉素是一极性物质，它完全不能进入脑组织。

Penicillin was compared to a miraculous care.

青霉素曾被比作灵丹妙药。

penile [ˈpiːnail] *a.* 阴茎的

The technical considerations for penile or digit reimplantation are very similar.

阴茎再造和断指再植在技术上的要求非常相似。

penis [ˈpiːnis]（*pl.* penises or penes [ˈpiːniːz]）*n.* ［拉］阴茎

The anatomy of the male genital system includes the penis, the scrotum and its contents and the prostate.

男性生殖系统的解剖学包括阴茎、阴囊及内容物和前列腺。

pentachlorophenol [ˌpentəˌklɔːrəˈfiːnəul] 五氯酚

Pentachlorophenol（PCP）is an organochlorine compound used as a pesticide and a disinfectant.

五氯酚（PCP）是一种有机氯化合物，用作杀虫剂和消毒剂。

Pentachlorophenol can harm the liver, kidneys, blood, lungs, nervous system, immune system, and gastrointestinal tract.

五氯酚能够损害肝、肾、血液、肺、神经系统、免疫系统和胃肠道。

pentamidine [penˈtæmidiːn] *n.* 喷他脒，戊双脒，双戊烷（抗感染药）

Pentamidine induces acute renal failure in 25%-95% of patients, usually during the second week of therapy.

喷他脒可在 25% ~95% 的病人中引起急性肾衰，通常在治疗的第二周出现。

Pentamidine is used for prophylaxis and treatment of pneumocystis carinii infections.
戊双脒已经用于卡氏肺囊虫感染的预防和治疗。
Intravenous pentamidine is also effective but is not often used because of toxic side-effects.
静脉注射双戊烷也有效但不常用,因有毒性副作用。

pentazocine [pen'tæzəsiːn] *n.* 镇痛新
Pentazocine is a mixed narcotic agonist and a weak antagonist.
镇痛新具有混合的麻醉激动剂和弱的拮抗剂作用。

pentobarbital [ˌpentəu'bɑːbitəl] *n.* 戊巴比妥(安眠药)
Pentobarbital is used to relieve insomnia and agitation and also as an anticonvulsant.
戊巴比妥用于解除失眠和焦虑不安,也用作抗惊厥剂。
Pentobarbital may be administered intravenously until adequate sedation and mild intoxication are achieved.
戊巴比妥可作静脉注射到(病人)充分镇静和轻度中毒为止。

pentosuria [pentəu'sjuəriə] *n.* 戊糖尿
Pentosuria can be observed in normal individuals if the dietary pentose intake is increased.
正常人如果食入戊糖过高,可以出现戊糖尿。
Pentosuria means increased concentration of pentose in urine.
戊糖尿是指尿中戊糖浓度增加。

pentothal ['pentəθəl] *n.* 硫喷妥钠(麻醉药)
Pentothal is given by intravenous injection to produce general anaesthesia or as a premedication prior to surgery.
硫喷妥钠用于静脉注射以产生全身麻醉,或作为外科术前用药。

pentoxifylline [ˌpentɔk'sifilin] *n.* 己酮可可碱
The effects of pentoxifylline on myocardial ischemia were observed on a model of acute myocardial infarction by a permanent ligation of left anterior descending coronary artery in rats.
通过稳定结扎大鼠左冠状动脉前降支制备的急性心肌梗死模型,已观察到己酮可可碱对缺血心肌的保护作用。

pentraxin [pen'træksin] *n.* 五聚环蛋白,正五聚蛋白,穿透素
Pentraxin are a family of acute-phase proteins formed of five identical subunits.
正五聚蛋白是由五个相同亚单位组成的一个急性期蛋白家族。

pepsin ['pepsin] *n.* 胃蛋白酶
The optimum pH of pepsin, an enzyme found in the gastric juice, is approximately 2.
胃液中的酶——胃蛋白酶的最适 pH 值是 2 左右。
When hydrochloric acid and pepsin appear in the absence of food to dilute and neutralize the secretions, ulceration of the stomach wall may result.
当盐酸和胃蛋白酶出现而无食物去冲淡和中和这些分泌物时,胃壁就可能形成溃疡。

pepsinogen [pep'sinədʒən] *n.* 胃蛋白酶原
Pepsinogen is a zymogen secreted by chief cells, which is converted into pepsin in the presence of gastric acid.
胃蛋白酶原是主细胞分泌的酶原,在胃酸存在时转变成胃蛋白酶。
This patient has a high level of the chemical pepsinogen Ⅰ in his blood.
这个病人的血液中有高水平的胃蛋白酶原Ⅰ。

peptic ['peptik] *a.* 消化性的
Peptic ulcers result from the corrosive action of acidic gastric juice on a vulnerable epithelium.
消化性溃疡是酸性胃液对易受损上皮侵蚀的结果。
Peptic ulcers and so-called nervous indigestion are examples.
消化性溃疡和所谓的神经性消化不良就是常见的例子。

peptide ['peptaid] *n.* 肽

These peptides can affect both vascular permeability and the movement of leucocytes.
这些肽类能影响血管的通透性和白细胞的运动。
These amino acids are linked together by peptide bonds into long chains.
这些氨基酸通过肽键相连形成长链。

peptidergic [ˌpeptaiˈdəːdʒik] *a.* 肽能的
Mast cells and peptidergic nerves have histo-morphologic relation in dorsal root ganglia.
在背根神经节内,肥大细胞与肽能神经存在着组织形态学上的关系。

peptomyosin [ˌpeptəˈmaiəusin] *n.* 胃蛋白酶解肌球蛋白
A second protein called peptomyosin has been isolated from beef skeletal muscle digested with pepsin.
称作胃蛋白酶解肌球蛋白的第二种蛋白质是从被胃蛋白酶消化过的牛骨骼肌里分离出来的。
It is planned to present relevant data on the properties of peptomyosin.
我们计划展示有关胃蛋白酶解肌球蛋白属性的相关数据。

perceive [pəˈsiːv] *v.* 感觉,察觉
The patient was perceived to have difficulty in standing and walking.
已经发觉病人的站立和行走都有困难。

percentage [pəˈsentidʒ] *n.* 百分比,比例
Febrile fits occur in 5 percent of the population of infants and, in approximately an equal percentage of these seizures may continue into adult life.
热性抽搐发作出现于5%的婴儿之中,又约有相等比例的抽搐婴儿可延续到成年期。
New mutations are very rare and appear to account for only a small percentage of all cases.
新的突变非常少见,看来仅占所有病例中的一小部分。

perceptible [pəˈseptəbl] *a.* 察觉到的
If the amount of blood in the spinal fluids is minimal, the intensity of staining of the supernatant may be barely perceptible.
如果脑脊液中血的含量很少,上清液着色的深浅几乎不能察觉。

perception [pəˈsepʃən] *n.* 知觉,感觉
An hallucination is a perception without an adequate external stimulation.
幻觉是无充分外部刺激而产生的知觉。
Depersonalization syndrome is a rare neurotic disorder with an unpleasant state of disturbed perception.
人格解体综合征是具有知觉紊乱不愉快状态的一种罕见神经性疾病。

perceptual [pəˈseptjuəl] *a.* 感性的,知觉的
Illusions and hallucinations are perceptual disorders.
错觉和幻觉是知觉疾病。

percolation [ˌpəːkəˈleiʃən] *n.* 渗滤,渗滤法
In physics, chemistry and materials science, percolation concerns the movement and filtering of fluids through porous materials.
在物理、化学和材料科学中,渗滤关系到液体通过多孔材料的流动和过滤。
In mathematics, percolation theory describes the behavior of connected clusters in a random graph.
在数学里,渗滤理论描述了随机图中相互关联的集群行为。

percolator [ˈpəːkəleitə] *n.* 过滤器
Accordingly, Fromm put forward some new categories including "social character", "social unconsciousness" and "social percolator".
因此,弗罗姆提出了"社会特性"、"社会无意识"、"社会过滤器"等新范畴。
The seeds were extracted with petroleum ether and 95% EtOH using a percolator.

我们通过过滤器分别用石油醚回流和95 %EtOH浸提等方法来提取种子。

percussion [pəːˈkʌʃən] *n.* 叩诊

The chest percussion note is normally resonant.

胸部叩诊声音正常。

The four classical techniques of the physical examination are inspection, palpation, percussion and auscultation.

体检四项传统技能是望诊、触诊、叩诊和听诊。

percutaneous [ˌpəːkjuˈteinjəs] *a.* 经皮的

Percutaneous liver biopsy is the most reliable means of establishing diagnosis.

经皮肝活组织检查是确定诊断最可靠的方法。

peregal [pəˈriːgəl] *n.* 平平加，脂肪醇聚氧乙烯醚

It has also been showed that the reaction can be carried in the solvent of PEG-1000 or peregal-15 without adding sodium hydrate or in the solvent of OP-10 with adding small amount of sodium hydrate.

研究也显示，反应可以在不加入氢氧化钠的PEG-1000或平平加-15溶剂中，或者仅加入少量氢氧化钠的OP-10溶液中进行。

Peregal P improves the levelness of exhaust dyeing with vat dyes on cellulosic fibres.

平平加P可提高还原染料对纤维素纤维浸染的匀染性。

perforate [ˈpəːfəreit] *v.* 穿孔，贯穿

The treatment of appendicitis by excision is much better than allowing a single appendix to perforate.

手术治疗阑尾炎比让阑尾穿孔要好得多。

Vomiting is not an important symptom of perforated duodenal ulcer.

呕吐不是十二指肠溃疡穿孔的重要症状。

perforation [ˌpəːfəˈreiʃən] *n.* 穿孔，贯穿

A gunshot wound of the head with perforations of the skull and brain can be accident, homicide, or suicide.

头部中弹受伤以致颅骨和脑部穿孔，可能是意外、他杀或自杀。

Early reoperation will avoid the complication of perforation and peritonitis.

早期再手术将避免穿孔和腹膜炎等并发症。

perforin [pəˈfɔːrin] *n.* 穿孔素

The membrane-attack complex of complement pathway and perforin are important tools deployed by the immune system to target pathogens.

补体途径的攻膜复合体和穿孔素是免疫系统用于消灭病原体的重要武器。

Perforin, as its name implies, is able to target cell membrane perforation of the material.

穿孔素，顾名思义，就是能够在靶细胞膜上穿孔的物质。

performance [pəˈfɔːməns] *n.* 施行，执行；成绩；表演

Their original paper described the performance of this operation in nine dogs and eight patients.

他们最早的论文记载了给9条狗和8个病人施行这个手术的情况。

Great care should be exercised in the performance of the microscopic fungus examination.

在显微镜下进行真菌检查应谨慎操作。

Perfomance is defined as the way in which a health care organization carries out or accomplishes its important functions.

一个卫生机构执行或完成其重要职能的情况即其成绩。

perfuse [pəˈfjuːz] *v.* 灌注；使充满

The primary goal of treatment for shock is to maintain an adequate circulating blood volume in order to perfuse vital organs.

治疗休克的首要目标是维持足够的循环血量，以保证重要器官的灌注。

Highly perfused organs such as the brain, heart, liver, and kidney receive most of the drug.
血灌流量高的器官如脑、心、肝和肾接受的药物最多。

Necrotizing fasciitis spreads along poorly perfused fascial and subcutaneous planes.
坏死性筋膜炎沿着灌注不良的筋膜和皮下组织扩散。

perfusion [pəˈfjuːʒən] *n.* 灌注(法);灌注液

The perfusion rate of small intestine is considerably higher than that of stomach.
小肠的灌注率比胃高得多。

In large vascular procedures adequate renal perfusion is essential.
在大血管手术中,需要充足的肾脏灌流。

periadenitis [ˌperiˌædiˈnaitis] *n.* 腺周炎

The diffuse cervical periadenitis of severe diphtheria must not be confused with mumps.
不要把重症白喉弥漫性颈部腺周炎和腮腺炎混淆。

periampullary [ˌperiˈæmpuˌləri] *a.* 壶腹周围的

Periampullary tumors are neoplasms that arise in the vicinity of the ampulla of Vater.
壶腹周围的肿瘤是指出现在肝胰管壶腹附近的肿瘤。

Periampullary carcinoma is one kind of malignant tumor in digestive system. It causes obstructive jaundice at early stage.
壶腹周围癌是消化系统中的一种恶性肿瘤,早期可引起梗阻性黄疸。

perianal [ˌperiˈeinəl] *a.* 肛周的

There are two types of perianal gland tumors, perianal gland adenomas, which are benign, and perianal gland adenocarcinomas, which are malignant.
肛周腺性肿瘤分两种:肛周腺腺瘤(良性)和肛周腺腺癌(恶性)。

The major clinical manifestations of the disease are perianal skin lesions, fistula and abscess, while some patients can also suffer from abdominal pain, fever and anemia.
该病的主要临床表现为肛周皮损,肛瘘或肛旁脓肿,部分患者合并腹痛、发热、贫血,等。

periarteriolar [periɑːˌtiəriˈəulə] *a.* 动脉周围的

The periarteriolar lymphoid sheath (PALS) is part of the inner region of the white pulp of the spleen, and contains mainly T cells.
动脉周围淋巴鞘(PALS)就是脾脏的白髓区内部主要包含 T 细胞的区域(部分)。

pericardial [ˈperiˈkɑːdiəl] *a.* 心包的

Pericardial effusion may be defined by physical examination or chest X-ray.
心包渗出液可通过体检或胸部 X 光照片检查出。

Pericardial effusion may develop toxemia if it is purulent.
心包积液如果是化脓性的则可发生毒血症。

pericardiectomy [ˌperiˌkɑːdiˈektəmi] *n.* 心包切除术

Pericardiectomy may be required if severe constriction is present.
如果发生严重缩窄,则须行心包切除术。

pericardiocentesis [ˌperiˌkɑːdiəusenˈtiːsis] *n.* 心包(放液)穿刺术

Emergency echocardiography can rapidly identify pericardial effusions, avoiding the need for blind pericardiocentesis.
急诊超声心动图检查可迅速诊断心包积液,避免盲目进行心包穿刺。

pericarditis [ˌperikɑːˈdaitis] *n.* 心包炎

Pericarditis is common within the first week of acute myocardial infarction.
心包炎常见于急性心肌梗死的第一周。

Cardiac compression also occurs in longstanding chronic constrictive pericarditis.
长期慢性缩窄性心包炎也会导致心脏压迫症状。

Serial changes occur in the electrocardiograms of patients with pericarditis.
心包炎患者的心电图出现一系列变化。

pericardium [ˌperiˈkɑːdiəm] *n.* 心包

There is calcification of the pericardium in 50% of the cases with constrictive pericarditis.

50%的缩窄性心包炎患者可有心包钙化。

perichondritis [ˌperiˌkɔnˈdraitis] *n.* 软骨膜炎

Perichondritis is inflammation of cartilage and surrounding soft tissues, usually due to chronic infection.

软骨膜炎是软骨及其周围软组织的炎症，通常是由慢性感染所致。

A sharp or irritating object lodged in the larynx will produce severe edema and later suppurative perichondritis.

尖而有刺激性的异物若停留在喉部会产生严重的水肿，继而成为化脓性软骨周围炎。

perichondrium [ˌperiˈkɔndriəm] *n.* 软骨膜

An infection of the perichondrium of the ear, is often accompanied by infection of the underlying cartilage of the pinna.

耳软骨膜感染常伴有耳廓(软骨膜)下面软骨的感染。

perihepatitis [ˌperiˌhepəˈtaitis] *n.* 肝周炎

Perihepatitis is inflammation of the liver capsule complicating pelvic inflammatory disease.

肝周炎是并发于盆腔感染性疾病的肝脏包膜炎症。

perilla [pəˈrilə] *n.* 紫苏属

You can find elements of lavender, rosemary and purple perilla in it.

你能在其里面发现薰衣草、迷迭香和紫苏的成分。

Purple perilla is a kind of oriental spices.

紫苏是一种东方香料。

perillaldehyde [ˌperiˈlældihaid] *n.* 紫苏醛

Synthesis of perillaldehyde via selective oxidation of perilla alcohol is discussed in this paper.

本文探讨了通过紫苏醇选择氧化合成紫苏醛。

Perillaldehyde is widely used as a kind of food additives for flavoring.

紫苏醛是一种广泛用于调味的食物添加剂。

perilous [ˈperiləs] *a.* 危险的，冒险的

Confusion and drowsiness are evidence of a perilous situation whatever the cause.

不论何种原因引起的意识模糊和嗜睡都是危急状态的表现。

perimenopausal [ˌperimenəuˈpɔːzəl] *a.* 围绝经的

Perimenopausal periods are a normal part of a woman's life that comes with advanced age.

围绝经期是女性随着年龄增长而出现的一种正常生命现象。

The purpose of this study is to evaluate the clinical effects of abdominal acupuncture for perimenopausal period syndrome.

本研究的目的是要评价腹针治疗围绝经期综合征患者的临床疗效。

perimesencephalic [periˌmesensiˈfælik] *a.* 中脑周围的

Patients with perimesencephalic hemorrhage run an uncomplicated course and invariably have excellent outcome.

中脑周围出血的病人病程经过简单，预后都是良好。

perinatal [ˌperiˈneitəl] *a.* 产期的

Intrauterine growth retardation is a major source of perinatal morbidity and mortality.

宫内生长迟缓是围产期发病率和死亡率的主要来源。

perinatology [ˌperinəˈtɔlədʒi] *n.* 围生医学，围产医学

Non-or micro-invasive diagnosis became the highlight in perinatology and genetics.

(寻找)无创或微创性产前诊断技术是围产医学及遗传学研究的热点之一。

In the recent years, with the improvement in perinatology, the survival of preterm infants has increased significantly.

近年来,随着围产医学技术的改进,早产儿的存活率大大提高了。

perineal [ˌperiˈniːəl] *a.* 会阴的

The mother is at risk for lacerations to the cervix, vagina, and perineal area during labor.

分娩时母亲有发生宫颈、阴道和会阴部裂伤的危险性。

One investigates carefully the genital and perineal regions, palpates the inguinal lymph nodes, and looks for any exanthem or enanthem.

应仔细检查生殖器和会阴部,触摸腹股沟淋巴结,并查看皮疹或黏膜疹。

perinephric [ˌperiˈnefrik] *a.* 肾周的

The clinical condition of perinephric abscess can present dramatically as an acute emergency or insidiously as a chronic condition.

肾周脓肿的临床情况差异很大,可以表现为急性重症,也可以是隐匿性的慢性过程。

Most infections of the perinephric space occur as a result of extension of an ascending urinary tract infection, commonly in association with nephrolithiasis or urinary tract obstruction.

大多数肾周组织的感染是泌尿道感染上行性蔓延的结果,通常伴有肾结石或尿道梗阻。

perinephritis [ˌperinəˈfraitis] *n.* 肾周围炎

The computed tomographic scan showed right hydronephrosis and perinephritis.

CT 扫描显示右侧肾积水和肾周围炎。

Similar effects were seen in hearts with left ventricular hypertrophy secondary to perinephritis-induced hypertension.

同样的效果可见于肾周围炎所致高血压引起继发性左心室肥大的心脏。

perineum [ˌperiˈniːəm] (*pl.* perinea [ˌperiˈniːə]) *n.* 会阴

The progress of the descent of the fetus head can be judged by watching the perineum.

观察会阴情况能判断胎头下降的进展。

perineural [ˌperiˈnjuərəl] *a.* 神经周的

In pathology, perineural invasion refers to cancer spreading to the space surrounding a nerve.

在病理学上,神经周浸润是指癌扩散至神经周围区域。

Unlike vascular invasion, perineural involvement is not associated with bone metastases.

与血管侵犯不同,神经周受累与骨转移之间没有联系。

period [ˈpiəriəd] *n.* 时期;月经

The last normal period began 12 days before the onset of the present symptoms.

末次正常月经开始于发病前 12 天。

periodic [piriˈɔdik] *a.* 周期的

Angioedema is characterized by periodic episodes of edema.

血管(神经)性水肿的特点是周期性的水肿。

periodontal [ˌperiəuˈdɔntəl] *a.* 牙周的

The periodontal disease is widespread and is the most common cause of tooth loss in old people.

牙周病广泛存在,是老年人牙齿脱落最常见的原因。

Gingivitis is an infection of the gums, the earliest form of periodontal disease.

齿龈炎是牙龈的感染,是牙周病最早的形式。

periorbital [ˌperiˈɔːbitəl] *a.* 眶周的;眶骨膜的

Bacterial infections of the periorbital tissues can be categorized according to location.

眶周组织的细菌性感染可根据部位而分类。

Periorbital edema noted on awakening often results from renal disease and impaired Na excretion.

起床后眼睑浮肿常提示肾脏疾病和排钠障碍。

periosteal [ˌperiˈɔstiəl] *a.* 骨膜的

If cortical erosions or periosteal thickening of adjacent bone is observed, it suggests pyogenic arthritis with osteomyelitis.

如观察到邻近骨皮质侵蚀或骨膜增厚,则提示为化脓性关节炎伴骨髓炎。

Periosteal inflammation may result from infection of underlying bone, subperiosteal hemmorrhage, or hypertrophic osteoarthropathy.
骨膜炎症可由其下面的骨感染、骨膜下出血或肥大性骨关节病引起。

periosteum [ˌperiˈɔstiəm] *n.* 骨膜
The outer layer of the periosteum is extremely dense and contains a large number of blood vessels.
骨膜外层非常致密，并含有大量血管。
Periosteum is a specialized connective tissue covering all bones of the body, and possessing bone-forming potentialities.
骨膜是覆盖在体内所有骨骼上的特殊结缔组织，并具有骨形成的潜力。

peripancreatic [ˌperiˌpænkriˈætik] *a.* 胰腺周的
Repeated ultrasound examination revealed mild hepatosplenomegaly and enlarged peripancreatic lymph nodes.
反复超声检查揭示轻度肝脾肿大和胰周淋巴结肿大。
All of the patients with peripancreatic infected fluid collections were treated with ultrasound or CT guided percutaneous catheter drainage.
所有胰周感染性积液病人均实施超声或 CT 引导下经皮穿刺置管引流治疗。

peripheral [pəˈrifərəl] *a.* 周围的，外周的
With the dissipation of the fever, peripheral vasodilatation occurs and heat loss ensues.
随着发热的消退，周围血管舒张，并产生失热。
In addition, atherosclerosis of peripheral arteries may take place.
另外，还可能发生外周动脉粥样硬化症。

periphery [pəˈrifəri] *n.* 外周（部），周围（部）
It will be evident that the most active growth of the tumour takes place at the periphery.
显然肿瘤生长最活跃的是周围部位。

periplasmic [ˌperiˈplæsmik] *a.* 胞质的，周质的
Peptidoglycan is separated from the cytoplasmic membrane by the periplasmic space.
肽聚糖层和胞浆膜之间由周质间隙分开。

perish [ˈperiʃ] *v.* 死亡；消灭；腐烂
The optimal conditions for gonococci lies at pH 7.2, and they perish at the normally prevailing vaginal pH values.
淋球菌生长所需的最佳 pH 值为 7.2，在正常的阴道 pH 值情况下淋球菌不易存活。

peristalsis [ˌperiˈstælsis] *n.*（肠）蠕动
Peristalsis is a type of muscular contraction characteristic of the gut.
蠕动是肠特有的一种肌肉收缩。
Visible peristalsis itself is not diagnostic of intestinal obstruction.
明显的肠蠕动本身不能作为诊断肠梗阻的依据。
As the disease progresses the obstructed lower esophagus dilates and peristalsis within the body of the gullet becomes less powerful.
随着病情发展，梗阻的食管下段扩张，食管主体的蠕动变得无力。

peristaltic [ˌperiˈstæltik] *a.* 蠕动的
Fiber will enhance the peristaltic movement of gastrointestinal tract.
纤维将加强胃肠道的蠕动。
Objective of the research was to observe gastrointestinal peristaltic function in premature infants in the supine or prostrate positions.
该研究的目的是观察早产儿在仰卧或俯卧时其胃肠蠕动的功能情况。

peritoneal [ˌperitəuˈniːəl] *a.* 腹膜的
The presence of free air in the peritoneal cavity is an important clue to the diagnosis.

腹膜腔中出现游离空气是进行诊断的重要线索。

Antibiotics are given to contend with the peritoneal infection.

给(病人)服抗生素,以抵抗腹膜感染。

peritoneoscope [ˌperiˈtəuniɔskəup] *n.* 腹腔镜(laparoscope)

By using peritoneoscope the surgeon enables to view the organs in the abdomen.

运用腹腔镜外科医生能够观察腹部内的器官。

peritoneum [ˌperitəuˈniːəm] *n.* 腹膜

Tuberculosis of the peritoneum is common in young children.

腹膜结核常见于年少的儿童。

The peritoneum was closed with interrupted sutures.

用断续缝合关闭腹膜。

peritonitis [ˌperitəuˈnaitis] *n.* 腹膜炎

Pain that suddenly becomes generalized and stay that way suggests peritonitis.

疼痛突然变为弥漫性并持续不止,提示为腹膜炎。

periumbilical [ˌperiʌmˈbilikəl] *a.* 脐周的

A 16-year-old girl with a history of irritable bowel syndrome was sent to the emergency department with stabbing periumbilical abdominal pain.

一个 16 岁曾有肠易激综合征病史的女孩,因脐周腹部刺痛被送到急诊科。

Internal hernias are silent if they are easily reducible, but the majority often causes epigastric discomfort, periumbilical pain, and recurrent episodes of intestinal obstruction.

腹内疝如果易于复位可无症状,但大多数会引起上腹不适、脐周疼痛和反复发作的肠梗阻。

periureteral [ˌperijuəˈriːtərəl] *a.* 输尿管周围的

Renal carcinoma may stimulate fibrosis such as that seen in periureteral fibrosis.

肾癌可刺激纤维增生,如可见于输尿管周围的纤维增生。

perivascular [ˌperiˈvæskjulə] *a.* 血管周围的

Pulmonary venous hypertension results in thickening of the walls of small pulmonary vessels and an increase in perivascular cell and fibrous tissue.

肺静脉高压引起小肺血管壁增厚,以及血管周围细胞和纤维组织增多。

Perivascular mononuclear inflammatory changes are often seen contiguous to the necrotic areas.

在坏死区附近常有血管周围的单核细胞炎性反应。

periventricular [ˌperivenˈtrikjulə] *a.* (心、脑)室周的

Congenital toxoplasmosis produces diffuse intracranial calcifications, and cytomegalovirus often produces periventricular calcification.

先天性弓形体病产生弥漫性颅内钙化,而巨细胞病毒感染常引起脑室周围钙化。

permanent [ˈpəːmənənt] *a.* 永久的,持久的

Exposure to cold, particularly to moist cold, can cause permanent local tissue damage.

暴露于寒冷,特别是暴露于湿冷,会引起永久性的局部组织损伤。

The secret to permanent weight control is not a diet at all.

持久的体重控制的秘密根本不是节制饮食。

There are two sets of teeth developed during life: the milk teeth and the permanent teeth.

人一生中要生长两副牙齿:乳齿和恒齿。

permanently [ˈpəːmənəntli] *ad.* 永久地,持久地

There occur each year about 10 million injuries of sufficient severity to be temporarily or permanently disabling or fatal.

每年要发生约一千万受伤病例,其严重程度足以暂时或终身致残,甚至致命。

The number of red cells sometimes is permanently increased above the normal as a result of disease.

红细胞的数量有时因疾病而持久地超过正常数。

A medical research company in the US has developed an implant which can permanently cure many eyesight problems with minimal surgery.

美国一家医疗研究公司已研制出一种能永久性治疗许多视力不佳而手术简便的植入物。

permanganate [pəː'mæŋgənit] *n.* 高锰酸盐

Permanganate has a deep purple color in aqueous solution and is a strong oxidizing agent.

高锰酸盐在水溶液中呈深紫色，是一种强氧化剂。

permeability [ˌpəːmiə'biliti] *n.* 渗透性，透过性

These peptides can affect both vascular permeability and the movement of leucocytes.

这些肽类能影响血管的通透性和白细胞的运动。

Such intracellular oedema may be the result of increased permeability of the surface membrane to sodium.

这种细胞内水肿可能是表面膜对钠的渗透性增加的结果。

permeable ['pəːmjəbl] *a.* 可渗透的

The capillaries become permeable to large and small molecules and to white blood celles.

大小分子和白细胞能渗透过此处毛细血管。

The membrane is relatively permeable to potassium.

此膜对于钾有较好的透过性。

permeate ['pəːmieit] *v.* 渗透

Pieces of tissue small enough to be permeated rapidly are promptly placed in fixative.

小到足以迅速渗透的组织块被迅速放入固定液中。

The lymph permeates all the tissues and bathes the individual cells.

淋巴液渗入到所有的组织内，并使每个细胞都沐浴其中。

permeation [ˌpəːmi'eiʃən] *n.* 渗透

The latter type of growth is known as lymphatic permeation and usually accounts only for local spread of the tumor.

后一生长类型称为淋巴管渗透，而且通常只会造成肿瘤的局部蔓延。

permission [pə'miʃən] *n.* 准许，同意

The patient asks for permission to leave hospital.

这位病人要求准许出院。

pernicious [pəː'niʃəs] *a.* 有害的，恶性的

Pernicious anemia is by far the most common B_{12} deficiency disease.

恶性贫血是最常见的维生素 B_{12} 缺乏性疾病。

peroral [pə'ɔːrəl] *a.* 经口的

There is no significant difference in inhibition between transdermal therapy and peroral therapy groups.

经皮给药治疗组与口服治疗组之间在抑制作用上无显著性差异。

Peroral endoscopic myotomy has been developed to provide a less invasive treatment for oesophageal achalasia compared to surgical cardiomyotomy.

已开发出经口内镜肌切开术，与外科手术贲门肌切开术相比，它提供的是对食管失弛缓症的一种微创治疗。

peroxidation [pəˌrɔksi'deiʃən] *n.* 过氧化

Free ion injures mitochondria, causes lipid peroxidation, and results in renal, tubular, and hepatic necrosis.

自由基损伤线粒体，引起脂质过氧化，导致肾、肾小管和肝脏坏死。

peroxide [pə'rɔksaid] *n.* 过氧化物

Peroxidase catalyses the dehydrogenation of various substances in the presence of hydrogen peroxide.

在过氧化氢存在时，过氧化物酶催化各种物质脱氢。

peroxisomal [pəˈrɔksisəuməl] *a.* 过氧化物酶体的

Primary hyperoxaluria refers to two peroxisomal enzyme deficiencies.

原发性高草酸尿涉及两种过氧化物酶的缺陷。

perpetuation [pəˌpetjuˈeiʃən] *n.* 永久，长期，连绵不断

Recent investigations have identified the part immunocompetent cells and their products play in the induction and perpetuation of chronic asthma.

近来一些研究肯定了某些免疫活性细胞及其产物在使慢性哮喘发生和缠绵不愈方面所起的作用。

perphenazine [pəˈfenəziːn] *n.* 羟哌氯丙嗪（安定药）；奋乃静

Perphenazine, a major tranquillizer, is used to relieve anxiety, tension, and agitation and to prevent nausea and vomiting.

羟哌氯丙嗪是重要的安定药，用于缓解焦虑、紧张和激动，并能预防恶心和呕吐。

per se [pəːˈsei] *n.* [拉] 自身，本身

Anything socially practical is good per se.

任何具有社会实用性的事物本身就是好东西。

Uremia per se is not an indication for salt restriction.

尿毒症本身并非限制食盐的指征。

perseverance [ˌpəːsiˈviərəns] *n.* 毅力；坚忍

Perseverance in treatment is essential, and the patient must continue to take the effective drug for at least 2 years after the attacks cease.

坚持治疗很有必要，病人应在发作停止后，至少继续服用有效药物 2 年。

perseveration [pəˌsevəˈreiʃən] *n.* 持续动作，持续症

Perseveration refers to the repetition of behavior or speech.

持续症指的是行为或语言的重复。

persist [pəˈsist] *v.* 持续

The longer the infection persists, the more numerous and prominent become the late complications.

感染持续时间越长，晚期并发症就越多越明显。

The tradition has persisted to this day.

那个传统一直保持到现在。

persistence [pəˈsistəns] *n.* 持续

Some doctors couldn't explain the persistence of the high temperature.

某些医生不能解释持续的高热。

Clinically, secondary pneumonia differs from primary pneumonia chiefly in its persistence.

临床上，继发性肺炎不同于原发性肺炎主要在其持久性。

persistent [pəːˈsistənt] *a.* 不断的，持续的，顽固的

The persistent cough is due to irritation of the bronchus by a growth.

持续的咳嗽是由生长物对支气管的刺激引起的。

He has persistent pneumothorax which stems from the rupture of small cysts, or blebs, on the surface of the lungs.

他患顽固性气胸，系由肺表面小囊肿或气泡破裂所致。

Women's exposure to pesticides, solvents and persistent organic pollutants may potentially affect the health of the fetus.

妇女暴露于杀虫剂、有机溶剂和持久性有机污染物可潜在影响胎儿的健康。

personal [ˈpəːsənəl] *a.* 个人的；本人的；亲自的

Dietary and personal hygiene should be strictly observed.

应当严格遵守饮食卫生和个人卫生。

She made a personal donation to the poverty stricken medical students.

她对贫困患病的医学生作了个人的捐款。

personality [ˌpəːsə'næliti] *n.* 个性;人格

The final stage is a complete disintegration of the personality.

最终结局是人格的完全分裂。

The term "cyclothymia" refers to personality disorders characterized by affective anomalies.

"周期性情绪波动症"这一术语是指以情感异常为特征的人格障碍。

personalized ['pəːsənəlaizd] *a.* 个性化的,个人化的

We strive to help physicians improve diagnostic accuracy and to optimize your patients' disease management through personalized therapy.

我们力图帮助医生提高诊断准确率和通过个性化治疗来优化对病人的疾病管理。

This discussion will explain the genomic basis of personalized medicine and explore its potential for good as well as its possible risks.

该讨论将解释个体化治疗的基因组基础,并探讨其潜在的益处与可能的危险。

perspective [pə'spektiv] *n.* 正确观察的能力,眼力;前景,展望;观点,看法

It is useful to outline a classification of inflammation so that our descriptions and interpretations may be kept in perspective.

对炎症进行大概的分类是有用的,从而我们才能恰如其分地进行描述和解释。

New perspectives on the evolution of the human gene material and of animal species will be gained.

将可获得人类遗传物质和动物物种进化的新视角。

Their perspectives were broader.

他们的眼界比较开阔。

a. 透视的

The simplest form of projection is a perspective projection.

最简单的投影形式是透视投影。

perspiration [ˌpəːspə'reiʃən] *n.* 出汗;汗

The patient has profuse perspiration.

病人大量地出汗。

Besides, some waste products are dissolved in the perspiration and eliminated.

此外,一些废物溶解于汗水排出体外。

perspire [pəs'paiə] *v.* 出汗

The pores of your skin are open and you begin to perspire.

你皮肤上的汗孔是开着的,并开始出汗。

persuade [pə'sweid] *v.* 说服,劝服,使相信

The patient was persuaded to receive surgical treatment.

患者已被劝服接受外科手术。

pertain (to) [pəː'tein] *v.* 从属;有关

Somatic delusions pertain to the functioning of one's body.

躯体妄想与人体功能有关。

The nutritious food pertains to the health of every person.

营养食物关系到每个人的健康。

pertinent ['pəːtinənt] *a.* 有关的,恰当的,中肯的

A client's pertinent assessment data included decreased dietary fiber and limited fluid intake.

病人有关的评估资料包括膳食中纤维的含量减少和有限的液体摄入。

Knowledge of the patient's age, health, occupation, hobbies, living conditions, and the onset, duration, and course of the disease may be pertinent.

了解患者的年龄、健康状况、职业、爱好、生活条件以及疾病的发生、持续时间和病程都是有必要的。

pertussis [pə'tʌsis] *n.* 百日咳

Local reactions as well as fever may occur after injection of pertussis vaccine.

在注射百日咳疫苗后,可发生局部反应和发热。

Encouraging results from two large scale tests of new-generation vaccines against pertussis are raising hopes for a generation of healthier and cough-free children.

新一代抗百日咳疫苗两项大规模的试验所取得的令人鼓舞的结果燃起我们培育新一代更健康又无咳嗽的儿童的希望。

perusal [pə'ruːzəl] *n.* 查阅,细读

Perusal of electronic medical records or insurance claims data would not be considered as direct patient interaction.

查阅电子病历或保险理赔数据不能视作是与病人的直接交流。

That medical dissertation deserves careful perusal.

那篇医学论文值得细读。

pervasive [pəː'veisiv] *a.* 蔓延的,遍布的

Feedback regulatory systems are pervasive in the field of endocrinology.

反馈调节系统在内分泌学领域内广泛存在。

pesticide ['pestisaid] *n.* 农药

Pesticides include fungicide, herbicide, insecticide, rodenticide, etc. All these agents are considerably toxic to man.

农药包括杀真菌剂、除莠剂、杀昆虫剂、灭鼠剂等。所有这些药剂对人均有较大的毒性。

pestis ['pestis] *n.* 鼠疫,黑死病

The natural reservoir for Yersinia pestis is species of rodents, including rats.

鼠疫杆菌的天然宿主是啮齿类动物,包括大鼠。

They infer that medieval Europe must have been invaded by two different sources of Yersinia pestis.

他们推断,中世纪欧洲很可能被两种不同来源的鼠疫杆菌入侵过。

PET(positron emission tomography) [pet] ['pɔzitrɔn i'miʃən təu'mɔgrəfi] *n.* 正电子发射体层摄影

Positron emission tomography (PET) is a nuclear medicine imaging technique that produces a three-dimensional image or picture of functional processes in the body.

正电子发射体层摄影是一种核医学成像技术,可以产生人体功能过程的三维影像或成像。

PET scans are increasingly read alongside CT or magnetic resonance imaging (MRI) scans, with the combination giving both anatomic and metabolic information.

正电子发射体层成像逐渐与 CT 或 MRI 图像相结合,从而可以提供解剖及代谢信息。

petechia [pi'tiːkiə] (*pl.* petechiae [pi'tiːkiiː]) [拉] *n.* 瘀点,瘀斑

Petechia is a pinpoint, nonraised, perfectly round, purplish red spot caused by subcutaneous or submucous hemorrhage.

瘀斑是皮下或黏膜下出血引起的针尖大小、非隆起、很圆的紫红色斑块。

Petechiae are characterized by extravasation of blood without significant inflammatory reaction.

瘀斑的特点是血液外渗而无明显的炎症反应。

petrolatum [ˌpetrəu'leitəm] *n.* 凡士林;矿脂

For moisture, some people swear by a product that has petrolatum, or lecithin, or silk.

为了保湿,有些人信赖包含有凡士林、卵磷脂或蚕丝的产品。

Cosmoline is a trademark used for a rust and corrosion preventive compound of petrolatum.

卡斯莫兰(防腐润滑油)是一种防锈抗腐矿脂化合物的商标。

petroleum [pi'trəuljəm] *n.* 石油

Several cohort studies have examined the association between exposure to petroleum products and/or gasoline and the risk of kidney cancer.

几项队列研究已对接触石油产品和(或)汽油与肾癌危险度之间的联系进行了调查。

Petroleum distillate are long-chain hydrocarbons such as those found in petrol and numerous household cleaning agents.

石油的蒸馏物和汽油及众多家用清洁剂一样,都是长链碳氢化合物。

Pfizer [ˈpfizəː] *n.* 辉瑞

Pfizer had the greatest number of blockbuster products in 2009 with 14, which includes five inherited through the acquisition of Wyeth.

辉瑞在 2009 年生产的拳头产品数量最多,有 14 个,其中包括收购惠氏公司得到的 5 个并购产品。

By the 1950s, Pfizer was established in Belgium, Brazil, Canada, Cuba, Iran, Mexico, Panama, Puerto Rico, Turkey and the United Kingdom.

截至 20 世纪 50 年代,辉瑞在比利时、巴西、加拿大、古巴、伊朗、墨西哥、巴拿马、波多黎各、土耳其和英国均建立了公司。

phaeohyphomycosis [ˌfiːəˌhaifəumaiˈkəusis] *n.* 暗色丝孢霉病

Phaeohyphomycosis is a heterogeneous group of mycotic infections caused by dematiaceous fungi.

暗色丝孢霉病是由多组暗色真菌引起的霉菌感染。

phage [feidʒ] *n.* 噬菌体

The virus that lyses bacteria is called phage.

能溶解细菌的病毒称作噬菌体。

Phage therapy has some theoretical advantage over antibiotic chemotherapy.

噬菌体疗法在理论上有许多胜过抗生素化疗的优越性。

phagocyte [ˈfægəsait] *n.* 吞噬细胞

These neutrophils are called the phagocytes.

这些嗜中性白细胞叫做吞噬细胞。

Some capsules even appear to be toxic for phagocytes.

有些荚膜甚至对吞噬细胞具有毒性。

phagocytic [ˌfægəˈsitik] *a.* 吞噬细胞的

The phagocytic activity of macrophages in acute inflammatory reactions has already been described.

急性炎症反应时巨噬细胞的吞噬活性已作过叙述。

Leucocytes are phagocytic, erythrocytes, on the other hand, are not.

白细胞具有吞噬作用,而红细胞则没有。

phagocytose [ˌfægəˈsaitəus] *v.* 吞噬

These cells phagocytose immune complexes and, in doing so, secrete numerous lysosomal enzymes.

这些细胞吞噬免疫复合物,并在这时分泌大量溶酶体酶。

phagocytosis [ˌfægəsaiˈtəusis] *n.* 吞噬(作用)

The capsule can protect the bacterium from ingestion by phagocytosis.

荚膜能阻止吞噬细胞对细菌的吞噬。

Macrophages are more involved in phagocytosis of microorganisms which are less acutely destructive and cause chronic infections.

巨噬细胞主要吞噬急性致病力不太强并可引起慢性感染的细菌。

phagosome [ˈfægəsəum] *n.* 吞噬体

Waves of increasingly acid solutions containing lytic enzymes are released into the phagosomes, killing the bacteria.

大量不断增强的含有溶解酶的酸性溶液进入吞噬体内,从而杀死细菌。

pharmaceutical [ˌfɑːməˈsjuːtikəl] *a.* 药学的,药物的,药用的,药剂(师)的

Most of the basic science and general education requirements must be completed before the

students can delve into the pharmaceutical sciences.
大多数基础科学和普通教育课程必须在学生钻研药学科学之前完成。

pharmaceutics [ˌfɑːmə'sjuːtiks] *n.* 药剂学

Pharmaceutics is the discipline of pharmacy that deals with all facets of the process of turning a new chemical entity(NCE) into a medication able to be safely and effectively used by patients in the community.
药剂学是一门研究将新化合物(NCE)转变为可安全、有效地用于患者治疗药物的学科。

Pharmaceutics is the study of relationships between drug formulation, delivery, disposition and clinical response.
药剂学是研究药物制剂、转运、分布和临床作用间相互关系的科学。

Pharmacia ['fɑːməsiə] *n.* 法玛西亚

Pharmacia is a pharmaceutical and biotechnological company in Sweden.
法玛西亚是瑞典的一个生物制药和生物技术公司。

Dextran-based products were to play a significant role in the further expansion of Pharmacia.
基于右旋糖酐的产品在法玛西亚的进一步扩大中发挥重要作用。

pharmacodynamics [ˌfɑːməkəudai'næmiks] *n.* 药效学

Pharmacodynamics may be defined as the study of the actions and effects of drugs on organs and tissues at cellular and subcellular levels.
药效学的定义是从细胞和亚细胞水平研究药物对器官和组织的作用和效应。

Pharmacodynamics discusses the sites of action, the modes of action, and the mechanisms of action of drugs.
药效学是讨论药物的作用部位、作用方式和作用机制的。

pharmacoepidemiology [ˌfɑːməkəˌepiˌdiːmi'ɔlədʒi] *n.* 药物流行病学

The Textbook of Pharmacoepidemiology provides a streamlined text for evaluating the safety and effectiveness of medicines.
药物流行病学教科书提供了一部评价药物安全性和有效性的简明教材。

pharmacogenetics [ˌfɑːməkəudʒi'netiks] *n.* 药物遗传学

Pharmacogenetics may be defined as the study of the hereditary variation in the handling of drugs.
药物遗传学可定义为对药物应用中遗传变异的研究。

pharmacogenomics [ˌfɑːməkəudʒi'nɔmiks] *n.* 药物基因组学

Pharmacogenomics employs tools for surveying the entire genome to assess multigenic determinants of drug response.
药物基因组学通过采用检测整个基因组的一些工具来评估药物反应的多基因决定因子。

pharmacokinetic [ˌfɑːməkəukai'netik] *a.* 药物动力学的

Pharmacokinetic principles discuss the absorption, distribution, binding, biotransformation, and excretion of drugs and their metabolites in the body.
药物动力学原理是讨论药物及其代谢产物在体内的吸收、分布、结合、生物转化和排泄过程的。

This report discusses the influence of dietary intake on metabolic and pharmacokinetic activity, genetic stability, molecular and physiologic processes, compound toxicity, and pathogenesis.
这一报告讨论摄入的食物量对代谢和药物动力学活性、遗传稳定性、分子与生理过程、化合物毒性以及致病机制的影响。

pharmacologic [ˌfɑːməkə'lɔdʒik] *a.* 药理的,药理学的

The pharmacologic effects of atropine in general are dose dependent.
阿托品的药理作用通常与剂量有关。

pharmacologist [ˌfɑːmə'kɔlədʒist] *n.* 药理学家

Li Shizhen has been recognized as(being) one of the world's greatest pharmacologists.

李时珍已被公认是世界上最伟大的药理学家之一。

pharmacology [ˌfɑːməˈkɔlədʒi] *n.* 药理学

Pharmacology is the discipline that studies the effects of a drug on the body both in animal and in man.

药理学是研究药物在动物和人体内的作用的学科。

The pharmacology of acetylsalicylic acid will be discussed in detail as a prototype drug.

对于水杨酸作为原型药物的药理学将要进行详细讨论。

pharmacopoeia [ˌfɑːməkəˈpiːə] *n.* 药典

The British Pharmacopoeia(BP) is the leading collection of standards for UK medicinal products and pharmaceutical substances.

英国药典(BP)是英国先进的医药产品和医药物质标准的集成。

The British Pharmacopoeia(BP) makes an important contribution to public health by setting publicly available standards for the quality of medicines.

英国药典(BP),通过设置公开可用的药品质量标准,对公众的健康做出了重要贡献。

pharmacotherapy [ˌfɑːməkəuˈθerəpi] *n.* 药物疗法

His chances of survival are greatly improved because of modern pharmacotherapy.

由于有了现代药物疗法,他的存活可能性大大增加了。

pharmacovigilance [ˌfɑːməkəˈvidʒələns] *n.* 药物警戒

Pharmacovigilance(PV) is defined as the science and activities relating to the detection, assessment, understanding and prevention of adverse effects or any other drug-related problem.

药物警戒的定义是指与发现、评价、理解和预防药物不良作用或其他任何可能与药物有关问题的科学研究与活动。

pharmacy [ˈfɑːməsi] *n.* 药学

Pharmacy is the health profession that links the health sciences with the chemical sciences and it is charged with ensuring the safe and effective use of pharmaceutical drug.

药学是将化学与健康科学联系起来的学科,其任务是确保安全和有效用药。

A Doctor of Pharmacy is a professional doctorate degree in pharmacy. In some countries, it is a first professional degree, and a prerequisite for licensing to exercise the profession of Pharmacist.

药学博士是药学专业博士学位。在一些国家,它是首要的专业学位,是取得药剂师执业资格的先决条件。

pharyngeal [ˌfærinˈdʒiːəl] *a.* 咽的

Each pharyngeal arch contains a cartilage, a cranial nerve, and a blood vessel.

每个咽弓含有软骨、脑神经和血管。

In infection with either of the viruses, there is pharyngeal erythema and edema.

在任何病毒引起的感染中,都有咽部充血和水肿。

pharyngitis [ˌfærinˈdʒaitis] *n.* 咽炎

In acute nonstreptococcal pharyngitis, sore throat and pain on swallowing predominate.

在非链球菌急性咽炎中,喉痛及吞咽时疼痛是主要症状。

pharynx [ˈfæriŋks] *n.* 咽

The tonsils may be seen at either side of the pharynx.

咽的两侧可见到扁桃体。

The esophagus receives the contents of the contracting pharynx and forces them on by peristalsis.

食管从收缩着的咽部接受食物,并通过蠕动将食物往前推动。

phase [feiz] *n.* 期;阶段;相

Antimicrobial agents should not be used during the acute phase of viral respiratory disease.

在病毒性呼吸道疾病的急性期不能使用抗细菌性制剂。

The biotransformations in the liver are commonly grouped into two phases.

肝脏中的生物转化通常分为两相。

phase-contrast ['feiz kən'træst] *a.* 相衬的；相差的；相差显微镜的

Under the phase-contrast microscope, mitochondria appear as minute rods.

在相差显微镜下，线粒体看似小棍棒。

phellodendrine [filəu'dendriːn] *n.* 黄柏碱

It is researched by specific conductance that ultrasound has an effect on yield of phellodendrine.

经采用特定电导率测试法研究表明超声对黄柏碱的产率有影响。

Studies on the chemical constituents and taxonomy of phellodendrine will be made.

将要进行有关黄柏碱的化学成分与分类学法的研究。

phenacetin [fi'næsitin] *n.* 非那西丁，乙酰对氨苯乙醚

The serious, but rare, side effects of phenacetin are met hemoglobinemia and hemolytic anemia.

非那西丁的严重而较罕见的副作用是高铁血红蛋白血症和溶血性贫血。

phenformin [fən'fɔːmin] *n.* 苯乙双胍，降糖灵

Phenformin is a drug that reduces blood sugar levels and is used to treat diabetes.

苯乙双胍是一种用于治疗糖尿病的降血糖药物。

phenobarbital [ˌfiːnəu'bɑːbitəl] *n.* 苯巴比妥

Phenobarbital tends to stimulate all enzymes.

苯巴比妥趋向于刺激所有的酶。

If cholestasis is prominent, initiation of treatment with phenobarbital and/or cholestyramine should be contemplated.

如果胆汁淤积显著，应仔细考虑采用苯巴比妥或（和）消胆胺来治疗。

phenobarbitone [ˌfiːnəu'bɑːbitəun] *n.* 苯巴比妥（抗惊厥及镇静催眠药）

The metabolism of phenobarbitone is reduced in old people.

苯巴比妥在老人体内的代谢减慢。

Phenobarbitone is a safe anticonvulsant acting as a depressant both for the cortex and reticular formation.

苯巴比妥是一种安全的抗抽搐剂，既是皮质的抑制剂也是网状结构的抑制剂。

phenol ['fiːnɔl] *n.* 酚，石炭酸

For example, benzene undergoes oxidation, a phase Ⅰ reaction, to form phenol.

例如，苯经过Ⅰ相反应氧化后生成酚。

Phenol is administered as solution, ointments, and lotions and is highly toxic if taken by mouth.

苯酚使用的剂型有溶液、软膏和洗剂，口服有剧毒。

phenomenon [fi'nɔminən]（*pl.* phenomena [fi'nɔminə]）*n.* 现象

The anti-inflammatory effect of steroids may be accompanied by the adverse phenomena of tissue atrophy and psychosis.

类固醇类的抗炎作用可能伴有组织萎缩和精神病等有害现象。

Souques' s phenomenon is seen in incomplete hemiplegia, consisting of involuntary extension and separation of the fingers when the arm is raised.

苏克氏现象见于不全偏瘫，当抬高手臂时有手指的不随意伸展和分开。

phenotype ['fiːnətaip] *n.* 表现型，表型

Phenotype is the observed result of the interaction of the genotype with environmental factors.

表现型是基因型和环境因素相互作用的结果。

The dominant phenotype is expressed whenever a dominant gene is present in the genotype.

每当显性基因在基因型中出现时，显性表型就表达出来。

phenotypic [ˌfiːnə'tipik] *a.* 表型的

Genomic polymorphisms can serve as the starting point to assess whether genomic variability translates into phenotypic variability.

基因组多态性能够充作评价基因组变异是否会导致表型差异的起始点。

phenoxybenzamine [fiˌnɔksiˈbenzəmiːn] *n.* 苯氧苯扎明，苯氧苄胺，酚苄明

Phenoxybenzamine is an alpha-adrenergic receptor blocking agent.

酚苄明是一种 α-肾上腺素能受体阻断剂。

phenylbutazone [ˌfenilˈbjuːtəzəun] *n.* 保泰松，苯丁唑酮

The antiinflammatory effect of phenylbutazone is greater than that of aspirin.

保泰松的抗炎作用大于阿司匹林。

As phenylbutazone is metabolized and excreted slowly, its the-rapeutic effect is therefore prolonged.

保泰松代谢及排泄慢，故药效较长。

phenylketonuria [ˌfenilˌkiːtəˈnjuriːə] *n.* 苯丙酮(酸)尿

Persons with phenylketonuria do not metabolize phenylalanine properly.

患有苯丙酮尿症的人不能进行苯丙氨酸的正常代谢。

Phenylketonuria is a condition in which phenylalanine to tyrosine conversion is diminished, because the enzyme phenylalanine hydroxylase is deficient.

苯丙酮酸尿症是由于苯丙氨酸羟化酶缺乏致苯丙氨酸转变成酪氨酸减少所致的一种疾病。

phenytoin [ˈfenitəuin] *n.* 苯妥英，二苯乙内酰脲

Phenytoin is absorbed primarily from the upper intestinal tract.

苯妥英主要从小肠上段吸收。

Phenytoin, a hydantoinate, appears to inhibit the spread of seizure discharges rather than prevent their initiation.

苯妥英是一种乙内酰脲盐，它的机制是抑制癫痫神经放电的扩散而不是预防其始动发作。

pheochromocytoma [ˌfiːəˌkrəuməsaiˈtəumə] *n.* 嗜铬细胞瘤

Pheochromocytoma is characterized of paroxymal episodes of headache, sweating, palpitations and a markedly increased blood pressure.

嗜铬细胞瘤的特征是阵发性发作的头痛、出汗、心悸和显著血压升高。

pheromone [ˈferəməun] *n.* 信息素

A pheromone is a chemical that elicits a specific behavioural response at a distance.

信息素是可以在远距离诱导出特定行为反应的一种化学物质。

The findings also add support to the existence of pheromone-like compounds in humans.

这些研究结果同时为人类也存在类似信息素样的化合物提供了支持。

phlebitis [fliˈbaitis] *n.* 静脉炎

The bedbound patient is at risk for developing joint contractures and phlebitis.

卧床病人有发生关节挛缩和静脉炎的危险。

phlebography [fliˈbɔgrəfi] *n.* 静脉造影(术)

Phlebography in lower limbs is a simple and direct way to supply doctors with dependable information to treat diseases surgically or medically.

下肢静脉造影检查是一种简捷、直观的诊断手段，为医生对疾病进行手术治疗或药物治疗提供了可靠的信息。

Radioisotope scanning of lung associated with same-time phlebography on the low extremity also has fairly high positive rate to diagnosing acute pulmonary thromboembolism.

对肺部进行放射性同位素扫描的同时行下肢静脉造影，也可获得对急性肺血栓栓塞症的较高诊断率。

phlebostenosis [ˌflebəustiˈnəusis] *n.* 静脉狭窄

We can predicate phlebostenosis by measuring venous drip chamber pressures.

我们可通过测量静脉滴室压来判断是否存在静脉狭窄。

The venacavographies can show the extent, degree of phlebostenosis or obstruction, and collateral vascular dilatation.

腔静脉造影可显示腔静脉狭窄或闭塞及侧支血管扩张的范围和程度。

phlebothrombosis [ˌflebəuθrɔm'bəusis] *n.* 静脉血栓

Venous thrombosis(phlebothrombosis) is almost invariably occlusive, with the thrombus forming a long cast of the lumen.

静脉血栓几乎无一例外是阻塞性的,在管腔内形成长长的固体质块。

Recent studies indicate that measurement of the global activity of the coagulation system may have useful clinical predictive value for recurrent phlebothrombosis.

近期研究表明,凝血系统总活性的检测有助于预测复发性的静脉血栓。

phlebotomy [fli'bɔtəmi] *n.* 静脉切开术,放血术

However no study has demonstrated an objective improvement in hemodynamics, lung mechanics, or gas exchange following phlebotomy.

但还没有研究资料表明静脉切开后可以客观地改善血流动力学、肺机械功能或气体交换。

phlegmon ['flegmɔn] *n.* 蜂窝织炎

Phlegmon, inflammation of connective tissue, may lead to ulceration.

蜂窝织炎是结缔组织炎症,可导致溃疡。

phobia ['fəubjə] *n.* 恐惧,恐怖(症)

Fear of humiliation and embarrassment is characteristic of social phobia.

社交恐惧症的特点是对羞辱和困窘的恐惧。

Animal phobia is a morbid fear of animals, most commonly small animals, e. g. mice and spider.

动物恐惧症是对动物的病态害怕,最常见者为小动物,如小鼠和蜘蛛。

pholcodine ['fɔlkəudain] *n.* 福尔可定

Patients can continue to take pholcodine-containing medicines and should contact their doctor or pharmacist if they have any questions.

病人可以继续使用含福尔可定的药物,但如果有任何不适,应与他们的医生或药剂师及时联系。

The methods of HPLC and TLC were established to determine pholcodine oral solution and its related substances, respectively.

建立了 HPLC 法和 TLC 法分别测定福尔可定口服液和有关物质。

phonation [fə'neiʃən] *n.* 发声,发音

Phonation, or the production of vocal sounds, is a function of the larynx.

发声,或者声音的发生,是属于喉的功能。

phonocardiography [ˌfəunəuˌkɑːd'ɔːgrəfi] *n.* 心音描记法

Phonocardiography records heart sounds and murmurs and may help to elucidate difficult problems of ausculation.

心音描记法记录心音和杂音并有助于解释听诊中碰到的疑难问题。

phonophoresis [ˌfəunəfɔː'resis] *n.* 超声透入疗法

Phonophoresis has been suggested by early studies to enhance the absorption of analgesics and anti-inflammatory agents.

早期研究表明超声透入疗法可提高止痛药和抗炎药的吸收。

Phonophoresis has been shown to be ineffective for some treatments, where it did not increase the efficacy of absorption of drugs, or did not improve the outcome more than the use of ultrasound alone.

超声透入疗法已经显示对某些治疗无效,它没有增加药物吸收效力,或者与单用超声相比并没有改善治疗结果。

phosgene ['fɔzdʒiːn] *n.* 光气

Phosgene is a highly toxic, irritating and corrosive gas.

光气是一种剧毒、刺激性和腐蚀性的气体。

Inhalation of phosgene can cause fatal respiratory damage.

吸入光气可引起致命的呼吸系统损伤。

phosphatase [ˈfɔsfəteis] *n.* 磷酸酶

The magnesium ion, Mg^{2+}, is an inorganic activator for the enzyme phosphatase.

镁离子(二价阳离子)是磷酸酶的无机活化剂。

Investigation shows a high alkaline phosphatase and usually a high bilirubin.

检查发现碱性磷酸酶升高,通常胆红素也很高。

phosphate [ˈfɔsfeit] *n.* 磷酸盐,磷酸酯

The calcium phosphate mineral hydroxyapatite is the constituent giving hardness to bones and teeth.

磷酸钙矿物质羟磷灰石是使骨和牙坚硬的要素。

Sea water contains about 0.07mg/litre of phosphate.

海水含磷酸盐约为 0.07mg/l。

phosphatidic-acid [fɔsfəˈtidik-æsid] *n.* 磷脂酸

Most of phospholipids contain glycerol such as phosphatidic-acid, phosphatidylcholine, phosphatidylglycerol, etc.

大多数磷脂含有甘油,如磷脂酸、磷脂酰胆碱和磷脂酰甘油等。

phosphatidylcholine [ˈfɔsfəˌtaidilˈkəuliːn] *n.* 磷脂酰胆碱

The membrane phospholipids include mainly sphingomyelin, phosphatidylcholine, phosphatidyl ethanolamine, phosphatidyl serine.

膜磷脂主要包括神经鞘磷脂、磷脂酰胆碱、磷脂酰乙醇胺、磷脂酰丝氨酸等。

Phosphatidylcholine, one of the main active components of pulmonary surfactant, is markedly higher during early ARDS.

磷脂酰胆碱是肺泡表面活性物质主要活性成分之一,在急性呼吸窘迫综合征(ARDS)早期有明显升高。

phosphatidylinositol [ˈfɔsfəˌtaidilaiˈnəusitɔl] *n.* 磷脂酰肌醇

The results suggest that reacylation of fatty acids into brain membrane phospholipids (especially phosphatidylinositol) is hampered during ischemia and hypoxia.

结果表明进入脑膜磷脂(特别是磷脂酰肌醇)中的脂肪酸再酰化在缺血及缺氧时受阻。

The purpose of this study was to test and verify the hypothesis that IGF-1 promotes survival of mouse granulosa cells through the phosphatidylinositol 3-kinase/Akt signal transduction pathway.

本研究的目的是验证 IGF-1 是通过磷脂酰肌醇 3 激酶/Akt 信号转导通路促进小鼠颗粒细胞存活的假说。

phosphokinase [ˌfɔsfəuˈkaineis] *n.* 磷酸激酶

Diagnosis of myocardial infarction is substantiated by electrocardiographic changes and elevated serum creatine phosphokinase levels.

心电图改变和血清肌酸磷酸激酶水平的增高可证实心肌梗死的诊断。

phospholipase [ˌfɔsfəuˈlipeiz; -ˈlaipeiz] *n.* 磷脂酶

Protein kinase C is a cytoplasmic phospholipase-dependent serine/threonine protein kinase.

蛋白激酶 C 是存在于细胞质内磷脂酶依赖的丝/苏氨酸蛋白激酶。

Phospholipase A_2 is a family of enzymes which catalyzes the hydrolysis of the specific ester bond of phospholipids.

磷脂酶 A_2 是一大类能催化磷脂特定酯键水解的酶。

phospholipid [ˌfɔsfəuˈlipid] *n.* 磷脂

The phospholipids are similar to those in the cytoplasmic membrane.

这种磷脂与胞浆膜中的磷脂相似。

Phospholipids are the major form of lipid in all cell membranes.

磷脂是所有细胞膜中脂质的主要形式。

phosphoric [fɔsˈfɔrik] *a.* 磷的，含磷的

In egg yolk the prosthetic group is phosphoric acid.

蛋黄中辅基是磷酸。

phosphorolysis [fɔsfəˈrɔlisis] *n.* 磷酸解，磷变分解

The phosphorolysis of glycogen represents an amplification system.

糖原的磷酸解有一放大的系统。

phosphorus [ˈfɔsfərəs] *n.* 磷

In addition, individual proteins may contain phosphorus, iodine, iron, copper, zinc, or other elements.

此外，个别蛋白质还含有磷、碘、铁、铜、锌或其他元素。

phosphorylate [ˈfɔsfərileit] *v.* 使磷酸化

However, phosphorylated glycogen synthetase is inactive.

但是，磷酸化的糖原合成酶是无活性的。

phosphorylation [ˌfɔsfəriˈleiʃən] *n.* 磷酸化

Oxidative phosphorylation is the formation of high-energy phosphate bonds by phosphorylation of ADP to ATP.

氧化磷酸化是通过 ADP 磷酸化为 ATP 而形成高能磷酸键。

phosphorylcholine [ˈfɔsfərilˈkəuliːn] *n.* 磷酸胆碱

Acetyl glyceryl ether phosphorylcholine (AGEPc) was originally known as platelet activating factor (PAF), it has also been shown to possess antihypertensive properties.

最初知道乙酰甘油醚磷酸胆碱是血小板活化因子，它还显示有抗高血压的特性。

photochemical [ˌfəutəuˈkemikəl] *a.* 光化学作用的，光化学的

Photochemical smog is a type of air pollution caused by reactions between sunlight and pollutants.

光化学烟雾是一种由阳光与污染物反应所引起的空气污染。

Photochemical oxidants are the products of reactions between NOx and a wide variety of volatile organic compounds (VOCs).

光化学氧化剂是氮氧化物与很多种挥发性有机物（VOCs）的反应产物。

photodegradation [ˈfəutəuˌdegrəˈdeiʃən] *n.* 光降解（作用）

This type of photodegradation is used by some drinking water and wastewater facilities to destroy pollutants.

一些饮用水和污水处理设施使用这种类型的光降解，以破坏污染物。

Photodegradation includes photodissociation, the break up of molecules into smaller pieces by photons.

光降解包括光离解，通过光子将分子打碎成更小的分子。

photometry [fəuˈtɔmitri] *n.* 测光法，光度学

The amount of hemoglobin in the blood is easy to measure by photometry.

血液中血红蛋白的含量，很容易用光度测定法测定。

photon [ˈfəutɔn] *n.* 光子

The quantum of light is called a photon.

光的量子称为光子。

A real or virtual photon may spontaneously annihilate.

一个实的或虚的光子可以自发地湮没。

photooxidation [ˌfəutəuˌɔksəˈdeiʃən] *n.* 光氧化

Photooxidation was one of the main degradation approaches of pesticides in environment.

光氧化是环境中杀虫剂的主要降解途径之一。

Diaminobenzidine (DAB) photooxidation is a method for conversion of fluorescent signals into electron-dense precipitates that are visible in the electron microscope.

二氨基联苯胺(DAB)光氧化是一种将光信号转变成电镜下可见的电子致密沉淀物的方法。

photophobia [ˌfəutəu'fəubjə] *n.* 畏光

The patient gives a history of feeling of roughness in the eyes and photophobia.

病人主诉眼内有粗糙感并且有畏光的历史。

The patient had conjunctivitis with swelling and photophobia.

病人结膜发炎肿胀,并且畏光。

photosensitivity ['fəutəuˌsensi'tiviti] *n.* 光敏性,感光灵敏度

Drug-induced photosensitivity refers to the development of cutaneous disease as a result of the combined effects of a chemical and light.

药物引起的光敏性是指化学药品和光联合作用而引起皮肤病的发生。

Patients with photosensitivity have an immunological response to light, usually sunlight.

光敏性患者会对光,通常是阳光产生免疫反应。

photosynthesis [ˌfəutəu'sinθəsis] *n.* 光合作用

Cyanobacteria carry out plant-like photosynthesis with the formation of oxygen.

蓝菌能进行植物样的光合作用,并伴有氧的产生。

phototherapy [ˌfəutəu'θerəpi] *n.* 光线疗法

Phototherapy, the use of fluorescent light, is used in the treatment of jaundice and speeds the elimination of bilirubin from the body, removing the danger of brain damage.

光线疗法利用荧光,可治疗黄疸,以及加速胆红素从体内排除以消除脑损伤的危险。

phototoxicity [ˌfəutəutɔk'sisəti] *n.* 光毒性

Photosensitivity may be phototoxic or photoallergic. Phototoxicity is much more common.

光敏性可以是光毒性的、或是光过敏性的。光毒性更加常见。

Long-term ultraviolet phototoxicity results in chronic sun damage and skin cancer formation.

长期的紫外光毒性可导致慢性日光损害和皮肤癌形成。

phthalate ['θæleit] *n.* 邻苯二甲酸酯(盐)

Phthalates are esters of phthalic acid and are mainly used as plasticizers.

邻苯二甲酸酯是一类酞酸酯,主要用作增塑剂。

Personal-care products containing phthalates include perfume, eye shadow, nail polish and liquid soap.

含有邻苯二甲酸酯的个人生活用品主要有香水,眼影膏,指甲油和液体皂。

phycoerythrin [ˌfaikəu'eriθrin] *n.* 藻红蛋白

The content of phycoerythrin(PE) was increased by the enrichment of ammonia only in the absence of UVR.

只有在无紫外辐射的情况下,藻红蛋白的含量才会随着氨的增多而增加。

C-phycoerythrin was isolated and purified from marine Pseudanabaena sp. using two step chromatographic methods.

C-藻红蛋白是从海洋假鱼腥藻中采用两步层析法分离和纯化的。

phyllode ['filəud] *n.* 叶状柄

We evaluated long-term outcome and clinical characteristics of malignant phyllodes tumors arising from fibroadenomas of the breast.

我们评价了起源于乳腺纤维腺瘤的恶性叶状肿瘤的长期预后和临床特征。

Patients with malignant phyllodes tumors who exhibit rapid growth within 6 months require aggressive treatment.

恶性叶状肿瘤患者近6个月肿瘤生长迅速,需要较为激进的治疗措施。

phyllodulcin [filə'dʌlsin] *n.* 叶甜素,叶甘素

In addition, extraction efficiency of the subcritical water extraction for phyllodulcin was compared with ultrasonic extraction with methanol.

另外，对叶甜素的亚临界水萃取法和甲醇超声波萃取法的萃取率做了比较。

Phyllodulcin and hydrangenol also showed significant inhibition for the antigen-induced degranulations.

叶甘素和绣球酚对抗原诱导的脱颗粒作用也显示出明显的抑制效应。

phylogenetic [ˌfailəudʒiˈnetik] *a.* 系统发育的，种系发生的

Phylogenetic trees have been used to depict evolutionary relationships graphically.

系统发育树已被用于图解描绘（生物的）进化关系。

Some phylogenetic trees are based on the morphological evidence.

某些系统发育树是基于形态学的证据。

phylotype [ˈfailətaip] *n.* 种系型

A phylotype is biological type that classifies an organism by its phylogenetic, that is, evolutionary relationship to other organisms.

种系型是根据其种系发生、即与其他生物在进化上的关系来分类一种生物的生物型。

phylum [ˈfailəm] *n.* （表示生物分类的）门（*pl.* phyla）

By Budd and Jensen's definition, phyla are defined by a set of characters shared by all their living representatives.

根据鲍德和金森的定义，所有共享一组生物学性状的代表性生物归为门。

In biology, a phylum is a taxonomic rank below kingdom and above class.

在生物学中，"门"是在"界"以下和"纲"以上的分类单位。

physical [ˈfiːzikəl] *a.* 有形的，实物的；物理的；身体的

Genes, which are carried on chromosomes, are the basic physical and functional units of heredity.

基因位于染色体上，是遗传的基本结构和功能单位。

His physical force was weak, but his mental and moral force was very great.

他体力很弱，可他的精神和道德力量却非常强。

physician [fiˈziʃən] *n.* 医生，内科医生

Consult your physician before beginning any diet or exercise programme.

在开始实施节食或锻炼方案之前要先征询医生的意见。

For the bacterial type of pharyngitis, penicillin in certain forms can be given by mouth very effectively in accordance with a physician's directions.

对细菌型咽炎，有些类型的青霉素遵照医嘱口服很有效。

The diagnostic tests upon which physicians often rely can also have false-positive or false-negative results.

医生所依赖的诊断性化验也有假阳性或假阴性的结果。

physicochemical [ˌfizikəuˈkemikəl] *a.* 物理化学的

Another important function of plasma proteins is a physicochemical one.

血浆蛋白的另一重要功能是物理化学方面的。

physiologic [ˌfiziəˈlɔdʒik] *a.* 生理的

Physiologic process cannot take place normally unless there is sufficient water.

如果水分不够，生理过程就无法正常进行。

physiology [ˌfiziˈɔlədʒi] *n.* 生理学

Physiology means the science of function in living organisms, and study of this subject goes a long way toward explaining life itself.

生理学是研究生物体功能的科学，学习该课程将大大有助于解释生命本身。

physiotherapy [ˌfiziəuˈθerəpi] *n.* 理疗

The patient responded well to the physiotherapy.

这个病人理疗的效果良好。

phytoestrogen [ˌfaitəʊˈestrədʒən] *n.* 植物雌激素

Phytoestrogen has the ability to cause estrogenic or/and antiestrogenic effects.

植物雌激素具有雌激素或(和)抗雌激素作用。

In human beings, phytoestrogens are readily absorbed in plasma and are excreted in the urine.

在人体内,植物雌激素很容易在血浆中吸收和从尿液中排出。

pica [ˈpaikə] *n.* 异食癖

Other causes of iron deficiency anemia may be decreased absorption of Fe after gastrectomy, upper small-bowel malabsorption syndromes, and occasionally some forms of pica (primarily clay).

缺铁性贫血的其他原因是胃切除后的铁吸收降低,小肠上段吸收不良综合征,间或有某些形式的异食癖(主要是黏土)。

picking [ˈpikiŋ] *n.* 贴片

Theoretic basis for production technique of Xilei picking is provided by studying its recipe, stability, adhesivity and release property.

通过研究其配方、稳定性、黏附性及释放特性,为锡类贴片制备技术提供理论基础。

The picking is composed of protecting, pressure-sensitive, release-controlling, drug-storing and liner layers.

贴片是由保护层、压力敏感、控制释放、药物储存和衬垫层组成。

picture phone [ˈpiktʃə fəun] *n.* 电视电话

It was called the picture phone.

这种电话称为电视电话。

Picture phone is becoming more and more popular nowadays.

电视电话越来越流行了。

pierce [piəs] *v.* 刺穿,穿孔

The strength of the laser can pierce very hard substances.

激光的力度能穿透极其坚硬的物质。

pigment [ˈpigmənt] *n.* 色素

If it were not for this pigment, our skin would be almost as white as paper.

若不是有这种色素的话,则我们的皮肤就会白得几乎像纸一样。

The liquor amnii and the fluid in all the serous cavities contain blood pigments.

羊水及所有浆液腔中的液体都含有血色素。

pigmentation [ˌpigmənˈteiʃən] *n.* 色素沉着,着色

Jaundice is the yellow skin pigmentation caused by elevation in serum bilirubin level.

黄疸是由于血清胆红素水平升高引起的皮肤黄染。

Chronic cases of aplastic anemia may show considerable brown skin pigmentation.

再生障碍性贫血的慢性病例可以有相当程度的皮肤棕色色素沉着。

pigmentosa [pigˈmentəsə] *n.* 眼点;色点

Around one million people in Britain suffer from two of the most common forms of blindness: macular degeneration and retinitis pigmentosa.

在英国大约有一百万人患有两种最常见的失明疾病:视网膜黄斑变性和色素性视网膜炎。

Retinitis pigmentosa is a degenerative disease in which light receptors in the retina, on the back of the eyeball, gradually cease to function.

色素性视网膜炎是一种退行性疾病,在眼球背面视网膜上的光受体逐渐失去其作用。

pile [pail] *n.* 堆;痔

In most cases there are three main pile masses, one is situated anteriorly, the others posterolaterally.

大多数病例有三个主要的痔块,一个位于前面,其余的位于后侧面。

pill [pil] *n.* 丸剂,药丸

Pill (pharmacy) refers to anything small and round for a specific dose of medicine.

药丸(药学)指小而圆且剂量特定的药物。

Pills is a nickname for the recreational drug MDMA, also known as ecstasy.
丸是消遣性毒品亚甲二氧甲基安非他明的昵称,又被称为摇头丸。

pilot [ˈpailət] *a.* 小型实验性的

Pilot studies have not proved that alkylating agents or immunosuppressive drugs are beneficial.
小型实验性研究尚未证明烷化剂或免疫抑制药物是否有用。

pilus [ˈpailəs](*pl.* pili [ˈpailai]) *n.* 毛,发

These pili are present in much smaller numbers per cell(fewer than 10).
这类菌毛在每个细胞上的数量要少得多(少于 10 根/细胞)。

pineocytoma [ˌpiniəusaiˈtəumə] *n.* 松果体细胞瘤

Pinealomas are divided into two categories, pineoblastomas and pineocytomas, based on their level of differentiation, which, in turn, correlates with their aggressiveness.
松果体瘤根据分化程度分为两大类:松果体母细胞瘤和松果体细胞瘤,相应的其侵袭能力也是不同的。

Although aggressive surgery in the pineal region carries the risk of neurologic injury, gross total resection should be attempted for pineocytoma.
尽管在松果体区侵袭性手术可能带来神经损伤的危险,但松果体细胞瘤仍需要最大限度地切除肿块。

pinhead [ˈpinhed] *n.* 针头

Amoeba is a single-celled animal which may be as large as a pinhead.
变形虫是一种像针头般大小的单细胞动物。

pinocytosis [ˌpainəsaiˈtəusis] *n.* 胞饮作用,吞饮作用

Numerous small vacuoles are constantly being formed by pinocytosis.
大量的小空泡通过胞饮作用不断形成。

Pinocytosis occurs in many white blood cells and in certain kidney and liver cells.
细胞吞饮作用在许多白细胞和某些肾和肝细胞中发生。

pinpoint [ˈpinpɔint] *v.* 查明;精确地找到;准确描述

Psychotherapy aims to help people pinpoint the relative contributors to their depression.
心理疗法旨在帮助人们找出导致他们抑郁的相对原因。

In many cases, your doctor may not be able to pinpoint the exact cause of your urinary incontinence.
在许多情况下,医生没法查明引起尿失禁的确切原因。

piperacillin [ˌpipəræˈsilin] *n.* 哌拉西林

Gram-negative bacterium was sensitive to imipenem and piperacillin/sulbactam.
革兰阴性菌对亚胺培南和哌拉西林/舒巴坦敏感。

The sensitive rate of the Pseudomonas aeruginosa to cefoperazone-sulbactam was 66.6% and to piperacillin-tazobactam 71.4%-76.9%.
铜绿假单胞菌对头孢哌酮-舒巴坦的敏感率为 66.6%,对哌拉西林-他唑巴坦的敏感率为 71.4% ~76.9%。

piperazine [piˈperəziːn] *n.* 哌嗪,驱蛔灵

Piperazines do not, as a rule, produce drowsiness.
哌嗪通常不引起瞌睡。

pipette [piˈpet] *n.* 滴管;吸管;移液管

Pipette is used in a laboratory for transferring or measuring small quantities of liquids.
移液管用于实验室转移或测量少量液体。

Attention is paid to teaching the staff to use the 0.1ml washout pipette as accurately as possible.
注意告诫工作人员尽可能精确地使用 0.1 毫升冲洗过的吸管。

pit [pit] *n.* 凹;窝;痘凹

In anatomy, pit is a hollow or depression on the surface of the body, such as armpit.

解剖学上把体表的凹陷部位叫窝，例如腋窝。

pitch [pitʃ] *n.* 螺距

Pitch refers to the bed moving distance as the tube rotates one circle.

螺距指的是球管转动一周时床移动的距离。

pitfall [ˈpitfɔːl] *n.* 陷井，缺陷

The pitfalls in both techniques are well documented.

这两种技术的缺陷，已有充分的文献证明。

pitting [ˈpitiŋ] *n.* 凹痕；凹陷

Pitting oedema is swelling of the tissues due to excess fluid in which fingertip pressure leaves temporary indentations in the skin.

凹陷性水肿是由于积液过多引起组织肿胀，用指尖按压时留下暂时性皮肤凹痕。

Pitting of nails is strongly associated with joint disease.

指甲凹痕与关节疾病有很强的联系。

pituicyte [piˈtju(ː)isait] *n.* 垂体（后叶）细胞

The neuroglial cells in the pituitary are called pituicytes.

垂体内的神经胶质细胞叫做垂体细胞。

Pituicyte is similar in appearance to an astrocyte, with numerous fine branches that end in contact with the lining membrance of the blood channels in the gland.

垂体细胞与星形胶质细胞的外形相似，有许多细小分支，其末梢与腺体内血管壁接触。

pituitary [piˈtjuːitəri] *a.* 垂体的

The pituitary gland is composed of two main lobes, the adenohypophysis (anterior lobe) and the neurohypophysis (posterior lobe).

垂体（腺）由两个主要部分组成，即腺垂体（前叶）和神经垂体（后叶）。

The posterior pituitary gland also produces the antidiuretic hormone.

脑垂体后叶也产生抗利尿激素。

n. 垂体

The pituitary has attracted attention since the time of Galen.

从盖仑时代起，脑下垂体即引起人们的注意。

There is evidence that some of the relationships between the pituitary and the ovary are dose-dependent.

有证据显示垂体和卵巢间的一些关系是量依赖性的。

pituitrin [piˈtjuːitrin] *n.* 垂体后叶素（商品名）

Pituitrin has the effects of stimulating the contraction of the pregnant uterus.

垂体后叶素有刺激妊娠子宫使之收缩的作用。

pivotal [ˈpivətəl] *a.* 中枢的，关键性的

This is the pivotal step in the process of complement activation.

这是在补体激活过程中的关键性步骤。

Controlling rejection while avoiding the adverse side effects of immunosuppressive agents is pivotal to successful transplantation.

控制排异反应，同时避免免疫抑制剂的有害副作用对成功的移植是关键性的。

pixel [ˈpiksəl] *n.* 像素

A CT image is composed of many small units according to matrix arrangement, these basic units are named pixel.

CT 图像是由按矩阵排列的许多小单位组成，这些基本单位叫像素。

The pixel data can be cached for faster access.

此像素数据可以缓存以便更快地访问。

The number of bits per pixel must be less than or equal to 32.

每个像素的位数必须小于或等于 32。

placebo [plə'siːbəu] *n.* 安慰剂,无效(对照)剂

Twenty-two received placebo, and 16 received imipramine.

22 人服用安慰剂,而 16 人服用丙咪嗪。

All placebo-treated children received the maximum 5mg/kg dose.

所有用安慰剂治疗的患儿均服用每公斤体重 5 毫克的最大剂量。

A placebo is a treatment that has no specific physical or chemical action but is given to affect symptoms by a psychologic mechanism.

安慰剂是对所治疾病并无特殊物理或化学作用的一种疗法,使用此剂是通过心理机制来影响症状。

placenta [plə'sentə] *n.* 胎盘

Certain observations made on placentas were described previously.

关于对胎盘所进行的某些观察,前面已经描写过。

Regular contractions then begin again and separate the placenta from the uterine wall and push it down into the vagina.

规则收缩又开始,使胎盘与子宫壁分离,并下降至阴道。

placental [plə'sentəl] *a.* 胎盘的

Placental function can be evaluated by assessing its ability to metabolize substances in the maternal circulation.

胎盘功能可通过测量母体血液循环中胎盘代谢的能力而获知。

plague [pleig] *n.* 鼠疫,瘟疫,祸害

In many places, and in many trades, asbestosis is a plague to come.

在许多地方和许多职业中石棉沉着病是即将来临的祸害。

The germ that causes bubonic plague is carried by rats and other rodents.

引起鼠疫的细菌是老鼠和其他啮齿动物传播的。

plain [plein] *a.* 清楚的,明显的

It is perfectly plain that now the laser makes delicate eye surgery possible.

十分明显现在激光使非常精细的眼科手术成为可能。

Now his voice is quite plain after the operation of his throat.

经过喉部手术后现在他的声音很清楚。

n. 平片

The suggestion that a kidney is large, small, or absent can often be made without injecting contrast material in the abdominal plains.

腹部平片通常可了解肾脏是大,是小或是缺如,而不需要注射造影剂。

planar ['pleinə] *a.* 平面的

All planar structures are represented by a strike line and dip angle.

一切平面构造均可用向线和倾斜角来表示。

The best chips on the market today use planar transistors that are 32 nanometers in size. The next generation will use 22-nanometer transistors.

当今市面上最好的芯片使用 32 纳米的平面晶体管,而下一代芯片将使用 22 纳米晶体管。

plane [plein] *n.* 平面

The two sphenoidal sinuses are separated by a bony septum which is usually not in the median plane.

两侧蝶窦由一骨性中隔分离,但该中隔不位于正中。

plaque [plɑːk] *n.* [法] 斑,斑块

The artery was completely occluded by an atheromatous plaque.

动脉被粥样硬化斑块完全阻塞。

The arterial walls were moderately dilated and showed scattered atheromatous plaques.

动脉壁中度扩张，并有粥样斑块散在。

plasma [ˈplæzmə] *n.* 原生质，原浆

The plasma cells can produce large amounts of antibody.

浆细胞可产生大量的抗体。

Both cell shape and numerous functions of the plasma membrane are dependent on the cytoskeleton.

细胞形态和胞浆膜的许多功能都依赖细胞骨架。

plasmablast [ˈplæzməblæst] *n.* 浆母细胞，成浆细胞，原浆细胞

A plasmablast is a B cell in a lymph node that already shows some features of a plasma cell.

浆母细胞是指淋巴结中已经表现出一些浆细胞特征的 B 细胞。

plasmacytoid [ˌplæzməˈsaitɔid] *a.* 浆细胞样的

Plasmacytoid dendritic cells are a distinct lineage of dendritic cells that secrete large amounts of interferon on activation by pathogens.

浆细胞样树突状细胞是一种与树突状细胞截然不同的细胞，该细胞受病原体活化后能分泌大量的干扰素。

Under the electromicroscope, many neoplastic cells in this case are plasmacytoid.

在电镜下，该病例中许多肿瘤细胞是浆细胞样的。

plasmapheresis [ˌplæzməfəˈriːsis] *n.* 去血浆法；血浆提取法

Plasmapheresis denotes a method of removing a quantity of plasma from the blood.

去血浆法指的是一种把血液中大量血浆除去的方法。

The child was given 316cc plasma intravenously obtained from plasmapheresis from his father on this visit.

这次就诊给患儿静脉输入了 316ml 以血浆提取法获得的其父亲的血浆。

plasmid [ˈplæzmid] *n.* 质粒

Plasmid is an extrachromosomal genetic element capable of autonomous replication.

质粒是位于染色体外的能自我复制的遗传成分。

Plasmid usually carry a few genes essential to the bacterium's survival.

质粒通常携带少许细菌生存必需的基因。

plasmocytoma [ˌplæzməsaiˈtəumə] *n.* 浆细胞瘤

Plasmocytoma or multiple myeloma is a malignant proliferation of abnormal plasma cells, which leads to the focal destruction of bone tissue.

浆细胞瘤或多发性骨髓瘤是异常浆细胞的恶性增生，它可导致骨组织的局部破坏。

plasmodial [plæzˈməudiəl] *a.* 疟原虫的

Immunity to malaria is a state of relative resistance to the plasmodial infection or to the adverse effects caused by it.

疟疾免疫是一种对疟原虫感染的相对抵抗力，或对其引起的有害作用的相对抵抗力。

plaster [ˈplɑːstə, ˈplæstə] *n.* 石膏；胶布

Usually there is no stiffness of joints as in cases with plaster casts.

通常没有像用石膏模型病例中常出现的关节僵硬。

Plaster is used as a bandage to keep a dressing in place.

胶布像绷带一样可用来固定敷料。

plastic [ˈplæstik] *a.* 成形的，整形的 *n.* (*pl.*)塑料

Successful penile reimplantations have been performed by plastic surgeons with microvascular technique.

整形外科医生用微血管技术成功地进行了阴茎再造术。

A contracted bladder may call for plastic enlargement.

挛缩的膀胱需要用整形外科手术加以扩张。

plasticizer [ˈplæstisaizə] *n.* 增塑剂

Plasticizers for wallboard increase fluidity of the mix, allowing lower use of water and thus reducing energy to dry the board.
墙板增塑剂提高混合物的流动性，降低用水量，从而减少墙板干燥所需的能量。
Plasticizers for concrete increase the workability of the wet mix, or reduce the water required to achieve the desired workability, and are usually not intended to affect the properties of the final product after it hardens.
混凝土增塑剂可增加湿拌的操作性，或减少操作所需水量，它通常不影响硬化后终产物的特性。

plastid [ˈplæstid] *n.* 质体
Mitochondria are plastids, capable of self-replication.
线粒体是质体，能自我复制。

plateau [ˈplætəu] *n.* 高地，高原
Plaques are lesions >5mm in diameter with a flat, plateau-like surface.
斑块是直径大于5mm，有一扁平隆起类似高地样的病损。

platelet [ˈpleitlit] *n.* (血)小板
In diameter the blood platelets are only one-third as large as the red blood cells.
血小板的直径只是红细胞直径的1/3。
Platelet repair of vascular openings is based on several important functions of the platelet itself.
血小板修复血管裂口是基于血小板本身的几个重要功能。

platinum [ˈplætinəm] *n.* 铂，白金
Studies in the metal-refining industry suggest that many workers regularly exposed to the complex salts of platinum develop disorders of the upper or lower respiratory tract.
冶金工业的研究指出：经常接触铂复合盐的工人可发生上呼吸道或下呼吸道疾患。

plausibility [ˌplɔːzəˈbiliti] *n.* 似乎有理，可信性
There is biological plausibility in inferring that breast-feeding protects against bed-wetting.
推断母乳喂养能防止尿床在生物学上似乎有理。

pleiotropic [ˌplaiəuˈtrɔpik] *a.* 多效性的；多向性的
Hepatocyte growth factor (HGF) is a pleiotropic cytokine.
肝细胞生长因子是一多效性细胞因子。
Interleukin 10 is a pleiotropic cytokine produced by many cells in human.
白细胞介素10是由人体内多种细胞产生的多效细胞因子。

pleiotropism [plaiˈɔtrəpizəm] *n.* 多向性，多效性
The sickle-cell gene is a typical example of one showing pleiotropism.
镰形细胞基因是显示多效性的典型例子。

plentiful [ˈplentiful] *a.* 大量的
Nitrogen is the most plentiful gas in the atmosphere.
氮是大气中含量最多的气体。

pleomorphic [pli(ː)əˈmɔːfik] *a.* 多形的(=pleomorphous [pli(ː)əˈmɔfəs])
A pleomorphic skin rash appears first over the trunk and spreads to involve the extremities.
多形皮疹首先发生在躯干，并播散累及四肢。

pleura [ˈpluərə] *n.* 胸膜
The tumor may spread widely throughout the lung and involve the pleura.
癌可能扩散到整个肺部并累及胸膜。
Pleura effusion is common, and is due to irritation of the pleura by spread of the tumor.
常见胸膜渗出物，这是因为癌细胞扩散刺激胸膜所致。

pleural [ˈpluərəl] *a.* 胸膜的
A collection of transudate fluid in the pleural cavity is called a hydrothorax.
胸膜腔中漏出液的积聚(现象)称为胸膜积水。

pleurisy ['pluərisi] *n.* 胸膜炎

Pleurisy is an inflammation of the pleura.

胸膜炎是胸膜的炎症。

Pain in the front and top of the shoulder is thus characteristic of diaphragmatic pleurisy.

肩前部和顶部疼痛是膈肌胸膜炎的特征。

Purulent pleurisy, or empyema, is an accumulation of pus in the pleural spaces.

化脓性胸膜炎或脓胸是脓液聚积在胸膜腔内。

pleuritic [pluə'ritik] *a.* 胸膜炎性的

Haemoptysis occurs in about 40 percent of the pleuritis cases, and pleuritic chest pain may occur, but is not common.

约有40%的胸膜炎患者咯血，胸膜炎性胸痛也会发生，但并不常见。

pleuritis [pluə'raitis] *n.* 胸膜炎

Pleural effusion may or may not be associated with pleuritis.

胸腔积液可能但也不一定都与胸膜炎有关。

Pleuritis and pericarditis may be present simultaneously, as in the setting of tuberculosis.

在患有结核病时，胸膜炎和心包炎可同时存在。

pleurodesis [ˌpluərə'desis] *n.* 胸膜固定(黏合)术

The objective is to investigate the clinical effects of pleurodesis with erythromycin and cisplatin on malignant pleural effusion.

目的是研究红霉素联合顺铂行胸膜粘连术对恶性胸腔积液的临床效果。

plexus ['pleksəs] *n.* (血管、淋巴、神经等)丛

Peristalsis is controlled mainly by intrinsic nervous action in the myenteric plexus in the gut wall.

蠕动主要受胃肠壁内肠肌丛中的内在神经控制。

pliable ['plaiəbl] *a.* 易弯的，柔韧的

The presence of an opening snap and loud first sound denotes a pliable valve.

开瓣音及响亮第一心音的存在表示有一柔韧性瓣膜。

plot [plɔt] *n.* 图

Gemstone CT can also use bulls-eye plot of the left ventricle segments to demonstrate the function condition of left ventricle in ischemic heart disease.

宝石 CT 也可以通过“牛眼图”来显示缺血性心脏病左心室的功能状况。

pluripotent [plu'ripətənt] *a.* 多能的

Pluripotent stem cells are found in the blood islands of the embryonic yolk sac, in the liver of the fetus during fetal development, and later in the bone marrow.

多能干细胞见于胚胎卵黄囊的血岛、胎儿发育期的肝脏，以后则见于骨髓。

pneumobilia [ˌnjuːməu'biliə] *n.* 气性胆汁，胆道积气

Pneumobilia, gas within the biliary tract, is due to an abnormal connection between the gastrointestinal tract and the biliary tract and is considered a serious pathology usually requiring surgical intervention.

胆道积气即胆道内出现气体，是由于胃肠道和胆道之间的连接异常所致，被认为是一种严重的病理状态，通常需要手术治疗。

Most cases of pneumobilia are related to gallstone disease, and spontaneous biliary-enteric fistula is reported to be the most common cause of pneumobilia.

多数胆道积气病例与胆石症有关，据报道自发性胆-肠瘘是胆道积气最常见的原因。

pneumococcus [njuːmə'kɔkəs] *n.* 肺炎双球菌

The pneumococcus is particularly dangerous to the splenectomised patient.

对脾切除患者，肺炎双球菌(感染)是特别危险的。

pneumoconiosis [ˌnjuːməkɔni'əusis] *n.* 肺尘埃沉着病，尘肺

Pneumoconiosis is lung damage in persons who have inhaled various of dust.

尘肺是吸入了各种灰尘的人的肺损伤。

Since most of the severe cases of advanced pneumoconioses with impaired lung function are detected easily with a chest X-ray, how to detect early cases of pneumoconioses became a matter of question.

鉴于绝大多数已有肺功能损害的严重晚期尘肺很容易用 X 线胸片检出，如何检出早期尘肺就成为实际问题。

pneumocystis [ˌnjuːməˈsistis] *n.* 肺孢子虫属

Definitive diagnosis of Pneumocystis pneumonia requires visualization of the organism in pulmonary secretions or biopsy material.

肺孢子虫性肺炎的明确诊断要求在肺组织分泌物或活检材料中见到病原体。

The species Pneumocystis carinii causes pneumonia in immunosuppressed patients.

卡氏肺囊虫种属对免疫受抑制病人可引起肺炎。

pneumocyte [ˈnjuːməsait] *n.* 肺泡上皮细胞

Alveolar epithelium is a continuous layer of two cell types: flattened, platelike type Ⅰ pneumocytes covering 95% of the alveolar surface and rounded type Ⅱ pneumocytes.

肺泡上皮是由两种细胞构成的连续细胞层：扁平的Ⅰ型肺泡上皮细胞覆盖约 95% 的肺泡表面，以及圆形的Ⅱ型肺泡上皮细胞。

In the organizing stage of acute lung injury, type Ⅱ pneumocytes undergo proliferation, and there is a granulation tissue response in the alveolar walls and in the alveolar spaces.

在急性肺损伤的机化期，Ⅱ型肺泡上皮细胞增生，肺泡壁和肺泡腔内有肉芽组织反应。

pneumonectomy [ˌnjuː məˈnektəmi] *n.* 肺切除术

Pneumonectomy should not be done until a tissue diagnosis of cancer has been established.

只有在癌肿的组织学诊断确立后，才可行肺切除术。

pneumonia [njuˈməunjə] *n.* 肺炎

Inflammation of the lung is traditionally pneumonia, not pneumonitis.

肺的炎症传统上称为 pneumonia，而不是称为 pneumonitis。

Three months later, she was rehospitalized because of bilateral pneumonia and congestive heart failure.

3 个月后她因患双侧肺炎和充血性心力衰竭而再次入院。

pneumonic [njuˈmɔnik] *a.* 肺炎的

The lung surrounding the pneumonic foci is edematous.

肺炎病灶周围的肺组织有水肿。

pneumonitis [ˌnjuːməuˈnaitis] *n.* 肺炎

The passage of larvae through the lungs may result in pneumonitis.

蛔蚴通过肺部可引起肺炎。

Chlamydia is the best-studied organism of those that cause the afebrile pneumonitis syndrome.

衣原体是引起无热肺炎综合征病原体中被研究得最全面的一个。

pneumoperitoneum [ˌnjuːməuˌperitəˈniəm] *n.* 气腹，气腹术

Before pneumoperitoneum, the HR and MAP of patients in the experiment were respectively reduced significantly and much lower than those before anesthesia.

气腹术前，实验组患者的心率和平均动脉压分别比麻醉前显著减慢和降低。

No obvious difference is found on the diameter of femoral vein, the velocity and the blood volume of two groups before the establishment of CO_2 pneumoperitoneum($P>0.05$).

在确立 CO_2 气腹前，两组患者的股静脉直径、平均血流速度及血流量均无明显差异($P>0.05$)。

pneumotachometer [ˌnjuːməˈtækəmitəː] *n.* 气流速度计，呼吸速度测定器

Flow signals can be collected at the airway opening using a mask/mouthpiece and pneumotachometer.

流率信号能在气道开口使用面罩/口罩和气流速度计收集。

pneumothorax [njuməu'θɔːræks] *n.* 气胸

Accumulation of air in the pleural space is named pneumothorax.

空气聚集在胸膜腔内称作气胸。

The term "closed pneumothorax" is used when there is no external wound in the chest.

"闭合性气胸"这一术语用于胸部无开放性创伤情况时。

podocyte ['pɔdəsait] *n.* 足细胞

The visceral epithelial cell, also known as a podocyte, is important for the maintenance of glomerular barrier function.

脏层上皮细胞也称为足细胞,在维持肾小球的屏障功能中起重要作用。

The morphological hallmark of primary FSGS is diffuse effacement of podocyte foot processes.

原发性局灶性节段性肾小球硬化的形态学标志是足突细胞的足突弥漫性融合。

poikilocytosis [ˌpɔikiləusai'təusis] *n.* 异形红细胞症

In addition to variations in size (anisocytosis), variations in shape (poikilocytosis) may be seen.

红细胞除大小的变异(红细胞大小不均)外,还可出现形态的变异(异形红细胞症)。

Poikilocytosis is particularly marked in myelofibrosis but can occur to some extent in almost any blood disease.

异形红细胞症在骨髓纤维变性中特别明显,但在几乎所有血液疾病中均能有某种程度的出现。

poison ['pɔizn] *n.* 毒,毒药,毒物

In the US, poison exposures result in an estimated 5 million requests for medical advice or treatment annually.

在美国,每年发生大约5百万毒物接触事件需要求医。

Public health workers are doing all they can to destroy malaria before the mosquitoes become resistant to the poisons.

公共卫生工作者正努力在蚊子变得对毒物有抵抗力之前消灭疟疾。

v. 毒害,中毒

Man is slowly poisoning his environment.

人类正在逐渐毒害自己的环境。

poisoning ['pɔizniŋ] *n.* 中毒

The third most important emergency is poisoning, which needs immediate medical attention.

第三种最重要的急症是中毒,需要立即进行医疗关注。

The combining of hemoglobin with carbon monoxide is likely to cause poisoning of the body.

血红蛋白和一氧化碳的结合很可能引起人体中毒。

Acute symptoms of oral cobalt poisoning include anemia, loss of appetite and weight loss.

经口钴中毒的急性症状有贫血、无食欲和体重减轻。

poisonous ['pɔiznəs] *a.* 有毒的,有害的

Most people are aware of the poisonous effects on the brain of alcohol.

大多数人已意识到酒精对大脑的毒害作用。

Nevertheless, deaths from the escape of poisonous gases from heaters still are all too common.

然而,取暖器产生的毒气外逸而致死的事故仍是十分常见。

polar ['pəulə] *a.* 极的

The smaller, non-yolk-laden polar bodies usually degenerate.

较小的、不含卵黄的极体通常会退化。

The first polar body may undergo the second meiotic division to form two additional polar body.

第一极体经过第二次减数分裂形成另外两个极体。

polarity [pəu'lærəti] *n.* 极向,极性

Loss of polarity, disturbed orientation of tumor cells is an important morphologic change of malignant neoplasia.

肿瘤细胞极向消失、排列紊乱是恶性肿瘤的重要形态学改变。

Loss of cell polarity, tissue disorganisation and excessive cell growth are hallmarks of cancer.

极向消失、组织结构破坏和细胞过度增生是癌症的特征。

pole [pəul] *n.* 极，胎极

Twins may be diagnosed by palpation of more than two fetal poles, and often two heads are clearly recgnized.

触诊到两个以上的胎极可诊断为双胎，而且常常两个胎头能清楚辨认。

polio [ˈpəuliəu] *n.* 脊髓灰质炎

Like measles, polio infection gives a life-long immunity.

像麻疹一样，感染脊髓灰质炎可获得终生免疫。

Paralysis of this sick child was caused by the polio virus invading the central nervous system.

这个病儿的瘫痪是由脊髓灰质炎病毒侵入中枢神经系统引起的。

poliomyelitis [ˌpəuliəuˌmaiəˈlaitis] *n.* 脊髓灰质炎

The clinical diagnosis of poliomyelitis is usually not difficult.

脊髓灰质炎的临床诊断通常并不困难。

The incidence of poliomyelitis is much lower than that of many other children's infections.

脊髓灰质炎的发病率比许多其他儿童传染病的发病率要低得多。

poliovirus [pəuliəuˈvaiərəs] *n.* 脊髓灰质炎病毒

Poliovirus is an RNA virus whose diameter is only 28μm.

脊髓灰质炎病毒是一种核糖核酸病毒，其直径仅 28 微米。

There is as yet no antibiotic or antiviral drug effective against poliovirus infections in humans.

至今尚无抗菌药物或抗病毒药物能有效地抵抗人体内的脊髓灰质炎病毒的感染。

pollen [ˈpɔlən] *n.* 花粉；蒲黄

We study the effect of compound pollen injection on the patients with postpartum hemorrhage of cesarean section.

我们探讨复方蒲黄注射液对剖宫产后出血的干预效果。

Pollen allergy is the most common form of seasonal respiratory allergic disease in Europe.

花粉过敏是欧洲最常见的季节性呼吸系统变态反应病。

pollinosis [ˌpɔliˈnəusis] *n.* 花粉病，枯草热

Hay fever(allergic rhinitis or pollinosis), is an allergy characterized by sneezing, itchy and watery eyes, a runny nose and a burning sensation of the palate and throat.

枯草热(过敏性鼻炎或花粉病)是一种过敏症，其特征是打喷嚏、发痒和流泪、流鼻涕以及腭部、咽喉的灼热感。

This kind of weather often brings pollinosis.

这种天气常常引起花粉病。

pollutant [pəˈluː tənt] *n.* 污染物

These pollutants emerged from under the water.

这些污染物质从水底下出现。

In industry, bioengineers are developing special genes to use against pollutants in water.

工业上，生物工程学家们正在开发特殊基因用以对抗水中的污染物。

pollute [pəˈluː t] *v.* 弄脏，污染

The embryos of the worm may gain access to the human host in polluted drinking water.

蠕虫胚胎可随污染了的饮水侵入人类宿主体内。

pollution [pəːˈljuːʃən] *n.* 污染

Air pollution can affect our health in many ways with both short-term and long-term effects.

空气污染可在很多方面影响我们的健康，既有短期的、也有长期的影响。

Light pollution is a side effect of industrial civilization.

光污染是工业文明带来的不良后果。

poloxamer [pəˈlɔksæmə] *n.* 泊洛沙姆

Poloxamer used for a range of oral, injection and topical pharmaceutical formulations is generally considered non-toxic and non-irritating.

泊洛沙姆应用于一系列口服、注射和局部使用的药物制剂，通常被认为是无毒无刺激性的。

Poloxamer is mainly used in pharmaceutical preparations as emulsifiers and plasticizers.

泊洛沙姆在药物制剂中主要用做乳化剂和增塑剂。

polyacrylamide [ˌpɔliəˈkriləmaid] *n.* 聚丙烯酰胺

Polyacrylamide (PAM), also called flocculating agent, the dry powder of which is not suitable for using, should be confected into aqueous solution to ensure its using effect.

聚丙烯酰胺(PAM)，也被称为絮凝剂，其干粉不宜使用，需配制成水溶液使用以确保效果。

An antistatic agent of polyacrylamide quaternary ammonium compound was designed and synthesized.

设计合成了一种聚丙烯酰胺季铵化合物的抗静电剂。

polyadenylation [ˌpɔliˌædiniˈleiʃən] *n.* 聚腺苷酸化

The polyA tail appears to increase the stability of the resulting polyadenylated RNA.

polyA 尾巴看起来可以增加由此产生的聚腺苷酸化 RNA 的稳定性。

The location of the polyadenylation point is specified in part by the sequence AAUAAA (or a variant of this).

聚腺苷酸化位点部分由 AAUAAA 序列(或者它的变体)所决定。

polyamine [ˌpɔliəˈmiːn] *n.* 多胺

A polyamine is an organic compound having two or more primary amino groups - NH2.

多胺是一种有机化合物，有两个或两个以上的伯氨基 - NH2。

Polyamines are also important modulators of a variety of ion channels, including NMDA receptors and AMPA receptors.

多胺也是多种离子通道的重要调节分子，包括 NMDA 受体和 AMPA 受体。

polyarthritis [ˌpɔliɑːˈθraitis] *n.* 多关节炎

Polyarthritis is any type of arthritis which involves 5 or more joints simultaneously.

多关节炎是指任何类型的关节炎同时累及 5 个或以上关节。

Rheumatoid arthritis (RA) is a common systemic autoimmune disease, which is characterized by chronic polyarthritis symptom.

类风湿性关节炎是一种常见的以慢性多关节炎症为主要表现的全身自身免疫性疾病。

polyarticular [ˌpɔliɑːˈtikjulə] *a.* 多关节的

The three onset patterns of juvenile rheumatoid arthritis are acute systematic, pauciarticular, and polyarticular.

幼年型类风湿性关节炎起病的三种类型是急性全身型、少发关节型及多发关节型。

polychondritis [ˌpɔlikɔnˈdraitis] *n.* 多软骨炎

Polychondritis, also called relapsing polychondritis, is a rare disease in which cartilage in many areas of the body becomes inflamed.

多软骨炎，又称复发性多软骨炎，是一种全身多处软骨发生炎症的少见疾病。

Relapsing polychondritis may be an auto-immune disease in which the human's body's immune system begins to attack and destroy the cartilage tissues in the body.

复发性多软骨炎可能是一种自身免疫疾病，患者免疫系统开始攻击和破坏身体软骨组织。

polychromatophilia [ˌpɔliˌkrəumətəˈfiliə] *n.* 多染(色)性，多染(性)细胞增多

Adequate marrow response to anemia is evidenced by reticulocytosis or polychromatophilia.

网织红细胞增多或多染红细胞增多是骨髓对贫血有充分反应的证据。

polycistron [ˌpɔliˈsistrɔn] *n.* 多顺反子

We found a micro RNA polycistron as a potential human oncogene.

我们发现一个微小 RNA 多顺反子有可能是一种人类原癌基因。

The polycistron adenoviral expression vector was successfully constructed.

该多顺反子的腺病毒表达载体已构建成功。

polyclonal [ˌpɔliˈkləunəl] *a.* 多克隆的，多元性繁殖系的，多细胞系的

The invention also relates to a monoclonal or polyclonal antibody.

本发明还涉及一种单克隆或多克隆抗体。

The results show the gold-probe possesses high selectivity and DIGFA is capable of measuring the specificity of polyclonal antibodies accurately and rapidly.

结果表明金探针具有很强的选择性，斑点免疫金渗滤法能准确快速地检测出多克隆抗体的特异性。

polycyclic [ˌpɔliˈsaiklik] *a.* 多环的

Pollutants in cigarettes called PAHs(polycyclic aromatic hydrocarbons) can cause genetic damage in minutes.

香烟中的污染物质 PAHs(多环芳烃) 能在几分钟内对基因造成损害。

Polycyclic aromatic compounds which are widespread in water, soil and atmosphere are harmful to human health.

多环芳香化合物广泛存在于水、土壤和大气中，危害人类健康。

polycystic [ˌpɔliˈsistik] *a.* 多囊的

The kidneys are large in polycystic disease.

多囊肾病患者的肾脏较大。

About 30% of patients with adult polycystic kidney disease have hepatic cysts, but disturbance of liver function is rare.

成人多囊肾病人中约 30% 有肝囊肿，但是肝功能紊乱罕见。

polycythemia [ˌpɔlisaiˈθiːmiə] *n.* 红细胞增多(症)

The chronic bronchitis tends to have polycythemia.

慢性支气管炎有发生红细胞增多的倾向。

Polycythemia may be due either to a decrease in the total volume of the plasma or to an increase in the total volume of the red cells.

红细胞增多症可能是由于血浆总量的减少也可能由于红细胞总量的增加。

polydactyly [ˌpɔliˈdæktili] *n.* 多指(趾)

The polydactyly gene shows different phenotypes in different affected people.

多指(趾) 基因在不同受累者中有不同的表现型。

Even a person affected with polydactyly usually has one or two normal limbs.

即便是多指(趾) 患者通常有一肢或两肢是正常的。

polydipsia [ˌpɔliˈdipsiə] *n.* 烦渴；多饮

Polydipsia and Polyuria are the main syndromes of central diabetes insipidus, which belongs to "xiaoke" in traditional Chinese medicine.

中枢性尿崩症主要表现为多饮、多尿，(与糖尿病) 同属中医学的"消渴"范畴。

Puncturing Fengfu acupoint can relieve polydipsia and polyuria syndromes effectively.

针刺风府穴能有效地减轻患者的多饮及多尿症状。

polyethylene [ˌpɔliˈeθiliːn] *n.* 聚乙烯

Polyethylene is a synthetic plastic material, it has been used in reparative surgery.

聚乙烯是一种合成塑料物质，已用于修复外科。

The use of a polyethylene device has simplified the technique of this procedure.

使用聚乙烯装置简化了此项操作的手续。

polygala [pəˈligələ] *n.* 远志，远志属

Polygala tincture can be used to treat chronic bronchitis.
远志酊可用来治疗慢性支气管炎。
Studies on the alkaloidal components of polygala tenuifolia were reviewed.
我们对远志生物碱成分的研究已进行了综述。

polygenic [ˌpɔliˈdʒenik] *a.* 多基因的
In polygenic inheritance the trait is usually continuous in distribution.
多基因遗传的性状通常是连续分布的。
Hypertension is a common polygenic disease.
高血压是一种常见的多基因病。

polyhydramnios [ˌpɔlihaiˈdræmniəs] *n.* 羊水过多
There is no satisfactory explanation for the cause of polyhydramnios in most cases.
在大多数病例其羊水过多的原因还无法满意地解释。

polymer [ˈpɔlimə] *n.* 聚合物
The starches and glycogen are both large polymers of glucose.
淀粉和糖原都是大的葡萄糖聚合物。
Many bacteria secrete large polymers that adhere to the external surface of the cell.
许多细菌可分泌大的聚合物,此聚合物黏附于细胞表面。
Called aroma scan, the tabletop instrument has a sensor array of 32 semiconducting polymers.
名为香味测检器的台式仪器内有一组由 32 个半导体聚合物排列成的感受器。

polymerase [ˈpɔliməreis] *n.* 聚合酶,多聚酶
RNA polymerase and DNA polymerase are also Zn metalloenzymes.
RNA 聚合酶和 DNA 聚合酶也是含锌金属酶。
RNA polymerase Ⅱ is responsible for the synthesis of mRNA.
RNA 聚合酶Ⅱ对信使 RNA 的合成起作用。

polymerization [ˌpɔliməraiˈzeiʃən] *n.* 聚合,聚合作用
In polymer chemistry, polymerization is a process of reacting monomer molecules together in a chemical reaction to form three-dimensional networks or polymer chains.
高分子化学中,聚合反应是通过化学反应将单分子聚集以形成三维网络或聚合物链的过程。
Other forms of chain growth polymerization include cationic addition polymerization and anionic addition polymerization.
其他形式的链增长聚合包括阳离子加成聚合和阴离子加成聚合。

polymorph [ˈpɔlimɔːf] *n.* 多形核白细胞
In man the important wandering phagocytic cells are the neutrophil polymorphs and the monocytes.
在人类,其重要的游走性吞噬细胞是嗜中性多形核白细胞和单核细胞。
Polymorphs ingest and kill organisms, and in dying liberate enzymes which liquefy the resulting dead tissue.
多形核白细胞吞噬并杀死微生物,并且在死亡时释放一些酶来液化所产生的死亡组织。

polymorphism [ˌpɔliˈmɔː fizəm] *n.* 多形性,多态现象
They will also learn the importance of genetic polymorphism for species survival.
他们也将了解遗传多态性对物种生存的重要性。

polymorphonuclear [ˌpɔliˌmɔːfəˈnjuːkliə] *a.* 多形核的 n. 多形核白细胞
Acute inflammations characteristically show large numbers of polymorphonuclear leukocytes.
急性炎症的特性是出现大量的多形核白细胞。
The white blood cell count was 12500 with 55% polymorphonuclear cells and 45% lymphocytes.
白细胞计数为 12500/mm^3,其中多形核白细胞占 55%,淋巴细胞占 45%。

polymyalgia [ˌpɔlimaiˈældʒiə] *n.* 多肌痛

Polymyalgia rheumatica is a condition that causes pain and stiffness in the muscles around the shoulders, neck, buttocks and hips because of inflammation.

风湿性多肌痛是导致肩、颈部、臀部、髋部周围肌肉疼痛、僵硬的一种疾病。

Studies are inconclusive, however, several somewhat common viruses were identified as possible triggers for polymyalgia rheumatica.

虽然尚无定论，但研究发现某些较为普通的病毒可能是风湿性多肌痛的诱因。

polymyositis [ˌpɔliˌmaiəˈsaitis] *n.* 多肌炎，多发性肌炎

Adult polymyositis occurs three times more frequently in women than in men.

成年女性患多肌炎是男性的三倍。

Polymyositis is an inflammatory condition of skeletal muscle in which muscle tissue is involved predominantly by lymphocytic infiltration.

多发性肌炎是一种由于肌肉组织主要受淋巴细胞浸润而引起的骨骼肌炎症。

polymyxin [ˌpɔliˈmiksin] *n.* 多黏菌素

Polymyxin B is usually administered by injection but is also taken by mouth or applied as a solution or ointment for ear and eye infections.

多黏菌素 B 通常注射给药，但也可以口服，为治疗耳和眼的感染则可配制成溶液或软膏使用。

Topical antibiotic ointments, such as neosporin, polymyxin, or gentamicin are helpful additions in the treatment of the moist type of interdigital lesions.

一些局部抗生素软膏，如新孢菌素、多黏菌素、庆大霉素，对于湿型趾间损害的治疗都是有帮助的。

polyneuritis [ˌpɔlinjuəˈraitis] *n.* 多神经炎

Diabetic polyneuritis is characterized by burning feet and shooting pain frequently during the night. In the late stage sensation of heat and pain is totally lost in the feet.

糖尿病性多神经炎的特征常常是夜间出现脚有烧灼感和刺痛，到了晚期，脚的热和痛的感觉完全丧失。

polyp [ˈpɔlip] *n.* 息肉

Thirty percent of adenomas and occasional hyperplastic polyps are associated with gastric malignancy.

有百分之三十的腺瘤和偶尔增生性息肉与胃癌的发生有关。

Gastric carcinoma, lymphoma, polyps, and other tumors of the stomach and small bowel are uncommon cause of GI hemorrhage.

胃癌、淋巴瘤、息肉以及胃和小肠的其他肿瘤是胃肠道出血的少见原因。

polypectomy [ˌpɔliˈpektəmi] *n.* 息肉切除术

Polypectomy is one of the examples of therapeutic techniques in endoscopy.

内镜下进行治疗的例子之一就是息肉切除术。

polypeptide [pɔliˈpeptaid] *n.* 多肽

Short chains of amino acids(6 to 30 residues) linked together by peptide bonds are referred to as polypeptide.

氨基酸(6 ~ 30 个残基)通过肽键连接形成的短链称为多肽。

The thalassemia syndrome is a group of disorders in which the synthesis of polypeptide chains is decreased.

海洋性贫血综合征是一组多肽链合成减少的疾患。

polyperforin [ˌpɔlipəˈfɔːrin] *n.* 多聚穿孔素

Polyperforin is capable of inducing damage to membranes that causes the release of proteins from target cells.

多聚穿孔素能诱导靶细胞膜损伤，导致蛋白从靶细胞释放。

polyphagia [ˌpɔliˈfeidʒiə] *n.* 多食症

L-arginine supplementation can partially improve polydipsia and polyphagia and increase plasma protein in diabetic rats.

补充 L-精氨酸可部分改善糖尿病大鼠多饮、多食症状,并增加血浆蛋白。

The diabetic rats developed obviously polydipsia, polyphagia, polyuria and loss of body weight.

糖尿病大鼠出现明显的多饮、多食、多尿及体重减轻现象。

polypharmacy [ˌpɔliˈfɑːməsi] *n.* 复方药剂,多味药物

The treatment of a patient with many drugs together is known as polypharmacy.

用多种药物一起来治疗病人叫复方药剂。

It is better to avoid polypharmacy in the first place than to attempt to withdraw drugs later.

从一开始即避免应用多种药物较用了以后再试图停药为好。

polyphosphate [ˌpɔliˈfɔsfeit] *n.* 多聚磷酸盐

Blue dyes, such as methylene blue, appear red when bound to nucleic acid or polyphosphate granules.

如美蓝这种蓝色染料结合于核酸或多聚磷酸盐颗粒时,则呈现红色。

polypoid [ˈpɔlipɔid] *a.* 息肉状的

Polypoid tumors of the small intestine usually turn out to be hamartomas.

小肠的息肉状肿瘤往往都证明是错构瘤。

polyposis [ˌpɔliˈpəusis] *n.* 息肉病

Carcinomas that appear to have a genetic basis resist analytic efforts to prove a single gene difference except for the familial polyposis syndromes.

除了家族性息肉病综合征外,难以通过分析证明似乎有遗传基础癌肿的单个基因差异。

polypropylene [ˌpɔliˈprəupiliːn] *n.* 聚丙烯

Polypropylene is normally tough and flexible, especially when copolymerized with ethylene.

聚丙烯通常是坚韧和有弹性的,尤其是与乙烯共同聚合时。

Like many plastics, polypropylene has virtually endless uses, and its development has not slowed since its discovery.

像许多塑料一样,聚丙烯的用途几乎是无止境的,自从发现以来其发展一直没有放缓。

polyreactivity [ˌpɔliriækˈtiviti] *n.* 多反应性

Some antibodies show polyspecificity, the ability to bind to many different antigens. This is also known as polyreactivity.

有些抗体具有多特异性,能够结合多种不同的抗原,这种特性也被称为多反应性。

polysaccharide [pɔliˈsækəraid] *n.* 多糖

The remainder of the wall comprises primarily cell wall polysaccharides.

细胞壁其余部分主要由细胞壁多糖组成。

polyserositis [ˌpɔliˌsiərəuˈsaitis] *n.* 多发性浆膜炎

Familial Mediterranean fever has been given various names including familial paroxysmal polyserositis.

家族性地中海热已被赋予不同的名称,包括家族性阵发性多浆膜炎。

In recent years, an infectious disease characterized by polyserositis, arthritis and high death rate appeared and lead great economical loss in many pig farms.

近年来,许多猪场出现了一种以多发性浆膜炎和关节炎以及高死亡率为特征、并带来巨大经济损失的传染病。

polysome [ˈpɔlisəum] *n.* 多核糖体

One mRNA molecule plus several ribosomes is called a polysome.

一个 mRNA 分子和几个核糖体一起称为多核糖体。

Most cellular protein are made on polysomes located free in the cytoplasm.

绝大多数细胞的蛋白质是在游离于细胞质中的多核糖体上合成的。

polysomnography [ˌpɔlisɔmˈnɔgrəfi] *n.* 多导睡眠图,多频道睡眠记录,多导睡眠描记术

These results were consistent with the polysomnography data.
这些结果和多导睡眠图数据一致。
The airflow measured was recorded on polysomnography.
被测量的气流记录在多导睡眠图上。

polysorbate [ˌpɔliˈsɔːbeit] *n.* 聚山梨酯,聚山梨醇酯
Polysorbates are a class of emulsifiers used in some pharmaceuticals and food preparation.
聚山梨酯是用于一些药品和食品制备的一类乳化剂。
Polysorbate 80 is a nonionic surfactant and emulsifier derived from polyethoxylated sorbitan and oleic acid, and is often used in foods.
吐温 80 是一种非离子表面活性剂和乳化剂,它是由聚氧乙烯山梨醇和油酸所得,经常被用于食品中。

polyuria [ˌpɔliˈjuəriə] *n.* 多尿(症),尿频
Polyuria and excessive thirst may go unnoticed for years.
多尿和过分的口渴,可持续多年而未被注意。

polyvalency [ˌpɔliˈveilənsi] *n.* 多价性
Polyvalency influences on the binding properties of antibodies.
多价性影响抗体的结合特性。

pons [pɔnz] (*pl.* pontes [ˈpɔntiːz]) *n.* 桥;脑桥
The cerebellum lies dorsal to the pons and medulla oblongata.
小脑位于脑桥和延髓的背侧。

pool [puːl] *v.* (血)郁积,把……集中一起用
This assists the return blood to the heart and prevents the pooling of blood.
这有助于血液向心回流并防止血液淤滞。
This is the first study to use an online system that was developed in Asian countries for pooling data from an international clinical trial.
这是使用联机系统的首次研究,该系统开发于亚洲国家,用来把国际临床试验中的数据集中起来。
n. 池,库
Gene pool is the totality of the genes possessed by all of the members of a population.
一群体中所有成员拥有的基因总额为基因库。

poorly [ˈpuəli] *ad.* 贫乏地;不良地,拙劣地
The patient responded poorly to digitalis.
病人对洋地黄的反应很差。

popular [ˈpɔpjulə] *a.* 流行的,大众喜爱的,通俗的,大众的
Home medical tests become popular.
家中体检开始流行。
Jogging is a popular form of exercise.
慢跑是一种人们喜爱的锻炼形式。
Saccharin finds its widest use in the preparation of popular low caloric beverage.
糖精在配制大众的低热量饮料中用途最广。

popularity [ˌpɔpjuˈlæriti] *n.* 普及,流行;得人心
One of the most important reasons for the great popularity of electronic instruments is their relatively cheap price.
电子仪器之所以如此普及的最重要的原因之一是其价格比较便宜。
More recently, some complicated operations being perfomed under a microscope have gained popularity.
最近,在显微镜下施行的一些复杂手术得到了大家的赞誉。

popularize [ˈpɔpjuləraiz] *v.* 使普及,推广

In popularizing family planning, much work has been done to improve women's health and to provide better maternity and child care.

在推广计划生育的过程中，已经做了很多工作来增进妇女的健康，并提供更好的妇幼保健。

population [pɔpju'leiʃən] *n.* 人口

Some people are quite concerned about the effects of continuing growth of human population.

一些人十分担心人口持续增长的后果。

Beneficial mutations tend to be spread throughout a population.

有益的突变很可能在整个人群中扩展。

We herein present this experience as a study of the long-term efficacy of kidney transplantation in this population.

本文提供的经验是对这类患者肾移植长期效果的一项研究。

porcelain ['pɔːsəlin] *n.* 瓷，瓷料；瓷器 *a.* 瓷制的

Dental porcelain is a type of porcelain used in dental restorations.

牙瓷料是一种用于牙修复的瓷料。

pore [pɔː] *n.* 孔，门

Bulk flow of water through these pores results from hydrostatic and/or osmotic pressure.

大量水在流体静压和(或)渗透压的作用下穿过这些孔道。

porosity [pɔː'rɔsiti] *n.* 孔，多孔

Porosity of unglazed porcelain filter(Chamberland filter) alone is not the only factor preventing the passage of bacteria.

未上釉瓷滤器(钱伯兰滤器)的小孔不是防止细菌通过的唯一因素。

porous ['pɔːrəs] *a.* 多孔的

The lymph capillaries are extremely porous so that large paricles can enter the lymph vessels and be transported by the lymph.

淋巴毛细管是多孔的，因此大颗粒能进入淋巴管并借助淋巴液运输。

porphyria [pɔː'fiəriə] *n.* 卟啉病

Acute intermittent porphyria is a metabolic disorder rarely seen in prepubertal children.

急性间歇性卟啉病是一种见于青春期前儿童的罕见代谢性疾病。

The objective of our study is to establish the method of quantitative analysis of porphyrins, and obtain the urinary porphyrin pattern for the diagnosis of porphyria.

本研究的目的是要建立卟啉类化合物的定量测定法，确定卟啉病诊断用的尿卟啉谱。

portable ['pɔːtəbl] *a.* 轻便的，手提(式)的

Such portable X-ray equipment is easy to manipulate.

这种手提式 X 线设备操作简便。

The portable X-ray apparatus is not heavy to lift.

这架手提式 X 线机提起来不重。

portal ['pɔː təl] *a.* 门静脉的

Cirrhosis accounts for 80% of the portal hypertension seen in Britain.

在英国 80% 的门静脉高压的原因为肝硬化。

The blood brought by the portal vein to the liver is rich in food materials but poor in oxygen.

从门静脉送进肝脏的血液，富于营养物质，但是含氧少。

portion ['pɔːʃən] *n.* 部分

Aphasia is a language disorder that results from damage to portions of the brain that are responsible for language.

失语症是一种语言障碍，由大脑支配语言的部分受损而引起。

pose [pəuz] *v.* 提出；造成

The presence of preeclampsia poses a significant threat to the fetus.

先兆子痫的出现对胎儿是一个严重的威胁。

The physician is often confronted with the problem posed by pregnancy.

医生经常碰到由于妊娠而引起的问题。

position [pə'ziʃən] *n.* 体位

Occipitoanterior position is a position of the fetus in cephalic presentation in labor.

枕前位是分娩时胎儿头先露的位置。

v. 把…放在适当的位置

It is important that the patient be positioned properly on the operating table.

将病人在手术台上置于恰当的体位是很重要的。

Immediate complications can result from improper positioning.

由于体位不当可立即产生并发症。

positional [pə'ziʃənəl] *a.* 位置的,定位的

The Duchenne muscular dystrophy gene is identified by positional cloning.

杜兴氏肌营养不良(DMD)基因是用定位克隆的方法鉴定的。

positive ['pɔzətiv] *a.* 确定的;积极的;阳性的

A positive result of urine sugar test suggests the presence of diabetes.

尿糖试验的阳性结果提示糖尿病的存在。

Of great interest was the positive correlation with age.

非常有趣的是这确实与年龄有关。

positron ['pɔzitrɔn] *n.* 正电子

Positron emission tomography is a non-invasive method to detect the distribution of radionuclide in vivo.

正电子发射断层摄影术是一种无创性的探测放射性核素在机体内分布的断层显像技术。

Positron emission tomography consists of two types, the dedicated positron emission tomography and the dual-head coincidence detection imaging.

正电子发射断层摄影分为两种类型:专用型正电子发射断层成像和双探头符合探测成像。

possibility [pɔsə'biliti] *n.* 可能性

An alert clinician must be aware of the possibility of myocarditis complicating any acute viral infection.

有警觉的医生应当知道任何急性的病毒感染都有可能并发心肌炎。

Entirely different diagnostic possibilities are raised by a patient who presents with the first severe headache.

当病人第一次出现严重头痛时,完全不同的诊断的可能性增大了。

postcondylare [pəust'kɔndilɛə] *n.* (枕骨)髁后点

Tumors of postcondylare are the most common problems.

枕骨髁后点的肿瘤最常见。

Postcondylare is posterior condyle of occipital bone.

枕骨髁后点就是枕骨后面的髁状突起。

posterior [pɔs'tiəriə] *a.* 后的,后面的

The heart is posterior to the sternum.

心脏在胸骨的后面。

posteriorly [pɔs'tiəriəli] *ad.* 在后面,在背后

A typical vertebra has a body anteriorly and a vertebral arch posteriorly.

一个典型的椎骨具有椎体和椎弓,其椎体朝前而椎弓朝后。

posteroanterior ['pɔstərə,æn'tiəriə] *a.* 后前位的

Posteroanterior chest film is the most commonly used radiography position.

后前位胸片是最常用的放射拍片体位。

Posteroanterior spinal mobilization is a commonly used technique among physical therapists to diagnose and treat lower back pain patients.
后前位脊柱松动术是理疗师常用的一种技术，用于诊断和治疗下背痛病人。

posterolaterally [ˌpɔstərəuˈlætərəli] *ad.* 后侧面地
In most cases there are three main pile masses, one is situated anteriorly, the others posterolaterally.
大多数病例有三个主要的痔块，一个位于前面，其余的位于后侧面。

postganglionic [ˌpəustgæŋgliˈɔnik] *a.* (神经)节后的
In the autonomic nervous system, fibers from the ganglion to the effector organ are called postganglionic fibers.
在自主神经系统，从神经节到效应器官的纤维被称为节后纤维。
When the product is used with postganglionic anticholinergic drugs(such as atropine, Propantheline, etc.), its role diminishes.
本品与节后抗胆碱药(如阿托品、普鲁本辛，等)合用，其作用减弱。

postgenomic [pəustdʒiːˈnɔmik] *a.* 后基因组的
In the postgenomic era, the genomics research will play a leading role in future development of the biomedicine.
在后基因组时代，基因组学研究在未来的生物医学发展中将起主导作用。

postgraduate [ˌpəustˈgrædjuit] *n.* 研究生
This medical university has established special scholarship for postgraduates.
这所医科大学为研究生设立了专门奖学金。
a. 大学毕业后的，研究生的
In some instances, training in a specialty is referred to as postgraduate education.
在某些情况下，专业培训指的是研究生教育。

posthemorrhagic [pəustˌheməˈrædʒik] *a.* 出血后的
The causes of posthemorrhagic anemia are numerous, and the manifestations differ widely.
出血后贫血的原因为数众多，其表现极不一样。

posthepatic [ˌpəusθiˈpætik] *adj.* 肝后性的
We expose as fully as possible for the hepatic venae and the posthepatic inferior vena cava injury, and adopt effective methods to stop bleeding and repair the injury.
我们应尽可能充分暴露肝静脉及肝后下腔静脉损伤，采用有效方法止血和修复损伤。
Our findings suggest that the normal diaphragm mainly develops from the posthepatic mesenchymal plate.
我们的研究结果表明，正常的横膈膜主要从肝后性的间充质板发展而来。

post hoc [ˈpəusthɔk] 在此之后，事后分析
Were the medical research objectives/hypotheses predefined or post hoc?
医学研究目标/假设是预先确定的还是事后确定的？
Digoxin and reduction in mortality in heart failure: A comprehensive post hoc analysis of the DIG trial.
地高辛与心力衰竭患者死亡率的降低：一项对 DIG 试验的综合性事后分析。

postmaturity [ˌpəustməˈtjuəriti] *n.* 过度成熟
Postmaturity is a developmental concept whereas prolonged pregnancy is a chronologic one.
过度成熟是一发育概念，而过期妊娠是一时间概念。

postmenopausal [ˌpəustmenəˈpɔːzəl] *a.* 经绝后的
Vaginitis in postmenopausal women was formerly termed senile vaginitis, but the term atrophic vaginitis is preferrable.
绝经后妇女的阴道炎过去称为老年性阴道炎，但萎缩性阴道炎这一名称更为可取。
Postmenopausal syndrome can occur between the ages of 44 and 55 and the standard definition is

when mentrual periods have completely stopped for more than 12 months.
绝经期综合征可以发生在 44 到 55 岁之间,标准定义为月经完全停止超过 12 个月。

postmortem [pəust'mɔː təm] *a.* 死后的;验尸的 *n.* 尸体解剖,验尸

Postmortem heat loss is accelerated in cold environments.
在寒冷环境中,死后尸体的散热可以加快。

postoperative [pəust'ɔpərətiv] *a.* 手术后的

In any case the patient should observe the postoperative restrictions of movement.
无论如何,病人应该遵守术后关于体力活动的各种限制。

Retention catheters are withdrawn on the fifth postoperative day.
保留导尿管于术后第五天拔去。

postpartum [ˌpəust'pɑːtəm] *a.* 产后的

Ergometrine is used for the treatment of postpartum haemorrhage after the uterus has been emptied.
麦角新碱用于治疗子宫排空后产后出血。

post-pericardiotomy [pəust-ˌperiˌkɑːdi'ɔtəmi] *n.* 心包切开术后

A few patients develop the post-pericardiotomy syndrome, but this is usually easily treated with steroids or salicylates.
少数患者发生心包切开术后综合征,但此征通常易于用类固醇或水杨酸治疗。

postpone [pəust'pəun] *v.* 延缓

The surgeon decided to postpone operating on that patient.
外科医生决定推迟给该患者动手术。

As that patient hasn't recovered yet, we will postpone his leaving hospital.
由于那位患者尚未康复,我们将让他延期出院。

postponement [pəust'pəunmənt] *n.* 延缓,延期

Acute respiratory disease necessitates postponement of anesthesia and surgery.
患有急性呼吸系统疾病时需要推迟麻醉和外科手术。

postprandial [pəust'prændiəl] *a.* 餐后的,食后的

Postprandial hypoglycemia most often occurs in patients with prior gastric resection or bypass.
餐后低血糖主要见于那些已行胃切除术或分流术的病人。

A blood specimen drawn 2 hours after a meal is known as a two-hour postprandial specimen.
进餐后 2 小时抽取的血标本被称为 2 小时餐后标本。

post-traumatic [ˌpəust-trɔː'mætik] *a.* 创伤后的

The clinical course of post-traumatic stress disorder in children and adolescents is variable.
在少年儿童身上,创伤后应激症的临床病程是多变的。

postulate ['pɔstjuleit] *v.* 要求;假定

Wideman has postulated that an ascorbic acid deficiency predisposes the membranes to rupture.
怀德曼推测抗坏血酸缺乏易使胎膜破裂。

Heredity has been postulated to play a role in the pathogenesis of ulcer disease in some patients.
经推测遗传在有些患者溃疡病的发病机制中起作用。

postural ['pɔstʃərəl] *a.* 体位的,姿势的

Postural hypotension sometimes occurs with a fixed heart rate and signs of central nervous system dysfunction.
体位性低血压有时伴随出现固定心率和中枢神经系统功能障碍的体征。

This proteinuria can be classified in two categories—intermittent or persistent and postural.
蛋白尿可分为两类:间歇性或持续性和体位性。

Muscles that serve to maintain the upright posture of the body against the force of gravity are called postural muscles.
对抗地心引力,维持身体直立姿势的肌肉便叫做姿势肌。

posture [ˈpɔstʃə] *n.* 姿势,体位

Poor posture will give you backache.

姿势不端正会使你腰酸背痛。

Upright posture can cause an increase in urine protein excretion in normal individuals.

在正常人中,直立体位可引起尿蛋白的排泄增加。

potassium [pəˈtæsjəm] *n.* 钾

The nerve impulse is also a wave of depolarization,with sodium flowing in and potassium out.

神经冲动也是一种去极化波,伴随有钠的流入和钾的流出。

The serum potassium of the patient ranged from 4.8 to 5.9 mEq/liter.

病人的血清钾水平为4.8~5.9毫当量/升。

potency [ˈpəutənsi] *n.* 效力;效价

The drug has lost its potency by being exposed to moisture.

这药因受潮而失效。

Potency is a measure of the dosage required to bring about a response.

效价是对产生反应所需的药物剂量的一种衡量方式。

Vitamin D potency is measured in terms of cholecalciferol units.

维生素D效价用胆钙化醇单位表示。

potent [ˈpəutənt] *a.* 有力的,有效力的

Tetracaine is about ten times as potent as procaine.

丁卡因的效力是普鲁卡因的10倍。

Two compounds may be equally efficacious but one could be more potent.

两种化合物可能具有同等的效应,但是其中一种可能作用更强。

This is a potent respiratory stimulant.

这是一种有效的呼吸刺激剂。

Besides job-related carcinogens,most people are exposed to several potent cancerous agents.

除了与工作有关的致癌物质外,大多数人接触到几种强有力的致癌因子。

potential [pəuˈtenʃəl] *a.* 潜在的,有可能性的

The potential application of laser as a therapeutic tool has been actively attempted since 1960.

把激光作为一种治疗工具进行应用的可能性,自从1960年以来一直在积极尝试。

A large number of diseases and disorders are a potential threat to people's health and life.

众多的疾病和身体失调是人民健康和生命的潜在威胁。

n. 潜力,潜能;电位

This article will not discuss the carcinogenic potential of items such as food additives and insecticides.

本文将不讨论诸如食品添加剂和杀虫剂等物的致癌潜力。

Action potential is the electrical activity developed in a muscle or nerve cell during activity.

动作电位是在肌肉或神经细胞活动时产生的电位。

Overall,these results indicate that heparin-DOCA may have potentials as therapeutic agent that prevents tumor metastasis and progression.

总之,这些结果显示heparin-DOCA有可能成为治疗药物,用于阻止肿瘤转移和进展。

potentially [pəuˈtenʃəli] *ad.* 潜在地,有可能性地

It is now recognized that potentially serious chronic congenital infections can present at birth with absent or minimal physical findings.

现已认识到潜在的严重慢性先天性感染,可在出生体检时表现为无异常或有轻微异常。

Potentially harmful exposure to soil can occur in industrial locations or waste sites.

在工业区或废物场地可出现接触土壤产生的潜在危害性。

poverty [ˈpɔvəti] *n.* 贫困

She had been worn down by poverty and illness.

贫困和疾病把她折磨倒了。

Contributing factors include inadequate water supplies, overcrowding and lack of personal hygiene, poverty, and lack of education.

有关因素包括水供给不足，过于拥挤和缺乏个人卫生，贫穷以及缺乏教育。

powder [ˈpaudə] *n.* 粉，粉末；粉剂

Plain talcum powder or antifungal powders are helpful in tinea cruris.

一般爽身粉或抗真菌扑粉都对股癣有效。

v. 使成粉末

Powdered plasma may be sent long distances easily and inexpensively.

粉末状的血浆可以简便而廉价地长途运输。

power [ˈpauə] *n.* 能力

Man now has the power to change and control these life processes.

人类现在有了改变和控制这些生命过程的能力。

powerless [ˈpauəlis] *a.* 无力量的，软弱的

There are some diseases against which the doctor was once powerless.

过去医生对一些疾病束手无策。

practicality [ˌprækti'kæliti] *n.* 实践性，实际性；实用性

Appeals to logic and practicality have often appeared in the literature.

文献中常要求注意逻辑性和实用性。

practice [ˈpræktis] *n.* 实践

Physicians who wish to practice medicine in the U. S. must complete an accredited residency training program in the U. S. or Canada.

想在美国开业行医的医师必须在美国或加拿大完成一项被认可的住院医生培训计划。

Hospital Authority has recently launched a series of Clinical Practice Guidelines (CPG) on several common diseases.

医管局最近发布了一系列有关几种常见病的临床实践指南。

practitioner [prækˈtiʃənə] *n.* 行医者，医师

Any practitioner may today be confronted by an unfamiliar imported disease.

今日任何一名医师都可能面临一种不熟悉的、自外传入的疾病。

General practitioner (GP) is a medically qualified doctor who practices general medicine as a family practitioner.

全科医师（或非专科普通开业医师）是医学上的合格医生，往往以家庭医生的方式行医。

Some general practitioners are also qualified in specialised medicine.

有些全科医生也是某一医学专科方面的合格医生。

practolol [ˈpræktələl] *n.* 心得宁

This patient receives practolol, 100 mg. four times a day.

这个病人服用心得宁，每天4次，每次100mg。

praise [preiz] *n.* 称赞，赞扬

He received praise from his colleagues for winning the prize.

他的获奖受到同事们的赞扬。

praziquantel [ˌpreiziˈkwɔntəl] *n.* 吡喹酮

Side effects of praziquantel are rare, usually mild and self-limiting.

吡喹酮的副作用少见而且常常较轻微和有自限性。

Praziquantel is well tolerated, and no long-term toxicity has been shown.

研究已经显示吡喹酮容易使人耐受，且无持久毒性反应。

preantral [priːˈæntrəl] *a.* 窦前的，腔前的

A serum-free culture system was used to study the in vitro culture of the preantral follicles from bovine ovaries.

用无血清培养系统研究了牛腔前卵泡的体外培养。

The observation that the rate of preantral follicle development may be under some degree of endocrine control in vivo has clinical significance.

窦前卵泡在体内发育速度受到体内内分泌调控的观察结果具有临床意义。

preattack [priːəˈtæk] *n.* (疾病)发作前

In asthma, there are the general signs of a "head cold", especially in children during a preattack period.

哮喘有"上感"的全身症状,发病前期的儿童尤其如此。

prebiotic [ˌpriːbaiˈɔtik] *n.* 益菌生

Prebiotics are non-digestible food ingredients that stimulate the growth and activity of bacteria in the digestive system.

益菌生是刺激消化系统细菌的生长和活性的不能消化的食物成分。

It is assumed that a prebiotic should increase the number and/or activity of bifidobacteria and lactic acid bacteria.

一般认为一种益菌生应当能增加双歧杆菌和乳酸菌的数量和(或)活性。

precancerous [priːˈkænsərəs] *a.* 癌前的,癌变前的

The lesions are considered to be precancerous, but the rate of malignant conversion is unknown.

这种病变被认为是癌前病变,但是恶性转变的比率尚不知道。

precarcinogen [ˈpriːkəˈsinədʒən] *n.* 前致癌物

Precarcinogens must be changed by enzyme systems in your body to become carcinogens.

前致癌物必须经过人体内酶系统的转换才能变成致癌物。

Nitrite is thought to be a precarcinogen for gastric cancer.

亚硝酸盐被认为是胃癌的一种前致癌物。

precaution [priˈkɔːʃən] *n.* 预防措施

Every precaution should be taken to ensure that vomiting will not occur.

必须切实注意保证不致发生呕吐。

Provided certain precautions are taken, cell suspensions and even small animals can be frozen without being killed.

如果采取某些预防措施,细胞悬液,甚至小动物,可加以冰冻而不会致死。

precede [priˈsiːd] *v.* 先于,位于…之前

Hemoptysis occasionally precedes the onset of productive cough.

咯血有时先于排痰性咳嗽。

In such circumstances the onset of heart failure is preceded by some unusual injurious event.

在这种情况下,心衰发生之前会有某种异常的损害发生。

precedence [priˈsiːdəns] *n.* 领先,优先于…

After the patient is admitted, treatment of shock and replacement of blood take precedence over delivery procedures.

病人入院后,应首先考虑治疗休克和补充血液,而不是分娩操作。

preceding [priˈsiːdiŋ] *a.* 在前的,在先的

If you compare these cells with those in the preceding figure, the morphological difference will be easily understood.

假如把这些细胞和前图中的细胞作一比较,形态上的不同就很清楚了。

Rheumatic fever does not occur without a preceding hemolytic streptococcal infection of the throat but the exact mechanism of causation is not known.

风湿热发生前总是先有咽喉部的溶血性链球菌感染,但其发生的确切机制不明。

precipitate [priˈsipiteit] *v.* 加速,促使;沉淀

Stress or exertion may precipitate angina or heart failure in a person suffering from coronary disease.

紧张或劳累可使冠心病患者诱发心绞痛或心衰。

The precipitating cause should be looked for and dealt with.

应该找出疾病的诱因，并加以处理。

Infection is one of the most frequent events precipitating acute respiratory failure.

感染是促成急性呼吸衰竭的一种最常见的疾患。

precipitin [pri'sipitin] *n.* 沉淀素

The antibody-antigen reaction is specific; the precipitin reaction is therefore a useful means of confirming the identity of an unknown antigen.

抗体-抗原反应是特异性的，因此，沉淀素反应对鉴定一种未知抗原是一种有用的方法。

The value of serum precipitin antibody titers in predicting systemic fungal disease is not known.

血清沉淀素的抗体滴定度对预测全身性霉菌疾病的价值目前还不清楚。

precise [pri'sais] *a.* 精确的，准确的

There is no precise information as to how long the virus is carried in the respiratory tract.

现在没有关于此种病毒在呼吸道能停留多长时间的准确资料。

A precise description of the local muscle weakness usually makes it possible to decide whether a peripheral nerve, cord, trunk or root is affected.

对局部肌无力的精确描述使得有可能确定是否周围神经，还是脊髓(神经索)、神经干或神经根受到侵害。

precisely [pri'saisli] *ad.* 精确地，明确地

The action of laser can be very precisely directed and controlled.

激光的活动能被十分精确地引导和控制。

These are precisely defined autosomal dominant diseases.

这些被明确划定为常染色体显性疾病。

precision [pri'siʒən] *n.* 精密

As a precision instrument, the laser also has obvious advantages for medical operations.

作为精密仪器，激光在医疗手术应用上也具有明显的优点。

However, the usefulness of medical tests is dependent on accuracy and precision.

然而，医学检验的实用性取决于其准确性和精确性。

Your clinical pathological report lacks precision.

你的临床病理报告不精确。

preclinical [priː'klinikəl] *a.* 临床前的，潜伏期的

Preclinical studies have provided valuable insights into the pathogenesis of radiation-induced cognitive impairment.

在辐射诱导的认知损伤的发病机制上，临床前研究已经提供了有价值的线索。

We have reviewed the preclinical evidences of type 2 diabetes.

我们回顾了 2 型糖尿病的临床前征象。

preclude [pri'kluːd] *v.* 排除，阻止

This potential danger should not preclude the administration of fibrinogen.

这一潜在的危险不应妨碍纤维蛋白原的给予。

The high percentage of disturbing side effects produced by these two hormonal regimens precluded their widespread use.

这两种激素治疗方案可引起高比例的失调副作用，妨碍了其广泛应用。

precondition [ˌpriːkən'diʃən] *n.* 先决条件

Good muscles are one of the preconditions of physical fitness.

结实的肌肉是身体健康的必备条件之一。

preconditioning [ˌpriːkən'diʃəniŋ] *n.* 预适应，预先准备

Ischemic preconditioning of the myocardium has a protective effects against a subsequent sus-

tained ischemia.
心肌的缺血预适应对以后的持续性缺血有保护作用。

precursor [priˈkəːsə] *n.* 先兆；先驱；前体

Bradycardia often constitutes an important precursor of ventricular fibrillation.
心动过缓往往是心室纤颤的重要先兆。

Pregnenolone is an important precursor for the synthesis of all steroids in the adrenal glands.
孕烯醇酮是肾上腺内所有类固醇合成的重要前体。

predecessor [ˈpriːdisesə] *n.* 前辈，祖先；前任

Each relies on the work of predecessors and contributes to the work of successors.
每个人既依赖前辈人的成果，又为后继者的工作做出贡献。

predialysis [ˌpriːdaiˈælisis] *n.* 透析前

The blood pressure of predialysis is not correlating to the diagnosis of hypertension in patients with maintenance dialysis.
对于维持血液透析的病人而言，透析前血压水平与高血压的诊断并不相关。

predictable [priˈdiktəbl] *a.* 可预言的，可预测的

Prognosis would not be predictable from a single lung function test in such an individual.
只根据一次肺功能试验不能预测这种病例的预后。

Most drug toxicity is predictable and attributable to excessive dosage of common drugs.
大多数药物的毒性是可预测的，其毒性是由于普通药物用量过度所致。

predictably [priˈdiktəbli] *ad.* 可预言地

Predictably, technology is another trend that continues to impact on the future of nursing.
可以预计，技术是另一个继续对护理工作的未来产生影响的趋势。

prediction [priˈdikʃən] *n.* 预测

The topology prediction of transmembrane protein is a hot in bioinformatics.
跨膜蛋白的拓扑结构预测是生物信息学的一个热点。

For some diseases, clinically usable risk prediction can be performed using classical risk factors such as body mass index, lipid levels, smoking status, family history and, under certain circumstances, genetics.
对于某些疾病，临床适用的风险预测可以通过使用一些经典的危险因子来完成，例如体重指数、脂质水平、吸烟状况、家族史，有些情况下还有遗传因素。

predilection [ˌpriːdiˈlekʃən] *n.* 偏爱，嗜好

Each kind of the lesions had its predilection site and ultrasonic features.
每种病变都有其好发部位和超声特征。

Swine influenza seems to have a predilection for young adults, as did its notorious ancestor, the 1918 Spanish influenza.
猪流感似乎更容易光顾年轻人，就像其臭名昭著的祖先——1918 年的西班牙流感一样。

predispose (to) [ˌpriːdisˈpəuz] *v.* 使易感染，诱发

Chromosomal defects that result from exposure to X-ray irradiation may predispose an individual to cancer development.
由于 X 线照射而导致染色体缺陷的患者易发生恶性肿瘤。

Influenza frequently predisposes to highly fatal secondary infections of the lungs.
流感常常容易诱发严重致命的肺部继发性感染。

predisposition (to) [ˌpriːdispəˈziʃən] *n.* 诱因；素质；易感性

An early age at onset is frequently associated with a strong genetic predisposition.
发病年龄早常与很强的遗传易感性有关。

All these factors increase a person's predisposition to coronary artery thrombosis.
所有这些因素促使一个人易患冠状动脉血栓形成。

prednisolone [predˈnisələun] *n.* 泼尼松龙，强的松龙

Orchitis can be relieved by prednisolone(40mg daily for 4 days).

睾丸炎可采用强的松龙而得到缓解(每日 40mg,共用 4 日)。

Short sharp courses of prednisolone given infrequently do have a part to play and may avoid the need to admit the child to hospital.

偶尔采用短暂而集中的泼尼松龙疗程确实可起一定作用,且可免去孩子入院治疗的需要。

prednisone [ˈprednisəun] *n.* 去氢可的松,强的松

Her urinary protein excretion was negative by the second week of prednisone therapy.

在强的松治疗的第二周她的尿蛋白转为阴性。

predominant [priˈdɔminənt] *a.* 占优势的,主要的

The acute reaction to stress may manifest a predominant disturbance of emotions.

急性应激反应可表现为突出的情绪障碍。

The patient with predominant bronchitis is often overweight and cyanotic.

以患支气管炎为主的患者常常超重并有发绀。

predominantly [priˈdɔminəntli] *ad.* 主要地,占优势地

It is not understood why the spinal cord is predominantly affected.

为什么脊髓是主要受累部位还不清楚。

These methods are still predominantly used in clinical practice throughout the world.

这些方法在全世界临床中的使用仍占优势地位。

predominate [priˈdɔmineit] *v.* 居支配地位,占优势

In acute nonstreptococcal pharyngitis, sore throat and pain on swallowing predominate.

在非链球菌急性咽炎中,喉痛及吞咽引起的疼痛为主要症状。

In older patients with chronic hypertension, arteriosclerosis and atheroma predominate.

在慢性高血压的老年患者中,以动脉硬化和粥样硬化最为突出。

Menstrual bleeding may be either arterial or venous, with the former predominating.

月经出血可能是动脉性或是静脉性的,但以前者居多。

preeclampsia [ˌpriːeˈklæmpsiə] *n.* 先兆子痫,子痫前期

Few women who show the signs of mild preeclampsia will develop the severer forms of the disease.

显示轻度先兆子痫体征的妇女很少会发生严重疾病。

The two most important signs of preeclampsia(hypertension and proteinuria) are usually not recognized by the patient.

子痫前期的两个最重要体征(高血压和蛋白尿)通常不为患者所知。

preemptive [priːˈemptiv] *a.* 抢先的,提前的

Our long-term results support preemptive liver transplantation at early stages of renal failure, and kidney-liver transplantation for those with advanced renal disease.

我们的长期结果支持早期肾衰的提前肝移植和晚期肾病的肾-肝联合移植。

preexist [ˌpriːigˈzist] *v.* 预先存在

Unfortunately, this patient died on the eighteenth postoperative day of preexisting renal disease.

不幸,此患者于术后 18 天因原有的肾病而死亡。

Preexisting other heart disease may fully account for cardiac manifestations if myocardities is not suspected.

如果不怀疑心肌炎,就可用已有的其他心脏病来充分解释其心脏表现。

preferable [ˈprefərəbl] *a.* 优越的;更好的;更可取的

Cold food would be preferable in this heat.

天这么热,冷的食物较合人意。

Valproate is preferable for epilepsy in children in the presence of developmental or other neurological abnormalities.

丙戊酸对患有发育或其他神经系统异常的癫痫病儿童来说可能更有用。

To prevent potassium depletion in patients receiving thiazide diuretics, the addition of a potassium-retaining diuretic may be preferable.
为避免接受噻嗪类利尿药的病人缺钾,最好加用保钾利尿药。

preferably [ˈprefərəbli] *ad.* 更好地;更可取地
Blood is preferably collected by venipuncture.
血液最好通过静脉穿刺来采集。
Patients encountered during the preliminary stages of fainting should be placed in a position which permits maximal cerebral blood flow, preferably in the supine position.
遇到处于最初阶段的晕厥病人时,应将其放置在容许脑血流量最大的体位,最好是仰卧位。

preference [ˈprefərəns] *n.* 偏爱;优惠
In treating such cases, most doctors give preference to medical over surgical management.
多数医生在治疗这种病例时,愿意使用内科治疗而不愿使用手术治疗。

prefrontal [priːˈfrɔntəl] *a.* 前额的,额叶前部的;*n.* 额前骨
Prefrontal cortex is smaller in children with ADHD.
注意缺陷多动障碍患儿的前额叶皮质要比正常小些。
Dopamine within the prefrontal cortex has been implicated in working memory.
前额皮质中的多巴胺与工作记忆有关。

preganglionic [priːgæŋgliːˈɔnik] *a.* (神经)节前的
Because sympathetic ganglia lie close to the vertebral column, sympathetic preganglionic fibers are generally short.
因为交感神经节位置靠近脊柱,交感神经的节前纤维一般较短。
Preganglionic fibers connect the ganglion to the central nervous system.
节前纤维将神经节连接到中枢神经系统。

pregnancy [ˈpregnənsi] *n.* 妊娠
During pregnancy and labour the fetus may be at risk of damage or death from many causes.
胎儿在孕产期可能要面临许多因素引起的损伤或死亡的危险。
The patient has gone through three pregnancies.
病人已经历过三次妊娠。

pregnant [ˈpregnənt] *a.* 妊娠的,有孕的
A pregnant woman needs four times as much vitamin D as an average woman.
孕妇对维生素 D 的需要量是普通妇女需要量的四倍。

preimplantation [ˌpriːimplænˈteiʃən] *n.* (子宫中)胚胎植入前的,着床前
Preimplantation factor appears to be essential for pregnancy to succeed.
着床前因子对成功妊娠显得很关键。
Preimplantation genetic diagnosis(PGD) is performed at some centers to screen for inherited diseases.
有些中心进行胚胎植入前遗传诊断(PGD)来筛查遗传病。

prejudice [ˈpredʒudis] *n.* 成见,偏见
In order to succeed in treating any disease doctors will need to overcome their prejudices.
为了有效治疗各种疾病,医生们必须克服他们的偏见。

preliminary [priˈliminəri] *a.* 开端的,初步的
The chairman made a preliminary speech before beginning the main business of the meeting.
主席在开始正题之前,先在会上作了简短的开场白。
Preliminary results indicated that lysine had no apparent effect on cholesterol levels.
初步结果表明:赖氨酸对胆固醇水平无明显作用。
Preliminary research indicates that regular aspirin use is associated with reduced rates of ischemic heart disease.

初步研究表明:缺血性心脏病发生率的降低与定期服用阿司匹林有关。

preload [ˈpriːləud] *n.* 前负荷

The amount of filling during diastolic phase is called preload of the heart.

心脏在舒张期的充盈量称为心脏前负荷。

The predominant factor influencing preload is venous return.

静脉回流是影响心脏前负荷大小的主要因素。

prelude [ˈpreljuːd] *n.* 先驱;前奏

His frequent depressions were the prelude to a complete mental breakdown.

他的经常性抑郁是精神完全崩溃的前奏。

premature [ˌpriːməˈtjuə;ˌpreməˈtjuə] *a.* 早熟的

Premature infants as a general rule are at high risk for the development of neurologic problems.

总的来说,早产儿发生神经疾病的危险性很高。

The response of the premature infants to certain drugs should be thoroughly understood.

应该全面了解早产儿对某些药物的反应。

It is premature to assume there is only one etiology for affective disorders in children.

假定儿童情感障碍只有一种病因还为时过早。

prematurity [ˌpriːməˈtjuəriti] *n.* 早熟,早产

Prematurity often leads to neonatal respiratory distress syndrome.

早产常引起新生儿呼吸窘迫综合征。

premedication [ˌpriːmediˈkeiʃən] *n.* 术前给药法,前驱给药法

The physician anesthesiologist, if responsible for anesthesia, will usually examine the patient and write the premedication order.

麻醉医生如果负责麻醉,通常要检查病人和书写术前用药医嘱。

Premedication usually comprises injection of a sedative, to calm the patient down, together with a drug, such as atropine, to dry up the secretions of the lungs.

术前用药通常包括注射镇静剂使病人安静和使病人肺分泌物减少的药物,如阿托品。

premise [ˈpremis] *n.* 前提;(*pl.*)房屋

This book is written on the premise of many years of practice in basic microsurgical techniques.

写这本书的前提是基本显微外科技术的多年实践。

The police detective examines and photographs the premises.

警察局的侦探对房屋进行检查和拍照。

premium [ˈpriːmiəm] *n.* 保险费;助长;重视

You should pay medical insurance premium on time.

你应当按期付医疗保险费。

The high risk of infection puts a premium on the use of sterile needles.

感染的严重危险性使人们重视用消毒针头。

premunition [ˌpriːmjuˈniʃən] *n.* 相对免疫;传染免疫;带虫免疫

Individuals who temporarily leave the endemic area may lose their premunition and develop clinical paroxysms on their return.

那些暂时离开疫区的人可能失去带虫免疫力,当他们返回时可出现疾病发作。

Premunition, also known as infection-immunity, is a host response that protects against high numbers of parasite and illness without eliminating the infection.

带虫免疫又称为传染免疫,是一种宿主反应,以便在不消除感染的情况下阻止大量寄生虫和疾病。

premutation [ˌpriːmjuˈteiʃən] *n.* 前突变

The premutation is unstable when transmitted.

前突变在传代过程中是不稳定的。

prenatal [priːˈneitəl] *a.* 产前的

Blood pressure should be recorded at every prenatal visit.
每次产前就诊必须记录血压。

preoperative [ˌpriːˈɔpərətiv] *a.* 手术前的

The patient's condition is better compared with the preoperative period.
病人的情况与手术前比较,有所好转。

An assessment of the role preoperative radiation in stages Ⅰ and Ⅱ was made.
对在第Ⅰ和Ⅱ期中术前放射的作用做出了评价。

preovulatory [priːˈɔvjulətəri,-ˈəu-] *a.* 排卵期前的

Although the induction of oocyte meiotic resumption by the preovulatory luteinizing hormone surge is well established, the processes involved are complex and inadequately defined.
虽然排卵前的促黄体素峰诱导卵母细胞减数分裂恢复已成定论,但是参与该事件的各种过程非常复杂,因而还没有完全搞清楚。

The stimulatory effects of FSH on antral and preovulatory follicles are well known, but controversial results have been reported regarding the FSH dependency of preantral follicles.
卵泡刺激素(FSH)对有腔卵泡和排卵前卵泡的促生长作用已被普遍接受,但关于其对腔前卵泡发育的作用报道结果仍有争议。

preparation [ˌprepəˈreiʃən] *n.* 准备,制备;制剂

Most candidates will require a minimum of 6 to 8 months of intense preparation for the examination.
大多数考生为考试至少需要 6 至 8 个月的紧张准备。

However, proper pre-endoscopic preparation is critical to successful use of endoscopy.
然而,内镜检查前恰当的准备对顺利完成内镜检查非常重要。

in such cases topical preparations containing lanolin or preservatives should be avoided.
在这些病例中一定要避免使用含有羊毛酯或防腐剂的局部用制剂。

prepartum [priːˈpɑːtəm] *a.* 分娩前的,产前的

A variety of prepartum tests have been developed to assess the well-being of the fetus.
已有多种产前检查试验用来测定胎儿安危情况。

A gain of about 1 kg. per week is often noted in the prepartum record of many toxemic patients.
在许多患毒血症病人的预产记录中常可注意到每周体重增加一公斤左右。

preponderance [priˈpɔndərəns] *n.* (数量、重量、力量、影响等上的)优势

A preponderance of the iron of the newborn is contained in the circulating hemaglobin.
新生儿的铁大部分存在于循环血液的血红蛋白中。

In multiple pregnancies the normal sex ratio at birth, with a slight preponderance of males, is altered to a female preponderance.
在多胎妊娠中出生时男性略多于女性的正常性别比例变为女性多于男性。

prepotency [priˈpəutənsi] *n.* 优势;优性;优生遗传

The result shows that the above behaviors have different genetic prepotency.
结果显示,上述行为有不同的遗传倾向。

We study the effect of occupational poison contact on women's prepotency and fine rearing.
我们探讨职业有毒接触对女性优生优育的影响。

prepubertal [priːˈpjuːbətəl] *a.* 青春期前的

At one time bipolar disorders were not believed to occur in prepubertal children.
曾有一段时间人们不相信双相疾病会出现在青春期前的儿童身上。

prerenal [ˌpriːˈriːnəl] *a.* 肾前的

Prerenal azotemia is encountered when there is hypoperfusion of the kidneys that impairs renal function in the absence of parenchymal damage.
当肾脏灌流不足损伤肾功能但肾实质无损伤时会出现肾前性氮质血症。

Prerenal contributions to renal dysfunction may be transient and reversible, as in volume depletion, or more persistent as observed with heart failure and liver disease.

肾前性因素导致的肾功能障碍可以是短暂而可逆的,如血容量减少,更多是持续性的,如见于心力衰竭和肝脏疾病。

prerequisite [ˌpriːˈrekwizit] *n.* 先决条件,前提

The prerequisite to the diagnosis of myocarditis is the awareness of its existence and alertness to its manifestations.

诊断心肌炎的先决条件是想到这一疾病,并对其临床表现有所警觉。

To gain understanding of microbial disease in a scientific and technologic sense is an essential prerequisite to the building and maintenance of a modern society.

从科学技术意义上理解微生物疾病是建立和维持现代社会的基本前提。

prescribe [prisˈkraib] *v.* 命令;指定;开处方

Finally the physician prescribed the treatment and write out a prescription.

最后医生提出治疗方案并开出处方。

Extreme care must be taken when prescribing drugs.

给病人开处方时必须非常小心。

Such medication must be prescribed only by a psychiatrist.

这种药物只能由精神病医生来开处方。

prescription [priˈskripʃən] *n.* 处方

Take this prescription to your local chemist's.

拿此处方到当地药店取药。

A doctor writes the prescription and a chemist makes it up for you.

医生开处方,药剂师为你调配。

Shotgun prescription is an irrational prescription that contains a number of ingredients given with the idea that one or more of them may be effective.

散弹式处方是一种含有许多药物成分的不合理处方,期望其中有一种或多种成分能奏效。

presenile [priːˈsiːnail] *a.* 早老的

Alzheimer disease is the most common of the presenile dementias.

阿尔茨海默病是最常见的早老性痴呆。

present [priˈzent] *v.* 提出;呈现

A 2-month-old male presented with jaundice since 1 week of age.

一名 2 个月的男婴,出生后 1 周开始出现黄疸。

Ameobic hepatitis is common on a world basis and usually presents as a hepatic abscess.

阿米巴肝炎是世界范围内的常见病,一般表现为肝脓肿。

Deciding whether breathlessness originates from disease of the lungs or of the heart often presents a problem.

要判定呼吸短促来源于肺部疾病还是心脏疾病常常是个问题。

presentation [ˌprezənˈteiʃən] *n.* 表现;先露,胎位

Frequently the diagnosis of preeclampsia is not made because of an atypical presentation.

常常因为不典型的表现而不能诊断为先兆子痫。

The fetal heart sounds are best heard over the back of the fetus in vertex and breech presentations.

头顶和臀先露时,胎心音在胎背处听得最清楚。

The patient is examined to confirm that the presentation remains satisfactory.

检查患者证实胎位正常。

presently [ˈprezəntli] *ad.* 现在,目前;一会儿,不久

These data are not presently available.

这些数据现在还没有得到。

His headache will be relieved presently.

他的头痛一会儿就会缓解。

preservation [ˌprezəˈveiʃən] *n.* 保存

The dead bodies were in an excellent state of preservation in this anatomical department.

尸体在此解剖科室保存得很好。

Indeed, the preservation of glomerulotubular balance seen until the terminal stages of chronic renal failure is fundamental to the intact nephron hypothesis.

诚然,慢性肾衰终末阶段所见的球管平衡的保存对完整肾单位假说十分重要。

Dissociation also occurs in syringomyelia, in which the fingers may have loss of pain and temperature sensation but preservation of tactile sensations.

感觉分离还可见于脊髓空洞症,这种患者的手指可有痛觉和温度感觉消失,但仍有触觉存在。

preservative [priˈzəːvətiv] *n.* 防腐剂

Exogenous substances include drugs, coloring agents, preservatives, and so on.

外源性物质包括药物、着色剂和防腐剂等。

preserve [priˈzəːv] *v.* 保存,防护,维持

If the nutritive medium is changed at the right time, it is possible to preserve the culture for many days.

如果在适当时间更换营养性培养基,那么就可能将培养物保存许多天。

Early diagnosis and treatment of optic nerve disorders are important to preserve vision.

早期诊断和治疗视神经疾患有助于保护视力。

Arterioles may be tightly constricted, as they usually are in shock, attempting to preserve arterial pressure.

小动脉处于休克时通常可以紧缩以维持动脉血压。

preside [priˈsaid] *v.* 主持;统辖,指挥

The liver presides over so many vital activities that even the slightest damage to it is fraught with serious consequences.

肝脏统管许多生命活动,以至对其非常微小的损伤也会带来严重的后果。

prespecified [priˈspesifaid] *a.* 预先定义的

A medical study may evolve out of a explicit prespecified research question and hypothesis.

一项医学研究可以从明确的预先已定义的研究问题和假设发展而来。

prespecify [priˈspesifai] *v.* 事先确定

When solicitation of adverse reactions (AR) is not prespecified in the registry ' s operating plans, the registry may permit AR detection by asking general questions to solicit reactions.

若注册登记操作计划中没有事先确定不良反应的征集,该研究可以通过询问一般性的问题征集反应信息。

presumably [priˈzjuːməbli] *ad.* 推测起来,大概

Presumably, maternal immunity reduces the virulence of the fetal infection.

据推测母亲的免疫力可降低胎儿感染的毒力。

The reflex is presumably activated when reduced venous return underfills the left ventricle.

当静脉回心血量减少使左心室不能完全填充时,此反射可能被激活。

For teenagers, a planned vegetarian diet is presumably healthy, but be mindful that their diet should include such elements as calcium, vitamin D, iron, zinc, etc.

对青少年来说,素食饮食计划可能是健康的,但一定要在他们的饮食中添加钙、维生素 D、铁、锌等元素。

presume [priˈzjuːm] *v.* 假定,推测

The pathogenesis of prolonged pregnancy is presumed to be placental insufficiency.

据推测过期妊娠的发病机制是胎盘功能不全。

The risk of recurrent ischemic stroke after presumed perinatal stroke and the risk factors for such

recurrence are rarely reported.
假设性围产期中风后复发缺血性中风的危险及其危险因素罕见报导。
Metabolic syndrome, also presumed as an early stage of type Ⅱ diabetes, greatly increases the risk of heart disease and stroke.
代谢综合征(也被推定为二型糖尿病早期)大大增加了心脏病和中风的危险。

presumption [priˈzʌmpʃn] *n.* 推测;预测
The article makes too many false presumptions.
此论文作了太多靠不住的推测。

presumptive [priˈzʌmptiv] *a.* 推定的;预期的
Failure to hear the fetal heart sounds after the 24th week on careful auscultation will be strong presumptive evidence of fetal death.
24 孕周后仔细的听诊听不到胎心音则有力提示胎儿死亡。

presurgical [priˈsəːdʒikəl] *a.* 手术前的
Mary, 46, was admitted one evening for presurgical evaluation and preparation for a hysterectomy.
46 岁的玛丽一天晚上被接收入院进行手术前的评估和做子宫切除术的准备工作。

presymptomatically [priˌsimptəˈmætikəli] *ad.* 症状出现之前地
Frequently the diagnosis is made presymptomatically on routine chest radiography.
本病往往是在症状出现之前,在常规胸部 X 线检查时诊断出来的。

presynaptic [ˌpriːsiˈnæptik] *a.* 突触前的
Presynaptic neuron across a tiny gap to bind to receptors on the postsynaptic neuron's cell membrane.
突触前神经元穿过微小间隙与突触后神经元细胞膜上的受体结合。
Parkinson's disease is associated with a loss of dopamine-containing neurons in the striatum, resulting in a loss of dopamine transporter in the presynaptic nerve terminals.
帕金森氏病与纹状体中多巴胺能神经元丢失有关,造成突触前神经终末多巴胺转运蛋白的丢失。

pretend [priˈtend] *v.* 假装,伪称
She pretended that she was sick.
她假装患病。
He pretended not to know how to solve the problem.
他假装不知道如何才能解决这一问题。

preterm [priˈtəːm] *n.* 未足月
Preterm labor is defined by an onset before 37 weeks of gestation.
孕 37 周以前分娩称为早产。

prevail [priˈveil] *v.* 胜(过);流行
Hallucinations may also prevail in paresis.
麻痹性痴呆患者也会经常出现幻觉。
The additional tests usually try to determine the severity of the infection as well as the prevailing condition of the liver.
额外的测试通常试图测定肝脏一般状况以及其感染的严重程度。

prevailing [priˈveiliŋ] *v.* 占优势的;流行的
The prevailing view is that dietary restriction slows aging by modulating one or more of these putative primary aging processes.
普遍的看法是膳食限制通过调整一个或多个那些假定的主要老化过程而延缓老化。

prevalence [ˈprevələns] *n.* 流行,盛行
In the days of widespread prevalence, 40% of the adult population of the city had been infected.
在广泛流行的日子里,城市成年人曾有 40% 受到感染。
The reported prevalence of depression in children varies widely.

关于儿童抑郁症的患病率,各种报道差别很大。

prevalent [ˈprevələnt] *a.* 普遍的,流行的

Infection with rhinoviruses is more prevalent among adults than among children.

鼻病毒感染在成人中比在儿童中更为流行。

Is malaria still prevalent in that country?

疟疾在那个国家仍然流行吗?

prevent [priˈvent] *v.* 防止,预防

β-blockade may help to prevent angina.

β-阻滞剂可有助于防止心绞痛。

Although a range of recombinant genes have successully prevented HIV replication in vitro, none have been used clinically until now.

尽管众多的重组基因已有效阻止 HIV 在体外的复制,但到目前为止无一用于临床。

Resting diseased joints in splints will reduce pain and prevent deformity.

将患病关节用夹板固定可减少疼痛并预防畸形。

preventable [priˈventəbl] *a.* 可防止的,可预防的

Highly effective drugs and vaccine have made TB a preventable and curable disease.

极为有效的药物和疫苗使结核病成为可预防和治愈的疾病。

As is true of many contagious diseases, mumps is now preventable by the use of a vaccine.

和许多传染性疾病一样,腮腺炎现在也可使用疫苗来预防。

prevention [priˈvenʃən] *n.* 预防

Prevention is better than cure.

预防优于治疗。

Primary prevention and screening are crucial elements in improving the health of women.

一级预防和普查对改善妇女健康是非常重要的因素。

Researchers are constantly searching for causes of cancer and means of prevention and cure.

科研工作者正不断地寻找癌肿的病因及其预防和治疗的方法。

preventive [priˈventiv] *a.* 预防的

Preventive measures mainly lie in eliminating the sources of infection.

预防措施主要在于消除传染源。

Rosenau defines the domain of preventive medicine in two parts: that which deals with the person (hygiene) and that which deals with the environment (sanitation).

Rosenau 把预防医学的范围规定为两部分:个人卫生和环境卫生。

previa [ˈpriːviə]【拉】*a.* 前置的,前位的

The records of 39 gravidas with placenta previa were reviewed retrospectively, and the outcomes were compared.

对 39 例前置胎盘孕妇的记录进行回顾性分析并比较了其预后。

(注:previa 系拉丁语形容词,修饰名词 placenta,位于其后。)

previously [ˈpriːvjəsli] *ad.* 以前

Acute glomerulonephritis results usually from an upper respiratory infection by the haemolytic streptococcus occurring 1 to 3 weeks previously.

急性肾小球肾炎通常是由于 1 ~ 3 周前发生上呼吸道溶血性链球菌感染所致。

The clinical approach to the diagnosis of subclinical myocarditis and its possible value have been discussed previously.

亚临床型心肌炎的诊断方法及其可能具有的价值前面已讨论过了。

primaquine [ˈpriməkwin] *n.* 伯氨喹(抗疟药)

Primaquine is used to treat malaria, usually in combination with other antimalarial drugs, such as chloroquine.

伯氨喹用于治疗疟疾,通常与其他抗疟药如氯喹合用。

Primaquine given in a dose of 15mg daily for 14 days produces a high percentage of cures.
若服用伯氨喹每日 15mg,共用 14 天,则其治愈率很高。

primarily [ˈpraimərili] *ad.* 主要地,基本地
The effects of ethanol on the nervous system are primarily those of a depressant.
乙醇对神经系统的作用主要是一种抑制剂的作用。

primary [ˈpraiməri] *a.* 最初的,主要的,原发的
The liver is the primary metabolic center.
肝为主要代谢中心。
Adjuvant treatment is sometimes used in addition to the primary treatment to insure the destruction of any cancer cells that may have spread.
辅助疗法有时用来补充基本疗法以确保能破坏可能已经扩散的任何癌细胞。
Symptoms appear from a few weeks to 30 years after a primary tuberculous infection.
可在原发性结核感染后数周到 30 年才出现症状。

prime [praim] *a.* 首要的,基本的,主要的
Reducing pollution in the workshop is the prime problem.
减少车间的污染是个首要问题。
Heat is a prime stimulus to increased sweating, but other physiologic stimuli, including emotional stress, are important as well.
热是增加出汗的一个主要刺激,但其他生理刺激,包括情绪紧张也起着重要的作用。

primigravida [ˌpraimiˈgrævidə] *n.* 初孕妇,初产妇
A 23-year-old primigravida patient at 39 weeks' gestation is seen for her routine prenatal visit.
一个 23 岁的初孕妇在 39 孕周做常规产前检查。

primiparous [praiˈmipərəs] *a.* 初产的,一次产妇的
The congenitally infected infant is often born to young primiparous mothers.
先天性感染的婴儿常为年轻的初产妇所生。

primitive [ˈprimitiv] *a.* 初级的,原始的
Microorganisms are living things of a very primitive order.
微生物是一类非常原始的生物。
The early 1990s saw the development of primitive multitest strips.
20 世纪 90 年代早期出现了最初的多种检测的试纸。

primordial [praiˈmɔːdjəl] *a.* 原始的,根本的,原生的
The human primordial germ cells are recognizable by the fourth week of development.
胚胎发育第四周即可分辨出人类原始生殖细胞。
Until now, the three germ layers formed, the three germ layers is the development of primordial matrix.
到现在为止,三胚层就形成了,三胚层是胎体发育的原基。
Scientists think the molecules making up the primordial ooze of life on Earth might have formed in such a disk.
科学家猜测,地球上孕育生命的原始浆液中的组成分子很可能就在这样一种圆盘中形成。

principal [ˈprinsəpəl] *a.* 主要的,最重要的
Proteins are chemical compounds which are the principal constituents of protoplasm.
蛋白质是化学化合物,是原生质的主要成分。
The principal form of carbohydrate found in the plasma is glucose.
碳水化合物在血浆中的主要形式是葡萄糖。

principally [ˈprinsəpəli] *ad.* 主要地
Each tooth is composed principally of dentin, which gives it shape and encloses a cavity, the pulp cavity.
每个牙齿主要由牙质构成,牙质赋予牙齿以形状,并围成一个腔,即牙髓腔。

In diastolic failure, the major clinical manifestations relate principally to an elevation of filling pressures.
舒张性(心力)衰竭中,一些重要临床表现主要与充盈压增高有关。

print [print] *v.* 印刷,出版,打印
This printer can print 40 pages in a minute.
这台打印机一分钟能打印 40 页。
You may use an online printer to print out the data.
你可以使用联机打印机把数据打印出来。

prion ['praiɔn] *n.* 蛋白侵袭子,蛋白病毒,朊病毒
Prions are "rogue" forms of normal proteins.
朊蛋白是正常蛋白质的"异常"形式。
Prion is a slow infectious particle that lacks nucleic acids; prions are the cause of Creutzfeld-Jakob disease.
朊病毒是不含核酸的慢感染性颗粒,它是克-雅二氏病的病原。
Prion disorders are very rare conditions that commonly produce dementia.
通常引起痴呆的朊病毒疾患是罕见的情况。

prior(to) ['praiə] *a.* 在先的,在前的;更重要的
Prior research shows that this drug also relieves allergies.
早先的研究表明此药也可减轻过敏反应。
This task is prior to all others.
这项任务压倒其他一切。
Low doses of heparin, given prior to the onset of thrombosis, are effective in preventing clotting and are less likely to produce hemorrhage.
在血栓形成发生之前给予小剂量肝素,能有效预防凝血,并很少有引起出血的可能。

priority [prai'ɔriti] *n.* 优先考虑的事
Severe bleeding has priority over everything else in case of an accident.
事故发生时,大量出血是首先要考虑的事情。
Environmental protection has become a national priority.
环境保护已成为国家优先考虑的大事。
The search for a new vaccine took priority over all other medical researches.
找出一种新疫苗比所有其它医学研究所占的位置都重要。

privacy ['praivəsi] *n.* 独处;私事;隐私
The right to privacy includes having the patient's body, record and care kept private.
隐私权包括对病人的身体、病案记录和治疗护理情况严守秘密。

proactive [ˌprəu'æktiv] *a.* 主动的,积极的
As part of a post-marketing requirement, prospective product and disease registries are increasingly being considered as resources for examining unresolved safety issues and/or as tools for proactive risk assessment in the post-approval setting.
作为上市要求的一部分,预期产品和疾病登记都越来越被认为是检查尚未解决的安全性问题的资源和(或)在产品批准后进行积极风险评估的工具。
Dr. Wang has good communication skill and is proactive and initiative in his work.
王博士有良好的沟通能力,在工作上很主动且有开拓精神。

proarrythmia [ˌprəuə'riðmiə] *n.* 致心律失常作用
Proarrhythmia is a new or more frequent occurrence of pre-existing arrhythmias, precipitated by antiarrhythmic therapy.
致心律失常作用是指抗心律失常治疗后发生新的心律失常或使已经存在的心律失常发生频率增加。
Drug-induced proarrhythmia is a major clinical problem.

药物诱导的致心律失常作用是一个重要的临床难题。

probability [ˌprɔbəˈbiliti] *n.* 可能性；概率，几率

Probability is one of the basic tools of genetics.

概率是遗传学的基本工具之一。

The 2-year survival probability was 79.7% in Canada and 63.2% in the United States.

在加拿大2年存活率为79.7%，在美国是63.2%。

Specific therapy must be determined by the probability of a diagnosis, the risk of not treating, and the risk of treatment.

是否进行特殊治疗取决于诊断的可能结果和治疗与不治疗的风险有多大。

probable [ˈprɔbəbl] *a.* 很可能的

It is probable that many children have nephritis in such mild form that it goes unrecognized.

可能许多儿童有未被察觉的轻型肾炎。

When tumor does occur, it is more probable that it will involve the digestive tract.

如肿瘤确有发生时，它影响的部位更可能是消化道。

probably [ˈprɔbəbli] *ad.* 很可能，或许

The overactive spastic type of constipation is probably much more common than the atonic lazy kind.

过度紧张痉挛型便秘很可能比无张力弛缓型便秘要多得多。

Your biological rhythms probably haven't adjusted to your new schedule.

你的生物钟也许没有调整到与你的新作息表相适应。

probe [prəub] *n.* 探针

Surface molecules of cells can be demonstrated using fluorescent antibodies as probes.

细胞表面分子可利用荧光抗体作为探针来显示。

Brain tumours could be cured by a tiny probe that heats cancer cells when inserted into the skull.

脑肿瘤可用极小的探针插入颅骨内给肿瘤细胞加热来进行治疗。

probenicid [prəˈbenisid] *n.* 丙磺舒

Amoxcillin, ampicillin and penicillin are to be accompanied by probenicid(1.0g orally).

羟氨苄青霉素、氨苄青霉素和青霉素都必须同时加用丙磺舒(1.0克口服)。

probiotics [ˌprəbaiˈɔtiks] *n.* 益生菌

Probiotics are live microorganisms thought to be beneficial to the host.

益生菌是被认为对宿主有益的活的微生物。

Probiotics are thought to beneficially affect the host by improving its intestinal microbial balance, thus inhibiting pathogens and toxin producing bacteria.

益生菌是通过改善肠道微生物平衡，因而抑制病原微生物或产毒素的细菌而对宿主起着有益作用。

This is an important topic: Benefits of probiotics in infancy.

这是一个重要的主题：益生菌对婴幼儿期的好处。

Does taking probiotics routinely with antibiotics prevent antibiotic-associated diarrhoea?

与抗生素一起常规性地服用益生菌是否可阻止抗菌相关性腹泻？

procainamide [prəˈkeinəmaid] *n.* 普鲁卡因酰胺

Great care must be taken when procainamide is used by the intravenous route.

当普鲁卡因酰胺用作静脉注射时应非常小心。

Other drugs such as procainamide are associated with the development of antinuclear antibodies.

其他如普鲁卡因胺一类的药物与抗核抗体的发生有关。

procaine [ˈprəukein] *n.* 普鲁卡因

The potency of tetracaine is ten times that of procaine.

丁卡因的效力是普鲁卡因的10倍。

procarcinogen [prəˈkaːsinədʒən] *n.* 前致癌物

A procarcinogen is a precursor to a carcinogen.
前致癌物即致癌物的前体。
The procarcinogen itself is not usually carcinogenic but is converted to the active carcinogen after it has been metabolized.
前致癌物自身通常是不致癌的，但是经过代谢后可转化为活性致癌物。

procedure [prə'siːdʒə] *n.* 程序，操作；手术
The patient may carry on normal work shortly after the procedure.
处理以后不久，病人就可以进行正常的工作。
Anderson procedure refers to reconstruction of the hypopharynx and cervical esophagus.
安德森操作是指咽下部和颈部食管的重建。

proceeding [prə'siːdiŋ] *n.* 程序；诉讼（复），会议录（复）
Venereal diseases are of medicolegal importance, they may affect proceedings for divorce.
性病具有法医学的重要性，它可能影响离婚诉讼。
Whatever impact the conference and proceedings have will reflect the enthusiasm, interest, and commitment of the presenters-authors and their collaborators and staffs.
不管这次学术会议和会议录具有什么样的影响，都反映出出席人员—作者及其合作者与工作人员—的热忱、兴趣和支持。

process ['prəuses] *n.* 工序，工艺；突，突起
He has invented a new process of dyeing.
他发明了一种染色新工艺。
The nerve cells vary in shape and have several processes.
神经细胞的形状不一，并有若干突起。
v. 加工，处理
We learned how to process medicinal herbs.
我们学会了怎样加工中草药。
We must process the polluted water from these factories.
我们必须处理这些工厂的污水。

proctoscope ['prɔktəskəup] *n.* 直肠镜
By using proctoscope the lower part of the rectum and the anus can be inspected and minor procedures carried out.
应用直肠镜可检查直肠下端和肛门以及进行小的手术（操作）。

prodromal ['prəudrəuməl] *a.* 前驱症状的
The onset of symptoms of tuberculous meningitis is insidious, and there is almost always a prodromal phase of vague ill health.
结核性脑膜炎的症状是不知不觉地发生的，几乎总有模糊不适感的前驱症状期。
General paresis has prodromal manifestations of headache, fatigability and inability to concentrate.
麻痹性痴呆的前驱症状是头痛、易疲劳性和精神不能集中。

prodrome ['prəudrəum] *n.* 前驱症状
A prodrome is a symptom indicating the onset of a disease.
前驱症状是疾病开始发作时的症状。

prodrug ['prəuˌdrʌg] *n.* 前体药物
A prodrug is administered systemically and is converted to its toxic form only in those cells containing the transgene, resulting in cell kill.
前体药物全身给药后，只在含有转基因的细胞中才转化为有毒形式而导致细胞死亡。
The approach involves a double prodrug that is activated first by azoreductases and then by cyclization triggering drug release.
这种方法涉及一种双前体药物，其可先由偶氮还原酶激活，然后再通过环化作用触发药物

释放。

product [ˈprɔdəkt] *n.* 产物,产品

FDA has approved only one stem cell product.

美国食品和药品管理局只批准了一种干细胞产品。

Secretory cells of exocrine glands release their products into ducts in three different ways.

外分泌腺的分泌细胞以三种不同方式将其产物释放至导管。

proenzyme [prəuˈenzaim] *n.* 酶原,前酶

Proenzymes or zymogens, usually digestive proteases, are activated to the active form by peptide bond hydrolysis.

酶原,如消化性蛋白酶,通过肽键的水解被激活为活性形式。

profession [prəˈfeʃn] *n.* 职业

The author of the guidebook is a doctor by profession.

那本参考手册的作者是一位职业医生。

professional [prəˈfeʃnl] *a.* 职业上的,专业的

The doctor was accused of professional misconduct.

那位医生被控告失职。

proficiency [prəˈfiʃənsi] *n.* 熟练,精通

These procedures can be cultivated until you reach a high degree of proficiency.

你们能逐渐掌握这些方法直到达到高度熟练。

He has acquired proficiency in English.

他已精通英语。

profile [ˈprəufail] *n.* 外形,轮廓;侧面图

Those who, from their metabolic profiles, are at highest risk of heart disease show the greatest benefit from very low fat diets.

那些根据其代谢状况处于心脏病高危期的人们,从极低脂肪饮食中受益最大。

profound [prəˈfaund] *a.* 深长的;极度的;深刻的

Both of these changes have particularly profound effects upon the nervous system.

这两种变化对神经系统都有极其深远的影响。

The symptoms of pernicious anemia are often more profound than would be expected.

恶性贫血的症状常比预期的更严重些。

profuse [prəˈfjuːs] *a.* 非常丰富的,大量的

The patient has profuse perspiration.

病人大量地出汗。

Profuse bleeding occurred during surgery in one of these cases.

这些病例中有一例在手术时发生大出血。

profusely [prəˈfjuːsli] *ad.* 极其丰富地;过多地

These patients may vomit profusely and become dehydrated and alkalotic.

这些病人可因大量呕吐而致失水和碱中毒。

progenitor [prəuˈdʒenitə] *n.* 祖先,前体

Red bone marrow contains stem cells, progenitor cells, precursor cells, and functional blood cells.

红骨髓由干细胞、祖细胞、前体细胞和功能性血细胞组成。

Even though these progenitor cells can take to their environment and initiate the generation of new tissue, they would still be subject to attack by the patient's own body.

即使这些前体细胞能融入环境并形成新组织,但是仍有可能遭受患者身体的排斥。

progeny [ˈprɔdʒini] *n.* 子孙,后代

These new viral subunits are then assembled into progeny virions and released from the cell.

这些新产生的病毒亚单位组装成子代病毒颗粒并从细胞内释出。

progesterone [prəuˈdʒestərəun] *n.* 孕酮,黄体酮

The presence of progesterone receptor further increases the likelihood of hormone sensitivity.
孕酮受体的存在进一步增加了激素敏感的可能性。
Blood levels of estrogens and progesterone vary with placental function.
血液中雌激素和黄体酮水平随胎盘功能而变化。

progestogen [prəu'dʒestədʒən] *n.* 孕激素(类)
Progestogens were widely used for the treatment of recurrent abortion with little success.
孕激素已广泛用于治疗复发性流产,但很少成功。
Synthetic progestogens may be taken by mouth but the naturally occurring hormone must be given by intramuscular injection.
(人工)合成的孕激素可口服,而天然生成者则必须肌内注射。

prognosis [prɔg'nəusis] *n.* 预后
Treatment should not be delayed,because the prognosis is very poor.
治疗必须及时,因为本病预后差。
The degree of associated renal damage directly influences the prognosis.
与之相关的肾脏损伤的程度直接影响预后。

prognostic [prɔg'nɔstik] *a.* 预后的
Surgery gives no prognostic improvement in mild angina regardless of the disease distributions.
对于轻型心绞痛,无论病变分布范围如何,手术治疗均不能改善其预后。

program ['preugræm] *n.* 节目;程序;计划;大纲
This research was supported by the High Technology Research and Development Program of China(863 Program)(No. 2004AA2Z3212).
本研究获得国家高技术研究发展计划(863 计划)资助。
The feedback from the computer enables us to update the program.
计算机的反馈能使我们更新程序。

progress ['prəugres] *n.* 进步,进展
As the disease progresses,restlessness and irritability may be followed by delirium.
随着病情进展,继烦躁和易怒之后可发生谵妄。
v. [ˌprəu'gres] 进展
The syndromes of acute coronary insufficiency do not progress to irreversible ischemic damage and necrosis.
急性冠状动脉功能不全综合征并不发展为不可逆性缺血性损伤和坏死。

progression [prəu'greʃən] *n.* 前进,进行
Studies may be performed to follow the course of the lesion and to determine whether there is progression with time.
可进行研究以追踪此种损伤并确定损伤是否随时间而进展。
Respiratory failure in patients with chronic obstructive lung diseases may occur as a result of progression of the disease process.
慢性阻塞性肺病患者的呼吸衰竭,可能是该病本身病情恶化的结果。

progressive [prəu'gresiv] *a.* 进步的,进行性的,前进的
Modifications of patterns of hospital care have been developed into systems of progressive patient care.
医院护理模式的改变已发展为分级护理制度。
The diagnosis of progressive primary tuberculosis with effusion was considered.
考虑诊断为进展型原发性肺结核伴胸腔积液。
The progressive clinical deterioration dominated the terminal phase of illness.
日益加重的临床恶化为此病晚期的突出症状。

progressively [prəu'gresivli] *ad.* 进行性地,渐进地

The students participate progressively in the diagnosis and treatment of patients.
学生逐步参与诊断和治疗活动。

These drugs have usually been given to progressively deteriorating patients not benefited by steroid administration.
这些药物常用于病情进行性恶化而对激素无反应的患者。

proguanil [prə'gwænil] *n.* 氯胍(抗疟药)

Clinical attacks of malaria may be preventable by drugs such as proguanil.
疟疾的临床发作可用药物预防,如用氯胍。

Pregnant and lactating women may take proguanil or chloroguine safely.
孕妇及哺乳妇女可以很安全地服用氯胍或氯喹。

prohibit [prə'hibit] *v.* 禁止,阻止

Selling drugs beyond the expiration dates on their labels is prohibited.
出售超过标签上有效日期的药物是被禁止的。

Sexual intercourse is prohibited until healing of venereal disease has been established.
性病痊愈未确定前禁止性交。

prohormone [prəu'hɔːməun] *n.* 激素原,激素前体

Procalcitonin is a prohormone of calcitonin that is secreted by numerous organs in response to systemic bacterial infection.
前降钙素是全身性细菌感染时多个器官分泌的降钙素前体。

Glucagon is produced in islet α-cells through processing by prohormone convertase 2 and exerts its action through the glucagon receptor.
胰高血糖素在胰岛 α 细胞中由激素原转化酶 2 处理后产生,并通过胰高血糖素受体发挥作用。

proinflammatory [prəuin'flæmətəri] *a.* 促炎的

Stay away from proinflammatory foods, which accelerate the aging process.
远离促炎性食品,这类食品可加速老化过程。

Insulin increases the release of proinflammatory mediators.
胰岛素可增加促炎介质的释放。

project [prə'dʒekt] *v.* 突出,伸出

The crown of a tooth projects beyond the level of the gums.
牙冠突出超出牙龈之外。

The apexes of the columnar cells project into the lumen of the gland and in histologic cross section appear as if they are being extruded.
圆柱形细胞的顶端突入腺腔中,在组织的横切面上它们像是被挤出来的。

projectile [prə'dʒektail] *a.* 喷射的

Vomiting becomes projectile eventually and is characteristically unaccompanied by nausea.
呕吐最后变成喷射式,其特点是不伴有恶心。

projection [prə'dʒekʃən] *n.* 投射,投影;突出

Films should be taken from both the lateral and the anteroposterior projections.
应同时从侧面和前后位投射进行拍片。

The molars have broad crowns with small, pointed projections.
(后)磨牙的牙冠较宽,在其上面长有小的尖突。

prokaryote [prəu'kæriəut] *n.* 原核生物

All prokaryotes are single-celled organisms.
所有原核生物为单细胞生物。

Prokaryotes do not undergo true mitosis and meiosis.
原核生物不进行真正的有丝分裂和减数分裂。

prolactin [prəu'læktin] *n.* 催乳激素

Elevation of plasma prolactin levels is a common finding and may arise from a variety of causes.

血浆催乳素水平增高是常见的现象，引起的原因也很多。

In both sexes excessive secretion of prolactin gives rise to abnormal production of milk (galactorrhoea).

女性和男性催乳素分泌过多可引起乳汁异常分泌。

prolapse ['prəulæps] *n.* 脱出症，脱垂

Complications of labour including malpresentations, prolapse of the cord and placenta praevia may occur.

可能发生分娩并发症，包括胎位不正、脐带脱垂和前置胎盘。

Prolapsed intervertebral disc must be differentiated from other cases of low back pain.

椎间盘脱出必须与其他腰痛病例加以鉴别。

proliferate [prəu'lifəreit] *v.* 增生，增殖

After a menstrual period the endometrium proliferates in preparation for the reception of a fertilized ovum.

月经期后子宫内膜增生，准备接受受精卵。

The genetically altered cell proliferates abnormally to form a large family or clone of similar cells.

遗传性改变的细胞异常增生，从而形成一大系或克隆的相似的细胞。

proliferation [prəuˌlifə'reiʃən] *n.* 增生，增殖

Proliferation of lymphocytes in lacrimal and salivary glands may cause bilateral painless enlargement.

泪腺和唾液腺淋巴细胞增生，可引起两侧腺体无痛性肿大。

Cytotoxic drugs usually interfere with cell proliferation and tend decrease the tensile strength of the surgical wound.

细胞毒性药物通常干扰细胞增殖并有可能降低手术伤口的张力强度。

proliferative [prəu'lifərətiv] *a.* 增生性的

BLOM is a proliferative disease of local humoral immunity mediated by B lymphocyte.

BLOM 是一种由 B 淋巴细胞介导的增殖性局部体液免疫反应疾病。

Several observations suggest that androgens may counteract the proliferative effects of estrogen and progestogen in the mammary gland.

数个资料表明雄性激素可能阻断乳腺中雌激素和孕激素的增殖效应。

prolong [prəu'lɔŋ] *v.* 延长

Enterohepatic circulation may sometimes prolong the half-life of a drug.

肝肠循环有时可延长药物的半衰期。

Measurable effects on body chemical processes occur only after prolonged malnutrition.

只有长时期营养不良才明显影响人体化学过程。

Secondary amyloidosis is uncommon but may follow prolonged chronic colitis.

继发性淀粉样变性并不常见，但可并发于迁延性慢性结肠炎。

prolongation [ˌprəulɔŋ'geiʃən] *n.* 延长

The treatment of aneurysmectomy may result in prolongation of life.

动脉瘤切除术的治疗方法可能会使生命延长。

Postmaturity means prolongation of development of fetus in the uterus.

过度成熟是指胎儿在子宫内发育超过正常时间。

promethazine [prəu'meθəziːn] *n.* 异丙嗪

Some antihistaminics such as promethazine and diphenhydramine have local anesthetic properties.

某些抗组胺药如异丙嗪和苯海拉明有局麻性质。

prominence [ˈprɔminəns] *n.* 隆凸，突出

The swelling is often mistaken for a bone prominence.

这类肿胀常被误认为是一种骨隆凸。

prominent [ˈprɔminənt] *a.* 显著的，突出的

Thrombosis of small vessels is often prominent.

小血管血栓形成通常很明显。

The thyroid cartilage of larynx on the front of the neck is prominent, which is called Adam's apple.

颈前面的喉部甲状软骨很凸出，称作喉结。

promise [ˈprɔmis] *n.* (有)指望，(有)前途

This scientific research gives promise of ultimate success.

这项科研有最终成功的希望。

He is a young medical research worker who shows great promise.

他是一位大有前途的青年医学研究人员。

promising [ˈprɔmisiŋ] *a.* 有希望的，有前途的

Intra-aortic counterpulsation is a most promising technique.

主动脉内反搏术是一项非常有前途的技术。

Promising therapeutic approaches with beta blockers and stellectomy are now available.

目前已有 β 阻滞剂和星状神经节切除术疗法，可获得良好的疗效。

promonocyte [prəˈmɔnəusait] *n.* 前单核细胞，幼单核细胞，原单核细胞

Promonocyte is a cell in an intermediate stage of development between a monoblast and a monocyte.

前单核细胞是一种介于成单核细胞与单核细胞之间发育中间阶段的细胞。

The present study has investigated the effect of PMA on HIV expression in a chronically infected promonocyte clone.

本研究探讨了在慢性感染的幼单核细胞克隆中，PMA 对 HIV 表达的影响。

promotion [prəˈməuʃən] *n.* 促进

Health promotion constitutes an important part of community healthcare service.

健康促进是社区医疗保健服务的重点内容之一。

She is responsible for health promotion and wellness program.

她负责健康促进和福利保障计划。

promotor [prəˈməutə] *n.* 促催化剂；启动子

Promoter is a DNA site to which RNA polymerase will bind and initiate transcription.

启动子是基因中 RNA 聚合酶与之结合的部位，结合后可启动基因转录。

promptly [ˈprɔmptli] *ad.* 立即，迅速

Latent tetany can be cured quite easily if it is treated promptly.

如及时治疗，潜在性手足搐搦是很容易治愈的。

A burn victim must be given the best of modern medical care as promptly as possible.

烧伤病人必须尽快得到最好的现代化医疗。

promutagen [prɔˈmjuːtədʒən] *n.* 前致突变剂，前诱变剂

The results showed that Lapachol is a promutagen.

结果显示拉帕醇是一种前致突变剂。

A promutagen requires chemical modification (activation) to become a mutagen.

前致突变剂需要化学修饰(活化)而变成致突变剂。

promyelocyte [prəuˈmaiələuˌsait] *n.* 早幼粒细胞

Promyelocyte, late promyelocyte cells and nucleated red blood cells may appear in the peripheral blood.

外周血中可出现早幼粒细胞、晚期早幼粒细胞及有核红细胞。

prone(to) [prəun] *a.* 易于…的

The elderly are prone to toxicity of numerous drugs.

老年人对许多药物易于中毒。

Venous thrombosis is also prone to occur in some disorders of the blood.

静脉性血栓形成也易见于某些血液疾病。

pronounce [prə'nauns] *v.* 发音;宣称

The "b" in "debt" is not pronounced.

debt-词中的 b 不发音。

The doctors pronounced that the patient was no longer in danger.

医生宣称那位病人已脱离了危险。

After five weeks, the patient was pronounced well enough to leave hospital.

5 周后病人被通知其身体恢复较好已可出院了。

pronounced [prə'naunst] *a.* 显著的,明显的

The effect of this drug may be more pronounced in the neonatal period.

这种药物的效果在初生婴儿阶段可能更为明显一些。

In both groups, there was a similar pronounced dependence of clearance on protein intake.

两组实验中,对摄入蛋白的清除(肌酐)率有相似的明显依赖性。

pronucleus [prə'njuːkliəs] *n.* 原核,前核

Pronucleus is the nucleus of a sperm or egg prior to fertilization.

原核是指精子或卵受精前的细胞核。

proof [pruːf] *n.* 证据

From a regulatory standpoint, finding of carcinogenicity in rodents is considered proof that the chemical of concern does have a carcinogenic potential in humans.

按常规观点,发现对啮齿动物有致癌性,就可作为证据,说明所测化学物对人具有致癌潜力。

proopiomelanocortin [prəuˌəupiəuˌmelənəu'kɔːtin] *n.* 阿片促黑皮质素原,前阿片促黑皮质素

Proopiomelanocortin is the precursor of adrenocorticotropic hormone, the lipotropins, the melanocyte stimulating hormones and endogenous opioid peptides.

阿片促黑皮质素原是促肾上腺皮质素、促脂素、促黑激素和内源性类阿片肽的前体。

propagation [ˌprɔpə'geiʃən] *n.* 繁殖;传播

On some occasions, propagation of infectious material was accomplished for a brief period.

有时,传染因子可以在短期内完成增殖。

There is no specific treatment directed against propagation of the rhinovirus.

对于鼻病毒感染尚无特效疗法。

propantheline [prə'pænθəliːn] *n.* 普鲁本辛

Anticholinergic drugs such as propantheline should be taken 1 hour before meals.

抗胆碱药如普鲁本辛应在饭前一小时服用。

propellent [prəu'pelənt] *n.* 抛射剂

Common chemical propellants consist of a fuel; like gasoline, jet fuel, rocket fuel, and an oxidizer.

常见的化学抛射剂包括一种燃料如汽油、喷气燃料、火箭燃料和一种氧化剂。

In aerosol spray cans, the propellant is simply a pressurized gas in equilibrium with its liquid.

在喷雾罐中,抛射剂仅仅是与其液体保持着平衡的一种加压气体。

propensity [prə'pensiti] *n.* 倾向;嗜好

Some drugs have a propensity to accumulate in select tissues.

某些药物具有在特定组织蓄积的倾向。

Neuroblastoma has more propensity to metastasize to the skeleton, bone marrow, liver and lymph nodes.

成神经细胞瘤更倾向于转移至骨骼、骨髓、肝和淋巴结。

properdin [prəu'pəːdin] *n.* 血清灭菌蛋白;备解素

Properdin is a positive regulator of alternative pathway complement.

备解素是补体替代途径的正向调节物。

Properdin deposition has been recognized in glomeruli of patients with acute and chronic nephritis and lupus nephritis.

在急性和慢性肾炎以及狼疮性肾炎病人的肾小球中,均发现有备解素沉积。

properly ['prɔpəli] *ad.* 适当地,正当地

No adverse effects are to be anticipated provided the dosage is properly regulated.

如果用药量调整得当,预计没有什么副作用。

property ['prɔpəti] *n.* 所有权

Related topics include issues of transparency in the operation of registries, oversight of registry activities, and property rights in health care information and registries.

相关主题包括注册登记运作的透明度、登记工作的监管以及卫生保健信息与注册的所有权等项目。

prophase ['prəufeiz] *n.* (细胞分裂)前期

During prophase of mitosis, spindle fibers appear as the nuclear membrane disappears.

在有丝分裂前期,核膜消失,纺锤丝出现。

prophylactic [ˌprɔfi'læktik] *a.* 预防的 *n.* 预防药

Dipyridamole is used only as a prophylactic measure and is not effective during an acute attack of angina.

潘生丁仅作为预防使用,对心绞痛的急性发作无效。

If the antibiotic sensitivities of the organisms vary, the choice of the prophylactic drug is a difficult one.

如果细菌对某抗生素的药敏作用改变,对其预防药物的选择就很困难了。

prophylactically [ˌprɔfi'læktikəli] *ad.* 预防地,预防上

Chemicals may be used prophylactically in preventing the transmission of diseaes.

化学药物可预防性地用于防止疾病的传播。

If the device is used prophylactically, many cases with spontaneous recovery will appear as successes for the device.

如果将此装置用于预防目的,那么许多自发痊愈的病例将被视为此装置的效果。

prophylaxis [ˌprɔfi'læksis] *n.* 预防

Removal of the cause of disease is named causal prophylaxis.

清除疾病的原因称作病因预防。

In this case, the sulfonamides were the agents of choice for both treatment and prophylaxis.

在这种情况下,磺胺类曾作为治疗和预防的选择用药。

Antibiotic prophylaxis has been shown to be of value in certain obstetrical and gynecologic procedures.

在某些妇产科的处理中,抗生素的预防性应用表明是有价值的。

propionic [ˌprəupi'ɔnik] *adj.* 丙酸的

The clinical finding that may differentiate this disorder from other organic acidemias, especially propionic acidemia, is the skin manifestations.

皮肤的临床表现可以区分该病与其他有机酸血症,尤其是丙酸血症。

Propionic acid is an important chemical raw material.

丙酸是一种重要的化学原料。

propionic acidemia [ˌprəupi'ɔnik, æsi'diːmiə] *n.* 丙酸血症

Propionic acidemia is an autosomal recessive disorder.

丙酸血症是常染色体隐性遗传病。

Propionic acidemia is an organic aciduria resulting from the deficiency of propionyl-CoA carboxylase.
丙酸血症是一种由于丙酰辅酶 A 羧化酶缺乏引起的有机酸尿症。

proportion [prəˈpɔːʃən] *n.* 比例,比率
In health the specific gravity of urine depends upon the proportion of solids and water.
健康时尿的比重决定于固体和水的比例。
After the treatment, the proportion of relapses in two months was 9 per cent.
治疗后 2 个月内复发率是 9%。
Polyhydramnios is found in a large proportion of diabetics about the 30th week in pregnancy.
孕 30 周左右的糖尿病孕妇中有很大部分出现羊水过多。
The amount of vitamin B_{12} retained by the body is in proportion to the amount given.
身体保有维生素 B_{12} 的量与所给予的量成比例。

proportional (to) [prəˈpɔːʃənəl] *a.* 成比例的,相称的
The body weight of individual infants was found to be proportional to the mass of pancreatic islet tissue.
每个婴儿的体重与胰岛组织的量成比例。
Food intake is directly proportional to body weight.
摄入的食物量直接与体重成正比。
He claimed that the compensation was not proportional to his injuries.
他宣称赔偿与其所受伤害不相称。

proposal [prəˈpəuzl] *n.* 建议
Various proposals were put forward for uniting the two universities.
提出了合并两所大学的各种建议。

propranolol [prəˈprænəlɔl] *n.* 心得安
Propranolol is a beta-adrenergic receptor antagonist.
心得安是一种 β-肾上腺素受体的拮抗剂。

proprietary [prəˈpraiətəri] *a.* 专利的,专卖的
"Jianmin" is a proprietary trade mark and may not be used by other pharmaceutical factories.
"健民"是专利商标名,其他药厂不得使用。
Proprietary drugs often contain certain potent substances such as hyoscine or vitamin B_{12}。
专卖药常含有某些强效物质,如莨菪或维生素 B_{12}。

propylthiouracil [ˌprəupilˌθaiəˈjuərəsil] *n.* 丙基硫氧嘧啶
Treatment of hyperthyroidism during pregnancy is difficult, propylthiouracil in dosages <300mg/d may be effective.
妊娠期甲状腺功能亢进症妇女的治疗比较困难,而用丙基硫氧嘧啶在剂量小于 300 毫克/日时可能有效。
Propylthiouracil reduces thyroid activity and is used to treat thyrotoxicosis and to prepare patients for surgical removal of the thyroid gland.
丙基硫氧嘧啶能降低甲状腺功能,用于治疗甲状腺毒症及行甲状腺摘除术病人的术前准备。

prospective [prəˈspektiv] *a.* 预期的,未来的
Prospective studies comparing acyclovir and adenoside arabinoside have not been completed.
对比无环鸟苷和阿糖腺苷的前瞻性研究尚未完成。
They recommend a prospective randomized trial to evaluate the utility of the technic.
他们提议进行前瞻性随机化试验,以估计这一方法的实用价值。

prostacyclin [ˌprɔstəˈsaiklin] *n.* 前列环素,前列腺环素
Prostacyclin (PGI_2) is a labile prostaglandin synthesized by endothelial cells lining the cardiovascular system. It inhibits platelet aggregation and serotonin release and causes vasodilation.

前列腺环素是一不稳定的前列腺素，由衬在心血管系统内的内皮细胞合成，它可抑制血小板凝集和血清素释放，并可引起血管扩张。

prostaglandin [ˌprɔstəˈglændin] *n.* 前列腺素

Prostaglandins are mostly used as abortifacients.

前列腺素主要用作流产药。

Locally activated macrophages produce a large amount of prostaglandins.

局部被激活的巨噬细胞产生大量的前列腺素。

prostate [ˈprɔsteit] *n.* 前列腺

The prostate is the largest secondary sex gland in adult men.

前列腺是成年男性体内最大的第二性腺。

Cancer of the prostate, the second most common malignancy in men, can be asymptomatic.

前列腺癌是男性第二位最常见的恶性肿瘤，可以没有症状。

prostatectomy [ˌprɔstəˈtektəmi] *n.* 前列腺切除术

Prostatectomy may be performed through an incision above the pubis and through the urinary bladder.

前列腺切除术可经切开耻骨上部和经膀胱进行。

For organ-confined prostate cancer, both radiation therapy and radical prostatectomy are equally viable options.

对于局限于前列腺的肿瘤，放疗或根治性前列腺切除术两者同样有效。

prostatic [prɔsˈtætik] *a.* 前列腺的

The patient was given prostatic massage.

给病人做前列腺按摩。

Benign prostatic hyperplasia mostly occurs in men at 60 to 80 years of age.

良性前列腺增生主要发生在 60～80 岁的男性。

prostatitis [ˌprɔstəˈtaitis] *n.* 前列腺炎

The infection of the prostate gland results in prostatitis.

前列腺的感染导致前列腺炎。

Gram-negative urinary pathogens also cause acute bacterial prostatitis.

革兰氏阴性泌尿系病原菌也可引起急性细菌性前列腺炎。

prostatodynia [ˌprɔstətəuˈdinjə] *n.* 前列腺痛症

The surgeon evaluated the effect of combined therapy on chronic abacterial prostatitis and prostatodynia.

这名外科医生评估了综合治疗慢性非细菌性前列腺炎和前列腺痛的疗效。

The patients with chronic abacterial prostatitis and prostatodynia should be treated by combined therapy.

慢性非细菌性前列腺炎和前列腺痛的患者应采用综合治疗。

prosthesis [prɔsˈθiːsis]（*pl.* prostheses [prɔsˈθiːsiz]）*n.* 假体；修复术

Prostheses replace body parts and may be a plastic eye or nose or a bionic substitute for a damaged organ.

假体代替身体的某些部分，可以是塑料的眼、鼻或者是一个受损器官的仿生代替物。

Aortic valve prostheses are more often infected than mitral valves.

人工主动脉瓣比二尖瓣更容易发生感染。

prosthetic [prɔsˈθetik] *a.* 修复的；假体的；辅基的（非蛋白基的）

Infected prosthetic joints should be removed and replaced after antibiotic therapy.

在给予抗生素治疗后被感染的人工关节应置换。

The non-protein component to which the protein is attached is called the prosthetic group of enzyme.

与蛋白质结合的非蛋白质成分称为酶的辅基。

prostrate [ˈprɔstreit] *v.* 使卧倒;使衰竭,使虚脱

The pain associated with pancreatitis has been described as prostrating.

胰腺炎引起的疼痛被描述为衰竭性疼痛。

prostration [prɔsˈtreiʃən] *n.* 虚脱,疲惫

In some cases prostration may be severe, and shock may occur.

有些病例,可能发生严重虚脱,而且可出现休克。

The patient usually has fever, chills, pleuritic chest pain, and prostration.

病人常有发热、寒战、胸膜疼痛与乏力。

protamine [ˈprəutəmiːn] *n.* 鱼精蛋白

The platelet count, thrombin time, and protamine test are useful in defining consumptive coagulopathy.

血小板计数、凝血时间和鱼精蛋白试验可用于诊断消耗性凝血病。

protean [prəuˈtiːən] *a.* 变化多端的

Symptoms in brucellosis are protean and nonspecific.

布氏杆菌病的症状有变化多端的特点,并无特异性。

protease [ˈprəutieis] *n.* 蛋白酶

Trypsin is a protease, breaking down proteins to proteoses, peptones and amino acids.

胰蛋白酶是一种蛋白酶,能分解蛋白质为蛋白际、蛋白胨和氨基酸。

proteasome [ˈprəutiːsəum] *n.* 蛋白酶体

Proteasome can degrade cellular proteins which have been tagged for breakdown by ubiquitination.

蛋白酶体能够降解细胞内被泛素化作用打上降解标签的蛋白。

Components in charge of this process include ubiquitin, its startup enzymes, and proteasome system.

负责该过程的组件包括泛素、其启动酶和蛋白酶体系统。

protection [prəˈtekʃən] *n.* 保护

Our nation is a developing country, currently faces the double missions of economic development and environmental protection.

我国是一个发展中国家,目前正面临着经济发展和环境保护的双重任务。

Environmental protection is a practice of protecting the environment, on individual, organizational or governmental level, for the benefit of the natural environment and(or) humans

环境保护是在个人、组织及政府层面上实施对环境的保护,让自然环境和(或)人类受益。

protein [ˈprəutiːn] *n.* 蛋白质

Proteins are required for the growth and repair of tissues.

组织的生长和修复需要蛋白质。

The cytoplasm is a jelly-like solution of salts, proteins, lipids and carbohydrates.

细胞质是一种由盐类、蛋白质、脂类和碳水化合物组成的胶状溶液。

proteinaceous [ˌprəutiːˈneiʃəs] *a.* 蛋白的

Proteinaceous drugs are destroyed in the stomach and naturally are not given orally.

蛋白类药物在胃中被破坏,自然不能口服给药。

proteinuria [ˌprəutiːˈnjuəriə] *n.* 蛋白尿(症)

Proteinuria is even more common in endocarditis.

在心内膜炎患者中,蛋白尿尤为多见。

Proteinuria may indicate disease anywhere in the urinary tract.

蛋白尿表明尿道某部分有病。

proteolysis [ˌprəutiˈɔləsis] *n.* 蛋白质水解,蛋白水解作用

Such structure makes fibrils resistant to proteolysis.

这种结构使原纤维可以抵抗蛋白水解作用。

Filamin A regulates the proteolysis of the matrix in macrophages.
在巨噬细胞内,细丝蛋白 A 可调节基质的蛋白水解作用。

proteolytic [prəutiə'litik] *a.* 蛋白分解的,蛋白水解的

Pepsin is a weak proteolytic enzyme requiring an acid medium in which to work.
胃蛋白酶是一种弱水解蛋白酶,需在酸性环境中起作用。
Immunoglobulin fragments may be produced by proteolytic cleavage.
免疫球蛋白的断片可由蛋白水解的分裂作用产生。

proteome ['prəutiəum] *n.* 蛋白组

The proteome is the entire set of proteins expressed by a genome, cell, tissue or organism.
蛋白组是指一个基因组、细胞、组织或机体表达的全部蛋白质。
The proteome varies with health or disease, the nature of each tissue, the stage of cell development, and effects of drug treatments.
蛋白组因健康和疾病状态、各组织的性质、细胞发育的阶段以及药物治疗的效果而不尽相同。

proteomics [ˌprəuti'ɔmiks] *n.* 蛋白组学

The next generation of real wealth is going to be produced in fields like proteomics, genomics and nanotechnology.
下一代真正的知识财富将产生于蛋白质组学、基因组学和纳米技术等领域。
Proteomics is the study of how proteins work, how they interact, and how their diversity and specialization evolve among the living organisms.
蛋白质组学的研究对象是蛋白质的工作原理、交互作用方式以及它们的多样化和专一性在生命有机体中的发展演变。

proteose ['prəutiəus] *n.* 蛋白胨

The terms proteose and peptone refer to protein breakdown products containing large polypeptides.
蛋白脎和蛋白胨是指含大分子多肽的蛋白质分解产物。

proteus ['prəutiəs; 'prəutju:s] *n.* 变形杆菌

Proteus morganii is associated with acute enteritis in children, and proteus vulgaris can cause urinary tract infections.
摩根变形杆菌与儿童急性肠炎有关,普通变形杆菌能引起尿路感染。
Infection due to proteus species was found to be associated with clearance of funguria.
变形杆菌感染常与霉菌尿的消失有关。

prothrombin [prəu'θrɔmbin] *n.* 凝血酶原

If the prothrombin time is as long as 20 to 30 seconds, the person can be expected to be a bleeder.
如果凝血酶原时间长达 20~30 秒,此人很可能是一个易出血者。
Prothrombin is a protein present in the plasma that is converted to thrombin by extrinsic converting factor.
凝血酶原是出现在血浆中的一种蛋白,可被外源性转换因子转变为凝血酶。

prothrombotic [prəuˌθrəum'bɔtik] *a.* 致血栓的,血栓前的

The risk of a drug-induced thrombosis is dependent not only on the use of prothrombotic drugs, but on genetic predisposition to thrombosis.
药物诱发血栓形成的风险不仅依赖于致血栓药物的使用,也依赖于血栓形成的遗传易感性。
Thrombosis is a frequent complication of cancer, so it follows that the presence of a tumour confers a prothrombotic state.
血栓是癌症的常见并发症,因此结论是肿瘤的存在可引起一种血栓前状态。

protist ['prəutist] *n.* 原生生物

Some protists have features which resemble neither plants nor animals.
有些原生生物具有的特征既不像植物也不像动物。

protocol [ˈprəutəkɔl] *n.* 草案,议定书,原始记录
Two protocols are proposed for the management of prolonged pregnancy.
对过期妊娠的处理,作者建议两种方案。
The investigators submitted their research protocols on patients treated with this new technic.
研究人员提交了用这一新方法治疗病人的研究记录。

proton [ˈprəutɔn] *n.* 质子
Side chains of enzymic molecule lose or gain protons with rise or fall(respectively) of pH.
酶分子侧链随 pH 升高或降低而失去或获得质子。

protoplasm [ˈprəutəplæzm] *n.* 原生质
The bodies of plants and animals are composed of a living substance called protoplasm.
植物体和动物体都是由一种叫做原生质的活物质组成的。
The different substances that make up the cell are collectively called protoplasm.
形成细胞的不同物质总称为原生质。

protoporphyrin [ˌprəutəuˈpɔːfirin] *n.* 原卟啉
Free erythrocyte protoporphyrin is measurably increased in circumstances of altered heme synthesis.
在血红素合成有改变的情况下,游离红细胞原卟啉可增加到可测出的水平。
Protoporphyrin Ⅸ is a constituent of haemoglobin, myoglobin, most of the cytochromes, and the commoner chlorophylls.
原卟啉Ⅸ是血红蛋白、肌红蛋白、多数细胞色素以及一般叶绿素的组成部分。

prototype [ˈprəutətaip] *n.* 原型;标准,模范
For over two decades, 21 trisomy has represented a prototype disorder for the study of human aneuploidy and copy-number variation.
20 多年以来,21 三体综合征已经成为研究人类非整倍体和拷贝数变异的典型疾病。
Metal-wheeled chariots are the prototype of the tanks of modern warfare.
金属轮战车是现代战争中坦克的原型。

protozoa [ˌprəutəuˈzəuə] *n.* 原虫,原生动物
The eucaryotic protists are comprised of algae, protozoa, fungi, and slime molds.
真核原生生物包括藻类、原虫、真菌以及黏液菌。

protozoal [ˌprəutəuˈzəuəl] *a.* 原生动物的,原虫的
Malaria is one of the world's most common protozoal diseases.
疟疾是世界上最常见的原虫性疾病之一。
For patients with a history of recent travel, the onset of gastrointestinal symptoms only after return suggests protozoal disease.
对于有近期旅行史的病人,胃肠道症状刚好发生在回家之后提示是原虫性疾病。

protozoan [ˌprəutəuˈzəuən] (*pl.* protozoa) *n.* 原虫(= protozoon)
Trypanosomiasis is produced by protozoans of the genus Trypanosoma.
锥虫病是由锥虫属原虫所引起。
Leishmaniasis is produced by protozoa of the genus Leishmania.
利什曼病是由利什曼属原虫所引起。
a. 原虫的
Medical microbiology is concerned with viruses, bacteria, fungi, and protozoan parasites as infectious agents.
医学微生物学涉及诸传染性因子,如病毒、细菌、真菌和寄生性原虫。

protract [prəˈtrækt] *v.* 拖长,延长
Although hepatitis A is generally a benign infection, it may have a protracted or relapsing course.

虽然甲型肝炎通常是一种良性感染,但可能有一个持续的或复发的病程。

The protracted use of chlorothiazide may give rise to hypokalemia.

氯噻嗪的长期使用可发生低钾血症。

protracted [prəˈtræktid] *a.* 延长的;长期的,持久的

Usually the course of the disease is protracted: it extends with acute exacerbations and remissions over weeks and months, and rarely over years.

通常病程延长:自急性加重到消退约需数周至数月,个别达到数年。

Protracted analgesic use or abuse with aspirin or phenacetin leads to uraemia because of renal papillary necrosis.

长期服用止痛药或滥用阿司匹林或非那西丁,可因肾乳头坏死而致尿毒症。

Other extrapulmonary manifestations of severe adenovirus infections include hemorrhagic tendencies with thrombocytopenia, anemia, peripheral edema, and protracted fever.

严重腺病毒感染的其他肺外表现包括血小板减少性出血倾向、贫血、外周水肿及持续发热。

protrude [prəˈtruːd] *v.* (使)伸出,(使)突出

Compound fractures include those in which the skin and other soft tissues are torn and the bone protrudes through the skin.

复合性骨折包括皮肤和其他软组织都被撕裂,骨头也穿出皮肤。

protrusion [prəˈtruːʒən] *n.* 前突,突出

Thumb-sucking can cause protrusion of the teeth.

吮吸拇指可引起牙齿前突。

protuberant [prəˈtjuːbərənt] *a.* 隆凸的

On physical examination, this man's abdomen was slightly protuberant with a spleen edge felt 8cm below the costal margin.

体检时,此人腹部轻度隆起,脾脏边缘可在肋缘下 8cm 处触及。

prove [pruːv] *v.* 证明,表明是

Statistics prove that the incidence of lung cancer is higher this year than last year.

统计数字证明今年的肺癌发病率比去年高。

Carrying out the public health task in some rural areas proved to be more difficult than we'd thought.

在某些农村地区开展公共卫生工作的确比我们想象的要更困难。

His attempt to bring the patient back to life by cardiac massage has proved successful.

他设法用心脏按摩来挽救病人,终于取得成功。

provide [prəˈvaid] *v.* 提供,供给

Patients are provided with a very healthful diet in our hospital.

我们医院为病人提供的饮食很有助于健康。

The public health bureau has provided this hospital with an ambulance.

卫生局向该医院提供了一辆救护车。

Medical reforms also advocate that essential services be equally provided to everyone.

医疗改革还提倡使人人享有基本的医疗服务。

province [ˈprɔvins] *n.* 省;(学术)领域,范围

These areas of preventive medicine were formerly the province of public health departments.

这些预防医学领域以前是公共卫生部门的所属范围。

provirus [prəuˈvaiərəs] *n.* 前病毒

A provirus is the DNA form of a retrovirus.

前病毒是逆转录病毒的 DNA 形式。

Another pathway of transgenic signal-regulating was to apply sectorial product of provirus.

调节转基因信号的另一个途径是运用可切割的前病毒产物。

provision [prə'viʒən] *n.* 供应,预备;规定,条款

The provision of opportunities for independent action is important for the patient' s full rehabilitation.

提供独立活动机会对于病人的完全康复是重要的。

We should make provision for the future.

我们应该为将来做好准备。

There are severe provisions in the law for drunken driving.

法律上对酒后驾车有严厉的处罚条款。

provocation [ˌprɔvə'keiʃən] *n.* 刺激;激发

Alcohol provocation test can induce ventricular arrythmia in some patients.

酒精激发试验能诱发某些患者室性心律失常。

provoke [prə'vəuk] *v.* 激发,引起

Treadmill testing is also not particularly helpful since most episodes are not provoked by exercise.

活动平板试验亦无特殊价值,因为大多数发作不是由运动诱发。

Vomiting may provoke acidosis in this situation.

在这种情况下,呕吐可引起酸中毒。

proximal ['prɔksiməl] *a.* 邻近的,近端的

Glucose and other food substances are completely reabsorbed in the proximal tubule.

葡萄糖和其他营养物在近端小管中被完全重吸收。

The carotid sinus is a slight dilation of the proximal part of the internal carotid artery.

颈动脉窦为颈内动脉近端的稍微膨大部分。

proximally ['prɔksiməli] *ad.* 最近地

Each phalanx consists of a base proximally, a body, and a head distally.

每一趾骨由近端的底、体和远端的小头所构成。

proximity [prɔk'simiti] *n.* 接触,接近

Close physical proximity or direct person-to-person contact is the usual requisite for infection.

密切的身体接触或人与人的直接接触,通常是感染的必要条件。

Wherever we can bring two strongly electronegative atoms into close proximity, we can establish a hydrogen bond.

只要能使两个强负电性的原子紧密靠近,我们就能建立一个氢键。

prudent ['pruːdənt] *a.* 谨慎的;深谋远虑的

It would seem prudent to limit the use of drugs known to cause chromosome damage.

似应谨慎规定限制使用已知能引起染色体损伤的药物。

It seems prudent that repeated blood cultures be obtained for several days after termination of therapy.

在治疗终止后几天中重复进行血液培养是深思远虑的做法。

pruritic [pruə'ritik] *a.* 瘙痒的

Pruritic wheals lesion disappears within hours, though new lesion may continue to appear.

瘙痒的风疹块病变在几小时内消失,不过新的病变可继续出现。

Elevated, white pruritic welts were noted intermittently throughout childhood starting at 9 months of age.

从 9 个月开始整个儿童期断断续续出现白色隆起有瘙痒感的条痕。

pruritus [pruə'raitəs] *n.* 瘙痒

Symptoms usually become less severe as jaundice appears although pruritus may develop.

当黄疸出现时虽然伴有瘙痒,但上述症状减轻。

Pruritus of sudden onset which is generalized and persistent demands a general medical investigation.

突然发作全身的和持续的瘙痒,则需作全身的医学检查。

psammoma [sæ'məumə] *n.* 砂状瘤

Psammoma bodies are concentric lamellated calcified structures, observed most commonly in papillary thyroid carcinoma, meningioma, and papillary serous cystadenocarcinoma of ovary.

砂粒体是同心圆层状的钙化结构，通常出现于甲状腺乳头状癌、脑膜瘤和卵巢乳头状浆液性囊腺癌。

Psammoma bodies may represent an active biologic process ultimately leading to degeneration/death of tumor cells and retardation of growth of the neoplasm.

砂粒体代表一种主动的生物学过程，最终导致肿瘤细胞变性/死亡，以及肿瘤生长的减缓。

pseudo ['sjuːdəu] *a.* 虚假的

In chronic inflammatory diseases, a pseudo iron deficiency state exists.

慢性炎症性疾病存在着虚假的缺铁状态。

pseudoallele [ˌpsjuːdəuə'liːl] *n.* 拟等位基因

Pseudoallele is tandem variants of a gene: they do not occupy a homologous position on the chromosome.

拟等位基因是基因的串联变异：它们在染色体上并不占据同源位点。

pseudoaneurysm ['psjuːdəu'ænjuərizəm] *n.* 假性动脉瘤

Pseudoaneurysms of the cystic artery are rare complications related to cholecystitis.

由胆囊炎造成的胆囊动脉假性动脉瘤罕见。

Arterial hemorrhage, pseudoaneurysms, and arterial-venous fistulas require prompt intervention with angiographic embolization.

对动脉出血、假性动脉瘤以及动静脉瘘需要立即进行血管造影栓塞治疗。

pseudoautosomal [ˌpsjuːdəuˌɔːtəu'səuməl] *n.* 假体染色体；拟常染色体

Pseudoautosomal regions of the X and Y chromosomes are essentially identical to one another and undergo homologous recombination in meiosis I, like pairs of autosomes.

X 和 Y 染色体的假体染色体区域是相同的并且可以像常染色体配对那样在减数分裂时进行同源重组。

The pseudoautosomal regions get their name because any genes located within them are inherited just like any autosomal genes.

假体染色体区域被这样称呼是因为这个区域内的基因的遗传方式就像常染色体上的基因一样。

pseudodementia [ˌpsjuːdəudi'menʃiə] *n.* 假(性)痴呆

Deprssive "pseudodementia" is characterized by variability in performance.

抑郁性的"假性痴呆"以行为反复无常为其特点。

Pseudodementia is a disorder resembling dementia that is not due to organic brain disease and can be reversed by treatment.

假性痴呆是类似痴呆的一种疾患，它不是由于器质性脑疾患引起，并且可以经过治疗而康复。

pseudogene ['psjuːdəndʒiːn] *n.* 假基因

Pseudogene have been identified in various other gene families.

在其他一些基因家族中已鉴定出假基因。

pseudoginseng [sjuːdəu'dʒinseŋ] *n.* 三七

The study involves the pharmacological action of pseudoginseng used in the treatment of coronary heart disease.

这项研究涉及用三七治疗冠心病的药理作用。

Researchers carried out experiments for studying the anti-inflammatory mechanisms of saponin of pseudoginseng(Sanqi).

研究人员做了研究三七总皂苷抗炎作用机制的实验。

pseudogout ['psjuːdəgaut] *n.* 假性痛风

Pseudogout is a joint disease that can cause attacks of arthritis.
假性痛风是一种能导致关节炎发作的关节疾病。
But in pseudogout, the crystals are formed from a salt instead of uric acid.
但是在假性痛风，其结晶是由一种盐而不是尿酸形成。

pseudomembranous [ˌ(p)sjuːdəu'membrənəs] *a.* 假膜的
Pseudomembranous colitis usually is caused by antibiotic-related changes in colonic anaerobic microflora, leading to Clostridium difficile overgrowth and overproduction of toxins.
假膜性结肠炎通常由结肠厌氧菌群的抗生素相关性改变引起，后者导致艰难梭状芽胞杆菌过度增生并产生过量毒素。
Bacillary dysentery is a kind of pseudomembranous inflammation that causes watery diarrhea followed by dysentery.
细菌性痢疾是一种假膜性炎症，可导致水样腹泻以及痢疾。

pseudomonas [ˌpsjuːdəu'mɔnæs] *n.* 假单胞菌
The patients suffered from blood disorder, COPD and injury were apt to suffer pseudomonas nosocomial infection.
发生血液疾病、慢性阻塞性肺病和外伤的患者易于遭受假单胞菌院内感染。
Pseudomonas aeruginosa is a common bacterium that can cause disease in animals, including humans.
绿脓假单胞菌是一种常见细菌，能导致动物包括人类疾病。

pseudomosaicism [ˌpsjuːdəuməu'zeisizəm] *n.* 假镶嵌现象
In laboratory studies, cytogeneticists attempt to differentiate between true mosaicism and pseudomosaicism.
在实验室研究中，细胞遗传学家需区分真镶嵌现象和假镶嵌现象。
In pseudomosaicism, the mosaicism probably arose in cells in culture after they were taken from the individual.
在假镶嵌现象中，镶嵌性可能产生于从个体取下后的培养细胞中。

pseudomyxoma [ˌpsjuːdəumik'səumə] *n.* 假黏液瘤
B mode ultrasound may be a useful tool to find the pseudomyxoma peritonei before the operation.
B 超是术前诊断腹膜假黏液瘤的一种有价值的检查。
The correlation between CT findings and their pathology basis of pseudomyxoma peritonei was investigated in the study.
该研究探讨了腹膜假黏液瘤的 CT 表现和其病理基础之间的相关性。

pseudopodium [ˌsjuːdəu'pəudiəm] (*pl.* pseudopodia [ˌsjuːdəu'pəudiə]) *n.* 伪足，假足
Pseudopodia are pleats of peripheral cytoplasm from which the nucleus and other organelles are excluded.
伪足是外周胞质形成的褶状皱起物，但核和其他细胞器不包括在内。

pseudopyloric [(p)sjuːdəupai'lɔːrik] *a.* 假幽门腺的
This study suggests that Pancreatic-duodenal homeobox 1 (PDX1) plays an important role in the development of pseudopyloric glands.
该研究提示，胰腺-十二指肠同源盒 1(PDX1)在假幽门腺的发育中发挥重要作用。
Pseudopyloric glands may reflect a condition associated with gastric carcinogenesis.
假幽门腺可能提示一种与胃癌发生相关的疾病状态。

pseudorabies [ˌpsjuːdəu'reibiːz] *n.* 假性狂犬病
Pseudorabies is an infectious disease that primarily affects swine, but can also cause a fatal disease in dogs with signs similar to rabies.
假性狂犬病是一种最初感染猪的传染病，但也可导致犬死亡，其症状类似狂犬病。
The experiment was conducted to evaluate immune function of the mice challenged with pseudorabies virus.

该实验用来评价小鼠受到假性狂犬病病毒感染后的免疫功能。

psittacosis [ˌsitəˈkəusis] *n.* 鹦鹉热

Psittacosis is an atypical pneumonia caused by chlamydia psittaci.

鹦鹉热是由鹦鹉热衣原体引起的一种非典型肺炎。

Psittacosis should be considered strongly in patients with acute pneumonitis and splenomegaly.

对于患急性肺炎和脾肿大的病人应高度怀疑鹦鹉热的可能性。

psoriasis [sɔˈraiəsis] *n.* 银屑病，牛皮癣

Psoriasis is one of the most common dermatologic diseases, affecting 1 to 2 percent of people.

牛皮癣是最常见的皮肤病之一，约影响百分之一到百分之二的人。

Gyrate patterns are formed in erythema gyratum repens, psoriasis, mycosis fungoides, and sometimes syphilis.

回旋状的皮疹可在匐行性回旋状红斑、银屑病、蕈样肉芽肿中以及偶尔在梅毒中形成。

psoriatic [ˌsɔriˈætik] *a.* 牛皮癣的 *n.* 牛皮癣患者

The sausage digit is a useful clue to the diagnosis of psoriatic arthritis.

腊肠指是诊断牛皮癣性关节炎的有用线索。

Psoriatic arthritis often affects small joints, such as the terminal joints of the fingers and toes, or the spine and sacroiliac joints.

银屑病性关节炎通常侵犯小关节，如指、趾末端关节或脊柱和骶髂关节。

psyche [ˈsaiki] *n.* 心灵，精神，心理

Daydreaming is a healthy and natural act of the human psyche.

白日梦是人类的一种健康的和自然的心灵活动。

Psyche denotes the mind or the soul, i. e. , the mental(as opposed to the physical) functioning of the individual.

心理是指精神或心灵，即个人的内心功能（与躯体功能相对应）。

psychiatric [saikiˈætrik] *a.* 精神病学的

Psychiatric consultations will be held for these patients.

我们将给这些病人进行精神病科会诊。

More men than women are admitted to hospitals for psychiatric disorders.

在因精神病而入院者中，男性比女性多。

psychiatrist [saiˈkaiətrist] *n.* 精神病医生，精神病学家

Some suggest to refer the patient to a psychiatrist but others prefer not to.

有些人建议将这病人转给精神病医生，另有些人则主张不转。

psychiatry [saiˈkaiətri] *n.* 精神病学

In US attention-deficit disorder has grown into one of the most used clinical concepts in child psychiatry.

在美国，注意力缺陷障碍已成为儿童精神病学中使用最多的临床概念之一。

psychoactive [ˌsaikəuˈæktiv] *a.* 对精神起显著（或特殊）作用的

Many psychoactive preparations have proven useful for treating the hyperkinetic syndrome.

许多精神药物被证实能有效治疗多动综合征。

psychoanalysis [ˌsaikəuəˈnæləsis] *n.* 精神分析，心理分析

Transference is a key concept in psychoanalysis and psychoanalytically-oriented therapy.

移情是精神分析和精神分析导向治疗的一个关键概念。

psychodynamic [saikəudaiˈnæmik] *a.* 精神动力学的，心理动力学的

According to the psychodynamic theory, depression results from actual or perceived loss of a love object.

根据精神动力学理论，抑郁源于所爱对象真正的失去或感到会失去。

psychogenic [ˌsaikəuˈdʒenik] *a.* 精神性的，心理性的，心因性的

We assessed the duration and severity of tremor in patients with psychogenic tremor.

我们对有心因性震颤病人的震颤持续时间和严重性进行了评估。

Psychogenic bodily reactions include such discomforts as tension headaches or stress-induced rashes.

心因性的躯体反应包括紧张性头疼或压力诱导的皮疹等不适。

psychologic [saikə'lɔdʒik] *a.* 心理学的

Breast feeding has both practical and psychologic advantages.

母乳喂养同时具有实用的和心理学上的优点。

psychologist [sai'kɔlədʒist] *n.* 心理学家

A psychologist who is engaged in the scientific study of the mind may work in a university, in industry, in schools, or in a hospital.

心理学家是从事心理科学研究的工作者,可在大学、企业、学校或医院内工作。

A number of psychologists blame television for the decline in interpersonal communication.

许多心理学家把个人之间交往减少归咎于看电视。

psychology [sai'kɔlədʒi] *n.* 心理学,心理

She is studying child psychology.

她在研究儿童心理学。

I can't understand that man's psychology.

我不能理解那个人的心理。

psychometric [ˌsaikəu'metrik] *a.* 心理测验的

Psychometric evaluation of anxiety symptoms in children is in a very early stage of development.

对儿童焦虑症状的心理测验评估还处在一个很早的发展阶段。

psychomotor [ˌsaikəu'məutə] *a.* 精神运动性的

Psychomotor retardation and functional impairment are uncommon.

精神运动性阻滞和功能性损伤不常见。

psychopathology [ˌsaikəupə'θɔlədʒi] *n.* 精神病理学,病理心理学

Melancholia is a subtype of depression that indicates more severe psychopathology.

忧郁症是抑郁症的一个亚型,表现出更严重的精神症状。

psychopathy [sai'kɔpəθi] *n.* 精神变态,精神病

Psychopathy is a disorder associated with antisocial behavior and deficits in responding to emotional stimuli.

精神病是一种与反社会行为有关的疾病,对情感刺激有反应缺陷。

We found that psychopathy is associated with impairments in identifying behaviors.

我们发现精神病与识别行为损害有关。

psychosensory [ˌsaikəu'sensəri] *a.* 精神(性)感觉的,心理感觉的

Avoid using light in a way that may startle the patient and cause a psychosensory dilation.

使用光刺激时要避免使病人受惊而引起精神感觉性(瞳孔)散大。

psychosis [sai'kəusis]、(*pl.* psychoses [sai'kəusiːz]) *n.* 精神病

Psychoses are also common among children in U. S.

在美国,精神病在小儿中也常见。

The anti-inflammatory effect of steroids may be accompanied by the adverse phenomena of tissue atrophy and psychosis.

类固醇类的抗炎作用可能伴有组织萎缩和精神病的副作用(不良现象)。

psychosocial [saikəu'səuʃəl] *a.* 社会心理的

In brief reactive psychosis, there must be a significant psychosocial stressor.

在短暂的反应性精神病中,必然有一种重要的社会心理的应激源。

psychosomatic [ˌsaikəusəu'mætik] *a.* 身心的,心身的

This disorder may merely reflect an abnormal psychosomatic effect on the heart.

这种异常可能只反映身心方面不正常对心脏的影响。

Several theories have been developed regarding the etiology of psychosomatic disorders.
出现了好几种有关身心疾病病因的理论。

psychostimulant [ˌsaikəuˈstimjulənt] *a.* 精神刺激剂
Methylphenidate (Ritalin) has become the most popular psychostimulant used in the United States.
哌醋甲酯(利他林)已成为美国使用最多的精神刺激剂。

psychotherapy [ˌsaikəuˈθerəpi] *n.* 精神治疗,心理治疗
The patient was offered psychotherapy to deal with his tendency toward depression.
对病人进行了心理治疗以解决其抑郁倾向。
If weekly psychotherapy sessions don't clear up the problem, adding medication often does.
如果每周一次的精神疗法不能解决问题,增加药物治疗常常能奏效。

psychotic [saiˈkɔtik] *a.* (患)精神病的 *n.* 精神病患者
Splitting is typical of borderline and psychotic states.
分裂是边缘状态和精神病状态的典型特征。
The first group of patients for this experiment includes what we call psychotic criminals.
这项实验中的第一类病人是那些被称为精神病罪犯的人。

psychotropic [ˌsaikəuˈtrɔpik] *a.* 治疗精神病的
Psychotropic medication is necessary for psychosis.
精神病药物治疗对精神病人来说是必需的。
It is well known that caffeine is the world's most widely used psychotropic substances.
大家都熟知咖啡因是世界上最普遍被使用的精神药物。

pterin [ˈpterin] *n.* 蝶呤
Dried blood spots are the best sample for the simultaneous measurement of amino acids and pterins.
干血斑是用于同时测量氨基酸和蝶呤的最好样品。

puberty [ˈpjuːbəti] *n.* 青春期
The maxillary sinuses are very small at birth and grow slowly until puberty.
上颌窦在出生时很小,青春期前生长缓慢。
This patient is free of symptoms from puberty to adult life.
此病人从青春期到成年没有该病的症状。

public [ˈpʌblik] *a.* 公共的
In order to protect the public water source from chemical herbicides pollution, biological method has been suggested to control the growth of this weed.
为了保护公共水源免受化学除草剂的污染,建议用生物防治方法来控制杂草的生长。
"Minamata disease" is a public nuisance disease which was firstly found in Japan.
"水俣病"是在日本首先发现的一种公害病。

publication [ˌpʌbliˈkeiʃən] *n.* 出版;公布
It was clear, even before publication, that this medical reference book would be a success.
在出版前就很清楚,这本医学参考书会获得成功。

puerarin [ˈpjuːərərin] *n.* 葛根素
It introduced the research progress on insulin combining with anisodamine, gentamicin, Kangfuxin, puerarin, rifampicin and so on to treat patients with diabetic foot.
该文介绍了胰岛素联合山莨菪碱、庆大霉素、康复新、葛根素、利福平等药物治疗糖尿病足的研究进展。
It is evident that the reduction of polarity favors the deprotonation of puerarin.
很明显葛根素的去质子化容易引起极性下降。

puerperal [pjuˈəːpərəl] *a.* 产后的;产褥期的
After delivery or abortion, bacteria may also invade the placental site, causing puerperal pyrexia.

在分娩或流产后，细菌也可侵入胎盘部位，引起产褥热。

Puerperal infection may precipitate acidosis in this situation.

在这种情况下，产褥期感染可引起酸中毒。

puerperium [ˌpjuːəˈpiəriəm] *n.* [拉] 产褥期，产后期

Pulmonary embolism is a major cause of death in the puerperium.

产褥期发生的肺栓塞是主要的致死原因。

The period of up to about six weeks after childbirth is known as puerperium, during which the size of the womb decreases to normal.

分娩后约 6 周这段时间叫产褥期，其间子宫收缩至正常大小。

puffiness [ˈpʌfinis] *n.* 浮肿，肿胀

Puffiness round the eyes is a sign of poor health.

眼睛周围的浮肿是身体不健康的征兆。

Usually, the initial symptoms of acute nephritis are puffiness of the face or grossly bloody urine or headache and vomiting.

通常，急性肾炎的最初症状是面部浮肿、肉眼血尿、头痛和呕吐。

pulmonary [ˈpʌlmənəri] *a.* 肺的

The differentiation of lung abscess from pulmonary tuberculosis is less difficult.

鉴别肺脓肿和肺结核的困难较小。

Only those patients with advanced pulmonary vascular disease will show isolated right ventricular hypertrophy.

仅仅那些具有晚期肺血管疾病的患者才显示单独的右心室肥大。

pulmonologist [ˌpʌlməˈnɔlədʒist] *n.* 呼吸科医生

A pulmonologist should have been consulted, proper care should have been started and the patient would have gotten better in 20 minutes.

本应咨询呼吸科医生，开始正确的治疗措施，患者就会在 20 分钟内好转。

pulp [pʌlp] *n.* 髓

There are two main types of splenic tissue: the red pulp and the white pulp.

脾脏组织分为两种主要类型：红髓和白髓。

Dental pulp is the richly vascularized and innervated connective tissue contained in the central cavity of a tooth and surrounded by dentin.

牙髓是富含血管和受神经支配的结缔组织，包含在牙齿的中央腔内并被牙质包围。

pulsate [ˈpʌlseit] *v.* 搏动

It is safer to consider a pulsating tumor an aneurysm until identified otherwise.

在证明为其他情况以前，把搏动性肿瘤当作动脉瘤是比较安全的。

pulsation [pʌlˈseiʃən] *n.* (心脏)搏动

X-ray screening may show abnormal pulsation and an abnormal cardiac contour.

X 线透视可见到不正常的心脏搏动及不正常的心脏外形。

pulse [pʌls] *n.* 脉搏，脉冲

Normally the pulse rate is the same as the heart rate.

在正常情况下，脉率和心率相同。

Emotional disturbances may increase the pulse rate.

情绪紊乱可加快脉率。

In many infections the pulse rate increases with the increase in temperature.

在许多感染中，脉率随体温升高而加快。

pump [pʌmp] *n.* 泵，唧筒

The heart is a muscular organ, which acts like a pump.

心脏是一个肌性器官，其作用像唧筒。

The heart is a kind of natural pump that moves the blood around the body.

心脏是一种自然泵，它使血液周身循环。

punch [pʌntʃ] *n.* 穿孔

Quantitative cultures of punch biopsies from the wound are much more precise indicators.

从伤口钻取活检物的定量培养是精确得多的指标。

punctate [ˈpʌnkteit] *a.* 点状的

Minute 1-to 2-mm hemorrhages into skin, mucous membranes, or serosal surfaces are called petechiae, shown as punctate hemorrhages.

皮肤、黏膜或浆膜表面的微小的 1 ~2mm 的出血被称为瘀点，表现为点状出血。

With more severe mucosal damage in acute gastritis, diffuse erosions and punctate hemorrhage develop.

急性胃炎黏膜损伤更严重时可出现广泛的糜烂和点状出血。

punctual [ˈpʌŋktjuəl] *a.* 准时的，守时的；精确的

Punctual imaging of the heart is the main development direction of CT.

精准心脏成像是目前 CT 发展的主要方向。

puncture [ˈpʌŋktʃə] *n.* 穿刺

Lumbar puncture should be made as soon as possible and before specific treatment is instituted.

腰穿刺应在进行特定治疗之前尽可能地早做。

v. 刺穿

Care must be exercised not to puncture the mass and thus spread tumor cells.

小心不要穿入包块而引起肿瘤细胞扩散。

The surgeon punctured the abscess and cleared out the pus.

外科医生刺破脓肿，排出脓液。

As high diving has been known to puncture the eardrum, one should exercise normal precautions.

因为已经知道从高处跳水能使鼓膜穿孔，人们应当做好正常预防。

pupil [ˈpjuːpl] *n.* 瞳孔

The pupil changes size according to whether one is looking at a near object or a distant one.

瞳孔改变的大小是按照看近的还是看远的物体而定的。

Examination found the child's pupils completely dilated.

检查发现这个小孩的瞳孔已完全散大。

pupillary [pjuːˈpiləri] *a.* 瞳孔的

Pupillary reflex is the reflex change in the size of the pupil according to the amount of light entering the eye.

瞳孔反射指瞳孔随进入眼内光线的量而改变大小的反射。

Pupillary signs must be evaluated with due regard to other signs and the state of consciousness.

评估瞳孔的体征时，必须对其他的体征和意识状态给予适当的考虑。

purgation [pəːˈgeiʃən] *n.* 催泻，通便

Purgation following administration of the drug is no longer recommended.

服药后不再需要导泻通便。

purification [ˌpjuərəfiˈkeiʃən] *n.* 净化，提纯

Many refugees can get clean water at purification centers.

许多难民在净化中心能获得干净的水。

Self-purification of water body can remove some undesirable chemicals and biological contaminants from contaminated water.

水体自净能去除污染水中的一些不良化学物质和生物污染物。

Distillation has been the major method for water purification.

蒸馏法已成为水提纯的主要方法。

purify [ˈpjuːrifai] *v.* 净化，提纯

You should purify the water before drinking it.

喝水前你应先把水净化一下。

After the serum is purified, it is injected into a person having diphtheria.

血清经过纯化后，注入白喉患者体内。

purine [ˈpjuərin] *n.* 嘌呤

Adenine(A) and guanine(G) are purine bases.

腺嘌呤和鸟嘌呤是嘌呤碱基。

The purine bases include adenine and guanine, which are constituents of nucleic acid, hypoxanthine and xanthine.

嘌呤碱包括腺嘌呤和鸟嘌呤，它们是核酸、次黄嘌呤和黄嘌呤的组成成分。

purple [ˈpəːpl] *n.* 紫色 *a.* 紫色的

A simple form of Wood's light is the 125-volt purple bulb.

一种简单型的伍氏灯是一个 125 伏的紫色灯泡。

purpura [ˈpəːpjurə] *n.* 紫癜

Purpura is a common sign of acute leukemia.

紫癜是急性白血病的常见体征。

There may be various kinds of hemorrhage such as bloody stool, uterine bleeding and purpura.

可能发生各种不同的出血，如便血、子宫出血和紫癜。

purpuric [pəːˈpjuərik] *a.* 紫癜的，红紫的

The most common presenting symptom complex of acute childhood leukemia is fever, pallor, lassitude, and purpuric lesions.

儿童急性白血病最常见的征候群是发热、苍白、倦怠和紫癜。

pursue [pəˈsjuː] *v.* 进行，从事，继续

She decided to pursue a two year course master program after obtaining her first degree.

她决定在获得学士学位后继续攻读两年的硕士课程。

In rare instances, infectious hepatitis may pursue a very rapid course and prove fatal.

在少有的情况下，传染性肝炎病程可能发展很迅速，并足以导致死亡。

purulence [ˈpjuərulәns] *n.* 脓性，脓，化脓

All forms of chronic bronchitis may be subject to acute exacerbations with increased volumes of sputum with or without purulence.

各种慢性支气管炎常会急性加重，脓性痰或非脓性痰大量增加。

This powder is used to spread on the wound for prevention of purulence.

这种粉末用来撒在伤口防止化脓。

purulent [ˈpjuərulәnt] *a.* 脓性的

The lesions may appear as septic infarcts that are yellow and purulent.

病变可表现为败血性梗死，呈黄色脓性。

There may be purulent discharge from the duct of the parotid gland.

腮腺导管可能有脓性排出物。

Purulent sputum suggests chronic bronchitis, pneumonia, or lung abscess.

脓痰提示慢性支气管炎、肺炎或肺脓肿。

pus [pʌs] *n.* 脓，脓液

The infarct becomes surrounded by a layer of pus.

梗死灶被一层脓液包绕。

In the kidney pus may be discharged into the renal pelvis or on to the surface of the kidney.

肾脏内脓液可能流入肾盂或波及肾的表面。

putrefaction [pjuːtriˈfækʃən] *n.* 腐败，腐化

Putrefaction is the decomposition of organic material by bacterial growth.

腐败作用是指由细菌生长造成的有机物质的分解。

putrefactive [ˌpjuːtriˈfæktiv] *a.* 腐败的

In the limbs or bowel, the necrotic tissue is exposed to putrefactive bacteria.
四肢和肠道的坏死组织可受腐败菌感染。

putrid [ˈpjuːtrid] *a.* 腐烂的，腐败的
In the case of lung abscess, the sputum production may initially be minimal but can become putrid or fetid.
肺脓肿病例，痰开始量很少，但可以变得有腐烂气味或恶臭味。

puzzle [ˈpʌzl] *n.* 谜；难题
Their reason for doing it is still a puzzle to me.
他们干那件事的原因对我仍是一个谜。
v. 苦苦思索
The teacher left the students to puzzle out the answer to the problem themselves.
老师让学生自己动脑筋想出那个问题的答案。

pycnometer [pikˈnɔmitə] *n.* 比重瓶，比色计
A pycnometer is a device that determines the density of small samples by measuring volume very precisely.
比重瓶是一种设备，它可以非常精确地通过测量体积来决定小样本的密度。
The bicapillary pycnometer is a tool for accurate determination of density.
双毛细管比重瓶是用于精确测量密度的一种工具。

pyelectasis [paieˈlektəsis] *n.* 肾盂扩张
This case of congenital megalourethra with renal pyelectasis was discovered prenatally.
这个先天性巨尿道合并肾盂扩张的病例是产前发现的。
Pyelectasis can be seen during routine ultrasounds.
肾盂扩张能被常规超声检查发现。

pyelocystitis [ˌpaiələsisˈtaitis] *n.* 肾盂膀胱炎
With the increased liability to infection, hypostatic pneumonia and pyelocystitis may occur.
随着对感染的易感性逐渐增加，可能发生坠积性肺炎和肾盂膀胱炎。

pyelography [ˌpaiiˈlɔgrəfi] *n.* 肾盂造影术
Infusion pyelography may be required if the urea is above 13mmol/L.
如果尿素高于 13mmol/L 则需要作注射肾盂造影。
In intravenous pyelography (excretion urography) the contrast medium is injected into a vein and is concentrated and excreted by the kidneys.
做经静脉肾盂造影术（排泄性尿路造影术）时，造影剂注入静脉内，然后经肾浓缩和排出。

pyelonephritis [ˌpaiələuneˈfraitis] *n.* 肾盂肾炎
The term pyelonephritis refers to immediate and residual effects of bacterial infection in the kidney.
肾盂肾炎一词系指肾脏遭受细菌感染的直接和遗留后果。
The criterion of cure of acute pyelonephritis is a sterile urine.
急性肾盂肾炎的治愈标准是尿中无菌。

pyelostomy [ˌpaiiˈlɔstəmi] *n.* 肾盂造口术
One patient was catheterized with pyelostomy tubes.
一位病人通过肾盂造瘘的导尿管导尿。

pyemia [paiˈiːmjə] *n.* 脓毒血症
The term pyemia means septicemia caused by pus-forming bacteria being released from an abscess.
术语脓毒血症是指从脓肿中释出的化脓性细菌引起的败血症。
Neonatal pyemia and necrotizing enterocolitis cause significant neonatal mortality and morbidity in spite of appropriate antibiotic therapy.
尽管使用合适的抗生素，新生儿脓毒血症和坏死性小肠结肠炎仍保持较高新生儿的患病

率和死亡率。

pyknosis [pikˈnəusis] *n.* 核固缩

Apoptosis is an active process of cell destruction, characterized by cell shrinkage, chromatin aggregation with extensive genomic fragmentation, and nuclear pyknosis.

凋亡是一种细胞毁灭的主动过程,其特征性改变为细胞固缩、染色体凝集伴有广泛的基因组片段化,以及核固缩。

Morphological changes in treated prostatic adenocarcinoma include loss of glandular architecture, cytoplasmic vacuolization, and nuclear pyknosis.

治疗后前列腺癌的形态学改变包括腺样结构的消失、胞浆空泡化和核固缩。

pyloric [paiˈlɔːrik] *a.* 幽门的

The pyloric valve is a ring-like muscle surrounding the end of the stomach.

幽门瓣是围绕在胃末端的一片环状肌肉。

The severe inflammation will, in all likelihood, develop into pyloric obstruction.

这种严重的炎症很可能发展成为幽门梗阻。

pyloroplasty [paiˈlɔːrəuplæsti] *n.* 幽门成形术

Pyloroplasty is incision of the pylorus and reconstruction of the pyloric channel to relieve pyloric obstruction.

幽门形成术是切开幽门,重建幽门通道解除幽门阻塞。

pylorus [paiˈlɔːrəs] *n.* 幽门

The scar tissue may contract to such a degree that obstruction of the pylorus is produced.

瘢痕组织可能剧烈挛缩而引起幽门阻塞。

pyogenic [ˌpaiəˈdʒenik] *a.* 生脓的

Unless there is superadded pyogenic bacterial infection, tuberculous lesions do not usually suppurate.

结核性病变一般是非化脓性的,除非外加化脓菌感染。

Among the pyogenic organisms the pneumococcus carries the highest mortality.

在化脓菌中,肺炎双球菌带来的死亡率最高。

If the cerebrospinal fluid is turbid it may be assumed that the meningitis is pyogenic.

如果脑脊液是混浊的,就可设想脑膜炎是化脓性的。

pyonephrosis [ˌpaiəneˈfrəusis] *n.* 肾盂积脓

Pyonephrosis is uncommon in adults as well as children and rarely reported in neonates.

肾盂积脓在成人和儿童一样不常见,罕见于新生儿。

The authors report a recently observed psoas abscess which developed 10 years after ipsilateral nephrectomy for pyonephrosis.

作者报道了最近发现的一例腰大肌脓肿,是在同侧肾盂积脓切除肾脏 10 年后发生。

pyothorax [ˌpaiəˈθɔːræks] *n.* 脓胸(=empyema)

Pyothorax is a life-threatening condition, which can usually only be relieved by surgical drainage of the pus.

脓胸是一种威胁生命的疾病,一般只有通过外科引流脓液而缓解。

pyquiton [piˈkwitʌn] *n.* 吡喹酮

Pyquiton has the positive effect in treating cerebral schistomiasis.

吡喹酮对治疗脑血吸虫病有肯定疗效。

If an early diagnosis can be made and pyquiton and hormone therapy is given, surgery can be avoided.

如果能早期诊断并给予吡喹酮和激素治疗,就能避免外科手术。

pyrazinamide [ˌpairəˈzinəmaid] (PZA) *n.* 吡嗪酰胺,对二氮[杂]苯酰胺(抗结核药)

Pyrazinamide is particularly useful in the treatment of tuberculous meningitis because it diffuses well into the cerebrospinal fluid.

吡嗪酰胺治疗结核性脑膜炎尤其有效,因为它易扩散于脑脊液中。

pyrexia [paiˈreksiə] *n.* 发热

Fever is the rule, though the degree of pyrexia varies.

照例有发热,尽管发热的程度可有不同。

Aseptic pyrexia is associated with aseptic wounds, presumably due to the disintegration of leukocytes and necrotic tissues.

无菌性发热与无菌伤口有关,可能是白细胞和坏死组织的分解所致的发热。

pyridoxine [ˌpiriˈdɔksi(ː)n] *n.* 吡哆醇,维生素 B_6

Nutritional encephalopathies occur in patients with B_{12}, thiamine or pyridoxine deficiency.

营养性脑病发生于维生素 B_{12}、B_1、或 B_6 缺乏的病人。

Pyridoxine, pyridoxal and pyridoxamine are collectively termed vitamin B_6.

吡哆醇、吡哆醛和吡哆胺统称为维生素 B_6.

pyrimethamine [ˌpiriˈmeθəmiːn] *n.* 乙胺嘧啶

Pyrimethamine can only be given orally: in adults an initial dose of 75mg is given, followed by 25mg daily.

乙胺嘧啶只能口服:成人首次剂量为 75 毫克,以后每日 25 毫克。

Pyrimethamine is a potential teratogen and should not be used in pregnant women.

乙胺嘧啶是一潜在性致畸剂,孕妇禁用。

pyrimidine [paiˈrimidin] *n.* 嘧啶

Thymine(T) and cytosine(C) are pyrimidine bases.

胸腺嘧啶和胞嘧啶是嘧啶碱基。

One important alteration is the formation of a pyrimidine dimer in which two adjacent pyrimidines become bonded.

一个重要的变化是两个邻近的嘧啶结合形成嘧啶二聚体。

pyrogen [ˈpaiərədʒən] *n.* 致热质,热原质

The agents that cause fever are called pyrogens.

引起发热的因子称为致热质。

It is necessary to test all solutions to be injected into humans to verify the absence of pyrogens.

凡是给人注射的溶液都须加以检验,以证实其中没有热原质。

pyrogenic [ˌpaiərəˈdʒenik] *a.* 致热的

Most bacteria, viruses, and fungi are pyrogenic.

大多数细菌、病毒和真菌都是致热的。

pyrola [ˌpaiəˈrəulə] *n.* 鹿衔草

Eight compounds have been isolated from the pyrola.

从鹿衔草中分离得到 8 种化合物。

Pyrola is a traditional Chinese medicinal plant, from which two chemical compounds were isolated.

鹿衔草是一种中药植物,从其中可分离得到两个化合物。

pyrosequencing [ˌpairəˈsikwənsiŋ] *n.* 焦磷酸测序

Pyrosequencing is a method of DNA sequencing based on the "sequencing by synthesis" principle.

焦磷酸测序是一种基于"合成测序"原理的 DNA 测序方法。

The pyrosequencing method is based on detecting the activity of DNA polymerase with another chemiluminescent enzyme.

焦磷酸测序法是基于用另一种化学发光酶来测定 DNA 聚合酶的活性。

pyrosis [paiˈrəusis] *n.* 胃灼热

Pyrosis is a sensation of warmth or burning located substernally or high in the epigastrium with radiation into the neck sometimes.

胃灼热是一种位于胸骨下或高位上腹部的发热或烧灼感,有时放射到颈部。

pyruvate [paiˈruːveit] *n.* 丙酮酸

In plant cells the principal precursor of alanine, as well as leucine and valine, is pyruvate.
植物细胞中丙氨酸、亮氨酸和缬氨酸的主要前体是丙酮酸。

In aerobic respiration, therefore, pyruvate is completely oxidized to carbon dioxide and water.
因此,在有氧呼吸中,丙酮酸被完全氧化成二氧化碳和水。

pyuria [paiˈjuəriə] *n.* 脓尿

The condition in which increased numbers of leukocytes are found in urine is termed pyuria.
尿中发现有数量增多的白细胞被称为脓尿。

The presence of pyuria is one of the most important indicators of bacterial urinary tract infection.
脓尿出现是细菌性尿路感染最重要的指征之一。

Renal tuberculosis presents as pyuria and hematuria with negative cultures.
肾结核可出现培养为阴性的脓尿和血尿。

Q

quack [ˈkwæk] *n.* 庸医，江湖医

Quack is one who fraudulently misrepresents his ability and experience in the diagnosis and treatment of disease.

庸医是诡称其具有诊断和治疗疾病的能力和经验的人。

quadrant [ˈkwɔdrənt] *n.* 四分之一圆；象限

In acute appendicitis, however, pain is referred to the right lower quadrant.

然而在患急性阑尾炎时，疼痛位于右下象限。

A much simpler division into four quadrants is now less frequently used.

另一种简单得多的把腹腔分为四个象限的区分法现在已用得较少。

quadrate [ˈkwɔdrit] *a.* 正方形的

The liver is divided by fissures into four lobes: the right (the largest lobe), left, quadrate, and caudate lobes.

肝凭借裂隙分为 4 叶：右叶（最大）、左叶、方形叶及尾形叶。

quadratipronator [kwɔˌdreitiprəˈneitə] *n.* 旋前方肌

Pronate quadratus is called quadratipronator.

旋前的方形肌肉称作旋前方肌。

quadriceps [ˈkwɔdriseps] *n.* 四头肌

Quadriceps is situated in the thigh and is subdivided into four distinct portions: the rectus femoris (which also flexes the thigh), vastus lateralis, vastus medialis, and vastus intermedius.

四头肌位于大腿，分为四个不同部分：股直肌（亦可使大腿弯曲）、股外侧肌、股内侧肌和股中肌。

quadriplegia [ˌkwɔdriˈpliːdʒiə] *n.* 四肢麻痹，四肢瘫痪

Injury and loss of neurologic function in the upper cervical area of the spinal cord results in quadriplegia.

脊髓上颈段区域受损和神经功能丧失导致四肢瘫痪。

quadruplet [ˈkwɔdruplit] *n.* 四胞胎；四胞胎之一

Fully monozygotic quadruplets are rare, representing only one in about 15 million pregnancies.

完全单卵四胎非常罕见，一千五百万妊娠中仅会出现一例。

Quadruplets can be fraternal (multizygotic), identical (monozygotic) or a combination of both.

四胞胎可以来自异卵（多合子）的，同卵（单合子）的或者两者的结合。

qualification [ˌkwɔlifiˈkeiʃən] *n.* 资格，条件；合格；限定

There are now special boards that review and certify the qualifications of doctors.

现在设有专门委员会来审查和证明医生的合法资格。

qualify [ˈkwɔlifai] *v.* 使合格，取得资格

An unofficial agency holds a qualifying examination for which medical students may enrol on a voluntary basis.

一个非官方机构主持一种资格考试，医学生可自愿报名。

His training qualifies him as a radiologist.

他受的训练使他有资格做一个放射科医生。

qualitative [ˈkwɔlitətiv] *a.* 性质的，定性的；品质的

Qualitative and quantitative changes in the corresponding white blood cell type are usually found.

往往可发现相应的白细胞类型的质和量的变化。

qualitatively [ˈkwɔlitətivli] *ad.* 性质上，质量上

The pharmacologic properties of oral anticoagulants are identical qualitatively.

各种口服抗凝剂的药理特性在性质上是相同的。

quality [ˈkwɔliti] *n.* 性质，特性；品质，质量

Our goal was to assess the quality of care of acute myocardial infarction(AMI) in a rural health region.

我们的目的是评价一个农村卫生区域急性心肌梗死的护理质量。

The air quality in the city is worse than in the countryside.

城市里的空气质量不如乡下。

The measurement of quality of life has become important in evaluating new treatments of cardiac disease.

生活质量测定在评估心脏疾病的新治疗手段方面已经变得重要起来。

quantifiable [ˌkwɔntəˈfaiəbl] *a.* 定量的，可以计量的

Beyond those considerations are less quantifiable factors such as the likely natural history of the tumor being treated, the patient's physical and emotional tolerance for side effects and so on.

除此之外要考虑的是一些较难定量的因素，如肿瘤治疗的可能性自然史、患者对不良反应的身体和精神耐受等。

quantify [ˈkwɔntifai] *v.* 用数量表示，确定…的数量

The subsequent operation must be quantified with regard to flow rate and interaction of substances in the body.

继之而来的操作须对人体内各种物质的流速及相互作用进行量化。

quantitate [ˈkwɔntiteit] *v.* 测定，定量

Laboratory tests quantitate the degree of the anemia and provide data to aid in understanding its cause.

实验室检查可测定贫血的程度并可提供资料以助了解其病因。

Urine glucose is less accurately quantitated than blood glucose.

尿糖定量的准确性不及血糖。

quantitation [kwɔntiˈteiʃən] *n.* 定量

At the age of 4 he had serum immunoglobulin quantitation which revealed low IgG, IgA, and IgM.

在 4 岁时，患儿做了血清免疫球蛋白定量测定，显示 IgG、IgA 和 IgM 均低。

quantitative [ˈkwɔntitətiv] *a.* 数量的；定量的

Here, only the most accurate quantitative methods for noninvasive evaluation are acceptable.

这里唯有用于非损伤性评估的最精确的定量方法可以采用。

Accurate measurement of protein in urine requires 24 hours quantitative determinations.

精确测定尿蛋白，需要有 24 小时的定量测定。

quantitatively [ˈkwɔntitətivli] *ad.* 在数量上

Drug metabolism is very deficient qualitatively and quantitatively in the newborn.

新生儿对药物的代谢，无论在质量上或数量上都非常不完善。

quantity [ˈkwɔntiti] *n.* 数量，大量

When we prepare smear, the quantity of cells should be carefully checked.

当我们制备涂片时，应仔细检查细胞的数量。

This system is very useful for the expression of proteins in high quantity.

该系统对大量的蛋白表达非常有用。

quarantine [ˈkwɔrəntiːn] *v.* 对…进行检疫；隔离

The patient should be quarantined for the sake of others.

为了他人，应对此病人进行隔离。

n. 检疫期;隔离

Quarantine is a period of detention of vessels, vehicles, or traverlers coming from infected or suspected ports or places.

检疫期是对来自传染病可疑港口或地区的船舶、车辆或旅行者隔离一段时期。

quartan [ˈkwɔːtən] *n.* 四日热 *a.* 每四日的

Another defining feature of P. malariae is that the fever manifestations of the parasite are more moderate relative to those of P. falciparum and fevers show quartan periodicity.

三日疟原虫的另一个典型特征是发热症状较恶性疟原虫缓和,且其热型表现为每第四天复发的周期性特点。

The incubatory period in tertian malaria lasts from 10 days to 11 months, in quartan malaria, from 21 to 42 days, and in tropical malaria, from 9 to 16 days.

间日疟的潜伏期持续 10 天到 11 个月,三日疟为 21 到 42 天,热带疟为 9 到 16 天。

quartz [kwɔːts] *n.* 石英,水晶

This quartz watch keeps good time.

这块石英表很准。

Today, quartz crystal clocks are generally used on the seismograph stations.

目前地震台站一般采用石英晶体钟。

quaternary [kwəˈtəːnəri] *a.* 四元的;四级的

Not all proteins have a quaternary structure.

并非所有蛋白质都有四级结构。

quest [kwest] *n.* 寻找,探索;调查

Transplantation is not only the quest of a new means of treatment, but also opens the doors to new vistas in medicine.

移植不仅是新的治疗手段的探索,而且打开了通向医学新前景的大门。

Man is fated to suffer many disappointments in his quest for truth.

人类为了寻求真理注定会遭受许多挫折。

v. 寻找,探索

Our goal is to quest ceaselessly for improvements.

我们的目标是不断追求完善。

questionaire [ˌkwestʃəˈnɛə] *n.* 调查表;问题单;调查问卷

This questionaire is used to stimulate personal thinking and to encourage class discussion of life expectancy.

此调查表用于激发个人思考以及鼓励有关预期寿命的课堂讨论。

The purpose of this study is to examine the amount of job stress and the mental health problems among permanent night workers by means of questionnaire.

本研究的目的是运用调查表了解长期夜班工人的工作负担与精神健康问题。

The registry may use forms such as a questionnaire or a case report form of adverse reaction to collect the information from providers or patients.

注册登记可以使用诸如调查问卷或不良反应案例报告表的形式,从提供者或病人收集信息。

quickening [ˈkwikəniŋ] *n.* 胎动感

The first recognizable movement of the fetus, appearing usually from the sixteenth to eighteenth week of pregnancy, is named quickening.

通常在怀孕的 16 ~ 18 周时出现最早可辨别的胎儿活动称之为胎动感。

quick-frozen [ˈkwikˈfrəuzən] *a.* 快速冰冻的

Quick-frozen section and intra-operation pathologic diagnosis is widely used in the surgery.

快速冰冻切片和术中病理诊断广泛用于外科临床。

Intra-operation quick-frozen diagnosis helps the surgeon to choose the appropriate operative methods.

术中快速冰冻诊断帮助外科医生选择合适的手术方式。

quiescent [kwaiˈesənt] *a.* 静止的，静息的

The cell in the G_0 phase of the cell cycle is quiescent and not dividing.

在细胞周期 G_0 期的细胞是静止的、不分裂的。

Stable cells are normally quiescent, but they can undergo rapid division in response to stimuli.

稳定细胞正常情况下是静止的，但受到刺激后他们能进行快速分裂。

quinidine [ˈkwinidin] *n.* 奎尼丁

Quinidine is rarely given parenterally.

奎尼丁极少用于注射给药。

quinine [ˈkwinin; kwiˈniːn] *n.* 奎宁

Quinine is considered a specific remedy against malaria.

奎宁是一种治疗疟疾的特效药。

Quinine kills the malaria parasite but does not injure the body tissues.

奎宁杀死疟原虫而不损伤人体组织。

quit [kwit] *v.* 放弃；停止

He has quit smoking.

他已经戒烟了。

Kate quit (her job) because her salary was too low.

凯特因工资太低而辞去了工作。

quota [ˈkwəutə] *n.* 限额，配额，定量

I never exceed my quota of two cups of coffee a day.

我从不超过每天两杯咖啡的规定量。

In most of these conditions the heart is called on to pump abnormally large quantities of blood in order to deliver the normal quota of oxygen to the metabolizing tissues.

在大多数情况下，心脏根据需要泵出异常大量血液向进行代谢的组织输送正常足够量的氧气。

quotient [ˈkwəuʃənt] *n.* 商数，商

The ratio of the volume of carbon dioxide given off by the body tissues to the volume of oxygen absorbed by them is respiratory quotient.

身体组织排出的二氧化碳量与吸收的氧气量的比率为呼吸商数。

The problem not only affects the physical size of the baby but also may adversely affect the development of a high intelligence quotient.

这一问题（吸烟）不仅影响婴儿的体重，也可能对其高智商的发育产生不利影响。

R

rabies [ˈreibiːz] *n.* 狂犬病

Cat rabies now is reported more frequently than dog rabies.

现在报道猫咬引起的狂犬病常比狗咬伤的狂犬病多。

Rabies is caused by a rhabdovirus which infects central nervous tissue and salivary glands.

狂犬病是由侵犯中枢神经组织及唾液腺的狂犬病毒引起的。

raceme [rəˈsiːm] *n.* 外消旋体

The results showed that (+/−)-5 and (+)-5 had a higher potency than nitrendipine, and (+)-isomer was 1.79-fold the raceme at a dose of 2mg/kg.

结果显示(+/−)-5 和(+)-5 比尼群地平有更高的效能,(+)-同分异构体在 2mg/kg 时效能是外消旋体的 1.79 倍。

The kinetic resolution of raceme is one of the important ways in the synthesis of chiral compounds.

外消旋体的动力学拆分是合成手性化合物的重要方法之一。

racemization [ˌræsimaiˈzeiʃən] *n.* 外消旋作用

Racemization is the process in which one enantiomer of a compound, such as an L-amino acid, converts to the other enantiomer.

外消旋作用是一种化合物的对映体,如 L-氨基酸,转换成其他对映体的过程。

The most reliable of the complex network of diagenetic reactions is amino acid racemization, which involves the interconversion of L-amino acids to their D-isomeric configurations.

最可靠的成岩反应复杂网络是氨基酸外消旋作用,它包括 L-氨基酸与 D 型异构体的相互转换。

radial [ˈreidjəl] *a.* 光线的;放射的;半径的;桡骨的

Crater formation with radial grooves may be produced.

可产生火山口形状伴放射状的沟纹。

The major difficulty with other surgical techniques, such as radial keratotomy, where the cornea is cut with a laser to flatten its curvature, is its irreversibility.

其他手术技能,例如:径向角膜切开术系用激光切开角膜使曲率变平,其主要难题是不可逆转性。

Radial nerve paralysis with wrist drop is due to prolonged pressure against the back of the arm.

桡神经麻痹伴有腕下垂,是由于长时间压迫臂的背面所致。

radiate [ˈreidieit] *v.* 放射,发射光线

The wave fronts radiating from the circus movement produce the tachyarrhythmia.

环形运动发射出的波阵面引起心动过速。

Stomach pain as a result of pancreatitis is characterized by sharp pain that stretches across the middle of the belly and may radiate to the back.

胰腺炎引起的腹痛的特征是横跨腹中部的剧烈疼痛,也可放射到背部。

radiation [ˌreidiˈeiʃən] *n.* 放射(疗法),辐射

The doctor advised him to have radiation therapy.

医生建议他进行放射治疗。

Radiation fallout is rich in carcinogenic agents.

放射性沉降灰含有大量致癌物质。

There is a radiation zone encircling the earth, called the van Allen Belt.
有一条辐射带环绕地球,叫做范艾伦辐射带。

radical [ˈrædikəl] *a.* 根本的

Radical surgery is reserved for treatment failures or recurrent disease.
根治性手术可用于治疗失败和复发病例。

If a tumor is palpable, the disease is very often too advanced for radical treatment.
如果肿瘤可以被触摸到,根治此病往往已为时太迟。

n. 基,原子团

Free radical is a radical extremely reactive and having a very short half-life which carries an unpaired electron.
自由基是一很活跃的基团,半衰期很短,带有一不配对的电子 。

radically [ˈrædikəli] *ad.* 在根本上

Vegetable albumin, such as that in cereals, is radically different from animal albumin.
植物白蛋白(如谷类的白蛋白)和动物白蛋白根本不同。

A new device, SPES (Sub Perception Electro Stimulation), should radically improve quality of life for many chronic pain sufferers.
一种叫做下知觉电刺激(SPES)的新型设备从根本上改善了许多慢性疼痛患者的生活质量。

radicular [rəˈdikjulə] *a.* 根的

Radicular pain is caused by stretching, swelling, or compression of a nerve root.
神经根受牵拉、肿胀或受压都可引起(神经)根痛。

radioactive [ˈreidiəuˈæktiv] *a.* 放射性的

He used a special instrument to show where in the body the radioactive material went.
他用一种特殊的仪器显示这种放射性物质移行到身体的什么部位。

Whether natural or artificial, radioactive elements are exceedingly important.
无论是天然的或人工的,放射性元素都是极其重要的。

Nuclear medicine uses very small amounts of radioactive materials or radiopharma ceuticals to diagnose and treat disease.
核医学利用微量放射性物质,即放射性药物,来诊断和治疗疾病。

radioactivity [ˌreidiəuækˈtiviti] *n.* 放射

There are several ways to determine the amount of radioactivity present in the double-stranded DNA species.
测定双股 DNA 放射量的方法有数种。

radiochemical [ˌreidiəuˈkemikl] *a.* 放射化学的

The determination of radiochemical activity concentration in a sample will always require a sample count and a background count.
测定样品中放射化学活性浓度总是要求样品计数和本底计数。

Direct counting guarantees the quantitive accuracy you need for important experiments and radiochemical purity measurements.
直接计数保证了重要的实验和放射化学纯度测量所需要的定量精度。

radiograph [ˈreidiəugrɑːf] *n.* 放射照片,X 线(照)片

Patients with suspected perforation should have an abdominal radiograph to look for free air and peritoneal fluid.
怀疑有肠穿孔的患者须作腹部 X 线检查以确定有无游离气体和腹腔内积液。

radiographer [ˌreidiˈɔgrəfə] *n.* 放射科技师

Diagnostic radiographers use x-rays, ultrasound and other forms of imaging technology to examine patients.
放射诊断技师利用 X 线、超声波和其他影像技术来检查病人。

A radiographer performs imaging of the human body for diagnosis or treating medical problems.

放射科技师进行人体成像检查用于诊断或治疗医疗问题。

radiography [reidi'ɔgrəfi] *n.* X 线照相(术)

Frequently the diagnosis is made presymptomatically on routine chest radiography.

本病常常是在症状出现之前,在常规胸部 X 线检查时诊断出来。

radioimmunoassay [ˌreidiəuˌimjunəu'æsei] *n.* 放射免疫分析法

Recent advances in reproductive endocrinology are primarily due to the development of radioimmunoassay.

生殖内分泌学的研究进展主要归因于放射免疫分析技术的发展。

Using a newly developed radioimmunoassay, we measured serum concentrations of leptin.

应用最新研发的放射免疫检测法,我们检测了血清瘦素的浓度。

radioimmunometric [ˌreidiəuˌimjunəu'metrik] *a.* 放射免疫测定的

Ferritin is an Fe-storage glycoprotein known to exist as tissue-specific isoferritins and measurable in the serum by radioimmunometric methods.

铁蛋白是一种储铁的糖蛋白,已知其以组织特异性的同功铁蛋白的形式存在,而且可用放射免疫测定法在血清中测得。

radioiodine [ˌreidiəu'aiəudiːn] *n.* 放射碘

After total thyroidectomy and radioiodine therapy, thyroid-stimulating hormone-stimulated thyroglobulin should be below the detection limit.

在施行甲状腺完全切除术和放射碘治疗后,促甲状腺激素刺激的甲状腺球蛋白应低于检测范围。

She was treated with radioiodine for the symptoms of hyperthyroidism.

她接受了放射碘对甲状腺功能亢进症状的治疗。

radioisotope [ˌreidiəu'aisətəup] *n.* 放射性同位素

A radioisotope used for diagnosis must emit gamma rays of sufficient energy to escape from the body and it must have a half-life short enough for it to decay away soon after imaging is completed.

用于诊断的放射性同位素必须发射充足能量的伽马射线以能逃离身体,并且它的半衰期必须足够短以便在成像完成后能很快衰减。

The team just unveiled a new photovoltaic energy conversion system that can be powered by heat, the sun' s rays, a hydrocarbon fuel, or a decaying radioisotope.

这个小组前不久推出一款由热量、阳光、烃类燃料或正在衰变的放射性同位素驱动的新型光伏能量转换系统。

radiolabel [ˌreidiəu'leibəl] *v.* 用放射性同位素给…示踪

Radiolabeled Fe transfers rapidly from plasma transferrin to the marrow, but it fails to reappear normally in circulating RBCs at a normal rate.

放射性元素示踪的铁迅速从血浆转运蛋白转往骨髓,但不能以正常速度正常地重现在循环的红细胞中。

radioligand [ˌreidiəu'laigənd] *n.* 放射配体

Radioligand binding assays have been the mainstay of drug discovery and drug development.

放射配体结合分析法已经成为药物发现和药物开发的主要方法。

Ligase activity was measured with a radioligand millipore filter technique.

采用放射性配体微孔过滤器技术来测定连接酶活性。

radiologic [ˌreidiəu'lɔdʒik] *a.* 放射学的 (= radiological)

From the radiologic point of view, the infiltrates in viral pneumonia tend to be diffuse, ill-defined and hazy.

从放射学的观点来看,病毒性肺炎的浸润往往是弥漫性的,界限不清而且模糊。

Such necrosis is usually more extensive than the radiological changes.

这样的坏死变化一般较 X 射线所见的变化要广泛。

radiologically [ˌreidiəu'lɔdʒikəli] *ad.* 用射线（诊断或治疗）

In most cases, the lesions are symptomless, being diagnosed radiologically.

在大多数情况下，病变没有症状，而是由 X 线诊断出来的。

radiology [ˌreidi'ɔlədʒi] *n.* 放射学

Members of the departments of internal medicine, radiology, and pathology participate jointly in these conferences.

内科、放射科和病理科的成员都参加了这些会议。

radiolucent [ˌreidiəu'ljuːsnt] *a.* 透射线的，可透 X 线的

Uric acid renal stones are radiolucent.

尿酸肾结石是透放射线的。

radionuclide [ˌreidiəu'njuːklaid] *n.* 放射性核素

Radionuclide techniques have shown aspiration of gastric contents in 45% of normal volunteers during sleep.

放射性核素技术表明：在正常志愿受检者睡眠时，发生胃内容吸入者约占 45%。

radiopaque [ˌreidiəu'peik] *a.* 不透射线的

Radiopaque material can be found in the abdomen after ingestion of heavy metals.

摄入重金属后可在腹腔发现不透射线物质。

There is a radiopaque density in the small bowel lumen on the right side of the abdomen.

在腹部右侧小肠腔内有不透射线密度影像。

radiopharmaceutical [ˌreidiəuˌfɑːmə'sjuːtikəl] *n.* 放射性药物

The radiopharmaceuticals used in nuclear medicine emit gamma rays that can be detected externally by special types of cameras.

用于核医学的放射性药物散发出能由专门类型摄影机从体外进行探测的伽马射线。

Radiopharmaceuticals are agents used to diagnose certain medical problems or treat certain diseases.

放射性药物是用于诊断某些医学问题或治疗某些疾病的制剂。

Radiopharmaceuticals are radioactive substances used to diagnose, treat, or prevent disease.

放射性药物是用于诊断、治疗或预防疾病的放射活性物质。

radiopharmaceutics [ˌreidiəuˌfɑːmə'sjuːtiks] *n.* 放射药剂学

Radiopharmaceutics targeting integrins have been considered for tumor imaging.

靶向整合素的放射药剂学被考虑用于肿瘤显像。

The radionuclides used for labelling the radiopharmaceutics have to meet high quality standards.

用于标记放射药剂学的放射性核素必须符合高质量标准。

radioprotector [ˌreidiəuprə'tektə] *n.* 放射保护剂

Radioprotectors are designed to protect normal cells.

放射保护剂用于保护正常细胞。

radioreceptor [ˌreidiəuri'septə] *n.* 放射性受体

A simple and sensitive radioreceptor assay (RRA) has been developed to measure melatonin levels in serum.

已经开发出一种简单、敏感的放射性受体分析法用于测定血清中褪黑素水平。

Radioreceptor Assay for the Estrogen Receptor (ER) is important in cancer diagnostic and drug designation.

雌激素受体的放射性受体分析在癌症诊断和药物选定方面十分重要。

radiosensitizer [ˌreidiəu'sensitaizə] *n.* 放射增敏剂

Radiosensitizers are agents that enhance the effect of radiation.

放射增敏剂能增加放射的效果。

radiotherapy [reidiəu'θerəpi] *n.* 放射疗法，放射治疗

Some Chinese medicinal herbs ease the side effects of chemotherapy or radiotherapy so as to make the whole course of therapy possible.

有些中草药可减轻化疗和放疗的副作用,以使整个疗程得以进行。

The decision as to whether external radiotherapy is required is based on the surgical and histological findings.

决定是否进行外部放疗基于手术和组织学结果。

radiotoxicology [ˌreidiəuˌtɔksiˈkɔlədʒi] *n.* 放射毒理学

These analytical capabilities have become an essential instrument for the management of radiotoxicology laboratories.

这些分析功能已经成为管理放射毒理实验室的必要工具。

Radiotoxicology is a science aiming to estimate the biological effects induced by radiation.

放射毒理学是评价由辐射引起的生物效应的一门学科。

radishseed [ˈrædiʃsiːd] *n.* 莱菔子

You could use glucosinolates from radishseed extract as substrate.

你可以用莱菔子提取物中的硫代葡萄糖甙作为底物。

The influence of arecoline and radishseed on contraction of isolated smooth muscle is tremendous.

槟榔碱及莱菔子对离体平滑肌的收缩有很大影响。

radium [ˈreidiəm] *n.* 镭

The discovery of radium by Madame Curie was a great event in modern medical science.

居里夫人发现镭是现代医学科学中的一件大事。

In concentrated form, radium and uranium are dangerous.

浓缩型的镭和铀是危险的。

radon [ˈreidɔn] *n.* 氡

Radon is a gas that comes from the radioactive decay of radium in rocks.

氡是一种气体,由岩石中镭的放射性衰变而产生。

When you breathe air containing radon, you can get lung cancer.

当你呼吸含有氡的空气时,会患上肺癌。

rage [reidʒ] *v.* 狂暴;肆虐

One monkey from the shipment was discovered last month with a raging fever and bloody diarrhea.

上个月发运的一只猴子发现患有高热病而且便血。

rale [rɑːl] *n.* 啰音,水泡音

There are a few rales at the lung bases in this patient.

这个病人的肺底可听到少量啰音。

The rale is produced when air passes through mucus-clogged bronchioles.

当空气经过黏液阻塞的细支气管时会产生水泡音。

raman [ˈrɑːmən] *n.* 拉曼

Raman scattering or the Raman effect is the inelastic scattering of a photon.

拉曼散射或拉曼效应是光子的非弹性散射。

Raman amplification can be obtained by using stimulated Raman scattering (SRS), which actually is a combination of a Raman process with stimulated emission.

拉曼放大可以通过使用激发的拉曼散射(SRS)获得,这实际上是拉曼过程与受激发射的组合。

rampant [ˈræmpənt] *a.* 蔓延的,猖獗的

The disease was rampant at one time in that area, but it has been brought under control now.

这疾病一度在那个地区很猖獗,但现在它已被控制住。

random [ˈrændəm] *a.* 随机的,任意的

Controls were obtained by stratified random sampling from a computer registry of the Stockholm

population.
对照组是通过分层随机抽样法从斯德哥尔摩居民的电脑登记簿中取得的。
Random sample is selected by a random process ensuring that each member of the universe has an equal chance of being included in the sample.
随机样本是用随机方法抽取,以确保总体的每个成员都有同等的机会被选入样本。

randomize [ˈrændəmaiz] *v.* 随机取样,使随机化
Whether a randomized clinical trial will ultimately be possible remains to be determined.
随机化的临床试验最后是否可能尚待确定。
In a clinical trial of a new hypnotic, each patient was given the hypnotic on one night and a placebo tablet on another, the order in which the hypnotic and the placebo were given being randomized.
在一种新安眠药的临床试验中,每个病人一天晚上服安眠药,另一晚上服安慰药,服用安眠药和安慰药片的顺序是随机的。

randomly [ˈrændəmli] *ad.* 随机地,任意地
The experimental animals were divided randomly into 3 groups.
这些试验动物被随机地分成三组。
These children were randomly assigned to imipramine or placebo.
这些患儿被随机指定服用丙咪嗪或安慰剂。
At the heart of the instrument is an electronic diode that produces a randomly varying voltage.
在仪器的中心部分有一个二极管,能产生随机变化的电压。

range [reindʒ] *v.* (在一定范围内)变动,变化
Pretreatment estrogen levels ranged from 6mg. to 41mg.
治疗前雌激素水平的变异范围为 6 ~ 41 毫克。
n. 范围,幅度
There is a wide range of variability in individuals.
存在有大范围的个体差异。

rank [ræŋk] *vi.* 列为,位居
Prostate cancer ranks first among the male-only cancers.
在仅男性罹患的癌症中前列腺癌的发生率位居第一。
Complex carbohydrates rank next to simple sugars in their ability to generate energy.
复合碳水化合物在其产生能量的能力方面仅次于单糖。
n. 秩
We used the Wilcoxon signed rank test to compare data, if the data were not normally distributed.
如果数据不服从正态分布,我们使用威氏符号秩次检验来比较数据。
For continuous variables, we used the Wilcoxon rank sum test; and for categorical variables, we used a χ^2 test.
对于连续变量,我们使用威氏秩和检验;对于分类变量,我们使用卡方检验。

rapamycin [ræpəˈmaisin] *n.* 雷帕霉素,纳巴霉素(抗真菌抗生素)
Rapamycin, or sirolimus, is an immunosuppressive drug that blocks cytokine action.
雷帕霉素,又名西罗莫司,是一种能阻断细胞因子活性的免疫抑制药物。
Rapamycin is a bacterial product originally found in a soil sample from Easter Island.
雷帕霉素是最初从复活节岛土壤样本中发现的一种细菌产物。

rapidity [rəˈpiditi] *n.* 迅速(程度)
The rapidity with which one breathes depends on the demand of the body for oxygen.
一个人呼吸的速度需视人体对氧的需要量多少而定。

rash [ræʃ] *n.* 疹
The rash broke out on both the trunk and the limbs.

疹子突然在躯干和四肢出现。
Red rash developed round the neck in the wake of two days' fever.
发热两天之后接着就在颈部周围出现红疹。

rate [reit] *v.* 评价;认为
Depression was rated as moderate to severe in these patients.
在这些病人身上,抑郁症被评估为中等程度至严重程度。
Depressed children are rated as less popular by their peers.
抑郁儿童在同伴眼中是不太受欢迎的。
n. 率
The follow-up rate was 98.4%.
随访率是98.4%。
Heart rate was significantly higher during work than at rest.
工作中的心率要明显高于在休息时的心率。

ratemeter [ˈreitˌmiːtə] *n.* 测速计
This can be done with an abdominal lead and an electronic ratemeter.
可以用一个腹部探头和一个电子测速计进行。

ratio [ˈreiʃiəu] *n.* 比,比率
The ratio of the pulmonary/systemic flow is greater than 2:1 in most instances.
在多数情况下肺血流与体循环血流之比大于2:1。
At birth the ratio of head size to total body size is about 1:4.
出生时,头部与整个躯体的比例是1:4。

rational [ˈræʃənəl] *a.* 合理的,有理性的
Accurate diagnosis is now and always will be the keystone of rational treatment.
准确的诊断现在以及永远将是合理治疗的关键。

rationale [ˌræʃəˈnɑːli] *n.* 基本原理
Research on the rationale of acupuncture analgesia is being carried on.
关于针刺止痛的基本原理的研究工作正在进行中。

rattle [ˈrætl] *v.* 哮鸣音,啰音
The child began to experience difficulty in breathing with a rattling in the chest.
患儿开始有呼吸困难伴胸部哮鸣音。

ravage [ˈrævidʒ] *n.* 创伤
Simple physical exercise could protect your brain from the ravages of old age.
简单的身体运动可保护大脑免受老年创伤。
The old man's body was debilited by the ravaging disease.
这位老人的身体因患损耗性疾病变得衰弱了。

reabsorb [ˌriːəbˈsɔːb] *v.* 重吸收
Less tissue fluid may be reabsorbed because of reduced osmotic pressure.
由于渗透压降低,重吸收的组织液更少。

reabsorption [ˌriːəbˈsɔːpʃən] *n.* 重吸收
Edema may be due to decreased reabsorption of tissue fluid.
水肿是由于组织液的重吸收减少而引起的。

reaction [ri(ː)ˈækʃən] *n.* 反应,感应
The reactions that develop in tissues in response to damage or infection are termed inflammatory reactions.
组织针对感染或损伤的反应称为炎症反应。
When hypoxia is long-standing, fatigue, delayed reaction time, and reduced work capacity occur.
当低氧血症长期存在时,会产生疲劳,反应迟缓和工作能力下降。

readily [ˈredili] *ad.* 迅速地,容易地,示意地

These two forms of respiratory hypoxia are usually readily correctable by inspiring 100% O_2.
这两种类型的呼吸性低氧血症通常可通过吸入 100% 氧气迅速纠正。
Living matter is made up of atoms and molecules that are readily identifiable.
生命物质是由一些很容易辨别的原子和分子构成的。
A generalized shotty adenopathy is most readily palpable in the posterior cervical, axillary, and epitrochlear areas.
全身淋巴结肿大在颈后、腋下和滑车上很容易触及。
The patient readily followed the doctor's advice.
这位病人乐意地遵循医生的指导。

reagent [ri'eidʒənt] *n.* 试剂;反应物
Heat, changes in pH, strong acids, alcohol, and alkaloidal reagents all can denature protein.
高热、酸碱度的改变、强酸、醇和生物碱试剂都能使蛋白质变性。

reaginic [ˌriːə'dʒinik] *a.* 反应素的
IgE, also called reaginic antibody, is present in serum in the lowest concentration of all immunoglobulins.
免疫球蛋白 E(IgE)也叫作反应素抗体,在血清内所有免疫球蛋白中,其浓度最低。

realgar [ri'ælgə] *n.* 雄黄(二硫化二砷);鸡冠石
People drink realgar wine to protect themselves from illness.
人们喝雄黄酒保护自己免于害病。
The study of the effects of the super-micronized realgar particles on tumor cells is a new direction for treating cancers.
超细微雄黄颗粒对肿瘤细胞作用的研究是治疗癌症的一个新方向。

realm [relm] *n.* 领域,范围
The benefits of radium in the realm of medicine are incalculable.
镭在医学领域里的重要作用是无法估量的。

real-world ['riəl'wəːld] *n.* 真实世界
Reporting of known rates of adverse drug reaction in the context of a drug safety evaluation provides useful information on real-world performance.
在药物安全性评估的背景下,为已知药物不良反应发生率的报告提供在真实世界实践中的有用信息。

reanimate [ri'ænəmet, riː'ænimeit] *v.* 使复活,使重新活跃
Scientists have been seeking a way to reanimate organism before biological death occurs.
科学家已在寻找一种能使机体在生物死亡发生前复苏的方法。

rearrangement ['riːə'reindʒmənt] *n.* 重排
Genome rearrangement is an important area of computational biology.
基因组重组是计算生物学的一个重要研究领域。

reasonable ['riːzənəbl] *a.* 有道理的;适当的;合理的
It would seem reasonable to suppose that the deep glands are set in action reflexly, though of this there is no proof.
人们认为深层腺体的活动是反射性的,这似乎有道理,尽管还没有得到证明。
It seems reasonable to assume that progesterone plays a part in its causation.
推断孕酮在病因上起一定作用看来是合理的。

reasonably ['riːznəbli] *ad.* 合情合理地,适当地
When this occurs, the patient may make a reasonably satisfactory recovery.
当出现这种现象时,病人会合乎情理地得到令人满意的恢复。

reassurance [ˌriːə'ʃuərəns] *n.* 解除疑虑,使安心
The patient needs considerable reassurance about symptoms and their implications.
应该尽可能使病人对症状及其所含意义消除疑虑。

The periods are likely to return spontaneously and reassurance is all that is required.
只要消除疑虑,月经往往会自然恢复。

reassure [ˌriːəˈʃuə] *v.* 使放心,使消除疑虑;再向…保证

Placental function test might be reassuring, and prevent the unnecessary hazard of premature delivery.
胎盘功能试验可能消除疑虑,并能预防不必要的早产危险的发生。

The doctor reassured her about her child's health.
医生对她的孩子健康再次作出保证。

recall [riˈkɔːl] *v.* 记得,回想起;收回;使恢复

He does this so that he may use the written record to help him recall exactly what happened.
他这样做的目的是他可以使用文字记录帮助他回想起究竟发生了什么事。

I recalled having met you at last year's party.
我记得在去年的聚会上见过你。

I recall seeing an advertisment for a computer programmer in a newspaper put by a medical research institute.
我记得在报纸上见过由一个医学研究所刊登的招聘计算机程序设计员的广告。

These capsules for relieving arthritis pain are being recalled by the manufacturer because of contamination.
缓解关节炎疼痛的这些胶丸因为有污染正由生产商收回。

The invalid could not be recalled to his former vitality.
那病人不可能恢复先前那样的活力了。

n. 回忆

This procedure can be assessed by measuring the secondary antibody response to specific recall antigens to which most normal adults are commonly immunized following reimmunization.
此法能通过检测对特异回忆抗原的二次抗体应答进行评估,即大多正常人在二次免疫后一般能获得免疫。

recanalisation [ˈriːˌkænəlaiˈzeiʃən] *n.* 再穿通

Providing thrombolytic agent may benefit recanalisation of the vessel blocked by thrombus.
给予血栓溶解药物对被血栓阻塞的血管再通有利。

recapitulate [ˌriːkæpitjuleit] *a.* 概括,摘要

It will be helpful to recapitulate them.
将它们概括一下也是有帮助的。

Neo-sex chromosomes in the black muntjac recapitulate incipient evolution of mammalian sex chromosomes.
黑麂的新式性染色体反映出哺乳动物性染色体的初期进化过程。

receptacle [riˈseptəkl] *n.* 容器,贮藏器

The large intestine has almost nothing to do with digestion but acts as a receptacle for waste matters coming from digestion.
大肠与消化作用几乎无关,但可作为容器来贮藏消化后的废物。

reception [riˈsepʃn] *n.* 接待

She is preparing rooms for the reception of guests.
她正准备房间接待来客。

Patients can ask the nurse at the reception desk about the information of the hospital.
病人们可向接待处(服务台)的护士询问医院的有关情况。

The Chinese medical delegation met with a warm reception in NewYork.
中国医学代表团在纽约受到热情的接待。

He was honoured by reception into the American Academy of Child Psychiatry.
他被光荣地接纳入美国儿童精神病学会。

receptive(to) [ri'septiv] *a.* 可以接受的;能迅速接受的

This disease is receptive to x-ray treatment.

这种疾病可以接受 X 射线治疗。

This young doctor has made great achievements in medical research because he is receptive to new ideas.

这位年轻医生在医学研究中取得了重大成就,因为他能迅速接受新的思想。

receptor [ri'septə] *n.* 受体;感受器

Receptors may be located on the plasma membrane of a cell.

受体可以位于细胞的质膜上。

The cytoplasm contains a variety of nutrient transport systems and receptors that are used in the intracellular communications.

细胞浆含多种营养运输系统和细胞内传递信息的受体。

recess [ri'ses] *n.* 凹,隐窝

A small empty space,hollow,or cavity is called recess,such as accessory recess of elbow.

一个小的空隙,穴或腔称作隐窝,如肘副隐窝。

The numerous lacunae and recesses of this region may become infected with gonococci.

在这一区域内无数的小凹和隐窝可能被淋球菌感染。

recessive [ri'sesiv] *a.* 退缩的;隐性的

A recessive gene appears to produce its effect only when the genotype is homozygous.

隐性基因只有在基因型是纯合子时才能发生作用。

Cystic fibrosis is an autosomal recessive disorder.

囊性纤维化是一种常染色体隐性遗传疾病。

This syndrome is inherited in an autosomal recessive manner.

此综合征以常染色体隐性方式遗传。

recessively [ri'sesivli] *ad.* 隐性地

Most disorders involving metabolic errors are recessively inherited.

大多数伴有代谢异常的疾病是隐性遗传的。

recipient [ri'sipiənt] *n.* 接受者

One recipient has survived for more than 15 years.

一位(器官移植的)接受者已存活 15 年以上。

Blood lymphocytes from the donor are mixed with serum from the recipient.

供者的血液淋巴细胞与受者的血清混合。

The aim of this study was to discuss the anesthesia management of recipients for different stages after liver transplantation.

本研究的目的是讨论对肝移植接受者术后各阶段的麻醉处理。

reciprocal [ri'siprəkəl] *a.* 相互的

A reciprocal relationship exists between them.

两者之间存在相互的关系。

Wolpe's technique of behavior therapy utilizes the principle of reciprocal inhibition.

沃尔普的行为治疗术运用了相互抑制的原理。

reckon ['rekən] *v.* 估计;认为

The company,Frost & Sullivan,reckons that sales of artificial organs and artificial skin will top $2 billion a year by 2002.

弗罗斯特和沙利文公司估计:到 2002 年人造器官和人造皮肤的销售额一年将超过 20 亿美元。

reclosure [ri'kləuʒə(r)] *n.* 再闭合,再关闭

Treatment of hematomas in most cases consists of evacuation of the clot under sterile conditions, ligation of bleeding vessels,and reclosure of the wound.

在大多数情况下,血肿的处理包括在无菌条件下清除血凝块、结扎出血的血管以及伤口再

闭合。

recognition [ˌrekəɡˈniʃən] *n.* 认出,识别

Early recognition and immediate treatment of acute myocardial infarction are essential.

早期识别和及时治疗急性心肌梗死十分重要。

Recognition of these hemolytic mechanisms helps in clinical approach to the renal lesion as well as anemia.

对这些溶血机制的了解有助于对肾脏损害和贫血的临床处理。

recognizable [ˈrekəgnaizəbl] *a.* 可识别的

In the second month the features of the embryo become more recognizable.

到了第二个月,胚胎的特征将变得更加清晰可辨了。

recognize [ˈrekəgnaiz] *v.* 认出,识别,辨认

Can you recognize your former patient from amongst the group in that photograph?

你能从那张照片上认出你过去的病人吗?

The hospital has changed so much that you can scarecely recognize it.

那所医院变化很大,你几乎认不出来了。

Invading organisms have antigens which are recognized by the immune system.

入侵的生物体具有被免疫系统识别的抗原。

Four blood types have thus been recognized and are referred to as the A,B,AB,and O types.

现已据此区分出四种血型,分别 为 A 型、B 型、AB 型和 O 型。

recombinant [riˈkɔmbinənt] *a.* 重组的

Recombinant follicle-stimulating hormone(FSH)is purified by proprietary chromatographic techniques.

重组卵泡刺激素可通过特有的色谱技术进行纯化。

This is the first reported case of the successful use of recombinant activated factor Ⅶ to control bleeding with subsequent right ventricular assist device function.

这是首次报道成功使用重组活化因子Ⅶ来控制出血并随后具有右心室辅助装置功能的例子。

Although a range of recombinant genes have successfully prevented HIV replication in vitro,none have been used clinically until now.

尽管众多的重组基因已能够有效地阻止 HIV 在体外的复制,但直到目前为止尚无一例用于临床。

recombination [ˌriːkɔmbiˈneiʃən] *n.* 重组,重组合

Gene change every day by natural mutation and recombination,creating new biological variations.

基因由于自然突变和重组每天发生变化,因而造成新的生物学变异。

Recombinations of linked genes could result from crossing-over.

连锁的基因可因交换而出现重组。

Recombination is more likely to occur between genes that are far apart on a chromosome.

重组更可能发生在一条染色体上相隔很远的基因之间。

recommend [ˌrekəˈmend] *v.* 推荐,介绍,建议

Herbert recommends culture of family members and caution regarding the sharing of potentially contaminated fomites.

赫伯特建议家庭成员都应进行培养,告诫人们注意潜在污染物的家庭传播。

In fact,the regimens recommended in 1950s should have allowed cure of approximately 95% of cases of pulmonary TB.

事实上,二十世纪五十年代推荐的方案应该可治愈大约 95% 的肺结核病人。

Many older people would need to take a calcium supplement to get the recommended daily amount.

许多年龄较大的人需服用钙增补剂来达到每日的建议量。

reconfirm [ˌriːkənˈfəːm] *v.* 再核实

Upon arrival in the operating room, the patient should be identified and the scheduled operation reconfirmed.

病人进入手术室时必须核对，并再次核实所安排的手术。

reconstitution [ˈriːˌkɔnstiˈtjuːʃən] *n.* 重构，重建

The mucosal effects of alkylating agents are particularly significant in high-dose chemotherapy protocols associated with bone marrow reconstitution.

烷化剂的黏膜作用在与骨髓重建有关的高剂量化疗方案中尤为显著。

reconstruction [ˌriːkənsˈtrʌkʃən] *n.* 重建；改造

Pregnancy rates after tubal reconstruction and vas deferens reconstruction have more than doubled.

输卵管和输精管重建后的怀孕率是过去的一倍多。

Prophylaxis of breast cancer is performed with simple mastectomy and reconstruction rather than subcutaneous mastectomy.

预防乳腺癌的方法是施行单纯乳腺切除术和乳房再造，而不是皮下乳腺切除术。

reconstructive [ˌriːkənsˈtrʌktiv] *a.* 重建的

It is not decided whether to subject this patient to reconstructive operation for the renal artery stenosis.

尚未决定是否对这个肾动脉狭窄病人施行重建手术。

recount [riˈkəunt] *v.* 详细叙述

The author recounts his views on the anatomy, physiology, and pathology of the varicose veins of the lower limb.

作者详细论述了他对下肢静脉曲张的解剖学、生理学和病理学三方面的见解。

recoverability [riˌkʌvərəˈbiliti] *n.* 可回收性，可恢复性

Complete recoverability is an important aspect of the work of a conservative force.

这种可完全恢复的性质是保守力起作用的重要表现。

Backup and restore capabilities are key to ensuring data recoverability for any database management system.

对于任何数据库管理系统来说，备份和恢复功能是确保数据可恢复性的关键。

recovery [riˈkvʌəri] *n.* 恢复

There can be considerable recovery of brain function after a small stroke.

轻度中风以后，大脑的功能仍能得到很大程度的恢复。

recreational [ˌrekriˈeiʃənəl] *a.* 休养的，消遣的，娱乐活动的

Recreational exercise has become one of the more frequently requested services of the rehabilitation specialists.

娱乐活动已成为康复专业人员常用的治疗手段之一。

recruitment [riˈkruːtmənt] *n.* 招募

Registry developers for health should specify and implement recruitment practices that protect patients against inappropriate influences.

卫生登记开发者应具体说明和执行招募原则以保护患者免受不适当的影响。

The integrin α4β1/VCAM-1 played an important role in the recruitment of lymphocytes in the pulmonary tuberculosis.

整合素 α4 β1/VCAM-1 在肺结核病淋巴细胞募集过程中发挥重要作用。

Increased expression of granulocyte colony-stimulating factor mediates mesenchymal stem cells recruitment after vascular injury.

粒细胞集落刺激因子表达增加可介导血管损伤后的间充质干细胞募集。

rectal [ˈrektəl] *a.* 肛门的，直肠的

The rectal temperature is much more accurate than the others.

肛门体温比其他部位测得的体温准确得多。

There was no tenderness on rectal examination.

直肠检查无压痛。

rectovaginal [ˌrektəuvəˈdʒainəl] *a.* 直肠阴道的

The rectovaginal examination should be performed last because it is usually the most uncomfortable.

由于直肠阴道检查通常引起较大不适，所以在最后进行。

rectum [ˈrektəm] *n.* 直肠

The rectum ends at the anus, where circular muscles surround it and close it off.

直肠止于肛门，有环形肌围绕，将其闭合。

recumbent [riˈkʌmbənt] *a.* 躺着的，斜卧的

Patients should change their recumbent positions frequently so as to prevent bedsore.

病人应常常改变躺卧位置以预防褥疮。

The abdomen is examined by inspection, palpation, percussion, and auscultation with the patient in the recumbent position.

检查腹部时病人取仰卧位，通过望诊、触诊、叩诊及听诊进行检查。

recuperation [riˌkuːpəˈreiʃən] *n.* 复原，恢复

After a six months' recuperation, he feels much better now.

他经过半年疗养，精神变得好多了。

This environmental psychology study suggests that being stuck indoors on vacation can limit mental recuperation.

这项环境心理学研究指出假期呆在家里可能会限制精神上的恢复。

recur [riˈkəː] *v.* 复发

Ulcers tend to recur when the drugs are stopped.

停药后溃疡有复发的倾向。

If edema and increased weight recur, the maintenance dose is doubled for several days.

如果再出现浮肿和体重增加，在以后几天中把维持剂量加倍。

recurrence [riˈkʌrəns] *n.* 再发，复发

A depressed child or adolescent is at high risk for recurrence of illness.

患抑郁症的儿童或青少年的疾病复发危险性很高。

His illness has a tendency to recurrence.

他的疾病有复发倾向。

recurrent [riˈkʌrənt] *a.* 复发的，经常发生的

One of late complications is recurrent pneumonitis.

晚期并发症之一为复发性肺部炎症。

Common and recurrent diseases have recently been investigated and studied.

最近对常见病和多发病进行了调查和研究。

Recurrent episodes of cholecystitis are usually associated with gallstones.

反复发作的胆囊炎，一般与胆石症有关。

redistribute [riːdiˈstribjuːt] *v.* 重新分布

Blood flow is redistributed so that the delivery of oxygen to vital organs is maintained at normal or near-normal levels.

血流重新分配以便释放到重要脏器的氧保持正常或接近正常水平。

redress [riˈdres] *v.* 纠正；重新调整

The object of the treatment is to redress the imbalance between elastase and α1AT.

治疗的目的是纠正弹性蛋白酶和 α1AT 之间的失衡。

n. 矫正

Health officials said they would "press vigorously for redress".

卫生官员说他们会“施以重压以达到矫正的效果”。

reduce [ri'djuːs] *v.* 复位;还原

An indirect hernia appears as an elliptic swelling that may not reduce easily.

斜疝呈现为一卵圆形膨出,不易回纳。

reduced [ri'djuːst] *a.* 减少的,缩减的

In myelophthisic anemia the WBC count may be normal, reduced, or increased.

骨髓病性贫血时白细胞计数可能正常、减少或增多。

reducible [ri'djuːsəbl] *a.* 可复位的;可还原的

Examination of the groin reveals a mass that may not be reducible.

检查腹股沟部位时发现一个不能回纳的肿块。

reduction [ri'dʌkʃən] *n.* 减少,降低;还原,复位

In aplastic anemia a WBC count ≤1500 is common, the reduction occurring chiefly in the granulocytes.

再生障碍性贫血时白细胞计数常为≤1500,减少的主要是粒细胞。

Patients with thyroid storm require rapid reduction in circulating thyroid hormone levels.

对于甲状腺危象的病人需迅速降低血液循环中甲状腺素的水平。

A cell's key metabolic reactions involve oxidation-reduction reactions.

细胞中关键的代谢反应均涉及氧化还原反应。

The manipulative reduction of a fracture or dislocation without incision is called closed reduction.

处理骨折或关节脱位的复位而不需切开(组织)称为闭合复位术。

redundancy [ri'dʌndənsi] *n.* 过多,过剩,重叠性,冗余性,裁员

This provides the necessary redundancy and safety.

这样可以提供必要的冗余和安全性。

Though this figure does not contain a complete list of functions or systems, it shows the redundancy of system functions in a typical healthcare environment.

尽管这个图表没有包含一个功能或系统的完整列表,但是它展示了在一个典型医疗环境中系统功能的冗余。

Genetic redundancy is a situation in which other genes with overlapping biological activities are expressed in a tissue and lessen the impact of the loss of function of the mutant gene to a subclinical level.

遗传冗余即生物学活性重叠的其他基因在一个组织中表达,使突变基因功能丧失的影响减弱至亚临床水平。

reemphasize [riː'emfəsaiz] *v.* 再次强调

It warrants reemphasizing that in addition to relief of pain, treatment designed to prevent and care for shock should not wait until the burn can be properly dressed.

有必要再次强调,除了缓解疼痛之外,防治休克的治疗亦不应拖到烧伤创面包扎好之后进行。

reentry [riː'entri] *n.* 折返

Most arrythmias is due to reentry mechanism.

大多数心律失常是由于折返机制所致。

reestablish [ˌriːis'tæbliʃ] *v.* 重建

Treatment of aspiration involves reestablishing patency of the airway and preventing further damage to the lung.

吸入的处理包括使气道重新通畅并防止进一步损害肺。

refer [ri'fəː] *v.* 转送

This patient was referred for coronary angiography and surgery.

患者被送去做冠状动脉血管造影和外科手术。

The patient was referred for further treatment.

这名患者被转送作进一步治疗。

referable(to) [riˈfəːrəbl] *a.* 与…有关的

Of the 88 patients,44 had no neurologic symptoms referable to the injury.

88 名患者中,44 人没有与损伤有关的神经症状。

reference [ˈrefrəns] *n.* 参考(书);涉及,关联

An encyclopedia is a reference tool that aims at compactly summarizing every branch of knowledge.

百科全书是一种参考工具书,旨在简洁地概括各学科的每一分支。

Reference to MIMS and the Prescriber' s Journal will often give valuable information about drugs not easily obtainable elsewhere.

参考 MIMS 和处方杂志常可得到在其他地方不易得到的、有关药物的有价值的资料。

The term exocrine has reference to glands that secrete to epithelial surfaces other than blood vessels.

外分泌腺指的是分泌到上皮表面而不是血管的腺体。

referral [riˈfəːrəl] *n.* 治疗安排;转诊

For the peasants,referrals should be made to obtain economic assistance.

对于农民的治疗安排应力求经济实用。

Some patients may require referral to a pain clinic.

部分病人需转至疼痛门诊治疗。

refine [riˈfain] *v.* 精炼,提炼,使纯,净化

Foods rich in carbohydrates are molasses, refined sugar, syrups, honey, rich desserts, patatoes, rice, bread, cereal, beans, corn, and carrots.

富含碳水化合物的食物有糖蜜、精糖、糖浆、蜂蜜、厚味甜食、马铃薯、米饭、面包、麦片、豆类、玉米和胡萝卜等。

All these methods have refined the assessment of therapeutic results.

所有这些方法改进了对治疗结果的评估。

refined [riˈfaind] *a.* 精确的,精细的

It seems to me that the treatment of allograft recipients could be much more refined than it is today.

我认为对同种异体移植受体的处理似乎能比现在更为精确。

refinement [riˈfainmənt] *n.* 改进;精炼

A further refinement is to record the spontaneous contractions of the uterus with a tocograph.

进一步的改进是用分娩力描记器记录自发性子宫收缩。

Future refinements will enable the system to recognize faces from a variety of distances and angles.

将来进一步的完善将能使此系统从不同的距离和角度来鉴别面孔。

reflect [riˈflekt] *v.* 反映

Cyanosis reflects differences in the oxygenation of the local or systemic blood supply without structural change.

发绀反映局部或全身血液供应在氧合作用上的不同,并无结构上的改变。

The two main pathways for complement activation reflect the innate and adaptive immune response.

补体活化的两个主要途径反映了先天性和获得性免疫应答的特点。

reflection [riˈflekʃən] *n.* 反射(作用);反映;思考,看法

The intensity of color is most likely a reflection of the number of fully melanized melanosomes produced by the melanocytes.

颜色的深浅大致与黑素细胞所产生的、充分色素化了的黑素体的数目的多寡有关。

On reflection it may be apparent that a focal cause for the attacks exists, or phychological and en-

vironmental factors may be responsible for poor control.
据认为,发作存在局部的原因可能是显而易见的,或者心理学因素和环境因素可能使其不易控制。

reflex [ˈriːfleks] *n.* 反射
Many functions of the nervous system are the result of reflexes.
神经系统许多功能是反射的结果。

reflux [ˈriːflʌks] *n.* 反流,回流
Vesicoureteral reflux may develop in some cases.
膀胱输尿管反流可在某些病例出现。
It gave rise to a large granuloma, causing dyspepsia and reflux of food into the trachea.
它引起一个庞大的肉芽肿,造成消化不良和食物逆流进入气管。

refraction [riˈfrækʃən] *n.* 折射作用(正常视力调节)
Large changes in blood glucose levels can affect refraction reversibly.
血糖水平的大幅度变化可对正常视力调节产生可逆性影响。

refractive [riˈfræktiv] *a.* 折射的,屈光的
Surgical procedures intended to reduce a person's dependency on glasses or contact lenses are called refractive surgery.
旨在减少人们对眼镜或隐形眼镜依赖的外科手术称为屈光手术。

refractory [riˈfræktəri] *a.* 难医的,难治疗的
Typically, the patient was initially benefited by antibiotics and subsequently became refractory or even worsened.
典型的情况是病人开始用抗生素时病情好转,随后则变得顽固难治甚至病情反而恶化。
If blood pressure proves refractory to drug therapy, work up for secondary forms of hypertension, especially renal artery stenosis and pheochromocytoma.
当药物控制血压效果不佳时,要检查有无继发性高血压,特别是肾动脉狭窄和嗜铬细胞瘤。

refresh [riˈfreʃ] *v.* 恢复精神
Sleeping 15 minutes to one hour in the early afternoon can reduce stress and make us refreshed.
午后不久睡十五分钟到一小时可降低紧张情绪并能使精力得到恢复。
Researchers have noted that certain scents, such as citrus and peppermint scents, help induce wakefulness by stimulating the trigeminal nerve and make people feel refreshed.
研究者们注意到某些气味,如柑橘和薄荷的气味,可通过刺激三叉神经让人清醒,而使人倍感精神。

refrigerate [riˈfridʒəreit] *v.* 使冷,冷冻
Under no circumstances should an anaerobic specimen be refrigerated.
厌氧的标本决不能冷冻。

refrigeration [riˌfridʒəˈreiʃən] *n.* 冷却,冷冻
The solution is sensitive to heat, store under refrigeration.
此溶液对热敏感,应冷冻贮存。

refutation [ˌrefju(ː)ˈteiʃən] *n.* 驳斥,驳倒
If you believe you really are symptomatic, see your physician for confirmation or refutation of the diagnosis.
如果你认为你确有症状,就找你的医生对这种诊断加以证实或否定。

refute [riˈfjuːt] *v.* 驳斥,反驳;否认…的正确性
The primary purpose of the passage is to refute the theory.
该段的主要目的是反驳这一理论。
Our data tend to refute a relationship between parity and placental weight.
我们的资料倾向于否定产次与胎盘重量之间的关系。

regenerate [riˈdʒenəreit] *v.* 新生,再生

Most important is the liver' s remarkable ability to regenerate itself in a short space of time.

最重要的是肝脏有显著的短时间内再生的能力。

Trials have shown that the patch encourages the patients own skin and blood vessels to regenerate.

试用表明贴片可促使患者本身的皮肤和血管再生。

regeneration [riˌdʒenəˈreiʃən] *n.* 新生,再生

Regeneration can restore lost parts in some animal species.

有些种类动物能通过再生恢复其失去的部分。

Regeneration is a special type of growth in adults.

再生是成熟个体具有的一种特殊的生长方式。

regime [reiˈʒiːm] *n.* 制度,体制

The patient should stop smoking and adopt whatever dietary regime which suits him best.

病人应戒烟,并采取最适合于他自己的食谱。

regimen [ˈredʒimen] *n.* (生活)制度,(治疗)方案

Ulceration in such a carcinoma may respond to some therapeutic regimen.

某种治疗方案可能对这类癌肿的溃疡有效。

The treatment regimen often combines surgery with radiotherapy or chemotherapy.

治疗方案常包括外科手术加上放射疗法或化学疗法。

region [ˈriːdʒən] *n.* 地区;范围

I have a pain in the lumbar region.

我腰部疼痛。

A 42-year-old woman complains of a burning pain in the upper middle region of her abdomen.

一位 42 岁的妇女主诉中上腹部灼痛。

regional [ˈriːdʒənəl] *a.* 地区的;局部的

Regional anesthesia can also be used for postoperative pain relief.

局部麻醉亦可用于术后镇痛。

Tumor recurrence in local, regional, or distant sites occurred in 30% of women given placebo.

用安慰剂的妇女,30%的人有局部、区域性或远部位肿瘤复发。

Tumors of the small intestine are less likely to cause fever than is regional enteritis or tuberculosis.

小肠肿瘤引起发热的可能性比局限性肠炎或结核病要小。

registrar [ˌredʒiˈstraː;ˈredʒistrɑː] *n.* 专科住院医师

A registrar is a senior hospital doctor being trained as a specialist or consultant who may work with one or more senior surgeons or physicians.

专科住院医师(英国)是被训练为专科医师或会诊医师的高级医院医师,他可与一个或几个高年外科医师或内科医师一起工作。

registration [redʒiˈstreiʃən] *n.* 注册,登记

Memory function includes registration, retention, stabilization, and retrieval.

记忆功能包括记录、保留、巩固和追溯。

regression [riˈgreʃən] *n.* 倒退,退化;(症状的)消退;回归

$PGF_{2\alpha}$ reduces progesterone output and causes regression of corpus luteum.

前列腺素 $F_{2\alpha}$减少孕酮分泌并引起黄体的退化。(PG=prostaglandin)

Sufficient antimicrobial therapy are given to permit regression of secondary anatomic changes.

给予足够的抗微生物治疗以使继发性的结构变化消退。

Data were analyzed by multivariate logistic regression.

采用多元罗吉斯回归法进行资料的分析。

regressive [riˈgresiv] *a.* 退化的,退行的;消退的

With younger children, there may be noticeable regressive behavior.
较幼小的患儿可出现显著的退化行为。
Osteoarthrosis is the result of regressive change of articular surfaces but without pain or apparent inflammation.
骨关节病是关节表面退行性变化的结果,但无疼痛或明显炎症。

regularity [ˌregjuˈlæriti] *n.* 规律性;正规;定期
The triple rhythm of pain-food-relief shows a remarkable regularity.
疼痛食物缓解这种三部曲表现了明显的规律性。

regularly [ˈregjuləli] *ad.* 有规律地,定期地,经常地
A thoracic pain that regularly appears on rapid walking suggests the diagnosis of angina pectoris.
在快速行走时有规律地出现的胸痛可认为是心绞痛。
Scratching regularly produces bleeding, or scars, or causes lichenification.
经常搔抓可导致皮肤出血或产生抓痕或出现苔藓样变化。

regulate [ˈregjuleit] *v.* 调整,调节
The heart regulates the rate at which the blood circulates.
心脏可以调节血液循环的速率。
The coordination of function of the various organs is regulated by the central nervous system.
各种器官功能的协调是由中枢神经系统调节的。

regulation [ˌregjuˈleiʃən] *n.* 调整,调节
Heat regulation is one of the important functions of the body.
热调节是身体的重要功能之一。
The matter of temperature regulation is complex and involves several parts of the body.
体温调节这个问题是复杂的、涉及人体好几个部分。
The safety regulations of the factory are very strict.
该厂的安全条例非常严格。

regulatory [ˈregjuleitəri] *a.* 调节的,调整的
Regulatory gene may cause the cell to produce transcription complexes.
调节基因可使细胞产生转录复合物。
Some regulatory proteins lack zinc fingers.
许多调节蛋白缺乏锌指结构。

regurgitant [riːˈgəːdʒitənt] *a.* 吐出的;逆流的;反胃的
Vomiting may be accompanied by some nausea and a maximum of regurgitant material.
呕吐可能伴有某种程度的恶心和大量吐出物。

regurgitate [riˈgəːdʒiteit] *v.* 回流;反胃
Trauma victims are particularly likely to aspirate regurgitated gastric contents when consciousness is depressed.
受伤患者,当意识模糊时,就特别可能吸入回流的胃内容物。

regurgitation [riˌgəːdʒiˈteiʃən] *n.* 吐出;反流;反胃
Total regurgitation of swallowed material without any nausea whatsoever suggests esophageal obstruction.
将吃进的食物全部吐出而不伴有任何恶心,提示为食管梗阻。
Regurgitation and vomiting of infants are frequent symptoms of overfeeding.
婴儿的反胃和呕吐常是喂食过多的症状。
Aortic regurgitation occurs when the aortic valve has been partially destroyed.
主动脉反流发生在主动脉瓣部分损伤时。
During menstruation, retrograde regurgitation of desquamated endometrium commonly occurs.
月经时脱落的子宫内膜常发生反向逆流。

rehabilitate [ˌriːhəˈbiliteit] *v.* 使复原,恢复,康复

The intraocular lenses rehabilitate the cataract patients.
人工晶体使白内障病人得以康复。

rehabilitation [ˌriːhəbiliˈteiʃən] *n.* 恢复,康复

The rigid system of traditional hospital care is not well suited to the patient's full rehabilitation.
医院里传统的刻板的护理制度不太适宜于病人的完全康复。

The addict was sent home with a lecture about the dangers of drugs and an offer of drug rehabilitation.
吸毒者被送回家中,向他讲解毒品的危害,并提供康复的药物(戒毒药物)。

rehabilitative [ˌriːhəbiliˈteitiv] *a.* 康复的

Rehabilitative facilities will help the elderly people to develop and maintain the functional ability so that they can live as independently as possible.
康复设施将帮助老年人发展和保持活动能力,使之尽可能地独立生活。

rehmannia [reˈmæniə] *n.* 地黄;地黄属

Taxonomy and phylogeny of rehmannia are required courses.
地黄属分类学与系统学是两门必修课。

The stability of fresh glutinous rehmannia pigment was studied.
对新鲜胶状地黄色素的稳定性进行了研究。

rehydration [ˌrihaiˈdreiʃən] *n.* 再水化(作用),补液

If rehydration is not achieved rapidly and maintained, acute renal failure may ensure.
如果补液不能迅速实现并维持的话,则可能出现急性肾功能衰竭。

reimplant [riimˈplɑːnt] *n.* 再植

A ureteral reimplant is an operation to fix a ureter that is not connected to the bladder properly.
输尿管再植是将没有正确连接到膀胱的输尿管进行修复的一种手术。

v. 再植

If possible, rinse the tooth with water only, then reimplant the tooth at the site and hurry to a dentist as quickly as possible.
如果可能的话,仅仅用水冲洗牙齿,然后将牙齿再植入原位,并尽快赶往牙医处。

reimplantation [ˌriːimplɑːnˈteiʃən] *n.* 再植(入)术

The technical considerations for penile or digit reimplantation are very similar.
阴茎再造和断指再植在技术上的要求非常近似。

reinfection [ˌriːinˈfekʃən] *n.* 再感染

Recurrent infections can be classified as relapses (a recurrence with the same strain) or reinfections (a recurrence with a new strain).
再发的感染可归为复发(由同一菌种引起)或再次感染(由新的菌种引起)。

reject [riˈdʒækt] *v.* 抵制,排斥,拒绝

Bone marrow is matched so the recipient's immune system will not reject the donor's marrow.
骨髓的选用需经配型,以便受体的免疫系统对供体的骨髓不会进行排斥。

The big question now was: Would Jamie's body reject the new liver?
现在最大的问题是杰米的身体会不会排斥新的肝脏呢?

His proposal was rejected by the committee.
他的建议被委员会拒绝。

rejection [riˈdʒekʃən] *n.* 排斥;抵制

Further experiments in this area lead us to conclude that the phenomenon is related to rejection.
这方面进一步的实验使我们得出结论:这一现象与排斥反应有关。

The immunologic rejection reaction results from the genetic dissimilarity between the donor and the recipient.
这种免疫排斥反应为供体与受体之间的遗传学差异所致。

rejoin [ˌriːˈdʒɔin] *v.* 再接合

In the face of all these difficulties our medical workers have successfully rejoined the patient's severed fingers.

面对着所有的这些困难，我们的医务工作者成功地接活了这病人的断指。

rejuvenate [ri'djuːvineit] *v.* (使)恢复青春

The discovery means that one day clumps of cells could be taken from a person, rejuvenated and returned to them.

这一发现意味着有朝一日可将一簇簇的细胞从一个人身上取出，使其恢复青春后再输送回去。

Sleep allows the body to rejuvenate and be ready for another day of physical exertion and activities.

睡眠可让身体复原，为第二天的体力付出和活动做好充分准备。

relapse [ri'læps] *n.* 复发

The relapse rate following modern chemotherapy is about 4%.

使用现代化疗后复发率约为4%。

In the past two weeks, he has had two relapses.

在过去的两周里，他的病复发过两次。

People who are subjected to frequent relapses of chronic appendicitis may benefit from surgery.

对经常反复发作的慢性阑尾炎患者，进行手术或许有益。

v. 复发，再发

It is usually insidious in onset but may be an acute or a chronic relapsing disease.

发病常隐匿，但可急性或慢性反复发作。

relatedness [ri'leitidnis] *n.* 关联性

Prior to marketing approval, relatedness is an additional determinant for reporting events occurring during clinical trials or preclinical studies associated with investigational new drugs.

药品获批上市前，对于报告与试验新药有关的临床试验或临床前研究过程中所发生的事件，关联性是又一个决定因素。

relationship [ri'leiʃənʃip] *n.* 关系，联系

The Practice of Medicine in its broadest sense includes the whole relationship of the physician with his patient.

行医，从其广义来讲，要包括医患之间的全部关系。

The amount of urea in the urine bears a direct relationship to the amount of protein in the diet.

尿中的尿素量与食物中的蛋白质量有直接关系。

relax [ri'læks] *v.* 使松弛；使轻松

These pills will relax you and make you sleep.

这些药丸将使你松弛并使你入睡。

The patient lies motionless with skeletal muscles relaxed.

此病人骨骼肌松弛，一动不动地躺着。

relaxant [ri'læksənt] *n.* 松弛剂 *a.* 松弛的

The severe muscular spasm occurring in tetanus is managed by a muscle relaxant.

患破伤风时出现的严重肌肉痉挛，可用肌肉松弛剂治疗。

Paralysis by muscle relaxants simplifies exposure of the operative site.

肌肉松弛剂所导致的麻痹使手术野易于暴露。

relaxation [ˌriːlæk'seiʃən] *n.* 松弛，放松

Relaxation of ligaments aids in producing deformities.

韧带松弛会助长畸形发展。

Relaxation of a muscle without shortening is called isometric relaxation.

肌肉松弛而没有缩短称为等长松弛。

Freedom from mental worry is as essential as bodily relaxation.

解除精神忧虑和进行体力休息是同样必要的。

release [ri'liːs] *v.* 释放;放松;免除;发行

Catecholamine can also release renin, and this effect is blocked by propranolol.

儿茶酚胺也能使肾素释放,其作用可被心得安所阻断。

After the pressure is released, color should rapidly return to normal.

放松压迫后,颜色应很快恢复正常。

The nurse is released from duty at seven o' clock.

这位护士7点钟下班。

Death at last released her from her pain.

死神终于解除了她的痛苦。

"A Selection of Medical Theses" will be released next month.

《医学论文选集》将在下个月发行。

n. 释放

The release of insulin is closely linked with the level of blood glucose.

胰岛素的释放与血糖的水平密切相关。

relevance ['relivəns] *n.* 有关,关联,重大关系

The immediate relevance of the new result is for muscular dystrophy.

与新结果直接有关系的是对肌营养障碍的治疗。

The effects of mild to moderate ischemia on myocardial cells need investigation not only for general interest, but because of their clinical relevance.

从轻度到中度缺血对心肌细胞的影响需要研究,这不仅是一般兴趣,而且因为与临床有关。

Rather, we are attempting to characterize hazards with regard to their relevance to humans.

当然,考虑到(有害因子)与人有关联,我们正试图描绘其危害。

relevant(to) ['relivənt] *a.* 有关的

They discussed the relevant clinical features, pathology, and methods of treatment.

他们讨论了有关的临床特征、病理和治疗方法。

This finding may be relevant to the etiology of the disease.

这个发现可能与该疾病的病因有关。

reliability [ri,laiə'biliti] *n.* 可靠性,信度

In cases of ectopic pregnancy a rapid pregnancy test of high reliability is of considerable value.

可靠而快速的妊娠试验对宫外孕的诊断具有极大的价值。

Reliability was measured by comparing data collected by using the telephone questionnaire on Day 1 and Day 6.

通过比较第1天和第6天电话问卷收集到的数据来测量信度。

reliable [ri'laiəbl] *a.* 可靠的,可信赖的,确实的

Vaccination has been generalized as a reliable method of protection against many pathogens.

疫苗被认为是一种保护机体抵抗多种病原体的可靠方法。

There is no reliable laboratory test for the early diagnosis of sepsis.

没有一项可靠的实验室检查可以早期诊断败血症。

reliance [ri'laiəns] *n.* 信任,信赖

The oncologist often places his reliance on histologic diagnosis by pathologist.

肿瘤学家常依赖病理学家的组织学诊断。

reluctant [ri'lʌktənt] *a.* 不愿的,勉强的

Many physicians are reluctant to use these agents because of the risk of inducing hemorrhage.

许多医生不愿用此药剂,因其有引起出血的危险。

Most food companies are reluctant to have their product categorised as a medicine.

大多数食品公司不愿把它们的产品归属为药品。

remainder [ri'meində] *n.* 剩余物,残余部分; 剩下的人

In the remainder of the body, symmetry is to be expected.

身体其余部分均应是左右对称的。

remarkable [ri'mɑːkəbl] *a.* 值得注意的,显著的

The intense involvement of the conjunctiva bulbi is remarkable.

球结膜严重受累是显而易见的。

The rest of the physical was not remarkable.

体检其余部分无明显体征。

remarkably [ri'mɑːkəbli] *ad.* 显著地,异常地

Remarkably, the pattern of past memories tends to be the same for everyone.

显然,每个人对过去记忆的模式都趋于一致。

The brain tissue is remarkably susceptible to ischemia.

脑组织对缺血异常敏感。

remedial [ri'miːdjəl] *a.* 治疗的; 补救的

Such practice initially imposes a heavy strain on the nursing and remedial staff.

这种做法开始会给护理和医疗人员施加很重的压力。

We have started a remedial reading class for college freshmen.

我们为大学新生开办了一个阅读补习班。

remedy ['remidi] *n.* 药物;治疗(法)

It is a specific remedy for influenza.

那是一种治疗流行性感冒的特效药。

Before the fungi can be actively attacked, it is often necessary to employ mild soothing remedies on acutely inflamed or denuded areas of skin.

在积极治疗真菌病之前,往往需要使用温和的安抚性药物于皮肤急性发炎或裸露的区域。

In spite of all this traditional doctors continued to practise and home remedies continued to be passed among the people.

尽管如此,中医医生继续行医,家传药方继续在民间流行。

v. 治疗

Several disabling pulmonary diseases will be remedied only by successful lung transplantation.

有几种致残的肺部疾患只有用有成效的肺移植法进行治疗。

reminiscence [ˌremi'nisəns] *n.* 回忆,追忆

From middle age on, most people have more reminiscences from their youth and early adult years than for the most recent years of their lives.

从中年开始,大多数人对其青年和成年早期往事的回忆较之最近几年生活中的往事要多。

reminiscent(of) [ˌremi'nisənt] *a.* 暗示…的;表明…的

The third sample had a brown color reminiscent of a previous intraamniotic bleeding.

第三例标本呈褐色,表明先前有血液进入羊水。

The huge muscles of the mice were reminiscent of the double muscling in some breeds of cattle.

这些小鼠身上大块肌肉使人联想起某些种类牛身上的发达肌肉。

remission [ri'miʃən] *n.* 缓解,减轻

The patient is now in complete remission.

病人现在处于完全缓解状态。

It is not uncommon for such abnormal bleeding of endocrine origin to undergo spontaneous remission.

起因于内分泌的异常出血常自然缓解。

The therapy must not be interrupted until a satisfactory clinical and hematologic remission occurs.

不到临床表现和血象开始好转,就不可停止此项治疗。

remittent [ri'mitənt] *a.* 间歇的;弛张的

During the first week there is a gradually increasing remittent fever.

第 1 周内,弛张热逐渐升高。

remodeling [ri'mɔdliŋ] *n.* 重构

AF seems to cause a variety of alterations in the atrial architecture and function that contribute to remodeling and perpetuation of the arrhythmia.

房颤似乎可引起心房的结构和功能的多种改变,促成心房重构和心律失常的维持。

Amiodarone may reverse electrical remodeling even when AF is ongoing.

即便发生房颤,胺碘酮也可逆转电重构。

remodelling [ˌriː'mɔdəliŋ] *n.* 重构;改造

Gap junction remodelling may be correlated with electrical remodelling and autonomic nerve activity.

缝隙连接重构与电重构和自主神经活性可能相关。

Airway remodelling refers to changes in the airway structure.

气道重构是指气道结构的改变。

removal [ri'muːvəl] *n.* 移动;迁移;切除;排除

The removal of wastes is known as excretion.

排除废物叫做排泄。

Removal of a diseased appendix is only a minor operation.

切除病变阑尾只是一项小手术。

Seventy-five to eighty percent of cataract removals are immediately followed by intraocular implants.

75% ~80% 的病人摘除白内障后,立即植入了人工晶体。

remove [ri'muːv] *v.* 切除,除去,排除,清除

The child's inflamed appendix was removed,and he was soon back in school.

发炎的阑尾被切除后不久,这男孩又回到了学校。

Doctors remove the blood clot in his skull in order to relieve the pressure on the brain.

医生们除去他颅内的血块以免除对脑的压力。

The cause of uremia is the inability of the kidneys to remove these poisonous substances from the blood.

尿毒症的病因是肾无法排除血液中的有毒物质。

The main role of "professional" phagocytic macrophages is to remove particulate antigens.

"专职的"吞噬细胞的主要功能是清除颗粒性抗原。

At the specific place,the scientists may or may not remove a gene; the next step is to add a new gene or group of genes from some other organism.

在这个特定位点,科学家们可删除一个基因也可不删除,下一步是加入一个或一组来自其他生物的新的基因。

It may be necessary to give several courses of griseofulvin therapy and to remove the patient from the hot and humid environment.

可能有必要给几个疗程的灰黄霉素,并让患者离开热和潮湿的环境。

renal ['riːnəl] *a.* 肾的

The clinical picture is out of proportion to impairment of renal function.

临床表现与肾功能损害不成比例。

The serum creatinine is not increased unless renal disease is also present.

如果没有肾脏疾患,血清肌酐水平一般不升高。

render ['rendə] *v.* 提供;致使;使变为

Coverage of physician's services,especially those rendered in the hospital,is also extensive.

医生服务的范围,特别是在医院里提供的那些服务,也是很广泛的。

A defect in the A-D-A gene leads to immune deficiency, rendering the body defenseless against infection.

A-D-A 基因的缺陷会导致免疫缺陷,使机体对感染丧失抵御能力。

Always an enigma, cancers, inflammations, and pseudo-cysts of the pancreas are rendered more diagnosable.

常令人费解的是,癌、炎症和胰腺内的假性囊肿反而更易被诊断出来。

renew [riˈnjuː] *v.* (使)更新,(使)恢复原状

Members of the medical team were soon back on the march, renewed in spirit.

医疗队的队员们又回到行进队伍中来,精神也恢复了。

renin [ˈriːnin] *n.* 肾素,血管紧张肽原酶

Drugs altering the renin level are able to alter blood pressure.

改变肾素水平的药物可影响血压。

Renin is also supposed to be formed in the chief cells of the gastric glands.

肾素据认为也是在胃腺的主细胞中形成的。

renogram [ˈriːnəgræm] *n.* 肾图

A renogram is a scan that enables medical staff to look at kidney function.

肾图是一种能使医务人员检查肾功能的扫描术。

A Nuclear Medicine Renogram is performed using a special radioactive material that, when injected into the blood stream, shows the kidney blood supply and filtering action of the kidneys.

核医学肾图是使用一种特殊的放射活性物质注入血流以显示肾脏的血供和肾脏的滤过功能。

renography [riˈnɔgrəfi] *n.* 肾造影(术)

Isotope renography may indicate obstruction to outflow.

同位素肾造影可显示排尿阻塞。

renovascular [riːnəˈvæskjulə] *adj.* 肾血管性的

Renovascular hypertension is a low prevalence and curable disease.

肾血管性高血压是一种低发性和可治性疾病。

Resistive index was used to estimate renovascular resistance.

阻力系数被用来评价肾血管阻力。

rent [rent] *n.* 裂缝,裂隙

If the rent in a vessel is small, the platelet plug by itself can stop blood loss completely.

如果血管上的裂缝很小,血小板栓子本身就可以完全阻止失血。

reoperation [ˈriːɔpəˈreiʃən] *n.* 再次手术

The high residual cancer rate after local mass resection of thyroid carcinoma necessitates the reoperation.

甲状腺癌行局部切除手术后残癌率高,再次手术是必要的。

Main surgical treatments of bile duct reoperation include lobar resection with Roux-en-Y hepaticojejunostomy and T-tube drainage.

胆管再次手术的主要外科治疗包括肝叶切除并 Roux-en-Y 胆管空肠吻合术及 T 管引流。

re-orientation [ˈriːɔːrienˈteiʃən] *n.* 重定方向,重新把重点放在…

What is chiefly required is a re-orientation of general practitioners towards a preventive rather than curative role.

首要的要求是重新把全科医生的作用由治疗转为预防。

reovirus [ˌriːəuˈvaiərəs] *n.* 呼肠孤病毒(属)

More detail is known about the structure and function relationships of the Reovirus capsid than most other viruses.

相比其他多数病毒,对呼肠孤病毒衣壳的结构与功能之间的关系了解得更为详细。

reperfusion [ripəˈfjuːʒən] *n.* 再灌注

In myocardial infarction reperfusion of blood may produce a large potassium efflux.

心肌梗死时，血液的再灌注可引起大量钾流出。

Autophagy might play a cell-killing role in the lung ischemia-reperfusionin in rats.

自噬可能在大鼠肺缺血再灌注中有细胞杀伤作用。

The integrated mechanism of lung ischemia reperfusion injury is multifold.

肺部缺血再灌注损伤的整体机制是多方面的。

repertoire [ˈrepətwɑː] *n.* 所有组成成分，字汇，全部节目，演奏曲目

We have reviewed the literature describing antibody sequences in chronic lymphocytic leukemia and have compared them with the ‘fetal’ repertoire.

我们综述了有关慢性淋巴瘤中抗体序列的文献，并将它们与胎儿抗体库进行了比较。

Shaoxing opera has a whole complete set of performing system and owns rich repertoire.

越剧表演艺术是一个完整的艺术体系，剧目丰富多彩。

repetitive [riˈpetitiv] *a.* 重复的

Confusion associated with repetitive stereotyped movements may indicate ongoing seizure activity.

意识模糊伴有重复的刻板动作可能表示癫痫活动在发展中。

replace [riˈpleis] *v.* 取代，以…代替

Some traditional drugs have been replaced by new ones.

有些传统药物已被新药代替。

Machines have replaced many of the manual procedures, particularly in larger medical institutions.

机器已取代了许多手工步骤，特别是在较大的医疗机构里，更是如此。

If incompetence is dominant the first sound may be softer and the opening snap replaced by a third heart sound.

如果以关闭不全为主时，第一心音可能较柔和，而开放的拍击音则被第三心音所取代。

replacement [riːˈpleismənt] *n.* 取代，置换；补充

The cornerstone of treatment is replacement of fluid and electrolyte losses.

治疗的基础是补充水和电解质的丧失。

The replacement of damaged blood vessels with artificial ones is one of many developments in modern surgery.

用人工血管替代受损伤的血管是现代外科许多进展之一。

replant [ˌriˈplɑːnt] *v.* 再移，移植

It is of practical significance to replant the amputated fingers for a worker with innovative spirit.

为一位具有创新精神的工人进行断指再植手术是有实际意义的。

At autopsy, there was neither gross nor microscopic evidence of rejection of the replanted lung.

尸检时，肉眼与镜下均未见移植肺被排斥的迹象。

replenish [riˈpleniʃ] *v.* (再)装满，(使)充满

In order to replenish the lost bile acid, cholesterol becomes converted to bile acid.

为了补充丢失的胆汁酸，胆固醇就变成胆汁酸。

Therapy of oral Fe should continue for 6 months to replenish tissue stores.

经口服铁的治疗应继续进行 6 个月以补足组织对铁的贮存。

replenishment [riˈpleniʃmənt] *n.* 新补给，补充

If significant malnutrition has occurred, a period of nutritional replenishment is preferable.

如已发生显著营养不良，最好进行一段时期的营养补充。

replicate [ˈreplikeit] *v.* 复制

There has so far been little difficulty in replicating any organ apart from kidneys.

到目前为止，复制除肾脏以外的任何器官困难不大。

replication [ˌrepliˈkeiʃən] *n.* 复制；再试验

Persistent replication of virus may result in further damage to certain organs.
持续的病毒复制可造成某些器官的进一步损害。
Telomerase is the enzyme that directs the replication of telomeres.
端粒酶是指导端粒复制的酶。
Again replication of these findings is necessary.
同样有必要对这些实验结果进行重复试验。

replicative ['replikeitiv] *a.* 复制的
The five viruses of hepatitis are distinct and show no homology of structure, virus family, or replicative cycle.
五种肝炎病毒的不同在于有不同的结构、属于不同的病毒类或不同的复制周期。

repolarization ['riˌpəulərai'zeiʃən] *n.* 再极化,极化恢复
We may be able to detect changes in the cellular function of the muscle by changes in the wave of repolarization.
通过复极波的变化我们可测出肌肉细胞功能的变化。

represent [ˌrepri'zent] *v.* 主张;代表;体现
Delayed cord clamping represents a change in routine practice that favours early contact between a mother and her new born baby.
推迟脐带钳夹是常规医疗操作的一个变革,有利于新生儿与母亲之间最早的接触。

representation [ˌreprizen'teiʃən] *n.* 描写;表现;代表
This book is a vivid representation of the cardiovascular system.
这本书是对心血管系统的生动描述。
The composition of the board reflects the representation of varous interested groups including government.
这个委员会的组成反映了各种利益集团包括政府的代表性。

representative [ˌrepri'zentətiv] *a.* 代表性的
These are two representative popular oral forms of estrogen.
这是两种有代表性的常用口服雌激素。
n. 代表
The medical high tech seminar was expanded to include representatives from a dozen corporations.
医学高新技术研讨会的范围扩大到包括十几家公司的代表参加。

reproduce [ˌriːprə'djuːs] *v.* 繁殖;复制
The zygote grows and reproduces, forming millions of cells which develop into tissues.
受精卵经过生长和繁殖,形成数以百万计的细胞并发展成各种组织。
Many features associated with fever, including back pain, anorexia, can be reproduced by infusion of purified cytokines.
许多与发热有关的特征包括背部疼痛、食欲缺乏,可通过注射纯化的细胞因子再现。

reproducibility [ˌriːprədjuːsə'biliti] *n.* 再现性,复验性
They chose slab gels rather than cylindrical gels because of their reproducibility and the ease in lining up multiple samples.
他们选择板状凝胶而不是柱状凝胶,是因为它们可以复验并便于排列多个标本。

reproduction [ˌriːprə'dʌkʃən] *n.* 生殖,繁殖
The genes control the specific chemical functions of the cell and also control the reproduction of the cells.
基因控制细胞的特殊化学功能,并且还控制细胞的增殖。
The young scientists are studying the reproduction of rabbits.
这些青年科学家正在研究家兔的繁殖。

reproductive [ˌriːprə'dʌktiv] *a.* 生殖的

A woman's reproductive cell carries only female or X chromosomes.
女性生殖细胞只带有雌性染色体，即 X 染色体。
Most doctors recommend reserving assisted reproductive technology (ART) as a last resort for having a baby.
大多数医生建议将辅助生殖技术作为得子的最后手段。
Today, assisted reproductive technology (ART) refers not only to IVF but also to several variations tailored to patients' unique conditions.
现今，辅助生殖技术不仅仅指体外受精，而且还有根据病人量身订做的各种技术。

repulsion [ri'pʌlʃən] *n.* 反式；排斥
Alleles on the different homologues are in repulsion (or trans).
位于不同的同源染色体上的等位基因呈反式。
Repulsion refers to the case where each homologous chromosome has one dominant and one recessive allele from the two genes.
反式是指每个同源染色体各有源自两个基因的一个显性的和一个隐性的等位基因。

require [ri'kwaiə] *v.* 需要，要求
Children require more sleep than adults, and less sleep is needed with advancing age.
儿童比成年人需要更多的睡眠，但随着年龄的增长，睡眠的需要减少。

required [ri'kwaiəd] *a.* 需要的，必需的
Cobalt is an essential element: a required component in vitamin B_{12}.
钴是一种必需元素，是维生素 B_{12} 的必要成分。

requisite ['rekwizit] *n.* 必要条件
Close physical proximity or direct person-to-person contact is the usual requisite for infection.
与物体的密切接触或人与人的直接接触，通常是感染的必要条件。

rescue ['reskju] *v.* 营救，抢救
To rescue the wounded, the doctors did the little that they could.
为了抢救伤员，医生们已经尽了自己的一份力量了。
n. 解救，营救
The mountain climbers survived the rescue.
经过营救，登山运动员们活下来了。

resect [ri'sekt] *v.* 切除
The primary cancer of the colon is usually resected.
原发性结肠癌通常应予切除。
The patient underwent an operation of resecting the obstructing muscle.
这病人曾做过切除梗阻肌肉的手术。

resectable [ri'sektəbl] *a.* 可切除的
Not every case of carcinoma is resectable.
并非每一例癌肿都能切除。

resection [ri'sekʃən] *n.* 切除(术)
Failure to heal, the most common complication, requires resection.
最常见的并发症为长期不愈，需做切除。
There are many methods by which gastric resection may be accomplished.
胃切除可以有许多方法。

resemblance [ri'zembləns] *n.* 相似性
The resemblance between inhibitor and substrate is clear.
抑制剂与底物之间的相似性显而易见。
The tumour cells have no resemblance to ordinary cells.
瘤细胞的外形与正常细胞不同。

resemble [ri'zembl] *v.* 像，类似

Systemic manifestations of anemias due to excessive hemolysis resemble those of other anemias.
由于溶血过度所致贫血的全身症状与其他贫血的症状相似。
As previously mentioned, in appearance, protoplasm resembles the white of an egg.
如前所述,原生质在外观上和鸡蛋白相似。
At the periphery of the lobules are several layers of cells that resemble basal cells of the epidermis and are called germinative cells.
在小叶边缘有数层细胞,类似表皮的基底细胞,称为生发细胞。
There are still other protists that have features which do not resemble either plants or animals.
还有一些原生物其特征既不像植物又不像动物。

reserpine [ˈresəpiːn, riˈsəːpin] *n.* 利血平
Reserpine is now prescribed infrequently in the treatment of schizophrenia.
利血平现在不常用于治疗精神分裂症。

reservation [ˌrezəˈveiʃən] *n.* 储备;保留;预定
There may be some reservations about the proliferation of phage-resistant mutants in the calf intestine.
对于小牛肠道内噬菌体抗性突变株的增殖可能有保留意见。

reserve [riˈzəːv] *n.* 储备;保存
The contraction stress test is a method of assessing placental reserve.
宫缩应激试验是检查胎盘储备能力的方法。
Since the marrow reserve is limited, anemia may result from any massive hemorrhage.
由于骨髓的储备有限,贫血可因任何大出血引起。

reservoir [ˈrezəvwɑː] *n.* 贮器,贮藏所
The bladder has no function other than that of a reservoir.
膀胱除了作为贮器外,别无其他功能。
The cell becomes a silent reservoir for potassium.
细胞成为钾的没有被发现的贮藏所。
Subsequent editions of the book will add further to our reservoir of useful textbooks in geriatric medicine.
此书的后续版本将进一步充实老年医学优秀教科书的内容。

reshaped [ˌriːˈʃeipt] *adj.* 改型的,重组的
Humanized antibody has developed from chimeric antibody and reshaped antibody to the present fully human antibody.
人源化抗体的形成是从最初的嵌合抗体、改型抗体等逐步发展为今天完全的人抗体。
As time passes, memories are consolidated, submerged, perhaps retooled and often entirely reshaped when retrieved later.
随着时间流逝,记忆会被整理、掩盖、或者改变,再次寻回时,常常已经重组。

reside(in) [riˈzaid] *v.* 存在于,位于
It is well established that the thermoregulatory center resides in the anterior hypothalamus.
人们已确认温度调节中枢位于下丘脑前部。
This antibody is induced by repeated exposure to the allergen, and resides in tissue cells.
这种抗体是反复与过敏原接触而引起的,并存留在组织细胞里。

resident [ˈrezidənt] *a.* 居住的
Foreign applicants resident outside the USA might find it impossible to fulfil these conditions.
居住在美国之外的外国报考者可能难以具备这些条件。
n. 居民;住院医师
Increasing numbers of state-supported schools give first priority to state residents.
越来越多的由州赞助的学校给予本州居民优先权。
A resident must receive more training in a speciality in a hospital.

住院医师必须在医院内接受更多的专业训练。

I served as chief resident of the department of internal medicine last year.

去年我曾担任内科的住院总医师。

All patients were operated on by the resident staff under supervision of four members of the attending staff.

所有病人的手术都是住院医生在四名主治医生指导下进行的。

residual [ri'zidjuəl] *a.* 残留的

Most patients recover without residual disability.

大多数病人可以恢复而无伤残后遗症。

Many patients are able to describe the character of the vomitus, and many will have residual vomitus about the face or on their clothing.

大多数病人都能描述呕吐物的特点，而很多人还可能把呕吐物残留在脸上或衣服上。

n. 残差；残渣

Residual analysis was used to check whether the models fitted well.

残差分析用来检验模型是否拟合得好。

The residual plot of this model is shown in Figure 5A.

图 5A 所示为该模型的残差图。

residue ['rezidjuː] *n.* 残留物，残渣；残基

Chemical contaminants include pesticides and drugs used in agriculture, residues of which may persist in food.

化学污染物包括农业上使用的杀虫剂和农药，其残余物可能存留于食物里。

Each chain appears to be so arranged that its hydrophobic residues are buried in the interior of the folded structure.

每条链似乎这样排列，使它的疏水残基被包埋在折叠结构的内部。

resign [ri'zain] *v.* 辞去(职务)；把…交托给

The professor is intending to resign from the committee of malpractice identification.

这位教授打算辞去医疗事故鉴定委员会中的职务。

The parents resign their child to your care.

这对父母亲委托你照顾他们的孩子。

resilience [ri'ziliəns] *n.* 复原力；回弹，弹性；回能

Resilience is the quality that allows us to "survive", and even gain strength from hardship.

复原力指那些能使我们生存下去甚至在困境中获得力量的品质。

resist [ri'zist] *v.* 抵抗，忍住，抗拒

This child can never resist dessert.

这孩子从不拒绝甜食。

Certain types of malaria-carrying mosquitoes have already learned to resist some of the sprays.

某些类型传播疟疾的蚊虫已能对抗某些喷雾剂。

resistance [ri'zistəns] *n.* 阻力，抵抗力；耐力

The increases in heart rate and in peripheral resistance tend to raise the blood pressure.

心率和外周阻力增加势必使血压升高。

Resistance is the general ability of the body to ward off pathogens.

抵抗力是机体阻挡病原体的综合能力。

Microorganisms show resistance to drugs by diversified mechanisms.

微生物可通过多种机制对药物产生耐受性。

resistant(to) [ri'zistənt] *a.* 有抵抗力的；耐药的

Squamous epithelium such as that of the adult vagina is resistant to infection by the gonococcus.

成人阴道的鳞状上皮对淋球菌感染具有抵抗力。

Thus far, no meningococci resistant to penicillin or chloramphenicol have been identified.

至今还没有发现过对青霉素或氯霉素有抗药性的脑膜炎双球菌。

resolute [ˈrezəluːt] *a.* 坚决的，果断的

Security or insecurity, the young physician was resolute to try the acupuncture on his own body.

安全也好，不安全也好，这位年轻医生坚决要在自己身上试着扎针。

resolution [ˌrezəˈljuːʃən] *n.* 消退；消除，消散

Resolution means the complete restoration of normal conditions after the cause of the acute inflammation is removed.

消散意指急性炎症的原因除去后，炎区完全恢复正常状态。

resolve [riˈzɔlv] *v.* 决心；解决；消除；消退

He resolved to do better work in the future.

他决定今后要把工作干得更好。

The nasal discharge was mucoid in character and profuse at the beginning of the illness but has now resolved.

鼻分泌物呈黏液性，在起病时量极多，但现已消失。

The effusion was absorbed after the pleurisy resolved.

胸膜炎痊愈后渗出液被吸收。

resonance [ˈrezənəns] *n.* 反响；叩响；共振，共鸣

Vesicular resonance is the normal pulmonary resonance.

肺泡性叩响是正常的肺部叩响。

The sound of ordinary speech as heard through the chest wall is vocal resonance.

平常讲话的声音可在胸壁听到称为语音共振。

The various harmonics are in resonance in the oral cavity to different degrees.

在口腔中，各种谐音的共鸣程度不同。

This young doctor works in the unit of nuclear magnetic resonance(NMR).

这位青年医生在磁共振室工作。

resonant [ˈrezənənt] *a.* 共鸣的，洪亮的

The chest percussion note is normally resonant.

胸部叩诊正常。

resorb [riˈsɔːb] *v.* 再吸收，重吸收

Small hematomas may resorb, but they increase the incidence of wound infection.

小的血肿可能重吸收，但增大了伤口的感染率。

The major portions of sodium and water in the glomerular filtrate are resorbed in the nephron tubules.

肾小球滤过液中的钠和水大部分在肾小管被重吸收。

resort [riˈzɔːt] *n.* 求助，凭借

In other cases there may be so much damage that replacement is the only resort.

在另一些情况下，(瓣膜)受损过于严重，仅能借助置换来解决。

resources [riˈzɔːsiz] *n.* 资源

Resources management is an important business skill.

资源管理是一项重要的经营技能。

It allows users to effortlessly connect to Internet and network resources.

它可以让用户不费力气就能接到因特网和网络资源上。

respect [risˈpekt] *n.* 尊敬；(*pl.*) 敬意；方面

Young men should always show respect to old people.

年轻人应永远尊敬老人。

I feel great respect for his profound knowledge of medicine.

我对他渊博的医学知识深感敬佩。

The manifestations are in some respects contrary to what are typical of the disease.

在某些方面，其表现与本病的典型表现相反。

v. 尊敬

This doctor is respected by the patients for his noble medical morality.

这位医生由于他高尚的医德而受到病人的尊敬。

respectively [ri'spektivli] *ad.* 分别地，各自地

By 1992, average life expectancy at birth was 73.2 and 79.8 years, respectively, for white males and females.

到 1992 年，白人男性和女性在出生时的平均预期寿命分别是 73.2 岁和 79.8 岁。

The four subclass of human IgG occur in the approximate proportions of 66%, 23%, 7% and 4%, respectively.

人类 IgG 的四种亚型所占的大致比例分别为 66%、23%、7% 和 4%。

respiration [ˌrespə'reiʃən] *n.* 呼吸

The average rate is 12 to 18 respirations per minute in a normal adult at rest.

正常成年人在休息时的呼吸速率是每分钟 12 至 18 次。

After about ten minutes of artificial respiration, the patient came back to life.

在进行大约十分钟人工呼吸后，病人复苏了。

respirator ['respəreitə] *n.* 呼吸器，呼吸机；呼吸罩

The nurse may also use a respirator when respiratory assistance is needed.

在需要协助病人呼吸时，护士还可使用呼吸机。

People are kept alive by respirators that supply oxygen to the lungs and then remove the carbon dioxide.

病人可以依靠呼吸机对肺提供氧气然后排出二氧化碳而继续活着。

respiratory [ris'paiərətəri] *a.* 呼吸（作用）的

In normal adults bronchopneumonia may follow respiratory viral infections.

正常成年人支气管肺炎可在呼吸道病毒感染之后发生。

Acute heart failure may bring about a serious impairment of respiratory exchange.

急性心力衰竭可引起呼吸道气体交换的严重障碍。

respite ['respait, ri'spait] *n.* 暂时的休息；缓解；延期

The noise went on all night without a moment's respite.

噪音一刻不停地持续了一整夜。

vt. 使缓解；使延期

Neck massaging can respite the pain on the neck and the shoulders.

按摩颈部可缓解颈部和肩部的疼痛。

respond (to) [ris'pɔnd] *v.* 回答，反应

Antigen-presenting cells are required by T cells to enable them to respond to antigens.

T 细胞对抗原的反应需要抗原呈递细胞的参与。

The illness quickly responded to the proper treatment.

疾病经适当治疗迅速好转。

T. rubrum infections usually do not respond well to local treatment.

红毛癣菌感染通常局部治疗无效。

responder [ris'pɔndə] *n.* 应答者，反应者

Plasma imipramine levels were significantly higher in responders than nonresponders.

血浆丙咪嗪水平在起反应者身上比不起反应者身上要高得多。

response [ris'pɔns] *n.* 应答，反应，效应

The response to a drug is determined by the unbound fraction that is in the plasma water.

药物的效应是由血浆中未结合部分决定的。

Of more importance is the constriction of pulmonary vessels in response to alveolar hypoxia.

更为重要的是肺泡缺氧可以引起肺血管的收缩。

responsible(for) [ris'pɔnsəbl] *a.* 应负责的，责任重大的

The nervous system is responsible for the coordination of bodily activities.

神经系统负责协调人体的活动。

Bacteria or their products are responsible for most instances of food poisoning.

大多数食物中毒都是由细菌或其产物引起的。

responsive (to) [ris'pɔnsiv] *a.* (对)…迅即感应的

Both organisms are usually responsive to either tetracycline or ampicillin.

这两种细菌通常对四环素或氨苄青霉素均很敏感。

restlessness ['restlisnis] *n.* 不安定，不安宁

Initially, there may be restlessness due to cerebral hypoxia.

开始，由于大脑缺氧，引起烦躁不安。

restoration [ˌrestə'reiʃən] *n.* 恢复；回复，复位

Early restoration of normal quadriceps function will prevent these changes.

股四头肌正常功能的早期恢复能阻止这些改变的发生。

restore [ris'tɔː] *v.* 恢复，修复

The task of medicine is to preserve and restore health and relieve suffering.

医学的任务是保持和恢复健康，解除痛苦。

The victim of shock will die very quickly unless something is done to restore circulation immediately.

如不设法立即恢复血循环，休克病人会很快死亡。

He is entirely restored to health.

他已完全恢复健康。

restraint [ris'treint] *n.* 抑制，制止；节制；约束

The cellular proliferation of a tumor is only relatively free from the usual restraints.

肿瘤细胞的增生只是相对来说不受一般抑制的影响。

Restraints should be used only when there is a reasonable expectation that the patient may harm himself or others.

只有当有理由地估计病人可能会伤害自身或他人时才应进行管制。

restrict [ris'trikt] *v.* 限制，约束

Immunosuppressive therapy has been effective, but its trial should be restricted to nonlimited or idiopathic cases.

免疫抑制疗法已表明有效，但对其试用应限于非受限的或特发性的病例。

T. megninii is probably restricted to Southwest Europe.

麦格毛癣菌很可能仅限于西南欧。

restricted [ris'triktid] *a.* 有限的，受限制的

Each antibody binds to a restricted part of the antigen called an epitope.

每种抗体只与称为表位的抗原有限的部位结合。

restriction [ris'trikʃən] *n.* 限制，控制

For this patient, rigid salt restriction is the most important measure.

对这个病人来说，严格的盐分控制是最重要的措施。

Restriction of the maternal blood flow through the placental site can have a serious effect upon fetal growth and development.

通过胎盘的母体血流的减少可能对胎儿生长和发育产生严重影响。

resume [ri'zjuːm] *v.* 恢复；重新开始

The patient should be allowed up and encouraged to resume normal activities gradually.

应当允许这个病人起床并鼓励他逐渐恢复正常活动。

Anticoagulant therapy may be resumed as early as 24 to 48 hours after most operations.

抗凝血剂疗法可早在大多数手术后24～48小时内恢复使用。

resumption [riˈzʌmpʃən] *n.* 恢复；再开始

The resumption of chemotherapy brought about rapid improvement.

重新使用化学疗法，使病情得以迅速改善。

resuscitate [riˈsʌsiteit] *v.* (使)复苏

The patient developed bradycardia and then had cardiorespiratory arrest and could not be resuscitated.

患者出现心动过缓，接着呼吸心跳停止，复苏无效。

resuscitation [riˌsʌsiˈteiʃən] *n.* 复苏，回生

All preparations should have been made for the resuscitation and special care of babies of low birth weight.

应做好一切准备，进行低出生体重儿的复苏和特殊护理。

A new cardiopulmonary resuscitation methodology has been developed recently.

最近开发出了一种新的心肺复苏术。

retain [riˈtein] *v.* 保持，保留

They retain the immunological memory of particular antigens.

它们保留了对某种特定抗原的免疫记忆。

Maternal IgG antibody may be retained in the infant for as long as 100 days.

母亲的 IgG 抗体可保留在婴儿体内长达 100 天。

retard [riˈtɑːd] *v.* 延缓；妨碍，阻止

The pelvis in rickets is small and continues to be retarded in growth.

佝偻病患者的骨盆狭小，发育一直缓慢。

Meals, especially those with high fat content, retard the absorption of drugs.

进食，特别是含高脂肪的食物能延迟药物的吸收。

Antibiotics consisted of substances that had the capacity to destroy or retard the growth of other microorganisms.

抗生素是能杀灭其他微生物或阻止其生长的物质。

retardant [riˈtɑːdənt] *n.* 阻滞剂

Retardant is a large class of hydrophobic fat and wax-like material, it can delay the dissolution and release process of water-soluble drug.

阻滞剂是一大类疏水性脂肪和蜡样材料，它可延滞水溶性药物的溶解和释放过程。

Enteric material is also a class of coating retardant, we use its dissolution characteristics to produce sustained release in the sustained-release formulations.

肠溶材料亦为一类包衣阻滞剂，在缓释制剂中，我们利用其溶解特性产生缓释作用。

retardation [ˌriːtɑːˈdeiʃən] *n.* 阻滞，迟缓，延迟发育

Mental retardation is one of the attendant complications of measles.

智力发育迟缓是麻疹的并发症之一。

A 15-year-old boy was referred for evaluation of growth retardation and delayed sexual development.

一名 15 岁男孩因生长迟缓和性发育延迟而就诊。

retardate [riˈtɑːdeit] *n.* 智力迟钝者

The moderate group make up about 12% of mental retardates.

在智力迟钝者中，中等程度者约占 12%。

retch [retʃ] *n.* 反胃，干呕

Retches and vomits are commonly lumped together in behavioral analyses.

在行为分析中，反胃和呕吐通常混在一起。

v. 反胃，干呕

If you retch only occasionally, it does not matter; if it is very often, then you must go to see a doctor in the hospital.

偶尔干呕没关系，如果是很经常，那么你应去医院看医生。

Excuse me, what illness can have such manifestations as coughing continuously with retching for a month?

一个月期间持续咳嗽并伴有干呕，请问这样的症状有可能会是哪种病的表现？

retention [riˈtenʃən] *n.* 潴留，停留；保留

Frequency and retention of urine may be caused by pelvic tumours.

尿频或尿潴留可由盆腔肿瘤引起。

Retention of urine is best managed by catheterization as required.

尿潴留在必要时最好通过导管插入予以处理。

Retention of normal ovaries in women after the menopause is still a matter of contention.

绝经期后妇女的正常卵巢是否保留仍然是个有争论的问题。

reticulocyte [riˈtikjuləuˌsait] *n.* 网织红细胞，网状细胞

Since reticulocytes represent a young cell population, it is an important criterion of marrow activity.

由于网织红细胞是幼年细胞，因而是判断骨髓活动的重要标准。

Reticulocytes are generally not increased until treatment is started.

在没有开始治疗之前，网织红细胞一般不增加。

reticulocytopenia [riˌtikjuləusaitəuˈpiːniə] *n.* 网织红细胞减少

There is a reticulocytopenia and a failure to compensate for the anemia with erythroid hyperplasia.

网织红细胞减少而不能以红细胞系增殖来对贫血进行代偿。

Production defects result in a relative or absolute reticulocytopenia.

生成不足可导致相对的或绝对的网织红细胞减少。

reticulocytosis [riˌtikjuləusaiˈtəusis] *n.* 网织红细胞增多（症）

Reticulocytosis is particularly prominent in hemolytic anemias and in acute and severe bleeding.

网织红细胞的增多在溶血性贫血和急性严重失血时特别突出。

Adequate marrow response to anemia is evidenced by reticulocytosis or polychromatophilia.

网织红细胞增多或多染红细胞增多是骨髓对贫血有充分反应的证据。

reticuloendothelial [riˌtikjuləuˌendəuˈθiːliəl] *a.* 网状内皮的

The phagocytic cells consist of polymorphonuclear leukocytes, phagocytic monocytes, i. e., macrophages, and fixed macrophages of the reticuloendothelial system.

吞噬细胞由多形核巨细胞、吞噬性单核细胞（即巨噬细胞）和网状内皮系统的固有巨噬细胞组成。

reticulo-nodular [riˌtikjuləu-ˈnɔdjulə] *n.* 粟粒样结节，网状结节

Nodular or reticulo-nodular opacities widely distributed in the lung fields, chiefly peripherally.

结节影或网状结节影广泛分布于肺野，主要是肺外周。

The typical features of PCP included diffuse reticulo-nodular changes and infiltration patch or ground glass opacification.

卡氏肺孢子虫肺炎（PCP）的典型特征为弥漫性网状结节性改变，和浸润斑或毛玻璃样混浊。

reticulum [riˈtikjuləm] *n.* 网状物，网

The outer of nuclear envelope is contiguous with the endoplasmic reticulum.

核膜的外层与内织网相连。

retina [ˈretinə] (*pl.* retinas 或 retinae [ˈretiniː]) *n.* 视网膜

Light reaches the retina after passing through the cornea, aqueous humor, lens.

光线穿过角膜、房水、晶状体到达视网膜。

The retina may become detached from the choroid and float into the vitreous body.

视网膜有可能脱离脉络膜，漂浮于玻璃体中。

Leukemic infiltrates of the retina and optic disc occasionally occur.
偶尔可发生视网膜和视神经盘的白细胞浸润。

retinal [ˈretinəl] *a.* 视网膜的

Causes of retinal disease include central retinal artery occlusion due to emboli.
视网膜病的病因包括由栓子引起的视网膜中央动脉堵塞。

Retinal hemorrhages are seen in some severely thrombocytopenic children.
一些严重的血小板减少患儿可出现视网膜出血。

n. 视黄醛;维生素 A 醛

In the rods of the eye, retinol is oxidized to retinal.
在眼部视杆细胞里,视黄醇被氧化为视黄醛。

Certain animal tissues or products, such as liver extracts or fish oils, are a direct source of retinal or retinol esters.
某些动物组织或制品,如肝脏提出物或鱼油,是视黄醛或视黄醇酯的直接来源。

retinitis [ˌretiˈnaitis] *n.* 视网膜炎

Cytomegalovirus retinitis is a major cause of blindness in AIDS.
巨细胞病毒性视网膜炎是引起艾滋病人失明的主要原因。

retinoblastoma [ˌretinəublæsˈtəumə] *n.* 视网膜母细胞瘤

Necrotic tumors, especially retinoblastomas, can induce iris neovascularization and glaucoma.
坏死性肿瘤,尤其是视网膜母细胞瘤可导致虹膜新血管形成和青光眼。

Retinoblastoma is the most common primary intra-ocular malignancy of children.
视网膜母细胞瘤是儿童最常见的原发性眼内恶性肿瘤。

retinochoroiditis [ˌretinəukrɔːrɔiˈdaitis] *n.* 视网膜脉络膜炎

Toxoplasma has been estimated to cause 20 to 35 per cent of cases of retinochoroiditis in children and adults.
据估计儿童及成人中弓形虫使 20% ~35% 的病例患视网膜脉络膜炎。

retinoid [ˈretinɔid] *n.* 维甲酸;类维生素 A

I see a huge difference in patients who have used a retinoid for years—they look younger than their counterparts, and their skin is smoother and more resilient.
我看到了使用了几年维甲酸治疗的病人的巨大差别,他们比同龄人看着年轻,他们的皮肤更光滑,更有弹性。

Investigations focused on 3 polymorphisms in retinoid X receptors RXRA and RXRB gene associations. The possible association of their variability with psoriasis was investigated.
研究集中在维甲酸类 X 受体 RXRA 和 RXRB 两个基因的 3 个多态性上,研究了这些多态性与银屑病的关系。

retinol [ˈretinɔl] *n.* 视黄醇、维生素 A

The toxic level of retinol is about 500 times the minimum requirement.
视黄醇的中毒水平大约为其最低需要量的 500 倍。

Our retinol products help stimulate cell regeneration.
我们的视黄醇产品有助于刺激细胞再生。

retinopathy [retiˈnəupəθi] *n.* 视网膜病变

Background retinopathy is evidence of increased capillary permeability.
眼底视网膜病变是毛细血管通透性增加的反应。

retraction [riˈtrækʃən] *n.* 缩回,退缩

Clot retraction is the drawing away of a blood clot from the wall of a vessel; it is a function of blood platelets.
血块凝缩是血凝块从血管壁离开,这是血小板的功能。

Slight skin or nipple retraction is an important sign.
轻微的皮肤或乳头内陷是重要的体征。

There was increased anterior-posterior diameter of the chest with marked retractions during expiration.
有胸部前后径增加,呼气时则明显回缩。

retrieval [riˈtriːvəl] *n.* 检索;取回;恢复

Data storage and retrieval is an essential aspect of application development.
数据存储和检索是应用程序开发的重要方面。

Testicular sperm extraction (TESE) is often an effective method of sperm retrieval for men with non-obstructive azoospermia.
睾丸精子抽吸术是非梗阻性无精症患者获得精子常用的有效方法。

The slowed-down thinking process associated with clinical depression makes the retrieval of memories more difficult.
与临床抑郁症有关的思维过程的衰退使记忆力的恢复更加困难。

retrieve [riˈtriːv] *v.* 取回; 检索

With computer capabilities, a doctor can quickly retrieve information on a certain patient.
借助计算机的功能,医生能很快地检索出某一病人的有关资料。

This code would enable the computer to immediately retrieve the person's stored thermogram for comparison.
这个密码可使计算机能立即检索出此人过去储存的热象图以便进行比较。

retrograde [ˈretrəgreid] *a.* 逆行的

Retrograde amnesia is a failure to remember events immediately preceding an illness or injury.
逆行性遗忘(亦称近事遗忘)是对患病或受伤前刚发生的事件失去记忆。

Retrograde pyelography is helpful when excretory urography is nondiagnostic or contraindicated.
当排泄性尿路造影不能诊断或有禁忌证时,逆行肾盂造影有助于诊断。

When the cannulation is made from other entry sites, the blood may actually flow retrograde.
若将插管插入其他入口则血液将逆向流动。

retrogress [ˈretrəugres] *v.* 倒退,退化

About 20 follicles start to mature, but normally only one matures fully and ovulates while the others retrogress.
约有 20 个卵泡开始成熟,但正常仅有一个卵泡完全成熟和排出,而其他则退化。

retroperitoneal [ˌretrəuˌperitəuˈniːəl] *a.* 腹膜后的

Retroperitoneal fibrosis may cause chronic renal failure.
腹膜后纤维化可引起慢性肾功能衰竭。

Intraabdominal abscesses can be either intraperitoneal or retroperitoneal and are
not associated with a specific organ in 74% of cases.
腹腔内脓肿可出现在腹膜内或腹膜后,而且有 74% 病人不局限于一个脏器。

The pancreas is a retroperitoneal organ extending from the "C" loop of the duodenum to the hilum of the spleen.
胰腺是腹膜后脏器,从十二指肠 C 环延伸至脾门。

retroperitoneum [ˌretrəuˌperitəuˈniːəm] *n.* 腹膜后腔

It is easier to enter retroperitoneum by the straight and closing method.
采用直接闭合式方法进入后腹腔,操作更简便。

We reported a rare case of spontaneous rupture of the biliary tree with biloma in the retroperitoneum.
我们报告了一起腹膜后胆汁瘤引起胆道系统自发性破裂的罕见病例。

retropharyngeal [ˌretrəufəˈrindʒiəl] *a.* 咽后的

However, chewing and swallowing difficulties occur in patients with juvenile rheumatoid arthritis, retropharyngeal abscesses and tetanus.
然而,幼年型类风湿性关节炎、咽后壁脓肿和破伤风患者都可发生咀嚼和吞咽困难。

retrospect [ˈretrəuspekt] *n.* 回顾,追溯

This changing condition is subtle and occasionally identified only in retrospect.

不过这种变化是细微的,仅在回顾性研究中偶尔发现。

retrospective [ˌretrəuˈspektiv] *a.* 回顾的,回想的,追溯的

Retrospective studies examine frequency of childhood loss among child and adult psychiatric patients.

回顾性研究旨在调查儿童和成年精神病人中童年期走失发生的频率。

retrotranslocation [ˌretrəuˌtrænsləuˈkeiʃən] *n.* 逆向转运

Retrotranslocation or retrograde translocation returns endoplasmic reticulum proteins to the cytosol.

逆向转运或逆梯度转运即将内质网蛋白归还到胞质溶胶中。

A membrane protein complex mediates retrotranslocation from the ER lumen into the cytosol.

膜蛋白复合物介导从内质网腔到胞质溶胶的逆向转运。

retrotransposition [retrəˌtrænspəˈziʃən] *n.* 逆转录转座

Retrorransposition involves transcription, generation of a DNA copy of the mRNA, and finally integration of such DNA copies back into the genome.

逆转录转座包括转录、产生 mRNA 的 DNA 拷贝,以及最终把这些 DNA 拷贝整合到基因组中。

Group Ⅱ introns can act as mobile factors spreading within a genome or invading new genomes through the mechanism of retrohoming and retrotransposition.

Ⅱ组内含子通过逆转录归巢和逆转录转座的机制,能够充当在基因组内扩散或者侵入到新基因组中的移动因子。

retroverted [ˌretrəuˈvəːtid] *a.* 后倾的

The lateral position is very useful for assessing descent of the anterior vaginal wall and for viewing the cervix when the uterus is retroverted.

侧位检查有助于评估阴道前壁的下垂程度,而且当子宫后倾时,便于检查宫颈。

retrovirus [retrəuˈvaiərəs] *n.* 逆转录病毒

It is becoming increasingly clear that HIV, the etiologic agent of AIDS, is a human retrovirus.

越来越清楚的是,人类免疫缺陷病毒(HIV),即艾滋病的病原体,是一种人类逆转录病毒。

Dr Caskey uses a certain type of virus, called a retrovirus, as the vehicle for the gene transfer.

卡斯基博士使用一种被称作为逆转录病毒的特定病毒作为基因转移的载体。

return [riˈtəːn] *v.* 恢复

After operation, the patient's digestive function returned to normal.

手术后病人的消化功能已恢复正常。

The patient's temperature has returned to normal.

患者的体温已恢复正常。

reuptake [riːˈʌpteik] *n.* (神经元)重新吸收(神经递质),重新摄取

Atomoxetine is a highly specific norepinephrine reuptake inhibitor.

托莫西汀是一种高度特异性的去甲肾上腺素重吸收抑制剂。

These antidepressants are known as selective seotonin reuptake inhibitors.

这些抗抑郁药物被称作选择性血清素再摄取抑制剂。

revascularization [ˌriˌvæskjuləraiˈzeiʃən] *n.* 再建血管,血管重新吻合

This study establishes a baseline of long-term CABG survival that could be used for comparison with other methods of surgical, or nonsurgical coronary revascularization. (CABG = coronary artery bypass graft surgery)

这项研究确立了冠状动脉旁路移植手术长期存活的基础,可用于与其他手术方法、或非手术冠状血管再形成的比较。

The objective of this study was to describe the results with drug-eluting stents in patients with left

main coronary artery stenosis who were poor candidates for surgical revascularization.
本研究的目的是为了描述左主冠状动脉狭窄而又不太适于外科血管重建术的病人使用药物洗脱支架的一些结果。

The ischemia time of the graft-the time from the actual death of the donor to the revascularization of the graft in the recipient-was 90 minutes.
移植物缺血时间—从供者实际死亡时起到移植物在受者内血管吻合完成—总共是 90 分钟。

reveal [ri'viːl] *v.* 展现,显示

Physical examination revealed a dehydrated,thin man with normal vital signs.
体检显示病人脱水消瘦,但生命体征正常。

Examination of the extremities revealed numerous bruises over the lower ones.
肢体检查显示两下肢有许多瘀斑。

A careful history will often reveal the underlying cause of this type of lower motor neurone lesion.
详细的病史常可揭示这种类型下运动神经损害的基本原因。

reveratrol [rə'verəˌtrɔːl] *n.* 白藜芦醇

Resveratrol may act on different levels of cell signaling.
白藜芦醇可在不同的细胞信号水平发挥作用。

Resveratrol might help to prevent development of obesity or might be suited to treating obesity.
白藜芦醇有助于预防肥胖,还可能适用于治疗肥胖症。

reverberation [riˌvəːbə'reiʃən] *n.* 回响

The muscular contractions that cause respiration are the result of a complex pattern of reverberation in the respiratory center of the brain stem.
引起呼吸的肌肉收缩是脑干呼吸中枢内复杂反射模式作用的结果。

reverse [ri'vəːs] *v.* (使)逆转,回复

Moderate doses may be required to suppress the symptoms,if not to reverse the permanent injury.
需要用中等剂量来抑制症状,即使不能逆转其永久性损害。

With a healthy fetus the change in heart rate is reversed immediately the contraction passes off.
宫缩一消失,健康胎儿的胎心率改变立即恢复原来状态。

a. 逆转的,倒转的

Reverse transcriptase is a RNA-directed DNA polymerase.
逆转录酶是 RNA 指导的 DNA 聚合酶。

Chickenpox may be contracted from a patient with shingles but not the reverse.
接触带状疱疹病人后可患水痘,但反之则不行(即接触水痘病人后不会使人患带状疱疹)。

reversibility [riˌvəːsə'biliti] *n.* 可逆性

The reversibility of biliary cirrhosis is obviously dependent on more than the establishment of bile flow.
胆汁性肝硬化的可逆性显然不只是依赖于胆汁流的建立。

reversible [ri'vəːsəbl] *a.* 可逆的

Anticholinesterases are classified as reversible and irreversible inhibitors.
抗胆碱酯酶药分为可逆性抑制剂和不可逆性抑制剂。

Most forms of reversible injury to surface membranes are not associated with demostrable structural lesions.
表面细胞膜多数形式的可逆性损伤,都不伴有明显的结构病变。

The constriction is reversible upon increase in alveolar PO_2 with therapy.
经治疗使肺泡 PO_2 升高后,这种收缩可以缓解。

reversibly [ri'vəːsəbli] *ad.* 可逆地

Large changes in blood glucose levels can affect refraction reversibly.

血糖水平的大幅度变化可对正常视力调节产生可逆性影响。

revert [ri'vəːt] *v.* 回复

A positive test is suggestive of active infection since serologies usually revert to negative in 6-12 months.

因为血清学检测结果常在 6 ~ 12 月后转为阴性,所以阳性表明现存感染。

review [ri'vjuː] *v.* 回顾;复习;复查

The clinical evidence must be carefully reviewed before deciding to induce labour.

在作出引产决定以前必须仔细复查临床资料。

Patients operated upon for ectopic pregnancies were reviewed.

做过宫外孕手术的患者均已经过复查。

n. 评论,综述

The reader is referred to recent comprehensive reviews of this subject for further details.

更详尽的细节,请读者参阅最近关于这一主题的广泛综述。

revision [ri'viʒən] *n.* 修订,修改

Major revisions in these clinical practice guidelines can be anticipated in the future.

可以预期将来会对这些临床医疗准则进行重大修改。

revive [ri'vaiv] *v.* (使)复苏,(使)回生

Manual CPR is successful in reviving a victim only 15 percent of the time, said a Johns Hopkins expert.

约翰斯·霍普金斯大学的一名专家说,人工心肺复苏术使患者复苏的成功率目前仅为 15%。

rewarding [ri'ɔːdiŋ] *a.* 值得做的

This area of study has been very rewarding to scientists.

这个研究领域对于科学家们来说是值得探讨的。

rhabdomyoblast [ˌræbdəu'maiəblæst] *n.* 横纹肌母细胞

The rhabdomyoblast is the diagnostic cell in rhabdomyosarcoma, and it contains eccentric eosinophilic granular cytoplasm rich in thick and thin filaments.

横纹肌母细胞是横纹肌肉瘤的诊断性细胞,其胞浆具有偏位的嗜酸性颗粒,富含粗细肌丝。

Rhabdomyoblasts may be round or elongate and may contain cross-striations visible by light microscopy.

横纹肌母细胞可以圆形、细长形,具有光镜可见的横纹。

rhabdomyoma [ˌræbdəumai'əumə] *n.* 横纹肌瘤

Rhabdomyoma is a benign tumor arising from striated muscle.

横纹肌瘤是起源于横纹肌的良性肿瘤。

Cardiac rhabdomyomas are the most common primary tumor of the heart in infants and children and are associated with tuberous sclerosis.

心脏横纹肌瘤是婴幼儿和儿童心脏最常见的原发肿瘤,与结节性硬化相关。

rhabdomyosarcoma [ˌræbdəuˌmaiəusɑː'kəumə] *n.* 横纹肌肉瘤

Rhabdomyosarcoma is histologically subclassified into embryonal, alveolar, and pleomorphic variants.

横纹肌肉瘤组织学上分为胚胎性、腺泡性和多形性三种。

Rhabdomyosarcoma, the most common soft-tissue sarcoma of childhood and adolescence, mostly occurs in the head and neck or genitourinary tract.

横纹肌肉瘤是儿童和青少年最常见的软组织肉瘤,大多数发生于头颈部和泌尿生殖道。

rheology [ri'ɔlədʒi] *n.* 流变学

Rheology studies the flow of unusual materials, particularly non-Newtonian fluids such as mayonnaise, paint, molten plastics, and foams.

血液流变学研究不寻常材料的流动，特别是非牛顿流体，如蛋黄酱、油漆、熔融塑料和泡沫。

Rheology is the study of the flow of materials that behave in an interesting or unusual manner.

流变学是研究材料的流动，这些材料以一种有趣的或不寻常的方式表现。

rheum [ˈriːəm] *n.* 大黄属

Among them, the acetone extract of Rheum showed the strongest inhibitory activity.

其中，大黄的丙酮提取物显示有最强的抑制活性。

rheumatic [ruːˈmætik] *a.* 风湿性的

Thirty per cent of patients with mitral stenosis give no history of rheumatic fever.

30%二尖瓣狭窄的患者无风湿热病史。

Rheumatic fever is a bacterial infection whose victims are usually children and adolescents.

风湿热是一种细菌性感染，其罹患者通常为儿童和青少年。

rheumatism [ˈruːmətizəm] *n.* 风湿病

Poisons from diseased tonsils may cause heart ailments and rheumatism.

患病的扁桃体分泌的毒素可以引起心脏疾患和风湿病。

Nodose rheumatism is also called rheumatoid arthritis.

结节性风湿病也称作类风湿关节炎。

The climate does not agree with a patient with rheumatism.

这种气候不适合风湿病患者。

rheumatoid [ˈruːmətɔid] *a.* 类风湿病的

In the early phase of rheumatoid arthritis the disease is characterized by remissions and relapses.

类风湿关节炎的早期特点是时好时坏。

Rheumatoid arthritis is an inflammatory disease which affects the general health.

类风湿关节炎是一种影响全身健康的炎症性疾病。

Examples of autoimmune disease are rheumatoid arthritis and pernicious anaemia.

自身免疫病的实例是类风湿性关节炎和恶性贫血。

rheumatologist [ˌruːməˈtɔlədʒist] *n.* 风湿病学家

Most rheumatologists favor oral prednisone in low doses with favorable response.

大多数风湿病学家赞成口服小剂量的强的松，有良好效果。

rheumatology [ˌruːməˈtələdʒi] *n.* 风湿病学

Rheumatology is a medical specialty concerned with the diagnosis and management of disease involving joints, tendons, muscles, ligaments and associated structures.

风湿病学是涉及关节、肌腱、肌肉、韧带和相关结构的疾病诊断和治疗的一门医学专业。

rhinitis [raiˈnaitis] *n.* 鼻炎

Acute nonstreptococcal pharyngitis is usually more severe than acute viral rhinitis.

非链球菌急性咽炎通常比病毒性急性鼻炎更为严重。

Allergic rhinitis is the most common cause of persistent or recurrent nasal discomfort.

过敏性鼻炎是持续性或反复发作性鼻部不适的最常见原因。

Seasonal allergic rhinitis is commonly caused by exposure to grasses, trees, weeds and molds.

季节性过敏性鼻炎通常由于接触草、树、种子和霉菌引起。

rhinoplasty [ˈrainəuˌplæsti] *n.* 鼻整形术

In fact, it is the preferred material for numerous grafts in modern rhinoplasty.

事实上，它是现代鼻整形术中众多移植物的首选材料。

Rhinoplasty is precise surgery in which the margin of error is measured in millimeters.

鼻整形术是非常精确的手术，误差范围以毫米衡量。

rhinorrhea [rainəˈriːə] *n.* 鼻(液)溢

A 9-week old female infant comes to the clinic with a 3-week history of rhinorrhea and a 2-week history of cough.

一个 9 周女婴，有流涕史 3 周、咳嗽史 2 周而来诊所。

rhinovirus [ˌrainəuˈvaiərəs] *n.* 鼻病毒

Rhinoviruses are clearly the most common cause of this syndrome in adults.

鼻病毒显然是成人中这种综合征的最常见原因。

Rhinoviruses are considered to be etiologically associated with the common cold and certain other respiratory ailments.

鼻病毒被认为是与感冒或某些其他呼吸道疾病的病因有关。

rhomboid [ˈrɔmbɔid] *n.* 菱形肌

Rhomboid help to move the shoulder blade backwards and upwards.

菱形肌帮助肩胛骨向后和向上活动。

rhonchus [ˈrɔŋkəs] （*pl.* rhonchi [ˈrɔŋkai]） *n.* 干啰音，鼾音

Rhonchi or scattered moist rales may be present as a manifestation of branchitis.

支气管炎的一个表现是出现干啰音或散在性湿性啰音。

rhythm [ˈriðəm] *n.* 节奏，节律

The patient's own heart rhythm becomes slower than the preset pacing rate of the artificial pacemaker.

病人自身的心脏节律变得比人工起搏器的预调起搏率慢。

rhythmic [ˈriðmik] *a.* 有节律的，有节奏的

The rhythmic contractions of the heart muscle cause the beat of the heart.

心肌有节律的收缩造成心脏的跳动。

The slow rhythmic contraction and relaxing of the muscles in the walls of the intestine is called peristalsis or peristaltic motion.

小肠壁肌肉缓慢而有节奏的收缩和松弛就称为蠕动。

rhythmically [ˈriðmikəli] *ad.* 有节奏地

Most cardiac muscle fibers are capable of contracting rhythmically.

大多数心肌纤维都能节律性地收缩。

rib [rib] *n.* 肋骨

These ribs are connected to the sternum by means of costal cartilages.

这些肋骨通过肋软骨与胸骨连接。

ribavirin [ˌraibəˈvaiərin] *n.* 利巴韦林（抗病毒药；商品名：virazole）

Ribavirin is used to treat severe virus pneumonia in infants and young children.

利巴韦林用于治疗婴儿和幼儿的重症病毒性肺炎。

To help clear up your infection completely, ribavirin must be given for the full time of treatment.

为了彻底消除感染，利巴韦林服药必须达到治疗全程。

riboflavin [raibəuˈfleivin] *n.* 核黄素，维生素 B_2

Riboflavin is a respiratory coenzyme.

核黄素是一种呼吸辅酶。

Riboflavin was first isolated in pure form from milk whey.

核黄素首先是从牛奶乳清中分离提纯而得。

ribonuclease [ˌraibɔˈnjuːklieis] *n.* 核糖核酸酶

Ribonuclease is an enzyme located in the lysosomes of cells, that splits RNA at specific places in the molecule.

核糖核酸酶是存在于细胞溶酶体中的酶，它可在分子的特殊位置上分裂 RNA。

ribonucleic acid [ˌraibəunjuːˈkliːik-ˈæsid] *n.* 核糖核酸

The cytoplasm contains protein molecules known as ribonucleic acids (RNA) and small granular structures called mitochondria.

细胞质含有称为核糖核酸（RNA）的蛋白质分子和称为线粒体的小颗粒结构。

ribonucleoprotein [ˈraibəuˌnjuːkliəuˈprəutiːn] *n.* 核糖核蛋白

Heterogeneous nuclear ribonucleoprotein A1 is an RNA-binding protein that modulates splice site usage, polyadenylation, and cleavage efficiency.
异质性核糖核蛋白 A1 是一种可以调节拼接位点使用、聚腺苷酸化和剪切效率的 RNA 结合蛋白。
The promoter of the gene of La ribonucleoprotein domain family (LARP2) was significantly hypermethylated in β-thalassemia.
在 β-地中海贫血中,La 核糖核蛋白域家族(LARP2)基因启动子呈现明显的高度甲基化。

ribosomal [ˌraibəˈsəuməl] *a.* 核糖体的
All bacteria possess ribosomal RNAs.
所有的细菌都有核糖体 RNA。

ribosome [ˈraibəsəum] *n.* 核糖体
These granules are called ribosomes.
这些颗粒被称作核糖体。
Electron micrographs reveal large numbers of ribosomes.
电子显微照片能见到大量核糖体。

ribozyme [ˈraibəzaim] *n.* 核酶
Such ribozymes have been used successfully to prevent HIV infection of cells in culture.
这样的核酶已有效地用于阻止培养细胞的 HIV 感染。

rich [ritʃ] *a.* 丰富的;富于脂肪的
The doctor suggests that the patient should not eat large amounts of especially rich foods.
医生建议这个病人不要吃大量特别油腻的食物。

rickets [ˈrikits] *n.* (用作单或复) 佝偻病
Rickets is benefited by an increase of calcium and phosphorus in the blood.
增加血液中的钙和磷对治疗佝偻病有益。
The most common symptoms of vitamin D deficiency are rickets in young children.
幼儿维生素 D 缺乏最常见的症状是佝偻病。

rickettsia [riˈketsiə] (*pl.* rickettsiae [riˈketsiiː]) *n.* 立克次体
Rickettsiae are like viruses, in that they grow only in living organisms.
立克次体像病毒,因为它们只有在生物体内才能生长。
Rickettsiae are larger than viruses and can be seen with light microscope.
立克次体比病毒大,可以在光学显微镜下看到。

rickettsial [riˈketsiəl] *a.* 立克次体的
The purpose of lumbar puncture is to determine the presence and nature of bacterial, spirochetal, viral, fungal, or rickettsial infection of the meninges.
腰椎穿刺的目的是判断脑膜是否被细菌、螺旋体、病毒、真菌或立克次体感染及感染的性质。

rickettsiosis [riˌketsiˈəusis] *n.* 立克次体病 (*pl.* -ses)
A rickettsiosis is a disease caused by intracellular bacteria.
立克次体病是由胞内菌引起的一种疾病。
Rickettsioses are usually transmitted to humans by arthropods.
立克次体病通常是由节肢动物传播给人类。

rid [rid] (of) *v.* 使摆脱,使去掉
Treatment is aimed at ridding the patient of edema and abolishing the proteinuria.
治疗的目的是要去掉病人的水肿和消除蛋白尿。

ridge [ridʒ] *n.* 嵴,脊,棱线
The neighboring portion of the nail becomes dark, ridged, and separated from its bed.
邻近的指甲部分变黑,有嵴,并与甲床分离。
The ridges of the annular syphilid are made up of minute flat-topped papules, the boundaries be-

tween which may be difficult to discern.
环状梅毒疹的嵴是由很小的平顶型丘疹融合而成,其分界不明显。

rifampin [ˈrifəmpin] *n.* 利福平
Rifampin is bactericidal and is effective against intracellular as well as extracellular tuberculous organisms.
利福平是杀菌剂,对细胞内、外结核菌均有效。
Rifampin is an antibiotic that inhibits prokaryotic RNA polymerase.
利福平是能抑制原核 RNA 聚合酶的一种抗生素。

rifamycin [ˈrifæmaisin] *n.* 利福霉素
Rifamycin is used as an antibiotic to treat certain infections, particularly tuberculosis.
利福霉素是用于治疗某种感染,尤其是结核病的一种抗生素。

rigid [ˈridʒid] *a.* 严格的,僵硬的
Sometimes the abdominal muscles become rigid over this area.
有时该区的腹部肌肉变得僵硬。
When hyponatremia is present in the presence of edema, rigid water restriction is also advised.
如果有水肿的同时又有低钠血症,则应严格控制水的摄入。

rigidity [riˈdʒiditi] *n.* 僵硬,坚硬
Calcification contributes to the rigidity of the valve.
钙化增加瓣膜的僵硬程度。
Cervical rigidity is present at an early stage in almost every case of meningitis.
几乎每一例脑膜炎的患者都在发病早期出现颈项强直。

rigor [ˈraigɔː, ˈrigə] *n.* [拉] 寒战,发冷;强直,僵硬
A rigor, a profound chill, is common in bacterial diseases and in influenza.
寒战,极度畏寒,常见于细菌感染性疾病和流感。
Rigors are also common with drug-induced fevers.
寒战也常见于药物所致的发热。

rigorous [ˈrigərəs] *a.* 严格的;严密的,精确的
The Mormons observe rigorous dietary restrictions.
摩门教徒遵守严格的饮食限制。
He made a rigorous investigation of the medicinal herbs in the area.
他对这个地区的中草药做了认真的调查研究。

ringworm [ˈriŋwəːm] *n.* 癣,癣菌病
Ringworm is highly contagious and can be spread by direct contact or via infected materials.
癣有高度接触传染性,能直接接触传染或通过被污染物而传播。
Ringworm that is moderately severe, that is unresponsive to topical therapy, or that involves the scalp and nails should be treated systemically.
较严重的癣病,或外用药无效,或侵及头皮和指甲,均应该全身用药治疗。

rinse [rins] *v.* 冲洗;脱色
After 60 sec, the iodine solution is washed off with water and the slide is rinsed with 95% alcohol for 15-30 sec.
60 秒钟后用水洗去碘液,标本片用 95% 的乙醇脱色 15 ~ 30 秒钟。

risk [risk] *n.* 危险,风险
Infants of the diabetic mothers are at increased risk for the respiratory distress syndrome(RDS).
糖尿病母亲的婴儿患呼吸窘迫综合征的危险性增加。
However, they might have had reduced risk of acute respiratory distress syndrome.
然而,它们可能已经降低了急性呼吸窘迫综合征的风险。

risky [ˈriski] *a.* 危险的,有风险的
Coronary arteriography is risky, especially in the very sick patients.

冠状动脉造影是有危险的,特别是对重病患者。

It is a risky thing to operate upon this baby.

给这个婴儿动手术是有风险的。

ritalin [ri'tælin] *n.* 利他林,盐酸哌醋甲酯

Ritalin is a mild central nervous system stimulant.

利他林是一种温和的中枢神经系统兴奋剂。

Over the past decade there has been an increase in pupils taking legal drugs, such as Ritalin, to help focus their mind and increase their alertness.

过去十年里,越来越多的学生使用如利他林这些合法药物来帮助他们集中注意力,提高敏感度。

RNA 核糖核酸

RNA(Ribonucleic acid) is a chemical found in the nucleus and cytoplasm of cells.

RNA(核糖核酸)是细胞核和细胞质中的一种化学物质。

RNA plays an important role in protein synthesis and other chemical activities of the cell.

RNA 在蛋白质的合成过程及细胞的其他化学活动中起重要作用。

There are several classes of RNA molecules, including messenger RNA, transfer RNA, ribosomal RNA, and other small RNAs, each serving a different purpose.

RNA 可分为几类,包括信使 RNA、转运 RNA、核糖体 RNA 和其他小分子 RNA,每类执行一种不同的功能。

robot ['rəubɔt, 'rəubət] *n.* 机器人; 遥控机械

In early November of 2002, American surgeons repaired the atrial septal defects for 17 patients using the robot for assistance.

2002 年 11 月初,美国的外科医生们利用机器人的辅助给 17 位患者修补了房中隔缺损。

Medical researchers praise robot-guided heart surgery which has many advantages for both patients and doctors,

医学研究人员盛赞机器人指引的心脏手术,它对患者和医生双方都有许多好处。

robotic [rəu'bɔtik] *a.* 机器人的

More and more patients will have their heart defects repaired in a robotic operation in the future.

将来愈来愈多病人的心脏缺损可以用机器人手术进行修补。

Robotic-assisted surgery takes nearly double the amount of time that a typical open-heart surgery takes.

机器人辅助手术所需的时间接近常规开心手术时间的两倍。

robotics [rəu'bɔtiks] (复) *n.* [用作单] 机器人学;机器人技术

As robotics develop, physically handicapped persons will have mechanical servants to aid them in seeing, speaking and moving about.

随着机器人技术的发展,生理上有缺陷的人将会有机器人侍者帮助他们看、说和走动。

robustly [rəu'bʌstli] *adv.* 坚定地、稳定地、明确地

The experiments confirm that this algorithm can segment the moving targets accurately and track them robustly among the image sequence of hundreds of frames.

实验证实,这种算法在数百帧的图像序列中,能准确地分割出运动目标,并稳定跟踪它们。

In some registries, comparison groups may be less robustly defined than in more formal observational designs.

在有些注册登记中,对照组的定义可能不如更为正式的观察性设计那样明确。

rod [rɔd] *n.* 杆,柱;视杆细胞

These organells in their fully developed form are rod-shaped with a vacuole at one end, and resemble a tennis racquet.

发育成熟的细胞器呈杆状,其一端有空泡,形状类似网球拍。

The human eye contains about 125 million rods, which are necessary for seeing in dim light.

人的眼睛有 1 亿 2 千 5 百万个在暗淡光线中看东西所需要的视杆细胞。

rodent[1] [ˈrəudənt] *n.* 啮齿动物

Rodent cells, which are more sensitive to cadmium than human cells, accumulate higher levels of cadmium in the nucleus.

啮齿动物的细胞比人的细胞对镉更敏感,其细胞核内蓄积有较高浓度的镉。

rodent[2] [ˈrəudənt] *a.* 侵蚀性的

Rodent ulcers occur in middle age or later; if untreated, they destroy skin, muscle, and bone but they do not spread to other parts of the body.

侵蚀性溃疡发生在中年或中年以后。若未经治疗,则可破坏皮肤、肌肉和骨骼,但不向身体其他部位扩散。

roentgen [ˈrɔntjən, ˈrɔntgən] *n.* 伦琴(X 线量单位)

Roentgen is the international unit of X-or γ-radiation.

伦琴是 X 或 γ 射线的国际单位。

Thanks to an absent-minded professor, medical science obtained one of its most useful tools: roentgen-ray.

多亏一位心不在焉的教授,医学科学获得其最有用的工具之一:X 射线。

If it is considered necessary, roentgen-ray examination is made too.

如果认为必要的话,还可做 X 线检查。

roentgenogram [ˌrɔntˈgenəgræm] *n.* X 线(照)片

This collapse of the lung can readily be recognized in the roentgenogram.

肺萎陷很容易在 X 线片上被识别出来。

An opaque foreign body in the neck will be clearly demonstrated on a lateral roentgenogram.

颈部的不透光异物可在 X 线侧位片上清楚地显现出来。

roentgenographic [ˌrɔntgənəˈgræfik] *a.* X 线照相术的

The diagnosis of rickets is finally confirmed by serum chemical determinations and roentgenographic examination.

佝偻病的诊断最后可通过血清化学测定和 X 线照片加以证实。

roentgenography [ˌrɔntgeˈnɔgrəfi] *n.* X 线照相术

Roentgenography of the gallbladder and biliary tract is the principal means of diagnosis of cholecystitis.

胆囊和胆管的 X 线照相是诊断胆囊炎的主要方法。

rosacea [rəuˈzeiʃiə] *n.* 酒渣鼻,红斑痤疮

Initially, individuals with rosacea demonstrate a pronounced flushing reaction.

起初,患酒渣鼻的人都有一个明显的脸发红的反应。

roseola [rəuˈziːələ, rəuziˈəule] *n.* 蔷薇疹,玫瑰疹

The early eruptions are symmetrical, more or less generalized, superficial, nondestructive, exanthematic, transient, macular roseolas.

早期皮疹是呈对称性的,或多或少是全身性的、表浅的、非残毁性的、发疹性的、暂时性的斑状玫瑰疹。

rosin [ˈrɔzin] *n.* 松香

Rosin can be used as a glazing agent in medicines and chewing gum.

松香可作为药物和口香糖的上光剂。

Rosin is an ingredient in printing inks, photocopying and laser printing paper, varnishes, adhesives (glues), soap, paper sizing, soda, soldering fluxes, and sealing wax.

松香是印刷油墨、复印和激光打印纸、清漆、黏合剂(胶水)、肥皂、造纸施胶、苏打水、助焊剂和封蜡的组成成分。

rotate [rəuˈteit] *v.* 旋转;使轮流,使交替

Tourniquet may be placed around three extremities and rotated every 15 minutes.

止血带可以每 15 分钟交替地在三个肢体上使用。

Student were required to rotate through in-patient and out-patient clinical departments in hospital.

学生们要在医院的住院部和门诊部各个临床科室轮回实习。

The internship may be of the rotating type, consisting of several months of service in medicine, surgery and paediatrics.

医生实习期可能为轮回类型,在内、外、儿科各实践几个月。

rotation [rəu'teiʃən] *n.* 旋转,轮换

Extension and lateral rotation of the neck may narrow the neural foramen and reproduce the symptoms.

颈部伸展和向一侧转动可使神经孔狭窄,重现一些症状。

When the appendix lies on the left side due to transposition of viscera or failure of normal bowel rotation during embryonic life, the symptoms occur on the left.

由于内脏移位或胚胎期肠道旋转异常,使阑尾位于左侧,阑尾炎症状就出现在左侧。

rough [rʌf] *a.* 粗糙的;粗略的;剧烈的

The surface of papules may be smooth or rough.

丘疹的表面或光滑或粗糙。

roughly ['rʌfli] *ad.* 粗略地,大致

These medical instruments are at a cost of roughly 2000 yuan.

这些医疗器械约值 2000 元。

Its severity increases with age and is roughly correlated with the degree of arteriosclerosis.

疾病的严重程度随着年龄增加,大致与动脉硬化的程度有关。

round-the-clock ['raund-ðə-'klɔk] *n.* 一昼夜

Purified oxygen at 2 atm. pressure is kept in the hyperbaric chamber for a round-the-clock period.

让处于两个大气压的纯氧在高压舱内保持 24 小时。

route [ruːt] *n.* 路线,途径

Plasma infusions can also be used to administer IgG by the i. v. route to patients with antibody deficiencies.

对抗体缺乏的患者,也可通过静脉途径输入血浆供给 IgG。

routine [ruː'tiːn] *n.* 常规,惯例;日常工作

These physical examinations are done as a matter of routine.

这些体格检查项目只是一种惯例的做法。

Making morning rounds is part of a doctor's daily routine.

早晨查房是医生日常工作的一部分。

a. 日常的,常规的

Without the history, the physical examination is simply a routine mechanical procedure.

没有病史,体检只不过是常规的机械操作。

The inquiry is followed by a routine examination.

问诊之后接着进行常规检查。

routinely [ruː'tiːnli] *ad.* 常规地

Enemas need not be given routinely.

灌肠不需要常规施行。

Indomethacin should not be used routinely and chronically as an analgesic and an antipyretic substance.

消炎痛不应作为镇痛和解热的常规和长期用药。

rubella [ru'belə] *n.* 风疹

Rubella is an acute contagious disease.

风疹是一种急性的接触传染病。

rubeola [ruːˈbiːələ] *n.* 麻疹

Rubeola is an acute febrile illness predominantly affecting children.

麻疹是主要影响儿童的急性发热性疾病。

Rubeola can also make a pregnant woman have a miscarriage or give birth prematurely.

麻疹也可能导致孕妇流产或早产。

rubor [ˈruːbə] *n.* 红,发红

These aspects of inflammation were known by the Latin terms rubor(redness),tumor(swelling), dolor(pain),etc.

古代拉丁语用红、肿、痛等词表达人们对这些炎症现象的了解。

rudimentary [ruːdiˈmentəri] *a.* 残遗的,已退化的

The sense of smell,though extremely highly developed in some lower animals,is almost rudimentary in man.

嗅觉虽然在某些低等动物中高度发达,在人却几乎是残留的。

rule(out) [ruːl] *v.* 排除,取消

Gastric carcinoma cannot be ruled out in this case.

对这个病例,不能排除胃癌的可能性。

rump [rʌmp] *n.* 臀部

The growth of crown-heel length,crown-rump length,head circumference and biparietal diameter of fetus was faster before the 28 gestational week than after it.

胎儿的顶踵长、顶臀长、头围、双顶径的生长速度在 28 周前要快于 28 周后。

rupture [ˈrʌptʃə] *n.* 破裂

Severe hemorrhage is due to rupture of a large artery in the base of the ulcer.

严重出血是由于溃疡底部的大动脉破裂。

Cases complicating rupture of a tuberculous cavity will also require treatment as for pneumothorax.

并发结核空洞破溃的病例需要像治气胸那样予以治疗。

v. (使)破裂

The mycotic aneurysms most commonly occur in the brain and they may rupture.

真菌性动脉瘤最常发生于大脑,并可破裂。

The necrotic wall of the intestine is likely to rupture and its contents escape.

坏死的肠壁很可能发生破裂而使肠内容物逸出。

rural [ˈruərəl] *a.* 农村的

People living in rural areas tend to have shorter lives and higher levels of illness and disease risk factors than those in major cities.

生活在农村地区的人往往比那些生活在大城市的人有更短的寿命和更高等级的疾病风险因素。

China will continue to improve medical services in rural areas.

中国将继续改善农村地区的医疗服务。

rust [rʌst] *n.* 铁锈

At first there is a hard,dry,painful cough which later on,in older children,produces a rust-colored sputum.

最初,有剧烈的干咳,咳嗽疼痛,继之,年龄较大的儿童吐铁锈色痰。

S

sac [sæk] *n.* 囊

The sac is filled with an exudate secondary to tumour or inflammation.

囊内充满了肿瘤或炎症的渗出液。

saccharin [ˈsækərin] *n.* 糖精

Saccharin finds its widest use in the preparation of popular low caloric beverage.

糖精在制备大众化的低热量饮料中用途最广。

saccharomyces [ˌsækərəuˈmaisiːz] *n.* 酵母菌

Any unicellular fungus of the genus Saccharomyces is called yeast.

酵母菌属的所有单细胞真菌都叫做酵母菌。

sacral [ˈseikrəl] *a.* 骶骨的

The sacral vertebrae are as many as the lumber ones.

骶椎和腰椎一样多。

Advanced syphilis may cause destruction of the sensory roots of the sacral nerves.

晚期梅毒可造成对骶骨神经感觉根的破坏。

X-ray therapy of these tumors may produce sacral pain from necrosis of tissue and injury to nerve roots.

用 X 线治疗这些肿瘤后,由于组织坏死和神经根受损可引起骶部疼痛。

sacroiliitis [ˌseikrəuˌiliˈaitis] *n.* 骶髂关节炎

Sacroiliitis and ankylosing spondylitis are commoner in patients with ulcerative colitis.

骶髂关节炎和强直性脊柱炎是溃疡性结肠炎患者的常见病。

sacrum [ˈseikrəm] *n.* 骶骨

His abdominal girth increased,accompanied by the development of edema in the sacrum and lower extremities.

他的腰围增大,伴有骶骨和下肢水肿。

The sacral vertebrae are fused together in the adult to form a single borne,the sacrum.

在成年人,多个骶椎被融合在一起成为一块较大的骨骼,即骶骨。

safeguard [ˈseifgɑːd] *n.* 保护措施,安全装置

She smeared her skin with sun-tan lotion as a safeguard against sun-burn.

她将皮肤搽上防晒剂以免阳光灼伤。

v. 保护

Effective measures have been taken to better safeguard the health of children.

已经采取了有效措施以便更好地保护儿童的健康。

safety [ˈseifti] *n.* 安全性

A growing attention has been recently paid to the safety and quality of drinking water due to its importance in people' s daily life.

由于饮用水在人们日常生活中的重要作用,它的安全性和质量已经越来越受到人们的关注。

The group says health and safety issues are an important part of the anti-counterfeiting message.

这个团队表示健康和安全问题是防伪信息的重要组成部分。

safflower [ˈsæflauə] *n.* 红花,红花染料

Safflower is a highly branched,herbaceous,it is commercially cultivated for vegetable oil extracted from the seeds.

红花是一种高度分支的草本植物，其商业化培育是为了从种子中提取植物油。

Safflower seed oil is flavorless and colorless, and nutritionally similar to sunflower oil. It is used mainly in cosmetics and as a cooking oil, in salad dressing, and for the production of margarine.

红花籽油无味无色，与葵花油营养类似。它主要用于化妆品和用作烹调油、沙拉酱调料和生产人造黄油。

sag [sæg] *v.* 下垂，松垂

As a result, the skin may sag.

结果，皮肤就松弛下垂了。

saikosaponin [ˌsaikəuˈsæpəunin] *n.* 柴胡皂苷

This paper reports the experiment of saikosaponin extraction using macroporous absorptive resin.

这篇文章报道了大孔吸附层析分离提取柴胡皂苷的实验研究。

Saikosaponin K, L, M, N, Q and T were discovered lately.

在柴胡属植物中新发现柴胡皂甙 K、I、M、N、Q、T。

salbutamol [ˌsælˈbjuːtəmɔl] *n.* 舒喘宁，舒喘灵，嗽必妥

If the child has not responded well to inhaled salbutamol, intravenous hydrocortisone is indicated.

如果患儿在吸入舒喘宁之后仍未奏效，则可采用静脉注射氢化可的松。

salicylate [sæˈlisileit] *n.* 水杨酸盐

Acute arthritis can be relieved with salicylates or with corticosteroids.

急性关节炎可用水杨酸类或皮质激素缓解病情。

Hippocrates understood the medical value of the leaves and tree bark which contain salicylates.

希波克拉底懂得含有水杨酸的树叶和树皮的药用价值。

saline [ˈseilain] *a.* (含)盐的，咸的

The patient received 3 liters of normal saline solution.

病人接受了三升普通盐水输液。

n. [səˈlain] 盐水

To prevent dehydration the patient was given an infusion of glucose and saline.

给病人输葡萄糖和盐水，以防脱水。

saliva [səˈlaivə] *n.* 涎，唾液

Moistened by the saliva in the mouth, the food is broken up into small pieces by the teeth.

食物在口中经唾液弄湿后，被牙齿嚼碎成小块。

Saliva contains mucin and the enzyme amylase.

唾液中含有黏蛋白和淀粉酶。

Sweat and saliva are also minor routes of excretion of toxicants.

随同汗液和唾液排泄也是毒物排泄较次要的途径。

salivary [ˈsælivəri] *a.* 唾液的

Proliferation of lymphocytes in lacrimal and salivary glands may cause bilateral painless enlargement.

泪腺和唾液腺淋巴细胞增生，可引起两侧腺体无痛性肿大。

salivate [ˈsæliveit] *v.* 大量流口水

A dog salivates when it sees a bone.

狗一看见骨头就流口水。

salivation [ˌsæliˈveiʃən] *n.* 分泌唾液

Pupillary reflexes of this shock patient are lost, and salivation and sweating are absent or diminished.

此休克病人的瞳孔(对光)反射消失，唾液分泌和出汗消失或减少。

A small but regular salivation is maintained to promote cleanliness in the mouth when food is not being eaten.

即使不是正在进食,少量规则的流涎仍存在,以促进口内清洁。

Morning sickness is characterized by nausea, vomiting, and salivation, usually in the first trimester, but not necessarily in the morning.

孕妇晨病的特征为恶心、呕吐和流涎,通常见于第一个三月期,但不总是在早晨发生。

salmonella [sælmə'nelə] (*pl*. salmonellae [sælmə'neliː]) *n*. 沙门氏菌

Typhoid fever is the classical example of enterical fever caused by salmonellae.

伤寒是由沙门氏菌引起的肠热症的典型实例。

salmonellosis [ˌsælmənə'ləusis] *n*. 沙门氏菌病

Ampicillin is an alternative drug for therapy of known salmonellosis.

氨苄青霉素为治疗已知的沙门氏菌疾病的替代药。

Many of the foodborne diseases have declined in recent decades, but salmonellosis and some others have defied all efforts to control them.

许多由食物传染的疾病近几十年来已有所减退,但对沙门氏菌病和其他一些疾病的控制却收效甚微。

salpingectomy [ˌsælpin'dʒektəmi] *n*. 输卵管切除术

The operation of salpingectomy involving both tubes is a permanent and completely effective method of contraception.

切除两侧输卵管的输卵管切除术是永久性和完全有效的避孕方法。

salpingitis [ˌsælpin'dʒaitis] *n*. 输卵管炎

The most common cause of ectopic pregnancy is salpingitis, untreated or inadequately treated.

输卵管炎未得到治疗或治疗不彻底是异位妊娠最常见的病因。

After infection of the cervix gonococcus may ascend to the endometrium and Fallopian tubes, causing acute salpingitis.

宫颈淋球菌感染后可以上行至子宫内膜和输卵管,引起急性输卵管炎。

salpingography [sælpiŋ'gɔgrəfi] *n*. 输卵管造影术

30 cases of follow up showed 8 intrauterine pregnancies (IUPs) and 1 ectopic pregnancy after recanalization and 5 IUPs after selective salpingography.

随访 30 例,输卵管再通术后有 8 例宫内妊娠和 1 例宫外孕,选择性输卵管造影术后有 5 例宫内妊娠。

Salpingography or liquid flowing test was performed 3 months after treatment, and the tubal patent rate was 90%.

治疗后 3 个月作输卵管造影或通液试验,输卵管通畅率达 90%。

salpingostomy [ˌsælpiŋ'gɔstəmi] *n*. 输卵管造口(引流)术,输卵管复通术

It must also be remembered that salpingostomy may merely allow the formation of another pregnancy in the damaged part of the tube.

应当记住输卵管造口术可能仅仅是使受损的输卵管发生再次妊娠。

salvage ['sælvidʒ] *n*. (疾病的)抢救

This measure improves fetal salvage to a significant degree.

这个措施在较大程度上提高了对胎儿的救治。

Measures for severe burns salvage are greatly improved in recent years.

严重烧伤抢救措施近年来有很大改进。

v. 抢救

The hospital is taking emergency measures to salvage these poisoned patients.

医院正在采取紧急措施抢救这些中毒病人。

The doctor will try to salvage the patient's leg.

医生将尽力保住这个病人的腿。

sample [ˈsɑːmpl] *n.* 样本,标本

A computer is used to reconstruct images from hundreds of thousands of X-ray data samples.

计算机可用来从成百上千个 X 线数据样本中重建影像。

Random sample is a sample chosen from a population in such a way that each choice is independent of the other choices.

随机样本是以不受其他选择约束的方式选择的一个样本。

Sodium concentrations in urine samples vary widely, and depend on the volume of urine excreted as well as the tubular reabsorption of sodium.

尿液标本中钠离子浓度波动很大,取决于尿量和肾小管对钠离子的重吸收。

sampling [ˈsɑːmpliŋ] *n.* 取样

Major limitations of renal biopsy include the risk and inconvenience of the procedure as well as the potential for sampling errors.

肾活检的主要局限性在于有危险性,操作过程不方便和有取样错误的可能 。

sanatorium [ˌsænəˈtɔːriəm] (*pl.* sanatoria [ˌsænəˈtɔːriə]) *n.* 疗养院

This patient will be transferred to a newly-built sanatorium.

这个病人将要转到一个新建的疗养院去。

The number of local sanatoria established by regional health departments is growing at a rapid rate.

由地区卫生部门建立的地方疗养院数量正在迅速增加。

sanguisorba [sænˈgaisɔːbə] *n.* 地榆,地榆属

Sanguisorba is a hemostatic agent in TCM.

地榆为中医常用止血药。

Sanguisorba has a great value in clinical medicine.

地榆有很高的临床药用价值。

sanitary [ˈsænitəri] *a.* 卫生的,保健的

The food, water, and sanitary facilities here are acutely substandard.

这里的食物、水和卫生设备都比一般标准低得多。

Conditions were not sanitary and many attendants were poorly trained if they had any training at all.

环境不卫生,而且许多服务人员即使受过任何训练的话也是很差的。

sanitation [sæniˈteiʃən] *n.* 卫生,卫生设备

One quarter of the world' s present population still lacks safe drinking water and proper sanitation.

现在世界上 1/4 的人仍缺少安全饮用水和适合的卫生环境。

saponin [səˈpəunin, ˈsæpənin] *n.* 皂苷

Owing to their low UV absorption, the triterpene saponins were detected by evaporative light scattering.

由于其较低的紫外吸收度,三萜皂苷可通过蒸发光散射来检测。

Phytochemical screening revealed the presence of alkaloids, flavonoids, anthrones and saponins in the aqueous fraction.

植物化学成分筛选显示水馏分中存在生物碱、黄酮类、蒽酮和皂苷。

saprophytic [ˌsæprəuˈfitik] *a.* 腐物寄生性的

Most fungi are saprophytic.

大多数真菌为腐物寄生性。

sarcoid [ˈsɑːkɔid] *n.* 肉样瘤,结节病

When seen on chest radiograph, this appearance is sometimes called "alveolar sarcoid," although the nodules are discrete and interstitial.

在胸片上这种表现被称为"肺泡型结节病",虽然结节其实散布于间质内。

Bilateral cervical adenopathy is also prominent in tuberculosis, coccidioidomycosis, sarcoid, lymphomas, and leukemias.
双侧颈部腺病在结核、球孢子菌病、肉样瘤、淋巴瘤和白血病中也很突出。

sarcoidosis [ˌsɑːkɔiˈdəusis] *n.* 结节病
A chest X-ray helps to exclude sarcoidosis and bronchial carcinoma.
胸部 X 线检查有助于排除结节病和支气管癌。
Sarcoidosis may be one of the potential causes of some unproven abnormalities in brain, spinal cord, cranial and peripheral nerves.
结节病可能是某些原因不明的脑、脊髓、颅神经及周围神经异常的潜在病因之一。

sarcoma [sɑːˈkəumə] (*pl.* sarcomas 或 sarcomata [sɑːˈkəumətə]) *n.* 肉瘤
Metastasis through blood vessels is the common route for sarcomas.
血管是肉瘤常见的转移途径。
Cases which have been described as recurrent fibromyomata were probably sarcomata.
曾被描述为复发性纤维肌瘤的病例可能即为肉瘤。

sarcomatoid [sɑːˈkəumətɔid] *n.* 肉瘤样的
Various carcinomas in the bladder may assume sarcomatoid growth patterns and be mistaken histologically for sarcomas.
膀胱的多种癌可呈现肉瘤样生长方式，组织学上会误诊为肉瘤。
Sarcomatoid mesothelioma is the rarest form of mesothelioma and is generally the most difficult to diagnose, however treatment options are available.
肉瘤样间皮瘤是最罕见的间皮瘤，通常最难以诊断，但有可供选择的治疗方案。

sarcomatous [sɑːˈkəumətəs] *a.* 肉瘤的
Sarcomatous change may be suspected if there is pain, with a rapid increase in size of the tumour.
如有疼痛且肿瘤迅速长大，可怀疑为肉瘤变。

sarcomere [ˈsɑːkəmiə] *n.* 肌(原纤维)节
The sarcomere is the basic contractile unit of skeletal muscle.
肌节是骨骼肌的基本收缩单位。

sarin [ˈsærin] *n.* 沙林毒气
Sarin may have more severe long-term effects on women than on men, according to a study of the victims of the infamous nerve gas attack on Tokyo's underground.
根据对臭名昭著的东京地铁神经毒气案受害者的研究，沙林毒气可能对妇女比对男人有更加严重的长期影响。

SARS [sɑːz] 严重急性呼吸系统综合征(severe acute respiratory syndrome 的缩略词)
Symptoms of SARS(severe acute respiratory syndrome) include high fever, aches, dry cough and shortness of breath.
严重急性呼吸系统综合征的症状有高热、疼痛、干咳和气短。
Experts have linked SARS to a new form of coronavirus, other forms of which usually are found in animals.
专家们认为 SARS 是由一种新型的冠状病毒引起，其他型的此种病毒通常存在于动物身上。

satellite [ˈsætəlait] *n.* 卫星；卫星病灶；卫星结节
Satellite pustules are scattered along the periphery of the main macule.
卫星样小脓疱分散地沿着主斑的周围分布。
Pseudochancre redux is distinguished from relapsing chancre chiefly by the absence of satellite glands and by a negative darkfield examination.
复发性假性下疳与复发性下疳的主要区别在于没有近卫淋巴结(肿大)，且(在镜下的)暗视野里找不到螺旋体。

satiation [ˌseiʃiˈeiʃən] *n.* 满足,饱满

"Obesity gene " really appears to be more of a "satiation gene".

实际上,"肥胖基因"似乎不仅仅是"饱食基因"。

satiety [səˈtaiəti] *n.* 饱满感(食欲或渴感),厌腻

Then wait 20 minutes, the time it takes the brain to register satiety signals.

然后等 20 分钟,这 20 分钟是大脑记录饱食信号所需的时间。

Satiety means full gratification of appetite or thirst, with abolition of the desire to ingest food or liquids.

饱足感的意思是食欲和口渴充分得到满足而消除了摄食和摄液体的欲望。

satisfactorily [ˌsætisˈfæktərili] *ad.* 令人满意地

Only a small amount of equipment is needed to assess satisfactorily the ocular status.

只需要少量设备,就可满意地测定眼睛的状况。

satisfactory [ˌsætisˈfæktəri] *a.* 令人满意的,良好的

Your recovery from typhoid fever is quite satisfactory.

你患伤寒恢复的情况很令人满意。

If the lesion is made to bleed, it is necessary to wait until free bleeding has stopped to obtain satisfactory plasma.

如损伤被弄出血,必须等待出血停止,再取适合用的血浆。

satisfy [ˈsætisfai] *v.* 满足

Angiotensin converting enzyme(ACE) inhibitors satisfy these requirements and have become the most useful and widely used vasodilators.

血管紧张素转化酶抑制剂满足了这些需要,已成为最有效和使用最广泛的血管扩张剂。

Some physicians are satisfied with a diagnosis of manifestations and treat without an etiological diagnosis.

某些医生满足于症状学诊断,并在没有病因诊断的情况下治疗。

saturable [ˈsætʃərəbl] *a.* 可饱和的

Secretion of uric acid is a saturable process that is blocked by some commonly used medications.

尿酸的分泌是一个可饱和的过程,可被一些常用的药物阻断。

saturate [ˈsætʃəreit] *v.* 使饱和

The rate of the reaction will increase until the available enzyme becomes saturated with substrate.

反应速度会加快直到所有参与反应的酶都达到饱和状态。

A high intake of saturated fats and Trans fats can increase the levels of bad cholesterol.

饱和脂肪与反式脂肪的高摄入会提高有害胆固醇的水平。

saturation [ˌsætʃəˈreiʃən] *n.* 饱和,饱和剂量

The binding sites of the protein are not unlimited and are subject to saturation.

蛋白结合的部位不是无限的,而是可以饱和的。

sausage [ˈsɔsidʒ] *n.* 香肠

Generally mitochondria are sausage-shaped.

通常情况下线粒体呈香肠状。

save[1] [seiv] *v.* 救;节省

Unfortunately, all efforts to save the patient were futile.

遗憾的是一切抢救病人的努力均无效。

This technical innovation will save us much time and labour.

这次技术革新可为我们节约大量时间和劳力 。

save[2] [seiv] *prep.* 除…以外

Chemotherapy should not, save in exceptional instances, be employed in the absence of a diagnosis.

除非在特殊情况下,没有确诊时不应采用化疗。

scab [skæb] *n.* 痂

Scab is a hard crust of dried blood, serum, or pus that develops during the body's wound-healing process over a sore, cut or scratch.

痂是由干涸的血、血清或脓结成的硬壳,是身体上疮口、刀伤或抓伤等创伤愈合过程中产生的。

scaffold [ˈskæfəuld] *n.* 支架,骨架

The scaffold can be in any size or shape so that blocks of bone can be produced.

支架可以是不同的大小和形状,以便产生不同的骨块。

Scaffold proteins are adaptor-type proteins with multiple binding sites for proteins, which bring together specific proteins into a functional signaling complex.

支架蛋白是接头型蛋白,具有多个蛋白质结合位点,可将特异性蛋白组装成功能性的信号复合物。

IKAP is a scaffold protein of the IκB kinase complex.

IKAP 是 IκB 激酶复合物中的一种支架蛋白。

scald [skɔːld] *v.* 烫伤

A pot of coffee fell from the stove and scalded his hand.

一壶咖啡从炉子上掉下来并烫伤了他的手。

The cut surface has a rather cloudy appearance, slightly opaque, as if scalded in hot water.

切面十分混浊,不太透明,仿佛是在热水中烫过一样。

n. 烫伤

A sunburn or a mild scald is an example of a first-degree burn.

晒斑及轻度烫伤是一度烧伤的实例。

scalding [ˈskɔːldiŋ] *n.* 烫伤;烧灼样痛

Burns from scalding or hot metals tend to be superficial and managed on an outpatient basis.

烫伤或热金属引起的灼伤往往比较表浅,在门诊处可处理。

scale¹ [skeil] *n.* 标度,刻度;等级;规模;量表

On a worldwide scale, gonorrhea is one of the most frequent infectious diseases.

就全世界范围来讲,淋病是最常见的感染性疾病之一。

Low down in the scale of life we find that there are simple animals consisting of only one cell.

在低等生命中,我们发现存在着只是由一个细胞构成的简单动物。

The scale was tested for its validity, reliability and responsiveness.

对量表进行了效度、信度以及反应度的检测。

scale² [skeil] *n.* 鳞片,鳞屑

Secondary lesions are of many kinds, of which the most important are scales, excoriations, fissures, crusts, erosions, ulcers and scars.

继发性损害有许多类型,其中最重要的是鳞屑、表皮剥脱、皲裂、痂、糜烂、溃疡和瘢痕。

v. 脱屑,生鳞(屑)

Pustules heal with scaling and scarring.

脓疱脱屑和结痂而愈。

In due course, continued exposure leads to dryness, scaling and fissuring.

持续接触一定的时间后可引起干燥、鳞屑和裂隙。

scalp [skælp] *n.* (人的)头皮

If head, neck and scalp muscles are held too tightly, a tension headache may result.

如果头、颈和头皮部位的肌肉绷得太紧,可使人产生张力头痛。

scalpel [ˈskælpəl] *n.* 解剖刀,手术刀

There are two scalpels and you may use either of them.

有两把手术刀,你可以使用其中任何一把。

The surgeon discards the scalpel he has used to cut through the outer skin.

外科医生将切开外层皮肤用过的手术刀扔在一边。

scan [skæn] *v.* 扫描

These lesions can be identified with a high degree of accuracy by CT scanning.

CT 扫描能够高度准确地识别这些病变。

scanner ['skænə] *n.* 扫描仪,扫描器

In the experiment, the addict inside the scanner signalled that he was enjoying himself.

实验中,扫描器里边的吸毒者用信号表示他感觉愉快。

New generation CT scanners are faster and have larger numbers of detectors, thus scan time is markedly shortened and images are rapidly constructed.

新一代的 CT 扫描器进行速度更快,而且拥有更多的探头,因此扫描时间明显缩短,图像形成得很快。

scanning ['skæniŋ] *n.* 断续言语

Scanning speech is caused by disease of the cerebellum or its connecting fibres in the brainstem.

断续言语是由小脑或其在脑干中连接纤维的疾患所致。

scant [skænt] *a.* 欠缺的,不足的

There is scant information on the adrenal histologic findings in this disorder.

目前关于这种类型疾患,肾上腺组织学所见的资料尚感不足。

scanty ['skænti] *a.* 不充足的,缺乏的;稀疏的

The distal colon has a scanty lymph drainage, and consequently spread of the malignant cells is slow.

远端结肠缺乏淋巴引流,因此恶性肿瘤细胞的扩散较慢。

scar [skɑː] *n.* 瘢痕,伤疤

Sometimes the necrotic area is replaced by scar that does not contract.

有时坏死区域由不能收缩的瘢痕所代替。

v. 结疤;愈合

Throughout history smallpox has killed or scarred millions of people.

天花在历史上曾使数百万人死去或留下瘢痕。

scarce [skεəs] *a.* 缺乏的,不足的

More recent experience with single-lung transplants for these patients has been satisfactory, thus utilizing scarce donors more effectively.

最近对这些病人进行单个肺移植的结果是令人满意的,因此能更有效地利用来源不足的供体。

In some skin sites such as the back, adnexa of all types are comparatively scarce.

在某些部位如背部的皮肤,各类型皮肤附属器相对缺少。

scarcely ['skεəsli] *ad.* 缺乏地,几乎没有

The rooms were packed so closely with beds that there was scarcely space to walk between.

房间里摆满了病床以致几乎没有空间供通行。

There is scarcely a place on earth which is naturally free of microorganisms.

世界上几乎没有一个地方是天然地没有微生物的。

The body ordinarily is constantly undergoing a scarcely perceptible desquamation in the form of tiny, thin epidermal particles.

机体通常不断地有几乎查觉不出的细小而薄的表皮颗粒脱落。

scarlet ['skɑːlit] *a.* 猩红的

Scarlet fever is frequently complicated by nephritis.

猩红热常合并肾炎。

n. 猩红色

Scarlet is much lighter than crimson.

猩红色比深红色要浅得多。

Biebrich scarlet, water-soluble, is an azo dye used as a plasma stain.
水溶性比布里希猩红是一偶氮染料，用于原生质染色。

scatter [ˈskætə] *v.* (使)分散，散布

Rhonchi or scattered moist rales may be present as a manifestation of bronchitis.
干性啰音或散在湿性啰音可能作为支气管炎的一种征象出现。

Scattered daydreamers are easily bored and distracted.
精神不集中式的白日梦者易厌烦和注意力分散。

scavenger [ˈskævindʒə] *n.* 清除剂；清扫工

Scavenger cell is a cell which absorbs and removes irritant products.
清除细胞是一种能吸收和清除刺激物的细胞。

scenario [siˈnɑːriəu] *n.* (行动的)方案，事态，局面

In this scenario, one best practice is to have a notification sent promptly to the sponsor's safety group when a case report form of a serious adverse drug reaction is submitted.
这一行动方案中，最好的做法是当一份严重药物不良反应的病例报告表提交后，要立即向申办方安全小组发出通知。

The many possible scenarios are well illustrated by examples at the medical theoretical extremes.
通过医学理论上一些极端实例可充分说明许多可能的场景。

schedule [ˈʃedjuːl, ˈskedʒuːl] *n.* 时间表

Our guests have taken time from busy schedules to come here to join us for these discussions.
我们的客人在繁忙的工作中抽出时间来参加这些讨论。

They accomplished the task on schedule.
他们按时完成了任务。

v. 排定，安排

The transplantation of the liver is scheduled for the 20th instant.
肝脏移植手术定于本月 20 日进行。

Certain goals should be scheduled for accomplishment in a short period.
某些目标应当安排在短期内完成。

schisandrin [ʃiˈsændrin] *n.* 五味子素

We establish a HPLC method for the determination of schisandrin in Shengmai tablet.
我们建立了高效液相色谱(HPLC)法来测定生脉片中五味子素的含量。

Antioxidant response induced by schisandrin B is partly mediated by cytochrome P-4502E1 catalyzed reaction in mouse liver.
五味子乙素的抗氧化效应部分由小鼠肝脏细胞色素 P-4502E1 的催化反应介导。

schistosome [ˈʃistəsəum] *n.* 血吸虫

Infection occurs during immersion in fresh water containing schistosome cercariae.
感染发生于人体浸入带有血吸虫尾蚴的淡水中时。

The schistosome species infecting humans all share the same basic life cycle.
感染人类的各种血吸虫的基本生活史都相同。

Man is the definitive host of schistosomes and snails are their intermediate hosts.
人是血吸虫的最后宿主，而钉螺是它们的中间宿主。

schistosomiasis [ˌʃistəusəˈmaiəsis] *n.* 血吸虫病

On the individual level, schistosomiasis may be prevented by avoidance of contaminated waters.
对个人来说，避免接触被污染的水可预防血吸虫病。

The spread of schistosomiasis has already been brought under control in this region.
这个地区血吸虫病的传播已经得到控制。

schizont [ˈskizɔnt] *n.* 裂殖体

Rupture of schizonts liberates toxic and antigenic substances which cause further damage.
裂殖体破裂释放出有毒物质和抗原性物质，它们会更进一步的造成损害。

schizophrenia [ˌskizəuˈfriːniə] *n.* 精神分裂症

The lifetime prevalence rate for schizophrenia is about 1%.

精神分裂症的终身发病率约为 1%。

Schizophrenia is perhaps the most puzzling of all mental illnesses.

精神分裂症或许是所有精神病中最令人迷惑的。

Schizophrenia occurs most commonly in temporal lobe epileptics.

精神分裂症最常见于颞叶癫痫病人。

schizophrenic [ˌskizəuˈfrenik] *a.* 精神分裂症的

It was found that schizophrenic disorder is more prevalent in the central area of a city.

人们发现精神分裂症在城市中心较为多见。

Certain drugs reduce the risk of relapse of schizophrenic disorders.

某些药物可减少精神分裂疾患复发的危险性。

n. 精神分裂症患者

The social networks of schizophrenics are smaller than those of normal people.

精神分裂症患者的社交网络比常人要小。

schizophreniform [ˌskizəuˈfrenifɔːm] *a.* 精神分裂症样的

Schizophreniform disorder meets all the criteria for schizophrenic disorder except for duration.

除了持续时间不同外,精神分裂症样疾病符合精神分裂症的所有标准。

scholarship [ˈskɔləʃip] *n.* 奖学金;学问

Does this university award scholarships to freshman?

这所大学给新生提供奖学金吗?

The book shows meticulous scholarship.

该书表现出做学问的缜密方法。

schwannoma [ˌʃwɑːˈnəumə] *n.* 神经鞘瘤

Schwannomas are benign nerve sheath tumors composed of Schwann cells.

神经鞘瘤是良性的神经鞘肿瘤,由施万细胞构成。

Schwannoma is composed of both a cellular Antoni A area and a loose paucicellular Antoni B area.

神经鞘瘤由细胞丰富的 Antoni A 区和少细胞的 Antoni B 区组成。

sciatic [saiˈætik] *a.* 坐骨的

Sciatic nerve runs down behind the thigh from the lower end of the spine; above the knee joint it divides into two main branches.

坐骨神经起自脊柱下部末端,沿大腿后面下行,在膝关节上方,分成两个主支。

sciatica [saiˈætikə] *n.* 坐骨神经痛

Sciatica is pain along the distribution of the sciatic nerve.

坐骨神经痛是指沿着坐骨神经分布区域的疼痛。

After operation the patient was free from right-sided sciatica for sixteen months.

手术后,病人长达 16 个月的右侧坐骨神经痛的折磨已被解除。

scintigraphy [sinˈtigrəfi] *n.* 闪烁扫描术,闪烁显像

Myocardial perfusion scintigraphy provides complementary data for assessing ischemic burden.

心肌灌注闪烁扫描术可为评估缺血负荷提供补充资料。

Most malignant tumors are cold on scintigraphy.

闪烁显像检查中恶性肿瘤多为冷显像。

scintillation [ˌsintiˈleiʃən] *n.* 闪烁

The radiation intensity through the motor is determined with a scintillation counter.

发动机的辐射强度可用闪烁计数器来确定。

Scintillation optical fiber is applied to ray imaging more and more widely.

闪烁光纤在射线成像方面的应用越来越广泛。

scirrhous [ˈsirəs, ˈski-] *n.* 硬癌的

Female breast scirrhous carcinomas have an abundant collagenous stroma and are stony hard.

女性乳腺硬癌具有丰富的胶原性间质，质地如石般坚硬。

Carcinomas of the gallbladder with infiltrating growth pattern are scirrhous and have a very firm consistency.

浸润性生长的胆囊癌是硬癌，质地非常坚实。

scissors [ˈsizəz] [复] *n.* 剪(刀)

When the lesion is a vesicle, it is clipped off close to the margin by small pointed scissors.

损害若为小水疱，可用小尖头剪刀沿着它的边缘剪取。

Boiling in a water bath is a traditional method of sterilizing instruments such as scissors, knives, syringes, etc.

在水浴锅中煮沸的传统方法可用来消毒剪刀、刀子、注射器等器械。

sclera [ˈskliərə] *n.* 巩膜

Leukemic nodules are occasionally found in the cornea and sclera.

白血病小结有时可发现于角膜和巩膜内。

The cornea is continuous at its periphery with the sclera.

角膜的外缘与巩膜是相连的。

sclerite [ˈskliərait] *n.* 骨片

We take sclerites of SD rats for cell culture.

我们取 SD 大鼠的骨片来进行细胞培养。

The symmetry of left and right sclerites proves a bilaterally symmetrical body of the animal.

左右骨片对称证实该动物身体两侧是匀称的。

scleritis [skliəˈraitis] *n.* 巩膜炎

Scleritis of patients with rheumatoid arthritis is rarer but more serious.

巩膜炎在类风湿关节炎病人中较罕见，如果有则更严重。

Scleritis is of unknown aetiology but is often associated with collagen disease.

巩膜炎的病因尚不清楚，但常与胶原性疾病有关。

sclerodactyly [ˌskliərəuˈdæktili] *n.* 肢端硬化(指端硬化)

The most classic symptom of scleroderma is a type of skin tightening called sclerodactyly.

硬皮病最典型的症状是一种皮肤发紧感，称为肢端硬化。

When sclerodactyly first starts to develop, a person may notice his or her fingers start to swell, but not subside over time.

当指端硬化最初开始进展时，患者可能注意到他或她的手指开始肿胀，且不随时间消退。

scleroderma [skliərəˈdəːmə] *n.* 硬皮病

Scleroderma, localized or systemic is a disease of unknown cause in which there is sclerosis of connective tissue.

硬皮病，局部的或全身的，是原因不明的疾病，疾病的特点是结缔组织硬化。

Scleroderma is complicated by atrophy, ulceration, calcinosis, and/or pain.

硬皮病的并发症为萎缩、溃疡、钙质沉积和(或)疼痛。

scleromalacia [ˌskliərəuməˈleiʃiə] *n.* 巩膜软化

Scleromalacia perforans is even less common and occurs in long-standing rheumatoid arthritis.

巩膜软化穿孔更为少见，可见于长期患类风湿关节炎的病人。

sclerosis [skliəˈrəusis] *n.* 硬化(症)

Patients with slowly progressive systemic sclerosis can lead productive and useful lives.

缓慢进行的全身性硬化患者，生活中可作出有贡献和有益的事情。

Hypertension is followed by sclerosis as man is followed by his shadow.

硬化症随高血压而来正如影子随人而行一样。

Vaccines for different types of cancers, HIV and multiple sclerosis could also be available.

还可获得针对多种癌症、艾滋病以及多发性硬化症的疫苗。

sclerotherapy [ˌskliərəuˈθerəpi] *n.* 硬化疗法

Sclerotherapy therefore leads to worsening of gastropathy.

硬化疗法因此导致了胃病恶化。

The esophageal varices of 45 cases with cirrhotic patients were treated by endoscopic sclerotherapy with non-water ethanol totalling 96 times.

对 45 例肝硬化并发食管静脉曲张的患者,在内镜下用无水酒精行总共 96 次硬化治疗。

scoliosis [ˌskɔliˈəusis] *n.* 脊柱侧凸

Scoliosis means lateral (sideways) deviation of the backbone, caused by congenital or acquired abnormalities of the vertebrae, muscles, and nerves.

脊柱侧凸指脊柱向侧面偏斜,由先天的或后天的脊椎、肌肉、神经异常所致。

Idiopathic scoliosis is the most common variety. A familial type is also reported.

特发性脊柱侧凸是最常见的类型,家族性的脊柱侧凸也有报道。

scopolamine [skəˈpɔləmiːn] *n.* 东莨菪碱

Scopolamine depresses the CNS and in therapeutic doses causes fatigue, hypnosis, and amnesia.

东莨菪碱可抑制中枢神经系统,其治疗量可引起疲倦、催眠和遗忘。

score [skɔː] *n.* 分数;得分;二十;许多

The volleyball team of our college won the match with the score of 5 to 3.

我们学院的排球队以 5 比 3 获胜。

The expected life span of three score and ten is simply not enough hereafter.

70 岁的预期寿命今后是完全不够的。

Scores of foreign scholars visited our hospital last year.

一大批外国学者去年参观了我们的医院。

scotoma [skɔˈtəumə] *n.* 盲点

All people have a scotoma in the visual field of each eye due to the small area of retina occupied by the optic disc.

所有人每只眼睛的视野内都有一个盲点,这是由于视网膜上这个小区被视神经盘占有而形成的。

scout [skaut] *n.* 定位

Before CT scanning, scout view can determine the scanning range, reasonable scout view can effectively control the radiation dose.

CT 扫描前,定位像可以确定扫描范围,合理的定位像能够有效控制照射剂量。

scrape [skreip] *v.* 擦,刮

When dry or scaly, the material is scraped off with a scalpel or curet.

若遇到干燥或者有鳞屑,则可用解剖刀或刮器刮下。

n. 擦伤

The leaves of the tree kill harmful bacteria in cuts and scrapes.

此树的树叶可杀死割伤和擦伤伤口中的有害细菌。

scratch [skrætʃ] *v.* 搔,抓

Itching is an unpleasant cutaneous sensation which provokes the desire to scratch or rub the skin.

痒是一种令人不快的皮肤感觉,它使人产生搔抓或者摩擦皮肤的欲望。

n. 擦伤,抓伤

A break in the skin resulting from an animal or insect bite, a burn, a scratch, or surgery allows the entry of pathogenic agents.

由于动物或昆虫叮咬、烧伤、擦伤或手术引起的皮肤破损使病原体进入人体。

screen [skriːn] *n.* 屏,幕

The interventional operation for this liver cancer patient is shown on the screen.

这位肝癌病人的介入手术显示在屏幕上。

v. 筛选;检查

New drugs are now carefully screened before release for general use.

目前,新药在仔细审查后才允许广泛应用。

Blood transfusion units now screen all donor blood for the presence of hepatitis B virus.

目前输血中心对所有的供血进行乙型肝炎病毒的检查。

Women 50 to 59 years of age who took part in a breast cancer screening program have a mortality rate 46% less than those who had not been screened.

50～59 岁年龄组的妇女加入乳腺癌的普查计划,其乳腺癌的死亡率比那些不参加普查的妇女低 46%。

screening [ˈskriːniŋ] *n.* 筛选;集体检诊,普查

Developmental screening tests alert clinicians to biological aspects underlying the behavioral disorder.

发育普查检验使临床医师们意识到行为疾病的生物学基础。

Theoretically, screening for infective agent-specific fetal antibody (IgM or IgA) should provide a more reliable diagnosis.

从理论上看,对特异胎儿抗体(IgM 或 IgA)的感染原的筛查应该是一种更为可靠的诊断方法。

scrotum [ˈskrəutəm] *n.* 阴囊

Around the time of birth the testicles normally descend from the abdominal cavity into the scrotum.

通常在出生前后,胎儿的睾丸自腹腔下降至阴囊。

The autotransplantation of the testicle to the scrotum for cryptorchidism is now being performed routinely.

将自体睾丸回纳到阴囊以治疗隐睾症,现在是常规手术。

scrub [skrʌb] *v.* (施行手术前)擦洗并消毒(手、臂)

A five minutes' scrubbing of the hands and forearms with soap and water is the routine for surgeons before operating.

在手术前用肥皂和水擦洗五分钟的手和前臂,对外科医生来说是常规。

scrutiny [ˈskruːtini] *n.* 细看,详察

Escherichia coli is the organism under closest scrutiny.

大肠杆菌是人们研究得极为仔细的生物体。

scurvy [ˈskəːvi] *n.* 坏血病

Acute deficiency of ascorbic acid intake leads to the classic disease of scurvy.

急性抗坏血酸摄入不足可导致典型的坏血病。

seal [siːl] *v.* 封,密封

Bleeding continues, if the blood does not clot to seal the wound.

如果血不凝固以致伤口不能封住,就会继续流血。

They (the lungs) are tightly sealed in the chest so that air cannot get into the chest cavity outside the lungs.

肺脏被严密地封闭在胸腔中,因此空气不能进入肺外的胸腔。

sealer [siːlə] *n.* 闭合器

Use of a dissecting sealer offered no substantial benefit over the clamp crushing method in reducing blood loss during hepatic resection.

在降低肝切除术中的失血方面,使用切割闭合器并不比挤压夹方法具有实质的优越性。

search [səːtʃ] *v.* 寻找,查找,搜寻

This young doctor usually searches for references in the medical library at his leisure.

这位年轻医生常在他空闲的时间去医学图书馆查找资料。

In a search to further his knowledge of the unknown, man has explored the earth, the sea and now

outer space.
为寻求对未知事物的进一步了解，人类探索了地球、海洋，现在又探索太空。
When a negative FTA-ABS and a positive STS are found，a search for the underlying cause other than syphilis must be made.
当 FTA-ABS 试验呈阴性，而梅毒血清试验反呈阳性时，则必须寻找梅毒以外的其他原因。

seasickness [ˈsiːsiknis] *n.* 晕船
The symptoms of seasickness are too familiar to require much description.
晕船的症状是大家熟悉的，不需要太多描述。

sebaceous [siˈbeiʃəs] *a.* 皮脂的
Benign teratomas are usually unilocular cysts containing hair and cheesy sebaceous material.
良性畸胎瘤通常是单房性囊肿，其中包含毛发和干酪样皮脂性物质。
The wall of dermoid cysts is composed of stratified squamous epithelium with underlying sebaceous glands，hair shafts，and other skin adnexal structures.
皮样囊肿的囊壁由复层鳞状上皮构成，其下可见皮脂腺、毛干和其他皮肤附属结构。

seborrhea [ˌsebəˈriːə] *n.* 皮脂溢；脂溢性皮炎
Infantile seborrhea usually clears by the age of 2 years.
婴儿的脂溢性皮炎通常在 2 岁左右会自行痊愈。
Seborrhea is excessive secretion of sebum by the sebaceous glands and is sometimes associated by a kind of eczema(seborrheic dermatitis).
皮脂溢是皮脂腺分泌过多的皮脂，有时伴有一种湿疹(脂溢性皮炎)。

secondary [ˈsekəndəri] *a.* 次要的；继发的
In such cases，treatment by drugs is only of secondary importance.
在这种情况下，药物治疗仅仅是次要的。
The major lymphoid organs and tissues are classfied as either primary(central) or secondary(peripheral).
主要的淋巴器官和组织可分为初级(中枢)和次级(外周)淋巴器官。
Hypertension may be classified as essential hypertension and secondary hypertension.
高血压可分类为原发性高血压和继发性高血压。
Empyema may also be secondary to an underlying carcinoma of the lung.
积脓也可继发于潜伏的肺癌。

second-choice [ˈsekənd-ˈtʃɔis] *n.* 次选，第二选择
Propranolol is generally a second-choice antiarrhythmic drug unless the arrhythmia is catecholamine mediated.
除儿茶酚胺引起的心律失常外，心得安通常作为心律失常的次选药物。

secretase [ˈsekriːteis] *n.* 分泌酶
Alpha secretases are a family of proteolytic enzymes.
α 分泌酶是一类蛋白水解酶。
By inhibiting an enzyme called gamma secretase，researchers hope to reduce amyloid production so that no new plaques will form.
研究人员希望通过抑制伽马分泌酶来减少淀粉样蛋白的生成而抑制新生斑块的形成。

secrete [siˈkriːt] *v.* 分泌
Activated macrophages secrete a large number of biologically active factors.
活化的巨噬细胞分泌大量生物活性因子。
The hormones are manufactured and secreted into the blood by the endocrine system.
激素由内分泌制造并被分泌到血液中去。

secretion [siˈkriːʃən] *n.* 分泌；分泌物
The internal secretion is circulated to all parts of the body.
内分泌物通过血液循环被送到人体各部。

Organic acids and bases and some drugs are eliminated by active processes of tubular secretion.
有机酸和有机碱及某些药物通过肾小管分泌这一主动转运过程被排泄。

secretory [si'kriːtəri] *a.* 分泌的,分泌作用的

They are interstitial cells that stain with silver stains and contain secretory granules.
它们是一些银染的间质细胞,并含有分泌颗粒。

section ['sekʃən] *n.* 切开(术);切面;切片

On section the fibromyoma is paler, harder and more fibrous than the uterine wall.
子宫纤维肌瘤切面较子宫壁苍白、质硬和含有更多的纤维组织。

Microscopic sections showed minimal interstitial nephritis and nephrosclerosis.
显微切片表明有极轻微的间质性肾炎和肾硬化。

Frozen section is a section cut by a microtome from tissue that has been frozen.
冰冻切片是被切片机从已冰冻的组织切下的切片。

sectional ['sekʃənəl] *a.* 断面的,截面的

A cross sectional image is reconstructed by computer calculation.
通过计算机计算重新构成交叉断面的图像。

secure [si'kjuə] *v.* 使安全;保险;获得

He has been secured against personal accidents.
他已经投保人身意外险。

The drop of secretion or pus swelling up out of the urethra is secured with a platinum loop and smeared on a slide and on a culture plate.
用铂环获取自尿道溢出的分泌物或脓滴,涂在玻片及培养皿上。

securing [si'kjuəriŋ] *a.* 落实的,固定住的

There are several key steps in planning a patient registry, including articulating its purpose, identifying stakeholders, defining the scope and target population, assessing feasibility, and securing funding.
在计划一个病历注册时有几个关键步骤,包括明晰注册登记的目的、确认利益相关者、定义范围和目标人群、评估可行性和落实研究经费。

security [si'kjuəriti] *n.* 安全,安全感

People have the security of a guaranteed pension.
人民由于养老金有保证而无忧无虑。

Researchers are testing an electronic sniffer which hopes to produce security systems that would recognize people by their body odors.
研究者们正在试验一种电子嗅觉探测器,希望能生产出借助身体的气味鉴别不同人的安全装置。

sedate [si'deit] *v.* 给…服镇静剂,镇静

Lithium has the advantage of being less sedating than neuroleptic drugs.
锂具有比精神抑制药物镇静作用小的优点。

sedation [si'deiʃən] *n.* 镇静;镇静剂

Sedation is the act of calming, reducing activity or excitement in an individual.
镇静是指引起个体活动减少或兴奋性降低的安定作用。

Sedation may depress respiration further and is contraindicated.
镇静剂可加重呼吸抑制,应禁用。

sedative ['sedətiv] *a.* 镇静的

Tobacco has a sedative effect on some people.
烟对于某些人有定神的效果。

n. 镇静药

After taking a sedative she was able to get to sleep.
服过镇静剂之后,她就能睡着了。

Sedatives and hypnotics depress the central nervous system.
镇静药和催眠药抑制中枢神经系统。

sedentary [ˈsedəntəri] *a.* 静坐的，需要久坐的
There is some connection between a sedentary life and hemorrhoids.
久坐的生活方式与痔有一定的关系。

sediment [ˈsedimənt] *n.* 沉淀物，沉渣
Urinary sediment is the deposit of solid matter left after the urine has been allowed to stand for some time.
尿沉渣是让尿液静置一段时间后沉积下来的固体物。
The identification of the organism is carried out on fresh urethral smears or preferably in urine sediment.
病原体的鉴定要做新鲜尿的涂片，更好的则是用尿沉渣物涂片。

sedimentation [ˌsedimenˈteiʃən] *n.* 沉淀作用，沉积，沉降
The erythrocyte sedimentation rate is usually elevated and falls in response to therapy.
红细胞沉降率通常加快，并且在治疗起效后减慢。
On admission the patient's erythrocyte sedimentation rate was 86mm/h.
患者入院时血沉为 86mm/h。

seemingly [ˈsiːmiŋli] *ad.* 表面上，外观上
Glassmaking was seemingly the first industry tobe brought from Europe to the United States.
玻璃制造业似乎是从欧洲传入美国的第一种工业。

segment [ˈsegmənt] *n.* 节，段；部分
Bronchopulmonary segment is one of the smaller subdivisions of the lobes of the lung.
支气管肺段是肺叶一较小的再分节段。
The patient's electrocardiogram showed ST-segment elevation.
患者的心电图显示 ST 段抬高。
The 75-year-plus group is the fastest growing segment of the U. S. population.
75 岁以上年龄组是美国人口中增长最快的年龄段。

segmental [segˈmentəl] *a.* 节的，段的，分节的
The segmental bronchi further divide the lobes of the lungs.
段支气管进一步划分肺叶。

segregate [ˈsegrigeit] *v.* 隔离；分开
Why should the handicapped be segregated from the able-bodied?
为什么把残疾人和身体健康的人分开？

segregation [ˌsegriˈgeiʃən] *n.* 分离，分异
Growth of membrane between attachment sites would bring about the segregation of the DNA copies.
附着位点间膜的生长会引起 DNA 拷贝的分离。
One meaning of segregation is the progressive restriction of potencies in zygote to the various regions of the forming embryo.
分异的一个含义是将合子中的潜能逐渐限制于胚胎形成的不同区域。

seize [siːz] *v.* (疾病等)侵袭；抓住，夺取
The boy was suddenly seized by an illness.
这男孩突然病了。
He was suddenly seized with an uneasy feeling in his stomach.
他忽然感到他的胃里不舒服。

seizure [ˈsiːʒə] *n.* 抓住；夺取；(疾病的)发作，癫痫发作
After the convulsive seizure, the patient may remain comatose for a long time.
惊厥癫痫性发作之后，病人可能长时间昏迷不醒。

It is on the spot that the doctor gave an emergency care for a patient during a seizure.
是在现场这位医生给一个正癫痫发作的病人施行急救。
Organic and hysterical seizures may coexist in the same patient and video monitoring may be necessary to make a full diagnosis.
器质性和癔症性的发作可并存于同一病人，为了作出完善的诊断而使用视频监测系统可能是必要的。

selectin [si'lektin] *n.* 选择素，选择蛋白
Selectins are expressed on leucocytes or activated endothelial cells.
选择素被表达于白细胞或活化的内皮细胞上。
To access an inflmmatory site, neutrophils must first adhere to the vascular endothelium in a process mediated in part by L-selectin.
为到达炎症部位，中性粒细胞必须首先黏附于血管内皮细胞上，这一过程部分是由 L-选择素介导的。
Binding of selectins to their carbohydrate ligands requires calcium.
选择素结合到它们的碳水化合物配体上需要钙。

selection [si'lekʃən] *n.* 选择，被挑选出的人或物
This process is referred to as "negative selection".
这个过程称为"阴性选择"。
Vegetable protein contains a selection of amino acids, but not all the essential ones.
植物蛋白质含有多种氨基酸，但并非全都是必需氨基酸。

selective [si'lektiv] *a.* 选择的，挑选的
The relief of pain by morphine is selective.
吗啡缓解疼痛的作用是有选择性的。

selectivity [silek'tiviti] *n.* 选择(性)
Some of the techniques have been used in clinical laboratories to determine the selectivity of urine protein.
其中一些技术已用于临床实验室以确定尿蛋白的选择性。

selenide ['selinaid] *n.* 硒化物
Selenium occurs mainly in the form of selenide minerals.
硒主要以硒化物矿物的形式存在。
Some selenides are reactive to oxidation by air.
某些硒化物易于发生空气氧化反应。

selenite ['selinait] *n.* 亚硒酸盐
Sodium selenite had strong inhibitory effect on the genotoxicity of cadmium chloride when the compounds interact on each other.
当这两种化合物相互作用时，亚硒酸钠对氯化镉的遗传毒性有很强的抑制作用。
Before we discuss the benefits of sodium selenite, we will briefly discuss this nutrient.
在我们讨论亚硒酸钠的益处之前，我们将简要讨论它的营养价值。

selenium [si'liːnjəm] *n.* 硒(化学元素)
Selenium is promoted as an anti-aging supplement.
硒被宣传为一种抗衰老的补充元素。
Selenium protects animals from a number of carcinogenic chemicals and viruses.
硒能保护动物不受多种致癌物和病毒的侵害。
Selenium sulfide lotion used as a shampoo in patients receiving griseofulvin therapy resulted in negative cultures at two weeks in 15 of 16 patients.
接受灰黄霉素治疗的同时将硫化硒洗剂作为洗发剂应用，在 16 位患者中有 15 位 2 周后培养转阴。

selenoprotein [siˌlənəu'prəutiːn] *n.* 硒蛋白

Selenium is a component of selenoproteins, some of which have important enzymatic functions.
硒是硒蛋白的组成部分,某些硒蛋白有重要的酶的功能。

self-contained [ˌself-kənˈteind] *a.* 自给自足的,设备齐全的

A transistorized, self-contained, implantable pacemaker was established in 1960 by Chardack et al.
查达克等人于 1960 年采用了带有自身动力的、可植入的半导体起搏器。

self-esteem [ˌself-isˈtiːm] *n.* 自尊心

Several studies have reported low self-esteem in depressed children.
好几项研究都报道抑郁儿童自尊心不强。

selfheal [ˈselfˌhiːl] *n.* 夏枯草

They studied the extraction process of the total triterpenes of selfheal.
他们探讨了夏枯草中总三萜类成分的提取工艺。
We need to observe the influence of selfheal capsule (SC) on the subsets of T lymphocyte of rats.
我们需要观察夏枯草胶囊对大鼠 T 淋巴细胞亚群的影响。

self-imposed [ˌself-imˈpəuzd] *a.* 自己施加的,自愿担负的

Anorexia nervosa(AN) is an eating disorder characterized by self-imposed starvation.
神经性厌食是一种饮食疾患,其特点是自我施加的挨饿。

self-renewal [self-riˈnjuːəl] *n.* 自我更新

Stem cells are characterized by their self-renewal properties and by their capacity to generate differentiated cell lineages.
干细胞的特征是具有自我更新和产生分化细胞的能力。
Cancer stem cells could arise from normal tissue stem cells or from more differentiated cells that acquire the property of self-renewal.
肿瘤干细胞可能起源于正常组织干细胞或分化的细胞,这些细胞具有自我更新的能力。

self-tolerance [ˈselfˈtɔlərəns] *n.* 自身忍耐性,自身耐受

Self-tolerance is the failure to make an immune response against the body's own antigens.
自身耐受是对自身抗原的免疫不应答。
Rather, immune cells and other body cells coexist peaceably in a state known as self-tolerance.
相反,免疫细胞和其他体细胞却能和平共存,该状态被称为自身耐受。

sella [ˈselə] *n.* 鞍,蝶鞍

The connecting line between bilateral carotico-optic recess was the projection of tuberculum sella.
两侧视神经-颈内动脉隐窝的连线是鞍结节的投影。
Empty sella syndrome is a radiological finding where spinal fluid is found within the subarachnoid space herniating into the pituitary.
空蝶鞍综合征是在蛛网膜下腔有脊髓液疝入垂体内,可通过影像学检查发现。

semaphorin [seˈmæfərin] *n.* 信号素

Semaphorin 6D may play an important role in the occurrence and development of gastric carcinoma.
信号素 6D 在胃癌的发生发展中起重要作用。
Plexin A is a neuronal semaphoring receptor that controls axon guidance.
Plexin A 是一种控制轴突导向的神经元信号素受体。

semen [ˈsiːmen] *n.* 种子,精液

The analysis of semen dates back as early as the 17th century.
精液分析最早可追溯至 17 世纪。
Medical research has shown that the virus also is present in human breast milk, saliva and semen.

医学研究表明病毒也存在于人奶、唾液和精液里。

Human immunodeficiency virus(HIV) is spread from one person to another by blood, semen and vaginal fluid.

人类免疫缺陷病毒通过血液、精液和阴道分泌物由一个人传播给另一个人。

semicoma [ˌsemiˈkəumə] *n.* 轻昏迷,半昏迷

Such a description is preferable to summary terms such as semicoma or obtundation.

这种描述优于使用半昏迷或迟钝等总结性的词语。

semicomatose [ˌsemiˈkəumətəus] *a.* 轻昏迷的,半昏迷的

Management of airways in semicomatose and comatose patients is essential.

使已经半昏迷或昏迷的病人保持其呼吸道的通畅是很重要的。

semiconservative [ˌsemikənˈsəːvətiv] *a.* 半保留的

DNA replication is semiconservative.

DNA 复制是半保留性的。

semi-liquid [ˌsemiˈlikwid] *a.* 半流动的;半液体的

The semi-liquid material surrounding the nucleus is known as the cytoplasm.

围绕着细胞核周围的半液状物质叫做细胞质。

semilunar [ˌsemiˈluːnə] *a.* 半月形的

The left ventricle then goes into contraction, opening the aortic semilunar valve as it does so.

左心室随之开始收缩,在此同时打开主动脉半月瓣。

seminal [ˈsiːminəl] *a.* 精液的

Each seminal vesicle consists of a single tube which is folded back upon itself over and over again.

每个精囊由一个反复自身折叠的小管构成。

Biochemical tests of the seminal fluid are also of value as they give an index of the function of the seminal vesicles.

精液的生化检查也有一定价值,因为它表明了精囊的功能指数。

seminar [ˈseminɑː] *n.* (学术)研讨会

There are thirty minutes of the seminar remaining.

研讨会还剩下 30 分钟。

seminiferous [ˌsemiˈnifərəs] *a.* 生精子的,输精子的

Most of the tissue in the testes consists of the seminiferous tubules.

睾丸的大部分组织由生精管组成。

seminoma [ˌsemiˈnəumə] *n.* 精原细胞瘤

Germ cell tumors are subdivided into seminomas and non-seminomas.

生殖细胞肿瘤再分为精原细胞瘤和非精原细胞瘤。

This article reviews some oncogenes, anti-oncogenes and apoptosis-related genes of seminoma.

本文综述了与精原细胞瘤相关的一些癌基因、抑癌基因以及凋亡相关基因。

semi-permeable [ˌsemiˈpəːmjəbl] *a.* 半渗透的

The walls of the blood capillaries of a single-layer of endothelial cells which constitute a semi-permeable membrane.

毛细血管壁由单层内皮细胞构成,后者形成一半透膜 。

The basement membrane zone is considered to be a "porous " semi-permeable filter.

基底膜带被认为是一种"多孔的"半透过滤器。

semisynthetic [ˌsemisinˈθetik] *a.* 半合成的

During the past few years a large number of semisynthetic penicillins have been developed.

近几年已研制出许多半合成青霉素。

semitransparent [ˌsemitrænsˈpɛərənt] *a.* 半透明的

A laser beam can also pass through skin, which is semitransparent, to kill skin cancer.

激光束也可以通过半透明的皮肤杀死皮肤癌(细胞)。

senegenin [siˈnedʒinin] *n.* 远志皂苷元

We study on quantitative determination of senegenin in radix polygalae by RP-HPLC.

我们对用反相高效液相色谱法测定远志根中远志皂苷元的含量进行了研究。

In a word, senegenin content and hemolysis characteristics are related to the climate regions in some degree.

可见,远志皂苷元含量和溶血特性与气候区有一定相关性。

senescence [siˈnesəns] *n.* 衰老

Senescence is a physiological process of growing older.

衰老是机体变老的生理过程。

She continues to play tennis for refusing to be overcome by senescence.

为了保持青春,她坚持打网球。

senescent [siˈnesnt] *a.* 衰老的,变老的

The pathophysiologic mechanism is that senescent RBC Fe fails to be released by the reticulum cells for Hb synthesis by the erythron.

病理生理机制为衰老的红细胞的铁不能从网状细胞释放出来供红细胞系合成 Hb。

senile [ˈsiːnail] *a.* 老年的,衰老的

Senile dementia is out in the open, recognized now as one of the great challenges to medical science in our time.

老年性痴呆已是众所知,现在已被认为是当代医学科学面临的重大挑战之一。

Senile pruritus is due mainly to dryness of the skin(xerosis).

老年性的皮肤瘙痒主要是由皮肤干燥(干皮症)所引起的。

senility [siˈniliti] *n.* 衰老,老迈

Multi-infarct dementia is the second most common reason for severe senility.

引起严重衰老的第二位最常见的原因是多发梗死性痴呆。

senior [ˈsiːnjə] *a.* 年长的;资格老的

He is ten years senior to me.

他比我大 10 岁。

The president of this university is a senior academician.

这所大学的校长是一位资深院士。

Such measures will further improve the quality of life in the senior population.

这些措施将进一步改善高龄人群的生活质量。

senna [ˈsenə] *n.* 番泻叶(用作通便剂)

Senna is used as an irritant laxative to relieve constipation and to empty the bowels before X-ray examination.

番泻叶是一种刺激性轻泻剂,用以减轻便秘或 X 线检查前排空大肠。

sensation [senˈseiʃən] *n.* 感觉,知觉

After the accident he had no sensation in his left thumb.

这次事故之后他的左手拇指一点知觉都没有了。

sensational [senˈseiʃənəl] *a.* 感觉的;激动人心的

Each passing year has brought more sensational results and victories in heart surgery.

每年在心脏手术方面都带来了许多激动人心的成果和胜利。

sensibility [ˌsensiˈbiləti] *n.* 感觉,敏感性

These end organs for deep sensibility are located in the subcutaneous and deeper tissues.

这些深度感觉的终端感觉器位于皮下和更深层的组织。

At friction surfaces, such as the palms and soles, eccrine secretion is thought to assist tactile sensibility and improve adhesion.

在掌、跖等摩擦面,外泌汗腺的分泌被认为有助于提高触觉的敏感性和增强附着力。

sensible ['sensəbl] *a.* 明智的;可感觉到的

Are you sensible of the hot weather?

你感到天气很热吗?

sensitive ['sensitiv] *a.* 敏感的

When your teeth are sensitive to hot and cold, you want an effective tooth paste.

当你的牙齿对冷热敏感时,你需要一种特效牙膏。

Mitochondrial RNA polymerase is sensitive to rifampicin.

线粒体 RNA 聚合酶对利福平敏感。

Nerve cells are more sensitive to certain poisons and drugs than other body cells are.

和身体其他细胞相比,神经细胞对于某些毒素和药物更为敏感。

sensitivity [ˌsensi'tiviti] *n.* 敏感(性),感受性

As has already been mentioned, patients differ in their tissue sensitivity.

如上所述,机体组织的敏感程度因病人而异。

Chlorpropamide increases the sensitivity of the tubules to ADH(antidiuretic hormone).

氯磺丙脲可增加肾小管对抗利尿激素的敏感性。

The causative organism should be isolated and antibiotic sensitivities determined.

必须分离致病菌并确定抗生素的敏感度。

sensitization [ˌsensitai'zeiʃən] *n.* 致敏(作用),敏化(作用)

A striking example of sensitization is sunburned skin in which severe pain can be produced by a gentle slap on the back or a warm shower.

晒伤的皮肤对轻拍一下后背或洗温水澡都会感到剧痛,这就是感觉过敏的典型例子。

Langerhans cells play a role in induction of graft rejection, primary contact sensitization and immunosurveillance.

朗格汉斯细胞在诱导移植物排斥、原发性接触性过敏反应和免疫监视中起着重要的作用。

sensitize ['sensitaiz] *v.* 致敏,敏化

Asthma may be caused by sensitizing substances.

哮喘可能由有致敏性的物质引起。

It has also been suggested that sensitized cells could bring about accelerated rejection.

也有人提出已致敏的细胞能引起加速性排斥反应。

sensor ['sensə(r)] *n.* 传感器

Smoke sensors warned us of the fire.

烟雾传感器帮助我们警戒火灾。

The sensor arm allows surgeons to watch their manoeuvres live in three dimensions on a video monitor.

这种传感臂可以使外科医生通过视频监视器现场直观其操作的三维图像。

sensorineural [ˌsensəri'njuərəl] *a.* 感觉神经的

The most important subtle effect of congenital cytomegalovirus is an increased incidence of sensorineural hearing loss, primarily in high frequencies.

先天性巨细胞病毒最重要的微细影响是感觉神经听力丧失的发生率增加,主要是对高频率音。

The occurrence of sensorineural hearing loss suggests that cytomegalovirus can exert its effects in very localized area.

出现感觉神经听力丧失提示巨细胞病毒可在极其局限的区域产生影响。

sensory ['sensəri] *a.* 感觉的

Lack of mental stimulation leads to a form of sensory deprivation.

思维刺激的缺乏导致某些形式的感觉丧失。

sentiment ['sentimənt] *n.* 情感;观点

Reason should not be guided by sentiment.

理智不应受情感的支配。

sentinel [ˈsentinəl] *n.* 前哨

In breast cancer, biopsy of sentinel nodes is often used to assess the presence or absence of metastatic lesions in the lymph nodes.

乳腺癌中，前哨淋巴结的活检常用于评估淋巴结转移性病变的存在与否。

A sentinel lymph node is defined as the first node in a regional lymphatic basin that receives lymph flow from the primary tumor.

前哨淋巴结被定义为从原发肿瘤回流至局部淋巴系统所到达的第一站淋巴结。

separable [ˈsepərəbl] *a.* 可分开的

The lower part of the pipe is separable from the upper part.

管子的下部可与上部分开。

separate [ˈsepəreit] *v.* 使分离；区分，使离析

The diaphragm is a large structure made up of muscles which separates the chest cavity from the abdominal cavity.

横膈膜是一个大的肌肉结构，将胸腔与腹腔隔开。

The perimeter of these valves is attached to the ring of fibrous tissues which separates the atria from the ventricles.

这些瓣膜周缘附着在分隔心房和心室的纤维环上。

Patients were separated into groups on the basis of age, number of "positive" axillary nodes, menopausal status, and extent of mastectomy.

根据年龄、腋下淋巴结数量、绝经情况及乳腺切除范围，把病人分成若干小组。

a. [ˈsepərit] 分开的

Compound microscopes have two separate lenses or sets of lenses.

复合显微镜有两个或两组分隔开的镜头。

separation [ˌsepəˈreiʃən] *n.* 分离，分开，离析

The separation of the centromere also separates the previously joined and identical chromatids.

着丝粒的分离使得原本相连的两条染色单体也彼此分开。

sepsis [ˈsepsis] (*pl.* sepses [ˈsepsiːz]) *n.* 败血症，脓毒症

The effects are due to local ischaemia and sepsis.

其后果是由于局部缺血和败血症所致。

Conversely, adrenal hemorrhage during bacterial sepsis may cause glucocorticoid production to cease.

相反，细菌性脓毒症感染时，肾上腺出血可导致糖皮质激素生成停止。

septal [ˈseptəl] *a.* 间隔的

Under the shadowless lamp of the operating room a surgeon opens up the heart of a 25-year-old woman suffering from a ventricular septal defect.

在手术室的无影灯下，外科医生将一位25岁患心室间隔缺损的女病人的心脏打开。

Other causes of early systolic murmurs include congenital ventricular septal defect.

引起收缩早期杂音的其他原因包括先天性室间隔缺损。

septation [sepˈteiʃən] *n.* 分隔

Echogram showed splenomegaly with multiloculated hypoechoic spaces without septation or internal echo.

超声回波图显示脾脏肿大，伴有多房性低回声无间隔腔隙或内部回声。

Varying degrees of uterine septation are demonstrated by echogram.

超声显示出不同程度的子宫分隔。

septic [ˈseptik] *a.* 败血性的，脓毒性的

In septic venous thrombosis, fragments of infected thrombus may break away.

在败血性静脉血栓形成时，感染的血栓断片可以脱离。

Dr Smith has used Protein C on 12 patients, each of whom was on the brink of death with septic shock and organ failure.

史密斯医生将蛋白质 C 用于 12 名患者，他们均因败血症性休克和器官衰竭而濒临死亡。

septicemia [ˌseptiˈsiːmiə] *n.* 败血症

Norman Bethune caught septicaemia while operating on a wounded soldier.

白求恩在给一个伤员做手术时感染了败血症。

Septicemia is an inexact term meaning the circulation of bacteria or their by-products(endotoxin or exotoxin) in the blood.

败血症是一个不精确的术语，其含义是细菌及其副产物（内毒素或外毒素）在血液中循环。

septum [ˈseptəm]（*pl.* septa [ˈseptə]）*n.* 中隔，壁隔

The hyphae are sometimes not separated by septa between the individual cells.

有的菌丝在各细胞之间无中隔分开。

sequel [ˈsiːkwəl] *n.* 后遗症

Complications and sequels are relatively infrequent.

合并症与后遗症比较不常见。

sequela [siˈkwilə]（*pl.* sequelae）*n.* 后果，后患，后遗症

The sequela of aplasia(ie, anemia) requires a duration longer than usually exists with the acute episode.

发育不良的后果（即贫血）需要比通常急性病发作更长的时间才能显现出来。

Epilepsy in infancy is an occasional sequela of meningitis.

婴儿期癫痫偶为脑膜炎的后遗症。

In severe cases, the patient undergoes a prolonged recovery, often leaving permanent sequelae.

严重病例中，病人经历漫长的恢复期，常留下终生的后遗症。

sequence [ˈsiːkwəns] *n.* 序列，顺序

The sequences of ribosomal RNAs have changed slowly since the time any two organisms diverged from a common progenitor.

任何两种微生物从一共同的祖先分支出来后，其核糖体 RNA 的序列一直变化得很慢。

The physical examinations will be carried out in a definite sequence.

体检各项目将按一定的顺序进行。

Prof. Smith has published a sequence of essays on artificial immunity.

史密斯教授发表了一系列关于人工免疫的论文。

v. 排序

Polypeptide chains are most commonly sequenced by the Edman reaction.

测定多肽链序列最常用的方法是埃德曼反应。

Furthermore, sequencing the cDNAs will not provide crucial information about regulatory sequences.

而且，对 cDNA 测序不能获得有关调控序列的重要信息。

sequencing [ˈsiːkwənsiŋ] *n.* 测序

Sequencing means the determination of the order of nucleotides(base sequences) in a DNA or RNA molecule or the order of amino acids in a protein.

测序是指测定 DNA 或 RNA 中核苷酸（碱基）的排列次序或者蛋白质中氨基酸的次序。

sequential [siˈkwenʃəl] *a.* 连续的，继续的，按顺序的

Under this condition the enzyme is ready to proceed by linking the following nucleotids in a sequential manner.

在这种情况下，该酶将继续起作用，把后续的核苷酸依次连接起来。

sequentially [siˈkwenʃəli] *ad.* 连续地

For practical reasons the suppressive and stimulatory maneuvers are performed sequentially on successive days.

根据实际需要抑制和刺激手段的采用要一连数日。

sequestration [ˌsikwe'streiʃən] *n.* 隔离症

Chest radiographs can provide a reasonable diagnostic clue to pulmonary sequestration.

胸部 X 线可以提供一个合理的肺隔离症的诊断线索。

seriousness ['siəriəsnis] *n.* 严重,危急,重要

There is little correlation between the severity of chest pain and the seriousness of its cause.

胸痛的剧烈程度和病因的严重性之间几乎无关。

In any event, the seriousness of hepatitis must not be discounted because of the possibilities of complications in later life.

在任何情况下,都不能忽视肝炎的严重性,因为以后可能发生并发症。

seroglobulin [ˌsiərəu'glɔbjulin] *n.* 血清球蛋白

A range of different globulins is present in the blood(the seroglobulins, including alpha(α), beta (β), and gamma(γ) globulins).

血液中有一系列不同的球蛋白,包括 α、β 和 γ 血清球蛋白。

serologic [siərə'lɔdʒik] *a.* 血清学的

Serologic classification is used very commonly to distinguish differences among species within a given genus.

血清学分类常用于区分某菌属中的不同菌种。

Serologic tests are more reliable in diagnosis of fungal diseases.

血清学化验在真菌病诊断上更为可靠。

serology [siə'rɔlədʒi] *n.* 血清学

Serology is helpful in the diagnosis of invasive amebiasis.

血清学方法有助于诊断阿米巴病。

Since that time, HIV serology and specific viral culture techniques have been developed.

从那时起,人类免疫缺陷病毒(HIV)的血清学和特定的病毒培养技术已经建立起来了。

seromuscular [ˌsiərəu'mʌskjulə; ˌser-] *a.* (肠道)浆肌层的

The authors explain that in a standard blow-hole colostomy, the omentum and seromuscular layers of the colon are sutured to the peritoneum and the rectus fascia.

作者说明了在标准的低位肠造瘘术中,将网膜和结肠的浆肌层缝合到腹膜和腹直肌筋膜上。

An endoscopic gastrointestinal stapler is used to perform a seromyotomy across the anterior portion of the stomach to divide all the vagal fibers crossing through the seromuscular layer.

内[窥]镜下胃肠闭合器用于将胃前部的浆肌层切开,以分开穿过浆肌层的迷走神经纤维。

serosa [si'rəusə, -zə] *n.* 浆膜;绒毛膜;卵膜

The results show that the digestive tract consists of 4 layers, including mucosa, submucosa, muscular coat, and serosa.

结果表明:消化道管壁包含黏膜层、黏膜下层、肌膜和浆膜四层。

Difference between rectum and colon is that most of the rectum lacks serosa.

直肠和结肠之间的差别是大部分直肠没有浆膜。

serosal [si'rəusəl, si'rəuzəl] *a.* 浆膜的,绒(毛)膜的

The gross appearance of the bowel may be normal from the serosal surface.

肠管肉眼所见,浆膜面可能正常。

serotherapy [ˌsiərəu'θerəpi] *n.* 血清疗法

Serotherapy is the use of serum containing known antibodies to treat a patient with an infection or to confer temporary passive immunity upon a patient at special risk.

血清疗法是应用含有已知抗体的血清,治疗某种感染的患者,或给予某一高危患者以暂时性被动免疫。

serotonin [ˌserə'təunin] *n.* 5-羟色胺,血清素

Carbohydrates increase the brain's production of the calming chemical serotonin.
碳水化合物能增加脑中具有镇静作用的化学血清素的生成。
In preliminary experiments, Koella found that giving serotonin to cats produced signs of sleep.
在初步试验中,柯纳发现给猫注射血清素产生睡眠迹象。

serotoninergic [ˌsiərəuˌtəuniˈnəːdʒik] *a.* 血清素能的
Within the brain, the serotoninergic system(5-HT) is activated by stress.
脑内的血清素能系统(即5羟色胺能系统)可被应激反应激活。

serotype [ˈsiərətaip] *n.* 血清型
Antibodies have been used in a diagnostic capacity for identifying serotypes.
抗体已被应用于确定血清型。
In 2008, a nine-fold increase in new cases caused by this serotype has been reported compared with the same period in 2007.
与2007年同期相比,2008年这一血清型病毒导致的新病例报告数目增加了9倍。

serous [ˈsiərəs] *a.* 浆液的;血清的
The malignant serous tumour is the commonest variety of primary ovarian cancer.
恶性浆液性肿瘤是原发性卵巢癌中最常见的一种。
Nerves and blood and lymph vessels are abundant in serous membranes.
浆膜中含有丰富的神经、血管和淋巴管。

serpin [ˈsəːpin] *n.* 丝氨酸蛋白酶抑制剂,酶抑制剂
Serpins are a large family of protease inhibitors.
丝氨酸蛋白酶抑制剂是蛋白酶抑制剂中的一个大家族。
The serpins are a widely distributed family of proteins with diverse functions.
丝氨酸蛋白酶抑制剂是一种广泛分布、功能各异的蛋白家族。

serratia [səˈreiʃiə] *n.* 沙雷菌属
The paper was published because Serratia marcescens infections are very rare.
该论文被发表是由于黏质沙雷氏菌感染是非常罕见的。
The purpose is to evaluate the therapeutic effect of serratia marcescens vaccine in treatment of malignant pleural effusion.
目的是评估黏质沙雷氏菌疫苗在治疗恶性胸腔积液中的治疗效果。

serum [ˈsiərəm] *n.* 血清
Human serum has come into extensive use.
人类血清已被广泛地使用。
The serum creatinine is not increased unless renal disease is also present.
如果没有肾脏疾患,血清肌酐水平一般不升高。

service [ˈsəːvis] *n.* 服务
Music therapy has been an established health service similar to physical therapy.
与物理治疗一样,音乐治疗已成为一种成熟的健康服务。
Nursing is an important part of medical and health service.
护理工作是医疗卫生服务的重要组成部分。

sesame [ˈsesəmi] *n.* 芝麻
We have ordered well-dried sesame of fine quality.
我们订的是晒好的上等芝麻种子。
Use the white sesame and black sesame to make the pancake.
用白芝麻和黑芝麻做小薄饼。

sessile [ˈses(a)il] *a.* 广基的,无蒂的
Polyps of the vocal cords are unilateral, smooth, rounded, sessile or pedunculated excrescences.
声带息肉是单侧发生的、光滑、圆形、无蒂或有蒂的赘生物。
Endocervical polyps vary from small and sessile to large masses that may protrude through the

cervical os.

宫颈管息肉大小不一,从小而无蒂到大的肿块,可从宫颈口突出至宫口外。

session ['seʃən] *n.* 会议;会期;一段时间

Judging from the level of participant interest in the present session, the subject is a timely choice.

从与会者的兴趣可判断出这次会议所选择的主题是合适的。

Hopefully, guest scientists will find these sessions informative and useful.

希望被邀请来的科学家们,会感到这些讨论会是促进信息交流和有所裨益的。

setting ['setiŋ] *n.* 安装;背景

Such evaluation is especially important in the setting of proposed cardiac or abdominal surgery.

这种评估对于打算进行心脏和腹部外科手术的病人特别重要。

If the management beautifies the dull setting, the factory will be much more productive.

如果厂方美化一下单调的环境,工厂的生产率就可以大大提高。

settle ['setl] *v.* 沉淀;定居;变平静

The gall bladder is removed 2-3 months later after the inflammation has settled.

在炎症消退后 2 ~3 个月施行胆囊切除。

Occasionally the red cells settle before coagulation occurs.

偶尔在血液凝固前,红细胞发生沉降。

sever ['sevə] *v.* 切断

These surgeons have successfully rejoined severed limbs for more than 200 patients.

这些外科医生为 200 多病人成功地接活了他们的断肢。

After a quick examination of the patient and his severed hand, the young surgeon decided on an operation.

年轻的外科医生很快地检查了病人及其断手之后,决定施行手术。

severe [si'viə] *a.* 严重的,严格的

Illness accompanying recurrent infections with a given virus are usually less severe and are more likely to involve the upper respiratory tract.

伴有某种病毒反复感染的疾病通常不重,而且多累及上呼吸道。

severity [si'veriti] *n.* 严重

Thus, a vicious cycle is established and the anemia gradually increases in severity.

这样就形成一个恶性循环,贫血也就逐渐加重。

Signs of aplastic anemia vary with the severity of the pancytopenia.

患再生障碍性贫血时的体征因全血细胞减少的严重程度而异。

sewage ['sjuːidʒ] *n.* 污水,污物

Hepatitis A has traditionally been controlled by sewage disposal and better hygiene.

控制甲型肝炎的传统方法是处理污水和改善环境卫生。

sex [seks] *n.* 性别,性

The number of chromosomes in normal individuals is 46, of which 2 are the sex chromosomes.

正常人有 46 条染色体,其中 2 条为性染色体。

In epidemics caused by T. tonsurans there is often equal frequency in the sexes.

在由断发癣菌引起的流行病中,两性的发病率常是相同的。

In a recent study, 40 percent of HIV patients did not inform a sex partner about their condition.

最近的一项研究显示,有 40% 的艾滋病人并没有把实情告诉他们的性对象。

The two most common major subgroups encountered during reference range determinations are age and sex.

在决定参考值范围的因素中,两种最常见的要求是年龄和性别。

sexual ['seksjuəl] *a.* 有性别的;性的

Most fungi produce both sexual and asexual molds.

大多数真菌既产生有性孢子,又产生无性孢子。

shadow [ˈʃædəu] *n.* 阴影

The heart shadow of a hypertensive patient on the X-ray film looks like a boot.

高血压病人在 X 线照片上的心脏阴影看起来像靴。

shallow [ˈʃæləu] *a.* 浅的

Faintness, dizziness, thirst, sweating, weak and rapid pulse, and rapid respiration (at first deep, then shallow) may occur.

昏厥、眩晕、口渴、出汗、脉快而弱、呼吸快(起初深,以后表浅)这些症状均可发生。

sham [ʃæm] *a.* 假的

It would be possible to create a small extracorporeal circulation with sham organ bearing the donor's antigens.

用一个带供体抗原的假器官引发一个小的体外循环是有可能的。

Histological examination revealed no necrotizing pancreatitis in the sham-operated group, while all animals with pancreatitis showed marked parenchymal necrosis and hemorrhage (Table 1).

组织学检查显示假手术组无坏死性胰腺炎,而患胰腺炎的所有动物出现明显的实质性坏死和出血(见表 1)。

n. 假冒,假装

Her illness was a sham to gain sympathy.

她患病是假装的,以便获得同情。

shave [ʃeiv] *v.* 剃,刮

He watched TV program while having his face shaved.

他一边修面一边看电视节目。

The white spots are so superficial that they may be easily shaved off.

这些白点非常表浅以致易于刮掉。

sheath [ʃiːθ] *n.* 鞘

The brain capillaries are tightly joined together and covered by a footlike sheath.

脑的毛细血管结构紧密地连接在一起并被足样鞘覆盖。

Arachnoid sheath is the delicate membrane between the pial and dural sheath of the optic nerve.

蛛网膜是视神经软鞘和硬鞘之间的细软膜。

shell [ʃel] *n.* 壳

The snail has completely rotted away inside its shell.

蜗牛已在壳中烂掉。

v. 剥,脱落

Many benign tumours can be shelled out of their ovarian beds, so leaving behind normal ovarian tissue which will continue to function.

很多良性肿瘤能从其卵巢床上剥出,而剩留的正常卵巢组织继续发挥作用。

shellac [ʃəˈlæk] *n.* 虫胶,虫胶清漆

In1907, shellac was commonly used to insulate the innards of early electronics—radios and telephones.

1907 年,虫漆已被广泛用于早期电子产品的内部元件绝缘,例如半导体和电话。

The purpose of this study is to envelope paracetamol in the matrix of CAP and shellac for masking the bitter taste of the drug.

本文研究用 CAP 和虫胶为骨架材料包埋对乙酰氨基酚,能较好地掩盖药物的苦味。

shift [ʃift] *v.* 变动,转换

The cause of death has shifted from the complications of renal failure to infections.

死亡原因已从肾功能衰竭并发症转变为感染。

Most bacterial infection produce an increase in the leukocyte count and a shift in the differential count.

大多数的细菌感染会造成白细胞计数的增加和白细胞分类计数的改变。

shigella [ʃiˈgelə] (*pl*. shigellae [ʃiˈgeliː]) *n*. 志贺菌

Clinical features vary with the four different species of shigella.

四种志贺菌引起的临床表现各不相同。

Inflammatory diarrhea caused by shigella is also referred to as bacillary dysentery.

由志贺菌引起的感染性腹泻也常称为细菌性痢疾。

shigellosis [ˌʃigəˈləusis] *n*. 志贺菌病，志贺细菌性痢疾

Shigellosis is usually limited to a few days.

志贺菌病的病程只有几天。

Diagnosis of shigellosis is based on the finding of fecal leukocytes and culture of the organism from stool.

诊断志贺细菌性痢疾的依据是在粪便中找到白细胞和粪便微生物培养的结果 。

shingles [ˈʃiŋglz] *n*. 带状疱疹

Shingles usually starts with pain along the distribution of a nerve (often in the face, chest, or abdomen), followed by the development of veiscles.

带状疱疹往往以沿神经分布（常见于面、胸或腹部）的疼痛开始，随后发生水疱。

Pain is the heralding symptom of shingles infection and may precede the development of lesions by 48-72h.

带状疱疹的先驱症状是疼痛，而且疼痛比局部病变约早 48～72 小时。

shiver [ˈʃivə] *v*. 寒战，颤抖

If the hypothalamus call for more heat, shivering process is triggered to increase heat production.

如果下丘脑需要更多热量，就会触发寒战过程以增加热量的产生。

shivering [ˈʃivəriŋ] *n*. 寒战，战栗

Shivering can increase the basal metabolic rate to approximately five times the normal rate.

寒战可将基础代谢率增加至约为正常的五倍。

The attack of malaria commonly begins with headache and violent shivering.

疟疾发作开始时，患者通常头痛，并有剧烈寒战。

shock [ʃɔk] *n*. 休克；震惊

It is not uncommon that a fright or a shock may bring on abortion.

由于恐怖或震惊引起的流产病例并不少见。

This condition often brings on shock and requires immediate treatment.

这种情况常引起休克，需要立即治疗。

shortage [ˈʃɔːtidʒ] *n*. 不足，缺少

There are other causes for anemia than a shortage of iron in the food.

贫血除了食物中缺少铁质外，还有其他原因。

shortcoming [ˈʃɔːtkʌmiŋ] *n*. 缺点

Indeed, none of the shortcomings of using serum creatinine as a marker of glomerular filtration rate are avoided by using inverse creatinine.

事实上，用血清肌酐作为肾小球滤过率标志的缺点中没有一个可用肌酐倒数加以避免。

shorten [ˈʃɔːtn] *v*. 缩短，减少

The improved care shortens the period of necessary hospitalization.

改善护理，缩短了必要的住院时间。

The longer the muscle fibres, the more they will shorten.

肌肉纤维越长，它们的收缩性就越大。

short-term [ˈʃɔːttəːm] *a*. 短期的

In 4000 cases at the Academy of Traditional Chinese Medicine since 1957, the short-term cure rate has reached 99 percent.

自 1957 年来，在中医研究所治疗过的 4000 病例中，短期治愈率已达到 99%。

Short-term complications of pyloroplasty were: postoperative gastric outlet obstruction, rebleeding

in the immediate postoperative period and prolonged ileus.
幽门成形术的近期并发症是术后胃排出障碍、术后再发出血以及长时间的肠麻痹。

shoulder [ˈʃəuldə] *n.* 肩

Shoulder is painful and tender to palpation, and both active and passive range of motion is restricted.
肩部疼痛、触痛，主动和被动的运动范围都受限。

The early manifestations are apt to be distributed over the face, shoulders, flanks, palms and soles, and anal or genital regions.
早期皮疹倾向分布于面部、肩部、肋腹、掌、跖和肛门或生殖器等处。

v. 肩负，承担

She shouldered the responsibility of raising the children.
她承担起抚养孩子的责任。

shower [ˈʃəuə] *n.* 淋浴

The cleaning soap and water bath or shower is an important part of good grooming and health.
用肥皂洗澡或淋浴是保持整洁和健康的一个重要部分。

shrink [ʃriŋk] *v.* 收缩，缩小

Chemotherapy can be used before surgery to shrink a large tumour and after surgery to destroy remaining cancer cells.
化疗能用于手术前将较大的肿瘤缩小，手术后摧毁残余的癌细胞。

Cataract surgery now requires only an overnight stay, and even that is shrinking.
现在白内障手术病人只需在医院过一夜，时间甚至还在缩短。

shrinkage [ˈʃriŋkidʒ] *n.* 收缩，皱缩

Irradiation produced marked temporary shrinkage.
经过照射，暂时有明显的缩小。

There is rapid shrinkage of the thickness of the endometrium with leucocytic infiltration.
子宫内膜厚度迅速皱缩，并有白细胞浸润。

shunt [ʃʌnt] *v.* (使)分流

Cerebrospinal fluid volume may be reduced by repeated spinal taps or by shunting.
通过反复腰穿或分流可减少脑脊液容积。

sibling [ˈsibliŋ] *n.* 同胞(兄弟姐妹)

Prophylaxis with rifampin at 20mg/kg/day is indicated for the susceptible sibling, the parents, and the child(patient).
对易感同胞、父母及患儿给予利福平每日 20mg/kg 以作预防。

Questions are then asked about hereditary factors, the state of health of parents and siblings.
然后再问关于遗传因素，以及其父母和兄弟姐妹的健康情况。

sibpair [ˈsibpεə] *n.* 同胞对

One type of model-free analysis is the affected sibpair method.
有一种不依赖模型的连锁分析称为患病同胞对法。

In the affected sibpair method, DNA of affected sibs is systematically analyzed by use of hundreds of polymorphic markers throughout the entire genome.
在患病同胞对法中，用全基因组的几百个多态性标记来系统分析患病同胞的 DNA。

sickbay [ˈsikbei] *n.* 船上医务室

The three passengers were soon sent to the sickbay for emergency treatment.
三位旅客立即被送到船上医务室进行急救处理。

sickle [ˈsikl] *n.* 镰刀

Sickle cell anemia is an inherited hemoglobin abnormality.
镰状细胞性贫血是一种遗传性血红蛋白异常性疾病。

sickle-cell [ˈsiklsel] *n.* 镰状细胞

The anemia in this case is most likely sickle-cell disease.
这一病例的贫血最有可能是镰状细胞疾病。
The distribution of malaria before the introduction of mosquito control programs paralleled the distribution of sickle-cell disease.
在灭蚊计划开展之前,疟疾的分布范围与镰形红细胞病的分布相似。

sickness [ˈsiknis] *n.* 疾病;恶心,呕吐
They were absent because of sickness.
他们因病缺席。
Sleeping sickness should be considered in any febrile patient from an endemic area.
任何从锥虫病流行地区来的发热病人都应考虑有锥虫病(昏睡病)。

side-effect [said iˈfekt] *n.* 副作用
The major side-effect of this drug is headache and as many tablets as necessary may be taken.
该药主要的副作用是头痛,用药的片数则应视病人的需要而定。
Side-effect is the adverse effect produced by a drug, especially on a tissue or organ system.
副作用是药物产生的不良作用,特别是对组织或器官系统的不良作用。

sideroblastic [ˌsidərəuˈblæstik] *a.* 铁粒幼(红)细胞的
Clinical correlates have been made in some cases of sideroblastic anemia, but clear etiologic and pathophysiologic mechanisms are unknown.
在铁粒幼细胞贫血的某些病例中已找到了临床上的关联,但明确的病因及病理生理机制仍然不明。
Sideroblastic anemias are due to inadequate or abnormal utilization of intracellular Fe for Hb synthesis.
铁粒幼细胞性贫血是由于不能充分或正常利用细胞内的铁以合成血红蛋白所致。

siderocyte [ˈsidərəsait] *n.* 铁粒红细胞,高铁红细胞
Siderocytes are nonnucleated erythrocytes containing iron granules.
铁粒红细胞是含有铁颗粒的无核红细胞。

siderosis [ˌsidəˈrəusis] *n.* 铁尘肺,肺铁末沉着病
In an occupational setting, inhalation exposure to iron oxide may cause siderosis.
在某种职业环境下,吸入接触氧化铁可能引起铁尘肺。
Siderosis is the deposition of iron oxide dust in the lungs usually occurring in haematite miners.
肺铁末沉着病是氧化铁尘末在肺内沉积,常见于赤铁矿矿工。

sieve [siv] *n.* 筛
It should be understood that these filters do not act as mere mechanical sieves.
应懂得这些过滤器的作用不仅仅是机械性的过筛。

sievert [ˈsiːvət] *n.* 希沃特(放射吸收剂量当量)
Doses greater than 1 sievert received over a short time period are likely to cause radiation poisoning, possibly leading to death within weeks.
在短时期内接受超过 1 希沃特的剂量可能会导致辐射中毒,并可能导致数周内死亡。
Two measurements are essential for radiation protection: the measurement of the dose of radiation absorbed by the body and the assessment of the risk associated with this absorbed dose. Two units were thus created: the Gray and the Sievert.
为了辐射防护,两种测量必不可少,即测量身体吸收的辐射剂量和评估这一吸收剂量有关的风险。因此创立了两种测量单位,即戈瑞和希沃特。

sigmoid [ˈsigmɔid] *a.* 乙状的
These are the sigmoid artery branches from the inferior mesenteric.
它们是来自肠系膜下动脉的乙状结肠动脉分支。
n. 乙状结肠
The sigmoid is a part of the colon located between the descending colon and rectum.

乙状结肠是结肠的一部分，位于降结肠与直肠之间。

sigmoidectomy [ˌsigmɔiˈdektəmi] *n.* 乙状结肠切除术

Sigmoidectomy is performed for tumours, severe diverticular disease, or for an abnormally long sigmoid colon that has become twisted.

作乙状结肠切除是因为有肿瘤、严重的憩室性疾病，或因乙状结肠过长而引起的肠扭转。

sigmoidoscope [sigˈmɔidəskəup] *n.* 乙状结肠镜

Sigmoidoscope is an instrument used to inspect the interior of the rectum and sigmoid colon.

乙状结肠镜是一种用来观察直肠和乙状结肠内部的器械。

Sigmoidoscopy can be carried out in the outpatient clinic using a 20cm rigid plastic sigmoidoscope.

在门诊，可采用一支20厘米长的硬制塑料的乙状结肠镜来进行乙状结肠镜检查。

sigmoidoscopy [ˌsigmɔiˈdɔskəpi] *n.* 乙状结肠镜检查

Sigmoidoscopy and barium enema may cause endocarditis.

乙状结肠镜检查与钡灌肠可致心内膜炎。

Sigmoidoscopy is required for completeness of evaluation when there are rectal or colonic complaints.

当有直肠和结肠方面的主诉时，需行乙状结肠镜检查以便有一个全面的评价。

signal [ˈsignəl] *n.* 信号

A red light is often used as a danger signal.

红灯常用作危险信号。

Because pain is understood as a signal of disease, it is the most common symptom that brings a patient to a physician.

由于疼痛被认为是疾病的信号，因此它是导致病人就医的最常见症状。

v. 发信号，显示

Earlobe dermatitis signals nickle allergy.

耳垂皮炎标志镍过敏。

signal-to-noise ratio (SNR) [ˈsignəːltəˈnɔizˈreiʃiəu] *n.* 信噪比

Signal-to-noise ratio is a very important parameter in assessment of CT and MRI image quality.

信噪比是评估CT和MRI图像质量的一个非常重要的参数。

In order to improve the signal-to-noise ratio, high voltage and mA are always used.

为了提高图像信噪比，通常采用提高管电压和管电流。

signature [ˈsignətʃə(r)] *n.* 签字

A doctor must put his signature to the prescription.

医生必须在处方上签字。

This agreement will come into force upon signature.

这份协议签字后立即生效。

signet-ring [ˈsignit-riŋ] *a.* 印戒的

Gastric adenocarcinomas with a diffuse infiltrative growth pattern are more often composed of signet-ring cells.

弥漫浸润性胃腺癌常常由印戒细胞构成。

Signet-ring cells can be recognized by their large cytoplasmic mucin vacuoles and peripherally displaced nuclei.

印戒细胞可从其大的胞质内黏蛋白空泡和偏位于外周的细胞核来识别。

significance [sigˈnifikəns] *n.* 重要性，意义

The director wanted to see him on a matter of great significance.

院长要见他，有十分重要的事与他商量。

Only a few of them are of possible clinical significance.

其中只有几个可能具有临床意义。

Telomere length has been reported to be of prognostic significance in chronic lymphocytic leukemia.
已有研究发现端粒的长度与慢性淋巴细胞白血病的预后相关。

significant [sig'nifikənt] *a.* 值得注意的，明显的，显著地
A significant delay was observed in arriving at a proper diagnosis.
可以看出，做出正确诊断时已有明显耽误。
On many occasions, stained nasal smears will reveal significant numbers of eosinophils in allergic rhinitis.
许多次染色的鼻液涂片显示过敏性鼻炎存在大量嗜酸性细胞。
There was no significant difference between the two groups before treatment ($P>0.05$).
治疗前两组之间没有显著差异($P>0.05$)。

silencer ['sailənsə] *n.* 沉默子
A silencer is a DNA sequence capable of binding transcription regulation factors termed repressors.
沉默子是一段 DNA 序列，它可以和一种被称为抑制子的转录调节因子结合。
Silencers are control regions of DNA that, like enhancers, may be located thousands of base pairs away from the gene they control.
沉默子是 DNA 上的调控区域，像增强子一样，它们的位置可以距离所调控的基因数千碱基对。

silent ['sailənt] *a.* 无症状的
Patients with clinically silent myocardial infarctions have a lower death rate.
临床上无症状的心肌梗死患者的死亡率较低。

silhouette [ˌsiluː'et] *n.* 轮廓；廓影，侧影
On radiographic examination the cardiac silhouette is somewhat enlarged.
X 线胸片上显现心影轮廓稍增大。

silica ['silikə] *n.* 硅(矽)，硅石
Silica dust is harmful to the lungs.
矽尘对肺部有害。

silicon ['silikən] *n.* 硅(化学元素)
Among trace metals are tin, nickel, vanadium, chromium, and silicon, which are needed for proper growth of bone and connective tissue.
微量元素中有锡、镍、钒、铬和硅，它们是骨骼和结缔组织正常生长所必需的。
Silicon is a non-metallic chemical element found combined with oxygen in quartz, sandstone and other rocks.
硅是非金属化学元素，与氧结合存在于石英、砂岩及其他岩石中。

silicone ['silikəun] *n.* (聚)硅酮
The magnet is mounted on a silicone disc, which rests right on the eardrum, held in place by a thin film of oil.
磁铁装在硅酮盘上，直接安放在鼓膜上，并用很薄的一层油将其位置固定。

silicosis [ˌsili'kəusis] *n.* 矽肺，硅肺，石末沉着病
Silicosis results from the inhalation of silica during mining or quarrying of rock.
患矽肺是由于在采矿或采石过程中吸入了硅石粉尘引起的。
Patients with silicosis are at higher than normal risk for tuberculosis.
矽肺病人患肺结核的可能性比正常人高。

similarity [ˌsimi'læriti] *n.* 相似，相似点
The spleen is as well discussed after the lymphatic system, for there are some similarities.
在淋巴系统之后又来讨论脾，因为它们有相似处。
Mast cells have structural and functional similarities to basophilic polymorphs.

肥大细胞的结构和功能类似于嗜碱性多形核粒细胞。

simplex [ˈsimpleks] *a.* 单一的,单纯的

Adenosine arabinoside is currently the only drug with proven efficacy for treating neonatal herpes simplex infections.

阿糖腺苷是目前惟一经证实对治疗新生儿单纯疱疹病毒感染有效的药物。

simplicity [simˈplisiti] *n.* 简单,简易

Because of their simplicity, many bacteria can divide in less than 30 minutes.

由于它们(结构)简单,许多细菌不到30分钟便能完成分裂。

As far as the simplicity is concerned, chemotherapy has its advantage.

就简易而言,化疗有化疗的优点。

simplify [ˈsimplifai] *v.* 简化,使易做

Such protocols simplify the task of those in charge of testing.

这些草案简化了那些负责试验的人员的工作。

The Rapid Plasma Reagin(RPR) card test was introduced in 1962 as a simplified nontreponemal test for use in field or clinical settings.

1962年开始使用了一种快速的血浆反应素卡片试验法,作为一种简化的非螺旋体试验方法用于现场或临床。

simulate [ˈsimjuleit] *v.* 模仿,模拟

Such papillary lesions may grossly simulate invasive carcinoma.

这样的乳头状病变肉眼看来类似浸润癌。

Drug rashes are common and may simulate closely the eruptions of measles, German measles or scarlet fever.

药疹颇为常见,它与麻疹、风疹和猩红热的发疹很相似。

Ovarian carcinoma may also become fixed to the uterus and simulate a fibromyoma.

卵巢癌也可能固定在子宫上,类似肌瘤。

simultaneous [siməlˈteinjəs] *a.* 同时发生的,同时存在的

The simultaneous occurrence of these syndromes occurs, or is reported, only rarely.

这些综合征的同时出现是极少发生也极少被报道的。

simultaneously [ˌsiməlˈteinjəsli] *ad.* 同时发生地

The fetal heart rate is recorded simultaneously with an indication of fetal movement.

记录胎动时同时记下胎儿心率。

A gain in weight and development of peripheral edema often occur simultaneously.

体重增加及周围性水肿常常同时出现。

single [ˈsiŋgl] *a.* 单一的;单身的

This substance can be reduced to a single chemical and oxygen by passing an electrical charge through it.

通电后,这种物质可以被分解为一种单一的化学制品和氧。

He remains single. (He is still living a bachelor's life.)

他还是单身。

single-blind [ˈsiŋgl-blaind] *a.* 单盲的(统计学)

In a single-blind trial the patients included in the experiment do not themselves know which treatment they are receiving—the trial treatment, the orthodox treatment or, perhaps, a placebo.

参加单盲试验的病人自己不知道他们所接受的治疗是试验治疗、正规治疗、或者也许是服用安慰剂。

sinus [ˈsainəs] *n.* 窦

The sinus node is richly supplied with autonomic nerves, both sympathetic and parasympathetic.

窦房结分布有丰富的自主神经,包括交感神经和副交感神经。

The valve of the coronary sinus is variable in size and form and lies to the right of its opening.

冠状窦瓣的大小和形状不一，位于窦口的右侧。

Sinus bradycardia is often found in healthy individuals, especially athletes.

窦性心动过缓在健康人尤其运动员中较为常见。

sinusitis [ˌsainəˈsaitis] *n.* 窦炎

The most common complication of upper respiratory disease in adults is maxillary sinusitis.

成人上呼吸道疾病的最常见的并发症是上颌窦炎。

In persistent sinusitis treatment may require the affected sinus to be washed out or drained by a surgical operation.

顽固性鼻窦炎治疗需作病窦的冲洗或手术引流。

Sinusitis may be complicated by serious intracranial infections.

鼻窦炎可并发严重的颅内感染。

siphon [ˈsaifən] *n.* 虹吸管，虹吸作用

At first the stomach is filled with water through a funnel and rubber tube, then the tube is bent downwards to act as a siphon and empty the stomach of its contents.

首先通过一个漏斗和橡皮管用水灌满胃，而后将橡皮管向下弯，起虹吸作用，把胃内容物排空。

siphonostegia [siˌfɔnəusˈtedʒiə] *n.* 阴行草，刘寄奴

All these compounds were isolated from siphonostegia for the first time.

所有这些化合物均为首次从阴行草植物中分离得到。

The article introduced the treatment of scleroderma by using siphonstegia.

本文介绍了运用阴行草治疗硬皮病的方法。

sitosterolemia [saiˈtɔstərɔˈliːmiə] *n.* 谷固醇血症

Many patients with sitosterolemia develop coronary heart disease at an early age.

许多谷固醇血症患者在年轻时就发生了冠心病。

This kind of effect on the sitostanol concentrations in the blood and tissues is relatively unknown, especially in patients with sitosterolemia.

对血液及组织中植物甾醇浓度的这种影响还不明确，特别是在谷固醇血症患者中。

situation [ˈsitjuˈeiʃən] *n.* 位置；情况；形势

In this situation a single oral dose of 3 gm of griseofulvin(preferably micronized) is given.

在这种情况下，应给予一次性口服灰黄霉素 3 克（微粒的最好）。

The pain produced by similar injuries is remarkably variable in different situations and in different people.

类似创伤引起的疼痛因情况不同和人的不同而有显著差异。

Obviously, such a situation calls for prompt medical attention.

显然，此病需要迅速就医。

skeletal [ˈskelitəl] *a.* 骨骼的

The adult skeletal system or skeleton consists of over 200 bones which form the supporting framework of the body.

成人的骨骼或骨骼系统包括 200 多块骨，组成人体的支架。

Deficiency in vitamin D results in imperfect skeletal formation, bone diseases and rickets.

维生素 D 缺乏可造成骨骼形成的缺陷、骨病和佝偻病。

skeleton [ˈskelitən] *n.* 骨骼

The skeleton supports the body as the steel construction supports the modern skyscraper.

骨骼支持人体，正如钢筋结构支撑摩天大楼一样。

skillful [ˈskilful] *a.* 巧妙的

The treatment of most cancer patients requires a skillful interdigitation of multiple modalities of treatment, including surgery and irradiation, with drugs.

多数癌症患者的治疗需要将多种治疗措施包括手术、放射治疗和药物治疗巧妙的结合。

skin [skin] *n.* 皮肤

Skin is the largest organ of the human body, our skin consists of two main layers, the Dermis and Epidermis.

皮肤是人体最大的器官,我们的皮肤包括两大层,即真皮和表皮。

The common side effects encountered were digestive tract reaction, suppression of bone marrow and skin damage.

遭受的常见副作用有消化道反应、骨髓抑制和皮肤损害。

skull [skʌl] *n.* 头颅(骨)

The flat bones of the skull are used as a covering for the brain.

头颅的扁骨可用作脑的覆盖物。

sleeplessness [ˈsliːplisnis] *n.* 失眠

Sleep disturbances are divided into patterns of excessive daytime sleepiness, sleeplessness and nocturnal arousals.

睡眠失调分为白天睡眠过多、失眠和夜间觉醒。

sleeptalking [ˈsliːpˌtɔːkiŋ] *n.* 梦呓

Sleeptalking and nocturnal leg cramps are normal behavioral responses, particularly during times of increased fatigue and stress.

梦呓和夜间腿痉挛都是正常的行为反应,特别是在非常疲乏和思想压力较重时易出现。

sleep-walker [ˈsliːpˌwɔːkə] *n.* 梦游者

The sleep-walker would get up in the night and dress himself and go out, if he were not stopped.

夜游症患者要是没有人阻止的话,会在夜间起床、穿衣、外出。

slide [slaid] *n.* 玻片,载片

To prepare bacteria for staining, a small amount of culture is dispersed in a drop of water on a glass slide.

制备染色片时,可将少量细菌培养物分散于玻片上的一滴水中。

slight [slait] *a.* 微小的,细微的,轻微的

Aneroid barometers are able to show much slighter changes in the atmosphere than mercury barometers.

空盒气压表比水银气压表更能测出大气中的细微变化。

In the classical glomerulonephritis the child wakes with malaise, headache and loin pain; there may be slight fever.

在典型的肾小球性肾炎,小孩常因不适、头痛和腰痛而惊醒,可能有微热。

In the central portion of the lesion ulceration may occur, while at the margins there may be slight acanthosis.

损害的中心部分可形成溃疡,在边缘可有轻度棘层增厚。

The pulse usually has a slight collapsing quality due to the shortening of systolic ejection.

由于收缩期射血时间缩短,脉搏通常略显充盈不足。

slightly [ˈslaitli] *ad.* 轻微地,少量地

These two bones are slightly dissimilar in shape.

这两根骨头在形状上略有不同。

Some of the sulfa drugs can have a slightly bad effect on the kidneys.

有一些磺胺药对肾脏有轻微的不良作用。

slim [slim] *a.* 苗条的,微小的

Ladies are trying to get fit and slim down.

女士们设法使身体健康并变得苗条。

There's only a slim hope of survival for the crash victims.

在飞机坠毁的受难者中,很少有希望能找到生还者。

slope [sləup] *n.* 斜率;斜坡

Antiarrhythmic agents can slow down the spontaneous discharge frequency of an automatic pacemaker by depressing the slope of diastolic depolarization.
抗心律失常药可通过降低自律细胞的舒张期去极化斜率从而减慢自发放电频率。
She did not dare to bike down the abrupt slope.
她不敢骑着自行车冲下陡峭的斜坡。

slough [slʌf] *n.* 脱落
All the skin lesions ulcerate with a foul slough.
所有的皮肤病变组织腐烂脱落而形成溃疡。
In deep burns the integument forms a slough which in due course is cast off, leaving an ulcer which unless skingrafted heals slowly and with much fibrosis and scarring.
在深度烧伤,皮肤形成一种经相当长的时间才能脱去的腐痂,并留下一片溃疡,除非进行皮肤移植,否则痊愈缓慢,并留下大量纤维化组织和瘢痕。

sludge [slʌdʒ] *n.* 淤泥
Fluid sludge can be sold to farmers for spreading on their fields.
液态污泥可以出售给农民,洒布在农田里。
There is lots of sewage sludge in sewage disposal course.
在污水处理过程中会产生大量污泥。

sluggishly ['slʌgiʃli] *ad.* 缓慢地;迟钝地;呆滞地
The channels widen as more and more erythrocytes move sluggishly through this inflamed area.
当越来越多的红细胞缓慢地流经炎症区域时,血管变宽。

slur [slə:] *v.* 含糊地发音
She was covered with hives, felt she could not breathe, had a tingling sensation in her tongue, and her speech was slurred.
患者全身出现荨麻疹,感觉呼吸困难,舌部有刺痛感,言语含糊不清。

smallpox ['smɔ:lpɔks] *n.* 天花
There seems to be greater susceptibility among children to the virus of smallpox.
儿童似乎更易感染天花病毒。
The World Health Organization has declared the world to be free of smallpox.
世界卫生组织宣布世界上已无天花。

smear [smiə] *n.* 涂片
Identification of the pathogen by smear and culture remains a cardinal step in therapy.
通过涂片和培养确定病因仍是治疗的主要步骤。
Smear of the sputum revealed numerous acid-fast organisms.
痰涂片找到了大量抗酸杆菌。
Bacteria are far more frequently observed in stained smears than in living state.
染色涂片观察细菌比观察活菌常用得多。
v. 以…作涂片
A few drops of bone marrow are smeared directly onto slides to be stained with metachromatic stains and examined under the microscope.
直接向载玻片上推几滴骨髓作涂片,用异染性染料染色,在显微镜下检查。

smog [smɔg] *n.* 烟雾
When the smog hangs heavy in the city, it is poisoning the population that breathes it.
烟雾密布于城市上空,毒害着吸入它的人们。

smooth [smu:ð] *a.* 平滑的;光滑的
The adrenaline provokes relaxation of the smooth muscles of these small blood vessels while the noradrenaline causes contraction.
肾上腺素刺激引起这些小血管的平滑肌松弛,而去甲肾上腺素引起收缩。
The heart and valves are lined with endocardium to provide a smooth surface so that blood will

not clot.
心脏和瓣膜由心内膜衬覆,提供了光滑的表面,使血液不致凝固。
v. 使光滑,把…弄平
She smoothed down the sheets on the bed before putting on the blankets.
她在铺上毯子之前把床单弄平。

smother [ˈsmʌðə] *v.* 窒息,闷死
Asphyxia caused by obstruction of the external orifices of the air passages constitutes smothering.
呼吸道外孔堵塞引起的窒息可以导致闷死。

snail [sneil] *n.* 蜗牛;螺
These organisms penetrate into snails, multiply, and develop into cercariae, the infective form for men.
这些毛蚴进入螺体繁殖和发育成对人类有感染性的尾蚴。

snakebite [ˈsneikbait] *n.* 蛇咬伤
He is ill from a snakebite.
他因毒蛇咬伤致病。
Approximately 45000 snakebites occur annually in the United States.
美国每年大约发生 45000 例蛇咬伤。

sneeze [sniːz] *v.* 打喷嚏
The patient began to sneeze and to complain of some nasal obstruction and a sore throat.
病人开始打喷嚏,并主诉有些鼻塞和喉痛。
Symptoms of secondary peritonitis include abdominal pain that increases with motion, coughing or sneezing.
继发性腹膜炎的症状表现 为腹痛,它可随活动、咳嗽或打喷嚏而加重。
n. 打喷嚏
A sneeze cannot be performed voluntarily, nor can it be easily suppressed.
打喷嚏不受意志引发,也不能轻易抑制。

sniff [snif] *v.* 嗅,觉察出
The device can sniff out some common bacteria.
这种装置可以嗅出一些普通的细菌。

snooze [snuːz] *n.* 打盹,(白天的)小睡
It is good to health to take a half-hour snooze after lunch every day.
每天午饭后小睡半小时对健康有益。

snore [snɔː(r)] *v.* 打鼾
Snoring resulting in a hoarse noise usually occurs during sleep.
打鼾产生噪声,常发生在睡眠时。
n. 鼾声
Loud snores from the other room kept her awake.
来自另一房间的响亮鼾声使她不能入睡。

snort [snɔːt] *v.* 鼻吸,喷出;*n.* 鼻息声
Amphetamine can be used by snorting and smoking.
苯丙胺可以用鼻腔和口腔吸入。

snowblindness [ˈsnəublaindnis] *n.* 雪盲(症)
Many people believe that glare from snow causes snowblindness.
许多人认为由雪反射的眩目的日光会造成雪盲症。

soak [səuk] *v.* 吸收;浸泡
Carpets, curtains and furniture also soak up water.
地毯、窗帘和家具也吸收水分。
n. 浸泡

Don't use boric acid soaks in treating large burns, because enough boric acid could be absorbed to be dangerous.

不要使用硼酸浸剂治疗大面积烧伤，因为硼酸可大量被吸收达危险程度。

soap [səup] *n.* 肥皂；脂肪酸盐

The affected parts should be bathed thoroughly in soap and water, and the healthy areas that are not epilated may be shaved or depped.

受累的部位要用肥皂和水彻底浸洗，未拔毛的健康区域可剃去或剪掉须毛。

sober-minded [ˈsəubəˈmaindid] *a.* 清醒的，严肃的

This is a sober-minded and ethically justifiable transplantation.

这是一台严肃和伦理上合理的移植手术。

Is it an unhealthy phenomenon or a sober-minded experiment?

这是一种不良现象，还是一种冷静的试验？

socioeconomic [ˌsəuʃiəuiːkəˈnɔmik] *a.* 社会经济学的

People of lower socioeconomic status experience poorer health and a higher morbidity rate.

社会经济地位较低的人们健康状态较差，发病率较高。

sociology [ˌsəuʃiˈɔlədʒi] *n.* 社会学

Sociology is the scientific study of the nature and development of society and social behaviour.

社会学是研究社会本质、发展及社会行为的学科。

sociopathy [ˈsəusiəupæθi] *n.* 对抗社会性病态人格

This is a case of sociopathy.

这是一个反社会人格的病例。

In this study, we report a patient who, following trauma to the right frontal region, presented with 'acquired sociopathy'.

在该研究中，我们报道一位在右额部受创伤后的病人，表现为"获得性的反社会人格"。

socket [ˈsɔkit] *n.* 槽，臼，窝

The root of a tooth consists of one to three fangs contained in the socket.

牙根部由藏在牙槽内的 1～3 个牙根构成。

A hollow or depression into which another part fits is termed socket, such as the eye socket.

一个中空或凹陷结构，其中有其他组织充填，叫窝，例如眼窝。

sodium [ˈsəudjəm] *n.* 钠

The enzyme cannot catalyse ATP (adonosine triphosphate) hydrolysis unless sodium and potassium are transported.

除非钠和钾被转运，否则酶不能催化三磷酸腺苷水解。

Sodium-poor albumin infusions may be helpful in inducing diuresis.

低钠白蛋白输入可能有助于利尿。

soften [ˈsɔfən] *v.* (使)软化

The hydrochloric acid in the stomach juice softens the connective tissue in meat.

胃液中的盐酸有软化肉类中的结缔组织的作用。

Other problems include softening of bone and growth retardation.

其他问题包括骨骼的软化和生长迟缓。

This material can repeatedly be softened and hardened.

这种材料可以反复地变软或变硬。

softener [ˈsɔfnə] *n.* 软化剂

Constipation has been treated with fiber supplements, stool softeners, and laxatives.

便秘一直是用纤维补给品、大便软化剂和缓泻剂来治疗的。

software [ˈsɔftwɛə] *n.* 软件

All of the software would be destroyed by such a virus.

这种病毒能毁坏整个软件。

What sort of software do you have a good command of?
你擅长什么软件?

soil [sɔil] *n.* 土壤

Some children exposed to lead-contaminated soil have experienced brain and nervous system damage.
有些儿童由于接触铅污染的土壤,已经遭受到脑和神经系统损害。

Heavy metals, pesticides, solvents and other man-made chemicals, lead and oil spills are some of the common contaminants that lead to soil pollution.
重金属、杀虫剂、有机溶剂和其他人造化学制品、铅和石油泄漏是导致土壤污染的一些常见污染物。

solapsone [səˈlæpsəun] *n.* 苯丙砜

Solapsone was formerly a common drug used for the treatment of Leprosy.
苯丙砜是过去用于治疗麻风病的一种普通药物。

solar [ˈsəulə] *a.* 太阳的

Solar energy is now in its infancy.
太阳能的应用现在还只是刚刚开始。

Solar urticaria characteristically occurs within minutes of sun exposure.
暴露于日光下几分钟就可发病是日光性荨麻疹的特征。

solarium [səˈlɛəriəm] *n.* 日光浴室

The new sports center has saunas and solariums.
新的体育中心有蒸汽浴室(桑拿浴)和日光浴室。

The Cancer Council Australia strongly supports the National Standard on solariums, giving an age limit of 18.
澳大利亚癌症协会积极支持使用日光浴室的国家标准,年龄限制在 18 岁以上。

sole [səul] *a.* 唯一的

We would rarely make a diagnosis with a real patient on the sole basis of a description of the illness provided by a third party.
我们很少以第三者提供的病情描述为唯一的根据来给真正的病人做诊断。

solely [ˈsəu(l)li] *ad.* 只,单独地

Study of the opened valve is a procedure most often done solely for the purpose of measuring valve anuli.
对切开瓣膜的观察这种方法通常只是为测量瓣膜环的目的。

Micropuncture studies of pregnant rats suggest that the increase in glomerular filtration rate (GFR) is solely a consequence of the increase in renal blood flow.
对妊娠大鼠进行微穿刺研究提示肾小球滤过率的增加仅仅只是肾血流量增多的结果。

solicitation [ˌsɔlisiˈteiʃən] *n.* 收集、征集

For adverse events of active solicitation of information from patients, the requirements for mandatory reporting include whether or not there is a reasonable possibility that the drug caused the adverse experience.
对于主动收集的病人信息中的不良事件,强制报告的要求包括该药物引起该不良体验是否具有合理的可能性。

This paper is the result of a research on the volunteer solicitation system.
这篇论文是一项对于志愿者征集制度研究的成果。

solid [ˈsɔlid] *a.* 固体的 *n.* 固体

Heavy metal is a secondary pollutant from municipal solid waste incineration system.
重金属是城市固体废弃物焚烧系统产生的二次污染物。

The traditional techniques, such as liquid-liquid extraction and solid-phase extraction, are time-consuming and labor-intensive.

传统技术如液-液萃取和固相萃取是既耗时又耗人。

solidification [ˌsəlidifiˈkeiʃən] *n.* 固化作用

Solidification is one of the oldest processes for producing complex shapes for applications ranging from art to industry, and remains as one of the most important commercial processes for many materials.

固化作用是从艺术到工业等领域中用以形成复杂形状的最古老工艺之一,至今仍是多种材料商业化过程中最重要的步骤。

At the solidification temperature, atoms of a liquid, such as melted metal, begin to bond together at the nucleation points and start to form crystals.

在凝固温度,液体的原子例如熔化的金属,开始在成核点结合并形成结晶。

solitary [ˈsɔlitəri] *a.* 孤立的,单独的

Solitary pulmonary nodules are peripheral circumscribed pulmonary lesions.

孤立性肺部结节是周围性局限性肺部病灶。

solubility [ˌsɔljuˈbiliti] *n.* 溶解度,溶解性

Vitamins are divided into two main categories on the basis of their solubility: water-soluble and fat-soluble.

维生素可根据其溶解性分为两大类,即水溶性和脂溶性的。

The urinary solubility of the sulfonamides decreases when the pH of the urine decreases.

尿液 pH 值降低时,尿中磺胺类的溶解度降低。

solubilization [ˌsɔljubilaiˈzeiʃən] *n.* 增溶作用

Solubilization, according to an IUPAC definition is a short form for micellar solubilization, a term used in colloidal and surface chemistry.

根据 IUPAC 的定义,增溶是在胶体和界面化学中的一个术语,是胶束增溶的缩写形式。

Solubilization is one of the modern high technique applied to food industry.

增溶作用是应用于食品工业中的现代高级技术之一。

solubilize [sɔˈljubilaiz] *v.* 溶解

It should be recalled that not all solubilized drugs are absorbed.

应提醒大家,不是所有溶解的药物都能被吸收。

Lipids may be solubilized by bile and other intestinal contents.

脂质可被胆汁和其他肠道内容物溶解。

soluble [ˈsɔljubl] *a.* 溶解的,可溶的

Soluble particles may be absorbed through the epithelium into the blood.

可溶性颗粒可以经上皮吸收进入血液。

One of the functions of fat in the body is to transport the fat soluble vitamins, which are A, D, E and K.

脂肪在体内的功能之一是运输脂溶性的维生素 A、D、E、K。

Sugar cannot pass through the membrane because its molecule is too large—even though it is readily soluble.

糖无法通过细胞膜,因为它的分子太大——尽管它很容易溶解。

solution [səˈljuːʃən] *n.* 解决(方法);溶液;溶解

Many specialists have attempted to find a solution to the problem of urinary tract infections.

许多专家试图对泌尿道感染这个问题找出一个解决办法。

Salt solutions are used in humidity standardization.

在湿度标准化中采用盐溶液。

solvent [ˈsɔlvənt] *n.* 溶剂,溶媒

Water is an important solvent.

水是一种重要的溶剂。

The granules are soluble in acetic acid and insoluble in lipid solvents.

这种颗粒溶于醋酸而不溶于如氯仿那样的脂类溶剂。

soma ['səumə] *n.* 体,躯体;体细胞

Anatomic lesions are lacking in the psychosomatic(Greek psyche, spirit and soma, body) diseases.

身心(希腊语心灵与躯体)疾病中无解剖病变。

Soma denotes the entire body cells excluding the germ cells.

体细胞指生殖细胞以外的整个身体的细胞。

somatic [səu'mætik] *a.* 躯体的,体的

Anxiety symptoms appear frequently as somatic complaints.

焦虑症状常表现为躯体疾病。

Radiation damage is known to cause chromosomal abnormalities in somatic cells.

据悉放射损伤可引起体细胞染色体异常。

somatization [səumətai'zeiʃən] *n.* 躯体症状化

Somatization disorder(or hysteria)is more likely to begin in females before age 25.

躯体症状化疾病即癔症较多地初发于 25 岁以下的女性。

somatomedin [ˌsəumətəu'miːdin] *n.* 生长调节素

Somatomedin is necessary for deposition of collagen and ground substance.

生长调节素为胶原和基质的沉积所必需。

somatostatin [ˌsəumətəu'stætin] *n.* 生长抑素

Somatostatin is a hormone with many inhibitory effects on the gastrointestinal system.

生长抑素是一种对胃肠系统具有多种抑制作用的激素。

somatotropin [ˌsəumətəu'trəupin] *n.* 生长激素

Somatotropin favors retention of protein by the body.

生长激素有助于身体保存蛋白质。

somesthetic [səumes'θetik] *a.* 躯体感觉的

The somesthetic sensations are those that arise from the body surface or from the deep tissues.

躯体感觉是那些产生于体表或深部组织的感觉。

somnipathy [sɔm'nipəθi] *n.* 睡眠障碍

Improvement of somnipathy is an effectively adjunctive treatment for antihypertensive therapy.

改善睡眠障碍是抗高血压治疗的一种有效辅助疗法。

The efficacy of traditional Chinese medicine in treating somnipathy in patients with hypertension is quite obvious.

中药在治疗高血压患者睡眠障碍中的疗效是十分明显的。

somnolence ['sɔmnələns] *n.* 思睡,困倦,嗜眠症

Dopamine-agonist-induced impulsivity and daytime somnolence are not uncommon.

多巴胺激动剂引起的冲动和白天思睡也不少见。

There have been only rare reports on travelers' insomnia and diurnal somnolence.

关于旅游者中的失眠症和白天思睡情况仅有极少报道。

sonogram ['səunəgræm] *n.* 语音图,声音图像,超声波扫描图

A renal sonogram showed no evidence of ureteral obstruction and minimal ascites.

肾超声波图像未显示输尿管阻塞和少量腹水的迹象。

sonography [sə'nɔgrəfi] *n.* 超声波检查法

Sonography is still much used for evaluation of both native and transplanted kidney.

超声波检查仍较多的用于评估本身和移植的肾脏。

It is important to complete emergency abdominal sonography rapidly(<3 minutes)and limit the views to specific regions where fluid collects.

在 3 分钟以内尽快完成急诊腹部超声探查并将超声视野限制在液体积聚特定区是重要的。

sophisticated [sə'fistikeitid] *a.* 复杂的,精密的

In some cases of functional dyspepsia, sophisticated testing of gastrointestinal electrical activity may reveal disturbances of gastrointestinal motility.

在某些功能性消化不良的病例中,有关胃肠道电活动的复杂的检查可能会显示胃肠道运动障碍。

More and more sophisticated machines are playing an important role in medicine.

医学上现在有越来越多的精密仪器发挥着重要的作用。

sophistication [səˌfisti'keiʃən] *n.* 复杂性,精密性

The complexity and sophistication of patient registry structures and operations vary widely.

患者注册架构和操作的复杂性与精细度变化很大。

soporific [sɔpə'rifik] *n.* 催眠药

Soporifics are used for insomnia and sleep disturbances, especially in mental illnesses and in the elderly.

催眠药用于失眠症以及睡眠紊乱,尤其用于精神病以及年长者。

sorbent ['sɔːbənt] *n.* 吸附剂,吸收剂

The sorbent was highly reactive towards SO_2 as compared with hydrated lime.

该吸收剂对二氧化硫的吸附性强于对氢氧化钙的吸附性。

Various calcium and sodium based reagents can be utilized as sorbent.

各种钙基和钠基的试剂可以被用来作为吸附剂。

sorbitol ['sɔːbitəl] *n.* 山梨糖醇

Sorbitol is used by diabetics as a substitute for cane sugar.

山梨糖醇被糖尿病患者用作蔗糖的代用品。

Sorbitols is additionally dangerous in patients with absent bowel sounds because profound distention may occur.

山梨糖醇对无肠鸣音的病人有附加的危险,因为可发生肠道膨胀。

sore [sɔː] *a.* 痛的

After an incubation period of 1-4 days, patients develop sore throat, fever and sometimes nausea, vomiting, and abdominal pain.

在 1 ~4 天潜伏期后,病人出现咽喉痛、发热,有时出现恶心、呕吐和腹痛。

The organism is pathogenic for the anthropoid apes and produces a primary sore and secondary skin eruption closely simulating the desease in man.

这种病原体可使类人猿致病,发生原发疮和二期皮疹,和人的发病十分相似。

Infection by the Ducrey bacillus and T. pallidum at the same time will produce a "mixed sore".

同时感染杜克雷杆菌和梅毒螺旋体,就会发生"混合性溃疡"。

soreness ['sɔːnis] *n.* 痛

The soreness of the sprained ankle made him frown.

足踝扭伤的疼痛使他皱眉。

sour ['sauə(r)] *a.* 酸的

The milk has turned sour.

牛奶变酸了。

Four classes of taste are recognized: sweet, salt, sour, and bitter.

人可辨别四种味道:甜、咸、酸、苦。

source [sɔːs] *n.* 来源,发源地

Legume food are a good source of protein for vegetarians.

对于素食者来说,豆类食物是蛋白质的理想来源。

Oil pollution is the first pollution source of the seas and oceans.

石油污染是海洋污染的首要来源。

There is no pollution source in the park and the environmental quality has met the evaluation

standard.
园区内无污染源,环境质量达到评估标准。

space [speis] *n.* 空间

Early shock is usually due to a decrease in blood volume, or an increase in the capacity of the vascular space, or both.
早期休克通常是由于血量减少,或血管腔容量增加,或二者同时存在所引起的。

span [spæn] *n.* 持续时间,跨度,全长

The average life span of a red blood cell is 120 days.
红细胞的平均寿命为 120 天。

v. 横跨,跨越

These particular proteins span the entire membrane.
这些特殊的蛋白质横跨整个膜。

spare [spεə] *a.* 备用的,多余的

They kept some spare blood for urgent operation.
他们保留一些备用的血液为紧急手术用。

sparganii [spaː'gænii] *n.* 三棱

There is a great influence of rhizoma sparganii on the hemorrheology of rabbits.
三棱对家兔血液流变学的影响很大。

Experimental study on compatibility of rhizoma sparganii and mirabilite is set out.
三棱与芒硝配伍的实验研究将要开始了。

sparse [spɑːs] *a.* 稀少的

In old scars the nuclei are sparse and small, and the bundles are smooth and hyalinized.
陈旧的瘢痕细胞核稀疏而小,纤维束是光滑和透明的。

sparsely ['spɑːsli] *ad.* 稀少地

In sparsely populated areas, proper measures are taken to help increase population.
在人口稀少的地区,则采取适当的措施增加人口。

spasm ['spæzm] *n.* 痉挛

Unlike peritonitis, renal colic induces spasm confined to the ipsilateral rectus muscle.
与腹膜炎不同,肾绞痛诱发的痉挛仅限于同侧腹直肌。

spasmodic [spæz'mɔdik] *adj.* 痉挛的,痉挛性的;间歇性的

Spasmodic dysphonia is a voice disorder characterized by involuntary movements or spasms of one or more muscles of the larynx during speech.
痉挛性发音障碍是一种语音障碍,其特征是讲话过程中一块或更多的喉肌发生非随意运动或痉挛。

Spasmodic torticollis is an extremely painful chronic neurological movement disorder causing the neck to involuntarily turn to the left, right, upwards, and/or downwards.
痉挛性斜颈是一种非常痛苦的慢性神经运动障碍,导致颈部不自主地转向左、右、向上和(或)向下。

spasmolytic [ˌspæzmə'litik] *a.* 解痉的

Esophageal barium meal examination made visible the smooth funnel-shaped narrow at the lower part of the esophagus, and the application of spasmolytic agents will enable it to expand.
食管钡餐检查可见食管下端呈光滑的漏斗型狭窄,应用解痉剂时可使之扩张。

n. 解痉药

The ache can often be alleviated temporarily by the spasmolytic.
疼痛多可被解痉药暂时缓解。

spastic ['spæstik] *a.* 痉挛的

On rectal examination, the anal canal may be tender and spastic.
直肠检查时,肛管可能有触痛和痉挛。

Spastic esophagus with severe substernal pain may be triggered by intense emotions such as extreme grief.
有严重胸骨后疼痛的食管痉挛，可由强烈的情绪如极度悲伤引起。

spasticity [spæs'tisiti] *n.* 痉挛状态；强直状态
Follow-up evaluation at 3 months reveals a minimal spasticity of the lower extremities.
三个月时的随访评价，发现双下肢有轻微痉挛。

specialist ['speʃəlist] *n.* 专家
The family physician may decide that a patient should consult a medical specialist or be cared for in a hospital.
家庭医师可以作出决定让病人去看医学专家或住院治疗。
A specialist usually devotes years of study on perfecting his skills in the diagnosis and treatments of certain diseases.
专家常用几年的时间致力于完善某些疾病的诊断和治疗方面的技术。

speciality [ˌspeʃi'æliti] *n.* 专业，特长
Chemistry is his speciality.
化学是他的专业。
If he practices a speciality, he should have credentials of training in that speciality.
如果他从事某一专科，他应有该专业的培训证书。

specialization [ˌspeʃəlai'zeiʃən] *n.* 特殊化，专门化，专业化，特化作用
An autotrophic, unicellular, green alga presents the minimum of specialization.
自养的单细胞绿藻表现出最小程度的特化。
Boys performed in a manner consistent with right hemisphere specialization as early as the age of 6.
男孩早在 6 岁就表现为一种以右大脑半球专业化的行为方式。

specialize ['speʃəlaiz] *v.* 使专门化；专门研究
A heart specialist is a doctor who specializes in heart diseases.
心脏病专家就是一位专门研究心脏病的医生。
Some hospitals specialize in the care of patients with mental illness and with tuberculosis.
有些医院专门负责精神病和结核病患者的诊疗。

species ['spiːʃiːz]（单复同）*n.* 物种，种
Each species of organism is associated with a large number of proteins typical of itself and itself alone.
每个物种的机体均与自身特有和仅为自身所有的大量蛋白质相联系。
Each species of dermatophyte tends to produce its own clinical picture, although several species may provoke identical eruptions.
每种皮肤癣菌倾向于产生它自身的临床特征，尽管几种可产生同样的皮疹。

specific [spi'sifik] *a.* 特定的，特异(性)的
Each of the bodily organs has its own specific function.
身体的每一器官都有其特有的功能。
The diagnosis is confirmed by a rise in specific antibody titre.
特异性抗体滴定度升高可确定诊断。
Specific immunity may be inherited to a certain degree.
特异免疫在一定程度上是可以遗传的。
n. 详细，细节，特性，特效药
The events of everyday life are unremittingly dull, and people have little memory for their specifics.
日常生活中的事情总是单调乏味的，人们对生活中的细节记得很少。
So far, there is no specific for this cancer.

到目前为止尚无这种癌症的特效药。

specifically [spiˈsifikəli] *ad.* 特别地，明确地，尤其

The physician will ask many searching questions to more specifically characterize information already given.

医生会提出许多询问，使以往得到的信息特征更加具体化。

Specifically, 31% of the 299 patients entered in the study had four or more involved nodes.

具体地说，列入研究的 299 个病例中，31% 有四个或更多淋巴结转移。

specification [ˌspesifiˈkeiʃən] *n.* 规范，说明书

A specification is an explicit set of requirements to be satisfied by a material, product, or service.

说明书是一套满足顾客需要的有关材料、产品或服务的明确规定。

The obscure charges against him lacked specification.

针对他的模糊指控缺乏详细说明。

specificity [ˌspesiˈfisiti] *n.* 特异性，特殊性，特异度

It should be emphasized that the different histamine storage sites show certain degrees of specificity.

应该强调指出，组胺的不同储存部位有一定程度的特异性。

Some enzymes have broader specificity and will accept several different analogs of a specific substrate.

一些酶有较宽的特异性，可接受一种特异性底物的几种不同类似物。

Sensitivity was low (0.56) and specificity was high (0.90) in female non-athletes.

在女性非运动员中，灵敏度低(0.56)而特异度高(0.90)。

specimen [ˈspesimin] *n.* 标本；样品

The biopsy specimens of the stomach of this patient are cancer-free.

这个病人的胃部活检标本找不到癌细胞。

Adenovirus was isolated from both specimens with the isolates confirmed by complement fixation.

两个标本均分离出腺病毒，并经补体结合试验证实。

spectacle [ˈspektəkl] *n.* 场面；景象；(*pl.*)眼镜

The heart transplant operation was a wonderful and never-to-be-forgotten spectacle.

这次心脏移植手术是一个奇妙的、令人永远难以忘怀的景象。

Contact lenses have made it possible for more than 20 million people to get rid of their spectacles.

隐形眼镜使 2000 多万人能够扔掉老式眼镜。

spectacular [spekˈtækjulə] *a.* 引人注意的，壮观的

Vagotomy may give spectacular therapeutic results for peptic ulcer.

迷走神经切断术对消化性溃疡产生特别的治疗效果。

The loss of blood from a cut artery may be rapid and unpleasantly spectacular.

因动脉切破而引起的大出血，可能极其迅速，场面十分惊人。

spectinomycin [ˌspektinəuˈmaisin] *n.* 大观霉素

Spectinomycin inhibits protein synthesis in gram-negative bacteria.

大观霉素可抑制革兰阴性细菌的蛋白质合成。

Spectinomycin is an antibiotic used to treat various infections, particularly gonorrhoea.

大观霉素是用以治疗各种感染，尤其是治疗淋病的一种抗生素。

spectral [ˈspektrəl] *a.* 光谱的

Recently, spectral analysis of heart rate variability has been used as a marker of automatic nervous activity.

近来，心率变异性的光谱分析已被用来作为评价自主神经的标志。

spectrometry [spekˈtrɔmitri] *n.* 分光术，光谱测定法

A mass spectrometry-based plasma biomarker was developed.

开发了一种以质谱分析为基础的血浆生物标志物。

A novel experimental technique for tandem mass spectrometry is presented.

展示了一种用于串联质谱分析法的新颖实验技术。

Spectrometry plays an important role in the determination of trace metal elements.

光谱测定法在微量金属元素的检测中发挥着重要的作用。

spectrophotometer [ˌspektrəufəu'tɔmitə] *n.* 分光光度计

Routine training should be given in the use of detecting instruments such as absorptiometer, titrator, and spectrophotometer.

使用检测仪器应作常规训练,如吸收比色仪,滴定计和分光光度计。

spectroscope ['spektrəskəup] *n.* 分光镜

The simplest spectroscope uses a prism, which splits white light into the rainbow colours of the visible spectrum.

最简单的分光镜是用一个棱镜把白光分离成彩虹七色的可见光谱。

spectrum ['spektrəm] *n.* 范围;光谱,波谱,谱

Some antibiotic drugs are called broad-spectrum antibiotics because they are effective against both gram-positive and gram-negative bacteria.

有些抗生素药物叫做广谱抗生素,因为它们对革兰阳性和阴性菌均有效。

The methods for managing patients with hypertension encompass a wide spectrum.

高血压患者的处理方法是很多的。

Sinoatrial conduction delays account for part of the spectrum seen in patients with the sick sinus syndrome.

窦房结传导延迟是病窦综合征病人症候的一部分。

speculate ['spekjuleit] *v.* 思索,推测

The researchers speculate that by reducing television viewing, childhood and adolescent obesity could be decreased.

研究人员推测,如果减少看电视,便有可能降低童年期和青春期的肥胖。

speculation [ˌspekju'leiʃən] *n.* 思索,推测

This remains the subject of considerable speculation.

这仍是一个具有相当推理性的题目。

speculum ['spekjuləm] *n.* 反射镜;扩张器

The vagina itself is often inadequately inspected because the speculum covers a large part of its surface.

由于大部分阴道表面被窥阴器遮盖,常使阴道本身不能充分暴露。

speed [spiːd] *n.* 速度

The speed of onset and distribution often provide a clear indication as to the site of the lesion and its possible cause.

发生的速度及分布范围常常提供明显的指征,表明损害的部位及其可能的原因。

sperm [spəːm] *n.* 精液;精子

If an X sperm enters the egg, the baby will be a girl.

如果带 X 染色体的精子进入卵内,就怀女孩。

spermatid ['spəːmətid] *n.* 精细胞,精子细胞

During meiosis, the diploid spermatogonia produce haploid spermatids.

减数分裂期间,二倍体精原细胞产生单倍体的精细胞。

spermatocyte ['spəːmətəusait, spəː'mæ-] *n.* [细胞] 精母细胞

Primary spermatocyte undergoes meiosis I to form two haploid secondary spermatocytes.

初级精母细胞经过第一次减数分裂形成两个单倍体的次级精母细胞。

One secondary spermatocyte divides and eventually grows into two sperm cells.

一个次级精母细胞分裂并最终产生两个精子。

spermatogenesis [ˌspəːmətəu'dʒenisis] *n.* 精子发生

Spermatogenesis begins to occur at the time of puberty.

精子发生从青春期开始。

spermatogonium [ˌspəːmətəu'gəuniəm] (*pl.* spermatogonia [ˌspəːmətəu'gəuniə]) *n.* 精原细胞

Sperm originate from spermatogonia.

精子源于精原细胞。

Spermatogonia undergo mitotic divisions to produce spermatocyte.

精原细胞经过有丝分裂产生精母细胞。

spermatoxin [ˌspəːmə'tɔksin] *n.* 精子毒素

The first human trials involving spermatoxins probably took place in 1925, undertaken by Russian researchers.

第一次涉及精子毒素的人体试验可能是在 1925 年由俄国研究人员进行的。

In 1938, researchers proposed funding a long-term spermatoxin study, but could not gather sufficient support from the research community.

在 1938 年,研究人员提议资助一项长期的精子毒素研究,但是这一提议没能获得研究委员会的足够支持。

spermatozoon [ˌspəːmətəu'zəuɔn] (*pl.* spermatozoa [ˌspəːmətəu'zəuə]) *n.* 精子,精细胞

In the uterus the spermatozoon fuses with the ovum.

精子在子宫内和卵融合在一起。

The antibodies can often be revealed in seminal plasma and their antifertility effect seems mainly to be due to hampered penetration of antibody-covered spermatozoa into cervical mucus.

这些抗体在精浆中常可以发现,它们的抗生育作用主要是抗体包被精子受阻不能穿过宫颈黏液。

spermine ['spəːmiːn] *n.* 精胺,精素

Spermine is a polyamine involved in cellular metabolism found in all eukaryotic cells.

精胺是一种参与细胞代谢的多胺分子,存在于所有真核细胞。

Crystals of spermine phosphate were first described in 1678, in human semen, by Anton van Leeuwenhoek.

1678 年,安东凡·吕文胡克首次描述了人精液中的精胺磷酸盐结晶体。

sphere [sfiə] *n.* 球,圆体;范围,领域

The child has a wide sphere of action.

这孩子有广大的活动范围。

spherical ['sferikəl] *a.* 球形的

The eye is a small, spherical organ.

眼睛是小的球形器官。

spherocytosis [ˌsfiərəusai'təusis] *n.* 球形红细胞症

Spherocytosis is the morphologic expression of these biochemical abnormalities.

球形红细胞症就是这些生化异常在形态学上的表现。

Hereditary spherocytosis must be differentiated from other congenital hemolytic states.

遗传性球形红细胞症必须与其他先天性溶血病鉴别。

sphincter ['sfiŋktə] *n.* 括约肌

The acid gastric juice is poured into the first part of the duodenum when the pyloric sphincter relaxes.

当幽门括约肌放松时,酸性胃液流入十二指肠的第一部分。

Cholecystokinin is released from the duodenal mucosa and stimulates the gallblader to contract and the sphincter of Oddi to relax.

缩胆囊素从十二指肠黏膜释放,可刺激胆囊收缩,奥狄括约肌即松弛。

sphygmomanometer [ˌsfigməumə'nɔmitə] *n.* 血压计

A sphygmomanometer is used with a stethoscope for measuring blood pressure.
血压计连同听诊器用来测量血压。
Blood pressure is measured by an instrument known as sphygmomanometer.
血压可用一种称为血压计的仪器来测定。

spider ['spaidə] *n.* 蜘蛛痣
Main signs of the patient consisted of hepatomegaly, emaciation, jaundice, ascites and spider angioma
该患者主要体征有肝肿大、消瘦、黄疸、腹水及蜘蛛痣。

spill [spil] *n.* 溢出，泄漏
Environmentalists say the long-term impact of the spill is being ignored.
环保人士表示，此次泄漏的长远影响被忽略了。
Low-molecular weight plasma proteins may spill over into the urine when they are present in high concentrations.
当低分子量血浆蛋白浓度高的时候，它们可以溢出进入尿液 。

spinal ['spainəl] *a.* 棘的；脊柱的
The nervous system comprises the central and peripheral nervous system, the former is composed of the brain and spinal cord and the latter includes all the other neural elements.
神经系统由中枢和外周神经系统组成，前者由脑和脊髓构成，后者包括所有的其他神经成分。
The concentration of chlortetracycline in spinal fluid is only one-fourth that in the plasma.
氯四环素在脑脊液中的浓度仅为血浆浓度的 1/4。

spine [spain] *n.* 棘，刺；脊柱
Tuberculosis of the spine has a special name: Pott' s disease.
脊柱结核病有一专门名称：波特氏病。
Cervical spine disease can cause shoulder pain.
颈椎病可引起肩膀疼痛。

spinnbarkeit ['spinbɑːkeit] *n.* 子宫颈黏液成丝现象，排卵黏线
Similar trends were observed with the spinnbarkeit.
我们观察到子宫颈黏液成丝现象的相似趋势。
Under the influence of drug treatment, pH value and spinnbarkeit of cervical mucus decreased.
在药物的影响下，宫颈黏液的 pH 值、拉丝度下降。

spinous ['spainəs] ,**spinose** ['spainəus] *a.* 棘状的，刺的，棘突的
The spinous processes of the cervical vertebrae are not so long as those of the thoracic vertebrae.
颈椎的棘突没有胸椎的棘突那样长。

spiral ['spaiərəl] *n.* 螺旋菌
Spirals are in curved forms.
螺旋菌是弧形的。

spiramycin [spaiərə'maisin] *n.* 螺旋霉素
Spiramycin is used as second-line treatment for toxoplasmosi.
螺旋霉素是对弓形体病的二线治疗药。
Other antibiotics such as spiramycin also kill Toxoplasma gondii in animals, but have not been studied in infants.
其他抗生素如螺旋霉素也可杀死动物体内弓形体，但尚未在婴儿体内进行研究。

spirillum [spaiə'riləm] (*pl.* spirilla [spaiə'rilə]) *n.* 螺旋菌
About one half the bacilli and almost all of the spirilla possess filaments.
约半数的杆菌和几乎所有的螺旋菌都具有鞭毛。

spirit ['spirit] *n.* 精神；[复] 情绪；烈性酒；酒精；酊剂
We should cultivate medical students the spirit of an unselfish devotion to the improvement of

people's health.
我们应当培养医学生为增进人民健康而无私奉献的精神。
The patient's subjective mood should be elicited by asking for a description of current spirits.
通过询问病人最近情绪如何来了解病人的主观心境。
Whisky, brandy, gin and rum are all spirits.
威斯忌、白兰地、杜松子酒和兰姆酒都是烈性酒。

spirochete [ˈspaiərəkiːt] *n.* 螺旋体
The spirochetes are long, thin, flexible helical organisms, shaped like a corkscrew.
螺旋体是细长、易弯曲的螺旋形微生物,形似螺锥。
In syphilis, the spirochetes enter the body at the point of contact through the genital skin or mucous membranes.
梅毒感染时,螺旋体从接触点先通过生殖器的皮肤或黏膜再进入体内。

spirochetemia [ˌspaiərəkiːˈtiːmiə] *n.* 螺旋体血症
In mice, spirochetemia was detectable between postinoculation days 3 and 13.
小鼠在接种后 3 到 13 天可以检测出螺旋体血症。
The time points of spirochetemia may vary from patient to patient.
螺旋体血症的时间窗可因病人不同而不同。

spirometer [ˌspaiəˈrɔmitə] *n.* 肺活量计
Spirometer can be used to record the flow of air into and out of the lungs.
肺活量计是用来记录流进和流出肺部气流的仪器。

spironolactone [ˌspaiərənəuˈlæktəun] *n.* 安体舒通;螺内酯
In addition, spironolactone is reported to inhibit binding of dihydrotestosterone to receptors.
另外,有报道认为螺内酯能抑制双氢睾酮结合到受体。
Spironolactone has a direct portal hypotensive effect in addition to its ability to reduce plasma volume by diuresis.
螺内酯除了通过利尿作用降低血浆容量外还能直接降低门静脉压力。

spit [spit](spat [spæt]) *v.* 吐(痰、唾沫等)
In many countries it is considered rude to spit in public.
在许多国家当众吐痰被认为是粗野无礼的。
The sputum coughed up and spat by a person carrying the organism dries out, and the bacilli carried about for long periods of time in the dust of the air are inhaled by other individuals.
带有这种细菌的人咳出并吐出的痰干后,细菌会长时间地附着在空气的灰尘中到处传播而被其他人吸入。

splanchnic [ˈsplæŋknik] *a.* 内脏的
The disease caused by fungi that encroach subcutaneous tissue and splanchnic tissue is called deep fungus disease.
侵犯皮下组织及内脏的真菌,所引起的疾病称为深部真菌病。
Fibers pass through the splanchnic nerves into the adrenal glands and make synaptic connections on the chromaffin cells of the adrenal medulla.
纤维通过内脏神经到肾上腺,使突触连接到嗜铬细胞的肾上腺髓质。

spleen [spliːn] *n.* 脾
The stomach and spleen lie in the left upper portion of the abdomen.
胃和脾位于腹腔左上部。

splenectomise [spliˈnektəmaiz] *v.* 做脾切除
The pneumococcus is particularly dangerous to the splenectomised patient.
对脾切除患者,肺炎双球菌(感染)是特别危险的。

splenectomy [spliˈnektəmi] *n.* 脾脏切除术
Splenectomy often leads to improvement of splenic anemia (Banti's syndrome), but is of little

value in relieving portal hypertension.
脾脏切除常导致脾脏性贫血(班蒂氏综合征)改善,但对缓解门脉高压作用不大。
Splenectomy does not appear to benefit such patients.
脾切除术似乎并不使这样的患者受益。

splenic ['splenik,'spli:nik] *a.* 脾的
Liver was moderately enlarged and the splenic tip was palpable.
肝脏中度肿大,脾脏尖端可触及。

splenomegaly [ˌspli:nəu'megəli] *n.* 脾(肿)大
Portal hypertension is marked in the tropical splenomegaly syndrome.
热带脾肿大综合征中有显著的门静脉高压。
Splenomegaly is the most common physical manifestation of leukemias.
脾肿大是白血病最常见的体征。
Patients with splenomegaly should restrict their involvement in sports to avoid traumatic rupture.
脾肿大的病人应限制参加体育运动,从而避免创伤性脾破裂。

splenorrhaphy [spli'nɔrəfi] *n.* 脾缝合术
Surgery,usually splenectomy or splenorrhaphy,is the only effective management.
外科治疗如脾切除术或脾缝合术是惟一有效的手术治疗。

splice [splais] *v.* 拼接(n. splicing)
A one-celled germ found in the colon,E. Coli,is frequently used in gene splicing experiments.
存在于结肠内的一种单细胞细菌(大肠埃希菌)常被用于基因拼接实验。
The so-called gene splicing or recombinant DNA(deoxyribonucleic acid),it is a way to redesign the genetic composition of an organism.
所谓基因拼接或重组 DNA(脱氧核糖核酸)是一种对生物基因成分重新设计的方法。

splicing ['splaisiŋ] *n.* 剪接
While the function of introns remains unclear,the mechanism of splicing is beginning to be understood.
虽然对内含子的功能仍不清楚,但对剪接的机制已有所了解。

splint [splint] *n.* 夹板,夹
The patient has his right leg in a splint.
病人右腿上了夹板。

split [split] *a.* 分裂的
The first heart sound was normal and the second sound was physiologically split.
第一心音正常,第二心音有生理性分裂。

spoil [spɔil] *v.* 损坏,破坏
Don't spoil your appetite by eating too much candy just before dinner.
不要在饭前吃太多的糖果而坏了你的胃口。
Trans fats have a higher melting point,which makes them less likely to spoil,and since trans fats are more solid than oil,they can be stored for longer periods without spoiling.
反式脂肪有更高的熔点,这使得它们不易受到破坏;因反式脂肪比油更坚实,它们可储存更长的时间而不受损。

spondylitis [ˌspɔndi'laitis] *n.* 脊柱炎
Sacroiliitis and ankylosing spondylitis are commoner in patients with ulcerative colitis.
骶髂关节炎和强直性脊柱炎更常见于溃疡性结肠炎的患者。
Ankylosing spondylitis has been thought to be a disease primarily of men.
强直性脊柱炎一直被认为主要是男性的疾病。

spondyloarthropathy [ˌspɔndiləuɑ:'θrɔpəθi] *n.* 脊柱关节病
Spondyloarthropathy is a disease that affects the spinal column and causes inflammation and in severe cases deformity.

脊柱关节病是一种影响脊柱的疾病,可导致炎症和严重病例的畸形。

There is no known cause of spondyloarthropathy, however, some studies seem to indicate there may be a link to a specific gene that is present in many patients or that the condition may in fact be hereditary.

脊柱关节病没有已知的原因,然而一些研究显示其可能与出现于很多病人的一种特定基因有关,或者该疾病事实上可能就是遗传性的。

spondylosis [ˌspɔndiˈləusis] *n.* (脊)椎关节强硬

Advanced lumbar spondylosis is frequently associated with low back pain.

晚期的腰椎关节强硬常伴有腰痛。

Magnetic resonance imaging (MRI) will reveal the full extent of the anatomic abnormalities in cervical spondylosis and cervical disk disease.

对于颈椎关节强硬和颈椎间盘疾病,磁共振成像可显示其解剖学异常的整个范围。

sponge [spʌndʒ] *n.* 海绵;(外科用)纱布

The sham organ is represented by a sponge in which allogeneic antigens have been fixed.

用已固定同种抗原的一块海绵充当假器官。

It seems that the surgeon has left a sponge in the patient.

外科医生似乎将一块纱布留在病人体内了。

spongiform [ˈspʌndʒifɔːm] *a.* 海绵状的

Prions cause transmissible spongiform encephalopathy.

朊病毒导致传染性海绵状脑病。

Accumulation of abnormal prion protein leads to neuronal damage and distinctive spongiform pathologic changes in the brain.

异常朊蛋白的聚集导致大脑神经元受损及特征性的海绵状病理改变。

spongy [ˈspʌndʒi] *a.* 海绵状的

As spongy masses of lymph tissue, the tonsils form a ring of protection around your throat and nasal passages.

扁桃体是一个海绵状的淋巴组织团块,它在咽喉与鼻腔通道的四周形成一个保护性环带。

sponsor [ˈspɔnsə] *v.* 主办,举办;赞助,资助

The symposium on geriatric diseases last month was sponsored by the Chinese Medical Association.

上个月举行的老年疾病专题讨论会是由中华医学会主办的。

The firm is sponsoring five medical students at the university.

这家公司正资助 5 名医学生在大学学习。

spontaneous [spɔnˈteinjəs] *a.* 自发的,自然的

Spontaneous intracranial hemorrhages of all types can be precipitated by hypertensive crises.

所有类型的自发性颅内出血都能由高血压危象所引发。

The patient was the product of a full-term pregnancy and spontaneous vaginal delivery.

此患者系足月妊娠经阴道自然分娩。

spontaneously [spɔnˈteinjəsli] *ad.* 自发地,自然产生地

Sudden heart failure frequently occurs spontaneously as a result of clinically unsuspected heart disease.

突然心衰常由于临床上漏诊的心脏病而自然产生。

sporadic [spəˈrædik] *a.* 散在的,散发(性)的;偶尔发生的

Sporadic case reports of this tumor have appeared.

已出现过有关这种肿瘤的零星病例报告。

Last night the pain was colicky in nature, periumbilical, and rather sporadic.

昨晚在脐部周围发生时有时无绞痛性疼痛。

sporadically [spəˈrædikəli] *adv.* 零星地;偶发地

Kelly says the parasite gains the upper hand when anti-malarial drugs are taken sporadically.
凯莉说，如果抗疟疾药物不是按时服用，疟原虫就会产生抗药性（占上风）。

Paragangliomas of head and neck are rare tumors that occur sporadically with the prevalence of about 1 in 30,000 of head and neck tumors.
头颈部副神经节瘤是一罕见偶发的疾病，其发病约为头颈部肿瘤的三万分之一。

spore [spɔː] *n.* 芽孢

Some spore can remain viable for years, perhaps centuries, under normal soil conditions.
一些芽孢在正常土壤环境下存活数年，或许达数个世纪。

When favourable conditions return, the spores start to grow and reproduce.
恢复到有利条件时，孢子就开始生长和繁殖。

sporotrichosis [ˌspɔːrəutri'kəusis, spɔ-] *n.* 孢子丝菌症

Sporotrichosis is a disease caused by the infection of the fungus Sporothrix schenckii.
孢子丝菌症是一种申克孢子丝菌感染引起的真菌性疾病。

Primary lesions of sporotrichosis develop at the site of implantation of the fungus, usually at more exposed sites mainly the limbs, hands and fingers.
孢子丝菌症的主要病灶发生于真菌植入的部位，通常在更暴露的部位如四肢、手和手指。

sporozoite [ˌspɔːrəu'zəuait] *n.* 子孢子，孢子体

Sporozoites inoculated by an infected mosquito disappear from human blood within half an hour and enter the liver.
被感染的蚊子将子孢子接种到人体，子孢子在半小时内从血流中消失进入肝脏。

Sporozoites may develop immediately in liver cells into thousands of individual merozoites.
子孢子立即在肝细胞内发育成数以千计的裂殖子。

sporozoon [ˌspɔːrəu'zəuɔn] (*pl.* sporozoa [ˌspɔːrəu'zəuə]) *n.* 孢子虫

Sporozoa that parasitize vertebrates are transmitted from host to host by invertebrates, which act as intermediate hosts.
寄生于脊椎动物的孢子虫则以无脊椎动物为中间宿主而从一宿主传播至另一宿主。

spot [spɔt] *n.* 点，斑点；地点

Either "spot" urine samples or 24-hour urine collections can be evaluated.
无论是"点"尿的标本或是收集的 24 小时尿液均可用来测定。

In smallpox all the lesions begin as red spots which become small lumps turning into blisters.
出水痘时，损害都始于红色斑点，演变成小丘疹，再转化为水疱。

Preliminary treatment should be given, if possible, on the spot before the patient is removed to a hospital.
如有可能，在把病人送到医院之前，应该就地给以初步的治疗。

spouse [spauz] *n.* 配偶，丈夫或妻子

It is preferable that the therapy for this woman is done in the presence of her spouse.
对这位妇女的治疗最好有其配偶在场。

He loses caring behaviors for the spouse, relatives, friends, pets and home.
他不再具有关心自己的配偶、亲戚、朋友、宠物和家庭的行为。

sprain [sprein] *n.* 扭伤

A sprain of a joint is a stretching injury of one or more ligaments.
关节扭伤是指 1 条或多条韧带因牵拉而受到损伤。

Sprains should be treated by cold compresses (ice-packs) at the time of injury, and later by restriction of activity.
扭伤可在损伤时用冷敷（冰袋）治疗，以后要限制活动。

spray [sprei] *n.* 喷雾；喷雾剂

Antidiuretic hormone is given by nasal spray, but the intention is to produce systemic effects.
抗利尿剂激素经鼻喷雾使用，但其目的却在于产生全身效应。

DDT(dichlorodiphenyltrichloroethane) and other sprays made it possible for WHO to declare total war on mosquitoes.
滴滴涕和其他喷雾剂使世界卫生组织有可能向蚊子全面宣战。

sprue [spruː] *n.* 脂肪痢；口炎性腹泻
The small intestinal mucosa at high magnification shows marked chronic inflammation in celiac sprue.
在高倍镜下，小肠黏膜显示脂肪痢有明显的慢性炎症。
Celiac sprue has a prevalence of about 1∶2000 Caucasians, but is rarely seen in other races.
脂肪痢在白种人中的发病率为1∶2000，但很少发生在别的种族。

sputum [ˈspjuːtəm] (*pl.* sputa [ˈspjuːtə]) *n.* 痰，唾沫
Sputum should be sent for culture and Gram stain before starting antibiotics.
在开始抗生素治疗之前应送痰培养及革兰染色检查。
This is to be distinguished from the coughing up of bloodstained sputum.
这与咳出沾染血液的痰有所不同。

squama [ˈskweimə] (*pl.* squamae [ˈskweimiː]) *n.* 鳞屑（指表皮的）
Squama denotes any of the scales from the cornified layer of the epidermis.
鳞屑指来自表皮角质层的任何一种皮屑。

squamomastoid [ˌskweiməˈmæstɔid] *a.* 颞鳞乳突的
Squamomastoid location is at the squamous and petrous portions of the temporal bone.
颞鳞乳突的位置处在颞骨的鳞状坚硬部位。
Temporal pain and bone disorder may be relevant to medical information for squamomastoid disease.
颞鳞乳突的疾病可能和偏头痛和骨病有关。

squamous [ˈskweiməs] *a.* 鳞状的
The most common type of lung cancer is squamous carcinoma.
肺癌最常见的类型是鳞状肺癌。
Squamous metaplasia is a medical term used to describe the changes occurring to the cells in certain tissues of the body.
鳞状上皮化生是一个用来描述机体特定组织细胞的变化的医学术语。

squeeze [skwiːz] *v.* 挤，压
The squeezing effects of muscular contraction upon the veins accelerate the return of the blood to the heart.
肌肉收缩对静脉的挤压作用，加速血液回流到心脏。
Chyme, a thick liquid processed in the stomach, is then squeezed into the small intestine where digestion continues so that the body can absorb nutrients into the bloodstream.
食糜，在胃中处理过的黏稠液状食物，被挤进小肠，继续消化后，身体就可将营养吸收进血流。

stability [stəˈbiliti] *n.* 稳定，稳定性
Synovial fluid acts as a lubricant to the joint and helps to maintain its stability.
滑液对关节起一种润滑剂的作用，并有助于保持其稳定性。
Information on the purity and stability of the chemical to be tested is essential.
有关待测化学物质纯度和稳定性的信息是必不可少的。

stabilize [ˈsteibilaiz] *v.* 稳定，安定
Exploration and repair of the injuries should be done as soon as the patient's condition stabilizes.
患者情况稳定以后，应立即探查并修复损伤。
His blood pressure stabilized, his mental status improved, and his urinary output rose to 100cm^3/sec.

他的血压稳定下来，精神状态好转，排尿量上升到 $100cm^3$/秒。

stable ['steibl] *a.* 稳定的

The patient's condition is stable now.

病人的病情现已稳定。

Isotopes may be stable and maintain a constant character.

同位素可以是稳定的，保持着不变的特性。

Blood pressure was stable at 95/70mmHg.

血压稳定在 95/70mmHg。

Certain chemically stable compounds can be converted to chemically reactive metabolites.

有些化学性质稳定的化合物可被转化为具有反应活性的代谢产物。

stack [stæk] *n.* 层积，堆积

The Golgi complex consists of stacks of smooth endoplasmic reticulum.

高尔基复合体由光面内织网膜堆叠而成。

stadium ['steidiəm] (*pl.* stadia) *n.* 期，病期

The stadium invasion is the period between exposure to infection and the onset of symptoms.

疾病侵袭期指从接触感染到症状出现之间的一段时间。

staff [stɑːf] *n.* 全体职员，全体教员

This university has a hard-working staff.

这所大学的教职员工工作十分勤奋。

All patients were operated on by the resident staff under supervision of four members of the attending staff.

所有病例都是住院医生在四名主治医生指导下进行手术的。

In this operation, the patient is under anesthesia longer and doctors and other staff must also work longer hours.

这种手术病人麻醉的时间更长，医生和其他人员工作的时间也要更长。

v. 为…配备职员

Women staffed field hospitals.

妇女成为野战医院的工作人员。

In 1968 a research group on T-RNA was established in Shanghai, staffed by scientists from the Institute of Biochemistry.

1968 年在上海成立了 T-RNA 研究小组，由生化研究所的科学家们组成。

stage [steidʒ] *n.* 阶段；产程

The first stage of labour is proceeding normally if the cervix is progressively dilating and the fetal condition is satisfactory.

如宫颈逐渐扩张，且胎儿情况良好，第一产程会正常进行。

staging ['steidʒiŋ] *n.* 分期

The staging of cancers is based on the size of the primary lesion, its extent of spread to regional lymph nodes, and the presence or absence of blood-borne metastases.

肿瘤的分期是根据原发肿瘤的大小、局部淋巴结的受累和是否存在血源性转移而确定的。

The TNM staging varies for each specific form of cancer, but there are general principles.

TNM 分期不同肿瘤是不一样的，但有总的原则。

stagnant ['stægnənt] *a.* 不流动的，停滞的

The amniotic fluid is by no means stagnant.

羊水决不是停滞不动的。

stagnate ['stægneit] *v.* 停滞，淤积

The secretions in the blocked part of the bronchus cannot escape and therefore stagnate.

支气管阻塞部分的分泌物不能排走，因而停滞下来。

Exposure to violet light is used to ease arthritis; however, excessive exposure to violet may stag-

nate and suppress emotions.
接触紫光可缓解关节炎，然而过度的接触紫色有可能让情感受到停滞和抑制。

stain [stein] *v.* 染色
This is routinely determined after staining the bacteria.
通常要在细菌染色后才能确定。
The cell contains deeply stained cytoplasm and prominent nuclei.
细胞含有着色很深的细胞浆及明显的细胞核。
n. 染料，染色
Hematoxylin-eosin stain is employed universally for routine examination of tissue.
苏木精伊红染色被广泛使用于常规组织检查。
The stain enables one to differentiate between different types of bacteria.
这种染色可以使我们鉴别不同类型的细菌。

staining ['steiniŋ] *n.* 染色法，染色
Without staining, bacteria are difficult to see at the magnification (400 to 1000×) required for their detection.
如果不染色，细菌即使放大 400 到 1000 倍也难以辨别。
During the period of medication old underclothes are worn because of the inevitable staining if fuchsin is used.
用品红涂剂期间，因不可避免地要染脏衣服，宜穿旧内衣。

stakeholder ['steikhəuldə] *n.* 利益相关者；有关方；有权益关系者
Stakeholders include patients, clinicians, providers, product manufacturers and authorization holders, and payers such as private, state, and national insurers.
利益相关者包括病人、医生、供应商、产品制造商和授权持有人以及支付者如私人、政府和国家保险公司。
The people responded enthusiastically to the healthcare reform plan and over 100 written submissions were received by the Health Bureau from different key stakeholder groups of the community.
民众对医改方案反应热烈，卫生局共接收 100 多份由社区各主要有关团体提交的意见书。

stale [steil] *a.* 不新鲜的，陈腐的
During asthma enough fresh, oxygen-carrying air cannot get into the lungs, as they are already partially filled with the stale, trapped air.
患哮喘时含氧的新鲜空气不能充分地进入两肺，因为部分的肺已被停滞在那里的不新鲜的空气占据了。

stamina ['stæminə] *n.* 精力；持久力
Fatigue and loss of stamina can occur through a separate effect on the tissues (perhaps cellular enzyme dysfunction).
通过对各组织的影响（也许是细胞酶的功能障碍）而出现疲劳、精力不足。

stammer ['stæmə(r)] *n.* 口吃；结巴
He has always had a slight stammer.
他总是有点结巴。
v. 口吃
Stammering is not a symptom of organic disease and it will usually respond to the re-education of speech by a trained therapist.
口吃不是器质性疾病的症状，由受过训练的治疗人员进行言语再教育，通常能有所改善。

standard ['stændəd] *n.* 标准 a. 标准的
Details of the theoretical background and practical technique are not included here but can be found in standard textbooks of cardiology.
详细的理论基础和实用技术在此不涉及，可查阅标准的心脏病教科书。

In 1960 an international conference was held in Denver to establish a standard numbering-system for human chromosomes.

1960 年在丹佛举行了国际会议制订了一个标准的人类染色体编号系统。

The living and health standards of Chinese people have been greatly elevated in the past twenty years.

近 20 年来，中国人民的健康和生活水平大大的提高了。

standardize [ˈstændədaiz] *v.* 使标准化

The recent use of standardized diagnostic techniques has made it easier to diagnose depression.

近来使用标准化的诊断技术使抑郁症的诊断较为容易。

Macrobiotic diet guidelines are standardized and may be individualized based on factors such as climate, season, age, gender, activity, and health needs.

这些长寿饮食指南已标准化，也可根据一些因素，如气候、季节、年龄、性别、活动及健康需求的不同，而个体化。

standpoint [ˈstændpɔint] *n.* 立场，观点

From the standpoint of the patient the essential feature is the presence or absence of a myocardial infarct.

从病人的立场来看，基本特征是是否出现心肌梗死。

standstill [ˈstændstil] *n.* 停顿

In patients with ventricular standstill or ventricular fibrillation, loss of consciousness occurs 8 to 10s later.

室性停搏或室颤的病人在 8 ~ 10 秒后意识丧失。

staphylococcal [ˌstæfiləuˈkɔkəl] *a.* 葡萄球菌的

The neurologic symptoms noted with botulism help differentiate it from staphylococcal food poisoning.

由肉毒中毒而产生显著的神经系统症状，这有助于与葡萄球菌性食物中毒相鉴别。

Staphylococcal pneumonia usually occurs either in the presence of a source of bacteremia or after a viral infection.

葡萄球菌性肺炎通常来源于菌血症或继发于病毒感染。

staphylococcus [ˌstæfiləuˈkɔkəs](*pl.* staphylococci [ˌstæfiləuˈkɔksai]) *n.* 葡萄球菌

The semisynthetic penicillins are useful in staphylococcus infections.

半合成青霉素对葡萄球菌感染有效。

The "toxin" type of food poisoning most often identified is due to staphylococcus aureus.

"毒素"型食物中毒时最常见的病原要属金黄色葡萄球菌。

starch [stɑːtʃ] *n.* 淀粉

We find in our liver a kind of starch, which is not very different from potato starch.

我们可以在我们的肝脏里找到一种与土豆淀粉没有很大差别的淀粉。

The starch found in potatoes, the fatty layer of tissue under the skin and the majority of drugs are organic compounds.

存在于土豆中的淀粉，皮下组织中的脂肪层和大多数药物都是有机化合物。

starchy [ˈstɑːtʃi] *a.* 淀粉的

Starchy foods can be changed into a form of sugar.

淀粉质食物可以转变成为一种糖。

stasis [ˈsteisis] *n.* 停滞，淤积

Stasis within the microcirculation has many results.

微循环的淤滞产生许多后果。

The liver is enlarged and smooth in extra-hepatic bile stasis.

肝外胆汁停滞使肝脏肿大而平滑。

static [ˈstætik] *a.* 静的

Ascitic fluid is not a static reservoir.
腹水并不是静止的一坛水。

statin ['steitin] *n.* 他汀类;抑制素
In many cases niacin is a good drug for reducing statin levels.
很多情况下尼克酸是降低抑制素水平一种很好的药物。
Statin therapy has been shown to play a fundamental role in the treatment of coronary heart disease.
他汀类药物在冠心病防治中起重要作用。
Statin therapy should be considered for all diabetic individuals who are at sufficiently high risk of vascular events.
应考虑让所有有血管疾病高风险的糖尿病患者服用他汀类药物。

stationary ['steiʃənəri] *a.* 停滞的,静止的;不变的,固定的
Some tumors remain stationary indefinitely, whereas others increase in size, or break down as a result of infection and necrosis.
有些肿瘤长期维持不变,而有些肿瘤体积不断增大,或由于感染和坏死而溃破。

statistical [stə'tistikəl] *a.* 统计(学)的
What we are discussing here is strictly statistical.
我们现在所讨论的事项是作过严格统计的。

statistically [stə'tistikəli] *ad.* 在统计学上,用统计学
His report statistically strongly indicated and supported the diagnosis of ventricular tachycardia.
他的报告从统计学上有力地提示并支持室性心动过速的诊断。
This figure is statistically significant.
这个数字是有统计学意义的。

statistics [stə'tistiks] *n.* 统计学;统计数字
He is a doctoral student in statistics at Virginia Tech University.
他是美国弗吉尼亚理工大学一名统计学的博士生。
Apart from statistics, it might be helpful to look at what smoking tobacco actually does to the human body.
除了统计数字,看一看吸烟对人体的实际影响或许是有帮助的。
Statistics indicate that twins occur in about 1 in every 80 to 90 births, varying somewhat in different countries.
统计数字表明,双胎率约为每 80 ~ 90 例生产中有一例,不同的国家略有差异。

stature ['stætʃə] *n.* 身材
It is thought that the protein intake should be 50 per cent animal protein until full stature is reached.
在身体发育完全之前摄入的蛋白质应该有 50% 是动物蛋白。

status ['steitəs] *n.* 状态,情况;体质
The trainee advances through the ranks from the status of intern to that of resident and so on.
接受培训者由实习医生向住院医生等等逐级提升。

steadily ['stedili] *ad.* 稳定地,稳固地
In intestinal obstruction inspection of the abdomen may show distension which is most marked in low obstructions and increases steadily.
患肠梗阻时对腹部望诊可以看到腹部隆起在低位肠梗阻时最为明显,并逐渐加重。

steady ['stedi] *a.* 稳定的
The production of medicines rose at a steady rate from January to July.
药品生产从一月到七月持续上升。
There has been a steady decline in the incidence of epidemic diarrhoea following the recognition that the infection was due to contamination of food by dirt organisms.

随着人们认识到感染是由肮脏的有机物污染食物引起的，流行性腹泻的发病率已稳步下降。

steatohepatitis [ˌstiətəuˌhepəˈtaitis] *n.* 脂肪性肝炎

Current biochemical studies of Non-Alcoholic Fatty Liver Disease (NAFLD) and Non-Alcoholic Steatohepatitis (NASH) suggest a new therapeutic approach.

目前对非酒精性脂肪性肝病和非酒精性脂肪性肝炎的生化研究表明对这两种病有一种新的治疗手段。

steatorrhoea [ˌstiətəuˈriːə] *n.* 脂肪痢

The intrahepatic cholestasis results in jaundice, pale stools, dark urine and steatorrhoea.

肝内胆汁淤积引起黄疸、大便色白而小便色深，同时可有脂肪痢。

steatosis [ˌstiəˈtəusis, ˈstiːə-] *n.* 脂肪变性

In many forms of toxic hepatitis, extensive panlobular microvesicular and macrovesicular steatosis can be seen.

在很多中毒性肝炎中可以见到广泛的全小叶性小泡性和大泡性脂肪变性。

HCV-infected livers frequently show lymphoid aggregates within portal tracts and focal lobular regions of hepatocyte macrovesicular steatosis.

HCV 感染的肝脏常表现出门管区淋巴组织聚集及局灶性小叶内肝细胞大泡性脂肪变性。

stellate [ˈsteleit] *a.* 星状的

The gonococci cover not only the folded, stellate mucous membrane of the urethra, but also infiltrate into the urethral glands.

淋球菌不仅侵犯尿道多皱的星状黏膜，而且也浸润到尿道腺。

stem [stem] *n.* 茎，干，梗

Stem cells are undifferentiated, primitive cells in the bone marrow that have the ability both to multiply and to differentiate into specific blood cells.

干细胞是指骨髓中没有分化的、原始的细胞，具有增殖和分化为特定血细胞的能力。

stenosis [stiˈnəusis] (*pl.* stenoses [stiˈnəusiːz]) *n.* 狭窄

Patients with heart disease should be assessed for aortic stenosis.

对有心脏病者，应进行主动脉狭窄程度的估计。

The repeat angiograms showed six recurrent stenoses.

反复血管造影显示有 6 例狭窄复发。

stenotic [stiˈnɔtik] *a.* 狭窄的

Balloon angioplasty can effectively dilate highly stenotic coronary vessels.

充气血管成形术可有效扩张高度狭窄的冠状动脉。

stent [stent] *n.* 支架

Many patients receive stents in the treatment of carcinoma of esophagus.

许多病人在治疗食管癌时使用支架。

New devices such as intracoronary stents have shown some promise in reducing restenosis.

一系列新装置如冠脉内支架已显示出能减少再狭窄率的作用。

stephanotis [ˌstefəˈnəutis] *n.* 千金子藤

Stephanotis has fragrant waxy flowers.

千金子藤长有芬芳的蜡质的花。

Ms Donaldson walked up the aisle carrying a bouquet of white roses with stephanotis highlights.

唐纳森女士手中捧着千金子藤点缀的白色玫瑰花束，走上教堂的走廊。

stepwise [ˈstepwaiz] *a.* 逐步的，分段的

The dose was raised to 5mg/kg/day in a stepwise fashion according to a predetermined schedule.

按照事先确定的计划将剂量逐步提高到每日每公斤体重 5mg。

ad. 逐步

If hypercapnia of significant magnitude occurs, supplemental oxygen should not be completely

discontinued, but decreased stepwise.
如果出现相当程度的高碳酸血症,氧的补充不应完全停止,而宜逐渐减少。

stereotyped [ˈstiəriətaipt] *a.* 固定不变的
The reaction in the first few hours after injury is stereotyped.
损伤后最初几小时内的反应是固定不变的。

sterile [ˈsterail] *a.* 不生育的;无菌的,消毒的
The terms sterile, sterilize, and sterilization therefore refer to the complete absence or destruction of all microorganisms.
因此,无菌、消毒和灭菌这些术语是指完全没有或彻底消灭了一切微生物。
The inflammatory cells appear in the exudate or in scrapings taken with a sterile platinum spatula from the anesthetized conjunctival surface.
从经麻醉的结膜表面取得的渗出液或用无菌铂药刀刮取的碎屑中可见炎性细胞。
Cultures are best taken by rubbing the lesion vigorously with a sterile cotton swab moistened with sterile water and then streaked over the agar surface.
培养物最好用沾有无菌水的湿棉签用力摩擦皮疹取得,然后在琼脂表面画线培养。

sterility [steˈriliti] *n.* 消毒,无菌
The time of operation to achieve sterility depends on the nature of the material being sterilized.
消毒时间取决于被消毒物品的性质。

sterilization [sterilaiˈzeiʃən] *n.* 消毒,灭菌;绝育
Sterilization is the process of rendering any material free of living microorganisms.
灭菌是使物质摆脱活的微生物的一种方法。
Boiling water cannot be used in the laboratory as a method of sterilization.
煮沸不能作为灭菌法用于实验室内。
The patient emphasized that on account of her age and obstetrical history she would welcome surgical sterilization if an operation became necessary.
鉴于年龄及曾有生育情况,患者强调若需手术治疗,她愿接受绝育手术。

sterilize [ˈsterilaiz] *v.* 消毒,使无菌;绝育
When the transfer needle is sterilized, care should be exercised to prevent spatting.
在进行接种针灭菌时,应注意防止溅污。
In some countries women are sterilized to reduce the birth rate.
在一些国家里,妇女进行绝育以降低出生率。

sterilizer [ˈsterilaizə] *n.* 消毒器,灭菌器
When you need an autoclave that will sterilize your instruments, Alfa is the source for all your autoclaves and sterilizers needs.
当您需要高压灭菌器来对您的仪器进行消毒时,阿尔法是你所需高压灭菌器和消毒器的来源。
We provide prestige medical autoclaves and prestige medical sterilizers with competitive prices, contact us and you can know more details.
我们提供具有价格竞争力的声誉较高的医用高压灭菌器和医用消毒器,与我们联系,您将了解更多的细节。

sternum [ˈstəːnəm] *n.* 胸骨
The heart is situated immediately behind the sternum.
心脏紧靠在胸骨之后。
A heavy lump seemed to be perching on his chest, and severe pain radiated from the sternum area to his left shoulder.
好像有一块很重的东西压在他的胸部,剧痛自胸骨区向左肩辐射。

steroid [ˈsterɔid] *n.* 甾类化合物,类固醇
The patient is now fully recovered and no longer takes any steroids.

病人现已完全康复,并且不再服用类固醇药物了。

Steroids suppress the inflammatory response.

类固醇抑制炎症反应。

sterol [ˈstiərɔl] *n.* 固醇,甾醇

Similar to animal cells, mycoplasmas are surrounded only by a plasma membrane containing sterols.

支原体与动物细胞相似,仅由含固醇类的浆膜包绕。

The chief action of ultraviolet rays is to convert sterols in the skin into vitamin D.

紫外线的主要作用是将皮肤里的固醇转化为维生素 D。

stethoscope [ˈsteθəskəup] *n.* 听诊器

With the stethoscope the physician determines whether the breath sounds are normal.

医生用听诊器测定呼吸音是否正常。

stevioside [ˈstiːviəsaid] *n.* 甜味菊糖苷,蛇菊苷

Stevioside, a diterpene glycoside, is well known for its intense sweetness and is used as a non-caloric sweetener.

菊糖苷,一种双萜苷,因其甜度强而出名,被用作无热量的甘味剂。

Stevioside (SVS) is a widely used sweetener with multiple beneficial effects for diabetic patients.

甜菊苷是一种被广泛应用的甜味剂,对糖尿病人有多种益处。

sticky [ˈstiki] *a.* 黏性的

Injury to the endothelial walls of the microcirculation renders the surface of the capillary cell sticky.

微循环内皮壁的损伤造成毛细血管细胞表面的黏连性。

stiff [stif] *a.* 硬的,僵硬的,强直的,不灵活的

The joints become stiff and contractures develop in elderly patients after prolonged immobilization.

老年人长期卧床不动使关节僵硬,发生肌挛缩。

They were talking about stiffer sentences for criminals.

他们谈论对罪犯施以更严厉的判决。

Some tetanus patients show stiff neck and opisthotonos among the early signs.

某些破伤风病人的早期症状中表现有颈部强直和角弓反张。

stiffen [ˈstifn] *v.* (使)僵硬,(使)强直

Rigor mortis is the stiffening of muscles that occurs after death.

尸僵是发生在死后的肌肉强直。

stiffness [ˈstifnis] *n.* 僵硬,强直

As the disease progresses, joint pain and swelling increase and muscular stiffness becomes even more marked.

随着病情恶化,关节疼痛和肿胀加剧,肌肉强直更为明显。

stigma [ˈstigmə] *n.* 斑

Follicular stigma is a spot on the surface of an ovary where the vesicular follicle will rupture and permit passage of the secondary oocyte during ovulation.

卵泡斑是排卵时卵巢表面囊状卵泡破裂并允许次级卵泡通过而形成的斑点。

stigmatization [ˌstigmətaiˈzeiʃən] *n.* 污蔑、贬损

Certain populations of patients may be vulnerable to social, economic, or psychological harms as a result of stigmatization of health condition.

某些患病人群可能因健康状况受到歧视,而导致其容易受到社会、经济或心理上的伤害。

stilbestrol [stilˈbestrɔl] *n.* 己烯雌酚

The dose of stilbestrol should be restricted to 1-3mg daily.

己烯雌酚的用量应限制在每日 1～3 毫克。

Stilbestrol is used to relieve menstrual disorders and symptoms of the menopause, to treat prostate and breast cancer.

己烯雌酚用于减轻月经紊乱和绝经期症状，治疗前列腺癌和乳腺癌。

stillbirth [ˈstilbəːθ] *n.* 死产

Prematurity, stillbirth and toxemia are frequent complications of mild kidney infections during pregnancy.

早产、死胎和毒血症往往是妊娠期间轻度肾感染的并发症。

The perinatal mortality was 3.01%, the fetal death was 35.75%, the stillbirth was 26.09% and the neonatal death was 38.16%.

围产儿病死率为 3.01%，死胎、死产和新生儿死亡率分别为 35.75%、26.09% 和 38.16%。

stillborn [ˈstilbɔːn] *a.* 死产的；流产的

Neuroblastoma occurs during fetal life and is usually found in 5% of stillborn infants.

成神经细胞瘤发生于胎儿期，通常见于 5% 的死胎。

stimulant [ˈstimjulənt] *n.* 兴奋剂，刺激剂

The patient should be immediately brought into fresh air and given stimulants.

应将病人立即转移到新鲜空气处，并给予兴奋剂。

If necessary, these stimulants may be repeated at 4 to 6 hour intervals.

必要时，每 4～6 小时重复这些刺激剂为宜。

stimulate [ˈstimjuleit] *v.* 刺激；促进，激发

The substance, if it is a large polypeptide, acts as an antigen and stimulates the body to form antibodies.

如该物质是大分子多肽，则作为抗原刺激机体产生抗体。

These studies stimulated investigations to determine the mechanism(s) by which metal and metalloid compounds are carcinogenic.

这些研究激发人们对确定金属和非金属化合物致癌性机制的探索。

A foot massage is good for stimulating blood circulation.

脚底按摩有助于促进血液循环。

stimulation [ˌstimjuˈleiʃən] *n.* 刺激，兴奋

Cholinomimetic agents mimic the effects of stimulation of cholinergic nerves.

拟胆碱药的作用与胆碱能神经兴奋的效应相似。

stimulator [ˈstimjuleitə] *n.* 刺激器

Residual activity of muscle relaxants should be assessed with a peripheral nerve stimulator.

肌肉松弛剂的残余作用可以用外周神经刺激器来估价。

stimulus [ˈstimjuləs] (*pl.* stimuli [ˈstimjulai]) *n.* 刺激

A patient initially developing a fever may have chills, the severity and length of which depend on the stimulus.

最初发热的病人可能出现寒战，寒战的严重程度和时间的长短取决于刺激。

Vertebrate animals have evolved such complicated systems to mediate their responses to injurious stimuli.

脊椎动物已进化到具有这样复杂的系统来介导他们对有损害的刺激的反应。

stippling [ˈstipliŋ] *n.* 点彩

The anemia is hypochromic and the film contains target cells and stippling.

贫血为低色素性，血片上可见靶细胞和点彩。

stipulate [ˈstipjuleit] *v.* 确定，规定

Infertility is the inability to achieve pregnancy within a stipulated period of time, usually stated as one year.

不孕症指的是在规定的时间内,通常为一年,不能达到受孕。

stitch [stitʃ] *n.* 缝线

It is often necessary to cut the stitch before it can be withdrawn.

在缝线抽出前常有必要将其剪断。

stock [stɔk] *n.* 存货,库存

We don't have the medicine you want in stock now.

你要的那种药现在没有存货了。

stoma ['stəumə] (*pl.* stomata ['stəumətə]) *n.* 口;造口

Stoma therapists are nurses specially trained in the care of these artificial openings and the appliances used with them.

造口术治疗师是指经过专门训练、能对人工开口进行护理及应用其用具的护士。

stomach ['stʌmək] *n.* 胃

Carbohydrate digestion which begins in the mouth stops in the stomach and protein digestion begins.

碳水化合物的消化始于口腔终于胃,而蛋白质的消化始于胃。

The pain in the stomach often occurs at noon in that patient.

该患者胃痛常发生在中午。

Most gastric carcinoids occur in the body of the stomach.

大多数胃类癌发生在胃体部。

stomatitis [ˌstəumə'taitis] (*pl.* stomatitides [ˌstəumə'taitidiːz]) *n.* 口炎

Aphthous stomatitis is the most common ulcerative condition of the oral cavity.

口疮性口炎是口腔最常见的溃疡性疾病。

Stomatitis has recently become a problem for people who use antibiotic types of lozenges.

口炎近来成了服用抗生素类锭剂者的一个大问题。

Vesicular stomatitis is a viral illness of animals that occasionally affects humans.

水泡性口炎是动物的一种病毒性疾病,偶尔传染人类。

stomatocytosis [ˌstəuməsai'təusis] *n.* 口形红细胞增多

Most hereditary stomatocytoses are quite mild anaemias and the patients can lead a normal life.

大多数遗传性口形红细胞增多症只有很轻微的贫血,病人能够正常生活。

Dehydrated hereditary stomatocytosis is a rare congenital hemolytic anemia with a dominant inheritance pattern.

脱水遗传性口形红细胞增多症是一种罕见的显性遗传的先天性溶血性贫血。

stomatology [ˌstəumə'tɔlədʒi] *n.* 口腔学

Stomatology is the branch of medicine concerned with diseases of the mouth.

口腔学是从事口腔疾病(防治)的医学分支。

Prof. Baker is the director of the Department of Stomatology.

贝克教授是口腔科的主任。

stool [stuːl] *n.* 凳子;粪(便)

The patient may not vomit, but may pass the blood in the stools.

病人可能不呕血,但血可经大便排出。

stopcock ['stɔpkɔk] *n.* 气流开关,活塞,开关

When the stopcock is opened, water flows from the top of the warmer column into the colder column.

当活塞打开时,水即由较热的水柱顶端流入较冷的水柱。

storage ['stɔːridʒ] *n.* 贮藏

Some chemicals degrade on storage.

有些化学物质在贮藏时可发生降解。

Plastids, in general, serve as places of formation and storage for cell products.

一般来说,质体(粒)是细胞产物形成和贮存的地方。

These gene enhance the storage of fat when food is limited.

当饮食受到限制时,这些基因便会增强脂肪的沉积。

storax [ˈstɔːræks] *n.* 苏合香脂;苏合香

The investigation on physicochemical properties of storax has been made.

我们对苏合香的物理化学性能进行了考察。

Effects of storax cultivated in Guangdong on hemorrheology in rats are greater.

广东栽培的苏合香对大鼠血液流变学的作用更大。

storehouse [ˈstɔːhaus] *n.* 仓库

The liver acts as a storehouse for minerals and vitamins.

肝脏是储存矿物盐和维生素的场所。

strabismus [strəˈbizməs] *n.* 斜视,斜眼

The patient also has severe dental caries and strabismus.

患者还患有严重的龋齿和斜视。

The diagnosis of strabismus can be made by examining the location of the pupillary light reflexes.

斜视的诊断可借助于检测瞳孔对光的反射点来作出。

straight [streit] *a.* 直的

In young children the eustachian tube is relatively short and straight and hence easily allows infection to ascend from the nose and throat into the middle ear.

幼儿咽鼓管相对地短而直,故容易使感染从鼻和咽喉上行蔓延到中耳。

Straight-leg raising also may be tested by having the patient extend the knee while seated.

让病人坐位时膝部伸直也称为直腿抬高试验。

The straight dermal portion of the duct is composed of a double layer of cuboidal epithelial cells and is lined by an eosinophilic cuticle on its luminal side.

导管垂直的真皮部分由两层立方形上皮细胞构成,并在管腔的内侧衬以嗜酸性护膜。

straightforward [streitˈfɔːwəd] *a.* 简单的,直接的

The distinction between S1 and S2 is usually a straightforward process but can be difficult in the setting of a tachyarrhythmia.

分辨第一心音和第二心音通常是一个简单易做到的过程,但矫正心动过速则很困难。

strain [strein] *n.* 劳损,过劳;菌株

The most common cause of low back pain is mechanical strain.

下腰背痛最常见的原因是机械性劳损。

None but this pathogenic strain was shown to be sensitive to the new preparation.

除了这一致病菌株之外,其他细菌对此新制剂都不敏感。

strand [strænd] *n.* 股,链

The mixed samples are heated to separate the strands of DNA.

将混合物加热使 DNA 股链解开。

strangulation [ˌstræŋgjuˈleiʃən] *n.* 窒息,绞窄;

Is acute alveolar dilation an indicator of strangulation homicide?

急性肺泡扩张是引向窒息杀人的一种提示吗?

Acute intestinal strangulation is a lethal emergency that needs immediate surgery.

急性肠绞窄是一种致死性的急症,需要立即手术。

strategy [ˈstrætidʒi] *n.* 策略;对策

Strategies for dealing with drug addicts vary from country to country.

对待吸毒上瘾的人各个国家都有自己的策略。

These advances form a foundation for new therapeutic strategies to delay the onset of aging-related disorders.

这些进展为推迟老年性疾患的发生制定新的治疗策略提供了基础。

stratification [ˌstrætifiˈkeiʃən] *n.* 分层,分群婚配

Standardization and stratification both pursue the same objective of obtaining a pooled estimate of the drug effect.

标准化和分层都是为了达到同样的目的——获得药物效应的合并估计值。

Stratification describes a population in which there are a number of subgroups that have remained relatively genetically separate during modern times.

分群婚配描述了一个人群中在现代社会中仍存在一些遗传相对独立的亚群的现象。

streamlined [ˈstriːmlaind] *a.* 简化的,有效率的

The processes for reporting of adverse drug reaction should be streamlined as much as possible.

药物不良反应的报告过程必须尽量简化。

The modern hospital introduces a streamlined operating system for routine medical examination of patients.

这所现代化医院引入一种有效率的操作系统用于患者的常规体格检查。

strengthen [ˈstreŋθən] *v.* 加强,巩固

Some Chinese medicinal herbs strengthen the patient' s constitution, reduce pain and prolong his life.

有些中草药可增强病人的体质,减轻疼痛乃至延长他的生命。

Which of the following would most strengthen the conclusion drawn by the psychological researchers?

下列哪一项最能加强心理学研究者得出的结论?

strenuous [ˈstrenjuəs] *a.* 紧张的

The patient should stop smoking, lose weight and take regular non-strenuous exercise.

病人应该停止抽烟,减轻体重,同时进行非紧张性锻炼。

streptavidin [strepˈtævidin] *n.* 链菌蛋白,链霉亲和素

Avidin and streptavidin conjugates are extensively used as secondary detection reagents in histochemical applications

亲和素和链霉亲和素标记物在组织化学应用中被广泛用作第二检测试剂。

Streptavidin coated microspheres can be used to capture biotinylated compounds.

链霉亲和素包被的微球能用于捕获生物素化的复合物。

streptococcal [ˌstreptəuˈkɔkəl] *a.* 链球菌的

Prevention can be achieved only by the prompt detection, diagnosis, and treatment of streptococcal pharyngitis.

只有通过及时发现和诊治链球菌性咽炎,才能做好预防工作。

streptococcus [streptəuˈkɔkəs] (*pl.* streptococci [ˌstreptəuˈkɔksai]) *n.* 链球菌

Streptococci are much more resistant, some survive weeks after being dried.

链球菌耐干燥的能力要强得多,有些在干燥后可生存数周。

The streptococci are usually very sensitive to penicillin G.

链球菌通常对青霉素 G 十分敏感。

streptokinase [ˌstreptəuˈkaineis] *n.* 链激酶

Streptokinase is a thrombolytic agent.

链激酶是一种溶栓剂。

Streptokinase is used in thrombolytic therapy as a plasminogen activator.

链激酶作为纤溶酶原的血浆激活物已用于溶栓治疗。

streptomycin [ˌstreptəuˈmaisin] *n.* 链霉素

In the early days only penicillin and streptomycin were available.

起初只有青霉素和链霉素可供使用。

Streptomycin is a drug of choice in plague and tularemia.

链霉素为治疗鼠疫和土拉菌病的优选药。

stress [stres] *n.* 紧张;压力;激惹

The stresses and strains of work made him ill.

工作上的压力和劳累使他病倒了。

Whether this stress is from the loss of amniotic fluid, subclinical infection, or compression of the fetus in utero, the result is the same.

不论激惹是来自羊水的丢失、亚临床感染或胎儿宫内受压,结果是一样的。

stressor [ˈstresə] *n.* 紧张性刺激物,应激源

Other features have been emphasized, one of which is the possibility of precipitation by psychosocial stressors.

还强调了其他特点,其中之一是心理社会应激源促使发病的可能性。

Following exposure to environmental stressors, stress proteins become involved with the protection and repair of proteins complexes.

接触环境应激物后,应激蛋白发生的改变牵涉到蛋白质复合物的保护和修复。

Environmental stressors have been shown to induce the heat shock response, including the induction of HSPs and the reduction of normal protein synthesis in workers.

环境应激物能产生热休克反应,包括提高工人的热应激蛋白和降低正常蛋白的合成。

stretch [stretʃ] *v.* 伸长,伸展

Arteries are long, tubular blood vessels which can bend and stretch.

动脉是长管形血管,能弯曲,能伸展。

One fibre from a nerve cell may stretch as long as three feet.

一根神经细胞的纤维可延伸 3 英尺长。

With the entry of air in the lungs, the lung tissue is extended and the alveoli are stretched.

随着空气进入肺部,肺组织伸展,肺泡扩张。

n. 伸展(肢体),牵张

Make light stretches of the arms and legs before you begin exercising.

先轻轻伸展四肢,然后开始锻炼。

The simplest stretch reflex is illustrated by the muscle stretch response.

最简单的牵张反射可用肌肉牵张反应来说明。

stretcher [ˈstretʃə] *n.* 担架

There were quite a few stretchers in the clinic.

诊所里有好几副担架。

An ambulance officer brought a stretcher for the injured woman.

一个救护车上的救护员为受伤的妇女送来一副担架。

stria [straiə] (*pl.* striae [ˈstraiiː]) *n.* 纹,条纹

The striae gravidarum are the lines that appear on the skin of the abdomen of pregnant woman, due to stretching and rupture of the elastic fibres.

妊娠纹是孕妇腹部皮肤上出现的条纹,系弹性纤维拉长、断裂所致。

striated [ˈstraieitid] *a.* 纹状的

Though usually single, the nucleus may be multiple, as in a skeletal striated muscle.

细胞核虽然通常是单个的,但也可以是多核的,如骨骼横纹肌细胞核。

strict [strikt] *a.* 严格的,严厉的;精确的

He gave us a strict interpretation of the facts.

他向我们解释了那些事实的确切含义。

In paroxysmal cold hemoglobinuria therapy consists of strict avoidance of exposure to cold.

对阵发性冷性血红蛋白尿,治疗方法包括严格避免接触寒冷。

strictly [ˈstriktli] *ad.* 严格地;精确地

Dietary and personal hygiene should be strictly observed.

应严格遵守饮食卫生和个人卫生。

stricture [ˈstriktʃə] *n.* 狭窄

Urethral stricture diminishes the caliber of the urinary stream.

尿道狭窄使尿线变细。

Any factor that causes strictures or adhesions of the tubal wall may predispose to ectopic pregnancy.

任何引起输卵管狭窄或粘连的因素均易导致异位妊娠。

stride [straid] *n.* 大步;进展

Cause-directed surgery for glaucoma is making rapid strides.

针对病因的青光眼手术正在广泛开展。

strike [straik] (struck, struck) *v.* (疾病)侵袭;撞击

An illness companed by a high fever struck her when she was still an infant.

当她还是婴儿的时候就患了一种疾病,还伴有高热。

striking [ˈstraikiŋ] *a.* 显著的,引人注目的;惊人的

A striking feature of post-war general practice has indeed been its preventive role.

战后一般医疗的一个显著特点确实是其预防作用。

Acid can act as a precipitating cause of pain, but in some patients this does not occur, the most striking example being when perforation of an ulcer occurs without any preceding pain.

酸能作为促发疼痛的原因,但有些病人却并非如此,最显著的例子是有时虽已发生溃疡穿孔,却无先驱的疼痛。

string [striŋ] (strung, strung) *v.* 捆扎,串起

DNA is the blueprint of any organism and is made up of genes that are strung together to form the DNA chain.

DNA 是所有生物的基础,由众多基因组成,它们串在一起构成 DNA 链。

stringent [ˈstrindʒənt] *a.* 严格的,严厉的

The device has been subjected to stringent tests.

此仪器经受了严格的检验。

stringy [ˈstriŋi] *a.* 纤维的;黏性的

The algae consumed waste products from the reef and under the intense artificial sunlight they proliferated stringy green mats.

藻类吸收利用珊瑚礁排泄物,并在强烈的人造阳光下迅速增殖成黏稠的绿色簇团。

strip [strip] *n.* 条,带

Urine pH is usually measured with a reagent test strip.

尿液 pH 值通常可用试剂试纸条测定。

strobolaryngoscope [ˌstrɔbəuləˈriŋgəskəup] *n.* 动态喉镜,回旋喉镜

The objective of this project is to study the surface anesthesia efficacy of nebulized lidocaine strobolaryngoscope.

这项课题的目标是研究利多卡因喷雾式动态喉镜的表面麻醉效应。

In this study, we used a strobolaryngoscope and remote-controlled X-ray unit to observe the mechanism of speech formation.

在这项研究中,我们使用动态喉镜和远程遥控 X 线元件来观察发声机制。

stroke [strəuk] *n.* 卒中,中风;心搏动

This teaching film teaches people how they can prevent heart attacks and strokes.

这个教学影片教给人们如何预防心脏病突发和脑卒中的知识。

Infarction of brain tissue is the commonest cause of a "stroke".

脑组织的梗死是"卒中"最常见的原因。

Exertional tachycardia suggests an inability of stroke volume to increase appropriately with exercise.

劳累性心动过速表示心搏出量不能随着运动而适当地增加。

stroma [ˈstrəumə] *n.* 基质，底质

The second principal component of the marrow is the stroma.

骨髓的第二种主要成分是基质。

There may also be edema of the conjunctival stroma.

也可能出现结膜基质水肿。

stromal [ˈstrəuməl] *adj.* 基质的，间质的

Patients with stromal invasion should undergo radical surgery.

癌症侵及间质的患者应行根治性手术。

The stromal elements of cystic nephroma show malignancy more often than epithelium.

囊性肾瘤的间质成分常常较上皮更容易恶变。

structural [ˈstrʌktʃərəl] *a.* 结构(上)的

However, cells do have some common structural characteristics.

然而，细胞的确具有某些共同的结构特征。

Instead they look upon the cell as both the structural and functional unit of all life.

相反，他们把细胞看作既是一切生物的结构单位又是功能单位。

structure [ˈstrʌktʃə] *n.* 结构

The nucleus is usually to be observed as a circular structure in the center of the cell.

通常可见核在细胞中心呈圆形结构。

Cardiac muscle is not under the control of the will but varies considerably in structure from involuntary muscle.

心肌不受意志支配，但在结构上与不随意肌有显著不同。

All toxic effects result from biochemical interactions between the toxicants and certain structures of the organism.

所有毒性效应都是毒物与机体一定结构之间的生化相互作用。

study [ˈstʌdi] *n.* 研究

Some studies suggest that the drinking water has been variably polluted by the endocrine disrupting chemicals.

一些研究显示饮用水已不同程度地被内分泌干扰物污染。

In medicine, a cohort study is often undertaken to obtain evidence to try to refute the existence of a suspected association between cause and effect.

在医学上，往往采用队列研究为试图反驳已存在的可疑因果关系提供依据。

stupor [ˈstjuːpə] *n.* 昏迷；木僵

A history of an episode of stupor or unconsciousness is often obtained.

本病往往有一段昏迷或不省人事的病史。

Sleep is easily distinguished from the lessened consciousness of stupor.

睡眠容易与意识降低的木僵状态区分开。

styrene [ˈstairiːn] *n.* 苯乙烯

This paper introduced the progress in studies on metallocene catalysts and their applications in the polymerization of ethylene, propylene, styrene and the like.

本文介绍了茂金属催化剂的研究进展及其在乙烯、丙烯和苯乙烯等聚合中的应用。

Styrene and styrene oxide-induced DNA damage in various organs of mice was detected using the comet assay.

采用彗星试验检测了苯乙烯和氧化苯乙烯所诱导的小鼠不同器官的 DNA 损伤。

subacute [ˈsʌbəˈkjuːt] *a.* 亚急性的

The inflammatory diseases of the thyroid are termed acute, subacute, or chronic thyroiditis.

炎性甲状腺疾病可称为急性、亚急性或慢性甲状腺炎。

In subacute or chronic closed-angle glaucoma there may be only an ache, the eye becoming gradually adapted to high intraocular pressure.

在亚急性或慢性闭角型青光眼，可能仅有疼痛，眼睛可逐渐适应增高了的眼内压。

subarachnoid [ˌsʌbəˈræknɔid] *a.* 蛛网膜下的

The proportion of erythrocytes to leukocytes is similar to that in whole blood in cases of subarachnoid hemorrhage.

在蛛网膜下出血的病例中，红细胞与白细胞的比例与全血中的比例相同。

sub-cellular [ˌsʌbˈseljulə] *a.* 亚细胞的

In fact sub-cellular organization is in many respects analogous to the kind of organization of a complex multicellular organism.

事实上，亚细胞结构在许多方面与复杂的多细胞有机体的结构相似。

subchronic [sʌbˈkrɔnik] *a.* 亚慢性的

The toxicity of sucralose has been evaluated in acute and subchronic toxicity studies.

三氯蔗糖的毒性已经在急性和亚慢性毒性研究中进行了评估。

Acute toxicity, subchronic, chronic, and reproductive tests are the principal experiments conducted in a toxicology laboratory.

急性毒性和亚慢性、慢性生殖测试是毒理学实验室进行的主要实验。

subclass [ˈsʌbklɑːs] *n.* 亚纲，亚类

Another genetically influenced condition, low density lipoprotein subclass pattern B influences the blood cholesterol response to a low fat diet.

另一种受遗传影响的情况，即低密度脂蛋白(亚纲 B 型)可影响血胆固醇对低脂肪饮食的反应。

The six main classes of enzymes were assigned subclasses and sub-subclasses.

六大类酶又分为亚类和亚亚类。

subclinical [sʌbˈklinikəl] *a.* 亚临床的

The early diagnosis of chronic intrauterine infections, particularly those with subclinical presentation, remains a problem.

慢性宫内感染的早期诊断，特别是对那些亚临床表现者，仍是一个问题。

The clinical approach to the diagnosis of subclinical myocarditis and its possible value have been discussed previously.

亚临床型心肌炎的诊断方法及其可能具有的价值前面已讨论过。

subcostal [sʌbˈkɔstəl] *a.* 肋骨下的

Here each ascending lumbar vein is joined by the subcostal vein.

在这里每条腰升静脉都与肋下静脉相连。

subcutaneous [sʌbkjuˈteiniəs] *a.* 皮下的

The skin is attached to the subcutaneous tissue.

皮肤连接在皮下组织上。

The subcutaneous route should not be used, because absorption is relatively slow.

皮下注射法不应采用，因为吸收太慢。

subcutaneously [ˌsʌbkju(ː)ˈteinjəsli] *ad.* 皮下地

Morphine sulfate is often administered subcutaneously in a dose of 10mg for a 70kg person.

对 70 公斤体重的人，硫酸吗啡常皮下注射 10mg。

subdivide [ˌsʌbdiˈvaid] *v.* 把…再分

The bronchioles divide and subdivide like the rootlets of a plant.

细支气管分支、再分支，就像植物的根须一样。

For the purpose of description, the stomach is usually subdivided into three portions.

为了描述方便起见，常把胃细分为三个部分。

subdivision [ˌsʌbdiˈviʒən] *n.* 再分，细分

The terminal hairlike subdivisions of the bronchioles are each surrounded by a group of alveoli.

细支气管末端毛发似的分支每根都由一群肺泡所围绕。

subdural [sʌbˈdjuːrəl] *a.* 硬膜下的

Subdural effusions occur frequently during the course of meningitis but their exact origin is not known.

脑膜炎病程中常产生硬膜下积液，但源自何处尚不清楚。

subendocardial [ˌsʌbendəuˈkɑːdiəl] *a.* 心内膜下的

Interstitial fibrosis was prominent in microsections of the subendocardial portion of the left ventricle.

左室心内膜下部分的切片中有明显的间质纤维化。

subendothelial [səbˌendəuˈθiːliəl] *a.* 内皮下的

Exposure of normal platelets to vascular subendothelial structures results, within a matter of seconds, in the formation of a haemostatic plug.

当正常血小板暴露于血管内皮下结构时，几秒钟内即可导致血栓的形成。

Atorvastatin can decrease the infiltration of lipids and lipoproteins into the subendothelial space, and can be thus used to prevent and ameliorate atherosclerosis.

阿托伐他汀平可减少血浆中脂类渗入血管内皮下，因此能阻止和改善动脉粥样硬化。

subfamily [sʌbˈfæmili] *n.* 亚科(生物分类)，亚类

There are several integrin subfamilies.

存在若干种整合素亚类。

subgroup [ˈsʌbgruːp] *n.* 亚群，子群；亚(血)型

Patients with atopic dermatitis and widespread tinea corporis form a significant portion of this subgroup.

患有异位性皮炎和广泛性体癣的患者构成此亚型的主要部分。

Marked variations in disease occurrence and survival exist among different subgroups of the US population.

疾病的发生率和存活率在美国不同人群中有着显著的差异。

subhealth [ˈsʌbˌhelθ] *n.* 亚健康

There is a high rate of subhealth among the highly qualified intellectuals.

亚健康在高级知识分子中发生率高。

Aging, smoking, being short of exercise, poor quality sleep and often working overtime are the main risk factors of subhealth.

衰老、吸烟、少锻炼、睡眠质量差、经常加班是亚健康的主要危险因素。

subinvolution [ˌsʌbinvəˈluːʃən] *n.* 子宫复旧不全

Subinvolution is delayed return of the enlarged uterus to normal size and function.

子宫复旧不全是指增大的子宫延迟恢复到正常的大小和功能。

Subinvolution is a medical condition in which after childbirth, the uterus does not return to its normal size.

子宫复旧不全是产后子宫不能恢复到正常大小的病况。

subject[1] [ˈsʌbdʒikt] *n.* 主题；学科；受治疗者，受实验者，病人，患者

All subjects were started on 25mg of imipramine at bedtime.

所有受试者都开始在就寝前服用25mg丙咪嗪。

The early hypertrophic changes are usually observed only in young hypertensive subjects.

早期的肥厚性变化通常见于年轻高血压患者。

The subject of depression and bipolar disorders in children and adolescents is not really new.

儿童和少年的抑郁症和双相疾病并非新问题。

a. 易受…的，服从(to)

He is subject to colds.

他容易感冒。

The open wound is subject to infection.

敞开的伤口容易受感染。

Acute as well as chronic rheumatic conditions are subject only to symptomatic treatment.

急性和慢性的风湿病都只能用对症疗法。

subject²(to) [sʌb'dʒekt] *v.* 使…受

Foods are subjected to hydrolysis.

食物可受到水解作用。

The patient was subjected to an operation yesterday.

病人昨天做了手术。

Air is liquefied by subjecting it to a high pressure at a low temperature.

空气受到高压和低温的作用就可以液化。

subjective [sʌb'dʒektiv] *a.* 主观的

The evaluation of lung radiolucency in the radiograph is highly subjective.

X 线照片上肺部通亮度的评定具有很大的主观性。

Subjective symptoms are those that the patient tells about.

主观症状是病人自己讲述的症状。

sublimation [ˌsʌbli'meiʃən] *n.* 升华(作用)

Sublimation is considered a "mature" defense mechanism.

升华被认为是一种"成熟"的防御机制。

sublingual [sʌb'liŋgwəl] *a.* 舌下的

Relief within 5 minutes by sublingual or buccal glyceryl trinitrate makes angina more likely.

舌下或口含硝酸甘油片使疼痛在 5 分钟内缓解的情况更支持心绞痛诊断。

sublingually [sʌb'liŋgwəli] *ad.* 舌下地

Nitroglycerin is given sublingually in angina pectoris.

硝酸甘油在治疗心绞痛时要经舌下给药。

subluxation [sʌblʌk'seiʃən] *n.* 不全脱位,半脱位

In traumatic arthritis X-ray may show a foreign body, fracture, or subluxation of the joint.

对于外伤性关节炎,X 线拍片可显示异物、骨折或关节半脱位。

submandibular [ˌsʌbmæn'dibjulə] *a.* 下颌下的

There are three pairs of salivary glands: the sublingual, submandibular, and parotid.

唾液腺有三对:舌下腺、下颌下腺和腮腺。

The sublingual and submandibular glands lie between the tongue in the floor of the oral cavity.

舌下腺和下颌下腺位于口腔底部舌下。

submaxillary [sʌb'mæksiləri] *a.* 颌下的

Some glands are of a mixed type, containing both serous cells and mucous cells, as in the submaxillary salivary glands.

有些腺体是混合型的,既含有浆液细胞,又含有黏液细胞,如颌下唾液腺。

Submaxillary gland is one of a pair of salivary glands situated below the parotid glands.

颌下腺是位于腮腺下方的成对唾液腺之一。

submerge [sʌb'məːdʒ] *v.* 浸没,浸泡

The unborn child lies within the amniotic sac, submerged in a fairly large quantity of fluid.

胎儿躺在羊膜囊内,浸泡在相当大量的液体中。

submetacentric ['sʌbˌmetə'sentrik] *a.* (染色体)亚中间着丝粒的

A submetacentric chromosome has an off-center centromere and two arms with clearly different length.

亚中着丝粒染色体有一个偏离中心的着丝粒,两臂长度明显不同。

Y chromosome has two types of polymorphism: metacentric (or submetacentric) and acrocentric chromosomes.

Y 染色体有两种类型的多态性,即中间着丝粒(或亚中间着丝粒)和近端着丝粒染色体。

submit [səbˈmit] *v.* 提交

The investigators submitted their research protocols on patients treated with this new technic.

研究人员提交了用这一新方法治疗的患者的研究记录。

submucous [ˌsʌbˈmjuːkəs] *a.* 黏膜下的

Our objective is to evaluate the effect of transcervical resection of submucous myomas in 36 patients.

我们的目的是评估 36 名患者黏膜下子宫肌瘤在经宫颈切除后的效果。

Hysteroscopy for post menopausal bleeding may enhance efficacy in identifying endometrial atrophy and submucous myoma.

宫腔镜检查绝经后出血，可提高对子宫内膜萎缩及黏膜下子宫肌瘤的诊断率。

subnanoemulsion [ˌsʌbnænəiˈmʌlʃən] *n.* 亚纳米乳

The subnanoemulsion can be used as a drug carrier, but at present the application in medicine is not too much.

亚纳米乳可以作为药物的载体，但目前在药品中不太常用。

Almost all intravenous injection of subnanoemulsion should join isotonic regulator, in which glycerol is the most commonly used.

几乎所有静注的亚纳米乳都应加入等张调节剂，其中甘油最为常用。

subnormal [sʌbˈnɔːməl] *a.* 低于正常的，正常下的

Some drugs have subnormal oral bioavailability.

有些药物口服的利用度低。

subnormality [ˌsʌbnɔːˈmæliti] *n.* 低常状态

Individuals with this level of subnormality, corresponding to an IQ level of 50 to 70, are educable.

具有这种低于正常水平（智商相当于 50 ~ 70）的个体是可教育的。

Mental subnormality is essentially an administrative concept, describing the state of those whose intellectual powers have failed to develop to such an extent that they are in need of care and protection.

精神低常状态主要是管理学概念，指那些智力发育不好达到了需要照料和保护的程度。

subordinate [səˈbɔːdinət] *a.* 附属的；次要的

He was always friendly to his subordinate officers.

他对他的下级官员总是友好相待。

All the other issues are subordinate to this one.

所有其他问题都不如这个问题重要。

subpopulation [ˌsʌbpɔpjuˈleiʃən] *n.* 亚群

There are several subpopulations of T cells, each of which may have the same specificity for an antigenic determinant.

T 细胞有几个亚群，每一个亚群对一个抗原决定簇有相同特异性。

subsequent [ˈsʌbsikwənt] *a.* 随后的，后来的

Subsequent observations were focused upon this point.

以后的观察都集中到这一点上。

Her subsequent fertility is questionable in this case.

该病人今后的生育力是成问题的。

There is a subsequent decrease in left ventricular stroke volume and systemic arterial pressure.

继之左心室搏出量减少，全身动脉压降低。

These findings are expected to help in the prevention of diabetic atherosclerosis and subsequent cardiovascular and cerebrovascular disease.

希望这些发现有助于预防糖尿病性动脉粥样硬化和继发的心血管和脑血管病。

subsequently [ˈsʌbsikwəntli] *ad.* 随后，后来

Her course subsequently was complicated by fever and joint pain.
随后她的病程中伴有发热和关节痛。

The typical patient becomes suddenly ill with vomiting and, subsequently, fever, diarrhea, and generalized malaise.
典型的患者是突然起病伴呕吐,接着发热、腹泻及全身不适。

subserous [sʌb'siərəs] *a.* 浆膜下的

According to our research plan, the next step is to study the CT characteristics and differential diagnosis of outprojecting subserous uterine myoma.
根据科研计划,我们下一步要探讨外突浆膜下子宫肌瘤的CT特点及其鉴别诊断。

This article summarizes the operative experience of subserous appendectomy in patients with appendicitis and its long-term therapeutic effects.
本文介绍了阑尾炎病人阑尾浆膜下切除的手术体会及该术式的远期疗效。

subset ['sʌbset] *n.* 亚型,亚类

Granulomatous inflammation is a subset of chronic inflammation.
肉芽肿炎症是慢性炎症的亚型。

Other criteria have been used to subdivide αβT cell subsets.
其他的标准也已用于区分αβT细胞的亚类。

subside [sʌb'said] *v.* 减退,消退

Acute chest pain subsided on treatment with morphine.
用吗啡治疗后,急性胸痛减退。

The acute reaction to operation and the residual effects of anesthesia are subsiding.
手术的急性反应和麻醉的残余作用正在消退。

Antibiotics are administered in all except mild, rapidly subsiding cases.
全部都用抗生素,只是轻症和正在迅速好转的病例除外。

subsidiary [sʌb'sidjəri] *a.* 次要的,附属的

Animal evidence suggests that the major influence is prolactin with ovarian steroids playing no more than a subsidiary role.
动物的证据表明,具有主要影响力的是催乳激素,而卵巢类固醇则只不过起辅助作用。

Besides these departments, there are also other subsidiary departments in our hospital.
在我们医院除了这些科室以外,还有一些其他附属科室。

substance ['sʌbstəns] *n.* 物质;实质

Some gases, such as nitrogen dioxide and ozone, release substances that damage the lung lining.
有些气体,例如二氧化氮和臭氧释放的物质能损害肺黏膜。

substantial [sʌb'stænʃəl] *a.* 实质的;富裕的

There are substantial numbers of women who have been immunized by previous pregnancies.
由于在以前妊娠过而获得免疫的妇女数量是相当多的。

The hemoglobin-synthesizing red blood cell precursors of rabbit contain substantial amounts of a 9S RNA.
家兔合成血红蛋白的红血细胞前体含有大量的9S RNA。

substantially [sʌb'stænʃəli] *ad.* 实质地;大量地

The area of drug research substantially feels the constraining influence of law and regulations.
药物研究这个领域可感受到法律和规章约束的实质性影响。

Patients with Beckwith-Wiedemann syndrome have a substantially increased risk for the development of tumors.
贝(克威思)-威(德曼)二氏综合征病人发生肿瘤的危险性显著增高。

substantiate [sʌb'stænʃieit] *v.* 证实,证明

Radioimmuno-diffusion studies substantiated the low antigenic fibrinogen levels.
放射免疫扩散法测定也证实了抗原性纤维蛋白原水平低。

Further studies are necessary to substantiate these findings.
为了证实这些发现必须进一步研究。

substantive [ˈsʌbstæntiv] *a.* 实质的；大量的
It is anticipated that some substantive changes will be made in this respect.
人们期待在这方面做出某些实质性的改变。

substernal [sʌbˈstəːnəl] *a.* 胸骨后的
Inflammation of the pericardium may produce chest pain which is situated in either the substernal area or the left mammary region.
心包的炎症可产生胸痛，疼痛部位可以在胸骨后或左乳房区。

substitute [ˈsʌbstitjuːt] *v.* 代替
She substituted for the manager during his absence.
经理不在时，由她来代理。
It is advisable to be cautious before substituting new drugs for established and safe ones.
用新药取代已知的和安全的药物时以小心为宜。
Amikacin may be substituted for gentamicin resistant organisms.
对庆大霉素有抗药性的细菌，可改用丁胺卡那霉素。
a. 代替的，代用的
Substitute valves made of plastic materials have proved to be a lifesaving measure for many patients.
用塑料制作的代用瓣膜已成功地挽救了许多病人的生命。
n. 代替，代用品
Dextran expands the volume of plasms, although it is not a substitute for blood.
葡萄聚糖尽管不是血的代用品，却能扩大血浆的量。

substrate [ˈsʌbstreit] *n.* 底物，酶作用物，基质
Often, of course, the substrate as well as the enzyme is ionizable.
当然，底物和酶一样常常是可离子化的。
A drug substrate to be metabolized binds to oxidized cytochrome P450.
一种即将代谢的药物底物与氧化型细胞色素 P450 结合。

subtle [ˈsʌtl] *a.* 精细的；微妙的；不易觉察的
Subtle bony changes of erosion or fracture are not seen on plain radiographs.
在 X 线平片上看不见极细微的骨侵蚀和骨折变化。
Particular attention should be given to the often subtle but physiologically important alterations of the organs essential for life support.
对支持生命的重要器官发生的改变应该特别重视，这些改变常常不易察觉，但在生理上却有重要意义。

subtract [səbˈtrækt] *v.* 减去
A constant correction factor could be subtracted from creatinine clearance determinations to yield a more accurate estimate of glomerular filtration rate (GFR).
从肌酐清除率的测定值中减去一个固定的校正因子，得出肾小球滤过率更准确的评估。

subtraction [səbˈtrækʃən] *n.* 减法；减少；减影
Digital subtraction angiography (DSA) is a new medical imaging technique springing up in 1980's.
数字减影血管造影(DSA)是 20 世纪 80 年代兴起的一门新的医学成像技术。
One of these is the subtraction of water from the ocean by means of evaporation-conversion of liquid water to water vapor.
其中之一是通过蒸发即把液态水转化为水蒸气来减少海洋中的水分。

subtype [ˈsʌbtaip] *n.* 亚型
Adrenergic receptors are classified into alpha and beta and their subtypes.

肾上腺素能受体分为 α 受体和 β 受体及其亚型。

Scientists have identified at least 10 subtypes of the AIDS virus.

科学家至少确认了艾滋病病毒的十个亚型。

No one knows how many more subtypes of HIV will sprout in the next 40 years.

没有人知道在今后 40 年里会产生多少人体免疫缺陷病毒的亚型。

subunit [ˈsʌbjuːnit] *n.* 亚基

The subunits in quaternary structure must be in noncovalent association.

四级结构中的亚基必须处于非共价键结合。

Each eukaryotic RNA polymerase has between six and ten protein subunits.

每种真核 RNA 聚合酶有 6 ~ 10 个蛋白质亚基。

suburb [ˈsʌbəːb] *n.* 郊区

As cities grew, people from those cities moved out into the new suburbs.

随着城市的发展，那些住在城市里的人迁出到新的郊区。

In 1990 to 1992, the age-adjusted death rate for residents of large cities in the United States was 19 percent greater than in suburbs around large cities.

1990 ~ 1992 年间，美国大城市居民年龄校正的死亡率比大城市周围郊区的居民高 19%。

subvert [səbˈvəːt] *v.* 破坏，搅乱

Once in the cell, the viral nucleic acid subverts the host's replication machinery.

病毒核酸一旦进入细胞即破坏宿主的复制机构。

succeed [səkˈsiːd] *v.* 成功

Medical science is doing all it can to extend human life and is succeeding brilliantly.

医学科学在尽力延长人的寿命并且不断取得成就。

I have endeavoured in each succeeding edition to remedy this by submitting to the criticism of my learned friends those sections in which notable advances have occurred.

每次再版修订时，我都尽力补救这一缺陷，按照那些博学的友人的批评，去修改内容已有显著进展的章节。

succession [səkˈseʃən] *n.* 连续

Stimulator emits electrical impulses of any desired voltage either singly or in rapid succession.

刺激器能发射需要任何电压的电冲动，包括单个的或快速连续性的。

Rarely two tumors arise, simultaneously or in succession, in different parts of the colon.

在结肠的不同部位，极少同时或连续长出两个肿瘤。

successive [səkˈsesiv] *a.* 连续的；后续的

In a series of 1000 successive medical outpatients it was the presenting symptom in 13 percent.

在一千例内科门诊的连续病例中，有此症状的占 13%。

Successive epidemics of bubonic plague in the 14th century killed more than one fourth of Europe's population.

在十四世纪，腺鼠疫的连续流行使四分之一以上的欧洲人丧生。

Those results were then confirmed in successive studies.

这些结果随之为后续的研究所证实。

successor [səkˈsesə] *n.* 继任者，继承人

Mr. White is the successor to the university president.

怀特先生是校长的继任人。

succinylcholine [ˌsʌksinilˈkəuliːn] *n.* 丁二酰胆碱，琥珀酰胆碱

Succinylcholine is a muscle relaxant.

琥珀酰胆碱是一种肌肉松弛药。

succumb [səˈkʌm] *v.* 屈服；患病；死

Once a person has reached his or her 90th year, the risk of succumbing to Alzheimer's disease gets less.

人活到 90 岁以后，患阿尔茨海默症的危险反而少些。

At the present time as many people succumb to chronic obstructive pulmonary emphysema as to cancer of the lung.

目前死于慢性阻塞性肺气肿的人和死于肺癌的人一样多。

All patients with end-stage renal failure succumbed to their illness.

所有晚期肾功能衰竭的病人都死于该病。

succus ['sʌkəs] (*pl.* succi) *n.* 液；汁

Succus entericus contains mucus and digestive enzymes, including enteropeptidase, erepsin, lactase and sucrase.

肠液中含有黏液和多种消化酶，包括肠激酶、肠肽酶、乳糖酶、蔗糖酶等。

suck [sʌk] *v.* 吸，吮

The mosquito sucks blood from an infected person.

蚊子叮吸患者的血。

sucker ['sʌkə] *n.* 吸管，吸盘

This tapeworm, which can reach 3 to 8m in length, inhabits the upper jejunum and has a scolex with four prominent suckers.

这种绦虫可达 3 到 8 米长，寄居在空肠上段，有一个拥有四个突出吸盘的头节。

sucrase ['sjuːkreis] *n.* 蔗糖酶

Sucrase in the brush border of the small intestine hydrolyses sucrose to glucose and fructose.

位于小肠刷状缘的蔗糖酶将蔗糖水解为葡萄糖和果糖。

sucrose ['sjuːkrəus] *n.* 蔗糖

The principal carbohydrates of the diet are starch, sucrose, and lactose.

饮食中主要的碳水化合物是淀粉、蔗糖和乳糖。

suction ['sʌkʃən] *n.* 吸引，吸气引液

Endotracheal suction should be performed immediately.

应立即使用气管吸引术。

The efficiency of drainage is improved by the addition of suction.

增用吸引术可使引流效果得到改善。

sudden ['sʌdən] *a.* 突然的，意外的

The sudden lowering of blood pressure is an important symptom of shock.

血压突然下降是休克的一个重要症状。

suddenness ['sʌdənis] *n.* 突然

Biliary colic usually arises with suddenness and takes the form of spasms.

胆绞痛通常突然发生，并呈痉挛性。

suffice [sə'fais] *v.* 足够；有能力；满足

One meal a day won't suffice a growing boy.

一天一顿饭不能满足一个正在发育中的男孩子的需要。

sufficient [sə'fiʃənt] *a.* 足够的，充分的

However, some chemicals can be absorbed through the skin in sufficient quantities to produce systemic effects.

但有些化学物质能够经皮肤吸收至足够的量而产生全身性效应。

In case of an eroded chancre a few vigorous rubs with dry gauze are usually sufficient.

糜烂下疳只须用干纱布用力擦数次，通常已足够。

The lack of sufficient attention to the public health problem of TB must also be viewed as a societal problem.

对结核病这个公共卫生问题缺乏充分的重视也应被视为一个社会问题。

sufficiently [sə'fiʃəntli] *ad.* 足够地，充分地

All of these bacteria are killed by boiling, many of them by a lower temperature if prolonged sufficiently.

用煮沸的方法可以杀死这些细菌,在稍低的温度下若延长足够的时间亦有很多细菌可被杀死。

suffocate [ˈsʌfəkeit] *v.* 窒息致死;窒息

The fireman was suffocated by the fumes.

那消防队员为浓烟窒息致死。

Large amounts of blood can fill the airways, not only seriously disturbing gas exchange but causing the patient to suffocate.

大量出血可充塞呼吸道,不仅严重干扰气体交换,同时还会引起病人窒息。

suffocation [ˌsʌfəˈkeiʃən] *n.* 窒息

A wound of the chest can kill a person by suffocation.

胸壁伤口可通过窒息使人致死。

suggest [səˈdʒest] *v.* 建议;提示;暗示

Serum folic acid levels <5ng/mL suggest a deficiency.

血清叶酸水平低于5ng/mL,则表明叶酸不足。

A lesion at the frenum always strongly suggests a chancre.

在系带处的损害总提示为下疳。

suggestion [səˈdʒestʃən] *n.* 提议;意见;暗示

The suggestion of a nerve root lesion by history and examination does not specify the underlying cause.

病史和体检提示神经根病变,不能说明潜在的疾病是什么。

In psychology, suggestion denotes the process of changing a person's beliefs, attitudes, or emotions by telling him that they will change.

心理学中,暗示是指通过告诉一个人将会发生什么变化,从而改变他的信念、看法或情绪的过程。

suggestive [səˈdʒestiv] *a.* 暗示的,示意的

These findings are highly suggestive of aging process.

这些发现有力地提示衰老过程。

A true pain is suggestive of an organic cause.

真性疼痛表明有器质性原因。

suicidal [sjuiˈsaidəl] *a.* 自杀的,危及性命的

Emergency medicine physicians are often the first to deal with patients who have either completed suicide, attempted suicide, or have suicidal ideation.

急诊室医生常常是最先接诊那些已经自杀、企图自杀或有自杀想法的人。

They should be asked about suicidal ideas; for example, "Do you ever feel that life is not worth living ?"

应询问他们关于自杀的想法,如"你曾否感觉到不值得活下去?"

suicide [ˈsjuːisaid] *n.* 自杀

A person who has committed suicide may appear to have been the victim of murder.

一个自杀的人看起来可以像被谋杀的一样。

Several experiments have attempted to introduce "suicide genes" into tumor cells to directly kill the cells or to sensitize them to later drug or radiation therapy.

几个实验已试图将"自杀基因"导入肿瘤细胞,直接将肿瘤细胞杀死,或使肿瘤细胞对药物、化疗敏感。

v. 自杀

The man suicided after he had been accused of the crime.

这个人在被指控犯有该罪行后自杀了。

suit [sjuːt] *n.* 起诉,诉讼

The presence of damages in the patient is essential for a malpractice suit.
病人受到损害的表现是对医疗事故进行诉讼的必要条件。

sulfacetamide [ˌsʌlfə'setəmaid]（缩写:SA） *n.* 乙酰磺胺

Sulfacetamide is a drug of the sulphonamide group that is used in eye drops to treat such infections as conjunctivitis.
乙酰磺胺是磺胺类药物的一种,用作滴眼剂治疗结膜炎等感染。

sulfamethoxazole [ˌsʌlfəme'θɔksəzəul]（缩写:SMZ） *n.* 磺胺甲异噁唑

Most of sulphonamides, including sulfamethoxazole and sulfaphenazole, are rapidly absorbed from stomach and small intestine and should be taken at frequent intervals.
多数磺胺药,包括磺胺甲基异噁唑和磺胺苯吡唑,在胃和小肠内迅速吸收,应当隔较短时间服用。

sulfapyridine [ˌsʌlfə'piridiːn] *n.* 磺胺吡啶

For example, acetylsulfapyridine, a metabolite of sulfapyridine, may block renal tubules.
例如,磺胺吡啶的代谢物乙酰磺胺吡啶可阻塞肾小管。

sulfate ['sʌlfeit] *n.* 硫酸盐

If taken by mouth, barium sulfate makes the esophagus, the stomach, and/or the small intestine opaque to the X-rays so that they can be "photographed".
硫酸钡经口服后可使食管、胃和(或)小肠不透 X 线,因而可被摄影拍片。

sulfide ['sʌlfaid] *n.* 硫化物

Simple methods to test for the production of characteristic metabolic end-products such as gas and hydrogen sulfide are available.
可用一些简单的方法检测其特征性的代谢终末产物,如气体和硫化氢。

sulfonamide [sʌl'fɔnəmaid] *n.* 磺胺,氨苯磺胺

Sulfonamides are active against both grampositive and gramnegative bacteria.
磺胺类药物对革兰阳性和革兰阴性细菌均有效。

All sulfonamide drugs are highly toxic and may produce severe reactions.
所有磺胺药物的毒性都很强,能引起严重反应。

The sulfonamides can be used although the reports as to their value are conflicting.
可以服用磺胺,虽然有的报告对它的使用效果有争议。

sulfur, sulphur ['sʌlfə] *n.* 硫(磺)

After leaving the pits every day, the miners are immediately given sulphur baths to prevent rheumatism.
矿工们每天离井后,立即洗一个硫磺浴,以防得风湿病。

Among the common toxic gases are sulfur dioxide, methane, the oxides of nitrogen, ammonia, hydrogen sulfide, and hydrogen cyanide.
常见的有毒气体有二氧化硫、甲烷、氧化氮、氨、硫化氢以及氰化氢。

sulfuric [sʌl'fjuːrik] *a.* 硫的

Sulfuric acid is often used in the preparation of other acids whose boiling points are lower.
硫酸常用于制备沸点较其为低的其他酸类。

sulfydryl ['sʌlfidril] *n.* 巯基

An even simpler example is the blockage of the sulfydryl group at the active sites of enzymes by heavy metals such as mercury.
一个更为简单的例子是酶活性部位的巯基被重金属如汞所阻断。

sulodexide [sjulə'deksaid] *n.* 舒洛地特

Currently, there is no relevant report that sulodexide can inhibit the accumulation of glomerulus extracellular matrix in DM.
关于舒洛地特抑制糖尿病患者肾小球细胞外基质积聚,目前尚未见相关报道。

sulphonylurea [ˌsʌlfənil'juəriə] *n.* 磺酰脲;尿素类

Sulfonylurea (sulphonylurea) derivatives are a class of antidiabetic drugs.
磺酰脲衍生物是一类降糖药。
Metformin and a generic sulfonylurea should be the basis of oral glucose-lowering therapy.
二甲双胍和一种磺脲类是口服降糖疗法的基础药物。

summarize [ˈsʌməraiz] *v.* 概括,总结
This paper summarizes the 20 years of liver transplantation in Brazil.
本文总结了巴西肝移植 20 年的历程。
The basic immune mechanism can be summarized as follows.
基本的免疫机制可以总结如下。
A list of points at the beginning of each chapter summarizes the central concepts that follow.
在每章开头列出要点概括了本章的中心概念。

summary [ˈsʌməri] *n.* 摘要,概括
Here is a summary of the case history.
以下是病历摘要。
And so I would say, in summary, that the operation has been a great success.
因此,我可以概括地说,这次手术已获得很大成功。
In summary, drugs act by stimulating or depressing cell activity, by irritation, by replacement, and by attenuation or killing.
总之,药物可通过兴奋或抑制细胞活性、刺激、替代以及减弱或杀灭而起作用。

sunburn [ˈsʌnbəːn] *n.* 晒斑,晒伤
A severe sunburn with blister formation is a second degree burn.
有水泡形成的晒斑是二度烧伤。
There are two general theories about the pathogenesis of the sunburn response.
关于晒伤的发病机制有两种常见的理论。
Many sunburn lotions are of dubious value.
许多防晒水的价值值得怀疑。

suncream [ˈsʌnkriːm] *n.* 防晒霜
However, there is research available now that shows that suncreams are already providing protection against pre-cancers.
然而,现在有研究表明,防晒霜已经能够提供对癌前期的保护。

sunstroke [ˈsʌnstrəuk] *n.* 日射病,中暑
Sunstroke is characterized by raised body temperature (pyrexia), absence of sweating, and eventual loss of consciousness due to failure or exhaustion of the temperature-regulating mechanism of the body.
日射病的特征是因人体体温调节机制衰竭引起的体温升高、不出汗以及最终意识丧失。

superantigen [ˌsjuːpəˈæntidʒən] *n.* 超抗原
The PF is a superantigen and it is secreted into liquid culture by E. coli.
PF 是一种超抗原,可由大肠杆菌分泌至液体培养基中。
Superantigen in very light concentration can cause an enormous change of immunocytes, cytokines and antibody, cause a series of pathological and physiological change in the body.
超抗原以极低的浓度就能引起机体免疫细胞、细胞因子和抗体的巨大变化,引起机体一系列病理生理过程。

supercooling [ˌsjuːpəˈkuːliŋ] *n* 超速冷冻
Supercooling, also known as undercooling, is the process of lowering the temperature of a liquid or a gas below its freezing point without it becoming a solid.
超速冷冻,或称过冷冻,是液体或气体降至凝固点以下而不致形成固体的过程。

superfamily [ˌsjuːpəˈfæməli] *n.* [生物] 总科,超科,超家族
The OR gene family is actually part of a much larger gene superfamily encoding a large variety of

what are called G protein-coupled receptors.

OR 基因家族实际上是一种编码多种被称为 G 蛋白偶联受体的超基因家族的一部分。

Tumor necrosis factor (TNF)-related apoptosis-inducing ligand (TRAIL) is a member of TNF superfamily, which induces the programmed cell death with binding to its receptors.

肿瘤坏死因子相关凋亡诱导配体(TRAIL)是肿瘤坏死因子(TNF)超家族的成员之一,通过与受体结合而诱导细胞程序性死亡。

superficial [ˌsjuːpəˈfiʃəl] *a.* 表面的

He had a superficial wound on his leg.

他腿上有外伤。

The usual differentiation from basal to superficial varieties is not evident.

从基底层向表层细胞的普通分化是不明显的。

superhuman [ˌsjuːpəˈhjuːmən] *a.* (在身材、力量、智慧方面)超人的

This scientist's intelligence seems almost superhuman.

这位科学家似有近乎超人的才智。

superimpose [ˌsjuːpərimˈpəuz] *v.* 添上;重叠

A major depressive episode may be superimposed on a dysthymic disorder.

严重抑郁发作可能会与精神抑郁症相重叠。

superinfection [ˌsjuːpərinˈfekʃən] *n.* 重复感染,双重感染

These superinfections should be treated appropriately with vancomycin and other drugs.

这些重复感染可使用万古霉素和其他药物进行适当的治疗。

superior (to) [ˌsjuˈpiəriə] *a.* 优于,胜过

This new procedure seems to be superior to any of the other methods now in use.

此新法优于现在使用中的任何其他方法。

n. 长辈;上级;优越者

Young people should respect their superiors.

年轻人应该尊敬长辈。

The young doctor often gets advice from his superiors.

这位青年医生常常得到上级医生的指点。

In giving lectures to students, he had few superiors.

在讲课方面他几乎是数一数二的。

superiority [sjuːˌpiəriˈɔriti] *n.* 优势,优越(性)

This constitutes his superiority to other people.

这就是他胜过别人的地方。

No one doubts the superiority of laparoscopic surgery over the conventional abdominal operation.

无人怀疑腹腔镜手术比传统的腹部手术要优越。

supernatant [ˌsjuːpəˈneitənt] *a.* 上层的

The supernatant fluid, which should not be coloured, is drawn up to 0. 1 ml mark.

将上层液体(应是无色的)吸到 0. 1 毫升标记处。

superovulation [ˌsjuːpər,ɔvjuˈleiʃən] *n.* 超排卵

Superovulation is a term used to describe the drug-induced production of multiple eggs for use during assisted reproductive technologies, such as IVF.

超排卵这个术语被用来描述在辅助生殖技术(如体外受精)中运用药物诱导使多个卵泡生成以供需用。

Sometimes the drugs used for superovulation work "too well" leading to a condition known as ovarian hyperstimulation syndrome. Superovulation can also lead to a multiple pregnancy.

有时用于超排卵的药物起效太好了以致产生卵巢过度刺激综合征。超排卵也可导致多胎妊娠。

superoxide [ˌsjuːpərˈɔksaid] *n.* 超氧化物

Superoxide dismutase (SOD) is an enzyme found in all cells of the human body.
超氧化物歧化酶(SOD)是存在于人体所有细胞中的一种酶。
Superoxide has been implicated in diseases ranging from Alzheimer's to diabetes.
超氧化物与阿尔茨海默症、糖尿病等多种疾病有关。

superoxide dismutase [ˌsjuːpəˈɔksaid-disˈmjuːteis] *n.* 超氧化物歧化酶(SOD)
Superoxide dismutase is an enzyme that repairs cells and reduces the damage done to them by superoxide, the most common free radical in the body.
超氧化物歧化酶是一种能修复细胞并降低由最常见自由基超氧化物所致损伤的酶。

superscan [sjuːpəˈskæn] *n.* 超级显像
Bone scan revealed diffuse skeletal metastases with superscan appearance.
骨扫描可以超级影像形式显示弥漫性骨转移。
Superscans on bone scintigraphy have been described mostly in metastatic and metabolic bone diseases.
骨闪烁显像的超级影像多用于描述转移性和代谢性骨病。

supersede [ˌsjuːpəˈsiːd] *v.* 代替,取代
Radiological methods of localization of the placental site have been superseded by ultrasonic techniques.
用放射学方法做胎盘定位已被超声技术所取代。
Ultrasound technique has superseded all others where the equipment and skilled personnel are available.
在有设备和专业人员的地方,超声技术已取代了所有的其他方法。

supersensitivity [ˌsjuːpəˌsensiˈtiviti] *n.* 超敏感性,过敏性
Denervation supersensitivity becomes especially pronounced following application of norepinephrine.
应用去甲肾上腺素后去神经超敏性的表现尤其显著。

superstition [ˌsjuːpəˈstiʃn] *n.* 迷信
Ignorance and superstition prevent them from benefiting from modern medicine.
无知与迷信阻碍了他们受益于现代医学。

supervene [sjuːpəˈviːn] *v.* 意外发生;并发
When infection supervenes, the clear or white secretion becomes purulent and yellow.
当并发感染时,清亮或白色分泌物变为脓性和黄色。

supervise [ˈsjupəvaiz] *v.* 监督,监护
This patient should be supervised most carefully by a physician, his condition being a serious emergency case.
这位患者应由一名医生加以精心监护,因为他的病情是一种严重的急症。
It is important that kids with autism should be well supervised in areas where there might be an open fire such as the kitchen or the fireplace.
在有明火的场所,如厨房或壁炉旁,对患有自闭症的儿童的监管很重要。

supine [sjuːˈpain] *a.* 仰卧的
Palpation is performed with the patient resting in a comfortable supine position.
触诊应在病人处于舒适的仰卧位时进行。

supplement [ˈsʌplimənt] *n.* 增补,补充;增刊
The physician prescribed him a vitamin supplement.
医生给他开了一种维生素作为补充。
Interferon will serve as a useful supplement to existing therapies for some cancers.
干扰素对于某些癌症的现有疗法将起着有益的辅助作用。
The magazine Lancet has a supplement about organ transplantation.
《柳叶刀》杂志出了一份关于器官移植的增刊。

v. [ˈsʌpliːment] 补充

In salivary glands, the two divisions of the autonomic nervous system supplement each other.

在唾液腺中，两类自主神经分支的作用相互补充。

In resistant cases it may be necessary to supplement this treatment with kanamycin or erythromycin.

耐药病例可能需用卡那霉素或红霉素作补充治疗。

supplementary [ˌsʌpliˈmentəri] *a.* 补充的

The result of the ongoing research of the experimental project of the Cancer Research Center of our Foundation will provide supplementary materials.

本基金会癌症研究中心实验项目的不断发展的研究结果将提供补充资料。

supplementation [ˌsʌplimənˈteiʃən] *n.* 补充，增补

Vitamin supplementation is preferable, particularly fat-soluble vitamins(A, D, K, E).

维生素的补充更为可取，特别是脂溶性维生素(A、D、K、E)。

K^+ supplementation of replacement fluids is rarely required unless sodium bicarbonate induces hypokalemia.

除非碳酸氢钠引起低钾血症，否则在补液时很少需要补充钾离子。

support [səˈpɔːt] *v.* 支持，支撑

An outer tunic is made of a supporting connective tissue.

外层由起支持作用的结缔组织构成。

One of the functions of fat in the body is to support certain organs of the body, for example, the kidneys and the eyes.

脂肪的功能之一是支撑身体的某些器官，例如肾和眼。

supportive [səˈpɔːtiv] *a.* 支持性的

This medical treatment is actually supportive in nature, if no specific cause can be ascertained.

如果未能查出特殊原因，这种治疗实际上是支持疗法性质。

supportively [səˈpɔːtivli] *ad.* 支持性地

In general, idiopathic cases must be managed supportively.

一般说来，特发性病例必须用支持疗法。

supposition [ˌsʌpəˈziʃən] *n.* 想象，假定，推测

There is no valid evidence to support this supposition.

没有确实的根据支持这个推测。

A supposition appears to explain a group of phenomena and is advanced as a basis for further investigation.

一种假定似乎能解释一组现象，并作为进一步研究的基础。

suppository [səˈpɔzitəri] *n.* 栓剂

A suppository is a drug delivery system that is insert into the rectum(rectal suppository), vagina (vaginal suppository) or urethra(urethral suppository), where it dissolves.

栓剂是通过直肠(直肠栓剂)、阴道(阴道栓剂)或尿道(尿道栓剂)给药并在其中溶解的药物传递系统。

Vaginal suppositories are commonly used to treat gynecological ailments, including vaginal infections such as candidiasis.

阴道栓剂常用于治疗妇科疾病，包括阴道感染，如念珠菌病。

suppress [səˈpres] *v.* 抑制，降低，平定

There is no clear explanation of why infections sometimes suppress immunity.

为什么感染有时会抑制免疫目前尚无明确的解释。

Suppressed plasma renin activity was added as an additional feature of primary aldosteronism.

血浆肾素活性降低成为原发性醛固酮增多症的一个附加特征。

Cough, when productive of sputum, should be encouraged and not suppressed.

咳嗽，有痰时应咳出，不应忍住不咳。

suppression [səˈpreʃən] *n.* 抑制

Drug-induced bone marrow suppression or drug-induced hemolysis should always be considered.

药物引起的骨髓功能抑制或药物引起的溶血必须经常加以考虑。

suppressive [səˈpresiv] *a.* 抑制的

For these cases, the drug is not accepted because of its suppressive action on oxidative metabolism.

对于这些病例，此药由于它对氧化代谢的抑制作用而不能采用。

suppurate [ˈsʌpjuəreit] *v.* 化脓

The small haemorrhagic lesions may suppurate.

小的出血性病变可能化脓。

It is true that suppurating inflammation is virtually always caused by bacterial infection.

诚然，化脓性炎症实际上总是由细菌感染引起的。

suppuration [ˌsʌpjuəˈreiʃən] *n.* 化脓

The wall of the artery weakened by suppuration may become locally dilated.

由于化脓变薄弱的动脉壁可局部扩张。

suppurative [ˈsʌpjuərətiv] *a.* 化脓的

Chronic inflammation supervening on acute is almost always suppurative in type.

由急性演变而来的慢性炎症几乎均为化脓性炎症。

supramolecular [ˌsjuːprəməuˈlekjulə] *a.* 超分子的（由许多分子组成的）

At present, supramolecular chemistry has developed rapidly, and becomes the focus of study which chemists pay attention to.

目前，超分子化学迅速发展，已成为化学家们关注的研究焦点。

suprapubic [ˌsjuːprəˈpjuːbik] *a.* 耻骨弓上的

Many physicians refer to significant bacteriuria associated with dysuria, frequency, urgency, and suprapubic pain as cystitis.

很多医生认为显著的菌尿若伴有尿痛、尿频、尿急及耻骨上痛则可能是膀胱炎。

Eight patients had indwelling urinary catheters, while two had suprapubic cystotomy tubes.

八例病人有留置导尿管，另两例有耻骨上膀胱造瘘插管。

supraventricular [ˌsjuːprəvenˈtrikjulə] *a.* 室上的

Atrial distension may provoke a variety of supraventricular arrhythmias.

心房的扩张可能引起各种室上性心律不齐。

supravesical [ˌsjuːprəˈvesikəl] *a.* 膀胱上的

Supravesical obstruction may be completely asymptomatic when it develops slowly over a period of several weeks or months.

当膀胱上梗阻发展缓慢时，经数周或数月可完全无症状。

Anomalies of mesenteric fixation may lead to abnormal openings through which internal hernias may occur. This is the likely mechanism of paraduodenal and supravesical hernias.

肠系膜的固定异常会导致异常的裂隙，从而产生腹内疝，这有可能就是十二指肠旁疝和膀胱上疝的发病机制。

surelease [ʃuəˈliːs] *n.* 乙基纤维素水分散体

Surelease provides dependable drug release characteristics and dissolution performance throughout its shelf life period.

乙基纤维素水分散体可在整个保质期里确保可靠的药物释放特性和溶解性能。

Surelease is used primarily as a barrier membrane for developing extended release dosage forms.

乙基纤维素水分散体主要作为屏障膜用于开发缓释剂型。

surface [ˈsəːfis] *n.* 表面 a. 表面上的，外表上的

The skin forms a large surface for radiating body heat to the air.

皮肤形成了一个宽阔的表面，把人体热量辐射到空气中去。

Abnormal increase in the quantity of melanin may occur either in localized areas or over the entire body surface.

黑色素量的异常增多可能仅局限于某些区域，也可能会遍及整个体表。

Surface molecules can be demonstrated using fluorescent antibodies as probes.

表面分子可用荧光抗体作为探针来标记。

The cells forming simple tubular glands form a single tube which opens directly on to the free surface.

构成单管腺的细胞形成一个单管，直接开口于游离面。

surfactant [sə:ˈfæktənt] *n.* 表面活性剂，表面活性物质

The alveoli of human and other mammalian lungs are lined with a thin layer surfactant, which regulates surface tension at the air-liquid interface.

人类和其他哺乳动物肺的肺泡有一薄层表面活性剂，它在空气液体界面处调节表面张力。

Other nonobstructive factors contributing to atelectasis include decreased functional residual capacity and loss of pulmonary surfactant.

引起肺不张的其他非阻塞性因素包括功能性肺残气量降低以及肺表面活性物质降低。

surge [sə:dʒ] *n.* 巨浪；汹涌；高峰

The level of luteinizing hormone in the blood is fairly constant except during the preovulatory surge.

除排卵前高峰外，血中黄体生成激素的浓度是相当恒定的。

surgeon [ˈsə:dʒən] *n.* 外科医生

The first human nephrectomy is attributed to a German surgeon in 1869.

第一例人类肾脏切除手术是一位德国外科医生于 1869 年实施的。

surgery [ˈsə:dʒəri] *n.* 外科，外科学，手术

Surgery is the medical department responsible for performing operations on patients.

外科是负责给病人施行手术的医疗科室。

The past 20 years saw tremendous strides in the development of surgery.

过去 20 年间外科学有突飞猛进的发展。

Different types of anesthesia may be given for elective or emergency surgery.

对择期手术和急诊手术应给予不同类型的麻醉。

surgical [ˈsədʒikəl] *a.* 外科的，外科手术的

Intensive surgical care can of course be provided on a regular nursing unit.

在常规护理病房当然可以提供外科加强护理。

These drugs tend to decrease the tensile strength of the surgical wound.

这些药物有降低手术伤口抗张强度的倾向。

surpass [sə:ˈpɑ:s] *v.* 超过，胜过

Chinese medical workers should make efforts to catch up with and even surpass the advanced world levels in many fields of medicine.

中国医学工作者应努力在医学的许多领域里赶上甚至超过世界先进水平。

surplus [ˈsə:pləs] *a.* 过剩的，多余的

Stress or nerves can also activate surplus insulin.

心理压力或神经紧张也可激活过剩的胰岛素。

This medical instrument is surplus to requirements.

这种医疗器械供过于求。

surrogate [ˈsʌrəgeit] *n.* 替代

The surrogate measures of arterial stiffness have additive predictive value.

动脉硬度的替代测量具有额外的预测价值。

surround [səˈraund] *v.* 包围，围住

A nuclear membrane surrounds the nucleus and separates it from the cytoplasm.
核膜包裹着核,将它与细胞质分开。
If we examine a cross-section of the spine cord, we may see that the gray matter is in the interior of the cord and the white matter surrounds the gray.
如果我们观察脊髓的横断面,就可看出灰质在脊髓内部,而白质围住灰质。
There is a great deal of controversy surrounding the issue of hormone replacement therapy after transplantation.
在有关(围绕)移植后激素替代治疗这一问题上,存在很大的争议。

surrounding [sə'raundiŋ] *a.* 周围的
If carbon monoxide exists in the surrounding air, it gets into the body as a result of the diffusion of gases.
如果在周围的空气中含有一氧化碳,它就会因气体扩散而进入人体。
In local anaesthesia, the drug is injected directly in the nearby surrounding tissues.
局部麻醉时药物直接注射于附近的周围组织。
n. (复数)周围的事物,环境
A thin covering called the cell membrane encloses the cell and separates it from its surroundings.
叫做细胞膜的一层薄膜包裹着细胞,将它与周围环境分开。
The oozing urethral opening shows the infection of the urethra, and flea-bite-shaped reddening of their surroundings indicates disease in Skene's ducts.
尿道口渗出表示尿道感染,周围的蚤咬状红斑表明尿道旁腺受染。

surveillance [səː'veiləns] *n.* 监视,监督
Hospitalization with careful maternal and fetal surveillance is indicated.
需要住院并对产妇和胎儿进行密切监测。
Surveillance should either stimulate appropriate action or be used to evaluate actions already instituted.
监测应激发合适的行动或用来评估已经开始的工作。
Active surveillance may provide important information about therapy.
积极的监测工作可为治疗提供重要信息。

survey ['səvei] *n.* 概况;调查
50 percent of working adults, in one survey, admitted to having a back injury each year.
在一项调查中,有50%的成年工人每年背部受伤。
Geographical survey should be included in the taking of the history when confronted with a sick visitor or immigrant to this country.
在为旅游者或移民检查病情时,须将地域概况一项列入病史采集的内容。
v. [sə'vei] 概括评述;调查
In this book, the author surveys recent developments in genetics.
在这本书里,作者概述了遗传学最近的发展概况。
Of the five hundred householders surveyed, 10% had a family history of cancers.
在调查的500户居民中,10%有癌症家族史。

survival [sə'vaivəl] *n.* 幸存,存活;残存者
The patient's chances of survival are greatly improved with drugs such as propranolol and lidocaine.
运用心得安和利多卡因之类的药物,病人的存活机会大大增加了。
These enzymes are vital to the survival of the organism.
此种酶对有机体的生存是重要的。

survive [sə'vaiv] *v.* 活下来,幸免于;比…活得长
He is the only man who survived after the accident.
他是这次事故中惟一活下来的人。

Do you know how many people survived the earthquake?
你知道有多少人在这次地震中幸存下来。
In both groups tuberculin positive subjects survived longer than those who were tuberculin negative.
两组中,结核菌素试验阳性病人存活时间长于阴性者。
Insurance statistics show that most wives survive their husbands.
保险统计表明大多数妻子比丈夫活得长。

survivin [sə'vaivin] *n.* 生存素
Recombinant pEGFP-C1-antisense survivin plasmid was cloned and transfected to gastric cancer cells.
复制 pEGFP-C1-反义生存素的重组质粒,并将其转染至胃癌细胞。

survivor [sə'vaivə] *n.* 幸存者,生存者,残存者
Of all the survivors none was free from a distressing sequela.
在所有这些幸存者中,无人能免于痛苦的后遗症。

survivorship [sə'vaivəʃip] *n.* 幸存,残存
Both industry and government have noted in the past several years the extent of rat survivorship at the end of 2-year toxicity and carcinogenicity studies has been decreasing.
工业界和政府两方面在过去几年间都注意到,两年的毒性和致癌性试验结束时,大鼠残存的已在减少。

susceptible(to) [sə'septəbl] *a.* 易感的,敏感的
The old are particularly susceptible to brain damage and are less likely to completely recover from it.
老年人特别容易遭受脑损害,而且不太可能完全恢复。
Some patients are susceptible to pain, but others tolerate it with impunity.
有的病人很怕痛,有的则能泰然处之。
Aminoglycosides are bactericidal and inhibit protein synthesis in susceptible microorganisms.
氨基糖甙类对敏感微生物具有杀菌作用,并抑制其蛋白质的合成。
n. 易感的人
Exposed susceptibles should be isolated from social groups until it is determined whether disease is present.
在确定本病是否存在之前,应将受暴露的易感者从社会人群中隔离开。

susceptibility(to) [səˌseptə'biliti] *n.* 易感性,敏感性
There seems to be greater susceptibility among children to the virus of smallpox.
儿童似乎更易感染天花病毒。
In addition, there are individual variations in the susceptibility to decompression sickness.
此外,还有对减压病易感性的个体差异。

susceptive [sə'septiv] *a.* 易感的,敏感的
Most swine influenza viruses are susceptive to the antivirus medicine.
大多数猪流感病毒对抗病毒药物很敏感。
Some people are more susceptive to hospital infections than others.
有些人比其他人更容易受到医院内感染。

suspect [səs'pekt] *v.* 怀疑,猜想
Viral etiology of the pneumonia was strongly suspected.
高度怀疑此肺炎的原因为病毒性的。
This makes possible for the doctor to suspect the diagnosis earlier.
这使得医生有可能较早地作出拟诊。
Three more suspected cases of SARS(severe acute respiratory syndrome) were found yesterday in that city.

该市昨天又发现 3 例 SARS 的疑似病例。

suspend [səˈspend] *v.* 延缓

Malignant cells with mutant or absent p53 fail to suspend cell-cycle progression, do not undergo apoptosis, and exhibit resistance to these drugs.

突变或缺乏 p53 的恶性肿瘤细胞不能延缓细胞周期进程,不会遭受凋亡,并对这些药物产生抗性。

suspense [səˈspens] *n.* 不安,焦虑

We waited in great suspense for the doctor's opinion.

我们非常焦急地等待医生的意见。

suspension [səsˈpenʃən] *n.* 悬浮; 悬浮液

More often employed nowadays are the insulin zinc suspensions.

近来更通常使用的是锌胰岛素混悬液。

suspicious [səsˈpiʃəs] *a.* 可疑的

The doctor is suspicious of the reliability of the history told by the patient.

医生怀疑病人所说病史的可靠性。

All suspicious areas must be biopsied.

必须从所有可疑的部位做活检。

suspiciousness [səsˈpiʃəsnis] *n.* 猜疑,多疑,疑心

Suspiciousness and hypersensitivity suggest a paranoid personality disorder.

多疑和过敏提示类偏狂人格疾病。

sustain [səsˈtein] *v.* 支持,维持

Fever may be high and sustains in severe cases.

严重病例可发高热,且持续不退。

If you don't get enough calcium in your diet, your body takes calcium reserves from your bones to sustain normal cell function. This can result in osteoporosis.

如果你不能从你的饮食中得到足够的钙,你的身体就会从你的骨骼中摄取钙储备来维持正常的细胞功能,这就会导致骨质疏松。

sustained [səsˈteind] *a.* 持续的,持久不变的

In arteriosclerosis heart disease, the heart is not capable of a normal amount of sustained work.

患冠心病时,心脏不能承担正常的持续性的活动。

Sustained or severe hypertension is unusual, if present, another etiology for the nephrotic syndrome should be searched for.

持久的或严重的高血压并不常见,若的确存在,就应寻找引起肾病综合征的其他原因。

suture [ˈsjuːtʃə] *n.* 缝合;缝线

The Ascaris adults may perforate a suture line or cause a bile or pancreatic duct obstruction.

成虫可穿破缝线或引起胆管或胰腺管阻塞。

Blood sometimes leaks through skin sutures.

血液还会经皮肤缝合处渗出。

swab [swɔb] *n.* 拭子;药签

Nasopharyngeal and rectal swabs were cultured for adenovirus.

鼻咽及直肠拭子作了腺病毒培养。

Non-absorbent cotton swab, moistured with saline, is suitable.

非吸收性棉拭子用盐水弄湿是适合的。

swallow [ˈswɔləu] *v.* 吞下,咽下

The patient found it easier to swallow fluid than solid food.

病人感觉吃液体食物比吞咽固体食物要容易。

About 20 to 60 percent of intestinal gas represents swallowed air.

约 20% ~60% 的小肠气体是吞下的空气。

sweat [swet] *n.* 汗,出汗

Sweat is similar in composition to plasma, containing the same electrolytes, though in a more dilute concentration.

汗液在成分上与血浆相似,含有相同的电解质,但浓度较低。

The evaporation of sweat from the surface of the body also helps to cool the body.

人体表面汗的蒸发,也有助于人体降温。

The amount of sweat produced is associated with the maintenance of normal body temperature.

排汗的量是与维持正常体温有关联的。

swell [swel] (swelled, swollen) *v.* 肿胀;增大

The gall-bladder swells as a result of the obstruction.

胆囊肿胀是由于阻塞的结果。

The tonsils of this patient are red and swollen.

这个病人的扁桃体是红肿的。

swelling [ˈsweliŋ] *n.* 肿胀,膨胀

There was some respiratory difficulty due to the swelling of the tonsils.

由于扁桃体肿大,呼吸有些困难。

swing [swiŋ] (swang [swæŋ], swung [swʌŋ]) *v.* 摇摆

There are the associated features of bacterial infection: a swinging fever, malaise, anorexia and sweating, and an accompanying polymorph leukocytosis.

细菌感染的有关特征:弛张热、不适、厌食、出汗,并伴有多形核白细胞增多。

switch [switʃ] *n.* 开关

In the electrical industry copper is used for the production of transmission wires, switches, generators, motors, transformers, and pipes.

在电力工业中,铜用于生产导线、开关、发电机、发动机、变压器和管材。

v. 改变;关闭

Do not switch off the power for the electrocardiograph.

不要关掉心电图机的电源。

swollen [ˈswəulən] *a.* 肿胀的

The swollen epithelium secretes excessive quantities of mucus which further increase the resistance to air flow.

肿胀的上皮分泌大量的黏液,后者又进一步增强对气流的阻力。

The adjacent cuticle is pink, swollen, and tender on pressure.

邻近的甲小皮为粉红色、肿胀、有压痛。

symbiosis [ˌsimbiˈəusis] *n.* 共生现象

There is the symbiosis between a plant and the insect that fertilizes it.

在植物和使之受粉的昆虫间有共生现象。

symbol [ˈsimbəl] *n.* 象征;符号

Hg is the chemical symbol for mercury.

Hg 是汞的化学元素符号。

symmetrical [siˈmetrikəl] *a.* 对称的

Enzymes are able to distinguish between two equivalent atoms in a symmetrical molecule.

酶能区别对称分子中两个相等原子。

The fever gradually decreased to low grade levels while she developed symmetrical polyarthritis.

当她出现对称性多发性关节炎时,体温逐渐下降至低水平。

sympathetic [ˌsimpəˈθetik] *a.* 交感(神经)的

The sinus node is richly supplied with autonomic nerves, both sympathetic and parasympathetic.

窦房结分布有丰富的自主神经,包括交感神经和副交感神经。

Pharmacologic tests also can be tested to confirm the presence of a lesion in the sympathetic path-

way.
药理学试验也可用于证实交感神经通路损伤的存在。

sympathize [ˈsimpəθaiz] *v.* 同情;赞同
I profoundly sympathized with you.
我对你深表同情。
Her mother does not sympathize with her ambition to be an engineer.
她母亲不赞同她当工程师的志向。

sympathomimetic [ˌsimpəθəumiˈmetik] *a.* 拟交感的
The clinical reports we have just obtained suggest that the drug displays sympathomimetic toxicity.
我们刚得到的临床报告提示该药存在拟交感神经毒性。
n. 拟交感神经药,类交感神经药
A sympathomimetic acts mainly by causing release of norepinephrine.
拟交感神经药物主要通过引发去甲肾上腺素的释放起作用。

sympathy [ˈsimpəθi] *n.* 同情;怜悯;交感作用
She expressed great sympathy when I was injured.
我受伤时,她表示极大的同情。
In physiology, sympathy means a reciprocal influence exercised by different parts of the body on one another.
在生理学中,交感作用指身体不同部分彼此间的影响。

symphysis [ˈsimfisis] *n.* 联合;融合
Examples of symphysis are the pubic symphysis (the joint between the pubic bones of the pelvis) and the joints of the backbone.
关节联合的例子有耻骨联合(骨盆两耻骨间的关节)和脊柱关节。

symposium [simˈpəuzjəm] *n.* 专题讨论会
We shall announce in advance the date of the symposium.
我们将事先宣布专题讨论会的日期。
The whole staff, not excepting the heads of departments, attended the symposium on molecular biology yesterday.
昨天全体人员包括各科负责人都参加了分子生物学专题讨论会。
A symposium on heart transplants was held in our hospital three months ago.
三个月前我们医院举行了一次心脏移植专题讨论会。

symptom [ˈsimptəm] *n.* 症状
A few days later, serious symptoms began to come about.
几天以后,严重的症状开始出现。
Of more specific symptoms, the most common is cough often with mucoid sputum.
较特异的症状以咳嗽最为常见,常咳黏液样痰。

symptomatic [ˌsimptəˈmætik] *a.* 症状的,根据症状的
Of symptomatic patients only half show abnormalities on the small bowel series.
在有症状病人中仅一半显示小肠(X 线)连续检查不正常。
The doctors are discussing about the symptomatic treatment of tuberculosis for this patient.
医生们正在讨论对这个患者结核病的对症治疗。
Heaviness in the cardiac region is symptomatic of coronary artery disease.
心区沉闷是冠状动脉疾病的症状。

symptomatology [ˌsimptəməˈtɔlədʒi] *n.* 症状学
Some patients are unable to describe their distress or atypical localization and symptomatology.
有些病人不会说明其疼痛情况或不典型的疼痛部位和症状。
The histological and functional changes of this disease may persist for 1-2 weeks after clinical

symptomatology disappears.
此病组织学的和功能的改变在临床症状消失后可持续 1 ~2 周。
Diagnosis of chronic cholecystitis is practically the same as cholelithiasis as far as symptomatology is concerned.
就症状学来说,诊断慢性胆囊炎和诊断胆石症几乎是相同的。

symptomless [ˈsimptəmlis] *a.* 无症状的
In the large majority of cases, the primary infection is symptomless.
在大多数情况下,原发性感染是无症状的。

synaeresis [siˈniərəsis, -ˈnεə-] *n.* 脱水收缩
Characteristic defects are of two main types, regression and synaeresis.
特征缺陷主要有两类:退化和脱水收缩。
The results showed that the product had high viscosity, constant viscosity, water-absorption capacity and good anti-synaeresis.
结果显示这个产品的高黏度、常黏性、吸水性以及很好抗脱水收缩性能。

synapse [ˈsinæps] *n.* 突触
Serotonin seems deficient in the synapse in some patients who are depressed.
有些抑郁症患者的突触内似乎缺乏 5-羟色胺(血清素)。
v. 联会
The chromosomes do not synapse in mitosis(except in certain flies).
有丝分裂过程中染色体不发生联会(某些蝇例外)。
During the first meiotic division the synapsed unit of four chromatids is known as a tetrad.
在第一次减数分裂过程中发生联会的四条染色单体形成四分体。

synapsis [siˈnæpsis] (*pl.* synapses [siˈnæpsiːz]) *n.* 联会(同源染色体配合成对的现象)
The pairing of homologous chromosomes is termed synapsis.
同源染色体的配合成对称为联会。
Synapsis of chromosomes occurs during meiosis.
染色体的联会发生在减数分裂过程中。

synaptonemal [siˈnæptəunemәl] *a.* 联会丝的
The synaptonemal complex is protein in nature.
联会复合体实际上是蛋白质。
The formation of a synaptonemal complex starts at the attachment plaque.
联会复合体的形成开始于附着板处。

synchronous [ˈsiŋkrənəs] *a.* 同时发生的
Synchronous lesions are excluded or treated.
排除或治疗共存的病变。

syncopal [ˈsiŋkəpəl] *a.* 晕厥的
Epinephrine may be administered intracordally in heart block with syncopal seizures.
在传导阻滞伴晕厥发作时,可以心内注射肾上腺素。

syncope [ˈsiŋkəpi] *n.* 晕厥
Syncope is a sudden transient loss of consciousness.
晕厥是指突然而短暂的意识丧失。
Repeated spells of unconsciousness(several per day or per month) in a young person suggest seizure rather than syncope.
年轻人反复发生意识丧失(每天或每月数次)表明是癫痫发作而不是晕厥。
The young patient experienced his first of syncopes after drinking alcohol at the age of 22.
这个年轻患者在他 22 岁时喝酒后首次发作晕厥。

syncytial [sinˈsiʃəl] *a.* 多核的;合胞体的
Respiratory syncytial virus is the most important pathogen of early childhood, especially in the

first 2 months of life.
呼吸性多核病毒是婴儿期,尤其在出生后两个月内,最主要的致病体。
The most common virus producing pneumonia in children in the UK and the USA is the respiratory syncytial virus.
引起英美儿童患肺炎的最常见的病毒是呼吸道合胞病毒。

syndrome [ˈsindrəum] *n.* 综合征
Syndrome is a set of symptoms which occur together, the sum of signs of any morbid state.
综合征是同时发生的一组症状,任何疾病状态体征的总和。
Acquired immune deficiency syndrome(AIDS) is an epidemic transmissible retroviral disease due to infection with human immunodeficiency virus(HIV).
获得性免疫缺陷综合征(艾滋病)是由人类免疫缺陷病毒(HIV)感染引起的一种流行的、可传递的逆转录病毒疾病。
Toxemia is a syndrome of hypertension, edema, proteinuria in late pregnancy.
妊娠毒血症是一种妊娠后期高血压、水肿、蛋白尿的综合病征。

synergism [ˈsinədʒizəm] *n.* 协同作用
The widespread synergism of plant virus is one of main factors leading to crop loss.
植物病毒广泛的协同作用是造成农作物减产的主要原因之一。
Synergism, in general, may be defined as two or more agents working together to produce a result not obtainable by any of the agents independently.
协同作用一般可以定义为二个或二个以上的物质共同作用所产生的效应不能通过其中任何一种物质单独作用获得。

synergist [ˈsinədʒist] *n.* 增效剂
However, relatively few combinations of insecticides and synergists lend themselves to practical use, either because the degree of improved performance is small or because too much of the expensive synergist is required, or both.
然而,杀虫剂和增效剂的混合制剂实际应用较少,其原因或是由于药效提高不多,或是由于价格昂贵的增效剂的需用量太大,或是两种原因都有。

synergistic [ˌsinəˈdʒistik] *a.* 协同作用的
Not all antibiotics have synergistic effects.
并非所有抗生素都有协同作用。

synergy [ˈsinədʒi] *n.* 协同作用
The correlated action or cooperation on the part of two or more structures or drugs is termed synergy.
两个或两个以上结构或药物的相互关联作用或合作作用称为协同作用。

syngeneic [ˌsindʒəˈniːik] *a.* 同源的,同基因的,同系的
A syngeneic graft is a graft between two genetically identical individuals. It is accepted as self.
同系移植是两个遗传背景完全相同的两个体之间的移植,移植物被当做自我一样的接受。

synonymous [siˈnɔniməs] *a.* 同义的
This kind of mental aberration is an incomplete form of schizophrenia, actually synonymous with schizoid personality disorder.
这类精神迷乱状态是不完全性精神分裂症,实际上与分裂样人格障碍是同义词。

synonymously [siˈnɔniməsli] *ad.* 同义地
Rostral is often used synonymously with anterior in descriptions of the brain.
在描述脑时,嘴侧常是前方的同义词。

synopsis [siˈnɔpsis] (*pl.* synopses[siˈnɔpsiːz]) *n.* 提要,概要
In the summary, you should contain a synopsis of the article that is several paragraphs long.
在你的摘要叙述中,它应当包含具有好几个段落长的文章的概要。
Below are brief synopses of the clinical aspects of major categories of movement disorders.

下面将简要介绍几种常见运动障碍的临床问题。

synostosis [ˌsinɔsˈtəusis] *n.* 骨连接,骨性结合

Posttraumatic synostosis between the thyroid cartilage and the cervical spine can cause dysphagia.

创伤后甲状软骨与颈椎间的骨性连接能够引起吞咽困难。

What are the effects of metopic synostosis on visual function?

额骨连接对视觉功能的影响是什么?

synovial [siˈnəuviəl] *a.* 滑膜的,滑液的

The synovial A cells line the synovial cavity.

滑膜 A 细胞衬于滑膜腔内。

Synovial fluid is found in the enclosed space surrounding the joints.

滑液存在于关节周围的封闭空间。

synovitis [ˌsinəˈvaitis] *n.* 滑膜炎

The dominant clinical feature is a chronic synovitis.

主要临床表现为慢性滑膜炎。

synteny [ˈsintəni] *n.* [遗]同线性;同线型

In classical genetics, synteny describes the physical co-localization of genetic loci on the same chromosome within an individual or species.

在经典遗传学中,同线性描述一个个体或物种中同一条染色体上几个遗传位点的物理共定位。

The synteny is the condition of two or more genes being located on the same chromosome whether or not there is demonstrable linkage between them.

同线性是指两个或多个基因定位于同一条染色体上而不论它们之间的连锁关系如何。

synthesis [ˈsinθisis] (*pl.* syntheses [ˈsinθisiːz]) *n.* 合成,综合

A hereditary chronic hemolytic anemia is caused by a biochemical defect in the synthesis of hemoglobin.

遗传性慢性溶血性贫血是由血红蛋白合成的生化缺陷引起的。

Microcytic-hypochromic RBCs provide evidence that the production defect results from defects in heme or globin synthesis.

小细胞性低色素性红细胞表明生成缺陷是由于血色素或珠蛋白合成的缺陷造成的。

synthesize [ˈsinθisaiz] *v.* 合成;综合

The body synthesizes approximately 2 gm of cholesterol per day.

机体每天合成约 2g 胆固醇。

The adrenal cortex synthesizes cholesterol and pregnenolone by a group of enzymatic reactions.

肾上腺皮质可通过一组酶反应合成胆固醇和孕烯醇酮。

synthetase [ˈsinθiteis] *n.* 合成酶

Leucyl-tRNA synthetase is a temperature-sensitive synthetase.

亮氨酰-转运核糖核酸合成酶是一种温度敏感性合成酶。

When the temperature of the cultures was shifted to 41℃, the synthetase mutant stopped growing.

当培养温度转变到 41℃时,该合成酶突变体停止了生长。

synthetic [sinˈθetik] *a.* 综合的;合成的,人造的

This pharmaceutical factory produces many kinds of synthetic drugs.

这家药厂生产许多种合成药物。

The synthetic vitamins are cheaper and purer.

合成维生素较便宜,且更纯。

A synthetic device has successfully substituted for the heart and lungs in the open-heart surgery.

一个人造装置在心脏直视手术中成功地代替了心肺。

syphilis ['sifilis] *n.* 梅毒

Untreated syphilis will cause serious systemic and visceral lesions and can be transmitted to offspring.

未经治疗的梅毒将会引起严重的全身性和内脏的病损,并能传给后代。

syringe ['sirindʒ, si'rindʒ] *n.* 注射器

A syringe is used to give injections, remove material from a part of the body, or to wash out a cavity, such as the outer ear.

注射器用于注射,从身体某部吸走物质,或冲洗腔室(如冲洗外耳)。

Sanamycin is a labile product and should not be mixed with other medicaments in the same syringe.

萨纳霉素为不稳定的制品,故不能在注射器内与其他药物混合应用。

syrup ['sirəp] *n.* 糖浆剂

Medicated syrups are aqueous solutions containing sugar and at least one water soluble active ingredient.

药用糖浆是含有糖和至少一种水溶性活性成分的水溶液。

Golden syrup is a by-product of the process of obtaining refined crystallized sugar.

金糖浆是制备精制结晶糖过程中的副产品。

system ['sistəm] *n.* 系统

Certain chemicals can induce undesirable changes in the nervous system.

某些化学物质能引起神经系统的不良改变。

The immune system is the body's defense system.

免疫系统是人体的防御系统。

systematic [sisti'mætik] *a.* 系统的,有次序的

All biochemists, and most publications make use of both trivial and systematic names.

所有的生化学家和大多数出版物都兼用俗名和系统名称。

systematically [ˌsisti'mætikəli] *ad.* 系统地

Unfortunately, it is difficult to test these hypotheses systematically.

遗憾的是很难系统地检验这些假说。

systemic [sis'temik] *a.* 全身的,体的

Bronchiectasis is more of a localized disease than a systemic disorder.

支气管扩张与其说是一种全身性疾患,不如说是一种局限性疾病。

Blood flow in the systemic circulation will increase and decrease because of varying pressures.

体循环的血流可因压力变动而增减。

systole ['sistəli] *n.* 收缩(期)

Blood pressure is at its maximum during systole.

心脏收缩时血压最高。

The first heart sound marks the onset of ventricular systole.

第一心音标志着心室收缩的开始。

systolic [sis'tɔlik] *a.* 收缩的

The systolic and diastolic pressures change with age.

收缩压和舒张压随年龄改变。

Systolic blood pressure increases more rapidly than diastolic blood pressure.

收缩压比舒张压上升快。

T

table [ˈteibl] *n.* 平板

Frontal sinuses are located between the outer and inner tables of the frontal bone, posterior to the superciliary arches.

额窦位于额骨内外板之间,眉弓的后方。

tablet [ˈtæblit] *n.* 药片,药剂

This drug can be supplied in the forms of tablets, capsules or liquids.

此药能以药片、胶囊或液体的剂型供应。

The crushed tablets may be taken in fluids, and the whole tablets may be swallowed.

压碎的药剂可放入液体中口服,而整个片剂可吞服。

Another suggestion: To improve absorption, take calcium tablets with meals, drinking plenty of fluids.

另一建议:钙片宜在进餐时服用,同时多喝水,以提高钙的吸收。

taboo [təˈbuː] *n.* 禁忌,禁止使用

In obstetrics, where X- rays or isotopes are taboo, the placenta previa and abnormalities are noted by ultrasound waves.

在产科方面,禁用 X 射线或同位素检查,前置胎盘及异常情况可用超声波做出判断。

tachyarrhythmia [ˌtækiəˈriθmiə] *n.* 心搏过速,心动过速

The wave fronts radiating from the circus movement produce the tachyarrhythmia.

环状运动放射的波峰可引起心动过速。

tachycardia [ˌtækiˈkɑːdiə] *n.* 心搏过速,心动过速

An abnormally fast heartbeat is called tachycardia.

异常的快心率称之为心动过速。

The patient is pale and sweating, and has a tachycardia and a fall in blood pressure.

病人面色苍白和出汗,并有心动过速和血压下降。

tachyphylaxis [ˌtækifiˈlæksis] *n.* 快速耐受

These results demonstrated that EGCG may have a novel pharmacologic effect to prevent steroid-induced tachyphylaxis.

结果表明,儿茶素可能具有阻止类固醇所致快速耐受的新奇药理作用。

The β(2)-adrenergic receptor agonists with reduced tachyphylaxis may offer new therapeutic agents with improved tolerance profile.

低快速耐受的 β(2)-肾上腺素能受体激动剂可在改善耐受性方面提供新的治疗药物。

tachypnea [tækipˈniːə] *n.* 呼吸急促,呼吸过速

Atelectasis is usually manifested by fever, tachypnea and tachycardia.

肺不张通常表现为发热,呼吸急促与心动过速。

Tachypnea may develop more slowly and be limited to lesser grade of severity only in some pneumoconioses.

仅仅在某些尘肺病例中,呼吸急促发生得较慢,其严重度限制在较轻的程度。

tachysterol [təˈkistirɔl] *n.* 速固醇

Irradiation transforms ergosterol into Vitamin D_2, with certain by-products such as tachysterol and lamisterol.

日光辐射使麦角固醇转化成维生素 D_2,并附有某些副产品如速固醇和速甾醇。

tacrolimus [tækrəu'laiməs] *n.* 他克莫司(一种免疫抑制剂)

Tacrolimus, or FK506, is an immunosuppressive polypeptide drug that inactivates T cell.

他克莫司,又称为 FK506,是一种能灭活 T 细胞的免疫抑制性多肽类药物。

Tacrolimus and cyclosporine A are the most commonly used immunosuppressive drugs in organ transplantation.

他克莫司和环孢霉素 A 是器官移植中最常应用的免疫抑制剂。

Average concentration of tacrolimus remained 3. 4-4. 7ng/ml in the period of treatment, presenting steadily fluctuation.

在治疗期他克莫司的平均浓度保持在 3.4 ~4.7ng/ml,呈平稳波动。

tactic ['tæktik] *n.* 策略

Refined diagnostic and treatment tactics are needed in such cases.

在这些病例中需要采用细化的诊断和治疗策略。

Reducing prices is a common tactic in sales.

降价是常用的销售策略。

tactile ['tæktail] *a.* 触觉的;可感觉到的

Various resuscitative measures have reportedly been successful, including different forms of tactile stimulation as well as mouth to mouth breathing.

据报道,各种复苏措施都很有效,包括各种形式的触觉刺激以及口对口呼吸。

tag [tæg] *n.* 标记,标签 *v.* 标示,加标签

^{125}I is the preferred isotope for tagging antibodies in radioimmunoassay.

^{125}I 是在放射免疫分析中用于标记抗体的首选同位素。

Researchers have been using green fluorescent protein for years, tagging molecules and cells to make them glow under certain conditions.

研究人员已经使用绿色荧光蛋白好多年,用于标记分子和细胞使它们在某些条件下发光。

tail [teil] *n.* 尾

The "tail" of pancreas lies in front of the lower spleen.

胰尾位于脾下部的前方。

talc [tælk] *n.* 滑石,滑石粉

Talc is a mineral, produced by the mining of talc rocks and then processed by crushing, drying and milling.

滑石是一种矿物质,经开采的滑石岩粉碎、烘干、碾磨而得。

Talc is found in a wide variety of consumer products ranging from home and garden pesticides to antacids.

滑石粉存在于多种消费品中,从家庭和花园用的灭虫剂到制酸剂。

tamoxifen [tə'mɔksifən] *n.* 他莫西芬,三苯氧胺

Tamoxifen is the most widely used hormonal agent in the treatment of patients with breast cancer.

他莫西芬是一种应用最广泛的治疗乳腺癌的激素类药物。

tamponade [ˌtæmpə'neid] *n.* 填塞,压塞

Cardiac tamponade develops when the pressure in the pericardial cavity rises to a level equal to that in the heart during diastole.

当心包腔压力上升至与心脏舒张期压力相等时会出现心包填塞症状。

tangential [tæn'dʒenʃəl] *a.* 切线的,正切的;离题的,扯远的.

Fracture of zygomatic arch or scalp mass often requires the use of tangential position radiography.

颧弓骨折或头皮包块,往往需要采用切线位拍片。

tap [tæp] *n.* 穿刺(放液)

Blood is obtained with the tap.

穿刺抽出血液。

Spinal tap is also called lumbar puncture.

脊髓穿刺也称作腰部穿刺。

tapasin [ˈtɑːpæsin] *n.* 甲硫蛋白

Tapasin, or the TAP-associated protein, is a key molecule in the assembly of MHC class I molecules.

甲硫蛋白,又称为 TAP 相关蛋白,是 MHC I 类分子组装过程中的一个关键分子。

tape [teip] *n.* 带;磁带

The nail is covered either with adhesive tape alone or with a "finger" cut from a plastic glove held in place with adhesive tape.

指甲上可单用胶布覆盖,或用一个从塑料手套上剪下来的"指套"套住并用胶布条固定。

tapeworm [ˈteipwəːm] *n.* 绦虫

Humans acquire tapeworm by eating undercooked beaf.

人通过食用未煮熟的牛肉而感染绦虫。

Echinococci are the smallest of all tapeworms.

棘球绦虫是所有的绦虫中最小的一种。

tar [tɑː] *n.* 焦油,柏油

This discovery led to more stringent controls of food colors derived from coal tar.

这一发现引起对来源于煤焦油的食品着色剂的控制更加严格。

There is also nicotine, which is a powerful poison and black tar.

同时还有尼古丁,这是一种有剧毒的黑色焦油。

target [ˈtɑːgit] *n.* 目的,靶

Middle aged people should be the main target for health promotion.

中年人应成为促进健康的主要对象。

v. 把…作为目标

Thus, many researchers have focused their attention on targeting adhesion molecules for developing therapeutic agents.

因此,很多研究者将他们的注意力集中在以黏附分子为靶点来开发治疗性药物。

Food handlers may also be a group to be targeted as they are often the source of outbreaks.

食品经营者也可能是一群需注意的对象,因为他们往往是疾病暴发的源头。

targeted [ˈtɑːgitid] *a.* 靶向的;定向的;有针对性的

Endostar is a well studied targeted medicine.

恩度是一种经过深入研究的靶向药物。

Targeted therapy is becoming a main approach to control cancer.

靶向疗法正在成为控制癌症的主要方法。

tarragon [ˈtærəgɔn] *n.* 龙蒿叶;茵陈蒿

The influence of exogenous substance on germination of tarragon seeds must be paid attention to.

必须注意外源物质对茵陈蒿种子发芽的影响。

They have set out to study the effect of Chinese medicine tarragon soup on the prevention and treatment for pregnancy-induced hypertension syndrome.

他们开始研究用中药茵陈蒿汤防治妊娠高血压症的效果。

tarry [ˈtɑːri] *a.* 柏油的,焦油状的

The patient had a history of tarry stools prior to admission.

病人入院前曾有黑便史。

tartrate [ˈtɑːtreit] *n.* 酒石酸盐

A tartrate is a salt or ester of the organic compound tartaric acid.

酒石酸盐/酯是指酒石酸与盐或酯形成的有机化合物。

Metoprolol tartrate is used for the treatment of hypertension, angina and acute myocardial infarction.

酒石酸美托洛尔可用于治疗高血压、心绞痛和急性心肌梗死。

taxane [ˈtæksein] *n.* 紫杉醇

The toxicity of cytotoxic agents is greater during the DNA synthetic phase of the cell cycle, while others, such as taxanes, block the formation of a functional mitotic spindle in M phase.

细胞毒药物的毒性作用在细胞周期 DNA 合成期较强，而其他药物如紫杉醇类则是阻断 M 期功能性有丝分裂纺锤体的形成。

taxonomic [ˌtæksəˈnɔmik] *a.* 分类学的，分类的

The structure, arrangement, and location of the developing spores provide data for a major taxonomic key.

发育中孢子的结构、排列和部位提供的资料是分类的关键。

taxonomist [ˌtækˈsɔnəmist] *n.* 分类学家

Taxonomists have devised methods for tracing the family trees of living and fossil organisms.

分类学家已设计出探索现存生物和化石生物的系统树的方法。

taxonomy [tækˈsɔnəmi] *n.* 分类学

Taxonomy reveals evolutionary relationship among organisms.

分类学揭示了生物之间的进化关系。

tear [tɛə] (tore, torn) *v.* 撕破，撕裂 *n.* 撕裂

Sometimes there is an associated cerebrospinal fluid rhinorrhea resulting from a tearing of the dura overlying the paranasal sinuses.

副鼻窦上方的硬膜撕裂有时可伴有脑脊液鼻漏。

Esophagogastric mucosal tear occurs in the region of the esophagogastric junction.

食管胃黏膜撕裂发生在食管胃连接部位。

technetium [tekˈniːʃiəm] *n.* 锝

Technetium is the chemical element with atomic number 43 and symbol Tc.

锝是原子序数为 43、符号为 Tc 的化学元素。

Technetium-99m has become the most widely used radioisotope for diagnosing diseased organs.

锝-99m 已经成为最广泛使用的、用于诊断患病器官的放射性同位素。

technic [ˈteknik] *n.* 技术，操作（法）

They first used this technic in a patient with ischemic heart disease in September, 1987.

他们于 1987 年 9 月首次将这一方法用于一名缺血性心脏病患者。

Western blot technic is used for analyzing and identifying protein antigen.

韦斯顿印迹技术是用来分析和鉴别蛋白抗原的。

technical [ˈteknikəl] *a.* 技术的，专业性的

The screening method must have acceptable technical performance, detecting the disease at an earlier stage.

普查方法应有可接受的技术方法，在疾病的早期将其查出。

The article is rather technical in places.

这篇文章有些地方专业性太强。

technician [tekˈniʃən] *n.* 技术员，技师

Robert Hooke was an accomplished technician as well as a biologist.

罗伯特·胡克是一位熟练的技师，也是一位生物学家。

When a technician takes X-ray photographs, he is protected by lead screens.

技术人员在拍摄 X 线片时，借助铅制隔板保护自己。

technique [tekˈniːk] *n.* 技术，操作（法）

Successful clinical trials had convinced specialists that the technique was a major advance.

临床试用的成功使专家们确信这项技术是一重大进展。

Immunologisits employ a number of techniques which are commom to other biological sciences.

免疫学家大量使用其他生物科学常用的技术。

A technique is now available that enables the geneticist to prepare a karyotype of an unborn fetus.

现在已有一种技术,使遗传学者能得到未出生胎儿的核型。

Southern blot technique is a technique for detecting specific DNA fragment.

索顿印迹技术是一种检测特异 DNA 片段的技术。

technologist [tek'nɔlədʒist] *n.* 技术专家,技术员

Variability between technologists has been examined and has been found to be relatively high.

技术员之间的差异经过检验,发现这种差异相对较高。

technology [tek'nɔlədʒi] *n.* 工艺学,技术

The technology has improved, and the indications have broadened.

该项技术已经改进,适应证的范围也扩大了。

Modern technology develops so quickly, however, that many applications for the power of the laser have now been found.

然而,现代技术发展如此迅速以致激光的威力在多方面的应用现在得以发现。

teenager ['tiːneidʒə] *n.* 十几岁的少年

Most adult smokers in the U. S. acquire their habit as teenagers.

美国大多数成年吸烟者在少年时期已养成了吸烟的习惯。

teichoic [tai'kəuik] *a.* 磷壁酸的

The teichoic acid molecules extend through the cell wall and constitute major surface antigens.

磷壁酸分子穿过细胞壁并构成主要的表面抗原。

Teichoic acids are a diverse group of anionic polymers that constitute a substantial portion of the cell wall of Gram-positive bacteria.

磷壁酸是一组多样的阴离子聚合物,是革兰氏阳性细菌细胞壁的主要构成成分。

telangiectasia [tiˌlændʒiek'teiziə] *n.* 毛细血管扩张

Hereditary hemorrhagic telangiectasia is an autosomal dominant vascular disease.

遗传性出血性毛细血管扩张病是常染色体显性遗传的血管疾病。

Hereditary hemorrhagic telangiectasia often manifests itself as epistaxis, telangiectasia, and arteriovenous malformations.

遗传性出血性毛细血管扩张病常表现为鼻出血、毛细血管扩张和动静脉畸形。

telangiectasis [tiˌlændʒi'ektəsis] *n.* 毛细血管扩张症

The patient presented with ivory white scars, telangiectasis, hyperpigmentation and ulcerations on the both lower legs.

患者的双侧小腿出现乳白色瘢痕、毛细血管扩张、色素沉着过度和溃疡。

Telangiectasis may develop anywhere within the body but can be easily seen in the skin, mucous membranes, and whites of the eyes.

毛细血管扩张可出现在身体的任何部位,但在皮肤、黏膜和巩膜更容易见到。

telangiectatic [tiˌlændʒi'ektætik] *a.* 毛细血管扩张的

Telangiectatic osteosarcoma lacks the fish-flesh appearance of the usual high grade sarcoma.

血管扩张性骨肉瘤缺乏通常高级别肉瘤的鱼肉样外观。

It is difficult to determine whether this lesion is an aneurismal bone cyst or telangiectatic osteosarcoma at low power magnification.

在低倍镜下很难确定该病变是动脉瘤样骨囊肿还是血管扩张性骨肉瘤。

telemedicine ['telimedisin] *n.* (通过遥测、电话、电视等手段求诊的)远距离医学

Patients from all over the world can get advice from skilled physicians through an Internet service offered by a telemedicine center in the U. S.

世界各地病人可以从美国一个远距离医学中心通过英特网得到高明医生的指导。

telephone ['telifəun] *n.* 电话

You can always reach me by telephone.

你可以随时用电话和我联系。

Controls under the age of 65 were chosen through a telephone sample of all telephone subscribers in the metropolitan area.

65 岁以下的对照组系经大城市市区电话用户的电话样本而选择的。

telocentric [ˌteləu'sentrik] *a.* [细胞] 具端着丝粒的

A telocentric chromosome has a centromere at one end and only has one arm.

端着丝粒染色体的着丝粒位于一端末尾,并只有一条臂。

Telocentric chromosome does not occur in the human karyotype.

端着丝粒染色体在人类核型中不存在。

telomerase ['teləməreis] *n.* 端粒酶

Introducing telomerase into normal cells caused them to divide for 20 additional generations.

将端粒酶引入正常细胞中可使它们的分裂增加 20 代。

Telomerase activity is higher expressed in acute leukemia than normal samples and decreased significantly after chemotherapy.

与正常样本比较,端粒酶的活性在急性白血病时表达要高,化疗后其表达明显下降。

Telomerase is a specialized form of a reverse transcriptase.

端粒酶是一种特殊形式的逆转录酶。

telomere ['teləmiə] *n.* 端粒

Telomeres are DNA sequences found at the ends of chromosomes.

端粒是染色体两端的 DNA 顺序。

Telomeres are required to maintain chromosome stability.

端粒是维持染色体稳定所必要的。

The shortening of the telomeres with each division is what causes human cells to grow older.

端粒随着每次分裂而缩短正是引起人体细胞老化的原因。

Telomere length has been reported to be of prognostic significance in chronic lymphocytic leukemia.

已有研究发现端粒的长度与慢性淋巴细胞白血病的预后相关。

Reduction in telomere length has been associated with aging of somatic cells.

端粒缩短与体细胞的衰老有关。

telophase ['teləfeiz] *n.* (细胞分裂)末期

In telophase, the nuclear membrane reappears.

在(细胞分裂)末期,核膜重新出现。

In the last stage, or telophase, of mitosis, the nucleus is reformed.

在有丝分裂的最后一个时期即末期,细胞核重新形成。

temperament ['tempərəmənt] *n.* 气质,性格

Resent research suggests that mothers' personality types may influence their babies' temperament.

最近的研究表明母亲的个性可能影响她们孩子的气质。

To be a good doctor, skill is not enough—you have to have the right temperament.

要想成为好医生,光有技术是不够的——你还得有好的性格。

temperate ['tempərit] *a.* 有节制的,(气候)温和的

The doctor advises that this patient should be temperate in eating and drinking.

医生建议这位病人应节制饮食。

Multiple sclerosis is more common in temperate climates.

多发性硬化在温带气候中更常见。

Dengue is mainly a disease of the tropics and subtropics, although it can also occur in temperate areas during warm weather.

登革热主要是热带及亚热带的疾病,但是在温带地区气候温暖时期亦能发病。

temperature ['tempəritʃə] *n.* 温度

During otitis media the body temperature may jump to as high as 105℉.
中耳炎时体温可升高到105℉。
Normal temperature of the human body in health is about 37℃ when measured orally.
健康人体正常温度的口腔测量约为37℃。
The other portion of the material is planted on Sabouraud's glucose agar or Mycosel agar and cultured at room temperature.
标本的另一部分种植于沙氏葡萄糖琼脂或菌原糖琼脂,在室温中培养。

template [ˈtemplit] *n.* 模板
The DNA acts as a template for mRNA.
DNA 可作为 mRNA 的模板。
Messenger RNA(mRNA) is the RNA that serves as a template for protein synthesis.
信使 RNA 是一种作为蛋白质合成模板的 RNA。

temporal [ˈtempərəl] *a.* 颞的
Temporal arteritis primarily affects people>50years old.
颞动脉炎多出现于 50 岁以上的人。
The brain suffers a generalized atrophy with circumscribed shrinkage of the frontal and temporal lobes.
脑部发生具有额叶和颞叶局限性皱缩的全面萎缩。

temporary [ˈtempərəri] *a.* 暂时的,临时的
Eruption of the temporary teeth is sometimes delayed and out of the normal order.
有时乳牙萌出推迟且排列不齐。

tendency [ˈtendənsi] *n.* 倾向,癖好,意向
A thrombotic tendency often accompanies the hemolysis.
溶血常伴有血栓形成的倾向。
There is some tendency for cells to be spherical or round shaped.
细胞有成为球形或圆形的倾向。
The patient with leukemia exhibits the general symptoms of anemia. In addition, he has a tendency to bleed easily.
白血病患者显示出贫血的一般症状,此外,还具有易于出血的倾向。

tender [ˈtendə] *a.* 触痛的,敏感的
Digital rectal examination reveals the tender swelling.
直肠指诊发现触痛性肿胀。
In pharyngitis, the body temperature may rise to 104℉, and the lymph glands along the sides of the neck may be enlarged and tender.
咽炎时,体温可升至104℉,两侧颈淋巴结可能肿大和有压痛。

tenderness [ˈtendənis] *n.* 触痛
In many instances no tenderness can be elicited.
许多病人不能查到触痛。
The patient has tenderness in the lower abdomen.
病人下腹部有压痛。

tendinitis [ˌtendiˈnaitis] *n.* 腱炎
Calcific tendinitis results from deposition of calcium salts in tendon.
钙盐沉积在肌腱上可引发钙化性腱炎。

tendon [ˈtendən] *n.* 肌腱
The tendon is often a cord-like or band-like structure.
肌腱往往是一种索状或带状结构。

tenesmus [tiˈnezməs] *n.* 下坠;里急后重
A 69-year-old female, suffering from tenesmus and bloody stool, was admitted to the hospital for

the treatment of a sigmoid cancer.

一例 69 岁女性,有里急后重及血便症状,已被收入院治疗乙状结肠癌。

Bacterial or viral infection of the intestine may result in explosive watery diarrhea, tenesmus, and abdominal cramping pain.

细菌性或病毒性肠道感染可出现暴发性水泻、里急后重及腹部绞痛。

tenet ['tiːnet] *n.* 原则,宗旨

Ethical tenet should be practiced by all physicians regardless of specialty.

不管从事什么专业,医生都应遵循伦理学原则。

A critical tenet in the management of anemias is that therapy should be specific, and this infers that a specific diagnosis be made.

治疗贫血的一个重要原则就是必须是特异性的,这就意味着必须有特异的诊断。

tenosynovitis [ˌtenəuˌsinə'vaitis] *n.* 腱鞘炎

The earliest manifestation of joint involvement is tenosynovitis of several joints asymmetrically.

关节受累的最初表现是不对称多关节的腱鞘炎。

Flexor tenosynovitis is usually minimally painful condition that affects the flexor tendon sheaths of the fingers.

屈肌腱鞘炎是累及手指屈肌腱鞘的炎症,通常只有轻微的疼痛。

tension ['tenʃən] *n.* 张力;紧张

Extracellular oxygen tension falls below about 30 mmHg.

细胞外氧张力降低至约 30mmHg 以下。

Tension and anxiety are common precipitating causes of angina pectoris.

紧张和忧虑是心绞痛的常见诱因。

tentative ['tentətiv] *a.* 试验性的; 暂时的

A tentative diagnosis can usually be made from the Gram-stained smear of the cerebrospinal fluid.

通常可以从脑脊液的革兰染色涂片做出拟诊。

As a guide to action, the doctor makes the diagnosis, which may be tentative or firm but which is always subject to revision.

医生作出诊断作为治疗的指南,这种诊断可能是初步的或确定的,但往往需要修正。

tentatively ['tentətivli] *ad.* 试验性质地

That receptors are protein in nature was first tentatively demonstrated by Lu(1952).

受体实际上是蛋白质这一事实最先由陆氏于 1952 年经试验证实。

tepid ['tepid] *a.* 微温的,温热的

The drug may be taken dissolved in tepid water.

可将本药用温水溶解后服下。

A tepid bath might bring the patient relief.

温水浴往往可以给病人带来舒适感。

teratogen ['terətədʒən] *n.* 致(胎儿)畸形药

In fact a major characteristic common to infants exposed to teratogens is specifically that of prenatal onset growth deficiency.

事实上,接触了致畸物的婴儿常见的主要特征是产前发生的生长不良。

teratogenesis [ˌterətəu'dʒenisis] *n.* 致畸作用

Susceptibility to teratogenesis depends on the genotype of the conceptus and the manner in which this interacts with adverse environmental factors.

致畸作用的敏感性取决于孕体的基因型以及其与不利环境因素相互作用的方式。

The nutritional status of the pregnant female would be expected to play an important role in teratogenesis.

怀孕女性的营养状况被认为在致畸作用中起到重要作用。

teratogenic [ˌterətəu'dʒenik] *a.* 致畸的

It is important to take a routine pregnancy testing during thalidomide administration to prevent in utero exposure of this known teratogenic compound.
服用沙利度胺期间的常规妊娠检测十分重要,从而避免这种已知有致畸作用的化合物的宫内暴露。

teratogenicity [ˌterətəudʒiˈnisəti] *n.* 致畸性
Some organic chloride such as trichlormethane and bromoform can induce teratogenicity.
一些有机氯化物如三氯甲烷和三溴甲烷具有致畸性。
Substances with known teratogenicity must be handled carefully.
具有致畸性的物质必须小心处理。

teratology [ˌterəˈtɔlədʒi] *n.* 畸形学
Teratology is a division of embryology and pathology which deals with abnormal development and congenital malformation.
畸形学是胚胎学和病理学的一部分,它论述异常发育和先天畸形。

teratoma [ˌterəˈtəumə] *n.* 畸胎瘤
Non gestational choriocarcinoma generally arises as a component of a solid teratoma.
非妊娠性绒毛膜癌一般来自实性畸胎瘤的一种成分。
Ten patients with intraspinal teratomas were confirmed by operation and pathology.
10 例脊柱内畸胎瘤均经手术及病理证实。

teratozoospermia [ˌterəˌtəuzuːˈspəmiə] *n.* 畸形精子症
Teratozoospermia has been correlated with poor outcome of in-vitro fertilization (IVF) and embryo transfer.
畸形精子症与体外受精胚胎移植的低出生率相关。

terbinafine [təbiˈnæfiːn] *n.* 特比萘芬(商品名: lamisil 兰美抒)
Terbinafine is used to treat fungal infections of the toenail and fingernail.
特比萘芬用于治疗趾甲和指甲的真菌感染。

terlipressin [ˈtəːlipresin] *n.* 特利加压素
The effects of terlipressin are more persistent, and safe for treating portal hypertension than pituitrin.
应用特利加压素治疗门脉高压比垂体后叶素更加持久有效和安全。

term [təːm] *n.* 学期;术语;期限;足月
The term "closed pneumothorax" is used when there is no external wound in the chest.
"闭合性气胸"这一术语用于胸部无外伤情况时。
As term approaches, there is a good possibility of complications.
随着预产期的接近,并发症的发病机会增多。
Although the fetus may be carried to term, it is usually removed abdominally as soon as it is diagnosed.
虽然胎儿可能达到足月,但往往一经诊断就进行剖宫产取胎。
v. 把…称为
Another form of inborn immunity is termed racial immunity.
先天性免疫的另一种形式叫做人种免疫。
Bladder or detrusor instability of neurologic origin is termed detrusor hyperreflexia.
神经源性的膀胱或逼尿肌不稳定被称作逼尿肌反射亢进。

terminal [ˈtəːminəl] *n.* 末端,终点;终端机
The posterior lobe consists mainly of modified nerve fiber terminals whose cell bodies lie in hypothalamus.
后叶主要由细胞体在下丘脑内部的变态神经纤维末端组成。
The terminal is off line while repairs are being made to the central computer.
在中央计算机修理期间,这台终端不能使用。

a. 末端的;晚期的

The two terminal phosphate bonds of ATP contain high energy.

腺苷三磷酸的两个末端有高能磷酸键。

There is considerable muscular hypotonia, a general flaccid paralysis is a terminal event.

有明显的肌张力减低,全身弛缓性瘫痪是末期表现。

The specified terminal connection driver is invalid.

指定的终端连接驱动程序无效。

terminate [ˈtəːmineit] *v.* 终止,结束

This has sometimes provided the opportunity to terminate pregnancy before the fetus is viable.

这有时提供了机会在胎儿成熟前终止妊娠。

These axons terminate in the dorsal horn of the spinal gray matter.

这些轴突终止于脊髓灰质背角。

Urinary excretion is one way of terminating the action of most drugs or poisons in the body.

尿的排泄是终止大多数药物或毒物在体内作用的一种方式。

termination [ˌtəːmiˈneiʃən] *n.* 终止,结局

Regardless of severity, the definitive therapy is termination of the pregnancy.

无论严重到何种程度,肯定性的疗法是终止妊娠。

The termination of the gestation depends largely on the location.

妊娠的结局主要根据部位而定。

terminology [ˌtəːmiˈnɔlədʒi] *n.* 术语(学)

For the sake of convenience, we will use this terminology in the chapter.

为方便起见,本章决定采用这一术语。

Medical terminology is the science which deals with the investigation, arrangement and construction of medical terms.

医学术语学是进行医学名词的研究、整理和构造的科学。

territory [ˈteritəri] *n.* 领土;管区

How much territory does this medical practice cover?

这种医疗业务覆盖多大的范围?

tertian [ˈtəːʃən] *a.* 隔日的;*n.* 间日热

Tertian malaria was diagnosed by peripheral blood smear and elevated antibody titer against Plasmodium vivax.

外周血涂片和间日疟原虫抗体滴度升高用于间日疟的诊断。

We report a case of tertian malaria in a 36-year-old Caucasian male complicated by spontaneous splenic rupture 2 months after returning from Kenya.

我们报告一例从肯尼亚回国两个月的36岁高加索男性间日疟患者并发自发性脾破裂。

tertiary [ˈtəːʃəri] *a.* 第三期的;三级的

The tertiary structure refers to the total three-dimensional structure of the polypeptide units of the protein.

三级结构指蛋白质多肽单位的所有三维空间结构。

test [test] *n.* 检验

Data were analyzed using chi-square test and t-test.

数据分析采用卡方检验和t检验。

In this test system, bromoform and chlorodibromomethane were also mutagenic whereas chloroform was not.

在本试验体系中,溴仿和氯二溴甲烷也有致突变性,而氯仿则无此效应。

A medical test is a kind of medical procedure performed to detect, diagnose, or monitor diseases, disease processes, susceptibility, and determine a course of treatment.

医学检查是用于检测、诊断或监测疾病、疾病过程、易感性以及确定治疗过程的一类医学

操作。

testicle [ˈtestikl] *n.* 睾丸

The testicles are the organs in which the male germ cells are formed.

睾丸是形成男性精子细胞的器官。

A painful or swollen testicle may indicate a tuberculous or malignant involvement.

疼痛或肿胀的睾丸表明与结核或恶性肿瘤有关。

testicular [tesˈtikjulə] *a.* 睾丸的

Bilateral testicular involvement occurs in 2 to 6 percent of patients with orchitis.

有 2% ~6% 的睾丸炎病人其炎症发生于双侧睾丸。

Men who are regularly exposed to polyvinyl chloride(PVC) may be more likely to develop testicular cancer.

经常接触聚氯乙烯的男性更易患睾丸癌。

testimonial [ˌtestiˈməunjəl] *n.* 证明书；介绍信

She sent a testimonial from her former unit when applying for the post.

她申请谋取这一职位时，寄来了原工作单位的鉴定书。

testis [ˈtestis] (*pl.* testes [ˈtestiːz]) *n.* 睾丸

The testes are the site of sperm production in the male reproductive system.

睾丸是男性生殖系统中产生精子的场所。

The testis itself is spared and is of a normal size, but frequently cannot be palpated through the surrounding swelling.

睾丸本身未受损，呈正常大小，但由于周围组织肿胀，常不易触及。

testosterone [tesˈtɔstərəun] *n.* 睾酮

Normal sperm production is dependent on both follicle-stimulating hormone(FSH) and testosterone.

正常精子的产生依赖于卵泡刺激素和睾酮。

However, a milder form may result in low levels of gonadotropins and testosterone.

但轻型者可导致低水平促性腺激素和睾丸素。

tetanus [ˈtetənəs] *n.* 破伤风

The doctor gave the patient an injection against tetanus.

医生给病人注射抗破伤风针。

The doctors used the tetanus vaccine in their test because it is safe for pregnant women.

医生在试验中使用破伤风疫苗，因为这种疫苗对孕妇是安全的。

tetany [ˈtetəni] *n.* 手足搐搦，(肌)强直

Tetany results from increased excitability of peripheral nerves.

外周神经兴奋性增高可引起手足搐搦。

Calcium gluconate is administered as a 10% solution in treating hypocalcemic tetany.

给予 10% 的葡萄糖酸钙溶液治疗低血钙性手足搐搦症。

tetrachloride [ˌtetrəˈklɔːraid] *n.* 四氯化物

Carbon tetrachloride can cause long-term damage other than cancer, such as liver, kidney, or lung damage.

四氯化碳不致癌，而引起长期(组织)损害，如肝脏、肾脏或肺的损害。

tetracycline [ˌtetrəˈsaiklin] *n.* 四环素

The tetracyclines should be taken orally 1 hour before or 2 hours after meals.

四环素类应在饭前 1 小时或饭后 2 小时口服。

Tetracyclines remain the drugs of choice for brucellosis.

四环素仍然是治疗布氏杆菌病的首选药物。

tetrad [ˈtetræd] *n.* 四个，四分体

A tetrad is a unit composed of four chromatids.

四分体是由四个染色单体组成的。

If a cell has a diploid number of four, the number of tetrads formed at synapsis is two.

如果一个二倍体细胞的染色体数是四,那么在联会时形成的四分体就是二。

tetrahydrobiopterin [ˌtetrəˌhaidrəˈbaiəupterin] *n.* 四氢生物蝶呤

The traditional treatment of severe disorders of tetrahydrobiopterin metabolism is based on the replacement therapy with BH4, 5-hydroxytryptophan, and l-dopa.

四氢生物蝶呤严重代谢障碍的传统治疗方法是基于用四氢生物蝶呤、5-羟色胺和左旋-多巴的替代疗法。

Elimination of tetrahydrobiopterin and nitric oxide may contribute to the aggravation of diabetic nephropathy.

清除四氢生物蝶呤和一氧化氮可能会引起糖尿病肾病的恶化。

tetralogy [teˈtrælədʒi] *n.* 四联症

The patient has suffered from tetralogy of Fallot for some years.

这个病人患法洛四联症已有多年了。

tetramer [ˈtetrəmə] *n.* 四聚体

Tetramer is a molecule (as an enzyme or a polymer) that consists of four structural subunits (as peptide chains or condensed monomers).

四聚体是一种由四个亚单位(如肽链或浓缩的单体)所组成的分子(如酶或聚合物)。

tetraplegic [ˌtetrəˈpliːdʒik] *n.* 四肢麻痹患者

Most individuals who experience this kind of pain are paraplegics and tetraplegics.

大多数经受这种疼痛的人是截瘫患者和四肢麻痹患者。

tetraploid [ˈtetrəplɔid] *n.* 四倍体; *a.* 四倍体的

Tetraploid is occasionally observed in clinical material.

四倍体在临床材料中偶尔可以见到。

A cell or organism containing four times the haploid number of chromosomes is called tetraploid.

具有四个单倍染色体组的细胞或生物体称为四倍体。

texture [ˈtekstʃə] *n.* 结构,质地

Tumours tend to have a different color, texture, and consistency from the tissue of origin.

肿瘤往往具有与发源组织不同的颜色、质地及硬度。

thalamus [ˈθæləməs] (pl. thalami [ˈθæləmai]) *n.* 丘脑

Thalamic hemorrhage is the most common lesion of the midline thalamus.

丘脑出血是丘脑中部最常见的病损。

The thalami are relay stations for all the sensory messages that enter the brain, before they are transmitted to the cortex.

丘脑是所有进入脑的感觉信息在传递到大脑皮层之前的中继站。

thalassemia [ˌθæləˈsiːmiə] *n.* 珠蛋白生成障碍性贫血,地中海贫血

The deficiency is genetically determined and results in α thalassemia and β thalassemia.

缺陷类型取决于遗传,分别形成 α 地中海贫血和 β 地中海贫血。

thalidomide [θəˈlidəmaid] *n.* 沙利度胺,反应停

In the late 1950s, thalidomide was widely used as a sedative.

在 20 世纪 50 年代末期,反应停作为一种镇静剂被广泛使用。

Many deformed children were born before the teratogenic danger of thalidomide was recognized.

在人们认识反应停引起畸形的危险性之前已出生了许多畸形儿童。

Some 4500 children in West Germany alone had thalidomide-induced deformities.

仅在西德就有大约 4500 名由于服用反应停造成畸形的儿童。

The drug thalidomide may slow the progression of prostate cancer in some patients.

药物沙利度胺可以减缓某些病人前列腺癌的病程进展。

thallium [ˈθæliəm] *n.* 铊

The symptoms of thallium poisoning are most evident in the gastrointestinal tract and in the central nervous system.

铊中毒的症状在胃肠道和中枢神经系统表现得最为明显。

A few toxicants, e. g. ,5-fluorouracil, thallium, and lead, are known to be absorbable from the intestine by active transport system.

已知少数毒物,如5氟尿嘧啶、铊和铅,可以通过主动转运系统而经肠道吸收。

theaflavin [θiəˈflevin] *n.* 茶黄素

This paper reports the theaflavin and the tea green pigment extract and manufacture technique from the tea ash.

这篇论文报道了茶灰中茶黄素和茶绿素的提取和制造技术。

We study extraction and concentration of theaflavin by integrating membrane processes.

我们研究通过膜融合技术浓缩提纯茶黄素。

Theaflavin is a kind of golden pigment of the black tea.

茶黄素是存在于红茶中的一种金黄色色素。

theater, theatre [ˈθiətə(r)] *n.* (医院的)手术室;教室;剧院

The patient is on her way to the operating theater.

病人正被送往手术室。

Theatre is a room or hall for lectures, etc. with seats in rows rising one behind another.

阶梯教室是一个房间或大厅供讲课等使用,其横排座位一排比一排高。

Microsporum audouini has been found in barbers' brushes, and on the backs of theater seats and in caps and hats.

奥杜安小孢子菌在许多理发店的须刷里、剧院座位的靠背上和各种帽子的衬里中都已被发现。

theme [θiːm] *n.* 主题;题目

The theme of our discussion was the pathogenesis of AIDS.

我们讨论的题目是"艾滋病的发病机制"。

thence [ðens] *ad.* 因此

Thence the digestive products enter the circulating blood to be transported and used wherever in the body they may be needed.

因此,消化产物(由该处)进入血液,并将被运输到身体可能需要它们的部位加以利用。

theophylline [ˌθiəˈfilin] *n.* 茶碱

Theophylline inhibits the activity of phosphodiesterase.

茶碱可抑制磷酸二酯酶的活性。

In patients already taking theophylline, the loading dose is reduced or withheld.

对于已经用过茶碱的病人,应减少或不用负荷剂量。

theoretical [θiəˈretikəl] *a.* 理论的

Details of the theoretical background and practical technique are not included here but can be found in standard textbooks of cardiology.

详细的理论基础和实用技术在此不涉及,但可参阅标准的心脏病学教科书。

The recommendations on route, site, and dosages for vaccination are derived from theoretical considerations, experimental trials, and clinical experience.

所推荐的免疫接种途径、部位和剂量是从理论上的考虑、实验的尝试和临床实践得出的。

therapeutic [ˌθerəˈpjuːtik] *a.* 治疗的,疗法的

Recent reports suggest that this figure is increased by better therapeutic management.

最近的一些报告指出,经过更好的治疗处理,可使此数字增大。

Unlike many medical advances, the therapeutic benefits of laughter have long been suspected by doctors and scientists.

和医学上许多进展不一样的是,长期以来,医生和科学家一直猜想笑有治疗效用。

The therapeutic index is median lethal dose(LD50) to median effective dose(ED50).
治疗指数是半数致死剂量与半数有效剂量之比。

therapeutically [ˌθerəˈpjuːtikəli] *ad.* 在治疗上
Such agents are considered as(being) therapeutically equivalent.
从疗效上看这类制剂是相等的。
The treated mice did not appear stronger because a 10 percent replacement is not therapeutically useful.
经治疗的小鼠并未显得健壮一些,因为10%的替代物在治疗上不起作用。

therapy [ˈθerəpi] *n.* 治疗,疗法
It is obvious that, if multiple metastases are present, local therapy will not cure the cancer.
很清楚,如果出现了多发性转移,局部疗法不能治愈此癌症。
Deep X-ray therapy carries a slight but real risk of leukemia.
深部X线疗法所带来患白血病的危险,虽然不大,但是确实存在。

thereby [ˌðɛəˈbai, ˈðɛəbai] *ad.* 因此,由此,从而
These cells actively reabsorb sodium, thereby modifying sweat from a basically isotonic solution to a hypotonic one.
这些细胞可以主动地重吸收钠,从而使基本上是等渗液的汗液变成了低渗液。

thermal [ˈθəːməl] *a.* 热的,温度的
Chemical burns produce dermal injuries by different mechanisms from thermal burns.
化学烧伤与热烧伤引起皮肤损伤的机制不同。
The stomach from early life is exposed continuously to various mechanical, chemical, thermal, bacterial, psychogenic and physiologic influences.
从生命的早期胃就不断受到机械的、化学的、温度的、细菌的、精神的以及生理的影响。

thermally [ˈθəːməli] *ad.* 在热量上;由热引起
Ninety percent of burns are thermally induced, with chemical and electric burns accounting for the rest.
烧伤中有百分之九十由热引起,其余的原因为化学性和电灼伤。

thermodynamic [ˈθəːməudaiˈnæmiks] *a.* 热力学的
In contrast to some physically active compounds, some fumigants are simply volatile chemical poisons active at thermodynamic levels far below 0.1.
与某些具有物理学活性的化合物不同,有些熏蒸剂是一些简单的挥发性化学毒物,在热力学水平远低于0.1时仍具有活性。

thermolabile [ˌθəːməuˈleibail] *a.* 不耐热的
Furthermore, some pesticides, e. g. Carbamates, are thermolabile and therefore difficult to volatilize without decomposition.
此外,一些农药比如氨基甲酸酯是不耐热的,因此难以在不分解的情况下挥发。
Many bacterial exotoxins are thermolabile and can be easily inactivated by the application of moderate heat.
许多细菌外毒素是不耐热的,通过采用适当加热即能轻易灭活。

thermometer [θəˈmɔmitə] *n.* 温度计
The temperature of the human body is usually measured by a thermometer placed in the mouth, axilla, or rectum.
人的体温通常用置于口腔、腋下或直肠的体温计来测量。
One of his important inventions was the thermometer which made it possible to measure temperature carefully.
他的重要发明之一是温度计,使仔细测定温度成为可能。

thermophile [ˈθəːməufail] *n.* 嗜热生物;*a.* 嗜热的
Thermophiles are microorganisms that live and grow in extremely hot environments.

嗜热生物是生活和生长在极热环境中的微生物。

As a prerequisite for their survival, thermophiles contain enzymes that can function at high temperatures.

作为其生存的先决条件，嗜热生物含有可以在高温时正常工作的酶。

thermoregulation [ˌθəːməuˌregjuˈleiʃən] *n.* 温度调节

In some species of animals, apocrine gland secretion is important in thermoregulation as well.

在某些种类的动物身上，顶泌汗腺的分泌在体温的调节上也很重要。

thermoregulatory [ˌθəːməˈregjuleitəri] *a.* 温度调节的

It is well established that the thermoregulatory center resides in the anterior hypothalamus.

人们已确认体温调节中枢位于下丘脑前部。

thermostat [ˈθəːməstæt] *n.* 恒温器

Your skin is your body's thermostat.

你的皮肤就是你身体的恒温器。

thiacetazone [ˌθaiəˈsetəzəun] *n.* 硫醋腙，结核安

Thiacetazone, which is cheap, is widely used in developing countries.

结核安，由于价廉，在发展中国家广泛用于治疗结核病。

thiamine [ˈθaiəmiːn] *n.* 硫胺素，维生素 B_1

The water-soluble vitamins include thiamine (vitamin B_1), riboflavin (vitamin B_2) and so on.

水溶性维生素包括硫胺素（维生素 B_1）、核黄素（维生素 B_2）等。

Thiamine is one of the B vitamins. It functions in cellular metabolism.

维生素 B_1 是维生素 B 族中的一种，它在细胞代谢上起作用。

In Australia, scientists want to place beer with thiamine to reduce the instance of Wernicke-Korsakoff syndrome.

澳大利亚的科学家们想在啤酒中添加维生素 B_1 以减少沃涅克-科萨科夫综合征的发生。

thiazide [ˈθaiəzaid] *n.* 噻嗪

Thiazide diuretics are extremely effective in small doses in essential hypertension.

小剂量噻嗪类利尿剂对原发性高血压非常有效。

thiazolidinedione [θaiəˌzɔlidinˈdaiəun] *n.* 噻唑烷二酮

Thiazolidinedione (TZD) can improve insulin resistance and decrease blood glucose level.

噻唑烷二酮（TZD）可改善胰岛素抵抗并降低血糖。

PPARγ has also been identified as the major functional receptor of thiazolidinedione.

发现 PPARγ 也是噻唑烷二酮的主要功能受体。

thiazolyl [θaiəˈzəulil] *n.* 噻唑基

This eliminates one technical difficulty associated with the thiazolyl blue assay—solubilization of colored product.

这一步骤消除了一项与噻唑基蓝测定法有关的技术困难，即呈色产物的溶解性问题。

thicken [ˈθikən] *v.* （使）变厚，增厚

The tumor has a thickened capsule.

此肿瘤有一层增厚的包膜。

thickness [ˈθiknis] *n.* 厚度

Sonograms are used to assess kidney size and cortical thickness.

超声波检查用于估计肾脏的大小和皮质的厚度。

All skin sites are composed of these 3 anatomically distinct layers, although there is considerable regional variation in their relative thickness.

尽管不同部位的皮肤其相对厚度有所差异，但在解剖学上所有的皮肤均由三个不同的组织层次所构成。

thigh [θai] *n.* 大腿

Large motor units, where one neuron supplies several hundred muscle fibers, are found in the

large trunk and thigh muscles.
在大的运动单位中，一个运动神经元支配着数百肌纤维，这种运动单位见于较大的躯干和大腿肌肉。

thin [θin] *a.* 薄的，细的
It is thinnest in the two atria as they are receiving chambers and merely have to squeeze the blood into the adjacent ventricles.
两个心房的心肌最薄，因为它们是接受腔，只需将血液压入相邻的心室。
The epidermis is very thin on the eyelids, where it measures less than 0.1mm.
眼睑的表皮非常薄，不到0.1mm。

thioguanine [ˌθaiəuˈgwɑːniːn] *n.* 硫鸟嘌呤
The concentration of the active thioguanine metabolites is inversely related to TPMT activity.
活性硫鸟嘌呤代谢产物的浓度与硫代嘌呤甲基转移酶(TPMT)活性呈负相关。

thiol [ˈθaiɔl] *n.* 硫基
The products of the reaction are ammonia, pyruvate and a reactive thiol that is capable of binding covalently to cellular macromolecules.
此反应的产物有氨、丙酮酸盐以及能和细胞大分子共价结合的活性硫基。

thiomersal [ˌθaiəuˈməːsəl] *n.* 硫柳汞
Thiomersal is a preservative used in vaccines routinely administered to infants and children.
硫柳汞是一种防腐剂，被用于婴儿和小孩常规给予的疫苗中。
Thiomersal has been used widely since the 1930s in a number of medicines.
自20世纪30年代，硫柳汞已广泛应用于许多药物。

thiopental [ˌθaiəuˈpentəl] *n.* 硫喷妥，戊硫巴比妥
Thiopental, a highly lipid soluble substance, distributes into the brain rapidly.
硫喷妥是一种高脂溶性物质，它迅速分布到大脑。

thiophosphoryl [ˌθaiəuˈfɔsfɔːril] *n.* 硫代磷酰
Thiotepa is composed of three ethyleneimine groups stabilized by attachment to the nucleophilic thiophosphoryl base.
塞替派由三个乙撑亚胺基团组成，后者通过连接到亲核的硫磷酰基而变得稳定。

thiopurine [ˌθaiəuˈpjuriːn] *n.* 硫嘌呤，硫基嘌呤
Erythrocyte thiopurine methyltransferase activity measurement confirms the diagnosis.
红细胞硫嘌呤甲基转移酶活性的测量证实了诊断。
We reported a case of severe neutropenia after kidney transplantation due to a thiopurine methyltransferase deficiency.
我们报告了一个肾移植术后由于巯基嘌呤甲基转移酶缺乏引起的严重嗜中性白细胞减少的病例。

thiotepa [ˌθaiəuˈtiːpə] *n.* 硫替派(抗癌药)
Thiotepa, a cytotoxic drug, is given by injection to treat cancer of the breast or ovary, lymphoma, and sarcoma.
硫替派是细胞毒性药物，用于注射治疗乳腺或卵巢的癌肿，淋巴瘤和肉瘤。

thiouracil [ˌθaiəuˈjuərəsil] *n.* 硫脲嘧啶，硫氧嘧啶(抗甲状腺药；治甲状腺功能亢进、心绞痛及充血性心力衰竭)
Thiouracil may reduce the synthesis of thyroid hormones.
硫氧嘧啶可减少甲状腺激素的合成。
Thiouracil is used in the treatment of overactivity of the thyroid gland; its side-effects include fever, skin reactions, jaundice, and agranulocytosis.
硫脲嘧啶用于治疗甲状腺功能亢进，其副作用有发热、皮肤反应、黄疸和粒细胞缺乏。

thiourea [ˌθaiəuˈjuəriə] *n.* 硫脲
Thiourea is a white crystalline solid.

硫脲是一种白色结晶体。
Thiourea has been identified as one of the metabolites in workers exposed to carbon disulfide
硫脲已被确认为是接触二硫化碳的工人的代谢物之一。

thirsty [ˈθəːsti] *a.* 口渴的;渴望的
Salty food makes you thirsty.
吃了咸的食物使你口渴。

thistle [ˈθisl] *n.* 大蓟,蓟
European thistle was naturalized in the United States and Canada many years ago.
很多年前欧洲大蓟就被引入到美国和加拿大了。
Traditional Chinese physicians often use thistle for stopping bleeding.
中医师经常用大蓟止血。

thixotropy [θikˈsɔtrəpi] *n.* 触变性
Thixotropy is found in our bodies, in many products we purchase and in nature.
触变性可见于我们体内,可见于我们所购买的很多产品,也可见于自然界中。
Thixotropy is the property of certain gels or fluids that are thick (viscous) under normal conditions.
触变性是某些凝胶或液体的特性,这些凝胶或液体在正常条件下是黏稠的。

thoracentesis [ˌθɔːrəsenˈtiːsis] *n.* 胸腔穿刺术(=thoracocentesis)
Thoracentesis was performed and 30cc of straw-colored fluid was obtained.
胸腔穿刺抽出了30ml 草黄色液体。
A diagnostic thoracentesis is indicated for any undiagnosed pleural effusion.
诊断性的胸腔穿刺术适用于任何诊断不明的胸腔积液。

thoracic [θɔˈræsik] *a.* 胸的,胸廓的
The liver lies in the right upper position of the abdomen, the stomach and spleen in the left upper, and on both sides these organs are covered by the thoracic cage.
肝脏位于腹腔右上部,胃和脾位于左上部,这些器官在两侧均为胸廓所覆盖。
The 33 or 34 vertebrae of a human being are the cervical, the thoracic, the lumbar, the sacral and the coccygeal vertebrae.
人的33 或34 个椎骨被称为颈椎、胸椎、腰椎、骶椎和尾椎。

thoracocentesis [ˌθɔːrəkəusenˈtiːsis] *n.* 胸腔穿刺术
Aspiration of pleural fluid by thoracocentesis may be necessary to relieve breathlessness.
胸腔穿刺抽出胸腔积液对缓解气喘是必要的。
Thoracocentesis should be performed as an early step in the evaluation of any pleural effusion of uncertain etiology.
对于任何原因不明的胸腔积液,都应首先进行胸腔穿刺来评估病情。

thoracotomy [ˌθɔːrəˈkɔtəmi] *n.* 胸廓切开术
Exploratory thoracotomy should be made to see if the tumor is malignant.
应做剖胸探查以查看肿瘤是否为恶性的。
This article describes the nursing care of patients with acute pulmonary embolism after thoracotomy.
本文描述了开胸手术后急性肺栓塞的护理。
Information support before operation can decrease the anxiety level of patients for thoracotomy.
术前信息支持能降低开胸手术病人的焦虑程度。

thorascope [θɔˈræskəup] *n.* 胸腔镜(=thoracoscope)
By using an instrument called thorascope, the pleural cavity can be inspected.
用一种叫做胸腔镜的器械可以检查胸膜腔。

thorax [ˈθɔːræks] *n.* 胸
The thorax is the upper part of the trunk between the neck and the abdomen.

胸位于躯干上部，在颈和腹部之间。

thorough [ˈθʌrə] *a.* 完全的，彻底的，详尽的

Infection is almost inevitable in the absence of thorough sterilization.

没有彻底的消毒，感染就几乎无法避免。

A thorough physical examination can provide important clues to the cause of chest discomfort.

全面的体格检查能对胸部不适的原因提供重要的线索。

threaten [ˈθretn] *v.* 威胁；预示…的凶兆

In status epilepticus the patient's life is always threatened until consciousness returns.

在癫痫持续状态时，病 人恢复意识以前，其生命总是受到威胁。

The differential diagnosis includes appendicitis, pelvic inflammatory disease, rupture of a follicle or corpus luteum cyst, and even threatened intrauterine abortion.

鉴别诊断包括阑尾炎、盆腔炎性疾病、卵泡或黄体囊肿破裂甚至先兆流产。

threonine [ˈθriːəniːn] *n.* 苏氨酸，羟丁胺酸

Isoleucine can be synthesized from threonine.

苏氨酸可以合成异亮氨酸。

Threonine is an amino acid derived from aspartic acid.

苏氨酸是由天冬氨酸衍生而来的一种氨基酸。

threshold [ˈθreʃhəuld] *n.* 门槛；界限；阈

Codeine raises the pain threshold without altering the patient's reaction to pain.

可待因提高痛阈而不改变病人对疼痛的反应。

The elevated level of glucose surpasses the renal threshold, and glucose may appear continuously in the urine.

血糖水平超越肾阈，葡萄糖就会不断在尿中出现。

thrill [θril] *n.* 震颤，激动

A murmur that is associated with a thrill is likely to have an organic cause.

伴有震颤的心脏杂音通常提示有器质性病因。

The thrill due to a ventricular septal defect is usually located in the third and fourth intercostal spaces near the left sternal border.

室间隔缺损的震颤可在胸骨左缘3、4肋间触及。

thrive [θraiv] *v.* 兴旺，茁壮成长

The infant does not appear to be particularly ill, and the onset of failure to thrive is gradual.

婴儿似乎无明显病状，生长发育不良是渐进性的。

throat [θrəut] *n.* 咽喉，喉

Open your mouth as wide as you can, let me examine your throat.

尽量把嘴张大，让我检查你的咽喉。

She complained of nasal obstruction and a sore throat.

她主诉鼻塞、喉痛。

Throat cultures are not indicated in the absence of fever or lymphadenopathy.

无发热或淋巴结病时不需要进行咽拭培养。

throbbing [ˈθrɔbiŋ] *a.* 悸动的

About 30 minutes later, she called her nurse to complain of a throbbing sensation in her chest.

约三十分钟后，她叫来护士告知她胸中有悸动的感觉。

If you feel throbbing or excessive pressure, loosen the bandage.

如果你感觉到跳动或者过压，放松绷带。

thrombasthenia [ˌθrɔmbəsˈθiːniə] *n.* 血小板无力症，血小板功能不全

It has now been established that different genetic mutations of either GPIIb or IIIa genes results in such a heterogeneity of thrombasthenia phenotype.

目前已经明确 GPIIb 或 IIIa 基因的不同基因突变导致血小板无力症表型的异质性。

thrombectomy [θrɔm'bektəmi] *n.* 血栓切除术

Time is only one of the many variables that may impact outcome of thrombectomy after proximal arterial occlusion strokes.

对近端动脉闭塞脑卒中后进行血栓切除术的效果来说，时间只是众多影响因素之一。

This article investigates the effect of surgical thrombectomy combined with thrombolytic therapy for deep venous thrombosis of lower extremities.

本文探讨取栓加溶栓联合治疗下肢深静脉血栓形成的疗效。

thrombin ['θrɔmbin] *n.* 凝血酶

A small amount of thrombin is formed all of the time in the circulating blood.

循环血液中经常形成少量凝血酶。

Thrombin is formed during clotting from prothrombin which converts fibrinogen to fibrin.

在凝血时，凝血酶从凝血酶原形成，它将纤维蛋白原转变为纤维蛋白。

thromboangiitis [ˌθrɔmbəuˌændʒi'aitis] *n.* 血栓性脉管炎

Thromboangiitis obliterans can cause claudication, pain at rest, and ischemic ulceration.

闭塞性血栓性脉管炎可引起跛行、休息时疼痛以及缺血性溃疡。

Thromboangiitis is a condition affecting the arteries, especially in the legs, of young male Jews who smoke cigarettes.

血栓性脉管炎是一种发生于男性吸烟犹太青年的动脉炎性疾患，多见于下肢。

thromboclasis [θrɔm'bɔkləsis] *n.* 血栓溶解

The drug accelerates the thromboclasis and improves the supply of oxygen and nutrients to the tissue.

这个药物促进了血栓的溶解，并能增进组织氧气和营养的供给。

Plasmin system is a vital enzyme family with the function of thromboclasis and remodeling the extracellular matrix.

纤溶酶系统是人体内重要的酶系，功能在于溶解血栓和重塑细胞外基质。

thrombocyte ['θrɔmbəsait] *n.* 血小板

Thrombocytes are cell fragments that play an important role in both hemostasis and blood coagulation.

血小板是血液中的块状细胞，在止血和凝血方面起重要作用。

Sanamycin hardly reduces the erythrocytes, leukocytes, and thrombocytes.

萨纳霉素不会引起红细胞、白细胞和血小板减少。

thrombocytopenia [ˌθrɔmbəuˌsaitəu'piːniə] *n.* 血小板减少(症)

Early occurrence of leukopenia and thrombocytopenia seems to suggest leukemia.

早期出现白细胞减少和血小板减少似乎提示有白血病。

Heparin-induced thrombocytopenia is seen in five percent of patients receiving more than five days of therapy.

肝素治疗五天后有百分之五的病人出现血小板减少症。

If a lumbar puncture must be performed in the face of severe thrombocytopenia, a platelet infusion should be given first.

如果在严重的血小板减少症情况下又必须进行腰穿时，应当首先给病人输入血小板。

thrombocytosis [ˌθrɔmbəusai'təusis] *n.* 血小板增多(症)

Thrombocytosis is frequently seen in juvenile rheumatoid arthritis and other chronic inflammatory diseases.

血小板增多常见于幼年型类风湿性关节炎及其他慢性炎症性疾病。

The platelets in secondary thrombocytosis function normally.

继发性血小板增多症时，血小板功能正常。

thromboembolism [ˌθrɔmbəu'embəlizəm] *n.* 血栓栓塞

Venous thromboembolism is a common vascular disease with clinically high morbidity and mortality.

静脉血栓栓塞症是一个常见血管性疾病，临床上有高发病率和高死亡率。

Atrial fibrillation is one of the most common arrhythmias in clinical practice and often causes the thromboembolism complication.

心房颤动是临床上最常见的心律失常之一，常引起血栓栓塞并发症。

thromboendarterectomy [ˌθrɔmbəuˌendɑːtəˈrektəmi] *n.* 血栓动脉内膜切除术

The aim is to summarize the treating experience of 7 patients undergoing pulmonary thromboendarterectomy.

目的是总结经受肺血栓动脉内膜切除术 7 例病人的治疗经验。

She then underwent urgent pulmonary thromboendarterectomy, during which she was found to have pale, lobulated tissue completely filling both pulmonary arteries.

然后，她接受了紧急肺血栓动脉内膜切除术，术中发现她的双侧肺动脉都完全充满了苍白分叶状组织。

thrombogen [ˈθrɔmbəudʒen] *n.* 凝血酶原

The mutation of thrombogen G20210A is unlikely to be an independent risk factor for coronary heart disease in Chinese han nationality people.

凝血酶原基因 G20210A 突变不太可能是中国汉族人群冠心病的主要致病因素。

The active components inhibit ADP-induced platelet aggregation and retard the effect of plasma thrombogen.

活性成分抑制了 ADP 诱导的血小板聚集，延迟了血浆凝血酶原作用。

thrombogenic [ˌθrɔmbəuˈdʒenik] *a.* 血栓形成的

Currently, there has been widespread concern over the thrombogenic potential of contraceptive pills.

目前，普遍关心的是避孕丸引起血栓的可能性。

thrombokinesis [ˌθrɔmbəukiˈniːsis; -kai-] *n.* 血栓形成；血液凝固

The complications of phlebeurysma include skin ulcers and thrombokinesis.

静脉曲张的并发症包括皮肤溃疡和血栓形成。

Moderate beer-drinking can help to prevent thrombokinesis and ischemic stroke.

适度喝啤酒有助于防止血栓形成及缺血性脑卒中。

thrombolysin [ˌθrɔmˈbɔlisin] *n.* 纤溶酶

The active extracts from earthworm mainly have the effects of thrombolysin as well as antitumor and antimicrobial effects.

从蚯蚓中提取的各种活性成分主要具有纤溶酶以及抗肿瘤和抗菌作用。

This study introduces the measuring methods of the fermentation and activity in thrombolysin derived from microorganism.

这个研究介绍了微生物来源的纤溶酶发酵及活性测定的方法。

thrombolysis [θrɔmˈbɔlisis] *n.* 血栓溶解，溶栓

Thrombolysis should be initiated as quickly as possible in the emergency room or coronary care unit(CCU).

在急诊室和心脏病监护病房应该迅速进行溶栓治疗。

Thrombolysis is used in the dissolution of a blood clot(thrombus) to treat phlebothrombosis or pulmonary embolism.

血栓溶解用于溶解血凝块(血栓)以治疗静脉血栓形成或肺栓塞。

thrombophlebitis [ˌθrɔmbəufliˈbaitis] *n.* 血栓性静脉炎

The extremities are examined for evidence of edema and thrombophlebitis.

检查四肢，以证实有无浮肿和血栓性静脉炎。

thromboplastic [ˌθrɔmbəuˈplæstik] *a.* 促凝血的

The thrombin has thromboplastic function in vessels, and can regulate thrombosis.

在血管内,凝血酶具有促凝功能,可调节血栓形成。

Many Chinese herbal medicines have thromboplastic function.

许多中草药具有促凝血的作用。

thromboplastin [ˌθrɔmbəuˈplæstin] *n.* 凝血活酶

For partial thromboplastin time and prothrombin time see Laboratory Tests in Ch. 99.

关于部分凝血活酶时间及凝血酶原时间见 99 章实验室检查。

thrombosed [ˈθrɔmbəust] *a.* 形成血栓的

The lesions are associated with thrombosed vessels.

病变与形成血栓的血管有关。

thrombosis [θrɔmˈbəusis] *n.* 血栓形成

Necrosis after frostbite is due to damage to capillaries, resulting in thrombosis.

冻伤后的坏死是由于损伤了毛细血管导致血栓形成。

Physical obstruction of vascular channels can be produced by clotting or thrombosis.

血凝块或血栓形成可引起血管的物理性阻塞。

thrombotic [θrɔmˈbɔtik] *a.* 血栓性的

Blood-borne bacteria or fungi can directly cause valve damage and induce the formation of large thrombotic masses on the endocardium, called infective endocarditis.

血源性的细菌或霉菌可直接损伤瓣膜,导致在心内膜上形成大的血栓性疣赘物,这被称为感染性心内膜炎。

Sterile vegetations can also develop on noninfected valves in persons with hypercoagulable states, so-called nonbacterial thrombotic endocarditis.

无菌性疣赘物也可形成于血液处于高凝状态的患者的瓣膜上,瓣膜未受感染,这被称为非细菌性血栓性心内膜炎。

thromboxane [θrɔmˈbɔksein] *n.* 血栓素

Thromboxane A_2, which is synthesized by platelets, enhances platelet aggregation.

血栓素 A_2 由血小板合成,可以促进血小板聚集。

The researchers found "significantly elevated levels" of thromboxane A_2 in smokers.

研究人员发现抽烟者的血栓素 A_2 水平明显升高。

thrombus [ˈθrɔmbəs] (pl. thrombi [ˈθrɔmbai]) *n.* 血栓

Calcification occurs very commonly in old venous thrombi which have not undergone organisation.

没有机化的陈旧性静脉血栓常发生钙化。

thumb [θʌm] *n.* 拇指

The part of your thumb where it joins your hand is its proximal region.

拇指与手掌相接的部分是拇指的近侧端。

The lesion is grasped firmly between the thumb and index finger.

将损伤紧紧捏在拇指和食指之间。

thymic [ˈtaimik, ˈθai-] *a.* 胸腺的

During adulthood the thymic production of T cells slowly declines as the organ atrophies.

在成年过程中,随着胸腺萎缩,胸腺产生的 T 细胞逐渐减少。

Isolated thymic cysts are uncommon lesions that are usually discovered incidentally postmortem or during surgery.

孤立的胸腺囊肿是不常见的,常常在死后或手术中偶尔发现。

thymocyte [ˈθaiməsait] *n.* 胸腺细胞

Thymocyte development appears to be completed in less than 4 days.

胸腺细胞发育显示出在四天内完成。

Thymocyte apoptosis is induced by p53-dependent and independent pathways.

胸腺细胞凋亡由 P53 依赖的和非依赖的途径所诱导。

thymoma [θaiˈməumə] *n.* 胸腺瘤

About 30% to 45% of thymomas are detected in the course of evaluating patients with myasthenia gravis.

约 30% 至 45% 的胸腺瘤是在对重症肌无力患者的评估过程中发现的。

Invasive thymoma refers to a tumor that is cytologically benign but locally invasive.

侵袭性胸腺瘤是指细胞学上良性但局部有浸润的肿瘤。

thymosin [ˈθaiməsin] *n.* 胸腺素

The thymus secretes a substance that has been given the name thymosin.

胸腺分泌的一种物质,已被定名为胸腺素。

Thymosin is a 12kD protein hormone produced by the thymus gland.

胸腺素是由胸腺产生的一种 12kD 的蛋白质类的激素。

thymulin [ˈθaimjuːlin] *n.* 胸腺素,胸腺因子

The activity of thymulin(a thymic hormone) is dependent on the presence of zinc in the molecule.

胸腺素(一种胸腺激素)的活性有赖于其分子中锌的存在。

thymus [ˈθaiməs] *n.* 胸腺

The thymus is most active during early life.

胸腺活动在幼年时期最为旺盛。

The thymus atrophies during adolescence and is often scarcely recognizable by adulthood.

胸腺在青春期萎缩,成年后常难以辨认。

T lymphocytes develop in the thymus, while B lymphocytes develop in the bone marrow.

T 淋巴细胞在胸腺发育,而 B 淋巴细胞在骨髓中发育。

thyrocele [ˈθairɔsiːl] *n.* 甲状腺肿

Thyrocele may be due to lack of dietary iodine, which is necessary for the production of thyroid hormone.

甲状腺肿可因饮食内缺乏生成甲状腺激素所必需的碘所致。

thyroglobulin [ˌθairəuˈglɔbjulin] *n.* 甲状腺球蛋白

Anti-thyroglobulin assays show poor concordance.

抗甲状腺球蛋白测试的一致性很差。

Thyroglobulin is a tumour marker of thyroid cancer.

抗甲状腺球蛋白是甲状腺癌的肿瘤标记物。

thyroid [ˈθairɔid] *n.* 甲状腺

The thyroid participates in defending the body against germs and toxins.

甲状腺参与机体的防御,抵抗细菌和毒素。

The thyroid was small, smooth, and nontender.

(此病人的)甲状腺小,表面平滑且无触痛。

The major function of the thyroid gland is to synthesize the hormones thyroxine(T_4) and triiodothyronine(T_3).

甲状腺的主要功能是合成甲状腺素(T_4)和三碘甲状腺氨酸(T_3)。

thyroidectomy [ˌθairɔiˈdektəmi] *n.* 甲状腺切除术

Treatment of thyroid tumor is by total thyroidectomy with removal of affected cervical nodes.

治疗甲状腺肿瘤可采用甲状腺全切术及受侵犯颈淋巴结的摘除。

As a therapeutic option, subtotal thyroidectomy is considered for patients with large compressive glands.

对于甲状腺肿大产生压迫症状的病人可考虑采取甲状腺次全切除术的方法来治疗。

thyroiditis [ˌθairɔiˈdaitis] *n.* 甲状腺炎

The thyroiditis is more common in women and occasionally causes dysphagia.

这种甲状腺炎在女性中很常见,偶尔引起吞咽困难。

thyrotoxic [ˌθairəu'tɔksik] *a.* 甲状腺毒性的

Thyrotoxic periodic paralysis(TPP) resembles the familial primary periodic paralyses.

甲状腺毒性周期性麻痹与家族的原发性周期性麻痹类似。

Thyrotoxic crisis is most commonly precipitated by infection in a patient with previously unrecognised or inadequately treated hyperthyroidism.

以前未发现或未充分治疗甲状腺功能亢进症的病人发生感染最易诱发甲状腺危象。

thyrotoxicosis [ˌθairəuˌtɔksi'kəusis] *n.* 甲状腺毒症(甲状腺危象)

Propranolol may control symptoms of thyrotoxicosis.

心得安可以控制甲状腺危象的症状。

Such a situation may be encountered when fever or thyrotoxicosis occurs in patients in whom the cardiac output is fixed.

病人出现发热或甲状腺毒症,其心输出量是固定的情况是可遇到的。

thyrotropin [θai'rɔtrəpin] *n.* 促甲状腺素(垂体激素类药)

Thyrotropin is used in a test to determine how well your thyroid is working.

促甲状腺素用于测定甲状腺功能的试验。

thyroxine [θai'rɔksiːn] *n.* 甲状腺素

The most important hormone secreted by the thyroid gland is thyroxine.

甲状腺所分泌的最重要的激素是甲状腺素。

Aspirin decreases the binding of thyroxine.

阿司匹林降低甲状腺素的蛋白结合率。

tibia ['tibiə] *n.* 胫骨

Skeletal syphilis occur most commonly on the head and face, then on the tibiae.

骨骼梅毒最常发生在头骨和颜面骨,其次是胫骨。

ticarcillin [ˌtaikə'silin] *n.* 替卡西林,铁卡霉素

In the granulocytopenic patient, the aminoglycoside should be combined with high doses of ticarcillin or mezlocillin.

粒细胞缺乏的病人,氨基甙类应与大剂量的替卡西林或美洛西林联合使用。

tick [tik] *n.* 蜱,壁虱

Tick bites can cause serious skin lesions and occasionally paralysis, and certain tick species transmit typhus and relapsing fever.

蜱叮咬可引起严重的皮肤损害,偶可造成瘫痪。有的蜱类传播斑疹伤寒和回归热。

Patients with tick fever are lethargic and have facial flushing, fever and tachycardia.

患有蜱热的病人有嗜睡和面颊潮红、发热、心动过速。

tight [tait] *a.* 紧的,透不过气的

During asthma, in many cases, there is a hard, tight cough.

当患者哮喘发作时,许多病例都会有难以忍受的和透不过气来的咳嗽。

timeline ['taimlain] *n.* 时间表

The chapter describes how timelines for data analysis can be built in at registry inception and how to determine when the registry data are complete enough to begin analysis.

本章描述在注册登记的起始阶段如何建立数据分析时间表以及如何确定注册登记数据什么时候完成得足以开始分析。

timely ['taimli] *a.* 及时的

This has been a timely reminder of the need for taking the medicine regularly.

这及时提醒了病人需要按时服药。

timing ['taimiŋ] *n.* 时间选择;计时,定时

For diabetics, the timing of exercise can also help control blood-sugar level.

对糖尿病患者来说,运动的计时也有助于控制血糖水平。

The timing of vaccination depends on the likelihood of infection.

疫苗接种的时间应根据感染的可能性进行选择。

The timing of film sequence during IVP is governed by the rate of injection of the contrast medium.

静脉肾盂造影(IVP)过程中,一系列摄片的时间安排由造影剂的注射速度控制。

tincture [ˈtiŋktʃə] *n.* 酊,酊剂

Cloth adhesive tape is used to cover the normal skin surrounding the affected nail plate after pretreatment with tincture of benzoin or Mastisol.

在治疗前先涂安息香酊剂或 Mastisol,然后用一块胶布覆盖在受染指甲背周围的正常皮肤上。

tinea [ˈtiniə] *n.* [拉]癣

Tinea is a chronic fungal infection of the skin, hair, or nails.

癣是一种慢性的皮肤、毛发或指甲的真菌感染。

Tinea capitis occurs chiefly in school-aged children.

头癣主要发生在学龄儿童。

tingle [ˈtiŋgl] *v.* 有刺痛感;兴奋,激动

His fingers tingled with the cold.

他的手指冻得有刺痛感。

Tenderness of the breasts, sensations of tingling or of fullness and sometimes obvious enlargement are early signs of pregnancy.

乳房触痛,感觉刺痛或发胀,以及有时有明显增大是妊娠的早期体征。

tinnitus [tiˈnaitəs] *n.* [拉]耳鸣

Tinnitus, a feeling of ear fullness, or hearing loss may occur.

可出现耳鸣、耳胀或听力丧失。

Cogan's syndrome is associated with vestibulo-auditory symptoms such as deafness, tinnitus, vertigo, nystagmus and ataxia.

科根综合征伴有前庭听觉的症状,如耳聋、耳鸣、眩晕、眼球震颤和共济失调。

tiny [ˈtaini] *a.* 微小的

Germ is a tiny form of life invisible to the naked eye.

细菌是肉眼看不见的微小的生命形式。

Our bodies are made of millions of tiny living cells.

我们的身体是由亿万个微小的细胞构成的。

tip [tip] *n.* 梢尖,末端

The tip of the thumb is its distal region.

拇指尖是拇指的远侧端。

The entire tip of the finger is now numb.

此时整个指端都失去知觉。

tiptoe [ˈtiptəu] *n.* 脚(趾)尖

The sick child's mother entered the ward on tiptoe.

病孩的母亲踮着脚走进了病房。

tissue [ˈtisjuː] *n.* 组织

A collection of cells specialized to perform a particular function is called a tissue, Aggregations of tissues constitute organs.

专门完成特定功能的集合细胞称为组织,组织的聚集构成器官。

Typical animal tissue are epithelium and connective tissue.

典型的动物组织是上皮组织和结缔组织。

titanium [taiˈteiniːəm] *n.* 钛

The most noted chemical property of titanium is its excellent resistance to corrosion.

钛最引人注目的化学性质是其优异的耐腐蚀性。

Titanium dioxide is a popular photocatalyst and is used in the manufacture of white pigments.

二氧化钛是一种常用的光催化剂，常被用来生产白色颜料。

titrate [ˈtaitreit] *v.* 滴定

Anesthetic drug dosages can be titrated according to the patient's requirements.

可根据病人的需要滴入麻醉剂。

titrator [ˈtaitreitə] *n.* 滴定度

Routine training is given in the use of other instruments such as the micro cell absorptionmeter, titrator and spectrophotometer.

也用其他器材作常规训练，如微量细胞吸收计、滴定计，以及分光光度计。

titre [ˈtaitə] *n.* 滴定度(=titer)

Antibody appears at the onset of the illness and a rising titre indicates recent infection.

疾病开始时即有抗体生成，因此抗体滴定度的升高表明近期有感染。

The diagnosis of viral pneumonia is confirmed by a rise in specific antibody titre.

特异性抗体滴定度升高可确定病毒性肺炎的诊断。

toad [təud] *n.* 蟾蜍

Compensatory renal hypertrophy has been studied in a variety of species, including rats, rabbits, cats, dogs and toads.

代偿性肾脏肥大已在多种种类的动物中进行了研究，包括大鼠、兔、猫、狗和蟾蜍。

tobacco [təˈbækəu] *n.* 香烟，烟草

The most common cause of lung cancer is long-term exposure to tobacco smoke.

长期吸入香烟烟雾是引起肺癌的最常见原因。

Although there is generally less cadmium in tobacco than in food, the lungs absorb cadmium more efficiently than the stomach.

尽管通常镉含量在香烟中比食物中少，但肺对镉的吸收却比胃对镉的吸收有效的多。

tobramycin [ˌtɔbrəˈmaisin] *n.* 妥布霉素

Tobramycin may be given if no site of primary infection is apparent.

如果未发现明显的原发性感染灶，可应用妥布霉素。

tocography [təuˈkɔgrəfi] *n.* 分娩力描记法，产力描记法

Internal tocography is rarely used because of its invasive nature.

由于分娩力描记法有创伤性所以很少应用。

tocopherol [təˈkɔfərɔl] *n.* 生育酚

Because of this, it is called tocopherol, from the Greek meaning "to bear offspring"

由此，它被称为生育酚，取自希腊语其语义为"养育后代"。

Tocopherol is an alcohol which has the properties of vitamin E; isolated from the oil of the germ of wheat kernel, or produced synthetically.

生育酚是一醇类，具有维生素 E 的特性，它是从小麦核胚芽的油中分离出来，或者由人工合成产生的。

toddler [ˈtɔdlə] *n.* 学步的儿童(通常指 1 至 2 岁半的孩子)

The patient was able to pick up her toddler the day after her surgery.

该病人手术后第二天就能从地上抱起自己的幼儿。

toe [təu] *n.* 脚趾

It takes about two square yards of skin to cover the average adult from head to toe.

从头到脚趾覆盖一个普通成人的皮肤约两平方码。

By using acupuncture, the doctor saved the right foot of a sportsman suffering from necrosis in his right toe, by reviving the function of the foot artery nerve.

一位运动员右脚趾患坏死症，医生用针刺，通过恢复脚动脉神经的功能，保全了他的右脚。

toilet [ˈtɔilit] *n.* 厕所；盥洗室

Can you tell me where the toilets are?

你能告诉我盥洗室在哪里吗？

tolbutamide [tɔl'bjuːtəmaid] *n.* 甲苯磺丁脲,甲糖宁(口服降血糖药)

Tolbutamide is used in the treatment of diabetes mellitus.

甲苯磺丁脲用于治疗糖尿病。

The tolbutamide tolerance test is a sensitive and specific test for the diagnosis of insulinoma.

甲糖宁耐受试验是诊断胰岛瘤的一个敏感而又特异的试验。

tolerability [ˌtɔlərə'biliti] *n.* 耐受性

Rimonabant appears to have a favorable safety and tolerability profile.

利莫那班似乎在安全性和耐受性方面更好。

The severity and reversibility of the adverse reaction in question are of paramount importance to its tolerability.

讨论中的不良反应的严重性和可逆性对决定其耐受性极为重要。

tolerable ['tɔlərəbl] *a.* 可耐受的

Toxic reactions of this drug were tolerable.

这种药的毒性反应是可以耐受的。

Their use has made life more tolerable for the patients.

它们的应用使病人生命的耐受性增强。

tolerance ['tɔlərəns] *n.* 忍受;耐(药)量;耐受性

No tolerance develops to morphine induced miosis or constipation.

(机体)对吗啡引起的缩瞳或便秘作用不会产生耐受性。

The glucose tolerance test showed a frankly diabetic curve.

葡萄糖耐量试验表示出一明显的糖尿病曲线。

tolerant ['tɔlərənt] *a.* 宽容的

I am a tolerant man but your behaviour is more than I can bear.

我是一个宽容的人,但你的行为使我不能忍受。

tolerate ['tɔləreit] *v.* 忍受,容忍;有耐(药)力

Much larger volumes of blood loss can be tolerated when hemorrhage is slow rather than rapid.

当出血不是快速而是缓慢时,更大量的失血都能忍受。

Patients with chronic renal failure tolerate anemia well.

慢性肾功能不全患者能耐受贫血。

tolerogen ['tɔlərədʒen] *n.* 耐受原

Tolerogen is a tolerogenic antigen.

耐受原是指能导致耐受的抗原。

Levels of peripheral T cell tolerance is induced by different doses of tolerogen.

外周 T 细胞的耐受水平可由不同剂量的耐受原所诱导。

toluene ['tɔljuiːn] *n.* 甲苯

Lymphoma and leukemias were increased among male and female rats treated with toluene and xylenes.

用甲苯和二甲苯处理的雄性和雌性大鼠,淋巴瘤和白血病都增加了。

tomatine ['tɔmətiːn] *n.* 番茄碱

The content of tomatine was 26.48% in crude tomatine after purification with above technologies.

番茄碱粗品经上述工艺纯化后,含量达到 26.48%。

tomogram ['təuməgræm] *n.* X 线体层照片,X 线断层照片

The visual record of tomography is called a tomogram.

体层照相术的可见记录叫 X 线体层照片。

Tomograms just prior to his discharge revealed a cavity in the left apex.

在他出院前拍的 X 线断层照片显示左肺尖有一个空洞。

tomograph ['təuməgrɑːf] *n.* X 线断层摄影机,X 线体层摄影机

Computed tomograph is an important diagnostic instrument.
计算机体层摄影机是一种重要的诊断工具。

tomography [tə'mɔgrəfi] *n.* X 线断层照相术

Computerized tomography of the brain has revolutionized neurodiagnosis.
脑的计算机断层 X 线照相术已使神经学诊断发生了一场革命。

P. A. (posteroanterior) and a lateral X-ray of the chest should be taken and, if needed, tomography.
应该做后前位和侧位胸部 X 线检查,如果需要的话,可以做断层摄影。

A computerised tomography is a technique which combines X-ray pictures to obtain a three-dimensional image of the interior of the body.
计算机断层扫描术是一种综合多个 X 线图像而获得的机体内部三维图像的技术。

tone [təun] *n.* 张力

Tone is the state of excitability of the nervous system controlling or influencing skeletal muscles.
肌张力是指影响或控制骨骼肌的神经系统的兴奋状态。

tongue [tʌŋ] *n.* 舌

The tongue and the walls of the pharynx are made of voluntary muscle with a lining of mucosa.
舌和咽壁由随意肌组成,表面覆盖着黏膜。

tonic ['tɔnik] *a.* 强直的

Convulsions are characterized by both tonic and clonic phases.
惊厥以既有强直性的也有阵挛性的时相为特征。

tonometer [təu'nɔmitə] *n.* 张力计;压力计(尤指血压计和眼压计)

Ocular pressure is measured with a tonometer after proparacaine instillation.
眼压是在滴注丙美卡因(眼科局麻药)之后再用眼压计来测量。

tonsil ['tɔnsl] *n.* 扁桃体

The tonsils are red and swollen, as are the fauces and soft palate.
扁桃体是红肿的,咽门、软腭同样如此。

Tonsils may become infected and removal of them for that reason is common.
扁桃体容易受到感染,为此而切除已是很普遍的事。

tonsillectomy [ˌtɔnsi'lektəmi] *n.* 扁桃体切除术

Acupuncture anesthesia is routine in many hospitals in operations such as tonsillectomy, thyroidectomy and caesarean section.
许多医院已常规应用针麻施行手术,如扁桃体切除术、甲状腺切除术及剖宫产术。

tonsillitis [tɔnsi'laitis] *n.* 扁桃体炎

This sick child has a recurrent attack of tonsillitis.
这个病孩的扁桃体炎又复发了。

tooth [tuːθ] (*pl.* teeth [tiːθ]) *n.* 牙

There is usually not an actual hole in the tooth, but there is some form of decay.
通常在牙里没有一个真的洞,但却有某种形式的腐烂。

Before you were born, teeth began to develop within your jaws in little sacs.
在你出生以前,牙齿在你上下颌的小囊里开始生长。

toothache ['tuːθeik] *n.* 牙痛

Your toothache is due to caries cavity.
你的牙痛是由龋齿空洞引起的。

tophus ['təufəs] *n.* 痛风石(*pl.* tophi)

Tophi are most likely to be found in soft tissues, including tendons and ligaments, around joints. Less commonly tophi appear elsewhere.
痛风石大多见于关节周围的软组织,包括肌腱与韧带,较少见于其他地方。

Although less common, the tophus can also form in the kidneys and nasal cartilage.

尽管很少见，但痛风石也能在肾脏和鼻软骨中形成。

topical [ˈtɔpikəl] *a.* 题目的；局部的

Usually such topical use of streptomycin is not recommended.

通常不推荐这种局部使用链霉素的方法。

topically [ˈtɔpikəli] *ad.* 表面地；局部地

Sulfonamides are also used topically in burn therapy.

磺胺类药物还可用于烧伤的局部治疗。

torture [ˈtɔːtʃə] *v.* 折磨；使痛苦

Angina pectoris tortured her again and again.

心绞痛一次又一次地折磨着她。

total [ˈtəutl] *a.* 总的，全部的

Does the patient's stomach need a total resection?

病人的胃要全部切除吗？

The voluntary muscles constitute approximately 40% of the total body weight.

随意肌约占身体总重量的40%。

totipotent [təuˈtipətənt] *a.* (细胞等)全能的

Totipotent cells can generate an entire organism.

万能细胞可以发育成完整的生物体。

They can develop into all cells and tissues, as well as other "extra-embryonic" tissues such as the placenta—they are "totipotent".

它们能够发育成所有细胞和组织，以及其他"超出胚胎"组织，如胎盘——它们的确是"全能的"。

tough [tʌf] *a.* 坚韧的

Cartilage is a tough, elastic connective tissue.

软骨是一种坚韧的有弹性的结缔组织。

Crusts may be thick, hard and tough as in third-degree burns.

痂很厚而且坚韧，常见于三度烧伤。

toughness [ˈtʌfnis] *n.* 坚韧，韧性

The sulphur bridges are strong and contribute to the toughness of certain proteins.

硫桥的作用力强，有助于增强某些蛋白质的韧性。

tourniquet [ˈtuənikei] *n.* [法]止血带，压脉器

Because they create whole-limb ischemia, tourniquets are usually more limb threatening than the extremity injury itself.

由于止血带会引起整个肢体缺血，所以它比肢体本身创伤更有危险性。

If other measures are not sufficient to stop bleeding, rotating tourniquets should be applied to the extremities.

如果其他方法仍不足以止血，应采用四肢轮换止血带。

towel [ˈtauəl] *n.* 毛巾

Peripheral irritation, such as dashing cold water on the face and neck or the application of cold moist towels, is helpful.

外周的刺激如将冷水泼在脸上和脖子上或敷用湿毛巾是有用的。

toxemia [tɔkˈsiːmiə] *n.* 毒血症

In the management of mild toxemia, bed rest is of great importance.

处理轻度毒血症时卧床休息是很重要的。

Any disease that causes high fever and toxaemia may cause fetal death.

任何引起高热和毒血症的疾病都可能导致胎儿死亡。

toxemic [tɔkˈsiːmik] *a.* 毒血症的

Hypertension is usually seen in toxemic patients.

（妊娠）毒血症病人常见的症状是高血压。

toxic [ˈtɔksik] *a.* 中毒的；有毒的

Acute toxic dilatation of the colon with bleeding and perforation still has a high mortality.

伴有出血和穿孔的急性中毒性结肠扩张，死亡率仍很高。

Penicillins, which are the safest antibiotics, produce few direct toxic reactions.

青霉素类是最安全的抗生素，极少产生直接毒性反应。

toxicant [ˈtɔksikənt] *n.* 毒物

Certain toxicants can be secreted by the cells of the proximal tubules into the urine.

某些毒物可以通过近球小管细胞分泌到尿液中去。

toxicity [tɔkˈsisiti] *n.* 毒性，毒力

Cyclosporin A has caused reversible hepatic toxicity and nephrotoxicity.

环孢霉素 A 曾经引起可逆性的肝毒性和肾毒性反应。

There is a minimum drug level compatible with control of the patient's epilepsy and an upper level, if exceeded, will cause unacceptable toxicity.

癫痫的治疗，有一种最低限度药物水平，如果超过其上限就会引起不可耐受的药物毒性反应。

toxicogenomics [ˌtɔksikəudʒiːˈneumiks] *n.* 毒理基因组学

Toxicogenomics research combines toxicology with genomics approaches in order to obtain more accurate understanding of toxicological processes.

毒理基因组学研究将毒理学和基因组学方法相结合，以便对毒理学过程获得更准确的认识。

Toxicogenomics can be defined as the application of "omics" techniques to toxicology and risk assessment.

毒理基因组学可以定义为将"组学"技术应用于毒理学和危险评估。

toxicokinetics [ˈtɔksikəukaiˈnetiks] *n.* 毒物代谢动力学；毒动学

Toxicokinetics is also used in environmental risk assessments in order to determine the potential effects of releasing chemicals into the environment.

毒物代谢动力学也用于环境风险评估，以便确定释放入环境的化学物的潜在有害作用。

This paper gives a detailed review related to the absorption, distribution, toxicokinetics, biotransformation, and excretion of phenobarbital in living body.

本文详细综述了苯巴比妥在机体内的吸收、分布、毒物代谢动力学、生物转化和排泄。

toxicology [ˌtɔksiˈkɔlədʒi] *n.* 毒理学，毒物学

The author was invited to lecture on basic toxicology.

作者被邀请作关于基础毒理学的演讲。

As a result, cytochrome P-450 plays a key roles in several areas of research including pharmacology, toxicology, physiology, and biochemistry.

结果是，细胞色素 P-450 在包括药理学、毒理学、生理学和生化学的几个领域内发挥着关键作用。

toxicosis [ˌtɔksiˈkəusis] *n.* 中毒

Toxicosis includes any disease caused by the toxic effects of any substances.

中毒包括由任何物质的毒性作用所致的任何疾病。

toxin [ˈtɔksin] *n.* 毒素

This appears to result from the action of bacterial toxins.

这种情况看来是由细菌毒素的作用所造成的。

Toxins produced by bacteria include exotoxins, endotoxins, enterotoxins, neurotoxins and toxic enzymes.

细菌产生的毒素有外毒素、内毒素、肠毒素、神经毒素和毒性酶类。

toxoid [ˈtɔksɔid] *n.* 类毒素

The detoxicated toxins are called toxoids.
脱毒的毒素称为类毒素。
Active immunization or vaccination refers to administration of a vaccine or a toxoid in order to elicit long-lasting protection.
主动免疫或接种疫苗是指用疫苗或类毒素来达到长期保护作用。

toxoplasma [ˌtɔksəuˈplæzmə] *n.* 弓形体
Toxoplasma infection is a world-wide zoonosis.
弓形体感染是遍布世界各地的动物性传染病。
Secondary toxoplasma infection can occur by transplacental transmission.
继发性弓形体感染可以通过胎盘传播。

toxoplasmosis [ˌtɔksəuplæzˈməusis] *n.* 弓形体病
Death due to toxoplasmosis in immunocompetent individuals is extremely rare.
免疫功能正常的人因弓形体病致死的极为少见。
Appropriate serological tests are indicated to diagnose congenital toxoplasmosis.
需要适当的血清学试验用以诊断先天性弓形体病。

trabecular [trəˈbekjulə] *a.* 小梁的
Osteomas contain a component of trabecular bone in which the intertrabecular spaces are filled with bone marrow.
骨瘤包含有骨小梁成分,小梁间的间隙由骨髓填充。
The trabecular plates become perforated, thinned, and lose their interconnections in the osteoporosis.
在骨质疏松症中,小梁状骨板出现孔洞,变薄并失去互相连接。

trace [treis] *n.* (痕)迹;微量
Only trace amounts of iron are lost in the urine.
仅有微量铁从尿中丢失。
Selenium is an essential trace element required for the action of glutathione peroxidase.
硒是一种谷胱甘肽过氧化物酶发挥功能所必需的微量元素。

tracer [ˈtreisə] *n.* 示踪器;示踪物
The level of direct bilirubin is a major factor in interpreting radionuclide biliary imaging examinations with all of the tracers.
直接胆红素水平是解释各种示踪物放射性核素胆道造影检查的一个主要因素。

trachea [trəˈkiə] *n.* 气管
The respiratory system comprises the nose, pharynx, larynx, trachea, bronchi, lungs, etc.
呼吸系统由鼻、咽、喉、气管、支气管、肺等组成。
The larynx is located in the anterior portion of the neck and extends from the root of the tongue to the trachea.
喉位于颈的前部,从舌根到气管。

tracheobronchial [ˌtrækiəuˈbrɔŋkjəl] *a.* 气管支气管的
Tracheobronchial tree includes the trachea, bronchi and their branching structures.
气管支气管树包括气管、支气管和它们的分支结构。
Severe perihilar fibrosis limits visualization of the tracheobronchial tree and bronchial angles.
严重的肺门周围纤维化,限制了气管支气管树和支气管角的可见性。

tracheobronchitis [ˌtreikiəbrɔŋˈkaitis] *n.* 气管支气管炎
Tracheobronchitis was the leading cause of hemoptysis in children.
气管支气管炎是儿童咯血最常见的病因。
The pulmonary infections were mainly acute tracheobronchitis(39.07%), seconded by pneumonia, chronic bronchitis and pulmonary tuberculosis, etc.
肺部感染类型以急性气管支气管炎为主(占39.07%),其次为肺炎、慢性支气管炎和肺结核等。

tracheostomy [træki'ɔstəmi] *n.* 气管切开插管术,气管造口术

Bronchial obstruction by endotracheal or tracheostomy tubes often occurs.

进行气管插管或气管切开插管常引起支气管阻塞。

Tracheostomy with artificial respiration can only be performed in specialized centres.

用于人工呼吸的气管造口术只能在专门治疗中心做。

Direct trauma to the trachea is one of the few indications for emergency tracheostomy.

对气管的直接创伤是急诊气管造口术的少数适应证之一。

tracheotomy [ˌtræki'ɔtəmi] *n.* 气管切开术

The doctor in charge proposed performing an immediate tracheotomy for this patient.

主治医生建议给这个病人施行紧急气管切开术。

To make an opening into the windpipe surgically is known as tracheotomy.

用外科方法作一个进入气管的切口,这种手术称为气管切开术。

trachitis [ˌtrə'kaitis] *n.* 气管炎 (=tracheitis)

Trachitis causes soreness in the chest and a painful cough and is often associated with bronchitis.

气管炎引起胸痛和疼痛性咳嗽,并常伴有支气管炎。

trachoma [trə'kəumə] *n.* 沙眼

Trachoma is highly contagious, particularly in the early stages.

沙眼的传染性很强,特别是在(发病的)早期阶段。

Trachoma is resulted from infection with chlamydia trachomatis.

沙眼是由沙眼衣原体感染所致。

tracing ['treisiŋ] *n.* 示踪,追踪

It may be that only by an E. C. G. (electrocardiogram) tracing can ventricular fibrillation or standstill be confirmed or ruled out.

可能只有用心电图自动记录的方法,才能证实或排除心室纤颤或心跳暂停。

tract [trækt] *n.* 束,道

Such infections usually begin in the respiratory or urinary tracts.

这类感染通常开始于呼吸道或尿道。

Urinary infection is the invasion of any part of urinary tract by microorganism, these infections are generally pyogenic or tuberculous.

尿路感染是微生物侵入尿道的任何部分,这些感染通常是化脓性的或是结核性的。

traction ['trækʃən] *n.* 牵引(术)

Headache may also occur as the result of traction or displacement of large intracranial veins.

头痛也可由大的颅内静脉受牵拉或移位所致。

Traction is the application of a pulling force as a means of counteracting the natural tension in the tissues surrounding a broken bone.

牵引术是应用拉力抵抗骨折周围组织的自然张力的方法。

tradition [trə'diʃən] *n.* 传统观念;传统做法

What one thinks and feels is mainly due to tradition, habit and education.

一个人的想法和感觉主要与传统、习惯和教育有关。

Yong doctors should keep up the fine traditions of the hospital.

年轻医生应当保持医院的优良传统。

traditional [trə'diʃənl] *a.* 传统的;惯例的

Traditional Chinese Medicine (TCM) is a well of medical knowledge gained from over 4,000 years of observation, investigation and clinical experience.

中医(中国传统医学)是从四千多年的观察、研究和临床实践中获得的丰富的医学知识。

Other countries have tried to reinforce the position of traditional birth attendants but this policy seems to be controversial.

其它国家已试图倡导传统临盆护理,但该措施似乎存在争议。

traditionally [trəˈdiʃənəli] *ad.* 在传统上;惯例地

Such a chronic inflammatory mass is traditionally called a granuloma.

这种慢性炎性肿块传统上称为肉芽肿。

traffic [ˈtræfik] *n.* 交通;交易;交往

The traffic is very heavy in the rush hour.

高峰时间交通非常拥挤。

The drugs traffic is increasing yearly.

毒品交易年年递增。

Traffic of cells into and out of the thymus occurs via high endothelial venules(HEVs) in this region.

输入或输出胸腺的细胞是通过此区域的高内皮静脉进行交流的。

tragacanth [ˈtrægəkænθ] *n.* 西黄蓍胶

Gum tragacanth is a viscous, odorless, tasteless, water-soluble mixture of polysaccharides obtained from sap which is drained from the root of the plant and dried.

黄蓍胶是从植物根流出的树液经干化后得到的一种黏稠、无臭、无味、水溶性的多糖混合物。

Commercial cultivation of tragacanth plants has generally not proved economically worthwhile in the West, since other gums can be used for similar purposes.

在西方,商业化种植的黄蓍胶植物通常没有经济价值,因为其他树胶也有同样的用途。

trait [treit] *n.* 特性;特质;性状

Many of the so called inborn errors of metabolism are inherited as a recessive trait.

许多所谓先天性代谢错误是作为一种隐性特质被遗传下来的。

A trait marker is positive or abnormal prior to the onset of illness.

在疾病发作之前,特性标志为阳性或不正常。

Unlike recessive traits, co-dominant traits are expressed visibly in the heterozygous form.

与隐性性状不同,共显性性状在杂合子中均显现出来。

trance [trɑːns] *n.* 迷睡,恍惚,迷睡性木僵

The hypnotic trance seems to be characterized by a gradual narrowing of attention.

催眠性的昏睡(迷睡)似乎是以逐渐缩小其注意力为其特征。

tranquilize [ˈtræŋkwilaiz] *v.* (使)安定,(使)镇静

Reserpine may tranquilize and lead to depression.

利血平有安定作用并可引起抑郁症。

Nicotine, a chemical you see in tobacco products, has a tranquilizing effect—and, ironically, an anti-depressive effect as well—in our nervous system.

尼古丁,一种见于烟草产品的化学物,对神经系统有镇静作用,但令人感到有讽刺意味的是,它也会产生抗抑郁的效果。

tranquilizer [ˈtræŋkwilaizə] *n.* 镇定剂

Alcoholic women are more likely than alcoholic men to abuse tranquilizers.

酗酒的女性比酗酒的男性更有可能滥用镇定剂。

Sedatives and tranquilizers used to treat insomnia, pain, or anxiety may cause confusion, memory loss, and lethargy.

用于治疗失眠、疼痛或焦虑的安定药和镇静药可引起意识模糊、记忆丧失和昏睡。

transabdominal [ˌtrænsæbˈdɔminəl] *adj.* 经腹的

This led to the development of the transabdominal preperitoneal (TAPP) repair method.

这(项技术)推动了经腹腹膜前修补术(TAPP)的产生。

Transvaginal sonography is significantly more accurate than transabdominal sonography, and its safety is well established.

经阴道式超声的准确度明显高于经腹超声检查,而且其安全性已被确认。

transactivate [træn'sæktiveit] *v.* 反式激活

The subtractive cDNA library of genes transactivated by HBX was constructed.

HBX 反式激活基因表达的 cDNA 消减文库已建立起来了。

transaminase [træns'æmineis] *n.* 转氨酶,氨基转移酶

In medicine, the presence of elevated transaminases, commonly the transaminases alanine transaminase(ALT) and aspartate transaminase(AST), may be an indicator of liver damage.

在医学上,出现转氨酶升高,通常是指丙氨酸转氨酶和天冬氨酸转氨酶,可能是肝损害的指征。

A GABA transaminase inhibitor is an enzyme inhibitor that acts upon GABA transaminase.

γ-氨基丁酸转氨酶抑制剂是作用于 γ-氨基丁酸转氨酶的一种酶抑制剂。

transcribe [træns'kraib] *v.* 抄写,转录

RNA polymerase I transcribes the large ribosomal RNAs.

RNA 聚合酶 I 转录大分子量的核糖体 RNA。

Less than 10% of human DNA is transcribed into mRNA.

不到 10% 的人类 DNA 可被转录成 mRNA。

transcriptase [træns'kripteis] *n.* 转录酶

RNA viruses that carry reverse transcriptase are known as retroviruses.

带有逆(反)转录酶的 RNA 病毒称作逆转录病毒。

transcription [ˌtræns'kripʃən] *n.* 转录

The messenger RNA is produced by transcription.

信使 RNA 是通过转录产生的。

Transcription is the process by which a single-stranded RNA with a base sequence complementary to one strand of a double-stranded DNA is synthesized.

转录是 DNA 双链中的一股按碱基序列互补而合成单链 RNA 的过程。

transcriptional [træns'kripʃənl] *a.* 转录的

Cell differentiation is most probably controlled at the transcriptional level.

细胞分化很可能在转录水平受到控制。

transcriptome [træns'kriptəum] *n.* 转录组

The transcriptome is the set of all RNA molecules, including mRNA, rRNA, tRNA, and other non-coding RNA produced in one or a population of cells.

转录组是指一个细胞或一群细胞中产生的全部 RNA 分子,包括 mRNA、rRNA、tRNA 以及其他非编码 RNA。

The use of next-generation sequencing technology to study the transcriptome at the nucleotide level is known as RNA-Seq.

应用新一代测序技术在核苷酸水平上研究转录组称为 RNA-Seq。

transcriptomics [ˌtrænskrip'tɔmiks] *n.* 转录组学

The study of transcriptomics, also referred to as expression profiling, examines the expression level of mRNAs in a given cell population.

转录组学(也称表达谱)研究,是研究如何检测一个特定细胞群的 mRNA 表达水平。

The new methods for transcriptomics are bringing new challenges in bioinformatics.

这些转录组学的新方法正带给生物信息学以新的挑战。

transcytosis [ˌtrænzsai'təusis] *n.* 胞(吞)转(运作用),转胞吞作用,跨细胞作用

The active transport of molecules across epithelial cells is called transcytosis.

分子穿越上皮细胞的主动转运称为胞转作用。

transdifferentiation [trænsˌdifərenʃi'eiʃən] *n.* 转分化

A change in the differentiation of a cell from one type to another is known as transdifferentiation.

转分化是指细胞分化方向的改变,从一种细胞类型变为另一种细胞类型。

There is little evidence that transdifferentiation of hemopoietic stem cells contributes to tissue renewal in normal homeostasis or tissue repair after injury.

造血干细胞的转分化有助于正常内环境稳定和损伤后组织修复过程中的组织更新，有关这方面的证据很少。

transduction [trænz'dʌkʃən] *n.* 转导，转换，换能

The reaction time included time for transduction in visual system, time for visual processing, etc.

反应时间包括视觉系统的转导时间，视觉的加工时间等。

In biology, signal transduction is any process by which a cell converts one kind of signal or stimulus into another.

在生物学上，信号转换是一个细胞将一种信号或刺激物转换成另一种信号或刺激物的过程。

transect [træn'sekt] *vt.* 横断；横切 *n.* 横断面

Now the doctor is down to the upper chest and he' ll transect the vessels.

现在医生分离到了胸腔上部，他要分离血管了。

Health status, health care utilization and expenses about the inhabitants are studied with the transect investigation in the area.

运用卫生服务横断面调查技术对该地区居民的健康状况、卫生服务利用与费用进行研究。

transfection [træns'fekʃən] *n.* 转染

Transfection is a method of artificial infection of animal or bacterial cells by uptake of DNA or RNA isolated from virus or bacteriophage resulting in the production of mature virus or phage particles.

转染是一种用从病毒或噬菌体分离而得到 的 RNA 或 DNA 进行人工感染动物或细菌细胞来导致成熟的病毒或噬菌体产生的方法。

transfer [træns'fəː] *v.* 转移

The remaining material in the distillation flask was transferred to an Erlenmeyer flask, and 50ml of anhydrous diethyl ether was added.

将蒸馏烧瓶内的残留物质转移到锥形瓶中，同时加入 50ml 无水二乙酯。

n. ['trænsfəː]转移，传输

The ability of the placenta to act as an organ of transfer is the important consideration.

胎盘作为一种运输器官的功能应予以重视。

In most mammalian species, timing of ovum transfer is critical.

在大多数哺乳类动物中，卵移送的时机选择是非常重要的。

transferase ['trænsfəreis] *n.* 转移酶

Methylation is catalyzed by methyl transferases.

甲基化反应由甲基转移酶催化。

Transferases catalyze the transfer of a group(e. g. , an amino, carboxyl, or methyl group) from one molecule to another.

转移酶催化某一基团(如氨基、羧基或甲基)从一个分子转移至另一分子。

transferrin [træns'ferin] *n.* 转铁蛋白

Transferrin is a true plasma transport protein that mediates iron exchange between tissues.

转铁蛋白是一种真正的能调节组织间铁交换的血浆转运蛋白。

The presumed mechansim is either absence of Fe-transport protein transferrin or the presence of a defective transferrin molecule.

据推测，其产生机制为缺乏运输铁的蛋白质转铁蛋白或存在有缺陷的转铁蛋白分子。

transfersome ['trænsfəːsəum] *n.* 传递体

In broadest sense, a transfersome is a highly adaptable and stress-responsive, complex aggregate.

在最广泛的意义上，传递体是一种具有高度适应性和压力反应性的复杂聚合体。

Transfersome technology is best suited for non-invasive delivery of therapeutic molecules across

open biological barriers.
传递体技术最适用于非侵入性传递穿越开放生物屏障的治疗性分子。

transform [træns'fɔːm] *v.* 转变,使变态

Certain bacteria are transforming themselves and developing increasing resistance to antibiotics.
某些细菌自身发生变态,并形成对抗生素越来越强的抗药性。

Purified DNA from S-Ⅱ cells transformed R-Ⅰ cells into S-Ⅱ cells.
从 S-Ⅱ型 细胞中提纯的 DNA 把 R-Ⅰ型细胞转化成 S-Ⅱ型 细胞。

transformation [trænsfə'meiʃən] *n.* 变化,变形,转形,转化

A second group of adrenocortical steroids favors the transformation of amino acids into glycogen in the liver.
第二类肾上腺皮质类固醇有利于在肝脏内把氨基酸转换为糖原。

Psoriasis is characterized by an abnormally rapid transformation of basal cells into horn cells.
银屑病是以基底细胞异常迅速地转变为角细胞为特征的。

transfusable [træns'fjuːzəbl] *a.* 可转输的,可输液的

There is a great need for transfusable blood.
(目前)非常需要可输用的血。

transfuse [træns'fjuːz] *v.* 输血

There is no need for that patient to transfuse whole blood.
那位患者不需要输全血。

Blood transfused from one group to the other would be rejected.
一种血型的人群输血给另一人群会导致排斥。

transfusion [træns'fjuːʒən] *n.* 输(血)

Blood transfusion may be needed during or after operation.
在手术中或手术后可能需要输血。

You had better give the patient a transfusion if situation should ask you to.
如果情况需要输血的话,你最好还是给这病人输一次血。

transgenesis [træns'dʒenisis] *n.* 转基因术

Foreign genes can be placed in the mouse genome by transgenesis.
外源基因可通过转基因术插入到小鼠的基因组中。

transgenic [træns'dʒenik] *a.* 转基因的,基因转移的

Transgenic food is a subject of dispute among the scientists.
转基因食物在科学家中是一个争论的问题。

The transgenic DNA can be expressed in the resulting animals and transmitted in the germ cells.
转基因 DNA 能够在转基因动物上表达并传至生殖细胞。

A transgenic animal can reproduce and pass its cloned gene to its offspring.
转基因动物能复制其克隆基因并传给下一代。

transgenome [ˌtræns'dʒiːnəum] *n.* 转移基因组,转基因组

The site of association of the human transgenome and host murine chromosomes was determined in several subclones of related transformed cell line.
人转移基因组与宿主小鼠染色体的联系位点是通过相关转化细胞系的几种亚克隆确定的。

Study showed only a single host (murine) chromosome was associated with the human transgenome.
研究证实,仅一种宿主(小鼠)染色体与人转移基因组有关。

transient ['trænziənt] *a.* 短暂的,瞬时的

Without such binding most drugs would elicit too transient an effect to be of much value.
若没有这种结合,大多数药物作用时间就太短而无多大价值。

Pleural effusions associated with viral pneumonias are usually transient and of minor significance.

病毒性肺炎所致的胸腔积液常为短暂的，且无临床意义。

In most cases, joint disease is transient and recovery is completed within the acute phase of illness.

往往，关节的疾患是一时性的，可在急性期内完全恢复正常。

transiently [ˈtrænziəntli] *ad.* 短暂地，仅持续片刻地

Catecholamines and aminophylline may transiently worsen the arrhythmias.

儿茶酚胺和氨茶碱可短时加剧心律不齐。

This can make the patient transiently more symptomatic.

这样可使病人症状暂时加重。

transition [trænˈsiʒən] *n.* 过渡（时期）；转变，转换

The early thirties form a transition to the middle adult years.

30 岁之后的几年是中年期前的过渡时期。

Recent years have seen a transition in our concept of AIDS.

近来人们对艾滋病的概念已有所转变。

transitional [trænˈsiʒənəl] *a.* 过渡的，转变的

Tumors of the renal plevis are usually transitional cell carcinomas.

肾盂肿瘤常常是过渡性的细胞癌。

As the growing phase ceases, the follicle goes into the catagen, or transitional phase of activity.

当生长期停止后，毛囊进入退行期，或称活动的过渡期。

transitory [ˈtrænsitəri] *a.* 短暂的，暂时性的

In the earliest stage of essential hypertension the blood pressure elevation is usually transitory.

在原发性高血压的最初阶段，其血压的升高往往是暂时的。

transjugular [trænsˈdʒʌgjulə] *a.* 经颈静脉的

Portosystemic shunting, whether surgical or transjugular intrahepatic, has been a cornerstone of therapy for Budd-Chiari syndrome.

无论是手术的还是经颈静脉肝内的门体分流术，都已成为治疗布-加综合征的里程碑。

Tense and refractory ascites should be treated with large volume paracentesis followed by plasma volume expansion or transjugular intrahepatic portosystemic shunt.

高张力顽固性腹水必须先以高流量腹腔穿刺治疗，然后以血浆扩容或行经颈内静脉肝内门腔静脉分流术。

translation [trænsˈleiʃən] *n.* 翻译；转译

In cell biology, translation denotes the manufacture of proteins in cytoplasm, which takes place at the ribosomes.

在细胞生物学中，转译指在细胞质内核糖体制造蛋白质的过程。

translational [trænzˈleiʃənl] *a.* 翻译的

Many of proteins may undergo chemical modifications at the translational level.

很多蛋白质可能会在翻译水平受到化学修饰。

The control of gene expression can also utilize translational mechanisms.

基因表达的调控也能利用翻译机制。

translocation [ˌtrænsləuˈkeiʃən] *n.* 易位，转移

The reaction mechanism is envisaged as a translocation of protons.

反应的机制可视为质子的易位。

translucent [trænsˈljuːsnt] *a.* 半透明的

Carcinomas may have a rolled edge and a translucent ‘halo’ around them.

癌肿可以有一个滚压的边缘并有一个半透明的“晕圈”环绕。

transluminal [trænsˈljuːminəl] *a.* 腔内的

Percutaneous transluminal coronary angioplasty (PTCA) is a new form of treatment for patients with coronary heart disease.

经皮腔内冠脉成形术是治疗冠心病的一种新方法。

transmembrane [ˌtræns'membrein] *a.* 跨膜的

The seven transmembrane domain family of receptors contain several hundred members.

含有七个跨膜区域的受体家族可包括几百个成员。

transmissible [træns'misəbl] *a.* 可传染的

The transmissible agent, or prion, consists principally of an abnormal isoform of a host-encoded protein.

可传染的生物或称朊病毒,主要由一种异常的宿主编码蛋白质同型体组成。

transmission [træns'miʃən] *n.* 传播,传染;传递

Transmission is through contact with articles belonging to the patient.

传播方式是通过接触属于患者的用品。

These are the realities of HIV transmission today.

这就是今日艾滋病蔓延的现实。

transmit [træns'mit] *v.* 传递,传送

This information is transmitted by transcription into RNA molecules.

此信息通过转录传递给核糖核酸分子。

The gene transmitting tallness is called dominant and that transmitting shortness is recessive.

传递高的基因叫显性的,而传递矮的基因则叫隐性的。

HIV is spread or transmitted from one person to another by bodily fluids such as blood, semen, and vaginal fluid.

HIV 是通过体液如血液、精液和阴道分泌物由一个人传播或传染给另一个人。

The activation signal is transmitted by second messengers.

活化信号系通过"第二信使"传递。

transmitter [træns'mitə] *n.* 传递质,介质

Alpha-methyldopamine and alphamethylnorepinephrine are called false transmitters.

α 甲基多巴胺和 α 甲基去甲肾上腺素被称为伪递质。

transmural [træns'mjuərəl] *a.* 透壁的

The diagnosis of acute transmural myocardial infarction does not ordinarily present any difficulties.

诊断急性透壁性心肌梗死,通常不存在任何困难。

Transmural pressure is the difference between the pressure in the lumen of a vessel and that of the tissue around it.

透壁压是一个血管腔和围绕它周围组织之间的压力差。

transoesophageal [ˌtrænsəiːˌsɔfə'dʒiːəl] *a.* 经食管的

Transoesophageal echocardiography has become a vital method for diagnosing the type and degree of heart valve disease.

经食管心脏超声术已成为诊断心脏瓣膜疾病类型和程度的重要手段。

During surgery, transoesophageal echocardiography can provide real-time assessment of ventricular function, intracardiac shunting, preload and valve function.

在手术期间,经食管心脏超声术可对心室功能、心内分流、心内预负荷和瓣膜功能提供实时的评估。

transparency [træns'pεərənsi] *n.* 透明性,透明度

The normal transparency of the conjunctiva may be clouded in conjunctitis.

患有结膜炎时,其结膜的正常透明度下降,以至呈云雾状混浊。

transparent [træns'pεərənt] *a.* 透明的,透光的

Normal urine is usually a yellow, transparent liquid.

正常的尿是一种黄色的透明液体。

Light rays pass through a series of transparent, colorless eye parts.

光线穿透一系列透明无色的眼的构成部分。

transplacental [ˌtrænsplə'sentəl] *a.* 经胎盘的

Transplacental infection, resulting in fetal death and abortion, has been reported.

曾有报道经胎盘传染可导致胎儿死亡和流产。

transplant [træns'plɑːnt] *v.* 移植

American scientists have successfully transplanted brain tissue in laboratory animals.

美国科学家已成功地给实验动物做了脑组织移植手术。

Surgeons, nephrologists, and immunologists can totally rehabilitate most transplanted patients.

外科医生、肾病学家和免疫学家能使大多数做了移植手术的病人得以完全恢复。

n. 移植;移植物

It is rarely possible to perform a transplant between a genetically identical pair.

在遗传学一致的一对供受体之间进行器官移植是不大可能的。

The rats with cortex transplants took only three days to finish the task.

做过脑皮层移植手术的大鼠只需 3 天就完成了这一任务。

transplantation [ˌtrænsplɑːn'teiʃən] *n.* 移植(术)

Transplantation of organs and tissues obeys essentially the same principles as transfusion of blood.

器官和组织的移植也必须遵守与输血相同的原理。

Renal transplantation can truly restore the patients to a normal life style.

肾移植能使这些病人真正恢复正常生活方式。

In this case, blood transfusion prior to transplantation is favorable.

在这种情况下,器官移植前输血是有利的。

transplanter [træns'plɑːntə] *n.* 移植者,移植机

Transplanters take the heart or the kidney of one person and give it to another.

器官移植者将一个人的心脏或肾脏取出然后植入另一个人体内。

transport [træns'pɔːt] *v.* 运输,输送

New molecules can be synthesized and transported to the cell surface.

新的分子可被合成并输送到细胞表面。

Neurosecretions from cells of the hypothalamus may be transported to the anterior lobe cells along this route.

下丘脑细胞的神经分泌可以沿着这一途径被输送到前叶细胞。

One of the functions of fat in the body is to transport the fat soluble vitamins, which are A, D, E and K.

脂肪在体内的功能之一是运输脂溶性维生素 A、D、E 及 K。

transportation [ˌtrænspɔː'teiʃən] *n.* 运输,输送

Ambulance is a vehicle of transportation for conveying the sick or injured person.

救护车是转运患病或受伤者的运输工具(车辆)。

Most of the cells have no contact with the external environment and are entirely dependent upon the transportation function of the circulatory system for supplies of oxygen and nutrients.

机体大部分细胞和外部环境都没有直接接触,并且完全依靠循环系统的运输功能来供给它们氧和营养物。

transporter [træns'pɔːtə] *n.* 转运体

For many proteins, including enzymes, transporters, and receptors, the mechanisms by which amino acid substitutions alter function have been characterized in kinetic studies.

对许多蛋白质(包括酶、转运体和受体)而言,氨基酸置换导致功能改变的机制已经在动力学研究中得到鉴定。

transposition [ˌtrænspə'ziʃən] *n.* 错位,反位

If the stomach is on the right side of the body, the condition is gastric transposition.

如果胃的位置在身体的右侧,这种异常状态称为胃错位。

Transposition of the great vessels, ventricular septal defect, and coarctation of the aorta were the most common cardiac malformations.

大血管错位、室间隔缺损和主动脉缩窄都是最常见的心血管畸形。

transposon [ˌtræns'pəuzɔn] *n.* 转座子

Transposon is a specific DNA sequence which can move from one position in the genome of an organism to another.

转座子是一般能从机体基因组上的一个位点转移到另一个位点的特异性的 DNA 序列。

transtentorial [ˌtrænsten'tɔriːəl] *n.* 小脑幕裂孔;经小脑幕的

Researchers found that diffusion tensor tractography is useful in evaluating the presence and the severity of corticospinal tract injury in patients with transtentorial herniation following traumatic brain injury.

研究者发现弥散张量纤维束成像可用于评估创伤性脑损伤后的小脑幕疝病人是否有皮质脊髓束损伤及其损伤的程度。

transudate ['trænsjudeit] *n.* 漏出液

The ascitic fluid in liver cirrhosis is almost a light straw colored transudate.

肝硬化时腹水几乎是淡黄色的漏出液。

Middle ear secretions can be serous transudate, but also can be a serous exudate and mucus.

中耳分泌物可以是浆液性漏出液,也可为浆液性渗出液和黏液。

transudation [trænsju'deiʃən] *n.* 漏出,渗出

Crepitant rales are produced by intra-alveolar transudation of fluid.

捻发音是由于液体漏入肺泡内而产生的。

Most of immunoglobulins in respiratory tract are synthesized locally by the plasma cells in the submucosa of the respiratory tract; only a small portion is derived from serum by transudation.

呼吸道中大部分免疫球蛋白是由呼吸道黏膜下层内的浆细胞在该处合成,只有小部分是来自渗出的血清。

transverse ['trænzvəːs] *a.* 横向的

The stomach is superior to the transverse colon.

胃位于横结肠的上方。

transversly ['trænzvəːsli] *ad.* 横向地

In the parous woman the external os is irregular or transversly lacerated.

经产妇宫颈外口呈不规则或横形裂痕。

transversion [træns'vəːʃən] *n.* (碱基的)颠换

In contrast, the replacement of a purine for a pyrimidine (or vice verse) is called transversion.

相反,一个嘌呤被一个嘧啶所取代(或者相反),称为颠换。

Among the nucleotides substitution of cytochrome b, transition is obviously higher than transversion.

在细胞色素 b 基因的核苷酸替换中,转换明显高于颠换。

tranylcypromine [ˌtrænil'saiprəmiːn] *n.* 反苯环丙胺

Tranylcypromine increases the concentrations of monoamines in the body.

反苯环丙胺可增加体内单胺类(化合物)的浓度。

trastuzumab [træ'stʌzjumæb] *n.* 曲妥单抗

Pretreatment testing to select patients for response to treatment has become standard practice for hormonal therapy of breast cancer and for treatment with antibodies such as trastuzumab.

对于乳腺癌的激素治疗和使用诸如曲妥单抗之类的抗体治疗,预治疗测试以选择对治疗有反应的病人已成常规作法。

trauma ['trɔːmə] *n.* 外伤,创伤

Dementia may be caused by brain trauma.

痴呆可由脑部损伤引起。

Severe trauma to a joint results in torn ligaments, a common injury in contact sports such as football.

关节严重外伤可使韧带撕裂,这是对抗性运动中(如足球运动)常见的外伤。

traumatic [trɔː'mætik] *a.* 创伤的,外伤的

Any shock produced by trauma is traumatic shock.

由创伤引起的任何休克称作创伤性休克。

Traumatic rupture of the uterus may occur during overvigorous attempts at external version or abortion.

损伤性子宫破裂可发生于粗暴的外倒转术或人工流产。

traumatize ['trɔːmətaiz] *v.* 使受外伤;使受精神创伤

Typically, traumatized children will try to suppress thoughts about what happened.

典型的是,精神受创伤的儿童通常会试图抑制回想有关他所遭遇的事件。

traverse ['trævəs] *v.* 横越,经过

In order to reach its site of action, a drug may have to traverse a succession of membrances.

药物要达到作用部位必须通过一连串生物膜。

The blood traverses two separate circuits, the pulmonary and the systemic.

血液运行于两个互不沟通的环路内:即肺循环和体循环。

tray [trei] *n.* 托盘

The nurse distributes the medicines on the tray to the patients.

护士用托盘将药品分发给病人。

treadmill ['tredmil] *n.* 活动平板

Treadmill testing is also not particularly helpful since most episodes are not provoked by exercise.

活动平板试验亦无特殊价值,因为大多数发作不是由运动诱发。

treasurehouse ['treʒəhaus] *n.* 宝库

Chinese medicine and pharmacology are a great treasurehouse.

中国医药学是一个伟大的宝库。

treatable [triːtəbl] *a.* 能处理的,能治疗的

Many of them are not only treatable but completely reversible.

他们当中的许多人不仅是可以治疗的,而且是完全可以恢复的。

Clinical depression is treatable.

临床抑郁症是可以治疗的。

treatise ['triːtiz] *n.* 论文,专题

This is a treatise on oncogenesis.

这是一篇关于肿瘤发生的论文。

treatment ['triːtmənt] *n.* 处理,治疗

The two treatment methods are sometimes used jointly.

这两种治疗方法有时可合并使用。

Treatment options are still broad.

治疗方案还有很大选择余地。

Modern burn treatment has been eminently successful in saving the lives of many people.

现代烧伤治疗,在挽救许多人的生命中取得了突出的成就。

tremor ['tremə] *n.* 震颤,发抖

Tremor refers to rhythmic oscillations produced by involuntary contractions of reciprocally innervated antagonistic muscles.

震颤是指交互神经支配的拮抗肌不自主收缩引起的节律性震动 。

Only a few weeks earlier, 17 monkeys they were studying had tremors, muscle rigidity and other

symptoms of Parkinson's disease.
就在几周前,他们研究的 17 只猴子就表现出震颤、肌肉僵直和帕金森病的其它症状。

tremorous [ˈtremərəs] *a.* 震颤的
The muscle stretch reflex is especially important to make the body movements smooth in character, rather than jerky and tremorous.
肌牵张反射在保持身体活动状况平稳而不呈痉挛或震颤式方面特别重要。

trend [trend] *n.* 倾向
The trend of the evidence has been consistent and indicates that there is a serious health risk.
这种结果的倾向是一致的,表明在健康上存在着严重的危险。

triad [ˈtraiəd] *n.* 三个一组,三联体
Clinically, a triad of memory loss, gait disturbance, and bladder incontinence is typical.
在临床上,记忆丧失、步态紊乱和尿失禁的三联征是很典型的。
Changes in the incisor teeth, opacities of the cornea, and eighth nerve deafness are known as the Hutchinson triad.
上门齿的改变、角膜的混浊和第八对脑神经的神经性耳聋共称为哈钦森氏三联征。

triage [triˈɑːʒ] *n.* 筛查; 伤员检伤分类
In accordance with the simple triage and rapid treatment system, the walking wounded would be identified first.
根据简单筛查和快速治疗原则,应首先分流出可自由活动的伤者。
With triage, critical patients were served first, however, non-emergent patients may wait.
筛查分类让急重症患者获得优先处理,而不危急的患者就有可能等候。

trial [ˈtraiəl] *n.* 试用,试验;考验
The clinical trial was quite a success.
临床试验非常成功。
These new drugs are just undergoing clinical trials.
这些新药目前正在进行临床试用。
Crossover trial is a clinical trial in which each patient is exposed first to one treatment and then to the other, but in random order.
交换试用是一种临床试验,即每一病人首先用一种治疗,以后用另一种,先后次序是随机的。

triamcinolone [ˌtraiæmˈsinələun] *n.* 去炎松;曲安奈德
Patients with small lesions may be injected with triamcinolone or methylprednisolone.
病人损伤很小时,可以注射曲安奈德或甲泼尼龙。
In particular, literature pertaining to glaucoma in response to intravitreal triamcinolone acetonide will be reviewed.
特别是有关玻璃体腔内注射曲安奈德而引起青光眼的文献将被重点回顾。

triangle [ˈtraiæŋgl] *n.* 三角形
Vesical triangle is a smooth triangular portion of the mucous membrane at the base of the bladder.
膀胱三角是膀胱底部黏膜的平滑三角部分。

triangular [traiˈæŋgjulə] *a.* 三角(形)的
The liver is triangular in shape.
肝的形状呈三角形。

tribute [ˈtribjuːt] *n.* 称赞,颂词;贡物
The capacity for sound clinical judgement is the ultimate tribute to a qualified physician.
做出准确临床诊断的能力是对一个合格医生的最高称赞。

trichilemmal [ˌtrikiˈleməl] *a.* 毛根鞘的,毛囊的
This paper discusses the diagnosis and treatment of 25 cases of trichilemmal cyst in the leg.

本文探讨了 25 例小腿毛根鞘囊肿的诊断与治疗。

TLC is a rare adnexal tumor related to the external hair sheath and distinct from proliferative trichilemmal tumor.

毛囊癌是一种罕见皮肤附属器官肿瘤，与毛发外鞘相关而不同于增殖性毛囊瘤。

trichinella [ˌtrikiˈnelə] *n.* 旋毛虫

Trichinella spiralis is one of the most widespread parasites which can infect human being and more than 150 species of other mammals.

旋毛虫是分布最广泛的寄生虫之一，可感染人及 150 多种哺乳动物。

Trichinella showed a certain inhibiting effect on the growth of HCT-8 cells in BALB/c mice.

旋毛虫对 BALB/c 小鼠体内的人结肠癌 HCT-8 细胞的生长有一定的抑制作用。

trichomonas [ˌtrikəˈmɔnəs] *n.* 毛滴虫属

Trichomonas vaginalis can inhabit the urogenital system of both males and females.

阴道毛滴虫能寄生于男性和女性的泌尿生殖系统内。

It is important to also consider other causes such as Trichomonas vaginalis, Mycoplasma, Chlamydia, Candida albicans, and also mixed infections.

重要的是考虑其他原因，如滴虫性阴道炎、支原体、衣原体、白色念珠菌感染，当然还有混合感染。

trichomoniasis [ˌtrikəməˈnaiəsis] *n.* 滴虫病

Candidiasis and trichomoniasis are uncommon in children, but infection may be carried from an adult if the family standard of hygiene is poor.

念珠菌病和滴虫病在儿童中不常见，如家庭卫生水平差可从成人获得传染。

Trichophyton [triˈkɔfitɔn] *n.* 毛癣菌属

The object is to observe the effects of dexamethasone on the phenotype of Trichophyton rubrum.

目的是观察地塞米松对红色毛癣菌表型的影响。

The object is to investigate the anti-Trichophyton mentagrophytes activity of three different fibers-hemp, flax and ramie fibers.

目的是研究韧皮纤维、亚麻和苎麻纤维这三种不同纤维的抗须毛癣菌活性。

tricuspid [treiˈkʌspid] *a.* 三尖的，三尖瓣的

The right atrium and ventricle for the time being may be thought of as a single chamber with the tricuspid valve open.

三尖瓣开着时，右房室暂时被看作是一个单独的腔。

The latter finding is indicative of functional tricuspid regurgitation.

后者提示功能性三尖瓣关闭不全。

tricyclic [traiˈsiklik] *a.* 三环类的

Tricyclic antidepressant overdose has many cardiac manifestations.

三环类抗抑郁药应用过量会有许多心脏方面的反应。

Tricyclic antidepressants have an 80%-90% effectiveness in treatment and prevention of spontaneous attacks.

三环类抗抑郁药对于治疗和预防发作有 80% ~90% 的疗效。

triethanolamine [traiˌeθəˈnɔləmiːn] *n.* 三乙醇胺

The main barrier for triethanolamine salicylate permeability was the epidermis layer of the skin.

三乙醇胺水杨酸盐渗透的主要障碍是皮肤的表皮层。

The release of triethanolamine salicylate from commonly used ointment bases and commercial ointment preparations was studied in vitro.

体外实验研究了普通药膏基质和商用软膏制剂中三乙醇胺水杨酸盐的释放。

trigeminal [traiˈdʒeminəl] *a.* 三叉神经的，三联的

Trigeminal neuralgia is always on the same side and is usually in the second or third division of the trigeminal nerve.

三叉神经痛常发生在相同部位，且多发于三叉神经的第二或第三分支。

trigger [ˈtrigə] *v.* 触发，引起

There may or may not be environmental events that trigger such behavior.

可能有，也可能没有环境事件触发这种行为。

This whole process is triggered by a substance that attracts the cells together.

这整个过程由一种能把细胞吸引到一起的物质所激发。

Artificial organs will trigger transplant boom.

人造器官将使器官移植兴盛起来。

triglyceride [traiˈglisəˌraid] *n.* 甘油三酯

Many eucaryotic cells possess lipid reserves in the form of triglycerides.

许多真核生物细胞以甘油三酯的形式贮存脂质。

trihalomethane [traiˌhæləuˈmeθein] *n.* 三卤甲烷

Trihalomethanes are chemical compounds in which three of the four hydrogen atoms of methane (CH4) are replaced by halogen atoms.

三卤甲烷是甲烷 4 个氢原子中的 3 个被卤素原子所取代而成的化合物。

Trihalomethanes are formed as a by-product predominantly when chlorine is used to disinfect water for drinking.

三卤甲烷是饮用水加氯消毒时形成的一种主要副产物。

triiodothyronine [traiˌaiədəuˈθairəniːn] *n.* 三碘甲状腺原氨酸

A positive correlation was found among the triiodothyronine, thyroxin and the gastrin from the study.

研究发现三碘甲状腺原氨酸、甲状腺素与胃泌素之间呈正相关。

Triiodothyronine is a thyroid hormone that plays vital roles in the body's metabolic rate, heart and digestive functions, muscle control, brain development and the maintenance of bones.

三碘甲状腺原氨酸是一种甲状腺激素，在身体的代谢率、心脏和消化功能、肌肉控制、脑发育和骨的维持上起重要作用。

trimester [traiˈmestə] *n.* 三个月，三月期

In the first trimester the embryo begins the delicate structural differentiations that will lead to its final form.

在头三个月里，胚胎开始出现可以最终导致胚胎成形的细微的结构演变。

Ultrasound is a useful method for dating a pregnancy in both the first and second trimesters.

在早、中期妊娠中，超声波估计受孕日期是一项有效的方法。

Gestational age at the time of infection may be a factor, however, fetal involvement has been documented in all three trimesters.

感染时胎龄可能是一个因素，但已证明胎儿在妊娠三期均可累及。

trimethoprim [traiˈmeθəprim] *n.* 三甲氧苄氨嘧啶(磺胺增效剂，抗菌增效剂)

Trimethoprim is also used for the treatment of respiratory tract infections.

三甲氧苄氨嘧啶也用于治疗呼吸道感染。

The initial treatment regimen usually consists of IV administration of trimethoprim and sulfamethoxazole for a total of 14-21 days.

开始的治疗方案通常是静脉内给予甲氧苄啶和磺胺甲基异噁唑 14～21 天。

trioxide [triˈɔksaid] *n.* 三氧化物

Acute inhalation of arsenic trioxide may result in rhinitis, pharyngitis and bronchitis.

急性吸入三氧化二砷可能引起鼻炎、咽炎和支气管炎。

tripeptide [traiˈpeptaid] *n.* 三肽

An important tripeptide is glutathione, γ-glutamyl-cysteinyl-glycine.

谷胱甘肽(γ 谷氨酰半胱氨酰甘氨酸)是一种重要的三肽。

triphalangia [triˈfæləndʒiə] *n.* 三指(趾)节畸形

Triphalangia is defined as malformation in which three phalanges are present in the thumb or great toe.
三指(趾)节畸形通常被定义为拇指或跗趾中有三个趾骨畸形。
Classical triphalangia of the lateral toes was observed in 1,440 cases.
在 1440 个病例中发现其脚趾有典型的三趾节畸形。

triphosphate [trai'fɔsfeit] *n.* 三磷酸盐
The ligand-receptor complex causes the regulatory protein to bind with guanosine triphosphate.
配体受体复合物促使调节蛋白与鸟苷三磷酸结合。

triple ['tripl] *a.* 三(倍)的,三层的,三联的
Molecular oxygen(O_2)in the triple ground state is a free radical.
分子氧(O_2)处于三基态时是一个自由基。
Immunosuppressive therapy regimens vary but usually include triple therapy with cyclosporine, azathioprine, and prednisone.
免疫抑制疗法方案各不相同,但通常包括环孢霉素、硫唑嘌呤和强的松的三联疗法。
v. (增至)三倍
In this country, the direct cost for burn care exceeds $100000000 annually, and indirect costs triple that figure.
这个国家每年烧伤造成的直接损失超过 1 亿美元,间接损失则是其三倍。

triplet ['triplit] *n.* 三胞胎中的一个;[复]三胞胎;三联体,三核苷酸
Triplets usually occur once in several thousand births.
三胞胎通常几千例中才有一次。
Last night in the 3rd ward, a woman gave birth to triplets.
昨晚第三病室有位妇女一胎生了三个孩子。
The severity and age of onset of myotonic dystrophy is highly correlated with the number of triplet repeats.
强直性肌营养不良的发病年龄、病情严重程度与三核苷酸拷贝数有关。
Expansion of triplet repeats has also been described in the fragile X syndrome.
三核苷酸拷贝数扩展已在脆性 X 综合征中有过描述。

triploid ['triplɔid] *n.* 三倍体;*a.* 三倍体的,三倍性的
A cell or organism containing three times the haploid number of chromosomes is called triploid.
具有三个单倍染色体组的细胞或生物体称为三倍体。
Triploid infants can be liveborn, but they do not survive long.
三倍体婴儿可以活产,但存活时间不会太长。

trisomy ['traisəmi] *n.* 三体性
Down syndrome is also called trisomy 21.
Down 综合征也称为 21 三体综合征。
Trisomy 18 occurs in about 1 in 5000 births.
18 三体综合征在新生儿中的发生率约为 1/5000。

trivalent [trai'veilənt] *a.* 三价的
The most common inorganic trivalent arsenic compounds are arsenic trioxide and sodium arsenite.
最常见的无机三价砷化合物有三氧化二砷和亚砷酸钠。

trivial ['triviəl] *a.* 轻微的,不重要的
This matter is too trivial to worry about.
此事无关紧要,不必操心。
A fear of cancer may be expressed as concerns over a trivial vaginal discharge.
恐癌(者)对阴道平常的分泌物可能表示过分关注。

trophoblast ['trɔfəblæst] *n.* 滋养层

Hydatidiform mole, a developmental anomaly of trophoblast, consists of grapelike vesicles without an embryo.
葡萄胎,一种滋养层发育异常,由没有胚胎的葡萄样小水泡组成。

trophoblastic [ˌtrɔfəuˈblæstik, ˌtrəu-] *a.* 滋养层的

The reported incidence of gestational trophoblastic disease from Europe and North America is significantly lower than the reported incidence of GTD from Asia and South America.
欧洲和北美报道的妊娠滋养细胞疾病发病率要比亚洲和南美报道的低得多。

Gestational trophoblastic tumors do not develop from cells of the uterus as cervical cancer or endometrial cancer does, but start in the cells that would normally develop into the placenta during pregnancy.
妊娠滋养细胞肿瘤并不像宫颈癌或子宫内膜癌那样源于子宫,而是起源于妊娠的胎盘。

trophozoite [ˌtrɔfəuˈzəuait] *n.* 滋养体(原虫)

Amebic colitis is characterized by flaskshaped ulcers that contain pus and amebic trophozoites.
阿米巴结肠炎的特征是烧瓶样溃疡,内含脓和阿米巴滋养体。

Trophozoites then disseminate via the bloodstream or lymphatics to infect any nucleated host cell.
然后滋养体通过血流或淋巴管感染宿主的有核细胞。

tropical [ˈtrɔpikəl] *a.* 热带的

Malaria is found throughout the tropical regions of the world.
疟疾出现于热带地区。

It is said that fever is a common presentation in people who have recently arrived in Britain from tropical areas.
据说刚从热带地区到达英国的人们常有发热的症状。

tropicssprangletop [ˌtrɔpikˈspræŋlətɔp] *n.* 热带千金子

Tropicssprangletop is attached to Leptochloa Beauv.
热带千金子归于千金子属。

Tropicssprangletop is the traditional herbs of China, and it can inhibit tumors.
热带千金子是我国的传统中药,可用于抗肿瘤。

troublesome [ˈtrʌblsəm] *a.* 令人烦恼的,讨厌的,困难的

Infection and osteoporosis are particularly troublesome in patients with rheumatoid arthritis.
令类风湿关节炎病人特别烦恼的是发生感染和骨质疏松。

truncal [ˈtrʌŋkəl] *adj.* 躯干的

The results showed a significant anabolic response, with an increase in fat-free mass and a decrease in fat, mainly truncal fat.
结果显示出显著的合成代谢反应,去脂体重明显增加,而脂肪(主要为躯干脂肪)明显减少。

Truncal sarcomas (including both chest and abdominal wall) account for about 10% of sarcomas.
躯干肉瘤(包括胸部和腹壁)约占肉瘤的 10%。

trunk [trʌŋk] *n.* 躯干

The neck contains vessels, nerves, and other structures connecting the head and the trunk.
颈部有脉管和神经以及连接头和躯干的其他结构。

Urticarial patches and erythema may appear, especially on the upper extremities and trunk.
可出现荨麻疹性斑片和红斑,特别是在上肢和躯干。

trust [trʌst] *n.* 信赖,信任

I have absolute trust in the skill of famous doctors.
我完全信赖名医的医术。

trypanosome [ˈtripənəsəum] *n.* 锥虫

African sleeping sickness is caused by trypanosomes conveyed to humans.

非洲嗜睡病是由锥虫传播给人引起的。

Trypanosomes undergo part of their development in the blood of a vertebrate host. The remaining stages occur in invertebrate hosts.

锥虫在脊椎动物宿主的血中进行部分生长,其余各期是在无脊椎动物宿主体内生长。

trypanosomiasis [ˌtripənəusəu'maiəsis] *n.* 锥虫病

East African trypanosomiasis follows a more acute course than West African trypanosomiasis.

东非锥虫病的病程进展比西非锥虫病快。

Several diseases are caused by protozoa, including malaria, amebiasis and trypanosomiasis.

原虫感染可引起多种疾病,包括疟疾、阿米巴病和锥虫病。

trypsin ['tripsin] *n.* 胰蛋白酶

Trypsin digests of a protein are often used as an analytical tool for protein identification.

蛋白质的胰蛋白酶酶解产物是蛋白质鉴定常用的分析工具。

trypsinogen [trip'sinədʒən] *n.* 胰蛋白酶原

Intra-acinar trypsinogen activation leads to acinar death during early stages of pancreatitis.

在早期阶段的胰腺炎,腺泡内胰蛋白酶原的激活可导致腺泡死亡。

Trypsinogen is a substance that is normally produced in the pancreas and released into the small intestine.

胰蛋白酶原是通常产生于胰腺并释放至小肠的一种物质。

tryptic ['triptik] *a.* 胰蛋白酶的

The amino acid composition and N-termini of each peptide derived from tryptic hydrolysis were determined.

测定了通过胰蛋白酶水解得出的每个肽段的氨基酸组成与 N-末端。

The results show that the pepsin is a suitable catalyst for the plastein reaction of using tryptic hydrolyzate of soy protein and of sesame protein.

结果表明胃蛋白酶对使用大豆蛋白和芝麻蛋白的胰蛋白酶水解产物进行合成类蛋白反应是一种适宜的催化剂。

tryptophan ['triptəfæn] *n.* 色氨酸

Milk contains tryptophan.

牛奶中含有色氨酸。

The essential amino acids are leucine, isoleucine, lysine, methionine, phenylalanine, threonine, tryptophan, and valine.

必需氨基酸包括亮氨酸、异亮氨酸、赖氨酸、蛋氨酸、苯丙氨酸、苏氨酸、色氨酸和缬氨酸。

tubercle ['tjuːbəkl] *n.* 结节;结核

Some organisms, e. g. the tubercle bacillus are particularly prone to produce chronic inflammation.

有些微生物,例如结核杆菌,尤其易于引起慢性炎症。

Montgomery tubercles look like bumps around the areolas that become larger when a woman is pregnant.

蒙氏结节看起来就像围绕乳晕的肿块,当女性妊娠时这些结节变得更大。

tuberculin [tjuː'bəːkjulin] *n.* 结核菌素

The only way the infection is detected is by a positive tuberculin skin test.

阳性结核菌素皮肤试验是查出感染的唯一途径。

tuberculoma [tjuːˌbəːkju'ləumə] *n.* 结核瘤

Tuberculoma is an isolated spherical focus of caseous necrosis, sharply defined by fibrous encapsulation.

结核瘤是孤立的球形干酪样坏死灶,具有纤维包裹,境界清楚。

Tuberculoma is usually single, located in the apices of the lung about 2-5cm in diameter.

结核瘤通常单发,位于肺的顶部,直径 2 ~ 5cm。

tuberculosis [tjuːˌbəːkjuˈləusis] *n.* 结核(病)

In the majority of cases, the initial lesion in primary tuberculosis is in the lung parenchyma.

原发性肺结核大部分病例的原发病损在肺实质。

The differentiation of lung abscess from pulmonary tuberculosis is less difficult.

鉴别肺脓肿和肺结核不太困难。

tuberculous [tjuˈbəːkjuləs] *a.* 结核性的

Tuberculous pericarditis is very rare and nonsuppurative.

结核性心包炎极罕见,并且是非化脓性的。

The presence of signs of severe tuberculous toxemia is a certain indication that the disease is active and progressive.

严重结核毒血症体征的出现是说明这病正在活动和进展的肯定指标。

tubular [ˈtjuːbjulə] *a.* 小管的,管状的

Arteries are long, tubular blood vessels which can bend and stretch.

动脉是长管形血管,能弯曲,能伸展。

The child's chest roentgenogram suggests possible tubular bronchiectasis.

患儿胸部 X 线片提示可能为管状支气管扩张。

tubule [ˈtjuːbjuːl] *n.* 小管,细管

From the nephron, the fluid moves to collecting tubules and into the ureter leading to the urinary bladder.

液体从肾单位流到集合管,并进入通向膀胱的输尿管。

A toxicant can also be excreted through the tubules into the urine by passive diffusion.

毒物也可以通过被动扩散经肾小管排泄到尿液中。

tubulin [ˈtjuːbjulin] *n.* 微管蛋白

Chemicals that bind to tubulin or actin impair the assembly and/or disassembly of these cytoskeletal proteins.

结合到微管蛋白或肌动蛋白上的化学物质能损伤这些细胞骨架蛋白的装配和(或)分解。

tubulovillous [ˌtjuːbjuləuˈviləs] *a.* 管状绒毛状的

This vulvar tubulovillous adenoma was identical to a tumor resected 6 months before from this patient's rectal wall.

该患者外阴的管状绒毛状腺瘤与 6 月前直肠壁切除的肿瘤完全一致。

This vesical tubulovillous adenoma occurred in a background of protracted chronic cystitis with intestinal-type glandular metaplasia.

这种膀胱管状绒毛状腺瘤发生于迁延性慢性膀胱炎伴肠型腺上皮化生的基础上。

tularemia [ˌtjuləˈriːmiə] *n.* 土拉菌病,兔热病

The diagnosis of tularemia is usually based on serologic tests rather than culture.

土拉菌病的诊断通常是根据血清学试验而不是培养实验。

Tularemia presents with several different clinical syndromes after a 2 to 5-days incubation period.

经 2 ~ 5 天的潜伏期后,兔热病可表现出各种不同的临床症状。

tumorigenesis [ˌtjuːməriˈdʒenisis] *n.* 肿瘤发生

The interaction of multiple genes plays an important role in tumorigenesis.

多基因的相互作用在肿瘤发生中起重要作用。

The activation of protein kinase C (PKC) is closely correlated with the tumorigenesis, development and metastasis.

蛋白激酶 C 的活化与肿瘤发生、发展和转移密切相关。

tumour [ˈtjuːmə] *n.* 肿瘤(=tumor)

Macrophages may also be responsible for killing tumour cells.

巨噬细胞可能也有杀伤肿瘤细胞的作用。

Tumor suppressor genes participate in growth control.

肿瘤抑制基因参与生长调控。

tunic [ˈtjuːnik] *n.* 膜,被膜

The eyeball has three separate coats or tunics.

眼球有三层相互分开的被膜。

The second tunic of the eyeball is known as the choroid coat.

眼球的第二层膜叫脉络膜。

turbid [ˈtəːbid] *a.* 混浊的

If the cerebrospinal fluid is turbid, it is then appropriate to administer antibiotics.

如果脑脊液混浊,则宜用抗生素治疗。

turbidity [təːˈbiditi] *n.* 混浊,浊度

Cloudy urine is not necessarily pathological as turbidity may be caused by mucin secreted by the lining membrane of the urinary tract.

混浊的尿不一定是病理现象,因为混浊可能是混有尿道内的黏膜分泌的黏蛋白所致。

turnover [ˈtəːnəuvə] *n.* 周转率,翻转,反转,逆转

The surgical department of this hospital has a rapid turnover of patients.

此医院外科部门的病人周转率很高。

Cathepsins have a vital role in mammalian cellular turnover.

组织蛋白酶在哺乳动物的细胞更新中起重要作用。

tutor [ˈtjuːtə] *n.* 导师

Her tutor says that she has accomplished her dissertation.

她的导师说她已完成了她的学位论文。

Tween [twiːn] *n.* 吐温

Tween 20 and Tween 80 are types of polysorbate detergents.

吐温 20 和吐温 80 是聚山梨酯洗涤剂的两种类型。

Tween 20 is commonly used as non-ionic detergent.

吐温 20 是常用的非离子型去垢剂。

twin [twin] *n.* 双生,双胎

Twin studies can help researchers determine the influence of environment on gene expression.

双生子研究有助于研究者确定环境对基因表达的影响。

Twins are born about once in every 90 human births.

双生的发生率约为 1/90。

twirl [twəːl] *v.* 快速转动,捻弄

The needle may be either retained or withdrawn after twirling for a few seconds.

捻针几秒以后或留针或退出。

twist [twist] *v.* 扭转;扭弯;扭伤;盘绕

In spiral fractures the bone has twisted apart.

在螺旋形的骨折中,骨头裂开但相互扭绞着。

Until the diastasis has closed, the woman should avoid exercises that rotate the trunk, twist the hips, or bend the trunk to one side.

直到(腹直肌)分离闭合后,产妇才应进行转动躯干、扭转臂部或向一侧弯躯的锻炼。

twofold [ˈtuːfəuld] *a.* 两倍的,二重的

There is twofold increase in hormone production.

激素的产生成倍增加。

This cell has a twofold function in reproduction.

这种细胞在生殖方面具有双重功能。

tympanic [timˈpænik] *a.* 鼓(面)的;鼓室的

HEENT examination revealed that both tympanic membranes were slightly dull, but had good movement.

头眼耳鼻喉检查显示两侧鼓膜色泽轻度发暗，但活动尚好。

tympany [ˈtimpəni] *n.* 鼓音

Tympany is heard if the chest contains free air or the abdomen is distended with gas.

如果胸部含游离的空气或腹部由于气体而膨胀，叩诊便可听到鼓音。

The classic physical examination findings of abdominal distension, tympany to percussion, and high-pitched bowel sounds suggest the diagnosis of intestinal obstruction.

标准的体检发现腹胀、叩诊鼓音和高亢的肠鸣音就提示肠梗阻的诊断。

typhoid [ˈtaifɔid] *n.* 伤寒

Several decades ago the killed bacilli of typhoid and other diseases were used for prophylactic active immunization.

几十年前，灭活的伤寒和其他疾病的杆菌被用于进行自动免疫预防疾病。

a. 伤寒的

Typhoid fever is the classical example of enteric fever caused by salmonellae.

伤寒是由沙门氏菌属引起的肠热症的典型实例。

typhus [ˈtaifəs] *n.* 斑疹伤寒

Endemic typhus has been reported in laboratory workers.

地方性流行性斑疹伤寒病已有实验员报道。

The most widespread disease caused by rickettsiae is typhus.

立克次体引起的疾病中流行最广的是斑疹伤寒。

typical [ˈtipikəl] *a.* 典型的，代表性的

The IgG molecule may be thought of as a typical antibody.

IgG 分子被认为是典型的抗体。

Typical bacillary diseases include tetanus, diphtheria, tuberculosis and typhoid fever.

杆菌引起的典型疾病包括破伤风、白喉、结核和伤寒。

typically [ˈtipikəli] *ad.* 典型地，有代表性地

Anorexia nervosa typically occurs during adolescence.

神经性厌食通常发生于青春期。

Death from fat embolism in such circumstances typically occurs 2 to 5 days after the original injury.

在这种情况下，由于脂肪栓塞引起的死亡一般均发生在原始损伤后 2 ~ 5 天。

typing [ˈtaipiŋ] *n.* 分型，定型

Typing of the HLA of both transplant donor and recipient can be done by antibodies or 'typing' cells.

可用抗体或分型细胞对移植供受双方的 HLA 进行分型。

typify [ˈtipifai] *v.* 作为…的典型，具有…的特征

Hypochondriasis is typified by unrealistic interpretations of physical sensations and unrealistic fears.

疑病的典型特征是对身体感觉的非现实的理解和非现实的恐惧。

tyramine [ˈtaiərəmiːn] *n.* 酪胺

Iproniazid inhibits monoamine oxidase and increases the cardiovascular effects of tyramine.

异丙烟肼抑制单胺氧化酶，能增强酪胺的心血管效应。

Tyramine, naturally occurring in cheese, has a similar effect in the body to that of adrenaline.

酪胺天然存在于奶酪中，在体内与肾上腺素有相似作用。

tyrosinase [taiəˈrəusineis] *n.* 酪氨酸酶

Thirty-three drug extracts were screened for their tyrosinase inhibitory activity.

33 种药物提取物被用来检测其酪氨酸酶的抑制活力。

tyrosine [ˈtaiərəsiːn] *n.* 酪氨酸

Catecholamines are synthesized from tyrosine.

儿茶酚胺系由酪氨酸合成。

The tyrosine kinase receptors represent a large family of receptors that are involved in many facets of cell growth responses.

酪氨酸激酶受体代表着涉及细胞生长反应诸多方面的受体的一大家族。

tyrosinemia [ˌtaiərəsiˈniːmiə] *n.* 酪氨酸血症

Tyrosinemia is a genetic disorder characterized by elevated blood levels of the amino acid tyrosine.

酪氨酸血症是一种遗传病,特点是血中氨基酸酪氨酸水平增高。

Type I tyrosinemia is an autosomal recessive condition that causes hepatic failure and renal tubular dysfunction.

I 型酪氨酸血症是一种常染色体隐性遗传病,会导致肝衰竭和肾小管功能失调。

tyrosinosis [ˌtairəusiˈnəusis] *n.* 酪氨酸代谢(障碍)病,酪氨酸代谢症

Tyrosinemia Type I includes tyrosinosis, hereditary tyrosinemia, hepatorenal tyrosinemia.

Ⅰ型酪氨酸血症包括酪氨酸代谢病、遗传性酪氨酸血症、肝肾型酪氨酸血症。

Tyrosinosis type II, is a recessive autosomal genodermatosis consecutive to a disorder of tyrosine metabolism.

Ⅱ型酪氨酸代谢病是由于酪氨酸代谢障碍所致的常染色体隐性遗传性皮肤病。

U

ubiquitin [juː'bikwitin] *n.* 泛素,泛激素

Ubiquitin is a small protein that can be attached to other proteins to target them for degradation in the proteasome.

泛素是一种小分子蛋白,它能黏附到其他蛋白质上使该蛋白被蛋白酶体降解。

Ubiquitin-proteasome pathway is a highly effective protein-degradation pathway in the eukaryotic cells.

泛素-蛋白酶体途径是真核细胞内一种高效蛋白降解途径。

ubiquitous [ju(ː)'bikwitəs] *a.* (同时)普通存在的,无处不在的

Mycoplasmas, which are ubiquitous in nature, are a group of unusual bacteria lacking rigid cell walls.

支原体是一种缺乏完整细胞壁的特殊的细菌,在自然界中广泛存在。

ulcer ['ʌlsə] *n.* 溃疡

No cause is usually found though duodenal ulcer is associated with gastric hypersecretion.

虽然十二指肠溃疡与胃酸分泌亢进有关,但通常找不到发病原因。

Tuberculous ulcers may develop in the intestine from infection by bacilli in swallowed sputum.

由于咽下带有细菌的痰而引起的肠道感染可发生结核性溃疡。

ulcerate ['ʌlsəreit] *v.* 溃烂,形成溃疡

In some cases the Ghon focus or hilar lymph nodes may involve and ulcerate into a bronchus.

在有些病例中,戈恩病灶(结核原发性病灶)或肺门淋巴结的病变可累及并溃破入支气管。

ulceration [ˌʌlsə'reiʃən] *n.* 溃疡(形成)

The onset is abrupt and consists of the sudden appearance of sore throat, fever, and ulceration.

该病起病突然,包括突然出现的喉痛、发热和溃疡形成。

Ulceration of the uvula and other parts of the throat may be seen in typhoid fever.

悬雍垂和喉的其他部分的溃疡形成可见于伤寒。

ulcerative ['ʌlsərətiv] *a.* 溃疡(性)的

Chronic recurrent ulceration in the colon is the chief manifestation of ulcerative colitis, the etiology is unknown.

溃疡性结肠炎的主要表现是结肠中有慢性复发性溃疡形成,其病因不清楚。

ulna ['ʌlnə] (pl. ulnas 或 ulnae ['ʌlniː]) *n.* [拉]尺骨

On a lateral plain film of the wrist, the ulna and radius are parallel.

在腕部的侧位平片上,尺骨和桡骨是平行的。

Epiphysitis, especially of the ulna, is common in early congenital syphilis.

早期先天梅毒中,骨髓炎常见,尤其多发于尺骨。

ultimate ['ʌltimit] *a.* 最远的,最后的,基本的

Hysterectomy is, of course, the ultimate solution to the problem of dysfunctional uterine bleeding.

当然,治疗功能失调性子宫出血最后的措施是子宫切除术。

This method is capable of showing a renal arterial tree regardless of the ultimate excretory function of the kidney.

若不考虑肾脏基本的排泄功能,这种方法可以显示肾动脉树。

ultimately ['ʌltimitli] *ad.* 最后,最终

The ideal vaccine would protect the individual and ultimately eliminate the disease.
理想的疫苗可保护机体并最终除去疾病。
As we saw, a prolonged destruction of nephrons can ultimately render a kidney completely useless.
正如我们所看到的，肾单位长期的破坏，最终能使肾功能完全丧失。

ultracentrifugation [ˌʌltrəsenˌtrifju'geiʃən] *n.* 超(速)离心法
Lipoproteins are usually separated out by ultracentrifugation.
脂蛋白通常可用超速离心法进行分离。

ultrafast [ˌʌltrə'fɑːst] *adj.* 超快的；超速的
The fifth generation CT scanner is also named ultrafast CT or electron beam CT.
第五代 CT 扫描机也称为超高速 CT 或电子束 CT。

ultrafiltration [ˌʌltrəfil'treiʃən] *n.* 超滤作用
In biological terms, ultrafiltration occurs at the barrier between the blood and the filtrate in the renal corpuscle or Bowman's capsule in the kidneys.
从生物学角度看，超滤现象发生在血液与肾脏中肾小体或肾小球囊滤液之间的屏障处。

ultralente ['ʌltrəlent] *a.* 超长效的
Ultralente or semilente insulin is used to eliminate nocturnal and early morning hyperglycemia.
长时间和中等时间作用的胰岛素，适用于消除夜间或清晨高血糖症。

ultramicroscope [ˌʌltrə'maikrəskəup] *n.* 超显微镜
Ultramicroscope is used for examining particles suspended in a gas or liquid under intense illumination from one side.
超显微镜在一侧光照下用于检查悬浮在气体或液体中的微粒。

ultrasonic [ˌʌltrə'sɔnik] *a.* 超声的
It seems ironic to spend large sums on biochemical, ultrasonic, and radionuclide tests to determine its nature, when a specimen obtained directly from the lesion will provide a rapid diagnosis.
当直接从病变部位获取标本可提供快速诊断时，花费大量费用进行生化、超声和放射性核素检查以确定其性质是可笑的。

ultrasonography [ˌʌltrəsə'nɔːgræfi] *n.* 超声探查
Straight abdominal X-ray and ultrasonography will reveal many stones.
正位腹部 X 线检查和超声探查可发现大部分结石。
Amebic liver abscesses have also been visualized by ultrasonography, gallium scanning, and computed tomography.
阿米巴肝脓肿也可通过超声波摄影、镓扫描及电子计算机体层摄影显示出来。

ultrasound ['ʌltrəsaund] *n.* 超声
Ultrasound imaging can be used to locate the placenta accurately.
超声显像可用作胎盘准确定位。
Renal ultrasound may be sufficient to obviate urograms.
肾脏超声检查已足够，不必做尿路造影。
Doppler ultrasound is a form of ultrasound that can detect and measure blood flow.
多普勒超声是检测血流的一种超声形式。

ultrathin [ˌʌltrə'θin] *a.* 超薄的
He proposed the idea of using ultrathin polymer membrane microcapsules for the immunoprotection of transplanted cells.
他主张将超薄多聚膜的微粒用于移植细胞的免疫保护。

ultraviolet [ˌʌltrə'vaiəlit] *a.* 紫外的
Ultraviolet rays from the sun change a form of cholesterol in the skin into Vitamin D.
阳光中的紫外线使皮肤中的胆固醇变成维生素 D。

The ultraviolet waves have powerful effects upon the body.
紫外线波对人体有强烈的作用。

ultravist [ˈʌltrəvist] *n.* 优维显

Iodinated contrast ultravist 370 was injected into the antecubital vein by using a dual-syringe injector with an 18-gauge needle or larger.
碘对比剂优维显 370 用一个 18 号或者更大的双筒注射器注入肘前静脉。

umbilical [ʌmˈbilikəl] *a.* 脐的

Adult worms have been described issuing from umbilical fistulas, and even from the nose or ear.
成虫自脐瘘钻出已有描写,甚至自鼻或耳钻出。

The pain in acute intestinal obstruction is visceral and is therefore felt centrally and usually in umbilical area.
急性肠梗阻的疼痛是内脏性的,因此会感觉在腹部中央疼痛,通常是在脐周围的区域。

umbilication [ʌmˌbiliˈkeiʃən] *n.* 中间凹陷

A white rounded lesion with umbilication suggests cancer.
白色圆形中间凹陷病变提示为癌肿。

umbilicus [ʌmˈbilikəs] *n.* 脐

The pain is generalized, and is mainly referred to the umbilicus.
此种疼痛范围广泛,但主要在脐部。

Pain around the umbilicus may be seen in acute diseases of pancreas, small intestine and appendix.
脐周围疼痛可见于胰腺、小肠和阑尾的急症。

umbra [ˈʌmbrə] *n.* 本影

This is a lighter area between the umbra and the edge of a shadow.
这是本影和阴影边缘之间较亮的区域。

The determination of the umbra and penumbra is a difficult task in general
区分本影和半影通常是一个困难的任务。

unacceptable [ʌnəkˈseptəbl] *a.* 无法接受的

Incomplete bladder emptying can be obviated by catheterization, but the discomfort, risk, and inconvenience often make it unacceptable.
可通过插管避免膀胱排空不完全,但不适、危险性以及不方便使其难以被(病人)接受。

In one such trial, 1 out of every 1000 persons vaccinated contracted the disease—an unacceptable risk.
在一次这种尝试中,每 1000 接种牛痘的人中有一人患病——这是不能接受的危险。

unaided [ˈʌnˈeidid] *a.* 未受帮助的,独立的

Some protozoa will reach diameters of 1 mm to 2 mm and thus be visible to the unaided eye.
有些原虫大至 1 ~2 毫米,以至肉眼可见。

unambiguous [ˌʌnæmˈbigjuəs] *a.* 不含糊的;清楚的;明白的

The answer was clear and unambiguous.
这个答案很明了,不含糊。

The results published in the journal Brain in 1999 were unambiguous.
发表在 1999 年的一期脑科学杂志上的研究结果很清楚。

unanimous [juˈnæniməs] *a.* 一致的,一致同意的

A unanimous conclusion has been reached by all investigators in regard to the effect of the type of leakemia on survival.
关于白血病类型对存活的影响,所有的研究者获得的结论是一致的。

unavoidably [ˌʌnəˈvɔidəbli] *ad.* 不可避免地

This condition is unavoidably associated with hemorrhage.
这个状态不可避免地与出血有关。

unaware [ʌnə'wɛə] *a.* (一般作表语)未认识到的;没有察觉的

Still many people are unaware that today many of the side-effects of anti-cancer drugs can be controlled or eliminated.

仍然有许多人未能认识到今天抗癌药物的许多副作用可得到控制,并被消除。

Observations should be done in such a way that the patient is unaware that a check is being made.

观察病人,应注意不要让病人感知正在进行这方面的检查。

unbelievable [ˌʌnbi'liːvəbl] *a.* 难以相信的

When living conditions are ideal, the organisms reproduce with unbelievable rapidity.

当条件合乎理想时,致病菌以令人难以相信的速度繁殖。

uncertain [ʌn'səːtn] *a.* 不确定的

Although faecal antigens have been described, their infectivity is uncertain.

虽然粪便抗原的特性已有记述,但其传染性仍未肯定 。

Therefore follow-up investigations are necessary in uncertain cases on the 2nd and 3rd day of menstruation.

因此,对于尚未确诊病例的跟踪检查必须在经期的第 2 和第 3 天进行。

uncertainty [ʌn'səːtnti] *n.* 不确知,不确定

Uncertainty frequently exists as to the diagnosis of this condition.

此种疾病的诊断常常存在不肯定性。

unchanged [ˌʌn'tʃeindʒd] *a.* 未改变的

The diseased prostate gland at first is not enlarged on rectal palpation, and form and consistency are unchanged.

开始时肛门指检,前列腺患部并不肿大,形状和硬度也无变化。

uncinariasis [ˌʌnsinə'raiəsis] *n.* 钩虫病

Uncinariasis is a cutaneous (skin) condition characterized by skin lesions that are erythematous macules and papules.

钩虫病是一种影响皮肤的疾病,其特征是皮肤损害表现为红斑和丘疹。

Hookworm disease (also called uncinariasis), a helminthic infection of the upper intestine, is chronic and debilitating. The disease's major sign is anemia.

钩虫病是上段小肠的一种蠕虫感染,是慢性并使人虚弱的疾病,该病的主要体征是贫血。

uncinate ['ʌnsineit] *a.* 钩状的

The uncinate process is a hook-like projection of the inferior aspect of the head of the pancreas.

钩突是胰头下方的一个钩状突起。

The uncinate fasciculus is a white matter tract in the human brain that connects parts of the limbic system such as the hippocampus and amygdala in the temporal lobe with frontal ones such as the orbitofrontal cortex.

钩束是人脑中的白质纤维束,它将部分边缘系统如颞叶的海马和杏仁核同额叶如眶额叶皮层连接起来。

uncommon [ʌn'kɔmən] *a.* 罕见的,不平常的

Acute severe hemolysis(hemolitic crisis) is uncommon.

急性的严重溶血(溶血危象)不常见。

During the acute stage of the disease, delirium is not uncommon.

在该疾病的急性期常有谵语。

uncomplicated [ˌʌn'kɔmplikeitid] *a.* 不复杂的;无并发症的

Pregnancy, labor, and delivery were uncomplicated.

妊期、产程及分娩均无合并症。

An uncomplicated urinary tract infection may be cured by 10 days' treatment with a sulfonamide.

无并发症的尿道感染用一种磺胺药物治疗 10 天就可能治愈。

unconscious [ʌnˈkɔnʃəs] *a.* 人事不省的；意识丧失的

The soldier was unconscious from loss of blood.

这个战士因失血而丧失了知觉。

He is in hospital in an unconscious state.

他已住院，处于失去知觉的状态。

unconsciousness [ʌnˈkɔnʃəsnis] *n.* 人事不省，意识丧失

Coma and unconsciousness result in loss of airway protection, which in turn may lead to aspiration pneumonia.

病人的昏迷和意识丧失使其呼吸道的保护功能丧失，可能引起吸入性肺炎。

A few clonic jerks of the limbs and face may occur in some patients shortly after the beginning of the unconsciousness.

肢体和面部少量阵发性抽搐在某些病人的意识丧失开始后很快发生。

uncontrolled [ˈʌnkɔnˈtrəuld] *a.* 不受控制的

Uncontrolled diabetes leads to diabetic acidosis.

未控制住的糖尿病会引起糖尿病酸中毒。

Through the uncontrolled use of insectcides, man has polluted the land, killing the wildlife.

由于杀虫剂的滥用，人类污染了土地，毒死了野生动物。

uncoordinate [ˌʌnkəuˈɔːdineit] *v.* 不协调；不调和

The growth of a tumor exceeds and is uncoordinated with that of the normal tissues.

肿瘤的生长超过正常组织的生长，并与正常组织的生长不协调。

uncorrected [ʌnkəˈrektid] *a.* 未改正的

The nasal airway obstruction is due to a nasal septal perforation or still uncorrected abnormality or sequelae.

鼻道阻塞可由鼻中隔穿孔、未矫正的畸形或后遗症所致。

undeniable [ˌʌndiˈnaiəbl] *a.* 不能否认的

It is an undeniable fact that parents have a striking influence on children.

不能否认的事实是父母对孩子有着极大的影响。

underdeveloped [ˈʌndədiˈveləpt] *a.* 不发达的；发育不全的；显影不足的

When the self-cleaning mechanisms are underdeveloped, disturbed, or absent, a true gonorrheal vulvovaginitis can develop.

当自我清洁机制降低、被扰乱或缺乏时，便可能发生真正的淋病性外阴阴道炎。

underestimate [ʌndərˈestimeit] *v.* 低估，看轻

The responsibility of pharmacists should not be underestimated.

决不能低估药剂师的责任。

The role of surgery for this disease was sometimes underestimated.

手术对于此种疾病的作用过去有时被低估了。

undergo [ˌʌndəˈgəu] *v.* 经历；经过；忍受

On the way light rays undergo a process of blending known as refraction.

一路上，光线经历一个叫做折射的屈光过程。

This patient will undergo a complicated heart surgery.

这位病人将经受一次复杂的心脏手术。

Within the cell the nutritive material undergoes changes and is absorbed.

在细胞内，营养物质发生变化并被吸收。

Everything in the universe undergoes continuous development and change.

宇宙万物不断发展与变化。

The early lesions of syphilis undergo involution either spontaneously or under treatment.

梅毒的早期损害可自行消退或经治疗消退。

underground [ˈʌndəgraund] *a.* 地(面)下的

Excessive use of fertilizers and pesticides could pollute underground water.

过度使用化肥和杀虫剂会污染地下水。

The main conclusions are that no link between the underground environment and health has been found.

主要结论是:没有发现地下环境与健康之间存在联系。

underlying [ˈʌndəˈlaiiŋ] *a.* 根本的,基础的;潜在的

Little is known of the underlying mechanism of this disorder.

关于这种疾病的基本机制知道得很少。

One must search for underlying disease.

必须做基础疾病的检查。

Empyema may also be secondary to an underlying carcinoma of the lung.

积脓也可继发于潜伏的肺癌。

Penicillin and sulphonamides are effective against any underlying active streptococcal infection.

青霉素和磺胺类药物对任何潜伏的活动性链球菌感染有效。

undermine [ˌʌndəˈmain] *v.* 逐渐削弱

The ethical issues may undermine achievement of the registry's objectives.

这些伦理学问题可能逐渐削弱注册目标的实现。

underneath [ˌʌndəˈniːθ] *prep.* 在…下面,向…下面

The outer surface of spleen is domed to fit underneath the diaphragm.

脾的外表面呈穹顶状,与膈的下部相适应。

The cortex of lymph node, located underneath the subcapsular sinus, receives the afferent lymph and serves as the major site of B-lymphocyte localization.

位于被膜下窦下面的淋巴结皮质接受流入的淋巴,成为 B 淋巴细胞定位的主要部位。

underproduction [ˈʌndəprəˈdʌkʃən] *n.* 生产不足

It has been suggested that the Cooley's anemia is due to an unbalanced hemoglobin synthesis rather than underproduction.

现已提出库利贫血是由于一种血红蛋白合成不平衡而不是由于生成不足所致。

undertake [ˌʌndəˈteik] *v.* 进行,从事

During respiratory obstruction the cause must quickly be removed or alleviated before any further measures can be undertaken.

呼吸道堵塞时,在采取任何进一步措施之前必须先迅速除去病因或使其缓解。

Seminal examination is the most important laboratory procedure to be undertaken in the male.

对于男性最重要的是进行精液检查。

undesirable [ˈʌndiˈzairəbl] *a.* 不合需要的

For this reason, excessive dosages are undesirable and may be dangerous.

由于这个缘故,不宜于给过大剂量,过量可能有危险性。

undetected [ˈʌndiˈtektid] *a.* 未被发现的,未被识破的

Environmental influences may be unknown, undetected, or subject to long periods of latency before exerting clinical expression of disease.

在疾病的临床表现产生前,环境影响可能是不清楚的,未发觉的,或是长期隐伏的。

On the other hand, when urine volume is high and the urine is dilute, a relatively large amount of protein can go undetected.

另一方面,当尿量多和尿液稀释时,较大量的蛋白可能检测不出来。

undrain [ˈʌnˈdrein] *v.* 未引流,未排出

If an abscess remains undrained, its fibrous wall becomes progressively thicker and more rigid.

如果脓肿未引流,其纤维性壁会不断地增厚、变硬。

undue [ˈʌnˈdjuː] *a.* 过度的,不适当的

Diets too high in carbohydrate are likely to cause undue fermentation in the intestine.
饮食中含有过高的碳水化合物可能引起肠内发酵过度。

undulant [ˈʌndjulənt] *a.* 波状的;起伏的,波浪形的
The disease is called undulant fever because the fever is typically undulant, rising and falling like a wave.
这种疾病被称为波状热是因为这种发热呈典型的波状,像波浪一样升高和下降。
Undulant fever (brucellosis) is an extremely variable disease.
波状热(布鲁氏菌病)是一种极其多变的疾病。

unduly [ʌnˈdjuli] *ad.* 不适当地,过分地
In some instances, a trip to the X-ray department will delay operation unduly and will constitute a hazard to the patient.
在有些情况下,让病人到放射科拍片可能耽误手术,因而给病人造成危险。

unequivocal [ˈʌniˈkwivəkəl] *a.* 不含糊的,明确的
The result of the examination was unequivocal.
检查的结果是无疑问的。

unequivocally [ˈʌniˈkwivəkəli] *ad.* 不含糊地,明确地
Causes of sudden deaths resulting from disease are always demonstrated unequivocally at autopsy.
由疾病引起的突然死亡的原因均可在尸检时明确显示出来。
The laboratory criteria for the diagnosis of Zn deficiency are not unequivocally established.
诊断锌缺乏的实验室标准尚未明确地建立。

unevenly [ʌnˈiːvənli] *ad.* 参差不齐地;不规则地;不稳定地
The cell is swollen so that it projects unevenly into the lumen of the renal tubule.
该细胞肿胀以至参差不齐地突出在肾小管的管腔中。

uneventful [ˈʌniˈventful] *a.* 平静的;没有事故的
The remainder of her postoperative course was uneventful.
手术后的其他经过是平稳的。
In most cases of atelectasis, the course is self-limited and recovery uneventful.
肺不张的病程大多数是自限的,且恢复顺利。

unexpected [ˌʌnikˈspektid] *a.* 非预期的
All adverse drug reactions that are previously unobserved or undocumented are referred to as "unexpected".
所有之前没有观察到或没有记录的药物不良反应都可称作"非预期的"。

unexpectedly [ˈʌniksˈpektidli] *ad.* 出乎意外地
Cancer has been an unexpectedly frequent companion of clinical transplantation.
癌症是临床器官移植意想不到的常见伴侣。

unfavorable [ʌnˈfeivərəbl] *a.* 不适宜的,不顺利的
Prognosis is unfavorable in neither case.
在两种情况下预后都不良。
The study found that the frequency of more severe and prognostically unfavorable arrhythmias was higher in the diabetes mellitus 2 subgroup.
研究发现2型糖尿病病人发生较为严重、并且预后不良的心律失常的频率更高。

unfortunately [ʌnˈfɔːtʃənitli] *ad.* 不幸地,令人遗憾地
Unfortunately protein foods are expensive, and poverty unbalances the diet by restricting the protein intake.
不幸的是蛋白类食物很昂贵,贫穷限制了蛋白质的摄入量,使膳食不能平衡。
Unfortunately, hyperthyroidism recurs in at least 50% usually within 2 years of stopping treatment.

令人感到遗憾的是,甲状腺功能亢进通常在停药后2年内至少有50%复发。

unhealthy [ʌn'helθi] *a.* 对健康有害的,不健康的

Mixing vitamins, minerals and other drugs can sometimes produce unhealthy interactions.

混用维生素、矿物质和其他药物有时会产生不利于健康的相互作用。

unicellular [ˌjuːni'seljulə] *a.* 单细胞的

Bacteria are very small, unicellular organisms.

细菌是极小的单细胞生物。

unidirectionally [ˌjuːnidi'rekʃənəli] *ad.* 单方向地

It was initially concluded that the duplication of DNA molecule proceeded unidirectionally.

起初的结论是:DNA 分子的复制是单向进行的。

uniform ['juːnifɔːm] *a.* 相同的,一致的;均匀的

When distributive equilibrium has occurred completely, the concentration of drug in the body will be uniform.

当分布达到完全平衡时,体内药物的浓度都是均匀的。

uniformly ['juːnifɔːmli] *ad.* 相同地,一致地

Drug therapy alone has been uniformly unsuccessful in controlling symptoms in patients with the sick sinus syndrome.

单纯用药物疗法控制病窦综合征病人的症状全都无效。

unilateral ['juːni'lætərəl] *a.* 单边的,单侧的

Rapid sequence films may demonstrate unilateral renal artery stenosis.

快速顺序拍片可证实单侧肾动脉狭窄。

It is important to know whether the tumor is cystic or solid, and unilateral or bilateral.

重要的是应知道肿块是囊性还是实性,单侧还是双侧。

uniovular [ˌjuːni'ɔvjulə] *a.* 单卵的

Uniovular twins are developed from a single ovum, which after fertilization has undergone divisions to form two embryos.

单卵双胎是由单个卵子受精发育,分裂形成两个胚胎。

uniparental [ˌjuːnipə'rentl] *a.* 单亲的

Uniparental disomy is a condition in which an individual has two copies of a chromosome but both copies derive from one parent.

单亲二体是指某一个体有一个染色体的复份,两条染色体来源于一个亲代。

unipolar [ˌjuːni'pəulə] *a.* 单极的,单相的

Evidence now indicates that children experience both unipolar and bipolar affective disorders.

现在有证据显示儿童可遭受单极和双极两种情感性疾患。

unique [ju'niːk] *a.* 唯一的,独一无二的

This case report is unique for two reasons.

鉴于两点理由,这个病例报告是很独特的。

Every person's body has a unique arrangement of veins and arteries.

每个人身体的静脉和动脉都有其独特的排列方式。

uniqueness [juː'niːknis] *n.* 唯一性

A technical assessment of electronic records for their uniqueness within any dataset of patient information is necessary to minimize the potential for reidentification.

为尽量减少重新识别的可能,有必要对所有患者信息数据集内的电子记录的唯一性进行技术评估。

Uniqueness is something very different from everything else.

唯一性是指某东西与其他东西很不相同。

univalent [ˌjuni'veilənt] *a.* 一价的,单价的

However, a small percentage of the molecular oxygen is univalent reduced and this reduction re-

sults in the formation of oxygen radicals.
然而,分子氧中一小部分是单价还原性的,这种还原作用导致氧自由基的形成。

univariate [ˌjuːniˈvɛərieit] *a.* 单变量的

A univariate analysis was performed to determine the relationship between the characteristics and the duration of the patients' survival.
采用单变量分析来测定患者的特征和生存期的关系。

It is now realized by researchers that univariate analysis alone may not be sufficient, especially for complex data sets.
现在研究者们已经意识到,单靠单因素分析可能是不够的,尤其是对于那些复杂的数据集。

universal [juːniˈvəːsəl] *a.* 普遍的,全身的;万能的

Some doctors recommend "universal" screening of all pregnant women with normal fasting blood sugar level.
一些医生建议对所有空腹血糖正常的妊娠妇女进行普查。

Universal erythroderma, generally accompanied by scaling, may be associated with malignancy, usually lymphoma.
全身性红皮病,一般伴有脱屑,可并发恶性肿瘤,以淋巴瘤为常见。

"My blood is type O. I am a universal donor".
"我的血是 O 型的,我是万能输血者"。

universally [ˌjuːniˈvəːsəli] *ad.* 全世界地,普遍地

This is a theory universally received by the scientists.
这是科学家们公认的一种理论。

universe [ˈjuː nivəːs] *n.* 世界,宇宙,全体

These medical specialists refuse to admit anything beyond or outside the five-sense universe.
这些医学专家拒不承认五种感觉(视、听、触、嗅、味)器官所感知的世界以外的任何事物。

Our world is but a small part of the universe.
我们的世界仅是宇宙的一小部分而已。

For common and highly communicable childhood diseases, the target population is the universe of susceptible individuals.
对通常的和高度传染性的儿童疾病,人群对象是所有易感个体。

unlikely [ʌnˈlaikli] *a.* 未必可能的;靠不住的

It is unlikely that an axial view of a thrombus will be seen in a single section.
从单一断面观察血栓的轴面是不大可能的。

In early syphilis that has been promptly and adequately treated, a positive spinal fluid is unlikely.
经过及时充分治疗的早期梅毒,其脑脊液检查不大可能出现阳性。

unnecessary [ʌnˈnesisəri] *a.* 不必要的

The use of enemas and so-called colonic flushings is unnecessary and should be discouraged for most persons.
使用灌肠剂和所谓的结肠冲洗都是不必要的,对大部分人来说不应该提倡。

Indeed, early and unnecessary hemodialysis may exacerbate renal hypoperfusion.
事实上,过早的、不必要的血液透析可能会加重肾脏低(血流)灌注。

unprecedented [ʌnˈpresidentid] *a.* 没有先例的,前所未有的

New antibacterial products are appearing at an unprecedented rate.
新的抗菌药品正以空前的速度在增长着。

Their subsequent discovery was unprecedented for its speed.
他们随后的发现速度之快是前所未有的。

unproductive [ˈʌnprəˈdʌktiv] *a.* 不生产的

Unproductive, distressing cough should be suppressed.
无痰而痛苦的咳嗽应设法控制。

unprotected [ˌʌnprəˈtektid] *a.* 无保护的

Rapid-sequence induction minimizes the time during which the trachea is unprotected.
快速序贯诱导能使气管不受保护的时间缩短至最低限度。

unrelated [ˌʌnriˈleitid] *a.* 无关的，不相关的

Are those merely a collection of unrelated conditions to which we have attached the word shock?
是不是我们集合了互不相关的一些症状，牵强附会地加上了“休克”一词？

Patients with scleroderma have dysphagia to solids that is unrelated to posture.
硬皮病患者对固体（食物）吞咽困难，这与体位无关。

unremarkable [ˌʌnriˈmɑːkəbl] *a.* 不显著的，不值得注意的

Past history of this patient was unremarkable.
此病人既往史没有什么值得注意的。

unremitting [ˌʌnriˈmitiŋ] *a.* 不间断的，持续的，不停的

The course of illness in these children was characterized as nonepisodic and unremitting.
这些儿童患者的病程特点为非发作性和持续性。

unresponsive [ˌʌnrisˈpɔnsiv] *a.* 无反应的

Dopamine can be used if patients have bradycardia unresponsive to atropine.
多巴胺可用于对阿托品无反应的心动过速患者。

unsettled [ˈʌnˈsetld] *a.* 未解决的

It remains unsettled whether this results from hormonal imbalance alone.
这是否只因激素不平衡所致，尚未解决。

unstabilized [ʌnˈsteibilizd] *a.* 不稳定的

There are a number of complications of poorly treated or unstabilized diabetes.
治疗不当的或不稳定的糖尿病人可产生许多并发症。

unstable [ʌnˈsteibl] *a.* 不稳定的

A 58-year-old man with a history of unstable angina was admitted to the coronary care unit.
一名有不稳定型心绞痛史 58 岁的男子被收进冠心病监护室。

unsuspected [ˈʌnsʌsˈpektid] *a.* 不受怀疑的

Unsuspected malignancy has been found in 6% of gastrectomy specimens.
在胃切除标本中已发现有 6% 的胃癌漏诊。

untoward [ʌnˈtəuəd] *a.* 不合宜的；麻烦的

It is advisable to be on the alert for untoward reactions which may not have been described before.
宜警惕以前没有记载过的不良反应。

These drugs may ameliorate the behavior problems but have untoward side effects such as sedation, rigidity, and dyskinesias.
这些药物可改善行为障碍，但会产生一些难对付的副作用，如镇静、僵硬和运动障碍。

untreated [ʌnˈtriːtid] *a.* 未经治疗的

The rats with untreated brain damage took more days to finish the task.
脑损伤未经治疗的大鼠需要更多的天数才能完成这一任务。

unusual [ʌnˈjuːʒuəl] *a.* 不平常的，异常的

Tonsillitis is not highly contagious and it is unusual to have more than one case in a family at the same time.
扁桃体炎的传染性并不强，在一个家庭里同一时间很少有一例以上的病人。

Many times an unusual skin eruption may be a clue to some internal disorder that may not be obvious.
一种不常见的皮疹经常可能是某种不明显的内脏疾病的一个线索。

The occurrence of repeated or unusual infections in a patient is a primary indication of immunodeficiency.
患者发生反复感染或异常感染是免疫缺陷的主要标志。

unwanted ['ʌn'wɔntid] *a.* 不需要的，讨厌的
Certain drugs given even in low dosage to geriatric patients may cause unwanted effects.
某些药物用于老年患者，即使剂量小也可能产生副作用。

unwarranted ['ʌn'wərəntid] *a.* 未经保证的，无根据的
In depth evaluation of the asymptomatic patient with sinus bradycardia is unwarranted.
深入评价无症状的窦性心动过缓病人没有必要。

unwind [ʌn'waind] *v.* 解链，解开
After the unwinding of the DNA, the new strands are made in short segments.
DNA 解链后，新链以一小段一小段方式合成。

update [ʌp'deit] *v.* 使现代化，更新；向…提供最新资料
The medical equipment of this hospital must be updated.
这所医院的医疗设备必需现代化。
The aims of this chapter are to update the gastrointestinal complications of HIV infection.
本章的目的是提供有关 HIV 感染的患者胃肠道并发症的最新资料。

upgrade [ʌp'greid] *v.* 升级，提高，改善
You have to upgrade your computer.
你的计算机需要升级.
I would like to know how much it would cost to upgrade my current system.
我想知道我现在的系统要升级需要多少费用?

uppsala ['ʌpsɑːlə] *n.* 淀粉微球
Uppsala is a new class of biodegradable materials, it is widely used in medical, food, chemical and other fields.
淀粉微球是一类新型的可生物降解材料，广泛用于医疗、食品、化工等领域。
Uppsala as a new drug carrier in drug delivery systems has shown broad prospects.
淀粉微球作为新型的药物载体在给药系统中已显示出广阔的前景。

upregulation [ʌpˌregju'leiʃən] *n.* 上调(效应)
MEM1 is an oncogene, and its upregulation influences metastatic potential.
MEM1 是致癌基因，它的上调影响癌细胞转移能力。
Cerebral ischemia may induce upregulation of ANG and GFAP expression in the ischemic brain areas.
脑缺血可诱导缺血脑区 ANG 和 GFAP 的表达上调。

upright ['ʌprait] *a.* 直立的
The upright glass tube is fixed to a millimeter scale.
直立的玻璃管被固定在一个毫米标尺上。
ad. 笔直
We must tell the patient to sit upright.
我们一定要叫这个病人坐直。

upset [ʌp'set] *v.* 使(肠胃)不适；搅乱
The medicine upsets my stomach.
这药使我的胃不舒服。
When the homeostasis of this system is upset, acute symptoms and sometimes chronic disease may result.
当该系统稳态被破坏时，会出现急性期症状，有时会导致慢性疾病。

uptake ['ʌpteik] *n.* 摄入，摄取
This patient should increase his water uptake.

这个病人应增加水的摄入。

The uptake and utilization of glucose in the peripheral tissue decrease.

外周组织对葡萄糖的摄取和利用减少。

The action of norepinephrine is terminated by "re-uptake" mechanisms.

去甲肾上腺素的作用因“再摄取”的机制而终止。

up-to-date ['ʌptə'deit] *a.* 现代化的，新式的；掌握最新信息的

The hospital is equipped with up-to-date apparatuses for diagnosing and treatment.

这所医院配备有最新式的诊断和治疗器械。

After remoulding and augment of modern equipment, this teaching hospital has become an up-to-date hospital.

经过改造和增加新的设备，这所教学医院已变成了一所现代化医院。

They are up-to-date on recent developments in artificial heart transplantation.

他们了解人工心脏移植术的最新发展。

upward ['ʌpwəd] *a.* 向上的，上升的

Increasing cumulative toxin exposure, estimated by the level and duration of exposure, displayed an upward trend in renal cancer risk.

通过接触的浓度和时间而估计的蓄积性毒物接触量的增加显示肾癌的危险度呈上升趋势。

ad. 向上，上升

As the proliferative cell moves upward through the epidermis, it changes morphologically.

当增生的细胞经表皮向上移动时，细胞的形态便会发生变化。

uragogue ['juərəgɔg] *n.* 利尿剂

Uragogue is an agent that increases production of urine.

利尿剂是一种增加尿量的药剂。

Some manufacturers add uragogue, excitant and hormone into the drugs.

一些生产商在药物中加入利尿剂、兴奋剂和激素。

urban ['əːbən] *n.* 都市的，城市的

The cardiovascular disease occurs whether subjects live in large urban environments or in rural villages.

无论居住在都市或居住在乡村的人均可发生心血管疾患。

Trichophyton tonsurans in 1978 was the major cause of tinea capitis in urban areas with a large Latin American population.

1978 年在城市地区的大量拉美居民中，头癣主要是由断发癣菌所致。

urea ['juəriə] *n.* 尿素

The blood urea may rise to 15-25 mmol/L due to absorption of protein from the gut.

由于肠道内蛋白被吸收，血清尿素可升高至 15～25mmol/L。

Urea is the major end product of protein metabolism presented for urinary excretion.

尿素是蛋白质代谢的主要最终产物，由尿液排泄。

uremia [juə'riːmiə] *n.* 尿毒症

Mortality from strokes and uremia is decreased if hypertension is treated.

若高血压得到治疗，可降低中风和尿毒症的病死率。

Sometimes the patient develops uremia, as occurs following loss of large numbers of nephrons.

患者有时随着肾单位大量流失而产生尿毒症。

uremic [ju'riːmik] *a.* 尿毒症的

Hemolytic uremic syndrome is a rare disease.

溶血性尿毒症是一种少见的疾病。

For instance, E. coli poisoning can cause hemolytic-uremic syndrome, a cause of kidney failure in children.

例如,大肠杆菌中毒可引起溶血性尿毒症,该病可进一步引起儿童肾衰竭。

ureogenesis [ˌjuəriəuˈdʒenisis] *n.* 脲生成,尿素生成

In the liver, the main function of argininosuccinate lyase is ureogenesis.

精氨基琥珀酸裂解酶在肝脏的主要功能是尿素生成。

Ethanol suppresses ureogenesis.

乙醇抑制尿素生成。

ureter [juəˈriːtə] *n.* 输尿管

Each ureter is about the thickness of a goose quill and from 14 to 16 inches long.

每根输尿管约有鹅毛管粗,14～16 英寸长。

ureteroneocystostomy [juˌriːtərəˌniəusisˈtɔstəmi] *n.* 输尿管膀胱吻合术

Urinary tract continuity is usually established by ureteroneocystostomy.

通常是通过输尿管膀胱吻合术建立尿路的连续性。

A few surgeons prefer ureteropyelostomy to ureteroneocystostomy, but it is associated with a higher incidence of urinary fistula.

少数外科医生倾向于输尿管肾盂吻合术而不是输尿管膀胱吻合术,但前者尿瘘的发生率较高。

urethra [juəˈriːθrə] (pl. urethras 或 urethrae [juəˈriːθriː]) *n.* 尿道

Inflammation of the urethra can occur in both sexes.

尿道炎症可发生于两性。

Examination of the prostate and external urethra is the first step in the evaluation of isolated hematuria.

对于单纯性血尿病人的病情评估首先要检查前列腺和外尿道。

urethral [juəˈriːθrəl] *a.* 尿道的

The patient may notice a little discomfort on micturition, with slight urethral and cervical discharge.

病人可能注意到排尿时稍有不适,尿道和宫颈有少量分泌物。

urethritis [ˌjuəriˈθraitis] *n.* 尿道炎

The symptoms of the urethritis in this patient decreased after 3-6 weeks.

该患者尿道炎的症状在 3～6 周后减轻了。

Quantitation and identification of bacteria in the urine are vital diagnostic procedures in urethritis.

诊断尿道炎时重要的程序在于对尿中的细菌的识别和定量。

urgency [ˈəːdʒənsi] *n.* 紧急,迫切;尿急

In HIV-infected individuals, examination of cerebrospinal fluid may be a matter of comparative urgency.

在被 HIV 感染的患者中,脑脊液的检查相对来说更为紧要。

Dysuria, frequency and urgency may result from prostatic hyperplasia, foreign bodies (catheters, stones), and bladder tumors.

前列腺增生,尿道异物(导管、结石)和膀胱肿瘤均可有尿痛、尿频和尿急。

urgent [ˈəːdʒənt] *a.* 急迫的

Reestablishment of breathing by artificial respiration is most urgent if the victim's life is to be saved.

如果要挽救受害者的生命,最为紧迫的就是用人工呼吸来恢复呼吸。

It is most urgent that the old man should be sent to the hospital.

最要紧的是马上送老人去医院。

Patient with ongoing active hemorrhage should undergo urgent endoscopy as soon as possible.

活动性出血的病人应尽可能早的进行急诊内镜检查 。

uric [ˈjuərik] *a.* 尿的

The major sources of uric acid in the body are purines derived from metabolism of nucleic acids.
体内尿酸的主要来源是核酸代谢时产生的嘌呤。
Uric acid stones occur when urine is saturated with uric acid in the presence of an acid urine PH and dehydration.
当出现酸性尿和脱水使尿液中尿酸达到饱和状态时，就会形成尿酸结石。

uricosuria [ˌjuərikəuˈsjuəriə] *n.* 尿酸尿
The long-term use of ascorbic acid in these doses can interfere with the absorption of vitamin B_{12} and cause uricosuria.
按此剂量长期服用抗坏血酸可以妨碍维生素 B_{12} 的吸收，引起尿酸尿。

uricosuric [ˌjuərikəuˈsjuərik] *a.* 促尿酸尿的
Probenecid is a uricosuric drug that inhibits the tubular secretion of penicillin.
丙磺舒是一种促尿酸排泄药，它能抑制肾小管分泌青霉素。
The alkylchain oxidation of the drug produces a metabolite with strong uricosuric property.
药物的烃链氧化作用产生一种有强促尿酸排泄性能的代谢产物。

urinalysis [ˌjuəriˈnæləsis] *n.* 尿分析
Patients receiving sulfonamides should have periodic urinalysis.
服用磺胺药的患者，应该定期查尿。
During treatment the blood picture should be watched, and routine urinalysis performed.
治疗期间应注意血象，并做尿常规分析。

urinary [ˈjuərinəri] *a.* 尿的，泌尿的
In urinary tract infection, summer episodes tend to be more severe.
尿道感染夏季发作比较严重。

urinate [ˈjuərineit] *v.* 排尿
The inability to urinate postoperatively starts a vicious circle.
术后尿闭引起恶性循环。

urination [ˌjuəriˈneiʃən] *n.* 排尿
The likelihood of pain being caused on urination is low.
排尿引起疼痛的可能性是低的。
There was in the patient a constant desire for urination.
病人总想小便。

urine [ˈjuərin] *n.* 尿
Waste products eliminated through the kidneys are carried away in water in the form of urine.
由肾排泄的废物随水以尿的形式排出。

urogenital [ˌjuərəuˈdʒenitəl] *a.* 泌尿生殖的
The urogenital tract is almost always invaded from the exterior via the urethra, vaginal or cervical mucosa.
外界侵入泌尿生殖道几乎总是通过尿道、阴道或子宫颈黏膜。
In anatomy, the genitourinary system or urogenital system is the organ system of the reproductive organs and the urinary system.
在解剖上，泌尿生殖系统包括生殖器官和泌尿系统。

urografin [juəˈrɔgrəfin] *n.* 泛影葡胺
The membranous sac filled with urografin was applied to produce an animal model of chronic spinal cord compression (L_2).
采用泛影葡胺填充膜囊来建立慢性脊髓（第 2 腰椎）压迫动物模型。
Urografin is an ionic contrast agent, due to a high rate of allergic reaction, the use scope is more and more small.
泛影葡胺是一种离子型造影剂，由于过敏反应发生率高，目前使用范围越来越小。

urography [juəˈrɔgrəfi] *n.* 尿路造影术

Urography is an X-ray examination used to check the kidneys and the tubes that drain them (ureters).

尿路造影术是一种 X 线检查,用于检查肾脏和排尿管道(输尿管)。

Intravenous urography is a test that uses X-rays and a special dye to help assess the kidneys, ureters, bladder and urethra.

静脉尿路造影术是用 X 线和一种特殊染料来帮助评估肾脏、输尿管、膀胱和尿道的一种检查方法。

urokinase [ˌjuərəu'kaineis] *n.* 尿激酶

Urokinase is an enzyme produced by and isolated from human kidney which has thrombolytic effect.

尿激酶是由人的肾脏产生并分离出来的具有溶栓作用的一种酶。

Immunoglobulin A and urokinase are also secreted by the renal tubule and appear in the urine in small amounts.

免疫球蛋白 A 和尿激酶也是由肾小管分泌的,在尿中有小量出现。

urolith ['juərɔliθ] *n.* 尿石

Urolith in the urinary tract are commonly composed of calcium oxalate and are usually visible on X-ray examination.

泌尿道中的尿石通常由草酸钙组成,X 线检查中可以看见。

urolithiasis [ˌjuərəuli'θaiəsis] *n.* 尿石病

Urolithiasis refers to the process of forming stones in the kidney, bladder, and/or urethra.

尿石病是指在肾脏、膀胱和(或)尿道形成结石的过程。

Urolithiasis, especially kidney stone, is usually manifested by severe spasms of pain and hematuria.

尿石病,尤其是肾结石,通常表现为剧烈的疼痛发作和血尿。

urologic [ˌjuərəu'lɔdʒik] *a.* 泌尿(学)的

Urologic symptoms, such as frequency, nocturia, urgency and dysuria, indicate the need for immediate investigation.

泌尿道症状如尿频、夜尿、尿急和尿痛表明需要作立即检查。

urologist [juə'rɔlədʒist] *n.* 泌尿科医生

The urologist tells me that this patient can be discharged tomorrow morning.

泌尿科医生告诉我说这个病人明天上午可以出院。

urology [juə'rɔlədʒi] *n.* 泌尿科学

Urology is the branch of medicine concerned with the study and treatment of diseases of the urinary tract.

泌尿科学是涉及尿路疾病研究和治疗的医学分支。

uropathy [juə'rɔpəθi] *n.* 尿路病

These patients have diabetes mellitus or obstructive uropathy or have undergone renal transplantation.

这些病人有糖尿病或梗阻性尿路病变,或者已做过肾移植。

uropenia [juərəu'piːniə] *n.* 尿过少

No drug is comparable with furosemide in relieving uropenia.

在缓解尿少现象上,没有药物可以和速尿相比。

urothelial [ˌjuərəu'θiːliəl] *a.* 膀胱上皮的

Steineck et al. (1990) reported an increased risk of urothelial cancer in Stockholm, Sweden following exposure to benzene.

Steineck 等(1990)的报告称,在瑞典斯德哥尔摩接触苯后的膀胱上皮癌危险度增加。

urticaria [ˌəːti'kɛəriə] *n.* 荨麻疹

This case of viral hepatitis was seen with acute urticaria in the preicteric phase.

这例病毒性肝炎在黄疸前期伴有急性荨麻疹。

Extensive urticaria may occur in large patches on various parts of the body.

全身皮肤可出现大量大块的荨麻疹。

usher [ˈʌʃə] *v.* 作为先兆

An abrupt attack of vomiting usually ushers in this disease, along with irritability, general weakness, and discomfort.

此病常以呕吐的突然发作为其先兆,并伴有激动、全身无力及不适。

uterine [ˈjuːtərain] *a.* 子宫的

Abdominal examination will also show the frequency and strength of the uterine contractions.

腹部检查也能显示子宫收缩的频率和强度。

About 10 days before ovulation, the uterine lining has begun preparation to receive a fertilized egg.

子宫内膜约在排卵前10天开始准备接受受精卵。

uterus [ˈjuːtərəs] (*pl.* uteri [ˈjuːtərai]) *n.* 子宫

If the egg is not fertilized, it passes through the uterus and is charged.

如果卵没有受精,则通过子宫排出。

Pain localized to the lower abdomen may arise from the uterus or vagina.

位于下腹的疼痛可由子宫或阴道疾患所引起。

utility [ju(ː)ˈtiləti] *n.* 效用,有用

The utility of this antibody depends on its specificity.

这种抗体的效用取决于其特异性。

utilization [ˌjuːtilaiˈzeiʃən] *n.* 利用

Sideroblastic anemias are due to inadequate or abnormal utilization of intracellular Fe for Hb synthesis.

铁幼粒细胞性贫血是由于不能充分或正常利用细胞内的铁以合成血红蛋白所致。

utilize [ˈjuːtilaiz] *v.* 利用

If the adrenal cortex is removed or is defective, body cells cannot properly utilize glucose.

如果肾上腺皮层被切除或有缺陷,体细胞就不能正常地利用葡萄糖。

The human body cannot utilize the atmospheric nitrogen, it must rely upon protein for its nitrogen.

人体不能利用大气中的氮,它必须依靠蛋白质供氮 。

utmost [ˈʌtməust] *a.* 极度的,极端的;最大的

Nucleic acids are macromolecules of the utmost biological importance.

核酸是具有极其重要的生物学意义的大分子。

At times the patient complains only of the eruption on the hands, and examination of the feet is of utmost importance in these cases.

有时患者仅陈述手的皮疹,而在这些病例中,检查足部是最为重要的。

uveitis [ˌjuːviˈaitis] *n.* 眼色素层炎,葡萄膜炎

Scleritis may lead to uveitis and glaucoma.

巩膜炎可导致葡萄膜炎和青光眼。

uvula [ˈjuːvjulə] (pl. uvulae [ˈjuːvjuliː]) *n.* 悬雍垂

That dangling thing in the back of your mouth is the uvula.

在你口腔后面有一个悬垂的小东西就是悬雍垂。

When you breathe the soft palate and the uvula are at rest.

当你呼吸时,软腭和悬雍垂静止不动。

V

vaccinate [ˈvæksineit] *v.* 接种疫苗,预防接种

She was vaccinated against smallpox as a child.

她小时候就接种了天花疫苗。

At home it began a program to vaccinate children against infectious childhood diseases.

在国内开展了接种计划,预防儿童传染病。

vaccination [væksiˈneiʃən] *n.* 种痘,接种

Vaccination makes one immune from smallpox.

接种牛痘,可使人对天花免疫。

At present vaccination and chemoprophylaxis are available for epidemic influenza only.

目前,接种和化学预防法仅对正在流行的流感有效。

vaccine [ˈvæksin] *n.* 疫苗

Despite their benefits to medicine, vaccines are not without risk.

尽管疫苗对医疗有益,但并不是没有风险。

Local reactions as well as fever may occur after injection of pertussis vaccine.

在注射百日咳疫苗后,可发生局部反应和发热。

vacuole [ˈvækjuəul] *n.* 空泡,液泡

The cells have a cell wall made predominantly of the polysaccharide cellulose, and a vacuole in addition to the cytoplasm.

细胞具有主要由纤维素多糖组成的细胞壁,另外,除细胞质外,还有液泡。

The dark fibrilar substance in the vacuole might be a mixture of various substances after digested from the cell.

液泡中深色的原纤维物质可能是细胞被消化后各种物质的混合物。

vacuum [ˈvækjuəm] (*pl.* vacuums 或 vacuua) *n.* 真空

Vacuum tubes containing EDTA may be obtained commercially.

含依地酸的真空试管市场有售。

Vacuum aspiration is the standard method of termination up to 12 weeks' gestation.

终止 12 周妊娠的标准方法是负压抽吸术。

vagal [ˈveigəl] *a.* 迷走神经的

The frequency of impulses in the vagus nerve depends upon the extent to which the vagal centers in the medulla are themselves excited or inhibited by nerve impulses from various places.

迷走神经冲动的频率取决于延髓迷走神经中枢所受的各种由不同部位来的神经冲动所引起的兴奋或抑制的程度。

vagina [vəˈdʒɑinə] (*pl.* vaginae [vəˈdʒɑiniː]) *n.* 阴道

If the bleeding is heavy the blood passes through the cervix and clots in vagina.

如果出血多,血液就会经宫颈流出在阴道中凝成血块。

vaginal [vəˈdʒainəl, ˈvædʒinəl] *a.* 阴道的 ;鞘的

The child was the product of a full-term pregnancy and spontaneous vaginal delivery.

这男孩出生时是足月妊娠并经阴道自然分娩。

Mucous patches are most common on the labia minora, the vaginal mucosa, and the cervix.

黏膜斑常发生于小阴唇、阴道黏膜和子宫颈处。

Treatment of vaginal carcinoma may pose a difficult problem because of the proximity of bladder

and rectum.
由于阴道接近膀胱和直肠，所以阴道癌的治疗很困难。

vaginitis [ˌvædʒiˈnɑitis] *n.* 阴道炎

In children and postmenopaual women the vagina may be less exposed to infection, vaginitis may still occur because of the loss of the acid barrier.
儿童和绝经后妇女阴道遭受感染可能较少，但由于酸性屏障丧失，阴道炎仍可发生。

The vaginal pH value of patients with atrophic vaginitis was significantly higher than the pH value of pre menopausal women.
患萎缩性阴道炎妇女的阴道 pH 值明显高于绝经前妇女。

vaginosis [ˌvædʒiˈnəusis] *n.* 阴道病

With the rapid assaying card for the bacterial vaginosis, the sensitivity of the vaginal secretions is 97.1%.
用细菌性阴道病快速检测卡检测，阴道分泌物的敏感性为 97.1%。

Bacterial vaginosis, also known as vaginal bacteriosis and bacterial vaginitis, is a bacteria-related problem observed in the vagina among women, particularly of child-bearing age.
细菌性阴道病也称为阴道细菌病或细菌性阴道炎，是一种与女性阴道内的细菌相关的疾病。

vagolytic [ˌveigəuˈlitik] *a.* 迷走神经阻滞的

Quinidine can increase the sinus node discharge rate and exert vagolytic effects.
奎尼丁可以增加窦房结的放电率，并可发挥迷走神经阻滞作用。

n. 迷走神经阻滞药

Drugs that inhibit the muscarinic cholinergic receptor such as atropine are called vagolytic.
抑制毒蕈碱胆碱能受体的药物如阿托品等被称作迷走神经阻滞药。

vagotomy [veiˈgɔtəmi] *n.* 迷走神经切断术

Vagotomy is one of the surgical treatments of duodenal ulcer.
治疗十二指肠溃疡常用的手术方法之一就是迷走神经切断术。

For duodenal ulcer the acid-secretory capacity of the stomach may be reduced by vagotomy.
对于十二指肠溃疡，迷走神经切断术可减少胃酸分泌量。

vague [veig] *a.* 含糊的，不明确的

The term cloudy swelling, a relic of the past, is about as vague and unsatisfactory as could be conceived.
混浊肿胀这个术语是过去沿用下来的，其概念之模糊和不能令人满意是可以想象的。

In appendicitis, initial symptoms may be vague and may include nausea or discomfort gradully localizing to the right lower quadrant.
阑尾炎首发症状不明显，可表现为恶心及渐进性右下腹不适。

vagus [ˈveigəs] (*pl.* vagi [ˈveidʒai]) *n.* 迷走神经

The vagus nerves always exert a restraining influence upon the action of the heart.
迷走神经对于心脏活动总是起着抑制的作用。

valence [ˈveiləns] *n.* 效价；价

The valence of an antibody is the number of antigenic determinants with which it can react.
一个抗体的效价就是能与其反应的抗原决定簇的数目。

valid [ˈvælid] *a.* 有效的，有充分根据的

The experiment proves valid as a means of producing experimental hypertension.
这个实验作为产生实验性高血压的一种方法是有效的。

These methods can give valid information if practised with great care.
这些（检验）方法如果做得非常仔细，可以提供有充分根据的资料。

validate [ˈvælideit] *v.* 确认，验证

There are models that absolutely require validation that are never validated.

有些模型绝对需要验证却从来没有被验证过。

This document describes how to validate data or create a drop down list of options in Microsoft Excel.

这个文档讲述如何在微软 Excel 中验证数据或创造下拉选项列表。

validity [vəˈliditi] *n.* 有效性，确实性，效度

These experiments were designed to study the validity of the procedure.

这些实验是为研究其方法的可靠性而设计的。

We begin this chapter by discussing the validity of the drug and diagnosis information used by clinician in the management of patients' care.

在本章，我们从讨论临床医师处治患者所用药物和诊断信息的有效性开始。

The purpose of this study was to evaluate the validity and reliability of this device.

本研究的目的是评价这个设备的效度和信度。

valine [ˈvæliːn] *n.* 缬氨酸

Valine is one of the essential amino acids.

缬氨酸是一种必需氨基酸。

Valine is broken down to yield succinyl CoA.

缬氨酸分解产生琥珀酰辅酶 A。

valium [ˈvæliəm] (diazepam) *n.* 安定

Valium is used to relieve anxiety and tension and in the treatment of epilepsy and muscular rheumatism.

安定用于解除焦虑不安和精神紧张，治疗癫痫和肌风湿病。

valproate-sodium [vælˈprəueit-ˈsəudjəm] *n.* 丙戊酸钠

For most seizures in children the drug of choice is valproate-sodium 20 to 30 mg per kg body weight per day in two divided doses.

儿童中大多数癫痫发作的选用药物是丙戊酸钠每日 20 ~ 30mg/kg 体重，分 2 次剂量服用。

value [ˈvælju] *n.* 价值，值

Cognition function of brain was simulated by artificial nerve network by changing threshold limit value of linking point.

人工神经网络可以通过改变连接点的阈限值来模拟大脑的认知功能。

Long time medicine-taking may create the addictive reliance, which will bring about complications when the concentrations of medicine reach its threshold limit value.

长期服药可能会导致药物依赖，当药物在体内的浓度累积到某个临界点时，会引起相应的并发症。

valve [vælv] *n.* 瓣膜

Valves in veins ensure that blood flows toward the heart by preventing backflow.

静脉里的瓣膜通过阻止血液倒流而确保血液流向心脏。

The heart is a four-chambered organ, each side divided into two chambers with a valve between them.

心脏是一个包含有四室的器官，即每侧分为两室，中间有瓣膜隔开。

valvotomy [vælˈvɔtəmi] *n.* 瓣膜切开术

Mitral valvotomy may alter the natural history of mitral valve disease.

二尖瓣切开术可以改变二尖瓣疾病的自然病程。

valvular [ˈvælvjuːlə] *a.* 瓣膜的

The development of pericarditis in a patient with signs of valvular injury signifies pancarditis.

当患者心包炎发展到出现心脏瓣膜损害时即表明已患有全心炎。

The acute rheumatic fever is of limited duration, but the carditis may lead to permanent valvular damage.

急性风湿热持续期有限，但心脏炎却导致永久性瓣膜损害。

valvuloplasty [ˈvælvjuləˌplæsti] *n.* 瓣膜成形术

In selected patients, without mitral regurgitation, percutaneous balloon valvuloplasty is frequently a successful alternative to surgery.

选择没有二尖瓣关闭不全的病人进行经皮球囊瓣膜成形术常可成功替代外科手术。

vancomycin [ˌvæŋkəuˈmaisin] *n.* 万古霉素

There have been some vancomycin resistant enterococci in some hospitals that are almost untreatable.

在某些医院一直存在一些对万古霉素有抗药性的肠球菌,几乎无法对付。

vanillylmandelic acid [ˌvænəlilmænˈdelik æsid] *n.* 香草基苦杏仁酸

Vanillylmandelic acid (VMA) is a principal catecholamine metabolite whose presence in excess in the urine is used as a test for pheochromocytoma.

香草基苦杏仁酸是儿茶酚胺的主要代谢产物,其过量出现于尿液中被用于检测嗜铬细胞瘤。

vanishing [ˈvæniʃiŋ] *n.* 消失;*a.* 消没的

Leukoencephalopathy with vanishing white matter (VWM disease) is an autosomal recessive neurological disease.

白质消融性白质脑病是一种常染色体隐性的神经系统疾病。

Gorham vanishing bone disease is a very rare skeletal condition of uncertain etiology.

Gorham 消失骨病是一种病因不确定的非常罕见的骨病。

vapor [ˈveipə] *n.* 蒸气

Here the air is full of water vapor that causes such things as clouds, rain, and fog.

这里空气中充满了水蒸气,从而产生云、雨和雾这类东西。

Each time gasoline is loaded or unloaded, gasoline vapors are released into the atmosphere.

装汽油或卸汽油时,汽油的蒸气就被释放到大气中。

variability [ˌvɛəriəˈbiliti] *n.* 变异性,易变,变化的倾向

Variability of plasma membrane composition is a common aspect of neoplasia.

胞浆膜组成的变异性正是肿瘤的共同特点。

The variability both between and within individuals is very obvious when one examines the course of spirometric tests.

当检查肺量测定试验的过程时,就可以看到无论是个体之间还是个体本身变化都是十分明显的。

variable [ˈvɛəriəbl] *a.* 易变 的,可变的

The speed of this electronic apparatus is variable.

这台电子仪器的速度是可变的。

There is a highly variable region, which differs greatly in length in different tRNAs.

tRNA 有一个高度可变区,其长度在不同 tRNA 中有很大差别。

n. 变量,变数

This marked variation may be due to a number of variables such as the exact diagnosis, definition of latent period, etc.

这种明显的差异可能是由于很多可变因素,诸如准确的诊断、潜伏期的定义等所造成。

Categorical baseline variables were summarized by frequencies and percentages.

用频数和百分比来概述基线分类变量。

variance [ˈvɛəriəns] *n.* 不一致,方差

One-way analysis of variance was used to detect differences.

使用单向方差分析来检测差异。

variant [ˈvɛəriənt] *a.* 变异的,不同的

Leucocyte is a variant spelling of leukocyte.

Leucocyte 是 Leukocyte 的另一种拼法。

Problems include such difficulties as changes of name and variant name forms.
问题包括名称的改变和不同的名称形式等困难。
n. 变异体，变型，变种
Classically defined childhood manic depression is simply an early onset variant of the disorder.
按传统方法诊断的儿童期躁狂抑郁症只不过是此病的一个发病期早的变型。
Ganglioneuroblastoma is a variant of neuroblastoma.
成神经节细胞瘤是神经母细胞瘤的变种。

variation [ˌvɛəriˈeiʃən] *n.* 变化，变异
Living things show variations.
生物具有变异性。
A basic feature of reproduction is that it results in variation.
生殖的一个基本特征是能产生变异。

varicella [ˌværiˈselə] *n.* 水痘
Varicella virus can occasionally cross the placenta in early pregnancy, and when this occurs it produces congenital malformations.
妊娠早期中水痘病毒偶尔可通过胎盘，如发生此情况，可导致先天性畸形。

varicocele [ˈværikəuˌsiːl] *n.* 精索静脉曲张
The incidence of varicocele in older adolescence varies from 12.4 % to 17.8 % with an average of 14.7 %, similar to the incidence in adult males.
青春后期精索静脉曲张发病率为 12.4 % ~17.8%，平均 14.7%，与成年男性相似。

varicophlebitis [ˌværikəufliˈbaitis] *n.* 曲张静脉炎
Varicophlebitis is the most frequent and important acute complication of a varicosed long and/or short saphenous vein.
曲张静脉炎是长/短隐静脉曲张后最常见和最重要的急性并发症。
In 2003, a total number of 40 limbs with ascending varicophlebitis were observed, among which 10 extremities underwent surgical treatment.
2003 年总共观察到 40 个肢体上行曲张静脉炎，其中 10 个肢体进行了手术治疗。

varicose [ˈværikəus] *a.* 曲张的(静脉)
Varicose veins is a condition in which the superficial veins have become swollen, tortuous and ineffective.
静脉曲张是指浅静脉扩张、扭曲和失去功能。
Varicose veins in the rectum are commonly referred to as piles, or more properly, hemorrhoids.
直肠区静脉曲张，俗称痔疮，更确切的名称是痔。

varied [ˈvɛərid] *a.* 不同的，各式各样的
Each of the illnesses that can cause chest discomfort may have varied presentations.
每一种引起胸部不适的疾病可有不同的临床表现。
To achieve the recommended daily intake of vitamins and minerals, a varied diet including fish, lean meats and vegetables is recommended.
要得到推荐的每日应摄取的维生素和矿物质，建议饮食多样化，包括鱼、瘦肉和蔬菜。

variety [vəˈraiəti] *n.* 多样化，变化，种类，每种
A blood transfusion may be indicated for a variety of reasons.
输血可能出于多种原因。
Microbes are spread about through an almost infinite variety of means.
微生物的传播方式很多，不胜枚举。
A wide variety of molecules are involved in the development of immune responses.
种类繁多的分子参与了免疫应答的发展过程。
There are two main varieties of aspiration pneumonia differentiated from each other by the type of

fluid aspirated and the circumstances in which it occurs.
吸入性肺炎根据吸入液体及得病的情况可分成两个主要类型。

various [ˈvɛəriəs] *a.* 各种各样的

Aspirin in various forms is sold under a wide range of trade names.
不同形式的阿司匹林以各种各样的商品出售。

In addition to a diet, she pursues various exercises.
节食以外她还做各种锻炼。

varix [ˈvɛəriks] (pl. varices [ˈvɛərisiːz]) *n.* [拉]静脉曲张

Some patients have hematemesis due to gastroesophageal varices.
有的病人因胃食管静脉曲张(破裂)而呕血。

The general term for these enlarged vein is varices.
静脉曲张是这些扩张静脉的统称。

Vitamin K should be given if bleeding has occurred from varices.
如果是静脉曲张出血则一定要给维生素 K。

vary [ˈvɛəri] *v.* 变化,不同,有差异

The shape of cells varies greatly.
细胞的形状差异很大。

Some organs, such as the urinary bladder, must vary a great deal in size during the course of their work.
某些器官,如膀胱,在工作过程中大小变化甚大。

Signs of aplastic anemia vary with the severity of the pancytopenia.
患再生障碍性贫血时的体征因全血细胞减少的严重程度而异。

vascular [ˈvæskjulə] *a.* 血管的,脉管的

Similar pain in younger person may indicate multiple sclerosis, aneurysm or vascular anomaly.
年轻人出现类似的疼痛提示可能有多发性硬化症、动脉瘤或血管异常。

Unfortunately, in a patient who has suffered a cerebral vascular accident, the protective autoregulatory system becomes inoperative.
不幸的是,大脑血管意外的病人,其保护性自我调控系统已不再起作用。

vascularity [væskjuˈlærəti] *n.* 血管分布,多血管(状态)

Subsiding papilledema may reveal some atrophy of the optic disc with diminution of vascularity.
消退中的乳头水肿可显示某种程度的视盘萎缩,伴有血管分布减少。

Chest X-ray revealed a moderate degree of cardiomegaly and increased pulmonary vascularity.
胸部 X 线片显示中等程度的心脏扩大及肺血管分布增多 。

vascularize [ˈvæskjuləraiz] *v.* 形成血管,血管化

Since the blood stream functions as a "duct" and carries off the secretory products, these glands are all richly vascularized.
因为血流的功能有导管一样的作用,可以将分泌物带走,所以这些腺体都有很丰富的血管。

vasculature [ˈvæskjulətʃə] *n.* 脉管系统,血管系统

Adult schistosome worms parasitize defined sites of the venous vasculature of humans.
血吸虫的成虫寄生在人体内的静脉中某个特定的位置。

vasculitis [ˌvæskjuˈlaitis] *n.* 脉管炎,血管炎

Swelling and congestion of the optic disc are found in cases of vasculitis with ocular involvement.
视盘的肿胀和充血可见于眼部受累的脉管炎病例。

Chronic leg ulcers result from skin necrosis secondary to vasculitis.
血管炎可引起皮肤坏死,导致慢性小腿溃疡。

vasculogenesis [ˌvæskjuləuˈdʒenisis] *n.* 血管新生,血管发生

The interaction of endothelial cells and pericytes with their microenvironment plays a crucial role during vasculogenesis and angiogenesis.

内皮细胞和血管周细胞与其微环境的相互作用在血管新生和血管生成中发挥重要作用。

Both vasculogenesis, the de novo formation of vessels, and angiogenesis, the growth of new vessels from pre-existing vessels by sprouting, are complex processes.

血管新生是重新开始的血管形成,而血管生成是已有血管发芽长出新血管,二者均是非常复杂的过程。

vas deferens [væsˈdefərenz] *n.* 输精管

Both ephedrine and noradrenaline increased the amplitude and frequency of spontaneous contraction of isolated vas deferens of mice.

麻黄碱和去甲肾上腺素均能增强离体小鼠输精管自发性收缩的幅度和频度。

vasectomy [vəˈsektəmi] *n.* 输精管切除术,输精管结扎

To improve on vasectomy, it would need to be reversible and have minimal side effects.

如果要对输精管结扎手术进行改良,它必须具有可逆转性,还要将副作用降到最低。

This study demonstrates that vasectomy leads to a decrease in the number of spermatogenic cells.

本研究证实了输精管切除术导致生精细胞减少。

vaseline [ˈvæsiliːn] *n.* 凡士林

While vaseline can be used as a lubricant, it is also a useful moisture insulator for local skin conditions characterized by tissue dehydration.

凡士林可以作为润滑剂使用,也是改善局部皮肤脱水症状的有效保湿剂。

Carbon powder and vaseline were used for the construction of the carbon paste biosensor.

碳粉和凡士林被用于制造碳糊生物传感器。

vasoactive [ˌveizəuˈæktiv, ˌvæsəuˈæktiv] *a.* 血管活性的,作用于血管的

These responses result partly from the release of vasoactive agents from platelets.

这些反应部分是由于血小板释放血管活性剂所致。

vasoconstricting [ˌveizəukənˈstriktiŋ] *a.* 血管收缩的

Angiotensin Ⅱ enhances the vasoconstricting effects of norepinephrine.

血管紧张素Ⅱ可增强去甲肾上腺素的缩血管效应。

vasoconstriction [ˌveizəukənˈstrikʃən] *n.* 血管收缩

Renal vasoconstriction must be considered as a possible cause of reduced renal blood flow.

肾血管收缩必须被认为是肾血流减少的一个可能原因。

The functions associated with alpha receptors are vasoconstriction, mydriasis, and intestinal relaxation.

与 α 受体有关的功能是血管收缩、瞳孔散大和肠道松弛。

vasoconstrictor [ˌveizəukənˈstriktə] *n.* 血管收缩药

Vasoconstrictor is an agent that causes the blood vessels to constrict.

血管收缩剂是能使血管收缩的一种药物。

Methoxamine is a long acting vasoconstrictor and does not cause cardiac stimulation.

甲氧胺是一作用持久的缩血管药,不兴奋心脏。

vasodilation [ˌveizəudaiˈleiʃən] *n.* 血管舒张(=vasodilatation)

Histamine produces vasodilation.

组织胺可产生扩血管作用。

With the dissipation of the fever, peripheral vasodilatation occurs and heat loss ensues.

随着发热的消退,周围血管舒张,并随后产生失热。

vasodilator [ˌveizəudaiˈleitə] *a.* 血管舒张的

Meanwhile, the vasodilator center of the vasomotor center is stimulated to increase activity.

同时,血管运动中枢中的血管舒张中枢受到刺激而活动力增强。

n. 血管舒张药

These vasodilators can successfully be used in conjunction with digitalis and diuretics.

这些血管扩张剂也能有效地与洋地黄和利尿剂合并使用。

vasodilatory [ˌveizəudai'leitəri] *a.* 血管舒张的

A reduction in vasodilatory prostaglandins also may play an important role in preeclampsia.

有血管舒张作用的前列腺素减少也在先兆子痫中起重要作用。

vasoligation [ˌvæsəuli'geiʃən] *n.* 输精管结扎术

The study was designed to provide morphological basis for vasoligation and anastomosis of spermatic duct.

这项研究为输精管结扎术和吻合术提供形态学基础。

We evaluated the rate, influence factors and treatment effects of variety subtypes of psychosomatic reaction after vasoligation.

我们评估了输精管绝育术后人群的各种类型的身心反应的发生率、影响因素和治疗效果。

vasomotor [ˌveizəu'məutə] *a.* 血管舒缩的 *n.* 血管舒缩药

Vasomotor tone is very important in the regulation of arterial pressure.

血管运动紧张度在调节动脉血压中很重要。

Vasomotor symptoms can almost always be relieved by treatment with estrogens.

用雌激素治疗常可减轻血管舒缩的症状。

vasopressin [ˌveizəu'presin] *n.* (后叶)加压素

Vasopressin may stimulate the contraction of the muscular tissue of the capillaries and arterioles, raising the blood pressure.

加压素可刺激毛细血管和小动脉的肌肉组织收缩,使血压升高。

vasopressor [ˌveizəu'presə] *a.* 血管加压的

In such case, the use of vasopressor drugs may aggravate the condition.

在这种情况下,血管加压药物的使用可使此病的病情恶化。

n. 血管加压药

Systolic blood pressure can be maintained by replacing fluid loss and, if necessary, by vasopressors.

通过补充已丢失的体液来维持收缩压,若有必要,亦可用血管加压药。

vasospasm ['veizəuˌspæzəm] *n.* 血管痉挛

It has been established that variant angina is caused by vasospasm.

已经证实变异型心绞痛是由血管痉挛所致。

vasovasostomy [ˌveizəuvæ'sɔstəmi] *n.* 输精管吻合术

The objective of this article is to observe the change of sperm ultrastructure after vasovasostomy.

本文的目的是要观察输精管吻合术后精子超微结构的变化。

There are 8 primary factors which affect repregnancy following micro-vasovasostomy, among which the SIT and spermatic viability are the factors of primary importance.

影响显微外科输精管吻合术后复孕的主要因素有 8 个,其中以术后的 SIT 和精子存活率最为重要。

Vaspin ['væspin] *n.* 丝氨酸蛋白酶抑制剂

Vaspin serum concentrations were significantly higher in females as compared to males.

对于血清丝氨酸蛋白酶抑制剂水平,女性显著高于男性。

Vaspin was identified as an adipokine with insulin-sensitizing effects, which is predominantly secreted from visceral adipose tissue in a rat model of type 2 diabetes.

丝氨酸蛋白酶抑制剂是一个胰岛素增敏性脂肪因子,从 2 型糖尿病大鼠内脏脂肪组织分泌出来。

vector ['vektə] *n.* 媒介物(尤指动物,常为节肢动物传病媒介);载体;矢量,向量

In the latter case, the insects, like houseflies, serve only as a vector in transmission.

在后一种情况下,如家蝇一类的昆虫在传播中仅仅是一种媒介。

Several features make plasmids an ideal vector.

质粒的几个特性使其成为一种理想的载体。

The vector must have an affinity for the reservoir host.

传播媒介必须与宿主发生联系。

Since the cardiac depolarization and repolarization waves have direction and magnitude, they can be represented by vectors.

因为心脏去极化和复极化波有方向和大小，所以可以用向量来表示。

vegetable [ˈvedʒitəbl] *a.* 植物的；蔬菜的

Carbohydrates come mainly from the vegetable kingdom.

碳水化合物主要来源于植物界。

He is interested in vegetable cultivation.

他对蔬菜栽培感兴趣。

n. 蔬菜；植物人

The patient has been in a coma for five months and has been reduced to the condition of a vegetable.

这个病人已昏迷5个月并已变成植物人。

vegetarian [ˌvedʒiˈtɛəriən] *n.* 素食者

A strict vegetarian is a person who never in his life eats anything derived from animals.

严格的素食者是一个在一生中从来不吃动物性食物的人。

Vegetarians who don't supplement their diet with vitamins are likely to get insufficient vitamin B_{12}.

不用维生素来补充饮食的素食者，可能得不到充足的维生素 B_{12}。

a. 素食的

He went on vegetarian diet for the benefit of his health.

他为了健康而吃素。

vegetation [vedʒiˈteiʃən] *n.* 赘生物，增殖物

Echocardiogram may demonstrate vegetations on the infected valves.

超声心动图可见到感染的心瓣膜上的赘生物。

The incidence of vegetations is high in the left side of the heart, where the pressure is greatest.

赘生物的发生率以压力最高的左心室为多。

The typical valvular lesion consists of inflammatory vegetations.

典型的瓣膜损害包括炎性的增生物。

vegetative [ˈvedʒitətiv] *a.* 植物性的，无性繁殖的，细菌繁殖的

In this persistent vegetative state, the mind is dead but the brain is not.

在这种持续的植物状态下，意识已消失，但脑尚未死亡。

Leaves and roots can give rise to new individuals through vegetative reproduction.

叶和根能通过无性繁殖产生新个体。

Vegetative cells are much more sensitive to heat than are spores.

细菌繁殖体比芽胞对热要敏感得多。

vehicle [ˈviːikl] *n.* 运载工具；车辆；媒介物

Milk is sometimes a vehicle of infection.

牛奶有时是传染疾病的媒介。

Many people are wounded by or even die from motor vehicle accidents.

许多人因交通事故而受伤甚至死亡。

vein [vein] *n.* 静脉

Blood poured from the cut vein.

血从割破的静脉血管中流出。

The arteries carry blood away from, and the veins carry blood to, the heart.

动脉把血运出心脏，静脉把血运回心脏。

velocity [viˈlɔsiti] *n.* 速度，速率

Velocity is the quotient of displacement and time.

速度是位移和时间的商。

Because the velocity of sound in soft tissue is constant, the depth is measured by the time.

由于波在软组织中的传播速度是恒定的，因此可用时间检测其厚度。

venereal [viˈniəriəl] *a.* 性交的；性病的

Gonorrhoea is the commonest venereal disease and is caused by infection with the gonococcus.

淋病是最常见的性病，由淋球菌感染而引起。

venipuncture [ˈveniˌpʌŋktʃə] *n.* 静脉穿刺

Blood is preferably collected by venipuncture.

血液最好是通过静脉穿刺采集。

The venipuncture site should be cleansed with an antiseptic such as 70% alcohol.

静脉穿刺位点应当用诸如70%酒精之类的消毒剂来使之清洁。

venoconstriction [ˌviːnəukənˈstrikʃən] *n.* 静脉收缩

Peripheral venoconstriction produced by sympathetic stimulation results in an increase in pulmonary blood volume.

交感神经兴奋所产生的周围静脉收缩导致肺循环血量增加。

venography [viˈnɔgrəfi] *n.* 静脉造影术

Hepatic venography revealed a tumor stain in 2 of 13 cases.

在 13 例病人中，通过肝静脉造影术发现了 2 例有肿瘤染色。

The imaging findings of venography in 80 side lower limbs were reviewed retrospectively.

回顾性分析了 80 例侧下肢静脉造影的影像学资料。

venom [ˈvenəm] *n.* 毒液

Sea snakes prey on small marine animals, and the powerful toxins in the venom quickly immobilize the prey before it can swim off.

海蛇捕食小型海洋动物，其毒液中的强力毒素可迅速使猎物在能游走之前丧失移动能力。

In addition, massive wasp stings can also produce a lethal dose of venom in most adults.

此外，大量黄蜂蜇伤也能在多数成人中产生致死剂量的毒液。

venous [ˈviːnəs] *a.* 静脉的

This venous blood enters and fills the right atrium and the right ventricle.

静脉血进入并充盈右心房和右心室。

Venous disease in the upper extremities is rare.

上肢的静脉疾病较少见。

Deep venous thrombosis is the more serious condition that may lead to pulmonary embolism.

深静脉血栓形成的情况较严重，可引起肺栓塞。

ventilate [ˈventileit] *v.* 使（空气）流通，使通风

If any choice is available, the room chosen for home confinement should be reasonably spacious, well lit and ventilated.

如有选择余地，所选家庭分娩的房间应是宽敞的、明亮的和通风的。

The pulmonary circulation is for the purpose of "ventilating" the blood.

肺循环的作用是给血液"通风"（即补充新鲜的氧）。

ventilation [ventiˈleiʃən] *n.* 通气，通风

The tube then blocks ventilation of the other main bronchus, and atelectasis may ensure.

此时阻塞了另一侧主支气管的通气，而产生肺不张。

For the patient to support effective spontaneous ventilation, mechanical dead space should be minimal.

为了让病人维持有效的自然通气，机械死腔应尽量减少。

ventilator [ˈventileitə] *n.* 通风器；呼吸机

"Smart" ventilators, helpful robots and gene therapy will be commonly used in ICU after 2000.
2000 年以后,漂亮的呼吸机,助人为乐的机器人和基因疗法将在重症监护病房中普遍使用。

ventral [ˈventrəl] *a.* 腹的;腹侧的,前侧的

At all levels of the cord, the efferent fibers in the ventral roots carry impulses out to the muscles.
在髓的所有平面,腹根的传出纤维将冲动传到肌肉。

The sclerosis of the ventral and lateral columns of the spinal cord may lead to spastic paraplegia.
脊髓前侧柱的硬化可导致强直性麻痹。

ventrally [ˈventrəli] *ad.* 前面地

The larynx projects ventrally between the great vessels of the neck.
喉在颈部大血管之间向前突出。

ventricle [ˈventrikl] *n.* 室;心室

Failure of only one ventricle is not common.
单侧心室衰竭少见。

Valves allow blood to pass from the auricles to ventricles, but not in the reverse direction.
瓣膜只能让血液从心房流到心室,而不能反向。

ventricular [venˈtrikjulə] *a.* 心室的

Ventricular rate in atrial fibrillation is controlled by digitalization.
房颤时的心室率可用洋地黄化控制。

ventriculostomy [venˌtrikjuˈlɔstəmi] *n.* 脑室造口术

Which is the best radiological technique to demonstrate spontaneous or endoscopic third ventriculostomy?
哪种是最好的放射技术可展示自发性或者内镜下第三脑室造口术?

Endoscopic third ventriculostomy (ETV) has now been accepted widely as a safe procedure for treatment of non-communicating hydrocephalus.
内镜下第三脑室造口术已成为公认的治疗阻塞性脑积水的安全手段。

venule [ˈvenjuːl] *n.* 小静脉

The smallest veins are called venules.
最小静脉称为小静脉。

As a result of endothelial damage to capillaries, fluid is lost across capillaries and venules into interstitial space.
由于毛细血管内壁损伤,体液通过毛细血管和小静脉进入间质空隙而失去。

verapamil [vəˈræpəmil] *n.* 维拉帕米,异搏定

Verapamil is the most widely used anti-arrhythmic drug in this class.
维拉帕米是此类抗心律失常药中最常用的。

Verapamil can result in bradycardia and AV block, so combination with beta blockers is generally avoided.
异搏定能引起心动过缓和房室传导阻滞,因此,一般来说,应避免与 β 受体拮抗剂联合使用。

verbal [ˈvəːbəl] *a.* 语言的

Patients experience a number of uncomfortable sensations related to breathing and use a large number of verbal expressions to describe these sensations.
病人感到许多与呼吸有关的不舒服的感觉,并使用许多语言词句来描述这些感觉。

verbatim [vəːˈbeitim] *a.* 逐字表述的,直接表述的

Since reporters may use different verbatim terms to describe the same adverse drug event, it is recommended that sponsors apply coding conventions to code the verbatim terms.
由于报告人员可使用不同的表述术语来描述同样的不良药物事件,建议申办方用编码规则对这些直接表述的术语进行编码。

verge [vəːdʒ] *n.* 边缘

The patient was on the verge of death.

病人危在旦夕。

This drove me to the verge of distraction.

这使我几乎陷入了精神错乱的境地。

verification [ˌverifiˈkeiʃən] *n.* 证实，验证

Pathologic verification of malignant tumors must be present before any therapy is instituted.

恶性肿瘤开始任何治疗之前，必须先有病理证明。

This finding is needed for the verification of the diagnosis.

这个发现对确诊是必要的。

verify [ˈverifai] *v.* 证实，验证

Later findings verified the scientist's theory.

随后的发现证实了那位科学家的理论。

The first step of our treatment of cystic disease is to verify the diagnosis.

我们治疗囊肿性疾病的第一步是确诊。

vermox [ˈvəːmɔks] *n.* 安乐士

Vermox is a tablet in dosage form which is quite effective in treating pinworm infection.

安乐士为片剂剂型，治疗蛲虫感染十分有效。

verruca [veˈruːkə] (*pl.* verrucae [veˈruːsiː]) *n.* 疣

There may be fresh verrucae superimposed on the healed lesions.

在已愈合的病变上，可以出现新的疣赘物。

versatile [ˈvəːsətail] *a.* 多方面的；通用的

Computed tomography has proven to be most versatile and is widely accepted and used.

计算机断层扫描术已证实具有多方面的用途，并得到了广泛的认可和采用。

versatility [ˌvəːsəˈtiliti] *n.* 多面性

The metabolic versatility of the cells will be greatly reduced.

细胞的各种代谢功能将会大大降低。

versed [vəːst] *a.* 熟练的，精通的

He is well versed in the science of optics.

他精通光学。

An artist should be versed in various spheres of art.

一个艺术家应该精通各个门类的艺术。

version [ˈvəːʃən] *n.* 版本，译本；（胎位）倒转术

This dictionary is available in electronic version.

这部词典有电子版。

It eliminates the need to save your work, automatically saving every version of every document.

它让你无需手动存储，而是自动保存每个文档的每个版本。

If the fetus is oblique or transverse, external version is immediately performed to bring one pole of the fetus over the cervix.

如果是斜产式或横产式，可立即行外倒转术，使胎儿的头或臀在宫颈上方。

vertebra [ˈvəːtibrə] (*pl.* vertebrae [ˈvəːtibriː]) *n.* 椎骨

The vertebrae are joined to one another by means of strong ligaments.

椎骨通过牢固的韧带互相连接起来。

vertebral [ˈvəːtibrəl] *a.* 脊椎的

Diving, falling from a height, and automobile crashes are the most frequent causes of vertebral fractures.

跳水、从高处跌落和撞车是脊椎骨折最常见的原因。

These cases are diagnosed after trauma to the vertebral column.

这些病例是在脊椎遭受外伤之后加以诊断的。

vertebrate ['vəːtibrit] *n.* 脊椎动物

In vertebrates, immunity is divided into two major categories: natural immunity and acquired immunity.

在脊椎动物中,免疫力分为两大类:自然免疫力和获得免疫力。

In vertebrates, the liver is the richest source of enzymes catalyzing biotransformation reaction.

在脊椎动物中,肝脏是那些催化生物转化反应的酶类的最主要来源处。

vertical ['vəːtikəl] *a.* 垂直的

The vertical axis in the graph represents arterial pressure.

曲线图中的垂直轴代表动脉压。

Vertical bars represent one standard deviation.

(图中)纵轴代表一个标准差。

vertigo ['vəːtigəu] (*pl.* vertigoes 或 vertigines[vəː'tidʒiniːz]) *n.* [拉]眩晕

Vertigo is characterized by a sensation or illusion of rotation of the surroundings or of the self.

一种感到自身或周围环境旋转的感觉或幻觉是眩晕的特征。

For example, vertigo may indicate the possibility of Meniere's disease.

例如,眩晕可提示患有梅尼埃氏病的可能。

verumontanum [ˌveru'mɔntənəm] *n.* 精阜

We reported the case of a 61-year-old man with a primary carcinoid tumor of the verumontanum.

我们报道了一起61岁男性精阜原发性类癌瘤的病例。

The absence of the verumontanum at voiding cystourethrography correlates with verumontanum and prostate hypoplasia.

排尿期膀胱尿道造影时精阜不显影与精阜和前列腺的发育不良有关。

vesical ['vesikəl] *a.* 膀胱的

All the 8 patients were diagnosed as vesical transitional cell carcinoma on cystoscopy and biopsy.

8例患者均经膀胱镜检查及活检证实为膀胱移行细胞癌。

Pudendal arteries can arise from the obturator, inferior vesical and superior vesical arteries.

阴部内动脉可以起源于闭孔动脉、膀胱下动脉和膀胱上动脉。

vesicant ['vesikənt] *n.* 起疱剂, *a.* 起疱的

The mustard gas is a potent vesicant, which caused a topical burn to skin, mucosa, eyes and lungs.

芥子气是一种强力起疱剂,能导致皮肤、黏膜、眼和肺的局部灼伤。

vesicle ['vesikl] *n.* 囊泡

The vesicle then breaks away from the cell membrane into the interior of the cell.

然后囊泡脱离细胞膜进入细胞内。

The vesicles are thought to contain the chemical transmitter substance.

医学研究认为水疱中含有化学介质。

vesicoureteral [ˌvesikəujuə'riːtərəl] *a.* 膀胱输尿管的

The underlying cause of vesicoureteral reflex, its importance, and its management have received extensive urologic attention and led to controversy.

膀胱输尿管反流的根本原因,其重要性和处理已受到泌尿学广泛关注并导致(学术上)争论。

vesicular [vi'sikjulə] *a.* 囊状的,泡状的;水疱的

Small raised vesicular lesions may appear on the buccal mucosa.

口腔黏膜会出现凸起的小水疱。

The vesicular eruption tends to spread by extension and, unless checked, may involve the entire sole.

水疱性皮疹如不加以控制则易播散累及整个足底。

Vesivirus [ˌvesiˈvaiərəs] *n.* 水疱疹病毒属

Pathogenic caliciviruses of the genus Vesivirus circulate in oceanic ecosystems and spread to and among terrestrial mammals.

水疱疹病毒属中的致病性杯状病毒在海洋生态系中循环，扩散到陆生动物并在其中又扩散。

These results justify further investigation of an association between Vesivirus infection and illness in humans.

这些结果进一步为水疱疹病毒与人类疾病关系的研究提供了佐证。

vessel [ˈvesl] *n.* 管，血管

Veins are the vessels along which the blood flows back to the heart.

静脉是血液沿着流回心脏的血管。

There is evidence that walking may actually open up narrowed areas in the coronary blood vessels.

有证据表明，散步可使业已狭窄的冠状血管变宽。

vestibular [vesˈtibjulə] *a.* 前庭的

If the induced vestibular sensation is the same feeling as the patient's symptom, it is of vestibular origin.

如果诱发出来的前庭知觉和病人症状有相同的感受，那么（疾病）就来源于前庭。

vestibule [ˈvestibjuːl] *n.* 前庭

Next to the oval window is the vestibule.

紧接着卵圆窗的是前庭。

In newborns and small children, the vestibule and the vagina still possess a form of columnar epithelium.

新生儿和幼儿的阴道和前庭还处在柱状上皮形成过程中。

vestibulopathy [vesˈtibjuləˌpəθi] *n.* 前庭疾病

Acute vestibulopathy is made worse by head movement, and reduced by absolute stillness.

急性前庭疾病由于头部活动加重，绝对的静止则可缓解。

veterinarian [ˌvetəriˈnɛəriən] *n.* 兽医

This veterinarian has twenty years' practical experience.

这位兽医有20年的实际经验。

via [ˈvaiə] *prep.* 经过，通过

Most roundworms are transmitted via excreta.

大部分的圆体虫是由粪便传播的。

A few cases of human-to-human rabies transmission via corneal transplantation have been reported.

据报道，少数人传人的狂犬病是通过角膜移植传播的。

viable [ˈvaiəbl] *a.* 能生存的，能活的

The tubercle bacillus dried in sputum remains viable for even longer period of time.

结核杆菌在痰中干燥后存活的时间甚至还要长些。

vibrate [vaiˈbreit] *v.* 颤动，振动

The sound waves enter the external auditory canal and cause the eardrum to vibrate.

声波进入外耳道引起鼓膜振动。

Testing the hearing by bone conductions is accomplished by placing the stem of a vibrating tuning fork in contact with the head.

测试骨传导听力可通过将振动的音叉柄与头部接触来完成。

vibration [vaiˈbreiʃən] *n.* 振动，颤动

These vibration are amplified by the ossicles and transmitted by them to the perilymph.

这些振动由小骨扩大并传送至外淋巴。

Physical factors such as cold, light, water, vibrations, and pressure can cause urticaria.
物理因素如寒冷、光、水、振动以及压力都可引起荨麻疹。

vibrio ['vibriəu] *n.* 弧菌

Vibrio cholerae can live on some species of plankton.
霍乱弧菌可以靠一些浮游生物生存。

It is estimated that more than 30,000 people have fallen ill with acute watery diarrhoea, among which 3,315 were identified as positive for vibrio cholerae.
据估计有 3 万多人患急性水样腹泻,其中 3315 例被鉴定为霍乱弧菌阳性。

vibriocidal [ˌvibriəu'saidəl] *a.* 杀弧菌的(尤杀霍乱弧菌)

Serologic diagnosis requires demonstration of rises in agglutinating or vibriocidal antibody titers.
血清学诊断需要观察凝集滴度或杀弧菌的抗体滴度的升高。

vibriosis [ˌvibri'əusis] *n.* 弧菌病

This paper discusses the progress of research in the prevention and cure of vibriosis in aquatic animals.
本文探讨了海水养殖动物弧菌病防治的研究进展。

Eel vibriosis is one of the main diseases detected during the eel culture with great risk and high mortality.
鳗鲡弧菌病是鳗鲡养殖中主要的疾病之一,危害大,死亡率高。

vicinity [vi'siniti] *n.* 附近,邻近,近处

The patients have resided for many years in areas that were in the vicinity of mines.
这些患者已在靠近矿的地区生活了多年。

The adult female moves outside to the vicinity of the anus to lay its thousands of eggs.
雌性成虫会爬到体外肛门附近处产下数以千计的虫卵。

vicious ['viʃəs] *a.* 有毛病的;恶性的

Blood viscosity is increased, therefore a vicious circle is established.
血液的黏滞度增加,因而形成恶性循环。

victim ['viktim] *n.* 受害者;牺牲者;患者

The victims of the accident were taken to the hospital nearby.
事故的受害者被送往附近医院。

Facial paralysis is a terrible affliction, for it deprives the victim of emotional expression.
面神经麻痹是一种可怕的折磨,因为它剥夺了患者的表情能力。

Many leucocytes fall victims to the bacteria's deadly poisons.
许多白细胞死于该细菌的剧毒。

videolaseroscopy [ˌvidiəuleizə'rɔskəpi] *n.* 激光影像镜检

The most remarkable thing about videolaseroscopy is its potential to make operations less invasive and costly.
用激光影像镜检做手术最显著的潜力是减少创伤,节省费用。

videotape ['vidiəuteip] *n.* 录像带

Since each operation was recorded on videotape, patients would get vivid records of their own internal organs.
由于每次手术都录在录像带上,病人可以看到他们自己体内现状的清晰记录。

view [vjuː] *v.* 看,仔细观察

To view the retina, one needs an ophthalmoscope.
观察视网膜需要借助于眼底镜。

The solution is viewed under bright illumination.
在照明灯下观察溶液。

n. 观点

From the radiologic point of view, the infiltrates in viral pneumonia tend to be diffuse, ill-defined

and hazy.
从放射学的观点来看，病毒性肺炎的浸润往往是弥漫性的，界限不清和模糊。

viewpoint ['vjuːˌpɔint] *n.* 观点
From a clinic viewpoint, the mixed lymphocyte response assay measures responses involved in graft rejection and graft-vs-host reactions.
从临床观点看，混合淋巴细胞反应测定法测得的反应包括移植排异反应和移植物抗宿主反应。

vigorous ['vigərəs] *a.* 精力充沛的，强有力的
A man of his age must be very vigorous.
像他这样年纪的人一定是精力充沛的。
It is not well to engage in vigorous exercise immediately following a meal.
饭后立即从事激烈的运动是不妥当的。
The blood flow may be increased by more rapid and vigorous heart action.
心脏活动加快和增强可使血流增加。
It is only after vigorous medical therapy has failed that operative removal should be considered.
只有在药物积极治疗失败后，才应考虑进行手术切除。

vigour ['vigə] *n.* 活力；健壮
Lack of vigour may show itself in the intellectual or emotional spheres.
在其自身理智和感情方面均可出现缺乏活力的现象。

villous ['viləs] *a.* 绒毛的，绒毛状的
Abnormality of villous epithelial cells was felt to be the major cause of the functional abnormality.
上皮细胞绒毛的异常被认为是这种功能异常的主要原因。

villus ['viləs] *n.* (*pl.* villi) [脊椎]绒毛，长茸毛
Chorionic villus sampling (CVS) is a test done during early pregnancy that can find certain problems with your baby (fetus).
绒毛膜绒毛取样是怀孕早期用来检测胎儿异常的一种检测方法。
Intestinal villi are tiny, finger-like projections that protrude from the epithelial lining of the intestinal wall.
小肠绒毛是从小肠壁上皮层突出的细小、指状突起。

vimentin ['vimentin] *n.* 波形蛋白
Vimentin, a major constituent of the intermediate filament family of proteins, is ubiquitously expressed in normal mesenchymal cells.
波形蛋白，中间丝蛋白家族的主要成分，广泛表达于正常间充质细胞。
Vimentin's overexpression in cancer correlates well with accelerated tumor growth, invasion, and poor prognosis.
波形蛋白在癌症中的过表达与肿瘤生长加速、浸润和预后不良相关。

vincristine [vin'kristiːn] *n.* 长春新碱
The child was induced with prednisone, vincristine sulfate and 6-mercaptopurine.
以强的松、硫酸长春新碱和6-巯基嘌呤对患儿做了诱导治疗。

violate ['vaiəleit] *v.* 违反，侵犯
Whoever violates this law will be subjected to difficulty.
谁违反这条规律，谁就会遭到麻烦。

violent ['vaiələnt] *a.* 猛烈的，由暴力引起的
If an injury of any sort causes or contributes to death, the manner of death is violent.
如果任何一种损伤引起死亡，则死亡的方式为暴力性的。

violet ['vaiəlit] *n.* 紫罗兰色，紫色
Commonly used basic dyes are crystal violet.

常用的碱性染料是结晶紫。

Gentian violet is a dye with antibacterial antifungl properties, applied topically in the treatment of infections of the skin and mucous membrane.

龙胆紫是一种有抗菌和抗霉菌特性的染料，用于局部治疗皮肤和黏膜的感染。

vipoma [viˈpəumə] *n.* 血管活性肠肽瘤

Vipoma is a very rare type of cancer that usually grows from cells in the pancreas called islet cells.

血管活性肠肽瘤是一种非常罕见的肿瘤，通常由称作胰岛细胞的胰腺内细胞发展而来。

The Vipoma syndrome is caused by excessive, unregulated secretion of VIP by the tumor.

血管活性肠肽瘤综合征是由于肿瘤不受调节的、过度的分泌血管活性肠肽(VIP)而引起。

viral [ˈvaiərəl] *a.* 病毒的

The cause of the persistence of viral infection in some cases is not known.

有些患者的持续性病毒感染的原因还不清楚。

For prevention patients with viral hepatitis should be isolated and treated promptly.

为了预防，患病毒性肝炎的病人应被隔离并进行及时治疗。

Viral encephalitis and meningitis are relatively common pediatric illnesses.

病毒性脑炎和脑膜炎是两种相对常见的儿科疾病。

viremia [vaiəˈriːmiə] *n.* 病毒血症

This virus typically infects infants during the first month of life producing a vesicular rash, viremia, and subsequent infection of multiple organs.

该病毒在出生后一个月内的典型感染可产生疱疹样皮疹、病毒血症和继之而来的多器官感染。

virgin [ˈvəːdʒin] *n.* 处女

The patient with atrophic vaginitis is a young virgin.

患萎缩性阴道炎的病人是一个年轻的处女。

virilescence [ˌviriˈlesəns] *n.* (女性的)男性化

The core of the spirit of Western culture is the rational spirit of virilescence.

西方文化精神的核心是女性男性化的理性精神。

Virilescence is a condition of some animals, especially of some fowls, in which the female, when old, assumes some of the characteristics of the males of the species.

雌性雄性化指某些动物，尤其是雌性禽类衰老时呈现出同类雄性的某些特征。

virilism [ˈvirilizəm] *n.* 男性化

The symptoms and signs are those of virilism, with deepening of the voice, hirsutes, acne and amenorrhoea.

症状和体征为男性化，表现为音调低沉、多毛、痤疮、闭经等。

virion [ˈvaiəriɔn] *n.* 病毒体，病毒颗粒

This provirus is capable of replication and production of new virions.

这种前病毒能复制、产生新的病毒体。

The morphologically complete(mature) infectious virus particle is called virion.

形态学完整的(成熟的)具有感染性的病毒颗粒被称为病毒粒子。

viroid [ˈvaiərɔid] *n.* 类病毒

Viroid are made of an RNA molecule only.

类病毒仅由一个 RNA 分子组成 。

Viruses are simple enough, but viroids are even simpler.

病毒已够简单，但类病毒更简单。

virology [ˌvaiəˈrɔlədʒi] *n.* 病毒学

Virology is a branch of microbiology which is concerned with viruses and viral diseases.

病毒学是微生物学的分支，它的内容涉及病毒和病毒性疾病。

virome ['vairəum] *n.* 病毒组

The genomes of all the viruses that inhabit a particular organism or environment are called virome.

寄居在一个特定机体或环境中的全部病毒的基因组称为病毒组。

All viral genomes in a human body would be collected in a database called the "human virome."

人体内的所有病毒基因组将被收集到一个被称为"人类病毒组"的数据库中.

virtually ['vəːtjuəli] *ad.* 实际上,事实上

Deficiencies in every enzyme reaction are virtually associated with a congenital hemolytic anemia.

每种酶反应的不足实际上都与先天性溶血性贫血有关。

Infectiousness of tertiary syphilis is virtually nil, even for a fetus.

三期梅毒实际上无传染性,即使对于胎儿也无传染。

The one period of life that virtually no one remembers is the years before the age about four.

一生中实际上没能记住的阶段是大约 4 岁以前的时光。

virtue ['vəːtjuː] *n.* 优点,美德

Among his many virtues are high responsibility, creative thinking and pioneering spirit.

他有许多美德,如高度责任感、创新思维和开拓精神。

The kidney is particularly vulnerable to nephrotoxic renal injury by virtue of its rich blood supply.

由于肾脏血供丰富,故特别容易发生肾毒性损害。

virucide ['vaiərəsaid] *n.* 杀病毒剂

Similarly, the terms fungicide, virucide, and sporicide refer to agents that kill fungi, viruses, and spores respectively.

同样,杀真菌剂、杀病毒剂和杀孢子剂等术语分别是指杀真菌、杀病毒和杀孢子的制剂。

virulence ['viruləns] *n.* 毒力,毒性

The capsule often acts as a virulence factor.

荚膜常可起毒力因子作用。

The character of the inflammation varies exceedingly according to the virulence of the pathogen.

炎症的性质依病原体毒性的大小而有很大的不同。

virulent ['virjulənt] *a.* 有毒力的,致病力强的

When the causative bacteria is highly virulent, a normal heart may be affected by endocarditis.

当病原菌毒力极高时,正常的心脏也可受到心内膜炎的影响。

They discovered that these germs gradually lost their virulent power upon exposure to the air.

他们发现这些细菌接触空气就会逐渐失去其致病的活力。

viruria [vaiə'rjuəriə] *n.* 病毒尿

The incidence of maternal infection at the time of delivery, as determined by viruria, is 3%-4%.

母体在分娩时的急性感染通过发现病毒尿可以确诊,发生率为 3% ~4%。

virus ['vaiərəs] *n.* 病毒

Viruses are extremely tiny microorganisms that cause disease.

病毒是能引起疾病的极小微生物。

Blood transfusion units now screen all donor blood for the presence of hepatitis B virus.

输血中心目前正对所有的供血进行是否含有乙型肝炎病毒的普查。

There was no history of contact with cases of virus hepatitis.

没有接触过病毒性肝炎患者的历史。

Infectious hepatitis is produced by an unidentified hepatitis virus A.

传染性肝炎是由一种尚未被鉴别的甲型肝炎病毒所引起的。

visceral ['visərəl] *a.* 内脏的

The pain in acute intestinal obstruction is visceral and is therefore felt centrally and usually in the umbilical area.

急性肠梗阻的疼痛是内脏性的，所以感觉在腹部中央，通常在脐的周围。

By means of somatic and visceral reflexes, we make moderately rapid adjustments of the body to environmental changes.

我们可以借助躯体反射和内脏反射两者来对身体周围环境的变化作出快速的调节。

viscid ['visid] *a.* 黏的

At all events the secretion emerging from the ducts is a viscid mucous fluid.

总之，从管道排出的分泌物是一种黏稠的液体。

viscoelasticity [ˌviskəuˌilæs'tisiti] *n.* 黏弹性

Viscoelasticity is the property of materials that exhibit both viscous and elastic characteristics when undergoing deformation.

黏弹性是材料发生变形时表现出的黏性和弹性特征的性质。

Viscoelasticity is a rheological parameter that describes the flow properties of complex fluids like blood.

黏弹性是描述复杂流体（如血液）的流动特性的一种流变参数。

viscosity [vis'kɔsiti] *n.* 黏（滞）度，黏（滞）性

An increase in vascular permeability and loss of plasma water raises the viscosity of the blood.

血管通透性增加和血浆水分丧失使血液黏稠度增高。

viscous ['viskəs] *a.* 黏的，黏性的

The exudate becomes viscous in the 6th-7th week of chronic urethral gonorrhea.

在慢性尿道淋病第 6 ~ 7 周，其渗出物有些黏稠。

viscus ['viskəs] (*pl.* viscera ['visərə]) *n.* 内脏

The cancer is low in malignancy if contrasted with those affecting viscera.

如与脏器癌相比，这种癌毒性低。

The pain of viscus is poorly localized and its borders are only vaguely delineated.

内脏的疼痛不易确定，其边界只能模糊地加以描述。

visfatin [vis'fætin] *n.* 内脏脂肪素

At the same time, their plasma visfatin and other relevant glycolipid metabolism indices in blood were tested.

同时，检测了他们血中内脏脂肪素的水平及相关糖脂代谢指标。

Visfatin is a newly discovered novel adipokine existing universally in visceral adipose tissue of humans and mice.

内脂素是新近发现的一种广泛存在于人和小鼠的内脏脂肪组织中的脂肪细胞因子。

visible ['vizəbl] *a.* 可见的，明显的

A 2 to 3mm corneal abrasion may be visible without magnification.

一个 2 至 3 毫米的角膜擦伤不用放大即可被看见。

Visible light can harm the eyes if it is too intense.

如果可见光过于强烈，它能伤害眼睛。

In chronic intestinal obstruction there may be recurrent colicky pain accompanied by visible peristalsis.

慢性肠梗阻时，可有反复的绞痛，并伴有明显的肠蠕动波。

vision ['viʒən] *n.* 视觉，视力，视敏度

These are the receptors for the sense of vision.

这些都是视觉感受器。

On occasion, leukemia may present as difficulty in vision.

白血病偶尔可表现为视觉障碍。

Patients with myopia have decreased distance vision, but good near acuity.

近视患者远距离视敏度降低，但近距离视敏度良好。

visual ['vizjuəl] *a.* 视觉的，视力的

Another rather common visual defect is astigmatism.
另一相当常见的视力缺陷是散光。
Visual loss can result from abnormalities anywhere from the front of the eye to the back of the brain.
从眼睛到大脑后方任何部位的异常都可引起视力丧失。
Routine physical examinations should include measurement of visual acuity.
常规体检应当包括视敏度的检查。

visualization [ˌvizjuəlai'zeiʃən] *n.* 显现，观看
Staining the bacteria is a procedure that permits the visualization of the general shape.
通过染色能观察到细菌的基本形态。
Visualization may be greatly enchanced by the use of these techniques.
使用这类技术能使可见度大为增加。

visualize ['vizjuəlaiz] *v.* 使可见，显现
It is our belief that the entire extrahepatic biliary system should be visualized at once during each injection.
我们认为在每次注入造影剂后，整个肝外胆管系统应该显示影像。

visuospatial [ˌvizjuəu'speiʃəl] *a.* 视觉空间的
Visuospatial functions represent the brain's highest level of visual processing.
视觉空间功能代表大脑视觉加工的最高水平。
Visuospatial construction processes enable you to reproduce drawings.
视觉空间的建立过程可使人进行图画再现。

vital ['vaitəl] *a.* 生命的，重要的，必不可少的
The patient' s vital signs were normal.
该患者的生命体征正常。
A flare-up of a syphilitic inflammation in a vital structure may have serious consequences.
有关生命器官的梅毒炎症加剧，会产生严重的后果。
The nucleus is vital for the continued life of the cell.
对于细胞的继续生存来说，细胞核是必不可少的。
It was vital that persons were aware of the symptoms of the illness and sought prompt advice from doctors if this was suspected.
人们注意到此病的症状，如果有所怀疑便迅速就医，这一点是至关重要的。

vitality [vai'tæliti] *n.* 活力，精力
With the decay of vitality, the thought of rest will be not unwelcome.
随着精力的衰退，退休的意图不见得不受欢迎。

vitamin ['vaitəmin, 'vitəmin] *n.* 维生素
Vitamins are organic compounds that found in the diet.
维生素是存在于食物中的有机化合物。
Vitamin needs vary among organisms.
不同生物对维生素的需求不同。
Vitamin D intoxication results from chronic ingestion of large doses of vitamin D.
长期摄入过量维生素 D 会引起维生素 D 中毒。

vitreous ['vitriəs] *n.* 玻璃体
Haemorrhage into the vitreous causes sudden blindness.
玻璃体内出血可造成突然失明。

vitrification [ˌvitrifi'keiʃən] *n.* 玻璃化冷冻
An important application is the vitrification of an antifreeze-like liquid in cryopreservation.
抗冻样液体的玻璃化冷冻是在低温保存中的一种重要应用。
Vitrification is a proven technique in the disposal and long-term storage of nuclear waste or other

hazardous wastes.
玻璃化冷冻是处理及长期保存核废料及其他有害废物的成熟技术。

vitro [ˈviːtrəu]【拉】*n.* 试管;体外

In this research, vitro tests of cytotoxicological method were used to evaluate mutagenicity of thallium.
在这项研究中,采用了体外细胞毒性方法来评估铊的致突变作用。
In vitro fertilization is the most common type of assisted reproductive technology.
体外受精是最常用的辅助生殖技术。

vitronectin [ˈviːtrəunektin] *n.* 玻璃体结合蛋白,玻璃体粘连蛋白

Vitronectin is a glycoprotein of blood plasma that promotes cell adhesion and migration and is similar to fibronectin.
玻璃体结合蛋白是血浆中的一种糖蛋白,可促进细胞粘连和迁移,与纤维连接蛋白相似。

vivo [ˈviːvəu]【拉】*n.* 活体;体内

With the advances of magnetic resonance technology, studies can be done in vivo about brain morphous and function.
随着磁共振技术的发展,已可以进行活体大脑形态和功能的研究。
In vivo RNAi experiments are more challenging than their in vitro counterparts.
体内 RNA 干扰实验比相应的体外实验更具有挑战性。

vocal [ˈvəukəl] *a.* 发声的;嗓音的;言语的

Vocal cords extend across the larynx.
声带横贯喉部。
Hoarseness is the earliest and principal manifestation of vocal cord tumor.
声音嘶哑是患声带肿瘤时最早、也是最重要的表现。

void [vɔid] *v.* 排泄,放出;使…无效

The patient should void before pelvic examination except when stress incontinence of urine is to be demonstrated.
除证明有张力性尿失禁外,盆腔检查前要排空膀胱。
a. 无效的
This prescription is void because the doctor did not sign it.
这张处方无效,因为医生没有在上面签字。

volatile [ˈvɔlətail] *a.* 易挥发的,挥发性的

Volatile anesthetics are eliminated by the lungs.
易挥发的麻醉剂经肺排出。
This is especially true for gases such as carbon monoxide and for vapors of volatile liquids such as benzene.
对于一氧化碳等气体和苯等挥发性液体的蒸气尤其如此。
The volatile oil occurs in aromatic plants to which it gives odor and other characteristics.
挥发油出现在芳香植物中,他们具有香味和其他特征。

volume [ˈvɔljuːm] *n.* 容量

There is general agreement that early shock is usually due to decrease in blood volume, or an increase in the capacity of the vascular space, or both.
一般认为早期休克通常是由于血量减少或血管腔容积增大,或二者并存所致。

voluntary [ˈvɔləntəri] *a.* 随意的

This muscle is known as voluntary because it is under the control of the will.
这种肌肉称为随意肌,因为它受意志的控制。
The motor area of one hemisphere controls voluntary movements of the other side of the body.
一侧大脑半球的运动区控制着对侧身体的随意运动。

volvulus [ˈvɔlvjuləs] *n.* 肠扭转

Colonic obstruction is, except in the case of volvulus, chronic.
结肠梗阻,除患有肠扭转的情况外,是慢性的。
Chronic gastric volvulus is rare but is probably underdiagnosed.
慢性胃肠扭转很少见,但也有可能被漏诊。

vomit [ˈvɔmit] *v.* 呕吐
Nausea and vomiting may occur with most abdominal disorders.
恶心和呕吐可见于大多数腹部疾病。
Gastric crisis with severe pain and vomitting is the most frequent symptom of tabes dorsalis.
脊髓痨最常见的症状是胃危象,其表现多为剧痛和呕吐。

vomiting [ˈvɔmitiŋ] *n.* 呕吐;呕吐物;催吐药
An abrupt attack of vomiting usually ushers in this disease, along with irritability, general weakness, and discomfort.
此病通常以呕吐的突然发作作为先兆,并伴有激动、全身无力以及不适。
The medulla oblongata controls respiration, swallowing, vomiting, and other basic physiological functions.
延髓控制呼吸、吞咽、呕吐及其他基本生理功能。

vomitus [ˈvɔmitəs] *n.* 呕吐物;呕吐
The absence of bile in the vomitus is a feature of pyloric stenosis.
呕吐物中无胆汁是幽门狭窄的特点。
Replacement of water and electrolytes lost in stool and vomitus is the basis of cholera therapy.
补充腹泻及呕吐所丢失的水和电解质是治疗霍乱的基础。

voxel [vɔkˈsəl] *n.* 体素
The matter density within every small unit can be expressed by 1 CT value, so these small units are named voxel which is a 3-D concept.
任一小单位内的物质密度由一个 CT 值表达,因此这些小单位就叫体素,体素是一个三维的概念。

vulgaris [ˈvʌlgəris] *a.* 寻常的,普通的
Acne vulgaris is a common and frequently encountered disease among the pubertal people.
普通痤疮是青春期人群的常见病和多发病。
Enhancing health education to patients with psoriasis vulgaris could reduce the morbidity of erythrodermic psoriasis.
加强对寻常型银屑病患者的健康指导能够降低红皮病型银屑病的发病率。

vulnerable (**to**) [ˈvʌlnərəbl] *a.* 易受伤的,易损的
Its toxins create more ischemic and vulnerable tissue.
其毒素造成更广泛的缺血组织和易损组织。
Malignant cells are also vulnerable to degeneration.
恶性肿瘤细胞也容易变性。

vulnerability [ˌvʌlnərəˈbiliti] *n.* 脆弱性;易患病性
There is clear evidence that genetic factors contribute to vulnerability to many physical conditions.
明显的证据显示,遗传因素造成对很多种身体疾病的易感性。

vulva [ˈvʌlvə] (*pl.* vulvae [ˈvʌlviː]) *n.* [拉]外阴,女阴
An understanding of the lymph drainage of the vulva is essential as a basis for treatment.
掌握外阴的淋巴回流是治疗的基础。
The anogenital area is especially susceptible: common problems are pruritus ani and pruritus vulvae or scroti.
肛门与生殖器区对痒特别敏感:常见的病症是肛门瘙痒症和女阴瘙痒症或阴囊瘙痒症。

vulvar [ˈvʌlvə] *a.* 外阴的

Squamous cell carcinoma is the most common histologic type of vulvar cancer.
鳞状细胞癌是外阴癌最常见的组织学类型。

Classic vulvar intraepithelial neoplasia is characterized by nuclear atypia of the squamous cells, increased mitoses, and lack of cellular maturation.
经典的外阴上皮内瘤变的特征是鳞状细胞核异型、核分裂增多和细胞成熟丧失。

vulvectomy [vʌl'vektəmi] *n.* 外阴切除术

The overall 5-year survival from radical vulvectomy in the best hands is 70%.
即使是最好的医生做的根治性外阴切除术，术后病人的5年存活率也只有70%。

vulvitis [vʌl'vaitis] *n.* 外阴炎

Because vaginitis in children is usually accompanied by secondary vulvitis, the term vulvovaginitis is often used.
由于儿童阴道炎常伴随继发性外阴炎，故常用外阴阴道炎一词。

vulvovaginal [vʌlvə'dʒainəl] *a.* 外阴阴道的

The incidence of vulvovaginal candidiasis (VVC) was significantly higher in pregnant women with gestational diabetes mellitus (GDM) than in the control group.
糖尿病妊娠妇女外阴阴道假丝酵母菌病发病率显著高于对照组。

W

wakefulness [ˈweikfulnis] *n.* 觉醒，不眠

Evidence demonstrates that the total synaptic weight is associated with circadian rhythm, with wakefulness and sleep.

证据显示总的突触权重与生理节律、觉醒和睡眠有关。

Prolonged wakefulness is associated not only with obvious changes in the way we feel but also with seizures and hallucinations.

持续觉醒不仅与我们的感受的明显变化有关，还与惊厥和幻觉有关。

walking [ˈwɔːkiŋ] *n.* 步行

Thus DNA vectors that are used to clone large pieces of DNA are particularly valuable in chromosome walking.

因而，用于克隆大片段 DNA 的 DNA 载体在染色体步移中特别有价值。

ward [wɔːd] *n.* 病房，病室

Dr. Smith is making ward round and he is to come back in two hours.

史密斯医生正在查房，2 小时后可以返回。

The first ward is on the second floor and the fourth, on the third.

第一病房在二楼，第四病房在三楼。

The patient was taken into the isolation ward.

该病人被送进了隔离病房。

warn [wɔːn] *v.* 警告，预告

The doctor warned me not to overstrain my eyes in watching TV.

医生告诫我不要因看电视而让眼睛过度疲劳。

Many nations have made enormous efforts to warn people of the dangers of smoking.

许多国家已尽了极大努力警告人们吸烟的危害性。

Common examples include warning patients of medical conditions that may be dangerous.

常见的例子如预先通知病人可能会出现的危险的情况。

warning [ˈwɔːniŋ] *n.* 警告，预先通知；前兆

The warnings outlined previously in this chapter regarding hepatic toxicity with ketoconazole, apply here.

关于酮康唑对肝脏的毒性影响本章前面已有所告诫，此处依然适用。

Renal failure with oliguria or anuria supervenes without the warning persistent hypotension.

随着少尿症或无尿症的发生，可在无前兆的持续性低血压的情况下出现肾功能衰竭。

warrant [ˈwɔrənt] *v.* 使…有理由，保证

It warrants reemphasizing that in addition to relief of pain, treatment designed to prevent and care for shock should not wait until the burn can be properly dressed.

有必要再次强调，不仅解除疼痛，而且防治休克的工作亦不应拖到烧伤创面包扎后进行。

Anticoagulant administration or a pronounced bleeding tendency warrants concern.

进行抗凝剂治疗或有明显出血倾向者应予以关注。

Every patient deserves and must be provided optimal care as warranted by the underlying medical institution.

就像基础卫生机构保证的那样，每位病人都应该得到最佳的照料。

wart [wɔːt] *n.* 疣

Most visible genital warts can be diagnosed clinically.
临床上可以诊断出大多数可见的生殖器疣。

washout [ˈwɔʃaut] *n.* 洗脱,消退
All of the patients with thyroid cancer had delayed washout contrast enhancement.
所有的甲状腺癌的患者都具有造影增强的延后消退。
The washout period lasted at least five half-lives according to the different psychotropic medications taken by the patients.
根据患者服用过的精神药物的不同,洗脱期持续至少 5 个半衰期。

waste [weist] *n.* 废物
The U. S generates about four billion tons of solid waste a year.
美国每年产生的固体废料约有 40 亿吨。
A reduced GFR leads to retention of nitrogenous waste products such as blood urea nitrogen and creatinine.
肾小球滤过率(GFR)降低导致产氮的废物如血尿素氮和肌酐蓄积。

wasted [weistid] *a.* 浪费的,消耗掉的
Whatever the clinical syndrome associated with chronic bronchitis and emphysema, there are to some degree increases in both wasted ventilation and wasted blood flow.
不论慢性支气管炎和肺气肿的临床表现如何,患者都有某种程度的无效通气和无效血流增加(的现象)。

wasteful [ˈweistfl] *a.* 浪费的,无用的
It's wasteful to keep so many medicines which you won't take all of them.
保存这么多药,你又不会都吃,这是一种浪费。
The transfer of electrons from nitrogenase to molecular nitrogen has an energetically wasteful side reaction.
从氮化酶转化成分子氮的电子传递过程伴有一种能量浪费的副反应。

wastewater [ˈweɪstˌwɔːtə] *n.* 废水,污水
The treatment of wastewater can be used to create energy and biodegradable plastics.
废水处理能够用于制造能源和可生物降解的塑料。
Wastewater, especially domestic wastewater, contains pathogens which can cause disease spread when not managed properly.
污水,特别是生活污水中含有病原体,如果不能正确管理可导致疾病传播。

wasting [ˈweistiŋ] *n.* 消瘦
Additional but inconstant features include muscle wasting, anemia, and vitamin B and C deficiency.
其他一些不是经常可以见到的表现包括肌肉消瘦、贫血、维生素 B 和 C 缺乏。

water [ˈwɔːtə] *n.* 水
Many measures are taken to control the water pollution.
已经采取许多措施来控制水污染。
Water is the largest component of the body, accounting for more than half of body weight.
水是身体最大的组成成分,占体重的一半以上。

water-borne [ˈwɔːtəbɔːn] *a.* 水传播的
Chloride is effective against the causative organisms of water-borne diseases.
氯对于消灭经水传播的病原细菌很有效。

water-soluble [ˈwɔːtəˈsɔljubl] *a.* 水溶性的
Vitamins are classified as either water-solube or fat-solube.
维生素可分为水溶性维生素和脂溶性维生素。
Lipid-soluble substances diffuse readily, while water-soluble substances do not diffuse, or diffuse poorly.

脂溶性物质易透过，而水溶性物质不透过或难以透过。

wavelet [ˈweivlit] *n.* 微波；子波

At present, mechanism of atrial fibrillation originates mainly from the multiple wavelet hypothesis and spin wave hypothesis.

目前认为房颤的发生机制主要源于多子波假说和自旋波假说。

For many years, the multiple-wavelet hypothesis was the dominant theory explaining the mechanism of AF.

多年来，多子波假说在解释房颤的机制中占主要地位。

weakness [ˈwiːknis] *n.* 无力，软弱

Muscle weakness or paralysis is the commonest symptom of interference with the motor system.

肌无力即瘫痪是运动系统障碍最常见的症状。

General symptoms include lassitude, weakness, fever, constipation and loss of weight.

一般症状包括倦怠、衰弱、发烧、便秘和体重减轻。

The loss of power on control of voluntary muscle is usually described by patients as "weakness".

病人常把随意肌控制能力的消失称为"虚弱"。

wean(from) [wiːn] *v.* 使断奶；使放弃(坏习惯)

The child has been "rashy" after she initially had dry skin at 6 months of age when she was weaned from the breast.

病儿在 6 个月断奶时开始有皮肤干燥，后患"皮疹"。

weary [ˈwiəri] *a.* 疲惫的，虚弱无力的

Her face looked strained and weary.

她的脸色显得憔悴疲惫。

The unaccustomed heat made him weary.

反常的炎热令他虚弱无力。

web server [web ˈsəːvə] *n.* 网络服务器

The web server is just one application.

网络服务器只是一个应用程序。

Every web server machine has an IP address.

每部网络服务器计算机有一个 IP 地址。

weigh [wei] *v.* 称；估量，权衡

The observed therapeutic benefits must be weighed against the serious side effects of the treatment.

应将所观察到的治疗效果与此种治疗的严重副作用权衡轻重。

weight [weit] *n.* 重量；体重

Environment seems to affect weight to a much greater extent than it does height.

环境对体重的影响似乎比对身高的影响大得多。

The amount an organism eats is strongly related to its weight.

生物的进食量与自身的体重密切相关。

well-being [ˈwel-biːiŋ] *n.* 健康；幸福；福利

Generally, eight hours of sleep are enough for the well-being of adults.

一般 8 小时睡眠对成年人的健康是足够的。

Exercise improves your circulation and general well-being.

锻炼可以改善和促进血液循环和全身健康。

well-known [ˈwelˈnəun] *a.* 众所周知的，熟悉的

Narcotic overdose is a well-known antecedent to pulmonary edema.

麻醉药过量是众所周知的肺水肿的原因。

Two well-known radioactive substances are radium and uranium.

镭和铀是人们熟悉的两种放射性物质。

wheal [hwiːl] *n.* 疹块,风团

Clothing which applies pressure to the skin appears to exacerbate the urticarial wheals.

使皮肤受压的衣着似乎能使荨麻疹风团加重。

wheelchair [ˈhwiːlˌtʃɛə] *n.* 轮椅,椅车

It is extremely important for the wheelchair to be properly fitted to the individual patient.

很重要的是轮椅必须完全适合每个病人使用。

wheeze [hwiːz] *v.* 喘息,喘鸣

At the age of 10 years frequent upper respiratory tract infection associated with cough and wheezing first began.

10 岁时开始频发上呼吸道感染伴咳嗽和喘息。

n. 喘息声,喘鸣

On auscultation, diffuse wheezes could be heard through both lung fields.

听诊时,两肺均可听到布满的喘鸣音。

whey [wei] *n.* 乳清,乳清蛋白

Whey constitutes about 70% of the volume of the milk used to make cheese.

用来制造奶酪的牛奶中,乳清约占其体积的 70%。

Milk's proteins (whey and casein) can make you feel more satisfied than sugary drinks.

牛奶蛋白(乳清蛋白和酪蛋白)比含糖饮料会使你觉得更满意。

whipworm [ˈhwipwəːm] *n.* (毛首)鞭虫

Infections with whipworm are common all over the world under unhygienic condition.

全世界卫生条件差的地方鞭虫感染很常见。

WHO 世界卫生组织

WHO (World Health Organization) is an international agency associated with the United Nations and based in Geneva.

世界卫生组织是一与联合国有关的国际机构,基地在日内瓦。

wholesome [ˈhəulsəm] *a.* 有利于健康的,有益于身心的

The things I like doing are mostly wholesome.

我所喜欢做的事情绝大多数是有益于健康的。

whooping-cough [ˈhuːpiŋkɔf] *n.* 百日咳

Whooping-cough is a highly communicable acute respiratory disease. The incubation period is 7-14 days and man is the only natural host.

百日咳是一高度传染性急性呼吸道疾病,潜伏期为 7～14 天,人是惟一的自然宿主。

Mumps, measles, and whooping-cough are all communicable diseases.

腮腺炎、麻疹和百日咳都是传染病。

widespread [ˈwaidspred] *a.* 广泛的,分布广的,普遍的

Shock is the state in which failure of the circulatory system to maintain adequate cellular perfusion results in widespread reduction in delivery of oxygen to tissue.

休克是一种由于循环系统不能维持足够的细胞灌流所致组织广泛的供氧减少的一种状态。

Trichophyton tonsurans is difficult to diagose clinically so it is probably far more widespread than is reported.

由于断发癣菌的临床诊断困难,所以它的蔓延很可能比报道的要多得多。

Currently, there has been widespread concern over the chrombogenic potential of contraceptive pills.

目前,普遍关心避孕丸引起血栓的可能性。

widow [ˈwidəu] *v.* 使丧偶

Some of the risk factors to be aware of include older divorced or widowed men, unemployment, poor physical health, past suicide attempt and psychosis.

需要警惕导致自杀的一些危险因素包括有年老离异或丧偶的男人、失业、疾病、曾有自杀企图和精神病。

wild [waild] *a.* 野生的

Injuries caused by wild animals, by fights, or by falls crippled and killed many people.

由于野兽、格斗或跌倒造成的种种损伤使许多人残废和送命。

wilfordine [wil'fɔːdin] *n.* 雷公藤碱(= wilforine)

The content of wilforine in these capsules was determined by the ultraviolet spectrophotometry.

采用紫外分光光度法对这些胶囊中雷公藤碱的含量进行了测定。

The insecticidal spectrum of wilfordine was studied.

对雷公藤碱的杀虫谱进行了研究。

wind [wind] *v.* 使喘气

People with asthma often find that physical activity leaves them winded.

患有哮喘的人经常感到体力活动使他们喘息不止。

windpipe ['windpaip] *n.* 气管

The larynx, or voice box, is located between the pharynx and the windpipe.

喉(发声部位)位于咽和气管之间。

The only means of saving life in a situation like this is to make an opening into the windpipe surgically.

在类似这种情况下,挽救患者的生命的惟一办法就是用外科手术的方法作气管切开(作一通入气管的切口)。

wire [waiə] *n.* 电线,线路,网

The daily Medical News wire is designed to help physicians, researchers and other medical professionals stay informed of developments in their field.

每日医学新闻网是用来帮助医师、科研工作者和其他医务人员保持了解医学科学领域的进展。

withdraw [wið'drɔː] *v.* 取出,收回

When the biopsy is completed, the sheath and needle are withdrawn together.

一旦完成活检,套管和针一起退出来。

withdrawl [wið'drɔːl] *n.* 撤消,退隐;停止服药;戒除

The borderline personality is not characterized by social withdrawal.

社交退隐并非边缘人格的特征。

A woman using hormonal contraception will typically experience withdrawal bleeding when she is not exposed to any hormones from her birth control method, which is usually during the fourth week of her cycle.

运用激素避孕的妇女在停止使用激素避孕后通常都会出现撤退性出血,往往发生在月经周期的第四周。

Abrupt withdrawal after discharge is likely to revert the activity of drug-metabolizing enzymes.

出院后突然停止服药,就会使药物代谢酶活性恢复。

Orthostatic hypotension is not uncommon in alcohol withdrawal.

直立低血压在酒精戒除时并非不常见。

withhold [wið'həuld] (withheld[wið'held]) *v.* 制止,阻止;拒绝

A state close to dyspnea results if the drug is withheld.

如果中途停药,就会出现近似呼吸困难的状态。

Passive euthanasia includes the withholding of medication for treating a terminal illness or providing medication such as to relieve pain but may have side effects of shortening one's life.

被动安乐死包括不给终期患者用药或只施用那些可能会缩短病人生命副作用的镇痛药物。

withstand [wið'stænd] *v.* 抵挡,反抗;经受住

This organism withstands exposure to many disinfectants, but it is vulnerable to sunlight.
这种微生物能抗拒多种消毒剂，但可受到阳光伤害。
Some patients withstand high arterial pressures without showing very many significant changes in their vascular systems.
有些病人能经受高血压，血管系统并不呈现很多明显的变化。

witness [ˈwitnis] *v.* 目睹；证明
Recent years have witnessed a considerable number of these cases.
近年来出现相当数量的此类病例。
At the UCCA School of Medicine, I witnessed a demonstration in which a man controlled his own heartbeat.
在洛杉矶加州大学医学院，我亲眼见到一个人能够自己控制自己心跳的表演。
The diagnosis is supported by a history of a seizure disorder, a witnessed seizure, or clearance of the mental status and the motor disorder in a matter of hours.
有癫痫病史，被证实的癫痫发作，数小时的意识丧失和运动障碍均可以支持诊断。

wolfberry [ˈwulfbəri] *n.* 枸杞
Wolfberry is a famous plant fruit which has medicinal, edible and healthy values.
枸杞是一种著名的具有药用、食用、养生三重价值的植物果实。
Wolfberry wine is said to be very refreshing, sweet, and of nutritional value.
枸杞酒据说是非常的清爽、甘甜，而且有营养价值。

womb [wuːm] *n.* 子宫；孕育处
"Womb" is a popular term of the technical term "uterus".
"Womb"是正规术语"uterus"的通俗用词。
The womb during this period grows larger and larger to accommodate itself to the growing fetus.
这一时期的子宫越长越大以适应成长中的胎儿。

workstation [ˈwəːkˌsteiʃən] *n.* 工作站
Use the server edition or workstation edition of this product at your own risk.
可以根据你的风险要求使用这个产品的服务器版本或工作站版本。
There is not enough memory to start the workstation service.
内存不足，无法启动工作站服务。

work-up [ˈwəːkʌp] *n.* 检查（指化验、X 线等）
Complete work-up should be done before a final diagnosis is made.
最后诊断之前应当做完所有的检查。

World Health Organization (WHO) 世界卫生组织
Cognizant of the importance of toxicology, WHO organized a toxicology course in China in 1982.
认识到毒理学的重要性，世界卫生组织于 1982 年在中国举办了毒理学培训。

worm [wəːm] *n.* 蠕虫，蛔虫
The worms compete with the host for nutrients.
蠕虫和宿主争夺营养。
Heavy loads of worms may particularly be associated with intestinal obstruction in children in an endemic area.
在蛔虫是地方病的地区，蛔虫大量寄生于儿童，时常可并发肠梗阻。

wormwood [ˈwəːmwud] *n.* 艾草
The effect of wormwood with the concentrations of 0. 30g/ml and 0. 45g/ml was more significant than that of wormwood with the concentration of 0. 15g/ml.
浓度为 0. 30g/ml 和 0. 45g/ml 苦艾与浓度为 0. 15g/ml 组相比，前者的效果比后者效果更显著。
Experiment must be done to study the effect of wormwood on mice infected with Plasmdium.
必须进行艾草对疟原虫感染的小鼠的抗疟效果的实验研究。

wornout [ˈwɔːnˈaut] *a.* 用坏的，不能再用的

Lysosomes can destroy wornout organelles within the cell.

溶酶体能破坏细胞中无用的细胞器。

worsen [ˈwəːsn] *v.* 变坏

If the patient's condition worsens, call for me immediately, please.

如果病人的情况恶化，请立即叫我。

worthwhile [ˈwəːθwail] *a.* 值得做的

It may someday be worthwhile to try to recover uranium from seawater, but at present this process is prohibitively expensive.

也许以后人们从海水中提取铀是值得的，但目前这种方法还是过于昂贵。

wrinkle [ˈriŋkl] *v.* (使)起皱纹

The skin is abnormally sensitive to sunlight, and may appear wrinkled.

这样的皮肤对阳光异常敏感，可出现很多皱纹。

n. 皱纹

The old lady has wrinkles in her face.

这位老妇人脸上有很多皱纹 。

wrist [rist] *n.* 腕

These lesions occur most frequently on the shins or wrists.

这些损伤最多见于胫部或腕部。

The rubber gloves must come well over the wrists.

橡胶手套必须把手腕完全盖住。

Tennis wrist refers to tenovaginitis of the tendons of the wrist in tennis players.

网球员腕病是指网球运动员手腕肌腱的腱鞘炎。

wrong [rɔŋ] *a.* 错误的，有毛病的

Doctors can now study people's chromosomes and find out if there is anything wrong with them.

医生现在能够研究人的染色体并查出它们是否有毛病。

X

xanthine [ˈzænθi(ː)n] *n.* 黄嘌呤

Allopurinol is a xanthine oxidase inhibitor.

别嘌呤醇是一种黄嘌呤氧化酶抑制剂。

The three derivatives of xanthine mostly used in medicine are caffeine, theobromine and theophylline and their derivatives.

在医药中用得很多的黄嘌呤的三个衍生物是咖啡因、可可碱和茶碱及其衍生物。

xanthoastrocytoma [ˌzænθəuˌæstrəsaiˈtəumə] *n.* 黄色星形细胞瘤

Pleomorphic xanthoastrocytoma is a rare primary brain tumor which occurs in children and young adults.

多形性黄色星形细胞瘤是一种少见的原发性脑肿瘤，发生在儿童和年轻人。

Pleomorphic xanthoastrocytoma is designated as low-grade astrocytoma (WHO Ⅱ), although an anaplastic variant and malignant potential have been described.

尽管间变性和恶性潜能变型已被发现，但多形性黄色星形细胞瘤仍被定名为低级别星形细胞瘤（WHO Ⅱ）。

xanthogranuloma [ˌzænθəugrænjuˈləumə] *n.* 黄色肉芽肿

Juvenile xanthogranuloma is one of the most common forms of non-Langerhans cell histiocytosis in children.

幼年性黄色肉芽肿是儿童非朗格汉斯细胞组织细胞增生最常见的形式。

Immunohistochemical study reveals positive immunoreactivity for CD68 in most juvenile xanthogranuloma cases.

免疫组化研究显示，大多数幼年性黄色肉芽肿病例的 CD68 免疫反应性为阳性。

xanthogranulomatous [ˌzænθəuˌgrænjuˈlɔmətəs] *adj.* 黄色肉芽肿性

She received nephrectomy on the left side kidney due to xanthogranulomatous pyelonephritis.

她曾因黄色肉芽肿性肾盂肾炎而接受了左肾切除术。

The objective is to study the diagnosis and treatment of xanthogranulomatous pyelonephritis (XGP).

目的是研究黄色肉芽肿性肾盂肾炎（XGP）的诊断和治疗。

xanthoma [zænˈθəumə] （*pl.* xanthomas 或 xanthomata [zænˈθəumətə]）*n.* 黄瘤

Biopsy specimens of xanthomas show collections of lipid-containing macrophages.

对黄色瘤进行活检取样显示标本有大量含脂质巨噬细胞。

With time, xanthomata may appear on the extremities, prompted by the serum lipid abnormalities.

血脂异常时，随着时间的推移，黄瘤可出现在肢端。

xenical [ˈziːnikəl] *n.* 赛尼可

Xenical is a new drug which is quite effective in treating obesity.

赛尼可是治疗肥胖十分有效的一种新药。

xenobiotic [ˌzənəubaiˈɔtik] *n.* 外原化合物（异生物），异生质

Free reactive electrophilic intermediates of xenobiotics can produce damage to important cellular constituents.

外原化合物游离反应性的亲电子中间体能对重要的细胞组分产生损害。

The body removes xenobiotics by metabolism, including the deactivation and the excretion of xenobiotics, which happens mostly in the liver.

机体通过代谢排除异生质,包括灭活和排泄,这种情况大多发生在肝脏。

xenogeneic [ˌzenəudʒiˈniːik] *a.* 异种的,异基因的

Animals of different species are xenogeneic.

不同种属的动物就是异基因的。

To overcome the shortage of human organs for transplantation,pigs are considered as xenogeneic donors.

为了克服人体移植器官的短缺,猪被认为是异种移植的供者。

xenograft [ˈzenəgrɑːft] *n.* 异种移植,异种移植物

Xenograft means that tissues or organs from an individual of one species are transplanted into or grafted onto an organism of another species,genus,or family.

异种移植是指将一种生物个体的组织或器官移植到另一种、属、科的个体。

Xenografts are now being considered as an alternative due to inadequate supplies of human donor organs/tissues.

由于人体供者器官或组织来源受限,异种移植现在仍被认为是一种替代方法。

In order to address the problem of the shortage of human organs for transplantation,the use of animal organs(xenografts)is under consideration.

为了解决供移植的人体器官短缺的问题,动物器官(异种移植)已在考虑中。

xenon [ˈzenɔn] *n.* 氙

Xenon possesses nine stable isotopes.

氙具有九种稳定的同位素。

Meteorites all carry this excess xenon.

所有的陨星都含有过多的氙。

xeroderma [ˌziərəuˈdəːmə] *n.* 干皮病

Xeroderma is a mild form of ichthyosis,marked by a dry,rough,discolored state of the skin.

干皮病是一种轻型的鱼鳞病,其特点是皮肤干燥、粗糙和褪色状态。

xerography [ziˈrɔgrəfi] *n.* 静电照相术

Edge enhancement is intrinsic in xerography.

边缘增强是静电照相术的固有特点。

It is widely used in rectifiers,as a semiconductor,and in xerography.

它被广泛应用于整流器(如半导体)和静电照相术中。

xerosis [ziˈrəusis] *n.* 干燥病

The prevalence of xerosis was 55.6% in these patients.

在这些病人中干燥病的患病率为55.6%。

Xerosis was significantly associated with older age,female sex.

干燥病与年长、女性明显相关。

xerostomia [ziərəˈstəumiə] *n.* 口腔干燥

Sjogren's syndrome,a chronic systemic disorder mainly affecting women of middle age,is characterized by keratoconjunctivitis sicca,xerostomia and inflammatory joint disease.

斯约格伦综合征,主要影响中年妇女的慢性疾患,其特征是干燥性角膜结膜炎,口腔干燥和关节发炎。

xiphisternum [ˌzifiˈstəːnəm] (*pl.* xiphisterna [ˌzifiˈstəːnə]) *n.* 剑突

The level of the fundus is accurately determined by using the ulnar border of the hand and moving it downwards from the xiphisternum.

用手的尺侧缘从剑突往下移动,正确测定宫底高度。

xiphoid [ˈzifɔid] *n.* 剑突

The cardiac impulse,if at all visible,is seen only in the xiphoid and subxiphoid regions.

心尖搏动,如果说能看得见的话,也只能在剑突或剑突下区见到。

XO syndrome XO 综合征

XO syndrome or Turner' s syndrome is a disorder of phenotype female that is characterized by short stature, sexual infantilism, XO indicates the presence of only one sex chromosome, the other X or Y chromosome being absent.

XO 综合征或特纳氏综合征是一种表型为女性的疾患,其特征是身材矮小,婴儿型性器官,XO 表明只有一个性染色体,另一 X 或 Y 染色体缺乏。

xylene ['zailiːn] *n.* 二甲苯

For this purpose one removes the oil used for microscopy with xylene.

为此,应用二甲苯去掉玻片上用于显微镜观察的油。

xylitol ['zailitɔl] *n.* 木糖醇

Xylitol is a sugar alcohol sweetener used as a naturally occurring sugar substitute.

木糖醇是一种糖醇甜味剂,用作天然糖分的替代品。

Xylitol is a sugar-alcohol sweetener found in many sugar-free candies, chewing gums, baked goods and other products.

木糖醇是一种糖醇甜味剂,可见于多种无糖的糖果、口香糖、烘焙食品和其他产品。

xylol ['zailɔl] *n.* 二甲苯

Xylol is as satisfactory as KOH and need not be warmed.

二甲苯无需加温,即可获得与氢氧化钾一样满意的效果。

xylose ['zailəus] *n.* 木糖,吡喃木糖

A pentose, D-xylose, is mainly absorbed from the jejunum and constant fraction of the amount absorbed is rapidly excreted into the urine.

戊糖,即 D 木糖,主要从空肠吸收,吸收总量中的一恒定部分很快被排入尿中。

xylulose ['zailələus] *n.* 木酮糖

L-xylulose dehydrogenase converts L-xylulose to xylitol.

左旋-木酮糖脱氢酶可使左旋-木酮糖转变成木糖醇。

Deficiency of L-xylulose dehydrogenase leads to increased concentrantion of L-xylulose in blood and urine.

左旋-木酮糖脱氢酶缺乏可导致左旋-木酮糖在血和尿中的浓度增加。

Y

yaws [jɔːz] *n.* 雅司病

Yaws, which is common in large parts of Africa, is rapidly cured with penicillin.

雅司病常见于非洲广大地区,用青霉素可以迅速地治好。

yeast [jiːst] *n.* 酵母菌

Yeasts are classified by the nature of the spore-forming structures.

酵母菌是根据形成孢子的结构特性来分类的。

The yeast and E. coli genome sequences are now complete.

酵母菌基因组和大肠杆菌基因组的测序工作现已完成。

yellowish [ˈjeləuiʃ] *a.* 淡黄色的

The yellowish colour of many fats and oils is due to their carotene content.

许多脂类和油类之所以呈淡黄色,是由于它们含有胡萝卜素的缘故。

Yersinia [jəːˈsiniə] *n.* 耶尔森菌属

The objective is to explore the sensitivity of Yersinia pestis along Qinghai-Tibet Railway.

目的是探讨青藏铁路沿线鼠疫耶尔森菌的敏感性。

Despite this advance, we should still avoid Yersinia pestis like the plague.

尽管有这些进展,我们还是得像躲瘟疫一样躲着鼠疫耶尔森菌。

yield [jiːld] *v.* 生产;产生(效果,收益等),带来

Hence each diatomic molecule of nitrogen yields two molecules of ammonia.

因此,每个双原子的氮分子生成两个氨分子。

Recent researches show that bone marrow can yield nerve cells.

新近研究表明骨髓能产生神经细胞。

The bacterial pneumonia yields rather readily to sulfonamide or antibiotic therapy, while the viral one does not.

细菌性肺炎用磺胺或抗生素治疗较易见效,而病毒性肺炎用此则无效。

yolk [jəuk] *n.* 蛋黄;卵黄

The fetus develops within the gestational sac, forming a yolk sac that looks like a ring.

胎儿在孕囊内生长,形成环状的卵黄囊。

Yolk sac tumors (YST) are rare and highly malignant tumors, occurring in children as well as in young adults.

卵黄囊瘤是一种十分罕见并且高度恶性的肿瘤,好发于儿童和青年。

youngster [ˈjʌŋstə] *n.* 年轻人

Another step to problem-solving is to help youngsters see laws of cause and effect.

解决问题的另一步骤是帮助年轻人认清因果关系的规律。

Z

zedoary [ˈzedəuəri] *n.* 莪术；片姜黄

We need determine the content of zedoary turmeric oil gelatin microspheres first.

我们需要首先测定莪术油明胶微球剂的含量。

Our study on the treatment of children' s intractable nephrotic syndrome with zedoary turmeric oil and centella appealed to many other researchers.

我们用莪术油联合雷公藤治疗小儿难治性肾病综合征的研究吸引了很多其他研究人员的关注。

zein [ˈziːin] *n.* 玉米朊，玉米蛋白

Zein is a class of prolamine protein found in maize.

玉米朊是从玉米中发现的一类醇溶蛋白。

Zein is the storage protein in corn kernels.

玉米朊是玉米粒的储存蛋白。

zinc [ziŋk] *n.* 锌

These patients have low amounts of zinc and sodium in their hair.

这些病人的毛发中锌和钠的含量偏低。

These transcription-activator proteins are called zinc finger proteins.

这些转录激活蛋白称为锌指蛋白。

zone [zəun] *n.* 区，区域，带

It may then be reconstituted by adding sterile water as it is needed in a war zone.

然后，当战区需要时，便可加入消过毒的水使其恢复原样。

Melanosomes are synthesized in the Golgi zone of the cell.

黑素体合成于细胞的高尔基区。

The junction of epidermis and dermis is formed by the basement membrane zone.

基底膜带把表皮和真皮联结起来。

zonula [ˈzəunjulə] *n.* 小带

Zonula adherens are small，spotlike junctions located near the apical surface of epithelial cells.

黏着小带是小的点状的细胞连接，位于上皮细胞顶端表面（游离面）附近。

Zonula adherens and desmosomes are mediated by calcium-dependent adherence protein cadherins and catenins.

黏着小带和桥粒均由钙依赖性的黏附蛋白钙黏蛋白和连环蛋白介导。

zoom [zuːm] *n.* 图像放大，（快速）变焦距

You can also specify the zoom for the slides.

您还可以设定幻灯片的缩放比例。

You may use a zoom or telephoto lens on your camera.

你可以在照相机上安装可变距镜头或摄远镜头。

zoster [ˈzɔstə] *n.* 带状疱疹

The child was exposed to chickenpox in his school and required zoster immune globulin.

患儿在学校接触了水痘，需注射带状疱疹免疫球蛋白。

zwitterion [ˈtsvitəˈraiən] *n.* 两性离子

Proteins themselves are complex zwitterion type structures.

蛋白质本身是复杂的两性离子型结构。

zygoma [zaiˈgəumə] *n.* [希]颧(骨)颧突;颧弓;颧骨

The zygoma is a frequently fractured bone because of its prominent position in the facial skeleton.

由于颧骨位于面部骨骼的突出部位,所以会经常发生骨折。

zygote [ˈzaigəut] *n.* 合子,受精卵

As a result of fertilization a zygote with a diploid set of chromosomes is formed.

经过受精作用形成含有两套染色体的合子。

Zygote is referred to as the diploid cell resulting from fertilization of haploid gametes.

合子是指单倍体的配子经过受精作用形成的二倍体细胞。

When a fertilized egg, or zygote, doesn't travel into the uterus but instead grows rapidly in the fallopian tube, this condition is known as ectopic pregnancy.

当受精卵没有在子宫着床而是在输卵管中快速发育时,这种状态称作宫外孕。

zygotene [ˈzaigəutiːn, ˈzi-] *n.* [细胞]偶线期

At zygotene stage, homologous chromosomes begin to align along their entire length.

在偶线期,同源染色体开始沿着全长配对排列。

Zygotene is the stage in prophase of meiosis during which homologous chromosomes become paired.

偶线期是减数分裂前期,在此阶段同源染色体配对。

zymogen [ˈzaimədʒən] *n.* 酶原

A zymogen requires a biochemical change (such as a hydrolysis reaction revealing the active site) for it to become an active enzyme.

酶原变成有活性的酶需要发生生化改变,例如水解反应以暴露其活性位点。

In F-cells plenty of rough endoplasmic reticulum and zymogen can be observed.

F 细胞含有丰富的粗面内质网及酶原颗粒。

zymolysis [zaiˈmɔlisis] *n.* 发酵;酶解(作用)

The advantage of chemical-enzyme synthesis is high enzyme specificity but the disadvantage is higher cost of zymolysis.

化学-酶合成的好处是酶的特异性高,但缺点是酶解成本更高。

Zymolysis is a process in which an agent causes an organic substance to break down into simpler substances.

酶解是一个(化学反应)过程,在该反应中一种试剂可引起一种有机物分解成为更简单的物质。

附　录

一、英语医学术语的特征

英语是受拉丁语影响较深的一种语言，特别是英语医学术语，不仅拉丁语的成分极多，而且还有希腊语的成分。许多医学术语是直接借用的拉丁词和希腊词，或由拉丁词、希腊词成分作词根加前后缀构成的。尽管其中有一部分术语已英语化了，一般人不易察觉，但仍有一部分术语保留着明显的拉丁语和希腊语词汇的某些特征。这些特征往往为一般英语学习者所不熟悉，而成为学习中的一种困难。了解了这些特征，可以帮助英语学习者更好地理解这些术语并记住它们。

（一）特殊的单复数

英语名词的复数形式一般是在单数名词词尾加 s 或 es 构成。但有一部分由拉丁语和希腊语借用来的医学名词的单复数形式较为特殊，仍保留拉丁语和希腊语的原来形式，发音也较特殊，简单举例如下：

1. a-ae：(L.) aorta[ə] -aortae[iː]　主动脉
   pleura-pleurae　胸膜
2. us-i：(L.) coccus[əs] -cocci[ai]　球菌
   bacillus-bacilli　杆菌
3. um-a：(L.) serum[əm] -sera[ə] (serums)　血清
   bacterium-bacteria　细菌
4. on-a：(G.) phenomenon[ən] -phenomena[ə]　现象
   criterion-criteria　标准
5. 元音+x-元音+ces：(L.)
   cortex[ks] -cortices[siːz]　皮质
   appendix-appendices　阑尾
   thorax-thoraces　胸廓
   辅音+x-辅音+ges：
   pharynx-pharynges[dʒiːz]　咽
   larynx-larynges　喉
6. is-es：(G.) crisis[is] -crises[iːz]　危象
   analysis-analyses　分折
7. ma-mata：(G.) trauma[mə] -traumata[mətə]　创伤
   haematoma-haematomata　血肿
8. men-mina：(L.) lumen[men] -lumina[nə]　(管)腔
   abdomen-abdomina　腹

许多来自拉丁语和希腊语的医学术语已完全英语化，失去了拉丁或希腊原来的词尾，复数形式按英语的方式变化。如：

artery-arteries(L. arteria)　动脉
abscess-abscesses(L. abscessus)　脓肿

acid-acids(L. acidum) 酸
dose-doses(G. dosis) 剂量

(二) 两种拼写形式

有一些来源于希腊语或拉丁语的英语医学术语有着两种拼写形式。对于这些术语,不同年代的书本或不同作者常采用其中不同的形式。往往一个已经学过的单词,由于另一拼写形式出现,我们却误以为是另一单词,重查词典,因而增加阅读中的困难。为了避免这种情况,现将较常见的两种拼写形式的医学术语举例如下:

A. 两种字母可以互相通用者

1. ae-e:
   haemorrhage-hemorrhage 出血
   aetiology-etiology 病因学
2. oe-e:
   oedema-edema 水肿
   oesophagus-esophagus 食管
3. ou-u:
   oulitis-ulitis 龈炎
   ouroscopy-uroscopy 尿检查
4. ph-f:
   sulphate-sulfate 硫酸盐
   sulphonamide-sulfonamide 磺胺(药物)
5. k-c:
   leukocyte-leucocyte 白细胞
   katabolism-catabolism 分解代谢
6. qu-ch:
   quinine-chinine 奎宁
   quinotropine-chinotropine 喹诺托品
7. y-i:
   syrup-sirup 糖浆
   bacilysin-bacillisin 枯草杆菌溶素
8. 其他:
   dochmiasis-dochmiosis 钩虫病
   odontoplast-odontoblast 成牙质细胞
   distension-distention 膨胀

B. 部分字母可有可无者

1. ta:
   dilatation-dilation 扩张
   vasodilatation-vasodilation 血管扩张
2. at:
   hematocyte-hemocyte 血细胞
   hematotoxin-hemotoxin 血毒素
3. al:
   adrenalinemia-adreninemia 肾上腺素血症
   adrenalopathy-adrenopathy 肾上腺病

4. i：
ammoniemia-ammonemia　氨血(症)
bacteriemia-bacteremia　菌血症

5. e：
osteitis-ostitis　骨炎
gasterectasis-gastrectasis　胃扩张
vitamine-vitamin　维生素
pepsine-pepsin　胃蛋白酶

6. 其他
multplicable-multipliable　可增殖的
pathogenetic-pathogenic　病原的
technical-technic　技术的
acaridiasis-acariasis　疥虫病
pharmaceutist-pharmacist　药学家、药剂师

C. 英国英语和美国英语的不同拼写形式

英	美	
-our	-or	
coulour	color	颜色
tumour	tumor	肿瘤
-re	-er	
centre	center	中心
metre	meter	米
-yse	-yze	
analyse	analyze	分析
paralyse	paralyze	使瘫痪
-xion	-ction	
connexion	connection	连接、联系
reflexion	reflection	反射
-mme	-m	
gramme	gram	克
kilogramme	kilogram	千克、公斤
-ogue	-og	
dialogue	dialog	对话
catalogue	catalog	目录
-c	-k	
disc	disk	圆盘
sceptic	skeptic	怀疑论者

（三）有趣的同族词

在一个简单的词或词根的基础上，通过加各种前缀和后缀可以构成含有同一词根、意义相近的许多词，这样产生的词叫派生词。这整个一组词就叫做同族词。前缀是加在单词或词根前面的构词成分，它只改变词的意义，但不改变词性。后缀是加在单词或词根后面的构词成分，它不仅具有一定的意义，而且往往改变原来的词性。在医学英语里同族词的现象甚为突出。了解了这种构词方式，对同族词的理解和记忆就容易多了。这里举三组词来说明这种情况。

A. Act

1. act	*v.*	行动,充当,发生作用
	n.	行为,动作
2. action	*n.*	动作,活动,作用
3. active	*a.*	动的,积极的,主动的
4. actively	*ad.*	积极地,主动地
5. activity	*n.*	活动
6. react	*v.*	反应,反作用
7. reaction	*n.*	反应,反作用
8. interact	*v.*	互相作用
9. interaction	*n.*	相互作用
10. overactivity	*n.*	活动过度
11. overactive	*a.*	活动过度的
12. activate	*v.*	使活化,使活动
13. activation	*n.*	活性化(作用)
14. activator	*n.*	活化剂

B. Digest

1. digest	*v.*	消化
2. digestant	*a.*	助消化的
	n.	消化药
3. digestible	*a.*	可消化的,易消化的
4. digestibility	*n.*	可消化性
5. digestion	*n.*	消化(作用)
6. digestive	*a.*	消化的
7. indigested	*a.*	未消化的
8. indigestible	*a.*	不消化的
9. indigestion	*n.*	消化不良
10. indigestive	*a.*	消化不良的

C. Immune

1. immune	*a.*	免疫的
	n.	免疫者
2. immunifaction	*n.*	免疫作用,免疫法
3. immunity	*n.*	免疫性
4. immunize	*v.*	使免疫
5. immunization	*n.*	免疫法,免疫作用
6. immunogen	*n.*	免疫体原
7. immunogenic	*a.*	产生免疫的
8. immunologic	*a.*	免疫的
9. immunological	*a.*	免疫学的
10. immunologist	*n.*	免疫学家
11. immunology	*n.*	免疫学
12. non-immune	*a.*	无免疫性的
13. autoimmune	*a.*	自体免疫的

此外,还可将 immuno 作为词根,与其他词构成许多双词根的词,如:

14. immunoreaction	*n.*	免疫反应

15. immunoprotein	*n.*	免疫蛋白质
16. immunochemistry	*n.*	免疫化学
17. immunotherapy	*n.*	免疫疗法
18. immunodeficiency	*n.*	免疫缺陷
19. immunodepression	*n.*	免疫抑制
20. immunogenetics	*n.*	免疫遗传学

（四）词根交替现象

从上一节可以看出，一般英语医学词都是在同一个词根（或根词）的基础上增加其他构词成分而形成意义相关的派生词的，但是，也有一部分词，在构成意义相关的派生词时，不采用原来的简单词为词根，而以具有同样词义的拉丁词或希腊词（它们在现代英语里不一定能够独立成词）为词根，加上其他构词成分组成新词，这种情况叫做词根交替现象。举例如下：

1. 名词（英语）→形容词（改用拉丁或希腊词根）

mouth　口-oral（L. os）　口的
tooth　牙齿-dental（L. dens）　牙齿的
tongue　舌-lingual（L. lingua）　舌的
ear　耳-aural（L. aurus）　耳的
nose　鼻-nasal（L. nasus）　鼻的
eye　眼-ophthalmic（GK. opthalmos）　眼的
skin　皮肤-dermal（GK. derma）　皮肤的
heart　心脏-cardiac（GK. cardia）　心脏的
liver　肝-hepatic（GK. hepar）　肝的
stomach　胃-gastric（GK. gaster）　胃的
lung　肺-pulmonary（L. pulmo）　肺的
kidney　肾-renal（L. ren）　肾的
neck　颈-cervical（L. cervix）　颈的
chest　胸-thoracic（GK. thorax）　胸的
brain　脑-cerebral（L. cerebrum）　脑的
nerve　神经-neural（GK. neuron）　神经的
rib　肋骨-costal（L. costa）　肋骨的
mother　母亲-maternal（L. mater）　母亲的
heat　热-thermal（GK. thermo）　热的

附：仍用原来词根

bone　骨-bony　骨的
saliva　唾液-salivary　唾液的
virus　病毒-viral　病毒的
respiration　呼吸-respiratory　呼吸的

2. 名词（英语）→有关炎症名称（改用拉丁或希腊词根）

joint　关节-arthritis（GK. arthron）　关节炎
kidney　肾-nephritis（GK. nephros）　肾炎
nerve　神经-neuritis（GK. neuron）　神经炎
liver　肝-hepatitis（GK. hepar）　肝炎
brain　脑-encephalitis（GK. encephalon）　脑炎
stomach　胃-gastritis（GK. gaster）　胃炎

附：仍用原来词根

artery　动脉-arteritis　动脉炎

bronchus　支气管-bronchitis　支气管炎

3. 名词(英语)→有关学科名称(改用拉丁或希腊词根)

heart　心-cardiology(GK. cardia)　心脏病学

eye　眼-ophthalmology(GK. ophthalmos)　眼科学

cell　细胞-cytology(GK. kytos-cyto)　细胞学

tumour　肿瘤-oncology(GK. onkos)　肿瘤学

disease　病-pathology(GK. pathos)　病理学

drug　药-pharmacology(GK. pharmakon)　药理学

附:仍用原来词根

parasite　寄生虫-parasitology　寄生虫学

bacterium　细菌-bacteriology　细菌学

4. 构成其他名词时

cell:　细胞(GK. kytos-cyto)

cytochemistry　细胞化学

cytometer　血细胞计数器

cytotoxin　细胞毒素

blood:　血(GK. haema)

haematuria　血尿

haemochrome　血色素

haemoglobin　血红蛋白

(五) 复杂医学术语的构词方式(包括常用词根、前缀、后缀及例词)

新的医学术语不断出现。它们往往是以希腊或拉丁成分作为词根构成。除由一个词根加后缀构成外,现在愈来愈多的是由两个词根结合再加后缀构成。这样的一些新词有的不易从现有医学词典或医学词汇中查到。有的也不需要去查,可以通过对其结构的分析而达到了解其含义。

1. 术语构词分析示例

例一:Gastr/o/enter/o/logy

词根 ↓ 词根 ↓ 后缀

连接性元音

(1) 词根 gastr 的意思是 stomach(胃)

(2) 词根 enter 的意思是 intestines(肠)

(3) 后缀-logy 的意思是 process of study(研究过程)

(4) 连接元音 o 连接词与词根,及词根与后缀。

因此,整个单词的意思是:

英语(要从后缀开始读到前面去):

the process of study of the stomach and intestines

汉语(顺着理解):胃肠(病)学

例二:Electr/o/cardi/o/gram

词根 ↓ 词根 ↓ 后缀

连接性元音

(1) 词根 electr 的意思是 electricity(电)

(2) 词根 cardi 的意思是 heart(心)

(3) 后缀 -gram 的意思是 record(记录图)

整个单词的意思是：the record of the electricity of the heart 心电图

例三：onc /o /gen / ic

```
      ↓  │  ↓    ↓
    词根 ↓ 词根  后缀
     连接性元音
```

（1）词根 onc 的意思是 tumour(肿瘤)

（2）词根 gen 的意思是 producing(发生)

（3）后缀 -ic 的意思是 pertaining to(关于,有关)

整个单词的意思是：pertaining to tumour producing 肿瘤发生的

注意：连接性元音(o)通常置于词根与后缀之间,这个词没有用它是因为后缀以元音字母开头。然而,两个词根之间,即使第二个词根是以元音字母开头,连接性元音也是必须用的。

例如：gastr /o /enter / ic 而不是 gastrenteric

```
      ↓   │   ↓     ↓
    词根  ↓  词根   后缀
     连接性元音
```

2. 术语词例：

（1）词根+o+后缀

arthr/o/tomy-incision of a joint　关节切开术

nephr/o/logist-one who specializes in the study of kidney　肾病专家

encephal/o/pathy-disease condition of the brain　脑病

gastr/o/scope-instrument to examine the stomach　胃镜

（2）词根+后缀

aden/oma-tumour of a gland　腺瘤

leuk/emia-blood condition of excessive numbers of white blood cells　白血病

gastr/ectomy-removal of the stomach　胃切除术

（3）词根+o+词根+o+后缀

electr/o/encephal/o/gram-record of the electricity in the brain　脑电图

ile/o/cec/o/stomy-anastomosis between the ileum and the cecum　回肠盲肠吻合术

trache/o/laryng/o/tomy-inciscon of the trachea and larynx　气管喉管切开术

（4）词根+o+词根+后缀

path/o/gen/ic-pertaining to disease producing　病原的

carcin/o/gen/ic-pertaining to producing cancer　致癌的

erythr/o/cyt/osis-abnormal condition(elevation in number) of red blood cells　红细胞增多

nephr/o/scler/osis-sclerosis or hardening of the kidney　肾硬化症

gastr/o/duoden/itis-inflammation of the stomach and duodenum　胃十二指肠炎

构词小结：要理解医学术语,必须记住下列三条重要规则：

1）理解术语时,英语要从后缀开始再往前面读,汉语则顺着读。

2）后缀如以元音字母开头,前面的连接性元音就省去不用。如 gastric 而不是 gastroic。

3）两个词根之间的连接性元音则总是要保留。

3. 连接性元音

连接性元音除 o 外,还有 i。英语医学术语绝大多数都是由 o 连接,仅有极少数系由 i 连接。例如：

acidimetry　酸定量法(acid/i/metry)

germicide　杀菌剂(germ/i/cide)

有些词根在不同的结合构词中,分别用 o 和 i 作连接元音。例如：

cervicodynia　颈痛(cervic/o/dynia)

cerviciplex　颈神经丛(cervic/i/plex)

dentoalveolitis 牙槽炎(dent/o/alveol/itis)
dentiform 牙形的(dent/i/form)

还有一些词根在某些构词中可同时用 o 或 i 作连接元音。例如：
alkalotherapy-alkalitherapy 碱疗法
renopuncture-renipuncture 肾穿刺术

4. 常用词根构词形式及词例(60 个)

aden/o 腺 adenalgia 腺痛
adenocyte 腺细胞
adren/o 肾上腺 adrenoxidase 肾上腺氧化酶
adrenotoxin 肾上腺毒素
amin/o 氨基 aminolysis 氨解(作用)
aminomycine 氨基霉素
arthr/o 关节 arthritis 关节炎
arthrotomy 关节切开术
audi/o 听 audiology 听觉学
audiometer 听力计
bacill/o 杆菌 bacillosis 杆菌病
bacilloscopy 杆菌检视法
bacteri/o 细菌 bacteriology 细菌学
bactericide 杀菌剂
bi/o 生,生命 biology 生物学
biosynthesis 生物合成
bronch/o 支气管 bronchitis 支气管炎
bronchospasm 支气管痉挛
carb/o 碳 carbohydrate 碳水化合物
carbohaemia 碳酸血症
carcin/o 癌 carcinogen 致癌物
carcinogenic 致癌的
cardi/o 心 cardialgia 心痛
cardiectasis 心扩张
cephal/o 头,颅 cephalopathy 头部疾患
cephalotomy 穿颅术
cerebro- 脑 cerebrum 大脑
cerebrospinal 脑脊髓的
chlor/o 绿,氯 chlorophyll 叶绿素
chloromycetin 氯霉素
chrom/o 色 chromosome 染色体
chromogenesis 色素形成
cyt/o 细胞 cytobiology 细胞生物学
cytotoxin 细胞毒素
dent/o 牙 dentalgia 牙痛
dentoalveolitis 牙槽炎
derm/o 皮 dermoplasty 皮肤成形术
dermat/o dermatomycin 皮霉菌素
electr/o 电 electrolysis 电解(作用)
electrophoresis 电泳
encephal/o 脑 encephaledema 脑水肿
encephaloma 脑瘤

enter/o　肠　enteritis　肠炎
　　enterococci　肠内链球菌
erythr/o　红　erythrocyte　红细胞
　　erythromycin　红霉素
fibr/o　纤维　fibroma　纤维瘤
　　fibroblast　成纤维细胞
fibrin/o　纤维蛋白　fibrinogen　纤维蛋白原
　　fibrinolysin　纤维蛋白溶酶
gastr/o　胃　gastroptosis　胃下垂
　　gastralgia　胃痛
glyc/o　糖　glycolipid　糖脂
　　glycosuria　糖尿
gynec/o　妇人　gynecology　妇科学
　　gynecopathy　妇科病
hem/o　血液　hemoglobin　血红蛋白
hemat/o　hematoma　血肿
hepat/o　肝　hepatitis　肝炎
　　hepatectomy　肝切除术
hist/o　组织　histology　组织学
　　histotherapy　组织疗法
hom/o　同种　homogeneous　同质的,同族的
　　homoplasty　同种移植术
hydr/o　水,氢　hydrolysis　水解(作用)
　　hydroquinine　氢化奎宁
immun/o　免疫　immunology　免疫学
　　immunotherapy　免疫疗法
leuk/o　白　leukocyte　白细胞
　　leukemia　白血病
lingu/o　舌　lingula　小舌
　　linguogingival　舌龈的
lymph/o　淋巴　lymphedema　淋巴水肿
　　lymphocyte　淋巴细胞
my/o　肌　myocarditis　心肌炎
　　myofibroma　肌纤维瘤
nephr/o　肾　nephralgia　肾痛
　　nephrosclerosis　肾硬化
neur/o　神经　neuroma　神经瘤
　　neuron　神经元
onc/o　肿瘤　oncology　肿瘤学
　　oncogenesis　瘤形成
ophthalm/o 眼　ophthalmocopia　眼疲劳
　　ophthalmorrhea　眼渗血
oste/o　骨　osteoma　骨瘤
　　osteomalacia　骨软化
path/o　病　pathogen　病原体
　　pathogenesis　致病原因
pharmac/o　药　pharmacology　药理学
　　pharmacopoeia　药典

physi/o 生理,物理 physiology 生理学
physiotherapy 物理疗法
pleur/o 胸膜 pleuralgia 胸膜痛
pleurocentesis 胸腔穿刺术
pneum/o 肺 pneumococcus 肺炎球菌
pneumothorax 气胸
psych/o 精神,心理 psychiatry 精神病学
psychology 心理学
pyr/o 热 pyrogen 致热原
antipyretic 解热剂
radi/o 放射 radioactivity 放射性
radiotherapy 放射疗法
ren/o 肾 renopathy 肾病
renography 肾 X 线照相术
rhin/o 鼻 rhinitis 鼻炎
rhinorrhea 鼻漏
scler/o 硬 scleroderma 硬皮病
sclerocataract 硬性白内障
巩膜 scleromalacia 巩膜软化症
sclerotomy 巩膜切开术
spir/o 呼吸 spirograph 呼吸描记器
spirometer 肺活量计
thorac/o 胸 thoracoscope 胸腔镜
thoracoplasty 胸廓成形术
thromb/o 血栓 thrombolysis 血栓溶解
thrombosis 血栓形成
血小板 thrombocyte 血小板
tox/o 毒 toxoid 类毒素
toxoglobulin 毒球蛋白
toxic/o 毒 toxicology 毒物学
toxicosis 中毒
trache/o 气管 tracheorrhagia 气管出血
tracheotomy 气管切开术
ur/o 尿 urology 泌尿学
uroscopy 尿检查法

5. 常用后缀及词例(30 个)

-algia 疼痛 arthralgia 关节痛
cephalgia 头痛
-blast 成…细胞 neuroblast 成神经细胞
(胚,芽) osteoblast 成骨细胞
-cyte 细胞 erythrocyte 红细胞
leucocyte 白细胞
-ectasis 扩大 gastroectasis 胃扩张
胀大 bronchiectasis 支气管扩张
-ectomy 切除术 appendectomy 阑尾切除术
duodenectomy 十二指肠切除术
-emia 血症 bacteremia 菌血症
leukemia 白血病

-gen 原 pathogen 病原体
glycogen 糖原
素 androgen 雄激素
estrogen 雌激素
-genic …性 pyrogenic 致热性
…原的 radiogenic 放射原的
-gram 图，描记图 hemogram 血象
electrocardiogram 心电图
-graphy 照相术 bronchography 支气管造影术
造影术 lymphangiography 淋巴管造影术
-iasis 病 ascariasis 蛔虫病
cholelithiasis 胆石病
-itis 炎症 bronchitis 支气管炎
encephalitis 脑炎
-logy …学 cytology 细胞学
ecology 生态学
-meter 表，计 pyrometer 高温计
测量器 spirometer 肺活量计
-oid …样 amoeboid 阿米巴样的
…状的 chyloid 乳糜状的
-oma 肿瘤 adenoma 腺瘤
osteoma 骨瘤
-osis 病，症 cirrhosis 肝硬化
mycosis 霉菌病
（血细胞）异常增多 erythrocytosis 红细胞增多（症）
leucocytosis 白细胞增多（症）
-penia 缺乏，减少 leucopenia 白细胞减少
thrombopenia 血小板减少
-plasm 形成物 protoplasm 原生质，原浆
neoplasm 新生物
-plasty 成形术 gastroplasty 胃成形术
dermatoplasty 皮肤成形术
-ptosis 落，下垂 nephroptosis 肾下垂
hysteroptosis 子宫下垂
-rrhage 出血，流出 hemorrhage 出血
lymphorrhage 淋巴溢
-rrhagia 出血，流出 gastrorrhagia 胃出血
pneumorrhagia 肺出血
-rrhaphy 缝术 cardiorrhaphy 心（肌）缝术
celiorrhaphy 腹壁缝术
-rrhea 流 diarrhea 腹泻
menorrhea 月经
-scope 检查镜 bronchoscope 支气管镜
otoscope 耳镜
-scopy 检查法 celioscopy 腹腔镜检法
gastroscopy 胃镜检法
-stomy 吻合术 colostomy 结肠吻合术
ileostomy 回肠吻合术

-tome 切刀 keratotome 角膜刀
neurotome 神经刀
-tomy 切开术 ovariotomy 卵巢切开术
tracheotomy 气管切开术

6. 常用前缀及词例(45 个)

a- 无,缺 asymptomatic 无症状的
anaemia 贫血
ante- 前 anteflexion 前屈
antenatal 出生前的
anti- 抗,防止 antibiotics 抗生素
anticoagulant 抗凝血剂
auto- 自己,独自 autoimmune 自体免疫
autoxidation 自身氧化
bi- 二,双 bicarbonate 重碳酸盐
bilateral 两侧的
contra- 反,逆,对 contraceptive 避孕剂
contraindication 禁忌证
counter- 对抗,反对 counteragent 对抗剂
counteraction 对抗作用
de- 除,脱,去 detoxication 解毒,去毒
decomposition 分解(作用)
di- 二,双 dioxide 二氧化物
diplegia 两侧瘫
dis- 分离,除去 disinfection 消毒
discolor 脱色
dys- 异常,障碍 dysfunction 功能障碍
dyspepsia 消化不良
endo- 内部 endocarditis 心内膜炎
endocrine 内分泌
epi- 上,表,外 epigastrium 上腹部
epidermoid 表皮样的
exo- 外 exocrine 外分泌
exotoxin 外毒素
extra- 外,额外 extracellular 细胞外的
extrahepatic 肝外的
hemi- 半,偏 hemicrania 偏头痛
hemiplegia 偏瘫,半身不遂
hyper- 上,过多 hypertension 高血压
hyperthyroidism 甲状腺功能亢进
hypo- 低,过少 hypotension 低血压
hypothyroidism 甲状腺功能减退
in1- 内,在内 inhalation 吸入剂
injection 注射,注入
in2- 无,不 invertebrate 无脊椎动物
insanitary 不卫生的
infra- 下,低 inframammary 乳腺下的
infrared 红外线
inter- 相互,间 intercellular 细胞间的

intermolecular　分子间的
intra-　内,内部　intracranial　颅内的
intravenous　静脉内的
macro-　巨,大　macrocyte　巨红细胞
macromolecule　大分子
mal-　不良,恶劣　malformation　畸形
malnutrition　营养不良
mega-　巨,大　megacardia　心肥大
(megalo-)　megalocyte　巨红细胞
micro-　小,微　microbiology　微生物学
microcyte　小红细胞
mono-　单,一　monocyte　单核细胞
mononucleosis　单核白细胞增多
multi-　多　multicellular　多细胞的
multinuclear　多核的
neo-　新　neomycin　新霉素
neoplasm　新生物,瘤
non-　不,非,无　non-immune　无免疫性的
non-infectious　非传染性的
para-　副,旁　paratyphoid　副伤寒
parathyroid　甲状旁腺
peri-　周围,附近　peritonsillitis　扁桃体周围炎
pericarditis　心包炎
poly-　多　polyplegia　多肌麻痹
polyuria　多尿症
post-　后　postnatal　出生后的
postoperative　手术后的
pre-　前　prenatal　出生前的
preoperative　手术前的
re-　再,回　reinfection　再感染
redistillation　再蒸馏
semi-　半　semicircular　半圆形的
semicoma　半昏迷
sub-　下,亚,不足　subabdominal　下腹的
subacute　亚急性的
super-　在…上　superficial　表面的,浅的
过度的　superlethal　超致死量的
supra-　上,超　supramaximal　极量以上的
supramaxillary　上颌骨的
tetra-　四,丁　tetracycline　四环素
tetracaine　丁卡因
trans-　转,传,移　transfusion　输血
transplantation　移植术
tri-　三　triceps　三头肌
trigeminus　三叉神经
uni-　单,一　unicellular　单细胞的
unipara　初产妇

了解了医学术语的构词方式,记住了上面介绍的常用词根、后缀和前缀以后,对于英语

医学术语词义和拼写的识别和记忆能力将大大提高，许多术语甚至不需查找有关词典即可认识，因而给扩大医学词汇提供了一个有效的科学方法。这里选出的60个常用词根与30个常用后缀和45个常用前缀通过排列组合构成的词可以达到数万个。当然，一个词根不可能与所有的后缀或前缀都能构成新词，但它们之间交叉组合能构成的词的数量仍是可观的，其中包括2000～3000常用的医学术语是没有问题的。因此，通过所给例词熟记这些有用的构词词素，增强认词和记词能力，无形地等于认识了（即扩大了）2000～3000单词，成为学习医学术语的一条捷径。

下面列举几个较长的医学术语，可能过去从未见过，但由于熟悉了它们借以组合成词所用的词根、后缀和前缀，其词义很容易就可分析出来：

hyperglycemia　血糖过高，高血糖
fibrinogenopenia　纤维蛋白原减少
neurofibromatosis　神经纤维瘤
microradiography　显微放射照相术
electroencephalogram　脑电图

学习了医学术语的结构以后，识记新词的能力增强。例如下面这一组词可以比较容易地记住：

hypocalcemia　血钙过少，低血钙
hypokalaemia　血钾过少，低血钾
hypoglycemia　血糖过少，低血糖
hypoproteinemia　血蛋白过少，低蛋白血（症）
hypoalbuminemia　血白蛋白减少
hypoaminoacidemia　血氨基酸减少，低氨基酸血（症）
hypoadrenalinemia　血肾上腺素过少，低肾上腺素血（症）

（注：类似的词还可继续举出20个左右，此处从略。）

（六）缩略词

医学术语不断出现，而且语言形式愈来愈复杂。一个术语单词往往很长，更多的术语是由二三个单词组成，使用起来很不方便。因此，医学等科技术语现在使用缩略词的形式日益增多。这种缩略方式既可便利读者阅读又节省书刊篇幅，应用日趋普遍，英语医学书刊中比比皆是，故对其构成方式必须有所了解。

1. 缩略词　从完整的词中略去一部分相连的字母，保留下来的部分同样也作为一个独立的单词看待，代替原来的单词，并按单词来拼读，叫做缩略词。

（1）保留词的前部，而将后部略去。如：

doc（=doctor）　医生
lab（=laboratory）　实验室
math（=mathematics）　数学
polio（=poliomyelitis）　小儿麻痹症

（2）保留词的后部，而将前部略去。如：

bus（= omnibus）　公共汽车
phone（= telephone）　电话

（3）保留词的中部，而将前后部均略去。如：

flu（= influenza）　流行性感冒

2. 缩写词　取完整单词的前几个字母，加一圆点，作为代替该单词的缩写形式，叫做缩写词。如：

ab. abortion　流产
acad. academy　学会，学院
alcoh. alcohol　酒精

caps. capsule　胶囊
diag. diagnosis　诊断
tinc. tincture　酊剂

3. 首字母缩略词　由词组表示的术语，取各词的首字母构成缩略词，一概大写，按字母名称读。有时，由一个单词表示的术语也可取构成该词各部分的首字母而形成缩略词。

（1）代表单个的词

RT	radiotherapy	放射治疗
SP	sulfapyridine	磺胺吡啶
SST	succinylsulfathiazole	琥珀酰磺胺噻唑
SDM	sulfadimethoxine	磺胺二甲氧嘧啶
SMP	sulfamethoxypyridazine	长效磺胺
ECG	electrocardiogram	心电图

（2）代表词组

1）	GP	gram positive	革兰氏阳性
	GN	gram negative	革兰氏阴性
	AAO	amino acid oxidase	氨基酸氧化酶
	ACH	adrenal cortical hormone	肾上腺皮质激素
	APH	anterior pituitary hormone	垂体前叶激素
	ASD	atrial septal defect	房间隔缺损
	BCG	Bacille Calmette Guerin	卡介苗
	BOR	bowels open regularly	大便规律
	MBP	mean blood pressure	平均血压
	MFD	minimum fatal dose	最小致死量
2）	ADH	antidiuretic hormone	抗利尿激素
	ANF	antinuclear factors	抗核因子
	RNA	ribonucleic acid	核糖核酸
	DNA	deoxyribonucleic acid	脱氧核糖核酸
	ATP	adenosine triphosphate	三磷酸腺苷
3）	GPD	glucose-6-phosphate dehydrogenase	6-磷酸葡萄糖脱氢酶
	ANT	2-amino-5-nitro-thiazol	2-氨基-5-硝基噻唑
	APL	anterior-pituitary-like substance	类垂体前叶物质
	ASLO	antistreptolysin-O	抗链球菌溶血素 O
	A/G ratio	albumin-globulin ratio	白蛋白-球蛋白比
	Ba enem	barium enema	钡灌肠
	Bl T	blood type	血型
	E coli	Escherichia coli	大肠杆菌

注：laser（LASER），原文为 light amplification by stimulated emission of radiation。汉译激光，全文为受激辐射光放大。这个首字母缩略词比较特殊，它相当于一个独立的单词，按单词拼读，念作[ˈleizə]。

（3）同一缩略词有时代表多种词组术语

Af	acid-fast	抗酸
	albumose-free（tuberculin）	无（结核菌素）
	atrial fibrillation	心房纤颤
	audio frequency	感音频率
SD	standard deviation	标准差
	streptodornase	链球菌脱氧核糖核酸酶
	systolic discharge	心输出量

BP	bed pan	便盆
	biotic potential	生物性电位
	birth place	出生地
	blood pressure	血压
	British pharmacopoeia	英国药典

这类多义的首字母缩略词,在阅读时要特别注意,可根据上下文确定其代表的术语意义。

二、医学阅读常用短语

(一) 常用英语短语(975 条)

医学阅读中的英语短语也是一个需要重视的问题。所谓英语短语是指两个以上的词根据习惯使用形成的一种固定组合。由于它们表达的是基本语义,加之结构简练,所以使用频率较高。英语短语数量较大,其中一部分可从字面意义获得理解(如 point out,with certainty,from beginning to end 等),另一部分则具有新的整体含义,而不是各个词表面意义的简单总和(如 take place,by no means,if at all 等)。这里提供的英语短语主要属于后一种情况,而且是医学书刊中经常使用的,一旦掌握这些短语,阅读过程也就会变得更加轻松自如了。圆括号"()"内的字是可有可无的或为注解;方括号"[ ]"内的字是可替换的。

a batch of 一束,一批
a bit of 一点,少量
a bundle of 一束,一包
a chain of 一连串的
a cloud of 大群,大量
a couple of 两个,一对;几个
a crowd of 许多
a fraction of 一小部分
a good few 不少,很多
a good while 好久,长久
a host of 一大群,许许多多
a particle of 一点儿,少量
a series of 一系列的
a set of 一套,一组
a variety of 种种的,各式各样的
a wealth of 大量的
a world of 许许多多,极大
abound in[with] 富于
above all 尤其是,首先是,最重要的是
above measure 过度,非常,极
access to 通向…的入口,接近
accessible to 可接近的
accord with 适合,相配,与…相符
account for 说明,是…的原因,占…
accustomed to 习惯于
act against 与…对抗
act as 充当,作为
act for 代理

act on[upon]　作用于…，对…起作用
adapt…to　使…适应于
add up to　（加起来的）总数为，累积成…
addiction to　对…的嗜好，对…成瘾
adhere to　附着于…上
adjacent to　邻近于，接近
advantage over　与…相比的优点
adverse to　不利于，与…相反
advisable for　对…适宜
affinity(of…)for　对…的亲和力
after all　归根结底，毕竟
again and again　再三
ahead of　在…前面，优于
ahead of schedule[time]　提前
alert to　对…警惕(警觉)
all at once　突然，一齐，急速地
all but　除…以外都
all over　到处，周身，整个
all through　从头到尾
all told　总计，合计
allied to　与…有关
amount to　合计；等于，达
(an)abundance of　许多的，充裕的
analogous to　类似(相似)于
and so forth[on]　等等，诸如此类
and the like　等等，诸如此类
and vice versa　反之亦然
and what is more　此外
apply to　适用于
arise from　起因于
as(a)consequence of　由于…的结果
as a result of　由于…结果，因为
as a(general)rule　通常，照例
as a whole　整个地，就总体来看
as above　如上
as against　与…对照
as far as　远到，到…程度
as far as…is concerned[goes]　就…而论
as far back as　远在，早在
as follows　如下
as it is　句首作“实际上”解，句末作“照原来样子”解
as it is known　众所周知
as it were　好像，可以说
as long as　只要，…之久
as of　根据…的资料
as regards[respect]　关于，至于
as such　照这样；本身
as the case may be　看情况而定

as to　至于，关于
as usual　照常，照例
as well　同样，也
as well as　像…一样，也，不但…而且…
as with　如同…的情况一样
as yet　现在还，迄今仍，到那时还
aside from　除…外，暂置不论
at a time　一次(多少)，同时
at all　完全，全然
at all costs　无论代价如何
at all events　无论如何
at all times　不论什么时候
at hand　邻近，在手边，所讨论的，不久
at large　充分，详细，整体
at length　终于，详细地
at(the)most　至多不过
at one's disposal　听凭…处理，供…使用
at random　无定向地，随机地
at risk　冒险
at(a)short notice　临时，即刻，忽然
at the expense of　以…为代价
at the initiative of　在…创议下
at the instance of　应…的请求，由于…建议
at the point　此刻，现在
at the risk of　冒…的危险
at will　随意，任意
attributable to　属于…
attribute…to　认为由…引起，把…归功于
aware of　知道，觉察到
be about+inf.　正要，打算
be it so　纵然如此，让它如此
before long　不久之后
before now　以前，从前
below consideration　不予考虑
beside the question　离题
beware of　留心，注意
beyond(all)doubt　无疑地
beyond all hope　没有希望
beyond reach[grasp]　够不着，力不能及
bit by bit　渐渐地，一点一点地
break down　破坏，分裂，分解
break down into[to]　分解[分裂]为
break out　暴发，打开，劈开
bring about　引起，产生
bring forward　提出
bring…into operation　使…投入生产
bring…to light　暴露，阐明
bring up　培养，抚养

broadly speaking　概括地讲
burst forth　忽然出现，冲出，喷出
but for　假使没有，要不是
by accident　偶然
by all means　无论如何，务必
by and large　大体上，基本上
by chance　偶然，意外地
by itself　单独地，独自
by mouth　口服
by no means　决不
by the way　且说（作插入语），顺便
by then　到那时，当时
by turn(s)　轮流地，时而…时而…
by virtue of　依靠…力量，由于
by way of　经由，通过…方法
call for　要求，需要
call forth　唤起，振起，引起
can but　只得，只能
cannot but　不得不，不禁
cannot help(+ing)　不禁（…），忍不住（…）
carry on　开展，继续进行
carry out　进行，实行
carry through　将…进行[坚持]到底
catch hold of　抓住
catch sight of　看见
catch the point of　领会…的要点
center in　以…为中心
certain of　确信，深信
characterized by　以…为特征
classified as　被分类为
classify…into　把…分类为
clear off　清除，理清
coincide with　与…一致（重合）
come about　发生
come forth　出来，出现
come into effect[force]　实行，生效
come into fashion　流行
come into operation　开始运转，生效
come into play　开始起作用，开始运行
come into[in] use　开始应用，采用
come to a conclusion that　得出结论如下
come to a decision　作出决定
come true　实现，成为事实
common to　与…共有
complain of　主诉
comply with　遵照…（行事）
concerned about　关心
concerned with　涉及，与…有关

conduce to 有助于
confer…on[upon] 把…给予
confine…to 把…限制在…上
conform to[with] 与…相符[一致]
confronted with[by] 面临,碰到
consist in 在于,存在于
consist of 由…组成
consist with 与…一致
contrary to 与…相反
contrast…to[with] 把…和…对比
cope with 对付,解决,竞争,针对
date from 起始于,溯源到
deal with 研究,讨论,涉及,处理
decompose into 分解为
depend on[upon] 依靠,取决于
dependent on[upon] 取决于,依赖于
deprive…of 使…失去,剥夺
despite all this 尽管如此
despite of 不管,任凭
devoid of 缺少[无]…的
differentiate…from 将…与…区别开
dispense with 没有…也行,节省
dispose of 处理,安排,解决
divisible into 可分成
do away with 除去,废除
do…harm 对…有害
do much 极有用
do one's best[utmost](+inf.) 尽力…
drain away 流出,排尽
drain off[away] 排除,排出
draw a conclusion 作结论,推断
draw forth 引出,引起
drop away 下降,渐减
drop by drop 一滴一滴地
dwell on[upon] 详述,细说,提及
each other 互相,彼此
eat away 侵蚀,蛀坏
eat up 消耗,消灭,侵蚀
elicit…from 从…中引出
employ in[on] 从事于
empty of 没有,缺少
engaged in 从事于,致力于
enveloped in 被包围住
equal to 等于,胜任
equivalent to 相当于,等于,与…等效
even if 即使…也,甚至
even then 甚至那时
even though 虽然,纵使,即使…也

even when　即使，甚至当…时
ever since　从那时起
every other　每隔一个，所有其他
every second[other]　day　每隔一天
except for　除了，若无
exert an effort　努力，出力
exert…on[upon]　施(力)于
exist in　存在于，处于
exposed to　易遭，暴露于
faced with　面临
fade away　消失，凋谢
fall behind　落后
fall into　分为(几类)，属于，落入
fall into disuse　停止使用
fall out　偶然发生，结果是
fall over　翻倒
far and near　到处，远处
far and wide　普遍，四面八方
far from　远离，远非，决不
figure on　指望，估计
figure out[up]　想出，算出，弄清
find application[use]in　在…方面得到应用
find fault in　看出在…方面的缺点
find out　找出，求出，发现
first of all　首先，第一
fix…to　把…固定于
fix up　安置，准备好
focus…on　集焦，聚焦在
follow the example of　以…为榜样
follow up　把…追究到底，继续，追踪
fond of　喜欢
for a time　一些时候，暂时
for a while　暂时，片刻
for all that　尽管如此
for an instant　一瞬间，片刻
for ever(and ever)　永远
for example　例如
for good(and all)　永远
for instance　例如
for long　长久
for short　简称，为简略起见
for the first time　首次，初步
for the good of　为…利益
for the moment　暂时，目前
for the present　目前，暂时
for the sake of　为了…起见
for the time to come　在将来
for the worse　恶化，每况愈下

for this reason 由于这个缘故,根据这个道理
for want of 因缺乏
free from[of] 无…的,免除…的
free of charge 免费
from first to last 始终
from now on 今后
from the point of view of 据…观点
from then on 从那时起
from time to time 经常,时而,定期
gain an advantage over[of] 胜过,优于
gain an insight into 透彻理解
gain in 在…方面增加
generally speaking 一般说来
get access to 接近,走近
get along with 在…方面有进展,进行,与…相处
get on with 在…方面有进展
get over 越过,渡过,完成,克服
get rid of[from] 摆脱,免除
get through 通过,结束,完成,到达
give(an)account of 解释,叙述
give birth to 生(小孩),产生
give full play to 充分发挥
give light on 使…明白[明显]
give off 放出,排出
give rise to 引起,导致
give up 放出,放弃
given that 假定,已知,给定
go abroad 去国外,出国
go after 跟随,去寻求[探找]
go against 反对,逆…而行
go beyond 超过,胜过
go down 降低,沉没,(风浪)平静下来,屈服,被记下
go in for 从事,为…而努力,参加,爱好,赞成
go into action(effect) 行动起来(实行,生效)
go into operation 开始运转,实行
go into the figures 检查数字
go into the question 调查问题
go on 进行,继续,发生(时日),过去
go over 检查,调查,复习,越过,渡过
go through 通过,经历,看完,审查,讨论
go without 没有…也行
go wrong with …发生故障
good at 善于
good for 适于
good for nothing 无用,无益
group…into 把…分类为
grow up 成长,长大,发生
guard against 提防,预防

had rather[sooner](+inf.)　宁愿(…)
hand down…to　把…留传给
hand in　交进
hand out…to　把…分发给
hand over…to　交出…给,转交给…
hands off　请勿动手,不许干涉
hardly ever　极难得,几乎从不
have a bearing on(upon)　对…有影响(有关)
have a high opinion of　对…评价高
have a low opinion of　对…评价低
have an advantage over　比…优越
have access to　可以接近[理解,看到,出入]
have much to do with　与…有很大关系
have nothing in common with　与…无共同之处
have nothing to do with　与…完全无关
have to(+动词原形)　不得不(…),必须(…)
headed by　以…为首,由…率领
hold back　退缩
hold down[in]　抑制,压制
hold good for　对…有效[适用]
hold…in place　使…保持在适当位置
hosts of　许许多多
hundreds of　数以百计的,许多
hundreds of thousands of　千万个(…),几十万的(…),无数(…)
identical with　与…相同
if at all　即使有(也极少)
if only　只要…就好了
if[unless]otherwise stated　除非另有说明
ignorant of　不知道
illustrative of　说明
in a broad sense　在广义上
in a narrow sense　在狭义上
in a planned way　有计划地
in a sense　在某种意义上
in a word　总而言之
in accord[accordance]with　与…一致,依照
in addition　另外,又
in addition to　除…外
in advance　在…前,预先,事先
in all　总计
in all respects[ways]　在各方面
in brief　简单说来
in bulk　大批,大量
in case　假如,在…时,万一
in case of　如果,在…时,在…情况下
in charge of　对…负责,主管
in common　共同
in common with　与…同样[有共同之处]

in conclusion 最后,总之
in conformity with[to] 和…符合[一致]
in consequence 因此,结果
in consequence of 由于…的结果
in detail 详细地
in direct proportion to 与…成正比
in dispute 争论中,争执中
in doubt 怀疑,迟疑不决
in due course 在适当时候,不久
in due time 在适当时候
in essence 实质上,大体上
in fashion 流行,风行
in favour of 有利于
in general 通常,一般(说来)
in good order 有条不紊,整齐,正常
in honour of 为纪念,向…表示敬意
in inverse proportion of 与…成反比
in itself 就其本性而言,本来
in large 大规模地
in nature 本质上,事实上,在自然界中
in no case 决不
in no time 立刻
in one word 总之,一句话
in operation 在运转中,开工,施行着
in order 有条理,正常
in other words 换言之
in outline 概括地
in place 在适当位置,在场
in preference of 在…之先,优先于
in principle 基本上,原则上
in progress 在进展中
in proper(definite,right)proportion 按适当(一定,适宜)的比例
in prospect 预料,在期望中
in public 公开地
in question 所述的,议论中的,成为问题的
in ratio of…to 按…和…的比例
in[with]reference to 关于,根据
in[with]regard to 关于,就…而论
in respect to[of] 关于,就…而论
in reverse 相反,反之
in review 在审查中,在检查中
in round numbers 约计,大略,就整数计
in search of 寻求
in series 串联,连续,成级数
in set terms 明确地
in short 简单地,总之
in situ 在原位置,在应有的位置,就地,在(施工)现场
in so far as…goes 就…所及的范围

in some way　有几分,在某方面
in spite of　尽管,不管,虽然
in stock　备有,存积,现有
in substance　实质上,实际上
in succession　连续,接连地
in summary　总括地说
in terms of　就…来说,根据,用…话来说
in the absence of　无…时,缺少…时
in the case of　就…而论,在…情况下
in the end　最后,终于
in the event of　万一,如果
in the final[last]　analysis　总之,归根结底
in the first place　首先
in the following　在下文中,在下面
in the gross　大体上,概括地,粗略地
in the light of　按照,鉴于
in the long run　从长远来看,终于
in the mass　整体地,大体上
in the meantime　其间,同时
in the name of　以…名义,代表
in the neighbourhood of　在…的附近,大约
in the original　用原文,在原文中
in the presence of　在有…参与(存在)情况下
in the same manner[way]　同样地
in the vicinity of　在…附近,靠近
in the way of　便利于,关于,在…方面
in this case　在该情况下
in this way　用这种方法
in(good)time　及时,按时
in times　时常
in truth　实际上,说实在的
in turn　依次,而(轮到),(本身)又
in vain　徒然,无益
in view of the fact that　鉴于…这一事实
in virtue of　由于,借助于
inclusive of　连…在内
incompatible with　与…不相容
inconsistent with　和…不一致
independent of　和…无关的,不依赖于,不决定于…的
independently of　与…无关地
inferior to　次于,劣于
inherent in　为…所固有的
inquire into　调查,追究
instead of　代替,而不是
inversely proportional to　与…成反比
involved with　与…联系,涉及
irrespective of　不拘,不顾,不问
it follows that　由此可见,从而,于是

it(so)happened that 偶然,碰巧
it is not the case 情况并非如此
it is out of the question 这是不可能的
it is the case 情况正是如此
it is time(+ing.) 该是(…)时候了
it makes no matter that 无关紧要
it matters little 无关紧要
it matters much 事关紧要
it occurred to(…)that 想到
it was not until[till]…that 直到…才
join in 参加,加入
joined in parallel 并联
joined in series 串联
judging from 由…推测[判断]
jump to[at]a conclusion 匆匆得出结论
just as it is 照原样
just as well 正因如此
just as with 正如同…一样
just now 刚才,还
just so 正是如此
just then 正在那时
keep a record 记录,保持记录
keep abreast of[with] 跟上,使…及时知道
keep an eye on 注意,注视
keep…from(+ing) 使…不(…),阻止…(…)
keep…in mind 记住
keep…in good order 保持…整齐[正常运转]
keep…in place 放好,使…固定不动
keep off 防止…接近
keep on(+ing) 继续(…)
keep pace with 同…齐步并进,跟上
keep to the point 抓住要点
keep to the tradition 保持惯例(传统)
keep up 使…继续下去(保持不衰减)
keep up with 跟上,不落后于
know of[about] 知道关于…的事情
known as 被称为,即,通称是
lack of 缺乏
lag behind 落后,迟滞
later on 后来,今后
launch(out)into 开始做…(另一事情)
lay a basis for 为…打基础
lay down 放下,制订,建造
lay emphasis on[upon] 强调
lay hold of[on] 抓住,利用
lay stress on[upon] 着重于,强调
lay up 贮蓄,闲置不用
lead to 导致,通往

least likely　不大可能
least of all　最不
leave out　把…放在外边,省去,忽视
leave room for　留下…的余地
let alone　更不用说…了
level with　跟…相齐,跟…同等
lie down　躺下
lie in　在于,处于
lie on[upon]　落在,随…而定
live on[by]　以…为生(为食)
long for[after]　渴望
long since　很久以前(早就)
look after　照管,监督
look ahead for[to]　为…预先作准备,预见,预期
look back to　回顾,追溯
look for　寻找,期待
look into　窥视,调查,往…里看
look like　看来像
look out　当心
look upon…as　把…看作
lose no time　不失时机
lose sight of　忽略,看不见
lots of　许多,大量
made after　仿照[模仿]…做的
made from　由…制成(构成)
made(out)of　由…制成[组成]
make a compromise　折衷,兼顾
make a contribution to[towards]　对…作出贡献
make a deduction　推论,推导
make a difference　有差别,很重要,产生影响
make a great step forward　向前跨一大步
make achievements　作出成绩[成就]
make adjustments　进行调节[调整]
make allowance(s)for　考虑,估计,为…留余地
make an attempt(+inf.)　企图[试图](…)
make application for　应用于
make certain　确定,弄明白
make certain of　把…弄清楚
make contributions to　对…作出贡献
make efforts(+inf.)　努力(…)
make inquiries　调查,询问,质问
make light of　轻视
make little of　不重视
make measurement　量度
make much of　重视
make no difference　无足轻重,并无影响
make notes[a note]of　做…笔记
make out　看出,证明,填写,开(清单等)

make progress 取得进步
make sure 弄清楚
make sure of[that] 查明,确信
make up 组成,捏造
make up for 补偿
make up one's mind 下定决心
make use of 利用
many a time 许多次
matter little to 对…无关紧要
matter much to 对…事关紧要
meet the needs of 满足…的需要
merge in[into] 并入
mistake…for 把…误认为
more often than not 时常,多半
more or less 或多或少,多多少少,…左右
more than once 不止一次
more than ever 更加,更多的
most likely(+inf.) 很可能…
most of all 尤其是,首先
much less 况且,何况,更不用说(用于否定句),少得多
name…after 以…命名
named in honour of 为纪念…而命名
near at hand 邻近
nearly all 几乎所有的
needless to say 用不着说的
never mind 没关系,不必介意
next to 次于,紧接于,紧挨着
next to nothing 几乎没有,极少
no alternative but 除…外别无选择
no…at all 一点也没有
no doubt 无疑,当然
no longer 不再,已不
no matter 不要紧,不重要
no more 不再
no more than 不过,仅仅
no sooner…than 刚一…就(…)
no wonder 不足为奇,难怪
none the less (虽然那样)还是,仍然
not…at all 毫不,一点也不
not in any way 无论如何不
not in the least 毫不
not infrequently 常常
not to mention[say] 不用说,更不必说
not to speak of 更不必讲…
noted for 以…著称
nothing but 仅是,不过是
now and again[then] 不时地
null and void 无效,作废

object to　反对，讨厌
obliged to　感谢
of no effect　无效，无益，不中用
on account of　因为，基于
on all accounts　无论如何，总之
on behalf of　以…名义，代表
on condition that　在…条件下，如果
on display　陈列，展出
on duty　值日，值班
on good grounds　完全有根据地
on principle　根据原则
on purpose　故意，特意
on record　留有记录的
on request　函索(即寄)
on sale　出售，上市
on schedule　准时，按预定计划
on the[an]average　平均计算
on the contrary　反之，相反地
on the ground that　基于，由于
on the one hand　一方面
on the other hand　另一方面
on the spot　就地，现场
on the subject of　关于…问题
on the verge of　将近，快要
on the whole　大体上，总的说来
on time　按时，准时
on trial　试用中，试验中
once and again　屡次，再三地
once(and)for all　只此一次，断然
one after another[the other]　一个接着一个，相继地
one another　相互
one by one　逐一，挨个地
open into[on,onto]　通到
or otherwise　或相反，或它的反面
or so　大约，左右
or the like　等等
other than　除了，不同于，而不是
out of balance　不平衡
out of control　失去控制
out of danger　脱险
out of date　不合时宜的，陈旧的，旧式的
out of proportion to　与…不成比例
out of question　无疑地
over again　再一次，重新
owing to　由于，因为
pack up　包装
parallel to[with]　平行于
participate[partake]in　参与，参加，分享

pass away　终止,(时间等)过去;去世
pass into　进入,变成
pass over　越过,渡过,忽视
pay attention to　重视,注意
penetrate into　透入,贯穿
per cent　每百
persist in　坚持,继续存在
pertain to　附属于…,为…固有
pertinent to　与…有关的
pick out　挑选,拣出,辨别出
place an order for　订购
place emphasis[stress]on　强调,着重于
place reliance[confidence]on　信赖
play a part[role]in　在…中起作用
plug in　插上插头
point of view　观点
pour out　注出,倒出
prevail against[over]　胜过
prevent…from(+ing)　阻止…(…)
prior to　在…以前
project from　从…突出(伸出)
project…on[into]　把…投射到
proportional[proportionate]to　与…成比例
put down　放下,记下,削减
put emphasis on[upon]　强调,着重
put forth　发出,长出,伸出,出版
put forward　提出,促进
put…in motion　开动,使…运转
put…into effect　实现,完成
put…into operation[production]　把…投入生产
put…into practice　使…付诸实践
put…into service　使…交付使用
put off　拖延,推迟,脱去
put on　穿上,盖上,增加
put…on trial　对…进行试验
put one's faith in　相信
put one's mind to[on]　专心研究
put…through　实行,完成,通过
put to use　利用
put up　提出,贴出,挂
put up with　忍住
qualflied for[as]　适于作,有担任…资格
question[matter]at[in]issue　悬案,未决的问题
quite a few[a little]　好几个,不少
range between　介于…范围[中间]
rank with　与…并列
rather than　而不是,宁可不
rather…than　与其说…倒不如说…

reach out　伸展
react on[upon]　对…起反应
react to　对…有反应
react with　与…反应
ready for　准备好
reason out　解释清,推论
reckon on[upon]　期望,凭借
reckon up　合计,总计
recognize…as　把…认定为
recover…from　从…中回收
refer to　涉及,指的是,参考
refer to…as　把…称作[指为]
regardless of　不顾,不管
relevant to　与…有关
relieve…from[of]　使…解除[免于,不受]
rely on[upon]　依靠,信赖
remind…of　使…想起
remove…from　从…移走(除去)
report on(upon)　就…提出报告
representative of　表示…的,代表…的特征
research into　调查
resistant to　对…有抗力的,耐…的
responsible for　对…负责,担负,引起
rest on(upon)　依靠,根据,建立在…上
rest with　系于,在于,归于
result from　起因于,由…引起
result in　导致,结果形成
rich in　富于
right away[off,now]　立即,即刻
round about　各方面,大约
round numbers　整数
rule out　消除,排除
run after　追寻,寻求
run down　停止,使…变弱
run into　流入,注入,碰上
run low　快用完,不够用
run out　用完,溢出
run parallel with　和…平行
run short　快用完,不够用
run through　穿过,遍及,略读
seal off[up]　密封,封闭
search after[for]　寻找,探求
search into　调查
second to　次于
see to　留心,照料
see(to it) that　设法使,务使
seeing that　鉴于,由于,考虑到
send for　派人取(请)

send forth 发出,放出
send out 发出,放射出
sensible of 知觉到,觉察
sensitive to 对…灵敏,易感受
serve as[for] 用作,担任,起…作用
serve the purpose of 可充当,可用作
set about 开始,着手
set aside 撇开,取消,放弃,保留
set down 卸下,放下,记下,制订
set forward 提出,促进
set free 被释放,被放出
set in 来临,开始
set up 建立,产生,引起,提出,设立,安装
settle down 安定下来,沉下,沉淀
settle out 沉淀出来
settle up 决定,解决
share…with 和…分享
shed light on[upon] 照亮,阐明
short of 缺少,不到
show interest in 对…表示关切[感兴趣]
show signs of 表明有…迹象
show up 显露出来
similar to 类似[相似]于…的
single out…from 从…中区分出[选拔出]
sketch out 拟订
slow down 减慢,减速
so far 至今,至此
so far as 就…来说,在…范围内,到…的程度
so far as we know 就我们所知
so long as 只要,假如
so to say[speak] 可说是
something wrong with …有毛病[不对头]
sooner or later 迟早
sort out 拣出,分类
speak of…as 把…说成
spread over 传遍,遍布,延续,覆盖
spread to 传到,波及
stand for 代表,支持,可用作
stand good 有效,始终如一
stand out 突出,出色
stand still 站着不动,搁置不动
stand to it 支持,竭力主张
stand up to 经受住,对抗
stem from 基于,出于
step by step 逐步地
stick to 粘住,坚持,固守
straight away[off] 立刻,马上
strangely enough 不可思议

strictly speaking　严格地说
strive for　争取，为…而努力
struggle against[with]　同…斗争
struggle for　为…而斗争
subject…to　使…受[服从，从属于]
subject to　蒙受，易受
substitute…for　以…代替
such as above[below]　如同上[下]述那样
such as it is[they are]　虽然如此
such is the case with　…的情况也是如此
suck in　吸收
suck out　吸出
suffice for　满足…的需要
sum total　总和
sum up　总结，总计
superior to　优于，胜过
susceptible to　对…敏感，易受…的
symmetric to　对称于，和…对称的
take a different view　持不同观点[见解]
take a view of　观察一番
take account of　考虑到
take(the) advantage of　利用，运用
take…as　把…看做
take care　注意，留神
take care of　照看，看管，留心
take charge of　负责
take down　记下，卸下
take effect　见效，生效
take example　用作榜样
take…for　把…当做
take…for example(instance)　以…为例
take…for granted　认为…理所当然的
take in　收进，吸收
take…into account[consideration]　考虑到
take measures　采取措施
take medicine　服药
take note[notice]　of　注意到
take part in　参加，参与
take place　发生，举行
take possession of　占有
take precaution against　预防
take priority of[over]　比…占先[优先]
take shape　成形，现形
take steps　采取措施[步骤]
take the lead　带头，领先
take the place of　代替，取代
take time　花费时间
take turns　轮流，换班

tear out 扯下
tell…from 把…和…区别开
ten to one 十之八九,很有可能,有…趋势
tend to[towards] 倾向于,趋向于
thanks to 由于,幸亏
that is 也就是说
that is to say 就是说,即
the former…the latter 前者…后者
the other day 那天,前几天,前些日子
the way out 解决办法,出口
the way to 通往…的道路
think light[little] of 认为…不重要
think much of 重视
think nothing of(+ing) 不把…放在心里,轻视
think of 想起,考虑
think of…as 把…认为是
think out 想出
think over 考虑
thousands upon thousands of 成千上万
throw(a)light on 帮助说明,阐明
throw doubt on 对…表示怀疑
thus much 只此,就这么多,到此为止
time and again 反复,多次
to and fro 往复,来回
to be more exact(precise) 更精确地说
to be short 简言之
to date 至今
to our knowledge 据我们所知[看来]
to say nothing of 更不必说
to the contrary 相反
to the disadvantage of 对…不利
to the end[last] 到底,至终
to the point 中肯,扼要
to the point of[that] 到…程度
to this end 为此目的
trade brand 商品牌子
trade mark 商标
try every means 用各种手段
try one's best(+inf.) 尽全力(…)
turn aside from 偏离,撇开…(不谈)
turn back 折回,返
turn down 翻,折,驳回
turn…from…to 把…由…转变为…
turn into 变成,使变成(译成)
turn out 生产,关闭,培养出
turn out(to be)+a. 结果弄清楚是…,原来是…
turn over 翻,翻转,倾覆
turn round[around] 绕…旋转

turn to　变成，转向，着手
turn up　发生，出现
under consideration　在考虑之中的
under construction　在建设中
under correction　待纠正
under development　正在研制（发展）中
under discussion　在讨论中
under investigation　在研究中
under no account　决不
under no circumstances　在任何情况下都不
under observation　在观察中
under repair　在修理中
under review　在考虑中，在研究中
under the operating rules　根据操作规程
under way　在进行中，在航行中
unless otherwise indicated[mentioned, noted, specified, stated]　除非另有陈述（提及、注释、规定、说明）
until now　迄今
until then　直到那时
up to　达到，归…负责
up to date　最新的，现代化的
up to now　到现在为止
up to the present　直到现在
up to this moment　至今
upside down　颠倒
used to　习惯于
vary(directly) with[as]　与…成正比
vary inversely as[with]　和…成反比
vary with[as]　随着…而变化
void of　没有[缺乏]…的
volumes of　大量的
warm up　变热，兴奋，做准备动作
wash well　耐洗
watch for　（留意）等待，注视，提防
watch out　注意
watch over　看守，保护
wear and tear　耗损，磨损
wear away　磨损，（时间）渐渐过去
wear off　磨掉，（渐）消逝，变小
wear out　用坏，变旧
wear well　耐用，耐磨
well above[over]　大大超过[高于]
what with…and what with　一则由于…再则由于
whatever the reason be　不论什么理由
wipe away[off]　擦掉，抹掉
wipe out　擦去，扫除，消灭
with a[the] view of[to]　以…为目的，为…起见，意在
with advantage　有利于，有效地

with care　小心地，仔细地
with due regard for　适当考虑到
with ease　容易地
with effect　有效地
with leaps and bounds　飞速地，很快地
with one accord　一致地
with reference to　关于，至于，参考
with regerd[relation]to　关于，对于，在…方面
with reserve　有保留地
with respect to　关于，对于
with the intention[object,purpose]of　打算，以…为目的
with the purpose that　为的是，为了
with the result that　结果就，从而
with this end in view　为此目的，因此
with vigour　朝气蓬勃地
within experimental error　不超过实验误差范围
within(one's)grasp　在…力所能及的范围内
within the province of　在…界限(领域)内
without avail　无益，无效
without controversy　无可争辩的(地)
without doubt　毫无疑问
without effect　无效
without reserve　无保留地
work at　从事于学习[工作，研究等]
work in with　和…协调[配合]
work on[away]　继续工作，继续努力
work on[upon]　影响，对…发生作用，靠…工作
work out　制订，做出，算出，解决，尽量开采
worthy of note　值得注意的
year after[by]year　一年一年地
year in and year out　一年到头，年年不断
yield to　听从于，让步于，受到…作用[影响]，陷入…(某种状态)
zealous for　热望，切望
zealous in　热心于

(二) 常用拉丁短语(81 条)

医学英语受拉丁语的影响不仅表现在医学术语上，而且也体现在拉丁短语的使用上。这里提供的拉丁短语除少数用于处方外，其余均可偶尔出现在现代英语，特别是医学英语书刊中，谨供读者学习或查阅。

a posteriori　后天的[地]，归纳的[地]
a priori　先天的[地]，演绎的[地]
ab antiquo　自古
ab extra　从外部，外来
ab initio　从开头，自始
ab intra　从内部，从里面
ad arbitrium　随意地，独断地
ad decubitum　临睡时用

ad effctum　直到有效
ad extremum　极端地，最后
ad finem　最后，最终
ad hoc　为此目的
ad infinitum　永远，无限
ad interim　临时，暂时
ad libitum　随意（量），任意（量）
ad usum　依照习惯
ad usum externum　外用
ad usum internum　内服
ad verbum　逐字地
alma mater　母校
ante caenam　晚饭前
ante cibum　饭前
ante horam decubitus　睡前
ante jentaculum　早饭前
ante meridiem（略 a. m. 或 A. M.）　上午，午前
bis in die　每天二次（服药）
curriculum vitae　（个人）简历
de facto　事实上（的），实际上的
de novo　从头，再
et al（et alia 的缩写）　等等
et cetera　以及其他等等
et sequentes　以及下列等等
ex abrupto　突然
ex more　照惯例，按照风俗
exmpli gratia（略 e. g.）　例如
grosso modo　大概地，大约地
homo sapiens　人类
id est（略 i. e.）　那就是，即
in abstracto　抽象的，理论上
in brevi　简言之，简略地
in die　每天，每日
in esse　实际存在的
in extenso　全部地，详尽地
in extremis　临终，到最后关头
in fine　末尾（指书页或书的篇章）
in natura　实在
in parvo　微不足道的数量
in perpetuum　永久地
in situ　原位
in toto　全部地，整个
in vitro　（活）体外，试管内
in vivo　（活）体内
ipso facto　依照事实本身
loco citato　从上述引文中
locus in quo　现场
nota bene（略 N. B.）　注意，留心

per annum 每年
per anum 经肛门
per capita 每人,按人口(计算)
per centum(略 per cent) 百分之…
per diem 每日,按日
per mensem 每月,按月
per os 经口,口服
per rectum 经直肠
per se 本身,本来,本质上
post factum 事后
post hoc 因此,由此
post meridiem(略 p. m. 或 P. M.) 下午,午后
post mortem 死后
post partum 产后
post scriptum(略 p. s. 或 P. S.) (信末)又及,附言
pro dosi 一次量
pro et contra(略 pro et con) 赞成与反对
pro forma 形式上(的)
pro narcosi 麻醉用
pro rata 按比例的[地]
pro re nata 必要时
pro tempore 当时(的),暂时(的)
punctum saliens 要点,重要情况
quantum libet (处方用)随意量
quantum sufficit (处方用)适量,足量
quaque die 每天一次
quaque nocte 每晚(睡前服)
quaque quarta hora 每四小时一次
quaque secundo die 每二天一次
quoad hoc 到此程度[范围]
quod vide 参阅
rigor mortis 尸僵,死后僵直
semper paratus 时刻准备
sine die 不定期(延期)
sine dubio 无疑地
sine qua non 必要条件
status quo 现状
sub finem 参见本章[本篇、本书]末
summa summarum 总计,合计
ter in die 每天三次
unum et idem 同样的东西
ut infra 如下所述
ut supra 如上所述,同上
vice versa 反之亦然
vide infra 参见下文
vide supra 参见上文

（三）常用缩写词(210 个)

英语缩写词是指一个完整单词取其第一个或前几个字母加圆点来代替原来的词，实际的语言应用逐渐将一部分缩写词末尾的圆点也省去。扩大来看，缩写词也可指取多词中每个词的首字母组合而成的形式，这类形式往往被称为首字母缩略词。附录第一部分"英语医学术语的特征"虽已提及缩写词，但主要为概念性介绍，举例不多。英语缩写词的数量也较大，这里提供的是医学书刊中经常使用的一部分。下面大致按内容集中分组，以便读者学习查找。

AMA　American Medical Association　美国医学会
BMA　British Medical Association　英国医学会
CMA　Chinese Medical Association　中华医学会
AJMS　American Journal of Medical Sciences　美国医学杂志
BMJ　British Medical Journal　英国医学杂志
JAMA　Journal of American Medical Association　美国医学会杂志
CMJ　Chinese Medical Journal　中华医学杂志
BP　British Pharmacopeia　英国药典
BPC　British Pharmaceutical Codex　英国药物处方
USP　United States Pharmacopeia　美国药典
CP　Chinese Pharmacopeia(Pharmacopeia of People's Republic of China)　中华人民共和国药典
UK　United Kingdom　联合王国(英国)
USA　United States of America　美利坚合众国(美国)
PRC　People's Republic of China　中华人民共和国
UN　United Nations　联合国
WHO　World Health Organization　世界卫生组织
vol. volume　体积，容积
Vol. Volume　卷，册
Chap. Chapter　章
Sec. Section　节
Parag. Paragraph　段
P. (p.) Page　页
pp. pages　页
L. (l.) Line　行
No. Number(L. Numero)　数，序号，编号
Abstr. Abstract　摘要，文摘
et al. et alii(=and others)　等等，等人
etc. et cetera(=and so on)　等等
ca(c.) circa　大约，前后
ib. (ibid.) ibidem　出处同上
Cf(cf.) confer　比较，参看
ref. reference　参考
c/o care of　由…转交
vs versus　对…，与…相比较
i. e. id est(=that is)　即
viz. videlicet　即，就是
e. g. exempli gratia(=for example)　例如
Fig. Figure　图
N. B. Nota Bene(=note well)　留心，注意

P. S. (p. s.)postscript （信末签名后的）附言
C. V. curriculum vitae （个人）简历
IQ intelligence quotient 智力商数(智商)
p. a. per annum 每年
a. m. (A. M.) ante meridiem 上午
p. m. (P. M.) post meridiem 下午
B. C. Before Christ 公元前
A. D. Anno Domini 公元
wt. weight 重量,体重
ht. height 高度,身高
BP Blood Pressure 血压
R. B. C. red blood cell count 红细胞计数
W. B. C. white blood cell count 白细胞计数
C. B. C. complete blood count 全血细胞计数
ECG electrocardiogram 心电图
EEG electroencephalogram 脑电图
BCG Bacille Calmette-Guerin 卡介苗(菌)
RNA ribonucleic acid 核糖核酸
DNA deoxyribonucleic acid 去氧核糖核酸
pH symbol for expression of hydrogen ion concentration 氢离子浓度,酸碱度
BaE barium enema 钡灌肠
BaM barium meal 钡餐
TB tuberculosis 结核
CA(ca) carcinoma 癌,cancer 癌
AIDS acquired immune deficiency syndrome 艾滋病
CT computerized tomography(CT Scan) 计算机化断层 X 线摄影
NMR nuclear magnetic resonance 核磁共振
MRI magnetic resonance imaging 磁共振成像
C/O complain of 陈诉,主诉
ENT ears,nose and throat 耳鼻喉
GI gastrointestinal 胃肠
GIT gastro-intestinal tract 胃肠道
ASD atrial septal defect 房间隔缺损
VSD ventricular septal defect 室间隔缺损
DIC disseminated intravascular coagulation 弥漫性血管内凝血
SLE systemic lupus erythematosus 系统性红斑狼疮
Hb haemoglobin 血红蛋白
HBP high blood pressure 高血压
LBP low blood pressure 低血压
CNS central nervous system 中枢神经系统
ICU intensive care unit 重症监护病房
CCU coronary care unit 冠心病监护室
OP out-patient 门诊病人
IP in-patient 住院病人
a. c. ante cibum 饭前
p. c. post cibum 饭后
b. i. d. bis in die 每日二次
t. i. d. ter in die 每日三次
q. i. d. quater in die 每日四次

q. d. quaque die　每日一次
q. n. quaque nocte　每晚
q. s. quantum satis　足量，适量
stat. statim　立即
p. r. n. pro re nata(=as required)　必要时
i. m. (I. M.)　intramuscular　肌内的(肌肉注射)
i. v. (I. V.)　intravenous　静脉内的(静脉注射)
Ⅳ　四
Ⅶ　七
Ⅸ　九
XIV　十四
XXI　二十一
LXX　七十
CI　一百零一
CC　二百
DC　六百
MM　二千
c. c. cubic centimeter　立方厘米
cm　centimeter　厘米
gm(g.)　gram　克
l　litre　升
lb　libra[L] =pound　磅(重量单位)
oz　ounce　英两
m　meter　米
ft　foot(feet)　英尺
in. inch　英寸
hr　hour　(小)时
min　minute　分
sec　second　秒
lab　laboratory　实验室
cal　calorie　卡(路里)
Cal　Calorie　千卡，大卡
C　curie　居里(放射单位)
R　roentgen　伦琴
dB　decibel　分贝
Hz　hertz　赫兹
W　watt　瓦特
V　volt　伏特
N　newton　牛顿
mp　melting point　熔点
atm　atmospheres　大气压
℃　Centigrade　摄氏温标
℉　Fahrenheit　华氏温标
Å　angstrom unit　埃(波长单位 $=10^{-8}$ 厘米)
IU　international unit　国际单位
sq　square　平方
cu　cubic　立方
kg　kilogram　千克
km　kilometer　千米

kw kilowatt 千瓦
kv kilovolt 千伏
mg milligram 毫克
ml millilitre 毫升
mm millimeter 毫米
mA milliampere 毫安
mC millicurie 毫居
mEq milliequivalent 毫当量
μg microgram 微克
μA microampere 微安
μsec microsecond 微秒
mph miles per hour 英里/时
approx. approximately 大约
max. maximum 最大量
min. minimum 最小量
Sun. Sunday 星期日
Mon. Monday 星期一
Tues. Tuesday 星期二
Wed. Wednesday 星期三
Thur. Thursday 星期四
Fri. Friday 星期五
Sat. Saturday 星期六
Jan. January 元月
Feb. February 二月
Aug. August 八月
Sept. September 九月
Oct. October 十月
Nov. November 十一月
Dec. December 十二月
wk week(s) 周
yr year(s) 年
B. A. Bachelor of Arts 文学士
B. M. Bachelor of Medicine 医学士
B. Med. Sc. Bachelor of Medical Science 医学士
B. Pharm. Bachelor of Pharmacy 药学士
B. Sc. Bachelor of Science 理学士
M. A. Master of Arts 文学硕士
M. Med. Master of Medicine 医学硕士
M. Pharm. Master of Pharmacy 药学硕士
M. Sc. Master of Science 理学硕士
M. D. [L.] Medicinae Doctor 医学博士
D. M. Doctor of Medicine 医学博士
D. Pharm. Doctor of Pharmacy 药学博士
D. Sc. Doctor of Science 理学博士
Ph. D. Doctor of Philosophy = (L.) Philosophiae Doctor 哲学博士
GP General Practitioner 非专科医生(通看各科的开业医生)
R. N. Registered Nurse 注册护士
Prof. Professor 教授
Dr. Doctor 医师;博士

Mr. Mister　先生
Mrs. Mistress　夫人
Ms. [miz]　代表 Miss 或 Mrs.　女士
Mme. [Fr.]　Madame(=madam)　夫人,女士,太太
CCTV　China Central Television　中国中央电视台
BBC　British Broadcasting Corporation　英国广播公司
VOA　Voice of America　美国之音
CAAC　General Administration of Civil Aviation of China　中国民用航空总局(CAAC 是前译名 Civil Aviation Administration of China 的缩写,现仍沿用)
CA　China Airline　中国航空公司
SE　standard error　标准误差
VAT　value added tax　增值税
SOS　Save our souls!(international distress signal)　国际通用的呼救信号
UFO　unidentified flying object　来历不明的空中飞行物,飞碟
Am. Eng. American English　美国英语
Brit. Eng. British English　英国英语
Dept. department　科,系,部
Co. company　公司
Ltd. limited　股份有限(公司)
£　pound(sterling)　英磅
$　American dollar　美元
¥　Renminbi yuan　人民币元
¢　cent　美分
E　east　东
S　south　南
W　west　西
N　north　北
rd　road　路
cnr corner　(街道)拐角
ad. advertisement　广告

(四) 双词医学术语的理解和汉译(270 条)

双词医学术语是指由两个英语词组成的具有固定含义的常用术语。这类术语是由"名词或形容词(包括动词变来的分词)+名词"构成,数量甚多。其中大多数可以从字面获得正确理解,如:blood analysis 血液分析,pathogenic bacteria 病原菌,cystic calculus 膀胱结石,latent heat 潜热,maintenance dose 维持(剂)量。但是,也有相当一部分在理解时会遇到一定困难,不能望文生义,如:surgical abdomen 急腹症,threatened abortion 先兆流产,chronological age 实足年龄。这类术语的确切含义,以及与之对应的汉语术语同英语术语的表面文字略有变化,因此在阅读碰到时需要加以注意。两者之间的差异常见的有下列一些情况:①中外不同表达习惯,如:daughter cell 子细胞; brown sugar 红糖。②含义略有扩展,如:horizontal position 平仰卧位; breast feeding 母乳喂养。③含义略有引伸或转弯,如:hunger edema 营养不良性水肿;mother abscess 原发脓肿。④出自典故,如:Adam's apple 喉结;cesarean section 剖腹产术。⑤词的多义用于不同搭配中,如:essential,specific 等。下面提供的 270 条这类术语均属常用,如能集中学习初步熟悉,今后在阅读英语医学文献时碰到它们就不致造成理解上的差错。为了便于读者学习和记忆,特将有相对含义的两个术语或紧密关联的术语连排。

abdominal hydrops　腹[腔积]水
abdominal breathing　腹式呼吸

abdominal epilepsy 腹性癫痫
abdominal delivery 剖腹产
absolute amenorrhea 完全经闭
absolute ether 纯乙醚
absolute idiocy 深度白痴
absolute immunity 绝对免疫
absorbent gauze 脱脂纱布(吸水纱布)
accelerative epilepsy 前奔性癫痫
acquired astigmatism 后天散光
congenital astigmatism 先天散光
acquired immunity 获得性免疫
active principle 有效成分
active stage 进行期,活动期
Adam's apple 喉结
advanced stage 晚期
advanced technology 先进技术
after birth 胞衣,胎盘胎膜
after care 术后疗法
after vision 遗后视觉,遗视
air quarantine 航空检疫
air sacs 肺泡
air tube 呼吸管,呼吸道
alarm reaction 紧急反应
alcohol group 醇基
alimentary anemia 营养性贫血
alimentary therapeutics 饮食疗法,营养疗法
alimentary toxicosis 食物中毒
altitude anoxia 高空缺氧
ambulant edema 移动性水肿
ambulatory plague 轻鼠疫,不卧床鼠疫
ambulatory typhoid 逍遥型伤寒
angina pectoris 心绞痛
ardent fever 高热
artificial labor 引产
attending physician 主治医师
attending nurse 随访护士
baby teeth 乳齿
bad breath 口臭
bay salt 海盐(食盐)
birth injury 产伤
birth paralysis 产伤麻痹
black juice 粗制甘草浸膏
blood group 血型
blue baby 青紫婴儿,发绀婴儿
blue jaundice 青紫色黄疸
body build index 体格指数
bottle feeding 人工喂养
bottle nose 酒渣鼻
breast feeding 母乳喂养

breast pump　吸乳器
bronchic cell　肺泡
brown sugar　红糖
bypass technique　分流术
camp fever　斑疹伤寒
candle power　烛光
cell organ　细胞器
certified pipette　检定吸管
cesarean section　剖腹产术
characteristic X-rays　标识 X 线
chest index　胸径指数
Chinese gelatin　琼脂
chronological age　实足年龄
circulating albumin　体液白蛋白
clinical jaundice　显性黄疸
closed fracture　无创骨折,单纯骨折
　open fracture　有创骨折,哆开骨折
closed gland　内分泌腺
　open gland　外分泌腺
coarse injection　大血管注射液
coated tablet　包衣片
coated tongue　舌苔
cold injury　冻伤
collateral inheritance　旁亲遗传
color index　血色指数
confirmatory incision　诊断性切开
constitutional jaundice　体质性黄疸
contact lens　隐形镜片
contrast medium　造影剂,对比剂
control animal　对照动物
critical hemorrhage　骤退期出血
critical temperature　临界温度
cross fertilization　异体受精
crucial bandage　十字绷带
culture medium　培养基
daughter cell　子细胞
daughter colony　子菌落
dead hand　呆手(由机器震动引起)
dead time　失效时间
deep percussion　重叩(诊)
devil' s grip　鬼抓风,流行性胸膜痛
differential diagnosis　鉴别诊断
differential growth　微分生长
direct astigmatism　循环性散光
　inverse astigmatism　反规性散光
direct embolism　顺行栓塞
diving goiter　游动性甲状腺肿
dominant heredity　显性遗传
elementary analysis　元素分析

emergency center 急救中心
emergency room 急诊室
emergency theory 应急学说
emergency tracheotomy 紧急气管切开术
equivalent weight 当量
essential asthma 特发性气喘
essential cause 基(本原)因
  secondary cause 辅因,继发性原因
essential dysmenorrhea 自发性痛经
exertion dyspnea 运动性呼吸困难
family planning 计划生育
field block anesthesia 区域麻醉
field hospital 野战医院
fine adjustment 细调整
fine injection 小血管注射液
first circulation 原始循环
first finger(=thumb) 拇指
  second finger 食指
  third finger 中指
  fourth finger(=ring finger) 无名指(环指)
  little finger 小指
first-aid station 急救站
fluid lung 肺水肿
focal lesion 局灶性损害
full diet 普通饮食
general anatomy 解剖学总论
  special anatomy 解剖学各论
general hospital 综合医院,普通医院
general immunity 全身免疫
germ area 胚区,胚盘
germ cell 生殖细胞
germ theory 生原学说
germ tube 芽管
gross lesion 肉眼损害
heart failure 心力衰竭
heart kidney 心形肾
horizontal position 平仰卧位
hunger edema 营养不良性水肿
immediate auscultation 直接听诊
  mediate auscultation 间接听诊
indifferent epithelium 未分化上皮
indirect hernia 斜疝(腹股沟)
initial heat 初热
intellectual aura 梦样先兆
internal organs 内脏
interrupted sterilization 间歇灭菌法
intra-uterine pneumonia 胎儿肺炎
invalid food 疗养食物
iron-wire suture 钢丝缝术

Jonston's alopecia　斑形脱发
jump graft　迁移移植片
life insurance　人寿保险
life span　寿命
loose stool　稀粪
lung field　肺野
major antigen　主要抗原
　minor antigen　次要抗原
major asynergy　步行协同不能(重度协同不能)
　minor asynergy　指向协同不能(轻度协同不能)
major hypnotism　深催眠状态
　minor hypnotism　浅催眠状态
major neuralgia　重性神经痛
　minor neuralgia　轻性神经痛
major variola　重型天花
　minor variola　轻型天花
manifest hyperopia　显性远视
march hemoglobinuria　步行性血红蛋白尿
masked epilepsy　假面性癫痫,隐性癫痫
masked gout　隐匿性痛风
masked hyperthyroidism　掩蔽性甲状腺功能亢进
mass infection　大量感染
mass reflex　总体反射
medicinal glue　阿胶
metabolic pool　代谢库
milky ascites　油(脂)性腹水
molecular death　细胞死亡
mother abscess　原发脓肿
negative anemia　非红细胞减少性贫血
negligible glycosuria　非病理性糖尿
Newton's alloy　铋铅锡软合金
noble cell　分化细胞
noble gas　惰性气体
normal allergy　普通变应性
normal gigantism　全面巨大发育
normal solution　当量溶液
nurse cell　营养细胞
nurse school　护士学校
nursing department　护理部
nursing mother　哺乳母亲
optic radiation　视辐射线
organic paralysis　器质性麻痹
organized enzyme　活性酶
pictorial aphasia　象形性失语
pigeon chest　鸡胸
plain film　平片
plain filter　普通滤器
plastic phlebitis　粘连性静脉炎
primary alcohol　伯醇

secondary alcohol　仲醇
tertiary alcohol　叔醇
primary amputation　早期切断术
secondary amputation　二期切断术
tertiary amputation　三期切断术
primary anesthesia　初期麻醉
primary assimilation　初次同化
secondary assimilation　二次同化
primary atom　第一级原子
primary cancer　原发癌
primary digestion　第一度消化(胃肠消化)
secondary digestion　第二度消化(乳糜管内消化)
primary glaucoma　原发性青光眼
secondary glaucoma　继发性青光眼
primary radiation　初级放射
secondary radiation　次级放射
primary sex characters　第一性征
secondary sex characters　第二性征(副性征)
primary urethra　原尿道
secondary urethra　后成尿道
primary wall　初生壁
secondary wall　次生壁
preclinical medicine　基础医学
prescribed rate　规定率
primitive kidney　原肾
productive bronchitis　增生性支气管炎
productive cough　咳痰(多痰的咳嗽)
nonproductive cough　干咳
prolonged labor　滞产
protective inoculation　防御接种
purified aloe　精制芦荟
railway catheter　槽式导管
regional surgery　局部外科
relative amenorrhea　月经减少
remote heredity　间接遗传,隔代遗传
remote infarct　陈旧梗死
rhythm method　安全期避孕法
rhythmic respiration　节律性呼吸
sandwich irradiation　夹入照射
second sight　视力再生,老年期视力回春
secondary culture　继代培养
secondary hypertension　继发性高血压
secondary receptors　第二级受体
section preparation　切片标本
sensible perspiration　显汗
insensible perspiration　不显汗
side effect　副作用
silent peritonitis　潜伏性腹膜炎
simple gingivitis　单纯性龈炎

sliding scale　计算尺
smallpox vaccine　牛痘苗
solid edema　实性水肿
solid vision　实体视觉
somatic antigen　菌体抗原
somatic death　整体死亡
specific gravity　比重
specific ionization　电离比度
specific irritability　特殊应激性
specific reaction　特异性反应
specific remedy　特效药
specific volume　比容
still birth　死产
stronger ether　加醇乙醚
subtotal gastrectomy　大部胃切除术
sudden death　猝死
surgical abdomen　急腹症
surgical kidney　外科肾(脓肾)
systemic circulation　体循环
table salt　食盐
teacher's node　结节性声带炎
terminal arteries　终动脉
terminal edema　临终时水肿
terminal infection　末期感染
terminal leukocytosis　濒死期白细胞增多
terminal nerves　末梢神经
tertiary compound　三元化合物
tested antitoxin　标准抗毒素
theatre nurse　手术室护士
thermal hammer　烙锤
thermal water　温泉水
thirst cure　节饮疗法
thirst enema　解渴灌肠剂
threatened abortion　先兆流产
type culture　标准培养(物)
ultimate analysis　元素分析
universal antidote　一般解毒剂
vegetable alkali　生物碱
virginal generation　单性生殖
visiting hours　探视时间
visiting physician　主治医师
visiting scholars　访问学者
vital capacity　肺活量
vital signs　生命体征
walking dysentery　轻型痢疾,逍遥型痢疾
wandering arthritis　游走性关节炎
war medicine　军事医学
washed clot　冲击性血块
weeping eczema　湿润性湿疹

weight-height formula　高重公式
wet brain　脑水肿
wet lung　肺积水
wet nurse　乳母,奶妈
white nevus　无色(素)痣
wind colic　气绞痛
withdrawal effect　脱瘾作用
zero gravity　失重

还有一部分双词术语,由于中心名词的多义,也常引起理解上的困难。这类名词虽然为数不多,但也需对它们有所了解,以便以后遇到时在理解上会容易些。

1. uterine appendages　子宫附件
   pituitary appendage　垂体
   atrial appendage　心耳
   vermicular appendage　阑尾
2. thermal balance　热平衡
   precision balance　精密天平
   platform balance　台秤
3. pleural cavity　胸膜腔
   fissure cavity　裂(龋)洞
   alveolar cavity　牙槽
   secretory cavity　分泌室
4. blood cell　血细胞
   bronchic cell　肺泡
   absorption cell　吸收池
   apoplectic cell　卒中性小房
5. nerve center　神经中枢
   ossification center　骨化中心
   health center　卫生院
   blood donor center　献血站
6. heart chamber　心腔
   anterior chamber　前房
   condensing chamber　冷凝室
   hyperbaric chamber　高压(氧)舱
7. essential element　重要成分
   chemical element　化学元素
   memory element　存储单元
   threshold element　阈元件
8. auditory field　听区
   radiation field　照射野
   magnetic field　磁场
   scientific field　科学领域
9. sulfa film　磺胺薄膜
   blood film　血膜
   plain film　平片
   x-ray film　X 线胶片
10. molecular formula　分子式
    antigen formula　抗原公式
    chemical formula　化学结构式
    decomposition formula　化学分解式

official formula　法定处方

11. asexual generation　无性世代
filial generation　子代
parental generation　亲代

12. coli group　大肠菌群
nitrogen group　氮族
functional group　机能簇
reference group　参考组
alcohol group　醇基
blood group　血型

13. health habit　卫生习惯
drug habit　药瘾
endothelioid habit　内皮样型
apoplectic habit　中风体型

14. color index　血色指数
icteric index　黄疸指数
subject index　标题索引
Index Medicus　医学杂志总索引
index finger　食指

15. artificial lens　人工晶状体
compound lens　复透镜
spherical lens　球面镜片

16. sub-cellular level　亚细胞水平
alcohol blood level　血酒精浓度
skin potential level　皮肤电位水准
speech interference level　言语干扰级
chronic threshold level　慢性阈值

17. medical library　医学图书馆
gene library　基因文库

18. intellectual life　精神生活
intrauterine life　宫内生命期
average life　平均寿命
reproductive life　育龄
half life　半衰期

19. fluorescent light　荧光
infrared light　红外线
revelation light　聚光灯(手术用)

20. peptide linkage　肽键
genetic linkage　遗传连锁
record linkage　记录联系

21. alignment mark　对线法标志
pressure mark　压痕
birth mark　胎痣
electric mark　电流斑
ligature mark　索沟

22. Mikulicz's mask　米库利奇氏手术口罩
gas mask　防毒面具
face mask　面罩
anesthetic mask　麻醉罩

23. achromatic mass　非染色质
    appendix mass　阑尾块
    pill mass　丸块
    epithelial mass　上皮团
    atomic mass　原子质量
24. crystalline material　晶体物质
    infective material　传染物
    raw material　原料
    reference material　参考材料
25. preventive medicine　预防医学
    internal medicine　内科学
    compound medicine　复方药物
    folk medicine　民间医药
    specific medicine　特效药
26. culture medium　培养基
    blood medium　血(液)培养基
    blocking medium　阻滞媒质
    clearing medium　透明介质
    contrast medium　造影剂,对比剂
27. muscle pattern　肌范型
    breathing pattern　呼吸型式
    amino acid pattern　氨基酸模式
    finger patterns　指纹花样
28. latent phase　潜伏期
    recovery phase　恢复期
    inhibiting phase　抑制相
    specific phase　特异相
29. foot plate　底板
    culture plate　培养皿
    cover plate　盖片
30. critical potential　临界电位
    disease potential　发病潜势
    reproductive potential　生殖潜力
    racial differentiation potential　种族鉴定能力
31. magnifying power　放大率
    high power　高倍(镜)
    bactericidal power　杀菌力
    candle power　烛光
32. preoperative preparation　术前准备
    pharmaceutic preparation　药物制剂
    stained preparation　染色标本
33. dominant principle　优势原则
    displacement principle　移位原理
    active principle　有效成分
    anti-anemia principle　抗贫血物质
34. costal process　肋突
    birth process　产程,分娩过程
    dry process　干处置法(片剂)
    photochemical process　光化作用

35. vacuum pump　真空泵
breast pump　吸乳器
stomach pump　胃唧筒
36. absolute scale　绝对温标
French scale　法国标度
ball scale　球码天平
hand scale　手秤
37. erythrocytic series　红细胞系
radioactive series　放射[系列]
aromatic series　芳香族
linear series　线形排列
statistical series　统计数列
38. embryonic shield　胚盾
eye shield　眼罩
protective shield　防护屏
antithermic shield　抗热防护物
39. perfumed spirit　香料酒精
nitroglycerin spirit　三硝酸甘油酯
turpentine spirit　松节油
40. cooling stage　冷却台
infective stage　传染期
first stage　第一产程
41. alimentary system　消化系统
crystal system　晶体系
medical system　医疗制度
metric system　米制,公制
oxygen system　供氧装置
42. humoral theory　体液学说
occlusion theory　闭塞理论
evolution theory　进化论
43. temperate zone　温带
parietal zone　壁带
incubation zone　潜伏区
hyperesthetic zone　感觉过敏区

三、英语医学词汇自我测试题
(A Test on Medical Vocabulary)

说明:为配合本辞典的学习和使用,特编写了这套医学词汇测试题,供读者进行自我测试,以检查自己在一定学习阶段后对医学词汇的掌握水平。具体方式如下:

1. 做题方式　做题过程中不翻阅本辞典前面内容,也不参阅其他任何有关书本或词典。

2. 做题时间　1.5 小时。

3. 评卷方法　自己评卷。评卷时可参考本辞典及其他书本或词典,要求仔细认真,进行客观批阅,按规定分数计分和统计。

4. 成绩评定　试题包括两部分,每部分的满分均为 100 分,成绩的计算方法是:(第一部分实得分数+第二部分实得分数)÷2=测试分数

PART ONE

DIRECTIONS: Give the Chinese equivalents of the following English words. (100 marks)

A

1. ulcer
2. vein
3. vomit
4. urine
5. virus
6. toxic
7. acute
8. protein
9. symptom
10. infection
11. intake
12. therapy
13. incidence
14. secretion
15. radiation
16. chronic
17. diagnosis
18. metabolism
19. gastric
20. hepatic

B

21. rickets
22. spleen
23. lesion
24. uremia
25. carditis
26. recurrence
27. etiology
28. pregnancy
29. serum
30. swelling
31. sarcoma
32. contraction
33. malignant
34. virulent
35. retardation
36. cholesterol
37. hospitalize
38. susceptibility
39. hypertension
40. streptomycin

C

41. antigen
42. psychology
43. susceptible
44. rheumatism
45. digitalis
46. analgesic
47. survive
48. molecule
49. constituent
50. hemorrhage
51. crisis
52. implantation
53. viscera
54. atrioventricular
55. diarrhea
56. diaphragm
57. glycogen
58. anesthetic
59. bronchospasm
60. ambulance

D

61. dermatitis
62. meningitis
63. mitral
64. tonsil
65. anticoagulant
66. gallbladder
67. prognosis
71. emphysema
72. diastole
73. albumin
74. abortion
75. syndrome
76. asthma
77. emesis

68. umbilicus
69. thrombosis
70. leucocytosis
78. dislocation
79. scanning
80. electroencephalogram

E

81. globulin
82. duodenum
83. cirrhosis
84. inoculation
85. allergy
86. hereditary
87. jaundice
88. hypothermia
89. isotope
90. puncture
91. stenosis
92. shrinkage
93. radium
94. vasoconstriction
95. fungus
96. splenomegaly
97. ultrasonography
98. premature
99. auscultation
100. myocardium

PART TWO

Ⅰ. In the following groups choose the correct combining form for each given word. (20 marks)

1. Brain
   a. cerebro- b. entero- c. cardio- d. cephalo-
2. Nerve
   a. nephro- b. neuro- c. uro- d. nuero-
3. Eye
   a. ortho- b. bio- c. ophthalmo- d. audio-
4. Intestine
   a. gastro- b. gyneco- c. entero- d. carcino-
5. Blood
   a. hepato- b. hemo- c. cardio- d. gyneco-
6. Kidney
   a. gastro- b. neuro- c. patho- d. nephro-
7. Life
   a. rhino- b. adeno- c. bio- d. lifo-
8. Head
   a. cephalo- b. cyto- c. cerebro- d. gnoso-
9. Stomach
   a. entero- b. geno- c. gastro- d. stomato-
10. Gland
   a. arthro- b. entero- c. adeno- d. geno-
11. Nose
   a. radio- b. uro- c. sectio- d. rhino-
12. Neck
   a. cervico- b. thoraco- c. thyro- d. circo-
13. Skull
   a. cerebro- b. osteo- c. myelo- d. cranio-
14. Female
   a. gyneco- b. hystero- c. leuko- d. hemato-
15. Ear
   a. audio- b. sono- c. oto- d. oro-

16. Rib
    a. costo- b. chondro- c. thoraco- d. vertebro-
17. Liver
    a. hemato- b. lacto- c. hepato- d. patho-
18. Tissue
    a. geno- b. hemato- c. glyco- d. histo-
19. Tumor
    a. scopo- b. onco- c. tomo- d. cephalo-
20. Cancer
    a. cardio- b. costo- c. carcino- d. adeno-

Ⅱ. Match the meanings in Column 2 with the prefixes, suffixes, and roots in Column 1.

(20 marks)

Column 1	Column 2
1. neo-	——interior
2. hyper-	——against
3. anti-	——new
4. endo-	——above
5. multi-	——single
6. semi-	——beneath
7. mono-	——large
8. mal-	——one half
9. hypo-	——many
10. macro-	——ill, bad

Column 1	Column 2
11. -oma	——pain
12. -gram	——blood condition
13. -itis	——disease, conditions
14. -algia	——paralysis
15. -osis	——tumor
16. -ectomy	——removal of
17. -penia	——inflammation of
18. -emia	——picture, mark
19. -plegia	——science of
20. -logy	——lack, decreased

Column 1	Column 2
21. arthro-	——cell
22. cardio-	——colour
23. hemo-	——blood
24. osteo-	——tissue
25. dermo-	——joint
26. patho-	——skin
27. chromo-	——heart
28. histo-	——hard
29. sclero-	——disease
30. cyto-	——bone

Column 1	Column 2
31. dento-	——red
32. pharmaco-	——mouth
33. linguo-	——urine

34. erythro-　　——drug
35. pneumo-　　——lung, breath
36. stomato-　　——tongue
37. pyro-　　——tooth
38. uro-　　——white
39. leuko-　　——poison
40. toxico-　　——fire, heat

Ⅲ. Select from the lettered words or phrases the one nearest in meaning to the word given. (20 marks)

1. ensue
   a. compel　b. remain　c. absorb　d. follow
2. accelerate
   a. surpass　b. cheer　c. quicken　d. transport
3. benign
   a. contagious　b. fatal　c. ignorant　d. kindly
4. credible
   a. believable　b. unbelievable　c. correct　d. suitable
5. crucial
   a. technical　b. decisive　c. ill natured　d. rude
6. tiny
   a. very swift　b. very strong　c. very small　d. very sharp
7. hazard
   a. danger　b. storm　c. battle　d. fire
8. fissure
   a. gesture　b. rupture　c. mission　d. project
9. drowsy
   a. hungry　b. friendly　c. ugly　d. sleepy
10. mute
    a. little　b. silent　c. hungry　d. angry
11. discard
    a. oppose　b. injure　c. throw away　d. find by accident
12. void
    a. empty　b. sound　c. different　d. weak
13. hypothesis
    a. falsehood　b. supposition　c. inferior　d. sorrow
14. ailment
    a. assistance　b. appearance　c. illness　d. landscape
15. obese
    a. free　b. foreign　c. fatal　d. fat
16. copious
    a. fortunate　b. abundant　c. desirable　d. proper
17. postulate
    a. assume　b. exceed　c. contribute　d. offend
18. transient
    a. transparent　b. transitional　c. temperate　d. temporary
19. confirmation
    a. trust　b. suspense　c. proof　d. encounter
20. controversial
    a. pleasant　b. debatable　c. ugly　d. talkative

Ⅳ. The word in capitals at the end of each of the following sentences can be used to form a word that fits suitably in the blank space. Fill in each blank this way. (20 marks)

Example: The patient on ADMISSION must be checked for serious bleeding. ADMIT

1. Vitamin A plays an important role in the chemical events associated with visual ________ . EXCITE
2. The mechanical obstru ~ ction resulted from previous ________ . ADHERE
3. If the swelling is not ________ and promptly treated, suppuration is bound to happen. ADEQUATE
4. ________ of infectious material into the lung is the most common cause of lung abscess. ASPIRATE
5. The ________ of a muscle to a bone occurs by means of a fibrous structure known as a tendon. ATTACH
6. Doctors have presumed that peptic ulcers are caused by both ________ and environmental factors. GENE
7. The piece of paper you get from the doctor and take to the chemist's to obtain medicine is called a ________ . PRESCRIBE
8. The reaction is readily ________ under physiological conditions. REVERSE
9. The passage of simple nutrients from the intestine into the bloodstream is called ________ . ABSORB
10. The blood flow may be increased by more rapid and ________ heart action. VIGOR
11. A benign ________ tumor weighing about 200 pounds was recently removed from a 30-year-old woman. OVARY
12. On admission, the patient had a high fever and complained of ________ pain. ABDOMEN
13. The ________ of typhoid fever is decreasing. MORTAL
14. They more frequently have another ________ disorder associated with their nephrotic syndrome. UNDERLIE
15. Don't eat your food so quickly! You'll get ________ . DIGEST
16. The disease usually runs a self-limited course and treatment is purely ________ . SYMPTOM
17. In the small intestine the process of digestion is completed by the action of bile and ________ juice. PANCREAS
18. Inoculation with this virus confers upon man more or less ________ against smallpox. IMMUNE
19. During the physical examination, the doctor noted the ________ of lymph nodes in the patient. ENLARGE
20. During the ________ of this drug, weekly blood counts should be made. ADMINISTER

Ⅴ. Mark the ONE correct answer to each question by circling the letter preceding it. (20 marks)

1. If you suffer from ________, your doctor may recommend taking sleeping tablets.
   a. anorexia b. insomnia
   c. dizziness d. epilepsy
2. When she broke her leg, she had to go around on ________ for several weeks afterwards.
   a. crutches b. armchairs
   c. stretchers d. sticks
3. She was in such a state when her son died that the doctor gave her a ________ to help calm her down.
   a. depressant b. stimulant

c. additive d. sedative

4. Although my father has ________ hearing, he still refuses to wear a hearing-aid.

a. reflexive b. infectious

c. defective d. affective

5. In the word hemoglobin the component globin means ________ .

a. blood b. oxygen

c. carbon dioxide d. protein

6. When tissue loses its normal flow of blood and thus becomes deficient of oxygen, it is said to be ________ .

a. anemic b. ischemic

c. aplastic d. hemolytic

7. The mediastinum is found within the ________ cavity.

a. cranial b. pelvic

c. spinal d. thoracic

8. The cells necessary for blood clotting are ________ .

a. thrombocytes b. monocytes

c. erythrocytes d. eosinophils

9. The medical term which means surrounding the heart is ________ .

a. pencardium b. precardium

c. paracardium d. pericardium

10. ________ is a condition in which there is a reduction in the number of erythrocytes or amount of hemoglobin.

a. Anemia b. Ischemia

c. Leukemia d. Erythremia

11. The ________ is the basic unit of heredity.

a. autosome b. gene

c. DNA d. gamete

12. The birth of the fetus through an incision into the uterus is termed a/an ________ .

a. episiotomy b. cesarean section

c. laparotomy d. salpingectomy

13. Paralysis of one side of the body is called ________ .

a. paresthesia b. paraplegia

c. hemiplegia d. quadriplegia

14. The main artery of the trunk is the ________ .

a. coronary artery b. pulmonary artery

c. vena cava d. aorta

15. The interior lining of the heart wall is the ________ .

a. myocardium b. endocardium

c. pericardium d. endosteum

16. A ________ is an abnormal sound in the heartbeat.

a. diastole b. flutter

c. systole d. murmur

17. ________ indicates an abnormally low white blood count.

a. Leukemia b. Leukopenia

c. Leukopoiesis d. Leukocytosis

18. The air sacs of the lungs are known as ________ .

a. bronchioles b. glomeruli

c. pneumococci d. alveoli

19. A slight or transient increase in the number of white blood cells is termed ________ .

a. leukocytopathy　　b. leukopenia
c. leukocytosis　　d. leukemia

20. White cells which absorb dead cells and tissues, and ingest bacteria are called ________.
a. phagocytes　　b. monocytes
c. reticulocytes　　d. lymphocytes

Key to the Test

Part One: (100 medical terms. Check by yourself.)

Part Two:

Ⅰ. 1. a　2. b　3. c　4. a　5. b　6. d
7. c　8. a　9. c　10. c　11. d　12. a
13. d　14. a　15. c　16. a　17. c　18. d
19. b　20. c

Ⅱ. Column 2, 1-10: 4, 3, 1, 2, 7,
9, 10, 6, 5, 8
11-20: 14, 18, 15, 19, 11,
16, 13, 12, 20, 17
21-30: 30, 27, 23, 28, 21,
25, 22, 29, 26, 24
31-40: 34, 36, 38, 32, 35,
33, 31, 39, 40, 37

Ⅲ. 1. d　2. c　3. d　4. a　5. b　6. c
7. a　8. b　9. d　10. b　11. c　12. a
13. b　14. c　15. d　16. b　17. a　18. d
19. c　20. b

Ⅳ. 1. excitement　2. adhesion　3. adequately
4. aspiration　5. attachment　6. genetic
7. prescription　8. reversible　9. absorption
10. vigorous　11. ovarian　12. abdominal
13. mortality　14. underlying　15. indigestion
16. symptomatic　17. pancreatic　18. immunity
19. enlargement　20. administration

Ⅴ. 1. b　2. a　3. d　4. c　5. d　6. b
7. d　8. a　9. d　10. a　11. b　12. b
13. c　14. d　15. b　16. d　17. a　18. d
19. c　20. a